Non-Invasive Ventilation and Weaning

Principles and Practice

Second Edition

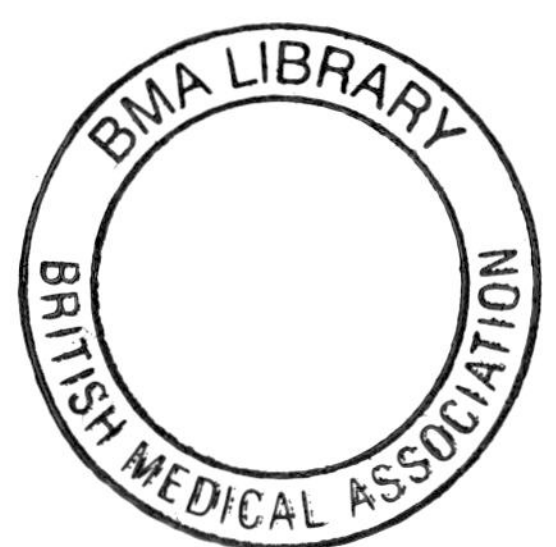

Non-Invasive Ventilation and Weaning

Principles and Practice
Second Edition

Edited by
Mark W. Elliott
Stefano Nava
Bernd Schönhofer

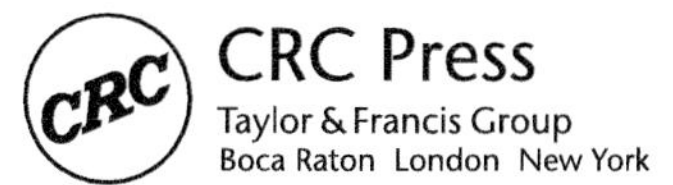

CRC Press is an imprint of the
Taylor & Francis Group, an **informa** business

CRC Press
Taylor & Francis Group
6000 Broken Sound Parkway NW, Suite 300
Boca Raton, FL 33487-2742

Printed on acid-free paper

International Standard Book Number-13: 978-1-4987-6476-6 (Pack–Book and eBook)

Visit the Taylor & Francis Web site at
http://www.taylorandfrancis.com

and the CRC Press Web site at
http://www.crcpress.com

Contents

Contributors **ix**

1 Non-invasive ventilation: From the past to the present 1
Dominique Robert and Barry Make

PART 1 THE EQUIPMENT **9**

2 Positive pressure ventilators 10
Dean R. Hess
3 Continuous positive airway pressure 22
Annie Lecavalier and Peter Goldberg
4 Emerging modes for non-invasive ventilation 30
Paolo Navalesi, Federico Longhini, Rosanna Vaschetto and Antonio Messina
5 Extracorporeal CO_2 removal 36
Lara Pisani and V. Marco Ranieri
6 Interfaces 43
Cesare Gregoretti, Vincenzo Russotto and Davide Chiumello
7 Quality control of non-invasive ventilation: Performance, service, maintenance and infection control of ventilators 55
Jordi Rigau and Ramon Farré
8 Humidifiers and drug delivery during non-invasive ventilation 63
Antonio M. Esquinas Rodriguez and Maria Vargas
9 How to start a patient on non-invasive ventilation 73
Raffaele Scala and Martin Latham

PART 2 THE PRACTICE – ACUTE NIV **84**

10 How to set up an acute non-invasive ventilation service 85
Paul K. Plant and Gregory A. Schmidt
11 Education programmes/assessment of staff competencies 95
Alanna Hare
12 Monitoring during acute non-invasive ventilation 101
Eumorfia Kondili, Nektaria Xirouchaki and Dimitris Georgopoulos
13 Troubleshooting non-invasive ventilation 111
Nicholas S. Hill, Mayanka Tickoo and Najia Indress
14 Sedation and delirium 122
Lara Pisani, Maria Laura Vega and Cesare Gregoretti
15 Timing of non-invasive ventilation 131
Stefano Nava and Paolo Navalesi
16 Why non-invasive ventilation works in acute respiratory failure? 139
Miguel Ferrer and Antoni Torres
17 Predicting outcome in patients with acute hypercapnic respiratory failure 149
Tom Hartley and Stephen C. Bourke
18 Use of NIV in the real world 157
Mihaela Stefan, Peter Lindenauer, Najia Indress, Faisal Tamimi and Nicholas S. Hill

PART 3 THE PRACTICE – CHRONIC NIV 164

19 Chronic ventilation service 165
Maxime Patout, Antoine Cuvelier, Jean-François Muir and Peter Wijkstra
20 Diagnostic tests in the assessment of patients for home mechanical ventilation 175
Michael Polkey, Patrick B. Murphy and Nicholas Hart
21 Ultrasound 190
Daniel A. Lichtenstein
22 Patient and caregiver education 200
Ole Norregaard
23 Discharging the patient on home ventilation 207
Joan Escarrabill and Ole Norregaard
24 Monitoring during sleep during chronic non-invasive ventilation 216
Jean-Paul Janssens, Jean-Christian Borel, Dan Adler and Jean-Louis Pépin
25 Continuity of care and telemonitoring 223
Michele Vitacca

PART 4 THE DISEASES 233

26 Pathophysiology of respiratory failure 234
Paul P. Walker and Peter M. Calverley

PART 5 COPD 246

27 Non-invasive ventilation for exacerbation of COPD 247
Martin Dres, Alexandre Demoule and Laurent Brochard
28 NIV in chronic COPD 258
Enrico M. Clini, Nicolino Ambrosino, Ernesto Crisafulli and Guido Vagheggini
29 Non-invasive ventilation in COPD: The importance of comorbidities and phenotypes 266
Jean-Louis Pépin, Jean-Paul Janssens, Renaud Tamisier, Damien Viglino, Dan Adler and Jean-Christian Borel
30 High-intensity non-invasive positive pressure ventilation 272
Sarah Bettina Schwarz, Friederike Sophie Magnet and Wolfram Windisch

PART 6 HYPOXAEMIC RESPIRATORY FAILURE 278

31 Home oxygen therapy in chronic respiratory failure 279
Jadwiga A. Wedzicha and Mark W. Elliott
32 Acute oxygen therapy 287
Mark W. Elliott
33 High-flow oxygen therapy: Physiological effects and clinical evidence 295
Nuttapol Rittayamai, Arnaud W. Thille and Laurent Brochard
34 Equipment for oxygen therapy 307
Jane Slough
35 Non-invasive ventilation for hypoxaemic respiratory failure 315
Massimo Antonelli and Giuseppe Bello

PART 7 CARDIAC FAILURE 325

36 Acute heart failure syndrome 326
Ross S. Archibald and Alasdair J. Gray
37 Ventilation in chronic congestive cardiac failure 341
Matthew T. Naughton

PART 8 NEUROMUSCULAR DISEASE 353

38 Muscle disorders and ventilatory failure 354
David Hilton-Jones
39 Pathophysiology of respiratory failure in neuromuscular diseases 364
Franco Laghi, Hameeda Shaikh and Dejan Radovanovic
40 Slowly progressive neuromuscular diseases 375
Vikram A. Padmanabhan and Joshua O. Benditt
41 Amyotrophic lateral sclerosis 388
Stephen C. Bourke and John Steer
42 Duchenne muscular dystrophy 399
Anita K. Simonds
43 Central sleep apnoea 408
Shahrokh Javaheri and Mark W. Elliott
44 Mouthpiece ventilation for daytime ventilatory support 419
Miguel R. Gonçalves and Tiago Pinto

PART 9 CHEST WALL DEFORMITY 425

45 Scoliosis 426
William J. M. Kinnear

PART 10 OBESITY 440

46 Pathophysiology of respiratory failure in obesity 441
Francesco Fanfulla
47 Acute non-invasive ventilation in obesity-related respiratory failure 452
Patrick B. Murphy and Nicholas Hart
48 Non-invasive ventilation in acute and chronic respiratory failure due to obesity 457
Juan Fernando Masa, Isabel Utrabo and Francisco Javier Gómez de Terreros

PART 11 OTHER CONDITIONS 469

49 Bronchiectasis and adult cystic fibrosis 470
Sean Duffy, Frederic Jaffe and Gerard J. Criner
50 Non-invasive ventilation in highly infectious conditions: Lessons from severe acute respiratory syndrome 474
David S. C. Hui
51 NIV in cancer patients 481
Raffaele Scala, Uberto Maccari, Giuseppina Ciarleglio, Valentina Granese and Chiara Madioni
52 Non-invasive ventilation in the elderly 487
Erwan L'Her and Corinne Troadec-L'Her
53 Post-surgery non-invasive ventilation 496
Maria Laura Vega and Stefano Nava
54 Trauma 504
Umberto Lucangelo, Massimo Ferluga and Matteo Segat
55 Spinal cord injuries 509
Sven Hirschfeld

PART 12 PAEDIATRIC VENTILATORY FAILURE 518

56 Equipment and interfaces in children 519
Alessandro Amaddeo, Annick Frapin and Brigitte Fauroux
57 Chronic non-invasive ventilation for children 525
Alessandro Amaddeo, Annick Frapin and Brigitte Fauroux

58 Non-invasive positive pressure ventilation in children with acute respiratory failure 533
Giorgio Conti, Marco Piastra and Silvia Pulitanò

PART 13 SPECIAL SITUATIONS 539

59 Bronchoscopy during non-invasive ventilation 540
Massimo Antonelli and Giuseppe Bello
60 Non-invasive positive pressure ventilation in the obstetric population 544
Daniel Zapata, David Wisa and Bushra Mina
61 Diaphragm pacing (by phrenic nerve stimulation) 547
Jésus Gonzalez-Bermejo
62 Tracheostomy 554
Piero Ceriana, Paolo Pelosi and Maria Vargas
63 Swallowing and phonation during ventilation 564
Hélène Prigent and Nicolas Terzi

PART 14 PROLONGED WEANING 570

64 End-of-life care and non-invasive ventilation 571
Christina Faull
65 Pathophysiology of weaning failure 582
Theodoros I. Vassilakopoulos
66 Non-invasive ventilation for weaning and extubation failure 591
Scott K. Epstein
67 Weaning strategies and protocols 607
Michele Vitacca and Luca Barbano
68 Specialised weaning units 615
Aditi Satti, James Brown, Gerard J. Criner and Bernd Schönhofer
69 Psychological problems during weaning 623
Amal Jubran

PART 15 THE PHYSIOTHERAPIST AND ASSISTED VENTILATION 631

70 Respiratory physiotherapy (including cough assistance techniques and glossopharyngeal breathing) 632
Miguel R. Gonçalves and João Carlos Winck
71 Rehabilitation 645
Rik Gosselink, Bruno Clerckx, T. Troosters, J. Segers and D. Langer

PART 16 OUTCOME MEASURES 655

72 Health status and quality of life 656
Wolfram Windisch

PART 17 THE PATIENT EXPERIENCE OF NIV 665

73 Psychological issues for the mechanically ventilated patient 666
Linda L. Bieniek, Daniel F. Dilling and Bernd Schönhofer
74 The patient's journey 690
Stefano Nava
75 A patient's journey: NIV 691
Jeanette Erdmann and Andrea L. Klein
76 A carer's journey 697
Gail Beacock and Patrick Beacock

Index 704

Contributors

Dan Adler
Division of Pulmonary Diseases
Geneva University Hospital
Geneva, Switzerland

Alessandro Amaddeo
Pediatric Noninvasive Ventilation and Sleep Unit
Hôpital Necker Enfants-Malades
and
Paris Descartes Faculty
Paris, France
and
Research Unit Inserm U 955
Créteil, France

Nicolino Ambrosino
ICS Maugeri IRCCS
Institute of Montescano
Pavia, Italy
and
University of Surakarta
Surakarta, Indonesia

Massimo Antonelli
Department of Anesthesia and Intensive Care
Fondazione Policlinico Universitario Agostino Gemelli
Università Cattolica del Sacro Cuore
Rome, Italy

Ross S. Archibald
Department of Emergency Medicine
Royal Infirmary of Edinburgh
Edinburgh, United Kingdom

Luca Barbano
Respiratory Unit and Weaning Centre
Fondazione Salvatore Maugeri
IRCCS
Lumezzane, Italy

Gail Beacock
Leeds, UK

Patrick Beacock
Leeds, UK

Giuseppe Bello
Department of Anesthesia and Intensive Care
Fondazione Policlinico Universitario Agostino Gemelli
Università Cattolica del Sacro Cuore
Rome, Italy

Joshua O. Benditt
Respiratory Care Services
University of Washington Medical Center
Seattle, Washington

Linda L. Bieniek
International Ventilator Users Network
and
Retired Certified Employee Assistance Professional
La Grange, Illinois

Jean-Christian Borel
HP2
Inserm U1042
and
EFCR Laboratory
Grenoble Alpes University Hospital
Grenoble, France
and
Association AGIR à dom
Meylan, France

Stephen C. Bourke
Northumbria Healthcare NHS Foundation Trust
North Tyneside General Hospital
North Shields, United Kingdom
and
Institute of Cellular Medicine
Newcastle University
Newcastle upon Tyne, United Kingdom

Laurent Brochard
Keenan Research Centre for Biomedical Science
Li Ka Shing Knowledge Institute
St Michael's Hospital
and
Interdepartmental Division of Critical Care Medicine
University of Toronto
Toronto, Canada

James Brown
Department of Thoracic Medicine and Surgery
Temple University Hospital
Philadelphia, Pennsylvania

Peter M. Calverley
Department of Respiratory Medicine
University Hospital Aintree
Liverpool, United Kingdom

Piero Ceriana
Pneumologia Riabilitativa e Terapia Subintensiva Respiratoria
IRCCS Istituti Clinici Scientifici Maugeri
Pavia, Italy

Davide Chiumello
U O Anestesia e Rianimazione
Dipartimento di Anestesia
Rianimazione (Intensiva e Subintensiva) e Terapia del Dolore
Milan, Italy

Giuseppina Ciarleglio
Pulmonology and Respiratory Intensive Care Unit
S. Donato Hospital
Arezzo, Italy

Bruno Clerckx
Department Rehabilitation Sciences KU Leuven
and
Division of Critical Care Medicine
Faculty of Kinesiology and Rehabilitation Sciences
University Hospitals Leuven
Leuven, Belgium

Enrico M. Clini
Department of Medical and Surgical Sciences
University Hospital of Modena
University of Modena and Reggio Emilia
Modena, Italy

Giorgio Conti
Intensive Care and Anesthesia Department
Pediatric Intensive Care Unit
Catholic University of Rome, Policlinico A Gemelli
Rome, Italy

Gerard J. Criner
Department of Thoracic Medicine and Surgery
Lewis Katz School of Medicine at Temple University
Philadelphia, Pennsylvania

Ernesto Crisafulli
Department of Medicine and Surgery
University Hospital of Parma
University of Parma
Parma, Italy

Antoine Cuvelier
Pulmonary, Thoracic Oncology and Respiratory Intensive Care Department
Rouen University Hospital
and
Normandie University UNIROUEN
and
Institute for Research and Innovation in Biomedicine (IRIB)
Rouen, France

Alexandre Demoule
Sorbonne Université and INSERM
UMRS1158 Neurophysiologie Respiratoire Expérimentale et Clinique
and
Intensive Care Unit and Respiratory Division
La Pitié Salpêtrière Hospital
Paris, France

Daniel F. Dilling
Loyola University Chicago Stritch School of Medicine
Maywood, Illinois

Martin Dres
Sorbonne Université and INSERM
UMRS1158 Neurophysiologie Respiratoire Expérimentale et Clinique
and
Intensive Care Unit and Respiratory Division
La Pitié Salpêtrière Hospital
Paris, France

Sean Duffy
Department of Thoracic Medicine and Surgery
Lewis Katz School of Medicine at Temple University
Philadelphia, Pennsylvania

Mark W. Elliott
Department of Respiratory Medicine
St James's University Hospital
Leeds, United Kingdom

Scott K. Epstein
Tufts University School of Medicine
Division of Pulmonary, Critical Care and Sleep Medicine
Tufts Medical Center
Boston, Massachusetts

Jeanette Erdmann
Lübeck, Germany

Joan Escarrabill
Master Plan for Respiratory Diseases PDMAR (Health Ministry)
Institut d'Estudis de la Salut
Barcelona, Spain

Antonio M. Esquinas Rodriguez
Intensive Care Unit
Hospital Morales Meseguer
Murcia, Spain

Francesco Fanfulla
Sleep Medicine Unit
Istituti Clinici Scientifici Maugeri
Istituto Scientifico di Pavia IRCCS
Pavia, Italy

Ramon Farré
Biophysics and Bioengineering Unit
School of Medicine
University of Barcelona
IDIBAPS
Barcelona, Spain

Christina Faull
Department of Palliative Care
LOROS Hospice and University Hospitals of Leicester
Leicester, United Kingdom

Brigitte Fauroux
Pediatric Noninvasive Ventilation and Sleep Unit
Hôpital Necker Enfants-Malades
and
Paris Descartes Faculty
Paris, France
and
Research Unit Inserm U 955
Créteil, France

Massimo Ferluga
Department of Perioperative Medicine
Intensive Care and Emergency
Cattinara Hospital
Trieste University School of Medicine
Trieste, Italy

Miguel Ferrer
Servei de Pneumologia
Institut Clinic de Respiratori
Hospital Clinic
IDIBAPS
Universitat de Barcelona
Barcelona, Spain
and
Centro de Investigación Biomedica En Red–Enfermedades Respiratorias
Instituto de Salud Carlos III
Ministerio de Ciencia e Innovación
Madrid, Spain

Annick Frapin
Pediatric Noninvasive Ventilation and Sleep Unit
Hôpital Necker Enfants-Malades
Paris, France

Dimitris Georgopoulos
Department of Intensive Care Medicine
University Hospital of Heraklion
Crete, Greece

Peter Goldberg
Department of Critical Care Medicine
McGill University Health Center
Montreal, Canada

Francisco Javier Gómez de Terreros
Pneumology Service
San Pedro de Alcántara Hospital
Cáceres, Spain

Miguel R. Gonçalves
Noninvasive Ventilatory Support Unit
Pulmonology Department
Emergency and Intensive Care Medicine Department
São João University Hospital
and
Instituto de Investigação e Inovação em Saúde (I3S)
Faculty of Medicine
University of Porto
Porto, Portugal

Jésus Gonzalez-Bermejo
Assistance Publique Hôpitaux de Paris
Groupe Hospitalier Pitié-Salpêtrière Charles Foix
Service de Pneumologie et Réanimation Médicale Département "R3S"
and
UMRS1158 Neurophysiologie Respiratoire Expérimentale et Clinique
Sorbonne Université
Paris, France

Rik Gosselink
Department Rehabilitation Sciences KU Leuven
and
Division of Respiratory Rehabilitation
and
Division of Critical Care Medicine
Faculty of Kinesiology and Rehabilitation Sciences
University Hospitals Leuven
Leuven, Belgium

Valentina Granese
Pulmonology and Respiratory Intensive Care Unit
S. Donato Hospital
Arezzo, Italy

Alasdair J. Gray
Department of Emergency Medicine
Royal Infirmary of Edinburgh
Edinburgh, United Kingdom

Cesare Gregoretti
Department of Biopathology and Medical Biotechnologies (DIBIMED)
Section of Anaesthesia, Analgesia, Intensive Care and Emergency
University Hospital Paolo Giaccone
University of Palermo
Palermo, Italy

Alanna Hare
Department of Ventilation and Sleep
Royal Brompton & Harefield NHS Foundation Trust
London, United Kingdom

Nicholas Hart
Division of Pulmonary, Adult Critical Care and Sleep
Lane Fox Respiratory Service
St Thomas' Hospital London
and
Centre for Human and Applied Physiological Science
School of Basic and Biomedical Sciences
King's College London
London, United Kingdom

Tom Hartley
Northumbria Healthcare NHS Foundation Trust
North Tyneside General Hospital
North Shields, United Kingdom
and
Institute of Cellular Medicine
Newcastle University
Newcastle upon Tyne, United Kingdom

Dean R. Hess
Massachusetts General Hospital
and
Harvard Medical School
Boston, Massachusetts

Nicholas S. Hill
Division of Pulmonary, Critical Care and Sleep Medicine
Tufts Medical Center
Boston, Massachusetts

David Hilton-Jones
Oxford Neuromuscular Centre
Department of Clinical Neurology
John Radcliffe Hospital
Oxford, United Kingdom

Sven Hirschfeld
BG Trauma Hospital Hamburg
Level 1 Trauma Centre
Spinal Cord Injury Department
Hamburg, Germany

David S. C. Hui
Department of Medicine and Therapeutics
Chinese University of Hong Kong and Prince of Wales Hospital
Shatin, Hong Kong

Najia Indress
Department of Internal Medicine
St Elizabeth's Hospital
Tufts University School of Medicine
Boston, Massachusetts

Frederic Jaffe
Department of Thoracic Medicine and Surgery
Lewis Katz School of Medicine at Temple University
Philadelphia, Pennsylvania

Jean-Paul Janssens
Division of Pulmonary Diseases
Geneva University Hospital
Geneva, Switzerland

Shahrokh Javaheri
Bethesda North Hospital
and
Division of Pulmonary, Critical Care and Sleep
University of Cincinnati College of Medicine
Cincinnati, Ohio
and
Division of Cardiology
The Ohio State University
Columbus, Ohio

Amal Jubran
Division of Pulmonary and Critical Care Medicine
Edward Hines Jr. VA Hospital
Hines, Illinois

William J. M. Kinnear
Home Ventilation Service
Nottingham NHS Treatment Centre Queens Medical Centre
Nottingham, United Kingdom

Andrea L. Klein
Cleveland, Tennessee

Eumorfia Kondili
Department of Intensive Care Medicine
University Hospital of Heraklion
Crete, Greece

Franco Laghi
Division of Pulmonary and Critical Care Medicine
Loyola University of Chicago Stritch School of Medicine
and
Edward Hines Jr. Veterans Administration Hospital
Hines, Illinois

D. Langer
Department Rehabilitation Sciences KU Leuven
and
Division of Respiratory Rehabilitation
Faculty of Kinesiology and Rehabilitation Sciences
University Hospitals Leuven
Leuven, Belgium

Martin Latham
Sleep Service
St James's University Hospital
Leeds, United Kingdom

Annie Lecavalier
Department of Critical Care Medicine
McGill University Health Center
Montreal, Canada

Erwan L'Her
Réanimation Médicale
CHU de Brest
and
LATIM INSERM UMR 1101
Université de Bretagne Occidentale
Brest, France

Daniel A. Lichtenstein
Intensive Care Unit
Hospital Ambroise-Pare
Paris-West University
Boulogne, France

Peter Lindenauer
Institute for Healthcare Delivery and Population Science
and
Department of Internal Medicine
University of Massachusetts Medical School–Baystate
Springfield, Massachusetts

Federico Longhini
Anesthesia and Intensive Care
Sant'Andrea Hospital
Vercelli, Italy

Umberto Lucangelo
Department of Perioperative Medicine
Intensive Care and Emergency
Cattinara Hospital
Trieste University School of Medicine
Trieste, Italy

Uberto Maccari
Pulmonology and Respiratory Intensive Care Unit
S. Donato Hospital
Arezzo, Italy

Chiara Madioni
Pulmonology and Respiratory Intensive Care Unit
S. Donato Hospital
Arezzo, Italy

Friederike Sophie Magnet
Department of Pneumology
Cologne Merheim Hospital
Kliniken der Stadt Köln
and
Faculty of Health
School of Medicine
gGmbH Witten/Herdecke University
Köln, Germany

Barry Make
COPD Program
National Jewish Health
and
University of Colorado-Denver School of Medicine
National Jewish Medical and Research Center
Denver, Colorado

Juan Fernando Masa
Respiratory Research Group
Centro de Investigación Biomédica en Red de Enfermedades Respiratorias (CIBERES)
Ministry of Science and Innovation
Madrid, Spain
and
Intermediate Respiratory Care Unit
Pulmonary Division
San Pedro de Alcantara Hospital
Cáceres, Spain

Antonio Messina
Anesthesia and Intensive Care
Maggiore Della Carità Hospital
Novara, Italy

Bushra Mina
Pulmonary Critical Care Fellowship
Lenox Hill Hospital
Northwell Health
Zucker School of Medicine at Hofstra
New York, New York

Jean-François Muir
Pulmonary, Thoracic Oncology and Respiratory Intensive Care Department
Rouen University Hospital
and
Normandie University UNIROUEN
and
Institute for Research and Innovation in Biomedicine (IRIB)
Rouen, France

Patrick B. Murphy
Lane Fox Respiratory Service
St Thomas' Hospital
and
School of Basic and Biomedical Sciences
King's College
London, United Kingdom

Matthew T. Naughton
Department of Respiratory Medicine
Alfred Hospital and Monash University
Melbourne, Australia

Stefano Nava
Respiratory Intensive Care Unit
Fondazione S Maugeri
IRCCS
Pavia, Italy

Paolo Navalesi
Intensive Care Unit
University Hospital Mater Domini
Department of Medical and Surgical Sciences
Magna Graecia University
Catanzaro, Italy

Ole Norregaard
Danish Respiratory Center West
Aarhus University Hospital
Aarhus, Denmark

Vikram A. Padmanabhan
Clinical Assistant Professor of Medicine
University of Washington School of Medicine
Seattle, Washington

Maxime Patout
Pulmonary, Thoracic Oncology and Respiratory Intensive Care Department
Rouen University Hospital
and
Normandie University UNIROUEN
and
Institute for Research and Innovation in Biomedicine (IRIB)
Rouen, France

Paolo Pelosi
Dipartimento Ambiente
Salute e Sicurezza
Universita' Degli Studi Dell'insubria
Varese, Italy

Jean-Louis Pépin
HP2
INSERM U1042
and
EFCR Laboratory
Thorax and Vessels Division
Grenoble Alpes University Hospital
and
CHU Grenoble
Grenoble, France

Marco Piastra
Pediatric Intensive Care Unit
Policlinico A Gemelli
Catholic University of Rome
Rome, Italy

Tiago Pinto
Noninvasive Ventilatory Support Unit
Pulmonology Department
São João University Hospital
Porto, Portugal

Lara Pisani
Respiratory and Critical Care Unit
Sant'Orsola Malpighi Hospital
Bologna, Italy

Paul K. Plant
Department of Thoracic Medicine
Aintree University Hospital
Liverpool, United Kingdom

Michael Polkey
National Heart and Lung Institute
Respiratory Biomedical Research Unit
Royal Brompton Hospital
Imperial College
London, United Kingdom

Hélène Prigent
Physiology Department and Home Ventilation Unit
Hopital Raymond Poincaré – GHU PIFO - APHP
Garches, France
and
UMR 1179 - End-ICAP (INSERM-UVSQ)
Université de Versailles-St-Quentin-en-Yvelines
Versailles, France

Silvia Pulitanò
Pediatric Intensive Care Unit
Policlinico A Gemelli
Catholic University of Rome
Rome, Italy

Dejan Radovanovic
Division of Pulmonary and Critical Care Medicine
Loyola University of Chicago Stritch School of Medicine
and
School of Respiratory Medicine
University of Milan
Milan, Italy

V. Marco Ranieri
Department of Anesthesia and Critical Care Medicine
Policlinico Umberto I
Sapienza Università di Roma
Rome, Italy

Jordi Rigau
Research, Development and Innovation Department
Sibel Group
Barcelona, Spain

Nuttapol Rittayamai
Division of Respiratory Diseases and Tuberculosis
Department of Medicine
Faculty of Medicine Siriraj Hospital
Mahidol University
Bangkok, Thailand

Dominique Robert
Claude Bernard University Lyon 1
and
ALLP
Lyon, France

Vincenzo Russotto
Department of Biopathology and Medical Biotechnologies
Section of Anaesthesia, Analgesia, Intensive Care and Emergency
University Hospital Paolo Giaccone
University of Palermo
Palermo, Italy

Aditi Satti
Department of Thoracic Medicine and Surgery
Temple University Hospital
Philadelphia, Pennsylvania

Raffaele Scala
Pulmonology and Respiratory Intensive Care Unit
S. Donato Hospital
Arezzo, Italy

Gregory A. Schmidt
Division of Pulmonary Diseases, Critical Care, and Occupational Medicine
University of Iowa Healthcare
Iowa City, Iowa

Bernd Schönhofer
Department of Respiratory and Critical Care Medicine
Klinikum Region Hannover, Oststadt-Heidehaus
Hannover, Germany

Sarah Bettina Schwarz
Department of Pneumology
Cologne Merheim Hospital
Kliniken der Stadt Köln
and
Faculty of Health
School of Medicine
gGmbH Witten/Herdecke University
Köln, Germany

Matteo Segat
Department of Perioperative Medicine
Intensive Care and Emergency
Cattinara Hospital
Trieste University School of Medicine
Trieste, Italy

J. Segers
Department Rehabilitation Sciences KU Leuven
and
Division of Critical Care Medicine
Faculty of Kinesiology and Rehabilitation Sciences
University Hospitals Leuven
Leuven, Belgium

Hameeda Shaikh
Division of Pulmonary and Critical Care Medicine
Loyola University of Chicago Stritch School of Medicine
and
Edward Hines Jr. Veterans Administration Hospital
Hines, Illinois

Anita K. Simonds
NIHR Respiratory Biomedical Research Unit
Royal Brompton & Harefield NHS Foundation Trust
London, United Kingdom

Jane Slough
Department of Respiratory Medicine
St James's University Hospital
Leeds, United Kingdom

John Steer
Northumbria Healthcare NHS Foundation Trust
North Tyneside General Hospital
North Shields, United Kingdom
and
Institute of Cellular Medicine
Newcastle University
Newcastle upon Tyne, United Kingdom

Mihaela Stefan
Institute for Healthcare Delivery and Population Science
and
Department of Internal Medicine
University of Massachusetts Medical School–Baystate
Springfield, Massachusetts

Faisal Tamimi
Department of Internal Medicine
Lahey Clinic Medical Center
Tufts University School of Medicine
Burlington, Massachusetts

Renaud Tamisier
HP2 Laboratory
INSERM U1042
University Grenoble Alps
and
EFCR Laboratory
Grenoble Alps University Hospital
Grenoble, France

Nicolas Terzi
Intensive Care Department
CHU Grenoble Alpes
and
INSERM, U1042
Université Grenoble-Alpes
Grenoble, France

Arnaud W. Thille
CHU de Poitiers
Réanimation Médicale
and
CIC 1402 ALIVE Group
University of Poitiers
Poitiers, France

Mayanka Tickoo
Division of Pulmonary, Critical Care and Sleep Medicine
Tufts Medical Center
Boston, Massachusetts

Antoni Torres
Servei de Pneumologia
Hospital Clinic
IDIBAPS
Universitat de Barcelona
Barcelona, Spain

Corinne Troadec-L'Her
Urgences Gériatriques
CHU de Brest
Brest, France

T. Troosters
Department Rehabilitation Sciences KU Leuven
and
Division of Respiratory Rehabilitation
Faculty of Kinesiology and Rehabilitation Sciences
University Hospitals Leuven
Leuven, Belgium

Isabel Utrabo
Intermediate Respiratory Care Unit
San Pedro de Alcantara Hospital
Cáceres, Spain

Guido Vagheggini
Auxilium Vitae
Volterra, Italy

Maria Vargas
Department of Neurosciences
Reproductive and Odonthostomatological Sciences
University of Naples Federico II
Naples, Italy

Rosanna Vaschetto
Anesthesia and Intensive Care
Maggiore Della Carità Hospital
Novara, Italy

Theodoros I. Vassilakopoulos
Department of Pulmonary and Critical Care Medicine
National and Kapodistrian University of Athens
and
3rd Department of Critical Care Medicine
Evagenideio Hospital, Medical School
Athens, Greece
and
McGill University
Montreal, Canada

Maria Laura Vega
Department of Physical Therapy
Fundacion Favaloro University Hospital
UCI
Buenos Aires, Argentina

Damien Viglino
HP2 Laboratory
INSERM U1042
University Grenoble Alps
and
EFCR Laboratory
Grenoble Alps University Hospital
Grenoble, France

Michele Vitacca
Respiratory Unit and Weaning Centre
Fondazione Salvatore Maugeri
IRCCS
Lumezzane, Italy

Paul P. Walker
Department of Respiratory Medicine
University Hospital Aintree
Liverpool, United Kingdom

Jadwiga A. Wedzicha
Academic Unit of Respiratory Medicine
University College London Medical School
London, United Kingdom

Peter Wijkstra
Department of Pulmonary Diseases/Home Mechanical Ventilation
University Medical Center Groningen
Groningen, the Netherlands

João Carlos Winck
Respiratory Medicine Unit
Alfena-Valongo and Braga Private Hospitals
Trofa Saúde Group
and
Northern Rehabilitation Centre Cardio-Pulmonary Group
CRN-SC Misericórdia do Porto
and
Instituto de Inovação e Investigação em Saúde (I3S)
Faculty of Medicine
University of Porto
Porto, Portugal

Wolfram Windisch
Department of Pneumology
Cologne Merheim Hospital
Kliniken der Stadt Köln
and
Faculty of Health
School of Medicine
gGmbH Witten/Herdecke University
Köln, Germany

David Wisa
Division of Pulmonary and Critical Care Medicine
Flushing Hospital Medical Center
Flushing, New York

Nektaria Xirouchaki
Department of Intensive Care Medicine
University Hospital of Heraklion
Crete, Greece

Daniel Zapata
Division of Pulmonary and Critical Care Medicine
Flushing Hospital Medical Center
Flushing, New York

1

Non-invasive ventilation: From the past to the present

DOMINIQUE ROBERT AND BARRY MAKE

HISTORY

Insights into the evolution of mechanical ventilation may be a useful starting point for further discussion of the current use and future directions of this therapy. The history of non-invasive (NIV) and of invasive mechanical (IMV) ventilation are intimately intertwined. The methods to deliver mechanical ventilation were initially described in the early twentieth century, and three main periods in the history of mechanical ventilation can be distinguished (Tables 1.1 and 1.2).

- *Negative pressure ventilation period:* During the earliest period of the use of mechanical ventilation, from 1928 to 1952, non-invasive negative pressure ventilation was the only available form of ventilation and was exclusively used, peaking with use in patients with poliomyelitis in the 1950s in both acute and chronic care settings.
- *Invasive ventilation period:* From 1953 to 1990, the use of invasive ventilation expanded rapidly and was the most common form of therapy used in acute care. During this period, the use of invasive mechanical ventilation was established as an important tool in critically ill patients. Negative pressure ventilation was used mostly in the home.
- *The modern era of mechanical ventilation – NIV via intermittent positive pressure ventilation/invasive ventilation period:* From 1990 to the present, the use of positive pressure NIV progressively increased in acute care. Moreover, NIV continuous positive airway pressure (NIV-CPAP) high-flow nasal cannula (HFNC) are now recognised as NIV methods. Even if these modalities do not deliver inspiratory support, they clearly interact with ventilation and require a flow generator device, circuit and facial interface, and are used to manage the same respiratory diseases as other forms of ventilator support.[1] NIV techniques are used in up to 30%–40% of patients in critical care units and up to 90% of patients receiving mechanical ventilation in the home.

During the first mechanical ventilation period, beginning in the late 1920s, NIV using negative pressure was found to improve survival compared with no ventilator assistance in patients with polio.[2] Many hospitals were equipped with such devices, including in the United States, where polio survivor President Roosevelt applied support for mechanical ventilation, and 'The March of Dimes' collected public donations. By the 1950s, due to the effectiveness of NIV intermittent negative pressure ventilation (NIV-INPV), the survival rate of patients with polio treated in specialised centres was about 98%.[3,4] This efficacy of NIV-INPV is underrecognised by healthcare professionals in the modern era. On the other side of the Atlantic, the mortality rate of polio patients needing mechanical ventilation was extremely high, reaching 94% at the beginning of the 1952 polio epidemic in Copenhagen. The explanation for this higher mortality was the lack of availability of ventilators (only one iron lung and six cuirasses in the city). The desperate inability to pursue the conventional use of NIV-INPV led to the necessity of using methods generally only practised during anaesthesia, that is, tracheostomy with cuffed tubes and handbag ventilation provided continuously for days or months. The success of the use of tracheostomy plus ventilation was immediately evident, and mortality decreased to 7% in polio patients receiving mechanical ventilation.[5,6]

The success of tracheostomy plus positive pressure ventilation combined with the ease of caring for the patient compared with treatment with the iron lung explains why the second mechanical ventilation period (invasive ventilation) proceeded rapidly. During the invasive ventilation period, tracheostomy or translaryngeal intubation and ventilation with automatic lung ventilator to replace handbag ventilation

Table 1.1 Types of mechanical ventilation

Invasive mechanical ventilation (IMV)
Using intermittent positive pressure (IMV-IPPV)
Non-invasive mechanical ventilation (NIV)
Using intermittent negative pressure around the thorax (INPV)
Using intermittent positive pressure delivered to the airway (NIV-IPPV)
Continuous positive pressure ventilation (NIV-CPAP)
High flow nasal cannula ventilation (NIV-HFNC)
Home mechanical ventilation (HMV)

spread rapidly, first in Europe and then in the United States. However, during the same time, an alternative form of NIV, namely intermittent positive pressure breathing (NIV-IPPB), was prescribed for other objectives: treatment of pulmonary atelectasis, aerosol delivery and short-term non-invasive ventilator support. But as controversies surfaced, the use of NIV-IPPB as a ventilator support technique fell into disfavour.[7] For chronic ventilator support in the home (HMV), few patients who remained ventilator-dependent over the long term received NIV-IPPV via mouthpiece while most patients used NIV-INPV.[8] HMV was also delivered via tracheostomy and IPPV ventilator not only for polio but also for patients with chronic respiratory insufficiency who remained ventilator-dependent after an episode of acute respiratory failure (ARF). Care for these patients was organised not only in intensive care unit (ICU) settings but also in chronic ventilator units leading to discharge.[9,10] During the invasive ventilation period, although HMV was recognised to significantly prolong life, it remained underutilised because of the difficulty in mobility with the iron lung and the invasiveness of tracheostomy.

The transition from the second to the third modern era of mechanical ventilation period gradually occurred between 1985 and 1990 and was driven by both the advances in sleep medicine and the practice of HMV. The sentinel event leading to the NIV-IPPV/invasive ventilation period of mechanical ventilation was the description in 1981 of the efficacy of nasal CPAP, replacing tracheostomy, in treating obstructive sleep apnoea.[11] Mimicking that experience, some teams working in HMV and to a lesser extent in ICUs began using NIV-IPPV. Treatment with nasal NIV-IPPV of chronic restrictive disorders related to neuromuscular (e.g. Duchenne muscular dystrophy) and chest disease (kyphoscoliosis, sequels of tuberculosis) proved to prevent recurrent hypoventilation and prolong life.[12–16] Furthermore, the non-invasive approach to treating patients with COPD presenting with acute-on-chronic respiratory failure managed in the ICU was successful.[17–21] Other advantages of NIV-IPPV were found to be clinically significant in these patients: fewer nosocomial infections, shorter duration of mechanical ventilation, lower intubation rate mortality.[20–22] Emphasising that successful story, other applications were progressively tried with some degree of success: acute pulmonary oedema due to cardiac failure, *de novo* ARF, difficult weaning from invasive ventilation, after surgery in patients at risk of pulmonary complications, before an intubation, during fibroscopy and care of the ventilator patient in a general ward or emergency room.[23–30] Strong reinforcement for the use of NIV-IPPV came from an increasing number of reports of complications of invasive mechanical ventilation and led to renewed interest in less aggressive, potentially less injurious ventilatory support techniques.[31,32] At the same time, small portable ventilators using flow generators (blower, turbine) primarily devised for HMV became available, affording at least comparable if not improved performance compared with ICU ventilators. The advent of algorithms to improve ventilator–patient interaction, especially in case of air leaks, further increased the utility of NIV-IPPV.[33]

Table 1.2 Three periods in the history of mechanical ventilation

Era	Non-invasive intermittent negative pressure ventilation	Invasive mechanical ventilation	Non-invasive positive pressure/ high nasal flow cannula/ invasive mechanical ventilation
Years	**1928–1952**	**1953–1990**	**1990–present**
Non-invasive negative pressure ventilation	*The only available mechanical ventilation* *Commonly used in poliomyelitis*	Rapidly decreasing use	Rarely used
Non-invasive ventilation using intermittent positive pressure	Not available	Not available	*Increasing use. Up to 30%–40% of ventilated patients in acute setting and 90% at home*
Invasive mechanical ventilation using intermittent positive pressure	Thoracic surgery	*Used almost exclusively*	Decreasing use. 60%–70% of ventilated patients in acute setting and 10% at home

Note: Italics represent the most notable feature of the era.

THE PRESENT TIME

Acute settings

The efficacy of NIV-IPPV has been substantiated over the past 25 years by randomised clinical trials. Based upon these results, recommendations can be developed to guide clinicians, even if newer trials will likely modify these in the near future (Table 1.3).

Regardless of the evidence supporting its efficacy in the research setting, a number of conditions must be met and important barriers overcome before NIV-IPPV can be used in everyday clinical practice. Results of surveys querying practitioners about their use of NIV and observational studies that document actual utilisation in clinical settings can help inform future directions for NIV. There are a few such peer-reviewed articles in the literature. The surveys have asked practitioners about their opinions on COPD,[48–50] all patients with ARF[39,51–53] and NIV as a 'ceiling' treatment.[43,54] Before 2002,[48,49] NIV was available in less than 50% of acute care settings, and the reasons for not using NIV were lack of equipment due to financial limitations and lack of training. Starting in about 2003, NIV has become available in the majority of hospitals which have been surveyed, although marked regional variations in the use of NIV have been found. For example, a large web-based survey collected responses from 2985 intensivists from Europe and the United States (41% in Europe and 19% in the United States).[53] Use of NIV was reported in >25% of cases of ARF by 68% of European physicians and 39% of physicians in the United States ($p < 0.01$). Sedation was more frequently advocated in the United States than in Europe (41% of respondents compared to 24%, $p < 0.01$). The most frequent indications for NIV were COPD exacerbations, heart failure and obesity hypoventilation. Although surveys can be valuable, a number of shortcomings of such studies need to be pointed out. The reported results are based on only the questionnaires that are returned (which in the studies mentioned above ranged from as high as 100% to as low as 27%) and only reflect limited subsets of healthcare providers. Because surveys report data from individual practitioners and institutions, and are not a randomly chosen sample of all potential respondents, their findings may not be relevant to other clinicians in different practice settings. And, importantly, these studies can only tell us what the institutions and individuals surveyed say they do, not what they actually do.

Table 1.3 Recommendations for NIV use in clinical settings

Strong positive evidence from multiple randomised controlled trials and meta-analysis

- Exacerbation of chronic obstructive pulmonary disease[34–36]
- Acute cardiogenic pulmonary edema[34–37]
- Acute respiratory failure in immunocompromised patients[35,36,38]
- Prevention of weaning failure in high-risk patients[34–36]

Strong negative evidence from multiple randomised controlled trials

- Established extubation failure[34–36,39]

Likely positive effect according to case control series or cohort study and no more than one clinical trial

- Prevention of weaning failure in low risk patients (NIV-HFNC)[40]
- Post-operative respiratory failure[35,36,41]
- Chest trauma[42]
- Acute respiratory failure in patients who do not wish to be intubated[43]
- Oxygenation prior to endotracheal intubation[44]
- Support during endoscopy[45]

Conflicting findings needing additional studies and clinical trials

- Acute lung injury and acute respiratory distress syndrome NIV-IPPV[35,36,46]
- Pneumonia[34–36]
- Extubation failure[39]
- Acute severe asthma[47]

Observational studies avoid some of these limitations since they document actual practice in the institutions in which they are performed. The caveats of such studies are that they reflect practice only at the time of the study, for the patients in the cohort and in the clinical setting evaluated. Two such reports are follow-up studies in which more recent NIV use is compared with the results of previous cohorts from the same groups of practitioners.[53,55–60] They are included in Tables 1.4 and 1.5, which summarise acute care use of NIV in adult patients, and reported use in the three main disorders in which NIV is commonly used: in acute-on-chronic respiratory failure, congestive heart failure and hypoxaemic ARF. In Table 1.5, one other observational study is reported.[60] The main findings in these studies were as follows: an increase in NIV use (10.2% to 17% of cases requiring mechanical ventilation), and similar distribution of aetiologies of respiratory failure, primarily in acute-on-chronic failure, and also in ARF. In a large study concerning all hospitalisations for COPD between 2001 and 2011 (723,560), initial NIV increased by 15.1% yearly (from 5.9% to 14.8%), and initial IMV declined by 3.2% yearly (from 8.7% to 5.9%); annual exposure to any form of mechanical ventilation increased by 4.4% (from 14.1% to 20.3%).[61] In Table 1.3, the overall failure of NIV (defined as the need for intubation) appears similar across the studies, about 37%. The proportion of patients with acute-on-chronic respiratory failure and ARF treated with NIV are quite similar (about 40% each), but the failure rate is much lower in acute-on-chronic failure (25%) than in ARF (50%). It is important to note that ARF includes many different clinical situations (pneumonia, acute respiratory distress syndrome, immunocompetent or immunocompromised, post-surgical respiratory failure), which do not have identical outcomes with NIV.

Table 1.4 Epidemiology of mechanical ventilation (MV) and non-invasive ventilation (NIV): multicentre follow-up observational studies conducted with the same methodology in the same environment at 5- and 6-year intervals

				Acute on chronic (AOC)		Cardiogenic pulmonary oedema (CPE)		Acute respiratory failure (ARF)	
Author	**Study year**	**MV all**	**NIV/MV all**	**Proportion of all patients on MV**	**Proportion of patients on NIV**	**Proportion of all patients on MV**	**Proportion of patients on NIV**	**Proportion of all patients on MV**	**Proportion of patients on NIV**
Carlucci[55]	1997	689	16%	15%	50%	7%	27%	48%	14%
Demoule[56]	2002	1076	23%	16%	64%	8%	43%	41%	22%
Esteban[57]	1998	5183	4.4%	13%	17%	10%	NA	57%	4%
Esteban[58]	2004	4968	11.1%	8%	44%	6%	NA	66%	10%
Schnell[59]	2014	3163	39%	33%	52%	36%	22%	31%	18%
Before	2000	5882	10.2%	14%	33.5%	8.5%	NA	52.5%	9%
After	2000	6044	17.5%	12%	54%	7%	NA	53.5	16%

Table 1.5 Non-invasive ventilation (NIV) use in respiratory failure and proportion of NIV by cause of respiratory failure

				Acute on chronic respiratory failure		Cardiogenic pulmonary oedema		Acute respiratory failure	
Author	**Study year**	**NIV total number**	**Proportion of NIV use**	**Proportion on NIV use**	**NIV failure**	**Proportion on NIV**	**NIV failure**	**Proportion on NIV**	**NIV failure**
Carlucci[55]	1997	110	40%	47%	NA	12%	NA	42%	NA
Demoule[56]	2002	247	44%	45%	NA	15%	NA	39%	54%
Esteban[57]	1998	228	31%	50%	NA	NA	NA	50%	37%
Esteban[58]	2004	551	35%	32%	26%	NA	NA	60%	NA
Schettino[60]	2001	458	39%	27%	31%	18%	16%	31%	60%
Schnell	2014	974	39%	33%	25%	36%	18%	31%	34%

Nevertheless, it is notable that these real-world effectiveness findings roughly confirm those observed in randomised controlled clinical trials in highly selected patients. In addition, data from follow-up studies[59,62] show an increasing use of NIV as the first-line mode for ventilation either before hospital admission (up to 13% of patients receiving mechanical ventilation) or at the time of admission (35% to 52% of patients receiving mechanical ventilation). There are few epidemiological data from observational studies reporting application of NIV as a post-extubation tool,[60,63] and with NIV as a 'ceiling' approach without the subsequent possibility of invasive ventilation – either at the patient's request (not to be intubated) or as a physician-imposed limitation.[43,54]

NIV improves survival in acute care settings as evidenced in a large meta-analysis of randomised controlled trials published in the last 20 years. Mortality was reduced when NIV was used to treat (14.2% vs. 20.6%; risk ratio = 0.72; $p < 0.001$; with survival improved in pulmonary oedema, chronic obstructive pulmonary disease exacerbation, ARF of mixed aetiologies and post-operative ARF) or to prevent ARF (5.3% vs. 8.3%; risk ratio = 0.64 [0.46–0.90]; with survival improved in post-extubation ICU patients), but not when used to facilitate an earlier extubation.[35,36]

Several studies emphasise on the risk of an increased mortality when NIV failed and subsequently required an intubation.[35,36,38,59,61,62,64] That statement pushes to identify factors predicting the success of NIV; the best remains a persistent improvement of the respiratory rate and of the $PaCO_2$ level (in case of hypercapnic respiratory failure).[59,61,65,66]

Home setting

Early limited experience with long-term HMV using either tracheostomy or negative pressure ventilation demonstrated that even patients with essentially no ventilatory function could be continuously supported, whereas individuals who retained partial ventilatory function could benefit from intermittent (e.g. during sleep) ventilatory assistance.[8] Since the 1990s, NIV has progressively obviated the requirement for tracheostomy and has led to the use of long-term HMV in a rapidly growing number of patients.[67] Among home ventilator users are patients presenting with relatively stable neuromuscular diseases or thoracic ventilatory restrictive disorders who gain a long extension of life with quite acceptable quality of life. Although there is no clear benefit in COPD,[68,69] long-term NIV is frequently prescribed in several countries.[67] In amyotrophic lateral sclerosis (ALS), most notably in those without bulbar involvement, NIV significantly prolongs survival for a few months and improves the quality of life.[70,71] It is now commonly accepted that in individuals with neuromuscular diseases who become dependent on nearly continuous ventilator assistance, additional techniques to assist coughing are necessary.[53] Two large epidemiological surveys in Europe and Australia–New Zealand have shown an overall incidence of home ventilation use of 10/100,000 people, with huge differences in regional medical practice.[67,72] Negative pressure ventilation required considerable technical expertise and infrastructure (e.g. to make custom-built cuirasses, maintain negative pressure ventilators, etc.). In the early days of NIV-IPPV, there were few masks made by industry, necessitating innovative approaches to customised 'homemade' interfaces, again requiring considerable technical back-up and expertise. These skills were not widely available. Furthermore, sleep-disordered breathing was not widely recognised by clinicians. With the increasing recognition of sleep-related abnormalities of breathing and their importance reflected in the training of physicians, the growth of respiratory sleep services and the easy availability of a wide variety of interfaces and ventilators, the provision of home ventilation is now possible from a much wider range of hospitals than was the case in the past. Demand is also rising because of increasing recognition of different groups of patients who might benefit from NIV and improved survival after critical illness, but with the patients needing ongoing ventilatory support, and, finally, changes in the population profile, the obesity epidemic and the ageing population.[72] All these factors combined will ensure that NIV will continue to expand in scope, and make its mark as one of the important advances in respiratory medicine in the past 30 years.[73,74] The cost effectiveness of HMV is quite obvious in restrictive cases (parietal or neuromuscular), but it remains uncertain in COPD.[75]

CONCLUSION

Finally, we must emphasise NIV properly applied saves lives in acute and in chronic respiratory failure.

REFERENCES

1. Papazian L, Corley A, Hess D. Use of high flow nasal cannula oxygenation in ICU adults: A narrative review. *Intensive Care Med.* 2016;42:712–24.
2. Drinker P, Shaw LA. An apparatus for the prolonged administration of artificial respiration: I. A design for adults and children. *J Clin Invest.* 1929;7.
3. Hodes HL. Treatment of respiratory difficulty in poliomyelitis. In Poliomyeliits: Papers and Discussion Presented at the Third International Poliomyelitis Conference. Philadelphia, 1955.
4. Becker LC. USPHS Polio survivors in the US 1915–2000 Age Distribution Data. 2006 (Updated October 2006; cited 21 December 2010). Available from: http://www.post-polio.org /PolioSurvivorsInTheUS1915-2000.pdf.
5. Lassen HCA. The epidemic of poliomyelitis in Copenhagen. *Proc R Soc Med.* 1954.
6. Severinghaus JW, Astrup P, Murray JF. Blood gas analysis and critical care medicine. *Am J Respir Crit Care Med.* 1998;157:S114–S122.

7. Murray JF. Review of the state of the art in intermittent positive pressure breathing therapy. *Am Rev Respir Dis*. 1974;110.
8. Splaingard ML, Frates Jr RC, Jefferson LS. Home negative pressure ventilation: Report of 20 years of experience in patients with neuromuscular disease. *Arch Phys Med Rehabil*. 1985;66.
9. Robert D, Gerard M, Leger. P. Permanent mechanical ventilation at home via a tracheotomy in chronic respiratory insufficiency. *Rev Fr Mal Respir*. 1983;11:923–36.
10. Stuart M, Weinrich M. Integrated health system for chronic disease management. *Chest*. 2004;125:695–703.
11. Sullivan CR, Berthon-Jones M, Issa FG, Eves L. Reversal of obstructive sleep apnea by continuous positive airway pressure applied through the nose. *Lancet*. 1981;1(8225):862–5.
12. Ellis ER, Bye PTP, Bruderer JW, Sullivan CE. Treatment of respiratory failure during sleep in patients with neuromuscular disease: Positive-pressure ventilation through a nose mask. *Am Rev Respir Dis*. 1987;135:148–52.
13. Kerby GR, Mayer LS, Pingleton SK. Nocturnal positive-pressure ventilation via nasal mask. *Am Rev Respir Dis*. 1987;135:738–40.
14. Bach JR, Alba AS, Mosher R, Delaubier A. Intermittent positive pressure ventilation via nasal access in the management of respiratory insufficiency. *Chest*. 1987;92:168–70.
15. Carrol N, Branthwaite MA. Control of nocturnal hypoventilation by nasal intermittent positive pressure ventilation. *Thorax*. 1988;43:349–53.
16. Leger P, Jennequin J, Gerard M, Robert D. Home positive pressure ventilation via nasal mask for patients with neuromuscular weakness or restrictive lung or chest-wall disease. *Respir Care*. 1989;334(2):73–7.
17. Meduri GU, Conoscenti CC, Menashe P, Nair S. Noninvasive face mask ventilation in patients with acute respiratory failure. *Chest*. 1989;95:865–70.
18. Brochard L, Isabey D, Piquet J. Reversal of acute exacerbations of chronic obstructive lung disease by inspiratory assistance with a face mask. *N Engl J Med*. 1990;323(22):1523–30.
19. Foglio C, Vitacca M, Quadri A. Acute exacerbations in severe COPD patients. Treatment using positive pressure ventilation by nasal mask. *Chest*. 1992;101:1533–8.
20. Bott J, Carroll MP, Conway JH. Randomised controlled trial of nasal ventilation in acute ventilator failure due to chronic obstructive airways disease. *Lancet*. 1993;341(8860):1555–7.
21. Brochard L, Mancebo J, Wysocki M. Noninvasive ventilation for acute exacerbations of chronic obstructive pulmonary disease. *N Engl J Med*. 1995;333:817–22.
22. Nourdine K, Combes P, Carton MJ. Does noninvasive ventilation reduce the ICU nosocomial infection risk? A prospective clinical survey. *Intensive Care Med*. 1999;25:567–73.
23. Mehta S, Jay GD, Woolard RH. Randomized, prospective trial of bilevel versus continuous positive airway pressure in acute pulmonary edema. *Crit Care Med*. 1997;25:620–8.
24. Sassoon CSH. Noninvasive positive-pressure ventilation in acute respiratory failure: Review of reported experience with special attention to use during weaning. *Respir Care*. 1995;40:282–8.
25. Nava S, Ambrosino N, Clini E. Noninvasive mechanical ventilation in the weaning of patients with respiratory failure due to chronic obstructive pulmonary disease: A randomized, controlled trail. *Ann Intern Med*. 1998;128:721–8.
26. Joris JL, Sottiaux TM, Chiche JD. Effect of bi-level positive airway pressure nasal ventilation on the postoperative pulmonary restrictive syndrome in obese patients undergoing gastroplasty. *Chest*. 1997;111:665–70.
27. Wysocki M, Tric L, Wolff MA. Noninvasive pressure support ventilation in patients with acute respiratory failure. A randomized comparison with conventional therapy. *Chest*. 1995;107:761–8.
28. Ferrer M, Esquinas A, Leon M. Noninvasive ventilation in severe hypoxemic respiratory failure: A randomised clinical trial. *Am J Respir Crit Care Med*. 2003;168:1438–44.
29. Plant PK, Owen JL, Parrot S. Cost effectiveness of ward based non-invasive ventilation for acute exacerbations of chronic obstructive pulmonary disease: Economic analysis of randomized controlled trials. *BMJ*. 2003;326:956–60.
30. Craven R, Singletary N, Bosken L. Use of bilevel positive airway pressure in out-of-hospital patients. *Acad Emerg Med*. 2000;7:1065–8.
31. Stauffer J, Silvestri RC. Complications of endotracheal intubation, tracheostomy, and artificial airways. *Respir Care*. 1982;27:417–34.
32. Tremblay LN, Slutsky AS. Ventilator-induced lung injury: From the bench to the bedside. *Intensive Care Med*. 2006;32:24–33.
33. Lofaso F, Brochard L, Hang T. Home versus intensive care pressure support devices. Experimental and clinical comparison. *Am J Respir Crit Care Med*. 1996;153:1591–9.
34. Keenan SP, Mehta S. Noninvasive ventilation for patients presenting with acute respiratory failure: The randomized controlled trials. *Respir Care*. 2009;54:116–24.
35. Keenan SP, Sinuff T, Burns KE. Clinical practice guidelines for the use of noninvasive positive-pressure ventilation and noninvasive continuous positive airway pressure in the acute care setting. *CMAJ*. 2011;183:195–214.

36. Cabrini L, Landoni G, Oriani A. Noninvasive ventilation and survival in acute care settings: A comprehensive systematic review and meta-analysis of randomized controlled trials. *Crit Care Med.* 2015;43:880–8.
37. Peter JV, Moran JL, Phillips-Huges J. Effect of noninvasive positive pressure ventilation on mortality in patients with acute cardiogenic pulmonary edema: A meta-analysis. *Lancet.* 2006;367:1155–63.
38. Amado-Rodríguez L, Bernal T, López-Alonso I. Impact of initial ventilatory strategy in hematological patients with acute respiratory failure: A systematic review and meta-analysis. *Crit Care Med.* 2016;44:1406–13.
39. Burns KE, Adhikari NK, Meade MO. A meta-analysis of noninvasive weaning to facilitate liberation from mechanical ventilation. *Can J Anesth.* 2006;53:305–15.
40. Hernandez G, Vaquero C, Gonzalez P. Effect of postextubation high-flow nasal cannula vs conventional oxygen therapy on reintubation in low-risk patients: A randomized clinical trial. *JAMA.* 2016;315:1354–61.
41. Jaber S, Lescot T, Futier E. Effect of noninvasive ventilation on tracheal reintubation among patients with hypoxemic respiratory failure following abdominal surgery: A randomized clinical trial. *JAMA.* 2016;315:1345–53.
42. Hernandez G, Fernandez R, Lopez-Reina P. Noninvasive ventilation reduces intubation in chest trauma-related hypoxemia: A randomized clinical trial. *Chest.* 2010;137:74–80.
43. Azoulay E, Demoule A, Jaber S. Palliative noninvasive ventilation in patients with acute respiratory failure. *Intensive Care Med.* 2011;37:1250–7.
44. Baillard C, Fosse JP, Sebbane M. Noninvasive ventilation improves preoxygenation before intubation of hypoxic patients. *Am J Respir Crit Care Med.* 2006;174:171–7.
45. Antonelli M, Conti G, Rocco M. Noninvasive positive-pressure ventilation vs conventional oxygen supplementation in hypoxemic patients undergoing diagnostic bronchoscopy. *Chest.* 2002;121:1149–54.
46. Frat JP, Thille AW, Mercat A. High-flow oxygen through nasal cannula in acute hypoxemic respiratory failure. *N Engl J Med.* 2015;372:2185–96.
47. Medoff BD. Invasive and noninvasive ventilation in patients with asthma. *Respir Care.* 2008;53:740–8.
48. Doherty MJ, Greenstone MA. Survey of non-invasive ventilation (NIPPV) in patients with acute exacerbations of chronic obstructive pulmonary disease (COPD) in the UK. *Thorax.* 1998;53:863–6.
49. Vanpee D, Delaunois L, Lheureux P. Survey of non-invasive ventilation for acute exacerbation of chronic obstructive pulmonary disease patients in emergency departments in Belgium. *Eur J Emerg Med.* 2002;9:217–24.
50. Drummond J, Rowe B, Cheung L. The use of noninvasive mechanical ventilation for the treatment of acute exacerbations of chronic obstructive pulmonary disease in Canada. *Can Respir J.* 2005;12:129–33.
51. Maheshwari V, Paioli D, Rothaar R. Utilization of noninvasive ventilation in acute-care hospitals: A regional survey. *Chest.* 2006;129:1226–33.
52. Devlin JW, Nava S, Fong JJ. Survey of sedation practices during noninvasive positive-pressure ventilation to treat acute respiratory failure. *Crit Care Med.* 2007;35:2298–302.
53. Crimi C, Noto A, Princi P. A European survey of noninvasive ventilation practices. *Eur Respir J.* 2010;36:362–9.
54. Sinuff T, Cook DJ, Keenan SP. Noninvasive ventilation for acute respiratory failure near the end of life. *Crit Care Med.* 2008;36(3):789–94.
55. Carlucci A, Richard JC, Wysocki M. SRLF collaborative group on mechanical ventilation. Noninvasive versus conventional mechanical ventilation: An epidemiologic survey. *Am J Respir Crit Care Med.* 2001;163:874–80.
56. Demoule A, Girou E, Richard JC. Increased use of noninvasive ventilation in French intensive care units. *Intensive Care Med.* 2006;32:1747–55.
57. Esteban A, Anzueto A, Frutos F. For the mechanical ventilation international study group. Characteristics and outcomes in adult patients receiving mechanical ventilation. *JAMA.* 2002;287:345–55.
58. Esteban A, Ferguson ND, Meade MO. VENTILA Group. Evaluation of mechanical ventilation in response to clinical research. *Am J Respir Crit Care Med.* 2008;177:170–7.
59. Schnell D, Timsit JF, Darmon M. Noninvasive mechanical ventilation in acute respiratory failure: Trends in use and outcomes. *Intensive Care Med.* 2014; 40:582–91.
60. Schettino G, Altobelli N, Kacmarek RM. Noninvasive positive-pressure ventilation in acute respiratory failure outside clinical trials: Experience at the Massachusetts General Hospital. *Crit Care Med.* 2008;36:441–7.
61. Stefan MS, Shieh MS, Pekow PS. Trends in mechanical ventilation among patients hospitalized with acute exacerbations of COPD in the United States, 2001 to 2011. *Chest.* 2015;147:959–68.
62. Chandra D, Stamm JA, Taylor B. Outcomes of noninvasive ventilation for acute exacerbations of chronic obstructive pulmonary disease in the United States, 1998–2008. *Am J Respir Crit Care Med.* 2012;185:152–9.
63. Thille A, Boissier F, Ben-Ghezala H. Easily identified at-risk patients for extubation failure may benefit from noninvasive ventilation: A prospective before-after study. *Crit Care.* 2016;20:48.

64. Corrêa TD, Sanches PR, Caus de Morais L. Performance of noninvasive ventilation in acute respiratory failure in critically ill patients: A prospective, observational, cohort study. *BMC Pulmon Med.* 2015;15:144–52.
65. Roberts CM, Stone RA, Buckingham RJ. Acidosis, non-invasive ventilation and mortality in hospitalised COPD exacerbations. *Thorax.* 2011;66:43–8.
66. Carrillo A, Gonzalez-Diaz G, Ferrer M. Non-invasive ventilation in community-acquired pneumonia and severe acute respiratory failure. *Intensive Care Med.* 2012;38:458–66.
67. Lloyd-Owen SJ, Donaldson GC, Ambrosino N et al. Patterns of home mechanical ventilation use in Europe: Results from the Eurovent survey. *Eur Respir J.* 2005 Jun;25:1025–31.
68. Wijkstra PJ, Lacasse Y, Guyatt GH et al. A meta-analysis of nocturnal noninvasive positive pressure ventilation in patients with stable COPD. *Chest.* 2003 Jul;124:337–43.
69. Köhnlein T, Windisch W, Köhler D. Non-invasive positive pressure ventilation for the treatment of severe stable chronic obstructive pulmonary disease: A prospective, multicentre, randomised, controlled clinical trial. *Lancet Respir Med.* 2014;2:698–705.
70. Andersen PM, Abrahams S, Borasio GD. EFNS guidelines on the Clinical Management of Amyotrophic Lateral Sclerosis (MALS) – revised report of an EFNS task force. *Eur J Neurol.* 2012;19:360–75.
71. Bourke SC, Bullock RE, Williams et al. Noninvasive ventilation in ALS: Indications and effect on quality of life. *Neurology.* 2003 Jul 22;61:171–7.
72. Garner DJ, Berlowitz DJ, Douglas J. Home mechanical ventilation in Australia and New Zealand. *Eur Respir J.* 2013;41:39–45.
73. Evans TW, Albert RK, Angus DC et al. Organized jointly by the American Thoracic Society, the European Respiratory Society, the European Society of Intensive Care Medicine, and the Société de Réanimation de Langue Française, and approved by ATS Board of Directors. International Consensus Conferences in Intensive Care Medicine: Noninvasive positive pressure ventilation in acute respiratory failure. *Am J Respir Crit Care Med.* 2001;163:283–91.
74. Sunwoo BY, Mulholland M, Rosen IM. The changing landscape of adult home noninvasive ventilation technology, use, and reimbursement in the United States. *Chest.* 2014;145:1134–40.
75. Dretzke J, Blissett D, Dave C. The cost-effectiveness of domiciliary non-invasive ventilation in patients with end-stage chronic obstructive pulmonary disease: A systematic review and economic evaluation. *Health Technol Assess.* 2015;19(81).

PART 1

The equipment

2 Positive pressure ventilators 10
Dean R. Hess
3 Continuous positive airway pressure 22
Annie Lecavalier and Peter Goldberg
4 Emerging modes for non-invasive ventilation 30
Paolo Navalesi, Federico Longhini, Rosanna Vaschetto and Antonio Messina
5 Extracorporeal CO_2 removal 36
Lara Pisani and V. Marco Ranieri
6 Interfaces 43
Cesare Gregoretti, Vincenzo Russotto and Davide Chiumello
7 Quality control of non-invasive ventilation: Performance, service, maintenance and infection control of ventilators 55
Jordi Rigau and Ramon Farré
8 Humidifiers and drug delivery during non-invasive ventilation 63
Antonio M. Esquinas Rodriguez and Maria Vargas
9 How to start a patient on non-invasive ventilation 73
Raffaele Scala and Martin Latham

2

Positive pressure ventilators

DEAN R. HESS

INTRODUCTION

Any ventilator can be attached to a mask or other interface for non-invasive ventilation (NIV). It is desirable to use a ventilator designed to compensate for leaks that occur with NIV (Box 2.1).[1,2] In this chapter, features of ventilators for NIV will be described. Because there are many different ventilators designed specifically, or in part, for NIV, and because the technical features of these ventilators are constantly changing, a generic approach will be presented.

CIRCUITS AND VENTILATORS

Circuits

For critical care ventilators, dual-limb circuits are used, and these have inspiratory and expiratory valves (Figure 2.1). The expiratory valve actively closes during the inspiratory phase, and the inspiratory valve closes during the expiratory phase. There are separate hoses for the inspiratory gas and the expiratory gas. In this configuration, there is segregation of the inspiratory and expiratory gases. In modern critical care ventilators, the exhalation valve is usually incorporated into the ventilator. For intermediate ventilators (Figure 2.1), a single-limb circuit is used with an exhalation valve near the patient. The expiratory valve is actively closed during the inspiratory phase to prevent loss of delivered tidal volume. During exhalation, the expiratory valve opens and the inspiratory valve is closed. Because the expiratory valve is near the patient, rebreathing is minimised. For bi-level ventilators, a single-limb circuit is used (Figure 2.1). A leak port, which serves as a passive exhalation port for the patient, is incorporated into the circuit near the patient or into the interface.

BOX 2.1: Considerations in the selection of a ventilator for NIV

- Leak compensation
- Trigger and cycle coupled to patient's breathing pattern
- Rebreathing
- Oxygen delivery (acute care)
- Monitoring
- Alarms (safety vs. nuisance)
- Portability (size, weight, battery)
- Tamper-proof
- Cost

Bi-level ventilators

These are blower devices that typically provide pressure support or pressure control ventilation. Some are able to provide volume-targeted pressure support/pressure control. Pressure applied to the airway is a function of flow and leak. For a given leak, more flow is generated if the pressure setting is increased. A single-limb circuit with a passive exhalation port is used. For a given pressure setting, more flow is required if the leak increases. Some modern bi-level ventilators can generate inspiratory pressures as high as 30–50 cm H_2O and flows >200 L/min. Evaluations of the performance of these ventilators have found that many perform well. In terms of gas delivery, some perform as well or better than sophisticated critical care ventilators.[3–16] However, the behaviour of bi-level ventilators is variable in response to different simulated efforts and air leaks, and this is unpredictable from the operating principles reported in the manufacturers' descriptions. This may be an issue during paediatric applications of NIV.[14] Most of these evaluations have been bench studies, and some caution is necessary in extrapolating such data to the clinical setting.

Intermediate ventilators

These ventilators are typically used for patient transport or home care ventilation. Many use a single-limb circuit

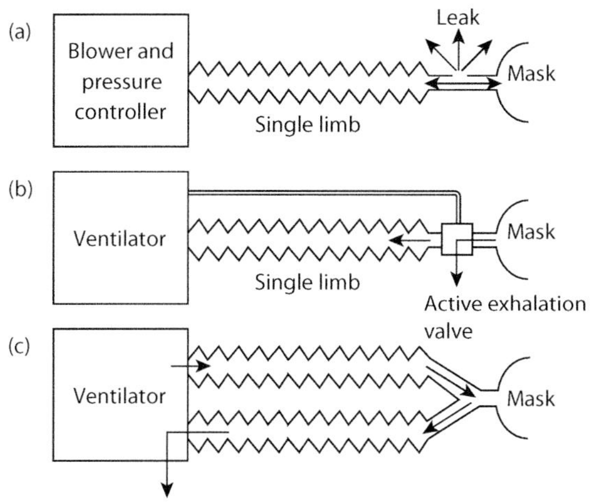

Figure 2.1 Circuits used with ventilators for non-invasive ventilation. **(a)** Single-limb circuit with passive exhalation port, such as that used with bi-level ventilators. **(b)** Single-limb circuit with active exhalation valve, such as that used with intermediate ventilators. **(c)** Dual-limb circuit with active exhalation valve, such as that used with critical care ventilators.

with an active exhalation valve near the patient, but some use a passive circuit. Nocturnal NIV in patients with neuromuscular disease typically uses these ventilators. Newer generations of these ventilators provide volume-controlled, pressure-controlled and pressure support ventilation. The current generation of these devices compensates well for leaks, and they may have an internal battery.

Critical care ventilators

These are sophisticated ventilators with a variety of modes and alarms. They are designed primarily for invasive ventilation, but can be used for NIV. Early applications of NIV for acute respiratory failure used critical care ventilators that were leak intolerant. Many current-generation critical care ventilators have NIV modes, and some compensate well for leaks.[15–18] Leak compensation, however, is variable among critical care ventilators, and thus it is important for the clinician to understand the leak compensation capability or the ventilators used in their practice.[19]

Rebreathing

An issue of concern with the bi-level ventilators, which use a passive exhalation port, is the potential for rebreathing. If the expiratory flow of the patient exceeds the flow capacity of the leak port, it is possible to exhale into the single-limb circuit and rebreathe on the subsequent inhalation. Ferguson and Gilmartin[20] reported that a bi-level positive airway pressure ventilator configured with the standard passive leak port resulted in no change in $PaCO_2$ in hypercapnic patients. When the ventilator was configured with a valve to minimise rebreathing (e.g. plateau exhalation valve), the $PaCO_2$ decrease was similar to that with a critical care ventilator. Lofaso et al.[10,21] reported that, compared with a critical care ventilator, a bi-level ventilator with passive exhalation port was associated with a greater tidal volume, minute ventilation and work of breathing. Patel and Petrini,[22] however, found no differences in work of breathing, respiratory rate, minute ventilation or $PaCO_2$ between a bi-level ventilator and a critical care ventilator. This finding is probably related to the higher pressures used by Patel and Petrini[22] compared with Lofaso et al.[21]

Although there is a potential for rebreathing with bi-level ventilators, there are several steps that can be taken to minimise that risk. Rebreathing is decreased if the leak port is in the mask rather than the hose,[23,24] if oxygen is titrated into the mask rather than into the hose,[25] with a higher expiratory pressure,[20] and with a plateau exhalation valve.[26] Major determinants of rebreathing are the expiratory time and the flow through the circuit during exhalation. Increasing the expiratory pressure requires greater flow and thus decreases the amount of rebreathing. Thus, the minimum expiratory pressure setting on many bi-level ventilators is 4 cm H_2O. Opening the ports on the interface increases leak, which increases the flow through the hose and flushes the hose to decrease rebreathing. Although it effectively decreases rebreathing, the plateau exhalation valve may increase the imposed expiratory resistance[10]; these devices are not commonly used. In a study by Hill et al.,[26] the plateau exhalation valve was compared with a traditional leak port in seven patients during nocturnal nasal ventilation. The plateau exhalation valve did not improve daytime or nocturnal gas exchange or symptoms compared with a traditional leak port. A nasal mask was used in that study, and it is unknown whether the results are applicable to patients using an oronasal mask. Patients found the plateau exhalation valve noisier and less attractive in appearance than the traditional leak port.

Leak

Leaks are a reality with NIV. The function of bi-level ventilators depends on the presence of a leak. Leaks comprise an intentional leak through the passive exhalation port as well as any unintentional leaks that may be present in the circuit or at the interface. The flow in the patient circuit represents the intentional leak as well as any additional leak related to a poorly fitting interface. If the inhaled tidal volume is greater than the exhaled measured tidal volume, the difference is assumed to be due to unintentional leak. However, the ventilator will underestimate the actual tidal volume if unintentional leak occurs during exhalation. Some bi-level ventilators allow the user to enter the interface that will be used to allow more precise identification of the intentional leak. This approach, however, requires the use of an interface provided by the manufacturer of the ventilator. Other bi-level ventilators allow the user to test the leak port as part of the pre-use procedure. Leak-detection algorithms must adjust for changes in leak with inspiratory and expiratory pressure changes, as well as changes that may occur breath-to-breath due to fit of the interface. Newer generations of bi-level ventilators use redundant leak estimation algorithms.

Leak compensation in some critical care ventilators rivals that of bi-level ventilators.[27]

Trigger

If the leak is great, the patient may breathe from the leak rather than producing a flow or pressure change that will trigger the start of the breath. On the other hand, the leak could produce a pressure or flow drop that produces auto-trigger. The ability of the ventilator to compensate for leaks thus has an important effect on triggering.

Triggers have traditionally assessed a pressure change or flow change at the proximal airway. Some ventilators are volume triggered, which is a variation on flow triggering. For example, with the Respironics bi-level ventilators, the inspiratory phase is triggered when patient effort generates an inspiratory flow, causing 6 mL of volume to accumulate. The Respironics bi-level ventilators also use a technique called Auto-Trak, in which a shape signal is created by offsetting the actual patient flow by 15 L/min and delaying it for a 300 ms period (Figure 2.2). A change in patient flow will cross the shape signal, causing the ventilator to trigger to inspiration (or cycle to exhalation). On some ventilators, such as the Respironics bi-level ventilators, the user cannot adjust the trigger sensitivity. On the ResMed bi-level ventilators, the user can choose trigger settings of HI (high), MED (medium) and LO (low), which relate to flow triggers

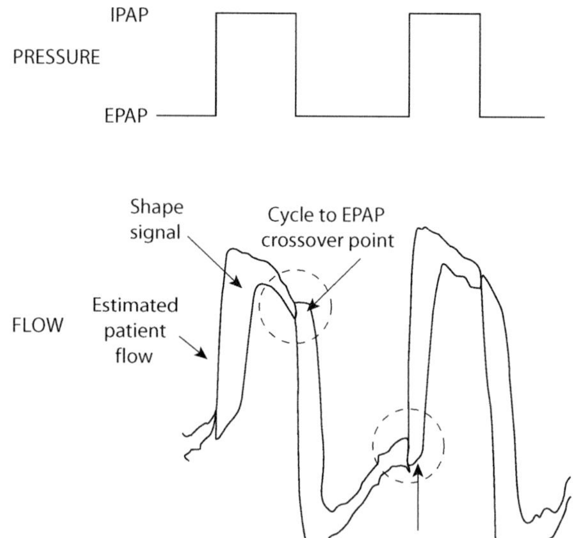

Figure 2.2 The shape signal used for triggering and cycling with Respironics bi-level ventilators is created by offsetting the signal from the actual patient flow by 15 L/min and delaying it for 300 ms. This intentional delay causes the shape signal to be slightly behind the patient's flow rate. A sudden change in patient flow will cross the shape signal, causing the ventilator to trigger to inspiration or cycle to exhalation. EPAP, expiratory positive airway pressure; IPAP, inspiratory positive airway pressure. (Courtesy of Respironics.)

of 2.5, 4.0 and 7.5 L/min, respectively. Some use redundant triggering mechanisms to improve sensitivity.

In eight patients recovering from chronic obstructive pulmonary disease (COPD) exacerbations and receiving NIV, Nava et al.[28] compared flow triggering and pressure triggering. Minute ventilation, respiratory pattern, dynamic lung compliance and resistance and changes in end-expiratory lung volume were the same with the two triggering systems. The oesophageal pressure drop during the pre-triggering phase (due to auto-positive end-expiratory pressure [PEEP] and valve opening) was higher with pressure triggering than with flow triggering. Auto-PEEP was lower during flow triggering in the pressure support mode. This not only suggests a benefit from flow triggering but also that triggering issues may often be related to the presence of auto-PEEP.

Borel et al.[29] reported that the level of intentional leak in seven commercially available masks ranged from 30 to 45 L/min at a pressure of 14 cm H_2O, which did not affect the trigger performance of bi-level ventilators. Miyoshi et al.[30] reported that bi-level ventilators triggered properly at all levels of unintentional leak (as much as 44 L/min), but uncontrollable auto-triggering occurred in the critical care ventilator when the gas leak was >18 L/min. Others have also reported a tendency for auto-triggering in the presence of a leak.[31] Using a lung model, Ferreira et al.[15] evaluated the ability of nine critical care ventilators in NIV mode and a bi-level ventilator to function in the presence of leaks. Most ventilators were able to adapt to an increase in the leak to 10 L/min without adjustments, but two of the critical care ventilators auto-triggered when the leak was increased, requiring changes in trigger sensitivity to achieve synchrony. At leaks of as great as 37 L/min, one critical care ventilator and the bi-level ventilators were able to adapt without adjustments. At leaks of 27 and 37 L/min, some of the critical care ventilators were unable to synchronise despite changes in trigger sensitivity. Vignaux et al.[16,17] conducted a lung model evaluation of critical care ventilators in NIV mode and found that leaks affected triggering, with marked variations among ventilators. In a bench and clinical study, Carteaux et al.[18] also found variations among ventilators in response to the effect of leaks on the trigger function.

Tidal volume

Pressure-controlled or pressure support ventilation may compensate for leaks better than volume-controlled ventilation. With volume control, flow and volume delivery from the ventilator are fixed. Thus, leak will reduce the inhaled tidal volume. A technique that can be used, with variable success, is to increase the tidal volume setting. However, this is variably successful because increasing the set tidal volume (and the associated pressure in the interface) may increase the leak. The ventilator targets a constant inspiratory pressure for pressure-controlled or pressure support ventilation. If a leak occurs, there will be a drop in pressure, at which point the ventilator increases flow to restore the pressure.

In a lung model with a leak, Smith and Shneerson[12] reported that the volume delivered by volume-controlled ventilators fell by >50% over most of the range of preset volumes. This decrease in tidal volume was associated with a fall in pressure of a similar magnitude. However, pressure control and pressure support compensated well for the leak. Mehta et al.[31] evaluated the leak compensating abilities of six different ventilators used for NIV in a lung model. Similar to Smith and Shneerson, they found that pressure control and pressure support maintained delivered tidal volume in the presence of leaks better than volume control. Borel et al.[29] found that the capacity of bi-level ventilators to achieve and maintain inspiratory positive airway pressure (IPAP) was decreased when intentional leaks increased, but maximum reduction in delivered tidal volume was only 48 mL.

Cycle

During volume- and pressure-controlled ventilation, the inspiratory phase is time cycled. For these breath types, the presence of a leak will not affect the inspiratory time. However, pressure support is usually flow cycled. If the leak flow is greater than the flow cycle criteria, the inspiratory phase will continue indefinitely.[32] Usually there is a secondary time cycle should this occur, which is fixed on some ventilators (e.g. 3 seconds) but adjustable on others.

If the inspiratory time is prolonged, expiratory time may be shortened, resulting in auto-PEEP. The presence of auto-PEEP makes triggering more difficult. If the patient fails to trigger, expiratory time will be prolonged, the amount of auto-PEEP decreases and the patient is then able to trigger. The result is variability in the respiratory rate provided by the ventilator. If auto-PEEP increases, the delivered tidal volume for a fixed pressure support setting is less. This results in variability in tidal volume delivery. Hotchkiss et al.[33,34] used a mathematical and lung model to explore the issue of leak on ventilator performance. They found that pressure support applied in the context of an inspiratory leak resulted in substantial breath-to-breath variation in the inspiratory phase, resulting in auto-PEEP if the respiratory rate was fixed, or in variability in respiratory rate, inspiratory time and auto-PEEP if the rate was allowed to vary. This was most likely to occur when the respiratory system time constant was long relative to the respiratory rate, as occurs in patients with COPD. A lung model study by Adams et al.[35] predicted a relatively narrow range for inspiratory flow cycle that provides adequate ventilatory support without causing hyper-inflation in patients with COPD.

Using an older-generation bi-level ventilator, Mehta et al.[31] reported that a large leak interfered with cycling of the ventilator and shortening of the expiratory time. Calderini et al.[36] compared the effect of time-cycled and flow-cycled breaths in six patients during NIV. In the presence of leaks, they found that time-cycled breaths provided better synchrony than flow-cycled breaths. Borel et al.[29] found that expiratory cycling was not affected by the level of intentional leaks in masks except in COPD conditions.

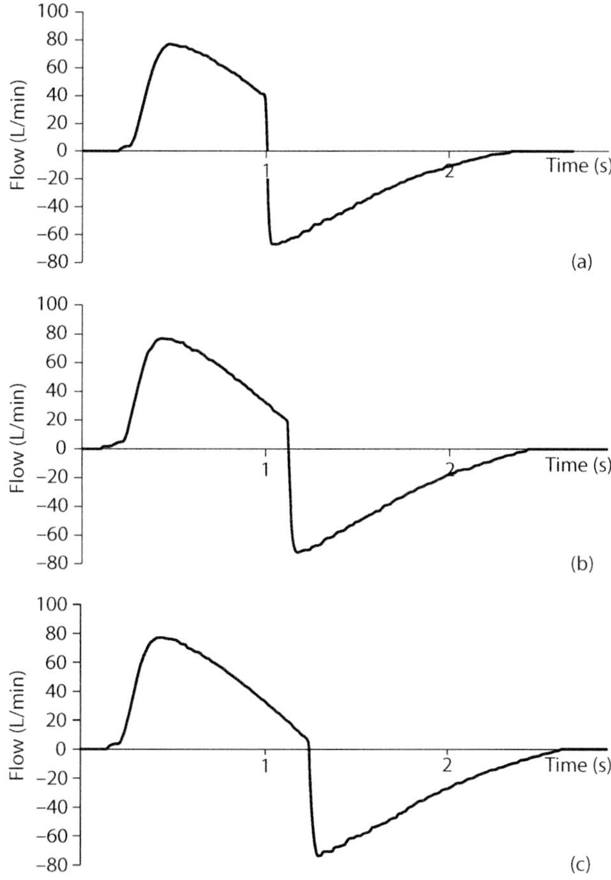

Figure 2.3 The effect of flow cycle adjustment on the inspiratory time. Note that a higher flow cycle shortens the inspiratory time. **(a)** Flow cycle at 50% of peak inspiratory flow. **(b)** Flow cycle at 25% of peak inspiratory flow. **(c)** Flow cycle at 10% of peak inspiratory flow.

However, Battisti et al.[11] reported delayed cycling in the presence of leaks with bi-level ventilators.

Several strategies can be used to address the issue of prolonged inspiration with pressure support. Unintentional leaks should be minimised, and use of a ventilator with good leak compensation is ideal. Some bi-level ventilators use redundant measures to determine end of inspiration. For example, the Respironics bi-level ventilators use the shape signal (Figure 2.2) and a method called spontaneous expiratory threshold. The spontaneous expiratory threshold is an electronic signal that rises in proportion to the inspiratory flow rate on each breath; when the spontaneous expiratory threshold and actual patient flow value are equal, the unit cycles to exhalation. The maximum inspiratory time is adjustable on some ventilators, and some ventilators allow the flow cycle criteria to be adjusted. Note that the effect of a higher flow cycle as a percentage of peak inspiratory flow translates to a shorter inspiratory time (Figure 2.3).

Oxygen delivery

For acute care applications, it is desirable to use a ventilator with a blender allowing precise administration of the fraction of inspired oxygen (FiO_2) from 0.21 to 1. Bi-level ventilators used outside the acute care setting generally do not have a blender, but rather provide supplemental oxygen by titration into the circuit or interface. This results in a delivered oxygen concentration that is variable, and only modest concentrations can be achieved (e.g. <60%). With oxygen titration, the FiO_2 is affected by the site of the oxygen titration, type of exhalation port, ventilator settings, oxygen flow, breathing pattern and leak. For some bi-level ventilators, oxygen titration can affect the displayed values of tidal volume.

Waugh and Granger[37] reported that with a bi-level ventilator and the leak port in the mask, the FiO_2 was higher when oxygen was added at the ventilator outlet instead of the mask and with lower IPAP and expiratory positive airway pressure (EPAP) settings. Thys et al.[25] reported that the FiO_2 was higher with lower IPAP and when oxygen was added at the mask than when added at the ventilator outlet. They also found that, although the FiO_2 was increased with a higher oxygen flow, it was difficult to obtain an $FiO_2 > 0.30$ without a very high oxygen flow. Schwartz et al.[38] reported that the oxygen concentration was significantly lower with the leak port in the mask, with higher IPAP and EPAP settings and with lower oxygen flow. With the mask leak port, the oxygen concentration was greater when oxygen was added into the circuit than into the mask, presumably because in the latter, much of the oxygen was exhausted out the exhalation port because of the close proximity of the oxygen entrainment site to the port. The highest oxygen concentration was achieved with the leak port in the circuit and oxygen added into the mask using lower IPAP and EPAP values. With a large unintentional leak, Miyoshi et al.[30] reported a reduction in the FiO_2 with a bi-level ventilator and oxygen titration into the circuit. Titration of oxygen into the circuit or interface may affect the monitored values of tidal volume, and high flows (>15 L/min) have the potential to affect ventilator performance.

MODES

Continuous positive airway pressure

With continuous positive airway pressure (CPAP), no additional pressure is applied during inhalation to assist with delivery of the tidal volume (Figure 2.4). With NIV, pressure applied to the airway during the inspiratory phase is greater than the pressure applied during exhalation. This provides respiratory muscle assistance, resulting in respiratory muscle unloading and increased tidal volume delivery in proportion to the amount of pressure assist. The most common use of CPAP mode is for the treatment of obstructive sleep apnoea.

Pressure support ventilation

Pressure support ventilation is used most commonly for NIV.[39,40] With a critical care ventilator, the level of pressure

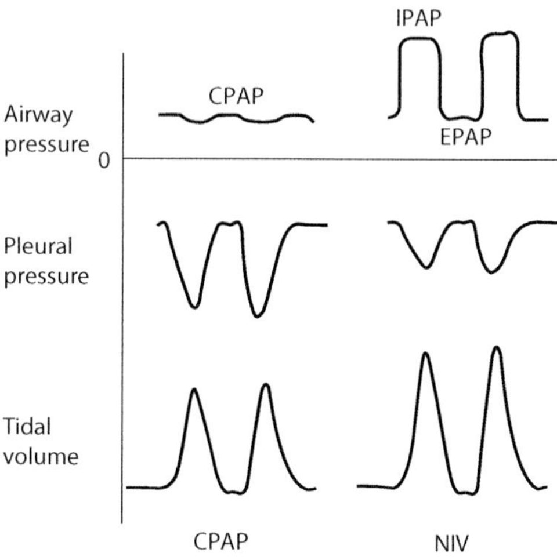

Figure 2.4 Comparison of continuous positive airway pressure (CPAP) and non-invasive ventilation (NIV). Note that no inspiratory support is provided with CPAP. EPAP, expiratory positive airway pressure; IPAP, inspiratory positive airway pressure.

support is applied as a pressure above the baseline PEEP. However, the approach is different with bi-level ventilators, where an IPAP and EPAP are set. In this configuration, the difference between the IPAP and EPAP is the level of pressure support (Figure 2.5). With pressure support, the pressure applied to the airway is fixed for each breath, but there is no backup rate or fixed inspiratory time (Table 2.1).

In 16 patients with acute respiratory failure, Girault et al.[41] reported that both pressure support and volume control provided respiratory muscle rest and similarly improved breathing pattern and gas exchange. These physiologic effects were achieved with a lower inspiratory work load, but at a higher respiratory discomfort, with volume control than with pressure support. Navalesi et al.[42] compared pressure support and pressure control in 26 patients with chronic hypercapnic respiratory failure. Compared with spontaneous breathing, NIV provided better ventilation and gas

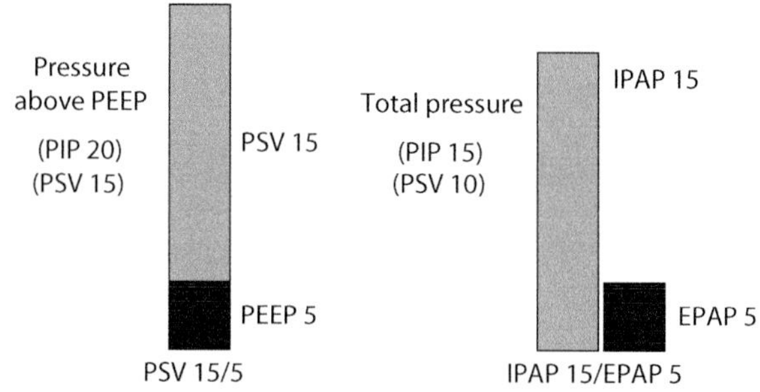

Figure 2.5 Comparison of pressure support ventilation (PSV), such as with critical care ventilators, and inspiratory positive airway pressure (IPAP) with a bi-level ventilator. Note that the IPAP is the peak inspiratory pressure (PIP) and includes the expiratory positive airway pressure (EPAP), whereas pressure support is provided on top of the positive end-expiratory pressure (PEEP).

Table 2.1 Comparison of various breath types that can be used during non-invasive ventilation

	VC	PC	APS	PS	PAV	NAVA
Tidal volume	Fixed	Variable	Minimum set	Variable	Variable	Variable
Inspiratory flow	Fixed	Variable	Variable	Variable	Variable	Variable
Airway pressure	Variable	Fixed	Variable	Fixed	Variable	Variable
Inspiratory time	Fixed	Fixed	Variable	Variable	Variable	Variable
Rate	Minimum set	Minimum set	Not set	Not set	Not set	Not set

Abbreviations: VC: volume control; PC: pressure control; APS: adaptive pressure support; PS: pressure support; PAV: proportional assist ventilation; NAVA: neurally adjusted ventilatory assist.

exchange irrespective of the ventilator mode. There were no differences between modes in tolerance of ventilation, gas exchange or breathing pattern. In patients with stable cystic fibrosis, Fauroux et al.[43] found that both pressure support and volume control decreased respiratory muscle unloading.

In the spontaneous mode on bi-level ventilators, IPAP and EPAP are set, but there is no backup rate. With the spontaneous/timed mode, the patient receives pressure support ventilation if the rate is greater than the set rate. However, if the patient becomes apnoeic, the ventilator will deliver flow-cycled or time-cycled breaths at the rate set on the ventilator. For critical care ventilators set for pressure support, backup ventilation and alarms occur if the patient becomes apnoeic. A backup rate is important to prevent periodic breathing. Central apnoea was found to be more prevalent with pressure support in normal subjects using a nasal mask,[44] in intubated patients[45] and in patients being evaluated in an outpatient sleep laboratory.[46] For these reasons, a backup rate is recommended during NIV, particularly with nocturnal applications.

Pressure-controlled ventilation

Pressure-controlled ventilation is similar to pressure support in that the ventilator applies a fixed level of pressure with each breath. Trigger and rise time are similar between pressure support and pressure control,[47] but there are two differences between them: there is a backup rate with pressure control, and the inspiratory time is fixed with pressure control. The backup rate is beneficial in the setting of apnoea or periodic breathing. The fixed inspiratory time of pressure control is beneficial when the inspiratory phase is prolonged during pressure support due to leak or lung mechanics (e.g. COPD). Vitacca et al.[48] found no difference in NIV success between volume control and pressure control. Schonhofer et al.[49] found that pressure control was successful in most patients after an initial treatment with volume control. However, a third of the patients who initially did well on volume control failed on pressure control. In chronic stable patients with neuromuscular disease, Chadda et al.[50] found that volume control, pressure control and pressure support had similar effects on alveolar ventilation and respiratory muscle unloading. Kirakli et al.[51] randomised 35 hypercapnic patients with COPD to 1 hour of pressure support or pressure control. They found that pressure control was as effective and safe as pressure support in carbon dioxide elimination with comparable side effects. Some bi-level ventilators have a timed mode. With this mode, the ventilator is triggered and cycled by the ventilator at the set rate and inspiratory time. This mode provides little interaction between the patient and the ventilator.

Proportional assist ventilation

With proportional assist ventilation (PAV), the applied pressure is determined by respiratory drive (i.e. inspiratory flow and tidal volume) and lung mechanics (i.e. resistance and compliance), and the proportion of assist is set by the user.[52] Because respiratory drive varies breath-by-breath and within the breath, the pressure assist also varies. With PAV, there is no backup rate or set tidal volume (Table 2.1). PAV has been used effectively with NIV and may improve patient tolerance during acute respiratory failure.[53–56] In patients with chronic respiratory failure due to neuromuscular disease and chest wall deformity, PAV with NIV may also improve patient comfort.[57–59] PAV may also improve sleep quality.[60] It is unclear whether PAV with NIV improves patient outcomes in either acute care or chronic care settings.

Neurally adjusted ventilatory assistance

With neurally adjusted ventilatory assistance (NAVA), the ventilator is triggered by electrical activity of a diaphragm.[52] The electrical activity of the diaphragm is measured by a multiple-array oesophageal electrode, which is amplified to determine the support level (NAVA gain). The cycle-off is commonly set at 80% of peak inspiratory activity. Schmidt et al.[61] reported that NAVA improved synchrony more than the use of NIV mode on a critical care ventilator. The combination of NAVA with the NIV mode seemed to offer the best compromise between good synchrony and a low level of leaks. They also found a high level of leaks with NAVA, probably as a result of the nasogastric tube. NAVA has been reported to improve synchrony during NIV,[62] but evidence is lacking regarding whether this translated into better patient outcomes. The need for a specialised nasogastric tube is an important barrier to the use of NAVA.

Volume-controlled ventilation

With volume-controlled ventilation, the ventilator delivers a fixed tidal volume and inspiratory flow with each

Table 2.2 Comparison of volume ventilator and bi-level pressure ventilator for NIV

Volume ventilator	Pressure ventilator
More complicated to use	Simple to use
Wide range of alarms	Limited alarms
Constant tidal volume	Variable tidal volume
Breath-stacking possible	Breath-stacking not possible
No leak compensation	Leak compensation
Can be used without PEEP	PEEP (EPAP) always present
Rebreathing minimised	Rebreathing possible

breath (Table 2.2). Usually, the inspiratory time is a function of the tidal volume, inspiratory flow and inspiratory flow pattern selected. However, some ventilators allow tidal volume, inspiratory flow and inspiratory time to be selected independent of one another. Volume control has been used during NIV primarily in the home setting with an intermediate ventilator.[63–66] It has also been used to provide mouthpiece ventilation.[67–77] A low-pressure alarm can be prevented during mouthpiece ventilation by producing enough circuit back pressure with sufficient peak inspiratory flow against the restrictive mouthpiece according to the set tidal volume.[72] The ventilator rate is also set at a low level to prevent an apnoea alarm. Some current generation ventilators feature a mouthpiece ventilation mode to address issues with this strategy using traditional modes. Carlucci et al.[73] reported that an appropriate alarm setting and combination of tidal volume and inspiratory time allowed the majority of the tested ventilators to be used for mouthpiece ventilation without alarm activation. Breath-stacking manoeuvres can be provided with volume-controlled, but not pressure-controlled or pressure support, ventilation. Martínez et al.[71] reported high rates of NIV tolerance in subjects with ALS receiving volume-controlled ventilation.

Adaptive pressure support

The adaptive pressure support modes average volume-assured pressure support (AVAPS) and intelligent volume-assured pressure support (iVAPS) adjust the level of pressure support to maintain a target tidal volume.[74] AVAPS maintains a tidal volume equal to or greater than the target tidal volume by automatically controlling the pressure support between the minimum and maximum IPAP settings. It averages tidal volume over time and changes the IPAP gradually over several minutes. If patient effort decreases, AVAPS automatically increases IPAP to maintain the target tidal volume. On the other hand, if patient effort increases, AVAPS will reduce IPAP. Alveolar ventilation is targeted by iVAPS using an estimation of dead space based on the height of the patient. A potential limitation of this approach is that dead space is increased in patients with lung disease, which is greater than that estimated by height. A limitation of both modes is that support is reduced if patient effort results in a tidal volume that exceeds the target. These modes also incorporate algorithms to adjust respiratory rate.[74] In a bench study, Luján et al.[75] found that the presence of dynamic unintentional leaks interfered with ventilator performance using adaptive pressure support modes. Inspiratory leaks resulted in a reduction in pressure support, with no guarantee of delivered tidal volume. Nicholson et al.[76] compared pressure support ventilation with AVAPS, and reported a more consistent tidal volume and better breathing pattern with AVAPS. Clinical studies, however, have reported mixed results with these modes,[76–80] and their role is yet to be determined.[81,82]

VENTILATOR OPTIONS TO IMPROVE TOLERANCE

In addition to selection of an appropriate mode, trigger, rise time and expiratory cycle, two other features incorporated into bi-level ventilators to improve patient tolerance are ramp and Bi-Flex.

Rise time

Rise time (pressurisation rate) is the time required to reach the inspiratory pressure at the onset of the inspiratory phase with pressure support or pressure-controlled ventilation.[31] With a fast rise time, the inspiratory pressure is reached quickly, whereas with a slow rise time, it takes longer to reach the inspiratory pressure. A faster rise time may better unload the respiratory muscles of patients with COPD, but this may be accompanied by substantial air leaks and poor tolerance.[83] In patients with neuromuscular disease, a slower rise time is often better tolerated. Rise time should be set to maximise patient comfort.

Expiratory pressure release

Expiratory pressure release provided a small pressure drop during the later stages of inspiration and the beginning part of exhalation (Figure 2.6). This feature, when used with CPAP in patients with sleep apnoea, was associated with similar outcomes to standard CPAP, but those with low compliance improved their adherence with this feature.[84] Evidence supporting the use of expiratory pressure release with NIV is lacking.

Ramp

Ramp reduces the pressure and then gradually increases it to the pressure setting. A ramp has been used primarily in patients receiving CPAP for sleep apnoea to allow the patient to fall asleep more comfortably. The role of a ramp during NIV is unclear, particularly for acute care applications, where it may be undesirable because it delays application of a therapeutic pressure.

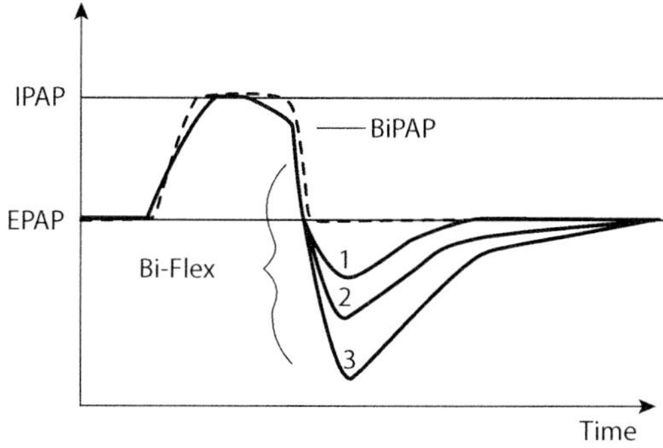

Figure 2.6 Bi-Flex inserts a small pressure relief during the later stages of inspiration and at the beginning of exhalation. BiPAP, bi-level positive airway pressure; EPAP, expiratory positive airway pressure; IPAP, inspiratory positive airway pressure.

Patient–ventilator synchrony

Failure of NIV to prevent intubation might relate, in part, to patient–ventilator asynchrony, although the relationship between asynchrony and NIV failure has not been well studied. Good NIV tolerance has been associated with success of NIV, and improved comfort has been associated with better synchrony. An asynchrony rate in more than 40% of patients has been reported to occur during NIV.[85] Asynchrony is commonly associated with leaks. A number of strategies might be used to correct asynchrony when it occurs during NIV (Table 2.3).[86]

Table 2.3 Strategies to improve synchrony with non-invasive ventilation

Trigger asynchrony
- Adjust trigger sensitivity for the best balance between trigger effort and auto-triggering
- Increase PEEP (expiratory positive airway pressure) to counterbalance auto-PEEP
- Minimise unintentional leak with appropriate fitting of the interface
- Treat underlying disease

Flow asynchrony
- Use pressure-targeted or volume-targeted ventilation per patient comfort
- Adjust inspiratory pressure with pressure ventilation; adjust flow and tidal volume with volume ventilation
- Adjust rise time (pressurisation rate) per patient comfort
- Minimise unintentional leak with appropriate fitting of the interface
- Reduce respiratory drive

Cycle asynchrony
- Minimise unintentional leak with appropriate fitting of the interface
- Use time-cycled (pressure control) rather than flow-cycled (pressure support) ventilation
- Adjust flow cycle setting
- Reduce pressure support setting
- Treat underlying disease process (e.g. bronchodilators to decrease airways resistance)

Mode asynchrony
- Use backup rate if apnoea or periodic breathing occurs

Source: Adapted from Hess DR, *Respir Care* 2011;56:153–65; discussion 165–7.

SAFETY

Alarms and monitoring

Alarms during NIV are a balance between patient safety and annoyance. The extent of alarms necessary depends on the underlying condition of the patient and the ability of the patient to breathe without support. For example, consider the patient with neuromuscular disease receiving near full support by NIV. This patient is unable to reattach the interface or circuit should it become disconnected. In this case, disconnect alarms and alarms indicating large leaks or changes in ventilation are desirable. Similar alarms are desirable in a patient with acute respiratory failure receiving NIV. On the other extreme, in the case of a patient using daytime mouthpiece ventilation, alarms may be an annoyance and techniques have been described to outsmart these alarms.[68,87] When a question of the extent of alarms is necessary, one should fault on the side of patient safety. Ventilators for NIV have increasing capability to monitor the patient's breathing. Display of tidal volume, respiratory rate and leak is useful for titrating settings. Many ventilators also display waveforms of pressure, flow and volume. These waveforms can be useful in titrating settings to improve patient–ventilator synchrony.

Battery power

Ventilators for NIV can be battery-powered for safety and portability. Some ventilators for NIV have an internal battery. Others can be powered with a battery or uninterruptable power supply (Figure 2.7). Many bi-level ventilators can be powered with a direct-current converter. The duration of the battery is determined by the size of the battery, ventilator settings, amount of leak and whether or not a humidifier is used. When using a battery, it is generally best not to use a humidifier to extend the life of the battery. It is also best to avoid use of the humidifier when the bi-level is made portable to avoid accidentally spilling water into the ventilator.

SUMMARY

A variety of options are available on positive pressure ventilators for NIV. Familiarity with these options allows the clinician to match the ventilator and its features to the needs of the patient who is receiving NIV.

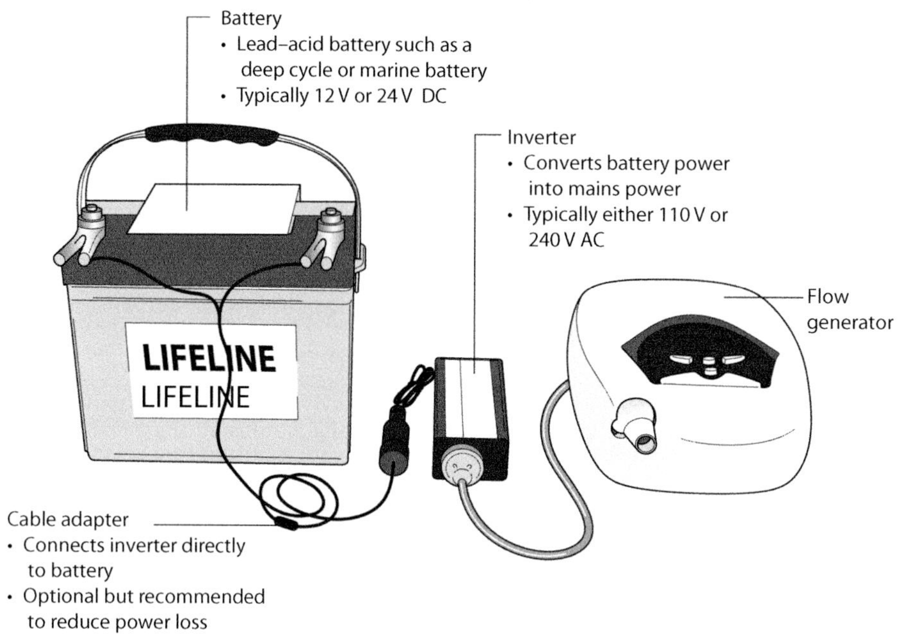

Figure 2.7 Configuration for use of a bi-level ventilator with a battery and inverter. (Courtesy of ResMed.)

REFERENCES

1. Chatburn RL. Which ventilators and modes can be used to deliver noninvasive ventilation? *Respir Care.* 2009;54:85–101.
2. Scala R, Naldi M. Ventilators for noninvasive ventilation to treat acute respiratory failure. *Respir Care.* 2008;53:1054–80.
3. Bunburaphong T, Imanaka H, Nishimura M et al. Performance characteristics of bilevel pressure ventilators: A lung model study. *Chest.* 1997;111:1050–60.
4. Stell IM, Paul G, Lee KC et al. Noninvasive ventilator triggering in chronic obstructive pulmonary disease. A test lung comparison. *Am J Respir Crit Care Med.* 2001;164:2092–7.
5. Highcock MP, Morrish E, Jamieson S et al. An overnight comparison of two ventilators used in the treatment of chronic respiratory failure. *Eur Respir J.* 2002;20:942–5.
6. Highcock MP, Shneerson JM, Smith IE. Functional differences in bi-level pressure preset ventilators. *Eur Respir J.* 2001;17:268–73.
7. Richard JC, Carlucci A, Breton L et al. Bench testing of pressure support ventilation with three different generations of ventilators. *Intensive Care Med.* 2002;28:1049–57.
8. Tassaux D, Strasser S, Fonseca S et al. Comparative bench study of triggering, pressurization, and cycling between the home ventilator VPAP II and three ICU ventilators. *Intensive Care Med.* 2002;28:1254–61.
9. Vitacca M, Barbano L, D'Anna S et al. Comparison of five bilevel pressure ventilators in patients with chronic ventilatory failure: A physiologic study. *Chest.* 2002;122:2105–14.
10. Lofaso F, Brochard L, Hang T et al. Home versus intensive care pressure support devices. Experimental and clinical comparison. *Am J Respir Crit Care Med.* 1996;153:1591–9.
11. Battisti A, Tassaux D, Janssens JP et al. Performance characteristics of 10 home mechanical ventilators in pressure-support mode: A comparative bench study. *Chest.* 2005;127:1784–92.
12. Smith IE, Shneerson JM. A laboratory comparison of four positive pressure ventilators used in the home. *Eur Respir J.* 1996;9:2410–5.
13. Scala R. Bi-level home ventilators for noninvasive positive pressure ventilation. *Monaldi Arch Chest Dis.* 2004;61:213–21.
14. Fauroux B, Leroux K, Desmarais G et al. Performance of ventilators for noninvasive positive-pressure ventilation in children. *Eur Respir J.* 2008;31:1300–7.
15. Ferreira JC, Chipman DW, Hill NS et al. Bilevel vs ICU ventilators providing noninvasive ventilation: Effect of system leaks: A COPD lung model comparison. *Chest.* 2009;136:448–56.
16. Vignaux L, Tassaux D, Jolliet P. Performance of noninvasive ventilation modes on ICU ventilators during pressure support: A bench model study. *Intensive Care Med.* 2007;33:1444–51.
17. Vignaux L, Tassaux D, Carteaux G et al. Performance of noninvasive ventilation algorithms on ICU ventilators during pressure support: A clinical study. *Intensive Care Med.* 2010;36:2053–9.
18. Carteaux G, Lyazidi A, Cordoba-Izquierdo A et al. Patient-ventilator asynchrony during noninvasive ventilation: A bench and clinical study. *Chest.* 2012;142:367–76.

19. Hess DR, Branson RD. Know your ventilator to beat the leak. *Chest.* 2012;142:274–5.
20. Ferguson GT, Gilmartin M. CO2 rebreathing during BiPAP ventilatory assistance. *Am J Respir Crit Care Med.* 1995;151:1126–35.
21. Lofaso F, Brochard L, Touchard D et al. Evaluation of carbon dioxide rebreathing during pressure support ventilation with airway management system (BiPAP) devices. *Chest.* 1995;108:772–8.
22. Patel RG, Petrini MF. Respiratory muscle performance, pulmonary mechanics, and gas exchange between the BiPAP S/T-D system and the Servo Ventilator 900C with bilevel positive airway pressure ventilation following gradual pressure support weaning. *Chest.* 1998;114:1390–6.
23. Schettino GP, Chatmongkolchart S, Hess DR et al. Position of exhalation port and mask design affect CO2 rebreathing during noninvasive positive pressure ventilation. *Crit Care Med.* 2003;31:2178–82.
24. Saatci E, Miller DM, Stell IM et al. Dynamic dead space in face masks used with noninvasive ventilators: A lung model study. *Eur Respir J.* 2004;23:129–35.
25. Thys F, Liistro G, Dozin O et al. Determinants of FiO_2 with oxygen supplementation during noninvasive two-level positive pressure ventilation. *Eur Respir J.* 2002;19:653–7.
26. Hill NS, Carlisle C, Kramer NR. Effect of a nonrebreathing exhalation valve on long-term nasal ventilation using a bilevel device. *Chest.* 2002;122:84–91.
27. Hess DR. Noninvasive ventilation for acute respiratory failure. *Respir Care.* 2013;58:950–72.
28. Nava S, Ambrosino N, Bruschi C et al. Physiological effects of flow and pressure triggering during non-invasive mechanical ventilation in patients with chronic obstructive pulmonary disease. *Thorax.* 1997;52:249–54.
29. Borel JC, Sabil A, Janssens JP et al. Intentional leaks in industrial masks have a significant impact on efficacy of bilevel noninvasive ventilation: A bench test study. *Chest.* 2009;135:669–77.
30. Miyoshi E, Fujino Y, Uchiyama A et al. Effects of gas leak on triggering function, humidification, and inspiratory oxygen fraction during noninvasive positive airway pressure ventilation. *Chest.* 2005;128:3691–8.
31. Mehta S, McCool FD, Hill NS. Leak compensation in positive pressure ventilators: A lung model study. *Eur Respir J.* 2001;17:259–67.
32. Hess DR. Ventilator waveforms and the physiology of pressure support ventilation. *Respir Care.* 2005;50:166–86; discussion 183–6.
33. Hotchkiss JR Jr, Adams AB, Stone MK et al. Oscillations and noise: Inherent instability of pressure support ventilation? *Am J Respir Crit Care Med.* 2002;165:47–53.
34. Hotchkiss JR, Adams AB, Dries DJ et al. Dynamic behavior during noninvasive ventilation: Chaotic support? *Am J Respir Crit Care Med.* 2001;163:374–8.
35. Adams AB, Bliss PL, Hotchkiss J. Effects of respiratory impedance on the performance of bi-level pressure ventilators. *Respir Care.* 2000;45:390–400.
36. Calderini E, Confalonieri M, Puccio PG et al. Patient-ventilator asynchrony during noninvasive ventilation: The role of expiratory trigger. *Intensive Care Med.* 1999;25:662–7.
37. Waugh JB, Granger WM. An evaluation of 2 new devices for nasal high-flow gas therapy. *Respir Care.* 2004;49:902–6.
38. Schwartz AR, Kacmarek RM, Hess DR. Factors affecting oxygen delivery with bi-level positive airway pressure. *Respir Care.* 2004;49:270–5.
39. Hess DR. The evidence for noninvasive positive-pressure ventilation in the care of patients in acute respiratory failure: A systematic review of the literature. *Respir Care.* 2004;49:810–29.
40. Hess DR. Noninvasive ventilation in neuromuscular disease: Equipment and application. *Respir Care.* 2006;51:896–911, discussion 911–2.
41. Girault C, Richard JC, Chevron V et al. Comparative physiologic effects of noninvasive assist-control and pressure support ventilation in acute hypercapnic respiratory failure. *Chest.* 1997;111:1639–48.
42. Navalesi P, Fanfulla F, Frigerio P et al. Physiologic evaluation of noninvasive mechanical ventilation delivered with three types of masks in patients with chronic hypercapnic respiratory failure. *Crit Care Med.* 2000;28:1785–90.
43. Fauroux B, Pigeot J, Polkey MI et al. In vivo physiologic comparison of two ventilators used for domiciliary ventilation in children with cystic fibrosis. *Crit Care Med.* 2001;29:2097–105.
44. Parreira VF, Delguste P, Jounieaux V et al. Effectiveness of controlled and spontaneous modes in nasal two-level positive pressure ventilation in awake and asleep normal subjects. *Chest.* 1997;112:1267–77.
45. Parthasarathy S, Tobin MJ. Effect of ventilator mode on sleep quality in critically ill patients. *Am J Respir Crit Care Med.* 2002;166:1423–9.
46. Johnson KG, Johnson DC. Bilevel positive airway pressure worsens central apneas during sleep. *Chest.* 2005;128:2141–50.
47. Williams P, Kratohvil J, Ritz R et al. Pressure support and pressure assist/control: Are there differences? An evaluation of the newest intensive care unit ventilators. *Respir Care.* 2000;45:1169–81.
48. Vitacca M, Rubini F, Foglio K et al. Non-invasive modalities of positive pressure ventilation improve the outcome of acute exacerbations in COLD patients. *Intensive Care Med.* 1993;19:450–5.

49. Schonhofer B, Sonneborn M, Haidl P et al. Comparison of two different modes for noninvasive mechanical ventilation in chronic respiratory failure: Volume versus pressure controlled device. *Eur Respir J.* 1997;10:184–91.
50. Chadda K, Clair B, Orlikowski D et al. Pressure support versus assisted controlled noninvasive ventilation in neuromuscular disease. *Neurocrit Care.* 2004;1:429–34.
51. Kirakli C, Cerci T, Ucar ZZ et al. Noninvasive assisted pressure-controlled ventilation: As effective as pressure support ventilation in chronic obstructive pulmonary disease? *Respiration.* 2008;75:402–10.
52. Sinderby C, Beck J. Proportional assist ventilation and neurally adjusted ventilatory assist: Better approaches to patient ventilator synchrony? *Clin Chest Med.* 2008;29:329–42, vii.
53. Fernandez-Vivas M, Caturla-Such J, Gonzalez de la Rosa J et al. Noninvasive pressure support versus proportional assist ventilation in acute respiratory failure. *Intensive Care Med.* 2003;29:1126–33.
54. Wysocki M, Richard JC, Meshaka P. Noninvasive proportional assist ventilation compared with noninvasive pressure support ventilation in hypercapnic acute respiratory failure. *Crit Care Med.* 2002;30:323–9.
55. Gay PC, Hess DR, Hill NS. Noninvasive proportional assist ventilation for acute respiratory insufficiency. Comparison with pressure support ventilation. *Am J Respir Crit Care Med.* 2001;164:1606–11.
56. Rusterholtz T, Bollaert PE, Feissel M et al. Continuous positive airway pressure vs. proportional assist ventilation for noninvasive ventilation in acute cardiogenic pulmonary edema. *Intensive Care Med.* 2008;34:840–6.
57. Hart N, Hunt A, Polkey MI et al. Comparison of proportional assist ventilation and pressure support ventilation in chronic respiratory failure due to neuromuscular and chest wall deformity. *Thorax.* 2002;57:979–81.
58. Porta R, Appendini L, Vitacca M et al. Mask proportional assist vs pressure support ventilation in patients in clinically stable condition with chronic ventilatory failure. *Chest.* 2002;122:479–88.
59. Winck JC, Vitacca M, Morais A et al. Tolerance and physiologic effects of nocturnal mask pressure support vs proportional assist ventilation in chronic ventilatory failure. *Chest.* 2004;126:382–8.
60. Bosma K, Ferreyra G, Ambrogio C et al. Patient–ventilator interaction and sleep in mechanically ventilated patients: Pressure support versus proportional assist ventilation. *Crit Care Med.* 2007;35:1048–54.
61. Schmidt M, Dres M, Raux M et al. Neurally adjusted ventilatory assist improves patient-ventilator interaction during postextubation prophylactic noninvasive ventilation. *Crit Care Med.* 2012;40:1738–44.
62. Sehgal IS, Dhooria S, Aggarwal AN et al. Asynchrony index in pressure support ventilation (PSV) versus neurally adjusted ventilator assist (NAVA) during non-invasive ventilation (NIV) for respiratory failure: Systematic review and meta-analysis. *Intensive Care Med.* 2016;42:1813–5.
63. Benditt JO. Full-time noninvasive ventilation: Possible and desirable. *Respir Care.* 2006;51:1005–12; discussion 1012–15.
64. Fauroux B, Boffa C, Desguerre I et al. Long-term noninvasive mechanical ventilation for children at home: A national survey. *Pediatr Pulmonol.* 2003;35:119–25.
65. Kerby GR, Mayer LS, Pingleton SK. Nocturnal positive pressure ventilation via nasal mask. *Am Rev Respir Dis.* 1987;135:738–40.
66. Leger P, Jennequin J, Gerard M et al. Home positive pressure ventilation via nasal mask for patients with neuromusculoskeletal disorders. *Eur Respir J Suppl.* 1989;7:640s–4s.
67. Bach JR, Alba AS, Bohatiuk G et al. Mouth intermittent positive pressure ventilation in the management of postpolio respiratory insufficiency. *Chest.* 1987;91:859–64.
68. Bach JR, Alba AS, Saporito LR. Intermittent positive pressure ventilation via the mouth as an alternative to tracheostomy for 257 ventilator users. *Chest.* 1993;103:174–82.
69. Toussaint M, Steens M, Wasteels G et al. Diurnal ventilation via mouthpiece: Survival in end-stage Duchenne patients. *Eur Respir J.* 2006;28:549–55.
70. Boitano LJ. Equipment options for cough augmentation, ventilation, and noninvasive interfaces in neuromuscular respiratory management. *Pediatrics.* 2009;123 Suppl 4:S226–30.
71. Martínez D, Sancho J, Servera E, Marín J. Tolerance of volume control noninvasive ventilation in subjects with amyotrophic lateral sclerosis. *Respir Care.* 2015;60:1765–71.
72. Boitano LJ, Benditt JO. An evaluation of home volume ventilators that support open-circuit mouthpiece ventilation. *Respir Care.* 2005;50:1457–61.
73. Carlucci A, Mattei A, Rossi V et al. Ventilator settings to avoid nuisance alarms during mouthpiece ventilation. *Respir Care.* 2016;61:462–7.
74. Johnson KG, Johnson DC. Treatment of sleep-disordered breathing with positive airway pressure devices: Technology update. *Med Devices (Auckl).* 2015;8:425–37.
75. Luján M, Sogo A, Grimau C et al. Influence of dynamic leaks in volume-targeted pressure support noninvasive ventilation: A bench study. *Respir Care.* 2015;60:191–200.
76. Nicholson TT, Smith SB, Siddique T et al. Respiratory pattern and tidal volumes differ for pressure support and volume-assured pressure support in amyotrophic lateral sclerosis. *Ann Am Thorac Soc.* 2017;14:1139–46.

77. Kelly JL, Jaye J, Pickersgill RE et al. Randomized trial of 'intelligent' autotitrating ventilation versus standard pressure support non-invasive ventilation: Impact on adherence and physiological outcomes. *Respirology*. 2014;19:596–603.
78. Murphy PB, Davidson C, Hind MD et al. Volume targeted versus pressure support non-invasive ventilation in patients with super obesity and chronic respiratory failure: A randomised controlled trial. *Thorax*. 2012;67:727–34.
79. Briones Claudett KH, Briones Claudett M, Chung Sang Wong M et al. Noninvasive mechanical ventilation with average volume assured pressure support (AVAPS) in patients with chronic obstructive pulmonary disease and hypercapnic encephalopathy. *BMC Pulm Med*. 2013;13:12.
80. Oscroft N, Ali M, Gulati A et al. A randomised crossover trial comparing volume assured and pressure preset noninvasive ventilation in stable hypercapnic COPD. *COPD*. 2010;7:398–403.
81. Hill NS. Noninvasive ventilation for COPD: Volume assurance not very reassuring. *COPD*. 2010;7:389–90.
82. Windisch W, Storre JH. Target volume settings for home mechanical ventilation: Great progress or just a gadget? *Thorax*. 2012;67:663–5.
83. Prinianakis G, Delmastro M, Carlucci A et al. Effect of varying the pressurisation rate during noninvasive pressure support ventilation. *Eur Respir J*. 2004;23:314–20.
84. Pepin JL, Muir JF, Gentina T et al. Pressure reduction during exhalation in sleep apnea patients treated by continuous positive airway pressure. *Chest*. 2009;136:490–7.
85. Vignaux L, Vargas F, Roeseler J et al. Patient-ventilator asynchrony during non-invasive ventilation for acute respiratory failure: A multicenter study. *Intensive Care Med*. 2009;35:840–6.
86. Hess DR. Patient-ventilator interaction during non-invasive ventilation. *Respir Care*. 2011;56:153–65; discussion 165–7.
87. Carlucci A, Mattei A, Rossi V et al. Ventilator settings to avoid nuisance alarms during mouthpiece ventilation. *Respir Care*. 2016;61:462–7.

3

Continuous positive airway pressure

ANNIE LECAVALIER AND PETER GOLDBERG

INTRODUCTION

Continuous positive airway pressure (CPAP) ventilation is a tool commonly used by respirologists for their outpatients as well as by critical care physicians in the intensive care unit (ICU). CPAP has varied uses, but a common physiology that benefits patients in different clinical settings. In this chapter, we review the history of CPAP, its physiology, its indications and contraindications, the equipment required and its patient tolerance.

HISTORY OF CPAP

Positive pressure breathing appears to have been first used clinically in the latter decades of the nineteenth century in the treatment of acute non-cardiogenic pulmonary oedema and asthma, and reports of its successful use in the treatment of cardiogenic pulmonary oedema first appeared in the 1930s.[1] However, it seems that the first systematic investigation of its use was made in its successful application in preventing hypoxemia in high-altitude pilots.[2]

It was not until the 1960s, however, that clinicians started to widely use CPAP in the treatment of hyaline membrane disease (HMD) of the newborn, then a major cause of neonatal mortality. The disease had been linked to low lung compliance and reduced functional residual capacity (FRC) as a result of a deficiency of pulmonary surfactant.[3] Dr George Gregory had documented that increasing minute ventilation often resulted in the inadvertent generation of positive end-expiratory pressure (PEEP) and improved blood gas values. Contrarily, reducing ventilation led to atelectasis and hypoxemia. As intriguingly, it had been clinically observed that the grunting exhibited by neonates with HMD was associated with improved oxygenation. Harrison and colleagues demonstrated, in their study into its physiological consequences, that grunting was indeed associated with improvements in oxygenation in that its elimination following endotracheal intubation was associated with the almost immediate onset of cyanosis.[4] In their set of elegant physiologic studies, the same investigators determined that grunting was associated with the generation of positive trans-pulmonary pressure during expiration which they attributed to the expiratory retention of air through a partially closed glottis. The authors then concluded that the mechanism responsible for the improvement in oxygenation was in fact the positive trans-pulmonary pressure generated during expiration, the resulting increase in lung volume and the latter's beneficial impact on the regions of low ventilation/perfusion (V/Q) mismatch and frank atelectasis inherent to this shunt-producing disease.[4] These findings were then followed by Gregory et al.'s seminal paper on CPAP that reported improved oxygenation and decreased mortality in 20 infants with HMD,[5] findings echoed by Llewellyn and Swyer who showed similar findings during that same period.[6]

At approximately the same time, investigators of the treatment of refractory hypoxemia in adult patients were similarly establishing the utility of increasing airway pressure during expiration. Both Asbaugh and colleagues, in their now classic paper describing the acute respiratory distress syndrome,[7] and Kumar et al.[8] demonstrated both the physiologic and clinical benefits of applying positive pressure during the expiratory phase of the respiratory cycle.

It was only several years later, in 1980 in Australia, that Dr Colin Sullivan had the idea of applying positive airway pressure through the nasal airway of an adult patient with very severe sleep apnoea, who was refusing the life-saving tracheostomy that had been recommended. This patient had a dramatically positive response to the newly fashioned device, even achieving rapid-eye movement sleep. Sullivan and his colleagues repeated the experiment in other patients and came to the conclusion that CPAP applied through a nasal mask provided a pneumatic splint for the nasopharyngeal airway and was a safe, simple treatment for the obstructive sleep apnoea (OSA) syndrome.[9]

PHYSIOLOGY

CPAP refers to the delivery of a continuous level of positive airway pressure, meaning a continually (but not constant) positive pressure during both inspiration and expiration to a spontaneously breathing patient. CPAP is not a true ventilator mode because it does not actively assist ventilation: the ventilator does not cycle during CPAP, and no additional pressure above the level of CPAP is provided by the breathing circuit to the patient (Figure 3.1).

CPAP should be considered analogous to the application of PEEP to the mechanically ventilated patient but, in the case of CPAP, as a means of providing positive pressure during the expiratory phase of respiration to the spontaneously breathing patient. In fact, in the following discussions, PEEP and CPAP will be used interchangeably when discussing the impact of positive expiratory pressure on cardiopulmonary physiology. Furthermore, it must be stressed that in providing positive pressure during expiration, it is critical that the inspiratory circuit be pressurised to approximately the same level so as to minimise the change in airway pressure during the respiratory cycle and avoid any increase in the work of breathing that would result, for example, from the pressurisation of the expiratory circuit alone.[10,11]

When considering CPAP, it is convenient to consider its application in two very separate and physiologically distinct clinical contexts: the first, its use in disease states in which low lung volumes, right-to-left shunt and significant hypoxemia are the predominant clinical concerns; and the second, in patients with hyperinflation in which intrinsic PEEP (PEEPi) is thought to play a major pathophysiological role. And it will be with these two manifestly different clinical settings in mind that the physiological effects of CPAP, on both the respiratory and circulatory systems, are to be considered.

Respiratory system

FRC is that lung volume determined by the balance between the inward recoil of the lung and the tendency of the chest wall to expand outwardly. A multitude of factors can decrease FRC, including the supine position, induction of anaesthesia, insertion of an endotracheal tube, breathing 100% oxygen, abdominal or thoracic surgery, restrictive chest disorders such as obesity, acute respiratory distress syndrome (ARDS), cardiogenic pulmonary oedema, pulmonary fibrosis, chest or abdominal trauma and atelectasis due to retained secretions. All these elements can result in airway closure, atelectasis, shunting and hypoxemia. In most instances, the application of CPAP increases FRC.[10]

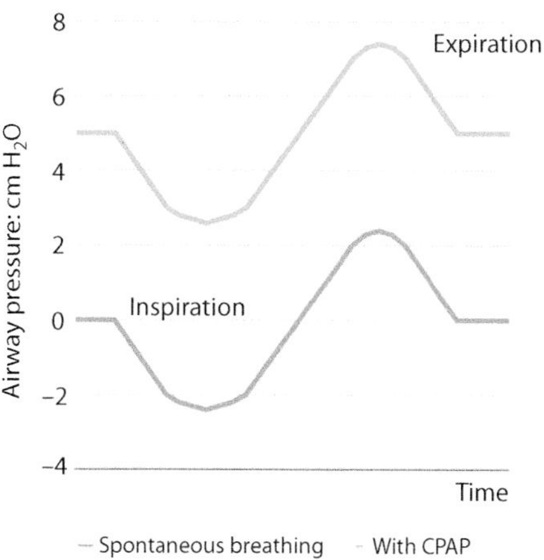

Figure 3.1 The respiratory cycle during spontaneous breathing and with CPAP support.

In those instances when CPAP does not result in an increase in lung volume, it is due to the presence of PEEPi and the presence of expiratory flow limitation, conditions encountered typically in patients with COPD.[12] In fact, clinically, the application of CPAP to patients with PEEPi has been shown, in a variety of clinical settings, to decrease the work of breathing by counterbalancing the additional elastic inspiratory load imposed by PEEPi.[13]

The increase in FRC when it does result may be due to recruitment of closed or atelectatic alveoli or may be due to alveolar overdistension.[14,15] Consistent with those variable mechanisms of increasing FRC, respiratory system compliance may either increase, decrease or remain unchanged.[14] Presumably, this variable response to the application of PEEP on respiratory and on pulmonary compliance, in particular, relates, in part, to the heterogeneity in the compliance characteristics of the millions of individual alveoli and to the specific volume history (tidal volume) to which the respiratory system has been exposed.[14] Additionally, mechanisms other than alveolar recruitment have been implicated in the increase in pulmonary compliance and include PEEP-induced decrease in pulmonary blood volume, release of surfactant and/or prostaglandins and a decrease in alveolar duct tone.[16]

The effect of PEEP on dead space (V_D/V_T) has been studied in both patients with normal lung function undergoing non-thoracic and non-abdominal surgery[15] and in patients with acute lung injury. In their study of patients with ARDS, Fengmei and colleagues noted a bimodal distribution of V_D/V_T, falling between zero end-expiratory pressure and 12 cm H_2O before rising again as increased PEEP levels were applied.[17] Maisch and coworkers, also using the Enghoff modification of the Bohr equation to calculate V_D/V_T, found much the same in normal subjects undergoing general anaesthesia during fascio-maxillary surgery.[15] In both patient groups, low levels of PEEP decreased V_D/V_T presumably by the increased efficiency of CO_2 elimination consequent to the decrease in right-to-left shunt, whereas higher levels of PEEP increased dead space through alveolar overdistension and conversion of more of the lung to West's zones I and II.[18]

The primary clinical goal in the application of PEEP is to improve oxygenation by decreasing right-to-left intrapulmonary shunt. However, similar to its effect on compliance, PEEP's impact on intrapulmonary shunt is variable, falling or increasing.[19] The fall has been attributed to the increase in FRC, a result of the recruitment of atelectatic and compressed areas of the lung,[8] whereas the increase is due to the overdistension of the more compliant regions of the lung with the resultant compression of its alveolar perfusion, and its re-direction to the more non-compliant diseased areas of the lung.[20] In this regard, Dantzker and colleagues[21] have demonstrated that a PEEP-induced fall in cardiac output (v.i.) may also result in a decrease in intrapulmonary shunt,[19] implying that any fall in right-to-left shunt following the application or increase in the level of PEEP must always be referenced to any accompanying change in cardiac output.

It has been shown that in COPD patients in acute respiratory failure (ARF), inspiratory work of breathing (WOB) is increased twofold when compared to normals, and most of that increased work is due to the presence of PEEPi and less, although significantly still, to the increase in airway resistance.[22] Given those findings, several groups have demonstrated that the application of PEEP to mechanically ventilated COPD patients and of CPAP to spontaneously breathing COPD patients weaning from mechanical ventilation decreases WOB, improves arterial blood gases, decreases oxygen consumption, improves breathing pattern and decreases the sense of dyspnoea.[13,23,24] Additionally, we were able to demonstrate that graded amounts of CPAP applied to non-intubated, spontaneously breathing COPD patients in ARF patients resulted in a decrease in inspiratory effort in a dose-response fashion, an improvement in the pattern of breathing and a decrease in the patients' sense of dyspnoea.[25]

However, the amount of externally applied PEEP ($PEEP_E$) in these circumstances is important and must be done with care given that when administered to patients even with PEEPi, end-expiratory lung volumes (EELVs) can nevertheless increase when $PEEP_E$ approaches or surpasses the amount of PEEPi present. The exact level at which hyperinflation begins to occur is uncertain, ranging in different studies from 85% to 100% ($PEEP_E$/PEEPi).

Although not studied as extensively, CPAP appears to decrease the WOB in patients with disease states characterised by decreases in FRC,[26] although the results have been variable and would be expected to differ depending on the presence or absence of PEEPi,[27] the variable effect of CPAP on lung compliance and airway resistance and the size of the accompanying tidal volume.[28]

Circulatory system

The application of CPAP can decrease cardiac output, leave it unaltered and, in some circumstances, result in an increase. The fall in cardiac output has been attributed to two mechanisms. The first implicates the transmission of the airway pressure increase to the pleural space and the consequential fall in venous return likely secondary to an increase in resistance to venous return. The second entails the possible increase in impedance to right ventricular output in response to a rise in pulmonary vascular resistance rises as CPAP converts more of the lung to West's zones I and II.

CPAP is thought to influence various autonomic reflexes at play on the pulmonary vessels and, more importantly, to alter pulmonary vascular tone through its effect on hypoxic pulmonary vasoconstriction. However, by far, the predominant effect of CPAP on pulmonary vascular resistance is secondary to its biphasic effect on lung volume, an effect attributed to the antithetical response of the alveolar and extra-alveolar vessels to the changes in lung volume.[29,30]

Clinically, these two mechanisms can be differentiated echocardiographically. In the first instance, in which an increase in pleural pressure is responsible for the fall in cardiac output, a decrease in right ventricular end-diastolic volume would be observed while an increase in right-ventricular afterload would manifest as a decrease in indices of right ventricular output including increases in both right ventricular end-systolic and diastolic volumes.[31]

Under normal conditions, changes in intrathoracic pressure have little effect on left ventricular output, but during large negative pressure swings as may occur in respiratory distress, changes in pleural pressure may have a significant adverse clinical impact on left ventricular output, particularly in the context of left ventricular dysfunction. For a given intracavitary (left ventricular) pressure, a coincident pleural pressure drop will increase the left ventricular wall stress and afterload by that same amount. Conversely, an increase in intrathoracic pressure through, for example, the application of positive airway pressure will have the opposite effect and decrease left ventricular afterload.

In the clinical context, a normally functioning and hence afterload-insensitive left ventricle will be little affected by swings in the surrounding pleural pressure. However, the afterload-sensitive, failing left ventricle may well respond positively to an increase in intrathoracic pressure and particularly to the attendant diminution in the degree of negative pleural pressure swings that often accompanies the relief of respiratory distress.[30,32]

Several investigators have examined the effect of increased intrathoracic pressure on coronary blood flow and have suggested that pressure may adversely affect the gradient for coronary perfusion through a variety of different mechanisms, thereby resulting in coronary ischemia, particularly in subjects with coronary artery disease.[30,32] These findings are made all the more relevant when considering the increased incidence of myocardial infarction in those patients suffering from cardiogenic pulmonary oedema that were treated with non-invasive bi-level mechanical ventilation (EPAP 5 cm H_2O; IPAP 15 cm H_2O) as compared to those patients treated with 10 cm H_2O of CPAP.[33] However, it must be added that subsequent studies have failed to demonstrate any such increase,[34] and a recent Cochrane analysis concluded that no such link was found to exist.[35]

In cases where CPAP is used at home for sleep-related disorders, its purpose is to splint the upper airway open in order to prevent airway collapse and periods of airway obstruction and apnoea episodes.

TYPES OF CPAP

Fixed CPAP delivers positive airway pressure at a level that remains relatively constant (within 1 to 2 cm of H_2O) throughout the respiratory cycle. The positive airway pressure splints the upper airway open, preventing upper airway collapse. No additional pressure above the level of CPAP is provided, and patients must initiate all breaths.

The optimal amount of positive airway pressure delivered by a fixed CPAP device is typically determined by titration. In cases of OSA, optimal fixed CPAP setting is typically the level of pressure at or above which obstructive events are eliminated for more than 90% to 95% of the time. This titration may be manually done in the sleep laboratory as part of a sleep study, or at home using an auto-titrating CPAP device. As opposed to a fixed CPAP, auto-titrating CPAP delivers an amount of positive airway pressure that varies during the night, in an attempt to provide the lowest level of airway pressure required to maintain the upper airway open. The variation in pressure is decided on by a software algorithm, which detects flow changes and increases the airway pressure until adequate airway patency is achieved. After a period of time, the pressure will be slowly decreased until airway obstruction is identified, at which point the pressure will be increased again. Auto-titrating CPAP may not function properly if a significant leak is present, since leaks can change airflow. Also, dependent on the device and algorithm used, central apnoeas may not be detected, if the patient exhibits any. Auto-titrating CPAP has been proposed for use in different situations: patients who don't tolerate the degree of fixed CPAP necessary to prevent respiratory events in all positions and stages, and patients subjected to factors that may vary their pressure requirements (such as the use of alcohol, nasal congestion from allergies or upper respiratory infections) and following a diagnosis made with home sleep apnoea testing and access to a laboratory titration of CPAP may be delayed or inconvenient. Many studies including meta-analyses have shown that there is little difference in use of fixed or auto-titrating CPAP with regards to efficacy or adherence in patients with uncomplicated moderate to severe OSA.

On the other hand, CPAP titration in the acute setting is usually performed by a respiratory therapist, and the goal is clinical improvement, as evidenced by improved oxygenation, lower respiratory rate and decreased WOB, while patient comfort and tolerance to CPAP is maintained.

INDICATIONS AND CONTRAINDICATIONS

CPAP and PEEP were initially used in premature infants with HMD, but their use have expanded greatly since the 1960s. The main indications for CPAP are obstructive sleep apnoea (OSA), obesity hypoventilation syndrome (OHS), cardiogenic pulmonary oedema, acute exacerbations of chronic obstructive pulmonary disease (COPD) and in instances of post-operative hypoxemia.

CPAP is generally the first-line treatment for most patients with OSA as it has been well studied, is readily available, is simple to use and is less costly than other options. It has been shown to be effective in reducing symptoms of sleepiness and improving the quality of life in moderate to severe OSA.[36] CPAP is also used in the treatment of OHS, usually when present concomitantly with OSA. Given that OHS patients may also suffer from a disordered control of breathing, not all patients with coexisting OHS and OSA will benefit from CPAP.[37] Hence, the failure of CPAP to eliminate nocturnal desaturation usually indicates a need for escalation to bi-level positive airway pressure ventilation.

The main goal in the use of CPAP in the acute setting is the avoidance of endotracheal intubation and mechanical ventilation and the latter's associated complications, most notably ventilator-associated pneumonia. While the indications for the use of CPAP in this context are varied, strong evidence exists for only a few.

The strongest evidence to support the use of CPAP in the acute hospital setting is, without a doubt, in cardiogenic pulmonary oedema. Several randomised trials have demonstrated its effectiveness.[38–42] In 2010, a meta-analysis of 13 trials found that patients who received CPAP plus standard care had a lower hospital mortality than standard care alone.[43] A Cochrane systematic review in 2013 concluded that non-invasive positive pressure ventilation, especially CPAP, when added to standard medical care is an effective and safe intervention for the treatment of adult patients with acute cardiogenic pulmonary oedema.[35]

In the post-operative setting, Squadrone et al. compared CPAP with supplemental oxygen alone in 209 patients with PaO2/FiO2 (P/F) ratio < 300 mmHg after abdominal surgery. The intubation rate was lower in the CPAP group (1% vs. 10%), and there was a reduction in the incidence of pneumonia and in the length of ICU stay.[44] A meta-analysis of 9 randomized controlled trials (RCTs) published in 2008 showed that CPAP significantly reduces the risk of postoperative pulmonary complications (risk ratio 0.66; 95% CI), atelectasis (risk ratio, 0.75; 95% CI) and pneumonia (risk ratio, 0.33; 95% CI), an analysis that supports its clinical use in patients undergoing abdominal surgery.[45]

Overall, the evidence for the use of CPAP in other indications is weaker. However, given the pathophysiologic role that PEEPi plays in an acute exacerbation of COPD, one would anticipate that CPAP could provide a therapeutic role. In 1993, Miro demonstrated that in seven COPD patients with hypercapnic respiratory failure, the CPAP significantly improved gas exchange and obviated the need for intubation in four of the seven patients.[46] The same year, De Lucas et al. showed similar findings in 15 COPD patients in acute respiratory failure. Using nasal CPAP, they showed that the respiratory rate decreased, the subjective sensation of dyspnoea improved as well as an improvement in both $PaCO_2$ and PaO_2.[47] To support these findings, Goldberg et al. evaluated the physiologic effects of CPAP in COPD patients. Ten patients with COPD who were admitted to the ICU in acute respiratory failure were treated with CPAP. They found that inspiratory effort and the pressure-time product for the diaphragm fell significantly with CPAP in a dose-dependent fashion. In addition, the pattern of breathing and level of dyspnoea improved, as did the gas exchange.[25]

The data regarding the use of CPAP in other aetiologies of hypoxemic respiratory failure remain unclear. One such study randomised 123 patients with acute lung injury (P/F ratio < 300 mmHg) to oxygen therapy alone vs. oxygen

Table 3.1 Indications and contraindications of CPAP

Indications	Contraindications
Obstructive sleep apnoea (OSA)	Cardiac or respiratory arrest
Acute cardiogenic pulmonary oedema	Inability to cooperate, protect the airway or clear secretions
Acute exacerbations of COPD	Severely impaired consciousness
Hypoxemic respiratory failure	Haemodynamic instability or unstable cardiac arrhythmia
Post-operative hypoxemia	Facial surgery, trauma or deformity
	High risk for aspiration, upper GI bleed
	Prolonged duration of mechanical ventilation anticipated
	Recent oesophageal anastomosis

Source: International Consensus Conferences in Intensive Care Medicine: Noninvasive positive pressure ventilation in acute respiratory failure. *Am J Respir Crit Care Med* 2001; 163:288. Copyright © 2001 American Thoracic Society.

therapy plus CPAP. The cause of the acute lung injury was felt to be pneumonia in 55% of cases and cardiac disease in 30% of cases. The use of CPAP improved oxygenation but failed to decrease the intubation or mortality rates.[48]

Other potential indications for the use of CPAP include the following: respiratory failure in the immunocompromised patient, asthma,[49] weaning from extubation, upper airway obstruction and trauma.[50,51] However, given that there are no convincing data to support the use of CPAP, the potential risks and benefits need to be weighed in deciding on a trial of CPAP in these patient groups.

Regardless of the setting in which CPAP is used, the contraindications remain the same as with any type of noninvasive ventilation (NIV) device. In the hospital setting, the need for emergent intubation constitutes an absolute contraindication to the use of NIV. Other contraindications are listed in Table 3.1.

CPAP EQUIPMENT

The CPAP equipment comprises the patient–device interface, often referred to as mask, the tubing and the motor or flow generator. The flow generator provides the airflow. The tubing consists of the hose connecting the flow generator to the interface. The patient–device interfaces are varied and include nasal masks, nasal pillows, full facemasks and oral interfaces. A helmet interface has been developed that may improve patient tolerance, but has yet to gain popularity.

The ideal interface is one that provides the best combination of comfort and efficacy. The optimal interface varies from patient to patient, and it is often recommended that trials of different interfaces should be done upon initial fitting and titration of the CPAP. The best interface is said to be 'the one that the patient will use'. Most CPAP circuits also allow for incorporation of humidification, mostly for comfort, as well as for addition of supplemental oxygen.

Also of interest is the fact that the cost of a piece of CPAP equipment is much lower than the cost of a piece of BIPAP equipment (approximately $1,500 for CPAP vs. approximately $20,000 for BIPAP), making CPAP a much more cost-effective treatment when used in the appropriate setting.

ACCEPTANCE AND TOLERANCE

In the outpatient setting, we know that non-adherence rates to CPAP therapy are quite high. The same issues that limit adherence to CPAP at home may be present in the hospital settings as well, notably mask discomfort, positive pressure non-tolerance and claustrophobia. Given that the main goal of CPAP being the avoidance of endotracheal intubation, it is of utmost importance that all efforts be made for optimal efficacy and that comfort to be instituted from the beginning of treatment. In the acute setting, the main factor likely responsible for such success relates to the skill and expertise of the healthcare worker (respiratory therapist) initiating the therapy. More specifically, the time taken to familiarise the patient with the interfaces, the stepwise increase in positive pressure and explanations and reassurance about the treatment itself surely play an immense role in patient adherence and tolerance. Close observation and frequent re-evaluation of the patient are primordial in this setting, thereby giving this treatment modality the best chance for success.

CPAP OUTSIDE THE HOSPITAL SETTING

CPAP is clearly beneficial for patients in the emergency department and in the ICU for certain types of respiratory failure. Given that early initiation of treatment is likely important for success, questions about the benefits of CPAP in the pre-hospital setting have emerged over the last decade. In 2009, Foti et al. used a helmet CPAP as the first-line pre-hospital treatment of 121 patients with presumed severe acute pulmonary oedema, with or without standard medical treatment. In both groups, CPAP significantly improved oxygenation, reduced the respiratory rate and improved haemodynamics, and no patient required pre-hospital intubation.[52] In this study, helmet CPAP appeared to be simple, efficient and safe in pre-hospital treatment of presumed acute cardiogenic pulmonary oedema. A meta-analysis conducted in 2013 showed a reduction in the number of intubations and mortality in 1002 patients with acute respiratory failure who received CPAP in the pre-hospital setting.[53] In contrast, two observational studies failed to show that the use of pre-hospital CPAP improved physiological variables, rates of intubation or mortality.[54,55] However, a literature review done in 2013, including 12 studies, concluded that pre-hospital CPAP led to improved patient vital signs, improvement in reduced short-term mortality and reduced rates of endotracheal intubation in patients with acute pulmonary oedema secondary to heart failure,[56] suggesting that this patient population may have a greater benefit from CPAP treatment than patients with undifferentiated acute respiratory failure. Interestingly, a meta-analysis performed in 2014 concluded that while pre-hospital CPAP reduced mortality and intubation rates, the effectiveness of pre-hospital BiPAP was uncertain.[57] Overall, CPAP in the pre-hospital setting appears to be a promising tool for acute respiratory failure, but further large, randomised controlled studies are needed to confirm these findings, better define the patient population that would benefit the most and how its implementation in emergency medical services can be achieved.

SUMMARY

CPAP is a simple, readily available, relatively inexpensive and NIV modality that has been used both in the inpatient and outpatient settings for several decades. In the acute in-hospital setting, CPAP is indicated as first-line therapy in patients with cardiogenic pulmonary oedema and in those with post-operative hypoxemia. Its primary goal is the avoidance of endotracheal intubation and mechanical ventilation. Familiarity and facility with CPAP equipment, a supportive approach by the healthcare team to optimise its acceptance by patients, and importantly, recognition of the contraindications to its use are all fundamental to its successful use at the bedside.

REFERENCES

1. Barach AL, Martin J, Eckman L. Positive pressure respiration and its application to the treatment of acute pulmonary oedema and respiratory obstruction. *Proc Am Soc Clin Investig.* 1937;16:664–80.
2. Ernsting, J. Some Effects of Raised Intrapulmonary Pressure in Man. The NATO Advisory Group for Aerospace Research and Development (doctoral thesis), 1966.
3. Smith CA. *The Physiology of the Newborn Infant.* Springfield, IL: Chas. C. Thomas, 1959; Nelson NM. Pulmonary function of the newborn infant; The alveolar–arterial oxygen gradient. *J Appl Physiol.* 1963;18:534–8.
4. Harrison VC, Heese H de V, Kline M. The significance of grunting in hyaline membrane disease. *Pediatrics.* 1968;41:549–59.
5. Gregory GA, Kitterman JA, Phibbs RH et al. Treatment of the idiopathic respiratory-distress syndrome with continuous positive airway pressure. *N Eng J Med.* 1971;284;1333–40.
6. Llewellyn MA, Swyer PR. Positive expiratory pressure during mechanical ventilation in the newborn. *Pediatr Res Progr.* 1970;224.
7. Ashbaugh DG, Bigelow DB, Petty TL, Levine BE. Acute respiratory distress in adults. Lancet. 1967;290:319.
8. Kumar A, Falke KJ, Geffin B et al. Continuous positive-pressure ventilation in acute respiratory failure – effects on hemodynamics and lung function. *N Eng J Med.* 1970;283:1430.
9. Sullivan CE, Issa FG, Berthon-Jones M, Eves L. Reversal of obstructive sleep apnea by continuous positive pressure applied through the nares. *Lancet.* 1981;1(8225):862–5.
10. Gherini S, Peters RM, Virgilio RW. Mechanical work on the lungs and work of breathing with positive end-expiratory pressure and continuous positive airway pressure. *Chest.* 1979;76:251.
11. Hillman DR, Finucane KE. Continuous positive airway pressure: A breathing system to minimize respiratory work. *Crit Care Med.* 1985;13:38–43.
12. Rossi A, Brandolese R, Milic-Emili J, Gottfried SB. The role of PEEP in patients with COPD during assisted ventilation. *Eur Resp J.* 1990;818.
13. Petrof BJ, Legaré M, Goldberg P et al. CPAP reduces the work of breathing and dyspnea during weaning from mechanical ventilation in severe chronic obstructive pulmonary disease. *Am Rev Resp Dis.* 1990;141:281.
14. Ranieri VM, Eisa NT, Corbeil C et al. Effects of positive end-expiratory pressure on alveolar recruitment and gas exchange in patients with ARDS. *Am Rev Resp Dis.* 1991;144:544.
15. Maisch S, Reissmann H, Fuellekrug B et al. Compliance and dead space fraction indicate an optimal level of positive end-expiratory pressure after recruitment in anesthetized patients. *Anesthesia/Analgesia.* 2008:175–181.
16. D'Angelo E, Calderini E, Tavola M et al. Effect of PEEP on respiratory mechanics in anesthetized paralyzed humans. *J Appl Physiol.* 1992;73:1736.
17. Fengmei GUO, Chen J, Liu S et al. Dead space fraction changes during PEEP titration following lung recruitment in patients with ARDS. *Respir Care.* 2012;57:1578–85.
18. Coffey RL, Albert RK, Robertson HT. Mechanisms of physiological dead space response to PEEP after acute oleic acid lung injury. *J Appl Physiol Respir Environ Exerc Physiol.* 1983;55:1550–7.
19. Horton WG, Cheney FW. Variability of effect of positive end expiratory pressure. *Arch Surg.* 1975;110:395.
20. Kanarek DJ, Shannon DC. Adverse effect of positive end-expiratory pressure on pulmonary perfusion and arterial oxygenation. *Am Rev Resp Dis.* 1975;112:457.
21. Dantzker DR, Lynch JP, Weg JG. Depression of Cardiac Output is a mechanism of shunt reduction in the therapy of acute respiratory failure. *Chest.*1980;77:636–42.

22. Coussa ML, Guerin C, Eissa NT et al. Partitioning of work of breathing in mechanically ventilated COPD patients. *J Appl Physiol.* 1993;75:1711.
23. Guerin C, Milic-Emili J, Fournier G. Effect of PEEP on work of breathing in mechanically ventilated COPD patients. *Intensive Care Med.* 2000;26:1207.
24. Reissmann H, Ranieri VM, Goldberg P, Gottfried SB. Continuous positive airway pressure facilitates spontaneous breathing in weaning chronic obstructive pulmonary disease patients by improving breathing pattern and gas exchange. *Intensive Care Med.* 2000;26:1764.
25. Goldberg P, Reissmann H, Maltais F et al. Efficacy of noninvasive CPAP in COPD with acute respiratory failure. *Eur Respir J.* 1995;8:1894–990.
26. Katz JA, Marks JD. Inspiratory work with and without continuous positive airway pressure in patients with acute respiratory failure. *Anesthesiology.* 1985;63:598.
27. Valta P, Takala J, Eissa NT, Milic-Emili J. Does alveolar recruitment occur with positive end-expiratory pressure in adult respiratory distress syndrome patients? *J Crit Care.* 1993;8:34.
28. Eissa NT, Ranieri VM, Corbeil C et al. Effect of PEEP on the mechanics of the respiratory system in ARDS patients. *J Appl Physiol.* 1992;73(5):1728–35.
29. Pinsky MR. Hemodynamics of ventilation. In: Scharf, SM, Pinsky, MR, Magder, S. Marcel Dekker Inc., eds. *Respiratory-Circulatory Interactions in Health and Disease.* New York, Basel, 2001.
30. Scharf SM. Pinsky MR, Magder S. *Lung Biology in Health and Disease.* Volume 57, Marcel Dekker, 2001.
31. Jardin F, Vieillard-Baron A. Right ventricular function and positive pressure ventilation in clinical practice: From hemodynamic subsets to respiratory settings. *ICM.* 2003;29:1426.
32. Scharf SM. Ventilatory support for the failing heart. In: Scharf, SM, Pinsky, MR, Magder, S. Marcel Dekker Inc., eds. *Respiratory–Circulatory Interactions in Health and Disease.* New York, Basel, 2001.
33. Mehta S, Jay GD, Woolard RH et al. Randomized, prospective trial of bilevel versus continuous positive airway pressure in acute pulmonary edema. *Crit Care Med.* 1997;25:620.
34. Bellone A, Monari A, Cortellaro F et al. Myocardial infarction rate in acute pulmonary edema: Noninvasive pressure support ventilation versus continuous positive airway pressure. *Crit Care Med.* 2004 Sep;32(9):1860–5.
35. Vital FM, Ladeira MT, Atallah AN. Non-invasive positive pressure ventilation (CPAP or bilevel NPPV) for cardiogenic pulmonary oedema. *Cochrane Database Systematic Review.* 2013 May 31.
36. Evans TW, Albert RK, Angus DC et al. International Consensus Conferences in Intensive Care Medicine: Noninvasive positive pressure ventilation in acute respiratory failure. *Am J Respir Crit Care Med.* 2001;163(1):283–91.
37. Banerjee D, Yee BJ, Piper AJ et al. Obesity hypoventilation syndrome: Hypoxemia during continuous positive airway pressure. *Chest.* 2007;131(6):1678.
38. Rasanen J, Heikkila J, Downs J et al. Continuous positive airway pressure by face mask in acute cardiogenic pulmonary edema. *Am J Cardiol.* 1985;55:296–300.
39. Vaisanen IT, Rasanen J. Continuous positive airway pressure and supplemental oxygen in the treatment of cardiogenic pulmonary edema. *Chest.* 1987;92:481–5.
40. Lin M, Chiang H. The efficacy of early continuous positive airway pressure therapy in patients with acute cardiogenic pulmonary edema. *J Formos Med Assoc.* 1991;90:736–43.
41. Bersten AD, Holt AW, Vedig AE et al. Treatment of severe cardiogenic pulmonary edema with continuous positive airway pressure delivered by face mask. *N Engl J Med.* 1991;325:1825–30.
42. Lin M, Yang Y, Chiany H et al. Reappraisal of continuous positive airway pressure therapy in acute cardiogenic pulmonary edema: Short-term results and long-term follow-up. *Chest.* 1995;107:1379–86.
43. Weng CL, Zhao YT, Liu QH et al. Meta-analysis: Noninvasive ventilation in acute cardiogenic pulmonary edema. *Ann Int Med.* 2010 May 4;152(9):590–600.
44. Squadrone V, Massimiliano C, Cerutti E et al. Continuous positive airway pressure for treatment of postoperative hypoxemia, a randomized controlled trial. *JAMA.* 2005;293(5):589–95.
45. Ferreyra GP, Baussano I, Squadrone V et al. Continuous positive airway pressure for treatment of respiratory complications after abdominal surgery, a systematic review and meta-analysis. *Ann Surg.* 2008;247(4).
46. Miro AM, Shivaram U, Hertig I. Continuous positive airway pressure in COPD patients in acute hypercapneic respiratory failure. *Chest.* 1993 Jan;103(1):266–8.
47. De Lucas P, Tarancon C, Puente L et al. Nasal continuous positive airway pressure in patients with COPD in acute respiratory failure: A study of the immediate effects. *Chest.* 1993 Dec;104(6):1694–7.
48. Delclaux C, L'Her E, Alberti C et al. Treatment of acute hypoxemic nonhypercapneic respiratory insufficiency with continuous positive airway pressure delivered by a face mask, a randomized controlled trial. *JAMA.* 2000 Nov 8;284(18).
49. Shivaram U, Miro AM, Cash ME et al. Cardiopulmonary responses to continuous positive airway pressure in acute asthma. *J Crit Care.* 1993 Jun;8(2):87–92.
50. Pettiford BL, Luketich JD, Landreneau RJ. The management of flail chest. *Thorac Surg Clin.* 2007 Feb;17(1):25–33.

51. Gunduz M, Unlugenc H, Ozalevli M et al. A comparative study of continuous positive airway pressure (CPAP) and intermittent positive pressure ventilation (IPPV) in patients with flail chest. *Emerg Med J.* 2005 May;22(5):325–9.
52. Foti G, Sangalli F, Berra L et al. Is helmet CPAP first line pre-hospital treatment of presumed severe acute pulmonary edema? *Intensive Care Med.* 2009 Apr;35(4):656–62.
53. Williams TA, Finn J, Perkins GD, Jacobs IG. Prehospital continuous positive airway pressure for acute respiratory failure: A systematic review and meta-analysis. *Prehosp Emerg Care.* 2013 Apr–Jun;17(2):261–73.
54. Cheskes S, Turner L, Thomson S, Aljerian N. The impact of prehospital continuous positive airway pressure on the rate of intubation and mortality from acute out-of hospital respiratory emergencies. *Prehosp Emerg Care.* 2013 Oct–Dec;17(4):435–41.
55. Aguilar SA, Lee J, Dunford, JV et al. Assessment of the addition of prehospital continuous positive airway pressure (CPAP) to an urban emergency medical services (EMS) system in persons with severe respiratory distress. *J Emerg Med.* 2013 Aug;45(2):210–9.
56. Williams B, Boyle M, Robertson N, Giddings C. When pressure is positive: A literature review of the prehospital use of continuous positive airway pressure. *Prehosp Disaster Med.* 2013 Feb;28(1):52–60.
57. Goodacre S, Stevens JW, Pandor A et al. Prehospital noninvasive ventilation for acute respiratory failure: Systematic review, network meta-analysis, and individual patient data meta-analysis. *Acad Emerg Med.* 2014 Sep;21(9):960–70.

4

Emerging modes for non-invasive ventilation

PAOLO NAVALESI, FEDERICO LONGHINI, ROSANNA VASCHETTO AND ANTONIO MESSINA

INTRODUCTION

Non-invasive ventilation (NIV) is generally delivered using pressure support ventilation (PSV). Unfortunately, however, PSV often fails to achieve optimal patient–ventilator interaction, resulting in poor patient comfort.[1] Consequently, the manufacturers have introduced several additional features in the attempt to facilitate patient–ventilator interaction.

A further challenging approach to improve patient–ventilator interaction is matching ventilator support and ventilator demand. Two modes, proportional assist ventilation (PAV) and neurally adjusted ventilatory assist (NAVA), have been developed for this purpose.[2]

Maintaining adequate ventilation, regardless of clinical variations over time, is another potential clinical goal. In PSV, the assistance delivered does not vary in the presence of modifications of the respiratory system impedance, secondary to changes in airway resistance and pulmonary and/or chest wall compliance, so that alveolar hypoventilation may occur. To overcome this drawback, volume-assured pressure support (VAPS) modes have been developed.[3,4]

NEW FEATURES OF PSV

The combination of PSV and positive end-expiratory pressure (PEEP) is the most common form of assistance for NIV application. When PEEP is applied to PSV, the preset inspiratory pressure is intended as an addition to PEEP, and the actual pressure applied during inspiration is the sum of inspiratory and expiratory preset pressures. When turbine-driven bi-level ventilators are used, the terms expiratory positive airway pressure (EPAP) and inspiratory positive airway pressure (IPAP) are generally used; in this latter case, IPAP is the total pressure applied during inspiration and, therefore, the inspiratory support is the difference between IPAP and EPAP.

When delivering NIV in PSV, air leaks may alter patient–ventilator matching, primarily by interfering with cycling-off of ventilator insufflation, as cycling from inspiration to expiration occurs when the flow drops below a preset threshold, which is in general a percentage of the peak inspiratory flow achieved at the onset of inspiration. Air leaks delay, and sometimes impede, the attainment of that threshold and cause asynchronies and discomfort, leading to NIV failure[1]; also, they affect inspiratory trigger function.[5] Ventilators capable of detecting and compensating for air leaks are necessary to achieve successful NIV.[6] Dedicated NIV ventilators allow better patient–ventilator synchrony than intensive care unit (ICU) ventilators equipped with dedicated software for NIV.[6]

Air leaks apart, the cycling-off threshold plays an important role in determining the quality of patient–ventilator synchrony and the patient's comfort during NIV. Most ventilators offer a specific function that allows modifying this threshold value, which should be set, in principle, in order to match as closest as possible the patient's own (neural) end of inspiration. When the ventilator stops the mechanical insufflations before the patient's effort ends, the inspiratory muscles keep contracting during the ventilator exhalation phase, causing double triggering and adding to the work of breathing (WOB).[7] In two studies performed in patients with acute respiratory distress syndrome (ARDS), a cycling-off threshold anticipating the end of mechanical insufflation with respect to neural inspiration caused a reduction in tidal volume, with an increase in respiratory rate and WOB.[8,9] In contrast, prolonging mechanical insufflation into the patient's own (neural) expiration may precipitate or worsen dynamic hyperinflation by reducing the time available for lung emptying, causing ineffective inspiratory efforts, recruiting the expiratory muscles and, overall, leading to patient discomfort.[10] Two studies performed in chronic obstructive pulmonary disease (COPD) patients found that anticipating the cycling-off threshold reduced dynamic hyperinflation and WOB.[11,12] During NIV, the presence of air leaks further complicates this complex interplay.[1]

In the past, most ventilators applied the inspiratory support with a fixed, usually the fastest, rate of pressurisation. Nowadays, aimed at improving a patient's comfort, most ventilators allow varying the rate of airway pressure rise to enhance the matching between the patient's demand and ventilator assistance. A faster rate of pressurisation generally corresponds to a higher and earlier peak inspiratory flow. Prinianakis et al.[13] studied 15 COPD patients recovering from an episode of hypercapnic acute respiratory failure (ARF), who underwent four trials of non-invasive PSV with different rates of pressurisation applied in random order. The authors found that increasing the rate of pressurisation progressively decreased inspiratory effort; at the same time, however, air leaks increased and patient tolerance to NIV worsened.[13] Noteworthy, arterial blood gases were not significantly affected by the different settings.[13] This study confirms that individual titration of this specific setting may help in improving WOB and comfort during NIV.

PROPORTIONAL ASSIST VENTILATION

During partial support, both the respiratory muscles and the ventilator contribute to the overall pressure applied to the respiratory system. While during PSV, a constant pressure is applied throughout inspiration regardless of the intensity of the patient's effort, with PAV, the ventilator generates pressure in proportion to the effort generated by the respiratory muscles.[2] With PAV, the ventilator instantaneously delivers positive pressure throughout inspiration in proportion to patient-generated flow and volume, and the patient retains control of both timing and size of the breath, without preset targets of pressure, flow or volume.

The effects of PAV have been investigated both in ARF and in chronic respiratory failure (CRF). In patients with stable hypoxaemic and hypercapnic CRF secondary to COPD or restrictive chest wall disorders, PAV delivered through a nasal mask was well tolerated, improved arterial blood gases[14] and decreased WOB.[15] Porta et al.[16] compared the short-term physiological effects of NIV delivery by PSV and PAV in clinically stable patients with CRF secondary to COPD or chest wall disease. PSV and PAV equally improved breathing pattern and reduced inspiratory muscle effort, compared to spontaneous unassisted breathing.[16] In 12 patients with severe cystic fibrosis and chronic hypercapnia, Serra et al.[17] studied the acute physiological response to NIV delivered by either PSV or PAV, both set according to patient comfort. The short-term NIV application of both modes had positive effects on minute ventilation, gas exchange and diaphragmatic effort; however, the mean inspiratory pressure was lower with PAV, as opposed to PSV.[17] In patients with CRF consequent to severe COPD, non-invasive PAV increased exercise tolerance.[18,19]

In a crossover study by Wysocki et al.,[20] 12 patients with ARF due to COPD exacerbation underwent NIV with both PAV and PSV. Compared to PSV, PAV was equally effective in unloading the respiratory muscles, while improving NIV tolerance. Gay et al.[21] compared PAV with PSV in a randomised pilot study including patients with mild to moderate ARF receiving NIV. They found PAV was feasible and, compared to PSV, better tolerated and associated with a more rapid improvement. In this study, however, PSV and PAV were delivered by two different ventilators, only one of which (PAV) incorporated algorithms for air-leak compensation.[21] A randomised controlled trial compared NIV with PSV and PAV in 117 patients with ARF of varied aetiologies.[22] The primary endpoints were rate of death and intubation, and the secondary outcomes gas exchange, respiratory rate, haemodynamics, dyspnoea, comfort and length of ICU and hospital stay.[22] Mortality and intubation rate were no different. Of the secondary outcome variables, only dyspnoea and comfort were significantly improved with PAV as opposed to PSV, with no other significant differences.[22] Rusterholtz et al.[23] compared PAV, combined with 5 cm H_2O of continuous positive airway pressure (CPAP), with CPAP 10 cm H_2O in the treatment of 36 patients with acute cardiogenic pulmonary oedema causing unresolving dyspnoea, tachypnoea and hypoxaemia despite maximal standard treatment. PAV+CPAP was not superior to CPAP alone.[23]

Air leaks hamper expiration during non-invasive PAV, because the ventilator keeps providing positive pressure related to the leaked flow and volume, which makes crucial the use of ventilators equipped with software for air-leak detection and compensation.[20] In addition, proper adjustment of PAV settings necessitates knowledge of the mechanical characteristics of the respiratory system.[2,24] This drawback has been overcome by a further development of PAV, i.e. PAV+, where resistance and elastance are constantly monitored through a non-invasive technique, and flow assist (FA) and volume assist (VA) are accordingly automatically adjusted.[25,26] This technique, however, requires a closed (leak-free) system and is not applicable for NIV.

In conclusion, PAV may improve patient comfort during NIV, but the extent of this improvement is rather small and the benefits not quite clinically relevant. In fact, in the last decade, no further study involving the use of non-invasive PAV has been published.

NEURALLY ADJUSTED VENTILATORY ASSISTANCE

NAVA was developed in an attempt to overcome some of the limitations of PAV, while maintaining the potential advantages.[27] With NAVA, triggering, cycling-off and assist profile are regulated by the electrical activity of the diaphragm (EA_{di}), whereas the amount of assistance depends on a user-controlled gain factor (NAVA level).[27,28] EA_{di}, obtained by transoesophageal electromyography, is the best achievable index of the neural respiratory drive.[27,29] The electrodes used to measure EA_{di} are mounted on a nasogastric feeding tube routinely used in critically ill patients. Because the ventilator is directly triggered by EA_{di}, the synchrony between neural and mechanical inspiratory time is guaranteed both at the onset and at the end of inspiration, regardless of the mechanical properties of the respiratory system, presence of dynamic hyperinflation and intrinsic-PEEP (PEEPi), variations in muscle length or contractility and air leaks (Figure 4.1).[27,28] As long as the respiratory centres, phrenic nerves and neuromuscular junctions are intact, the amount

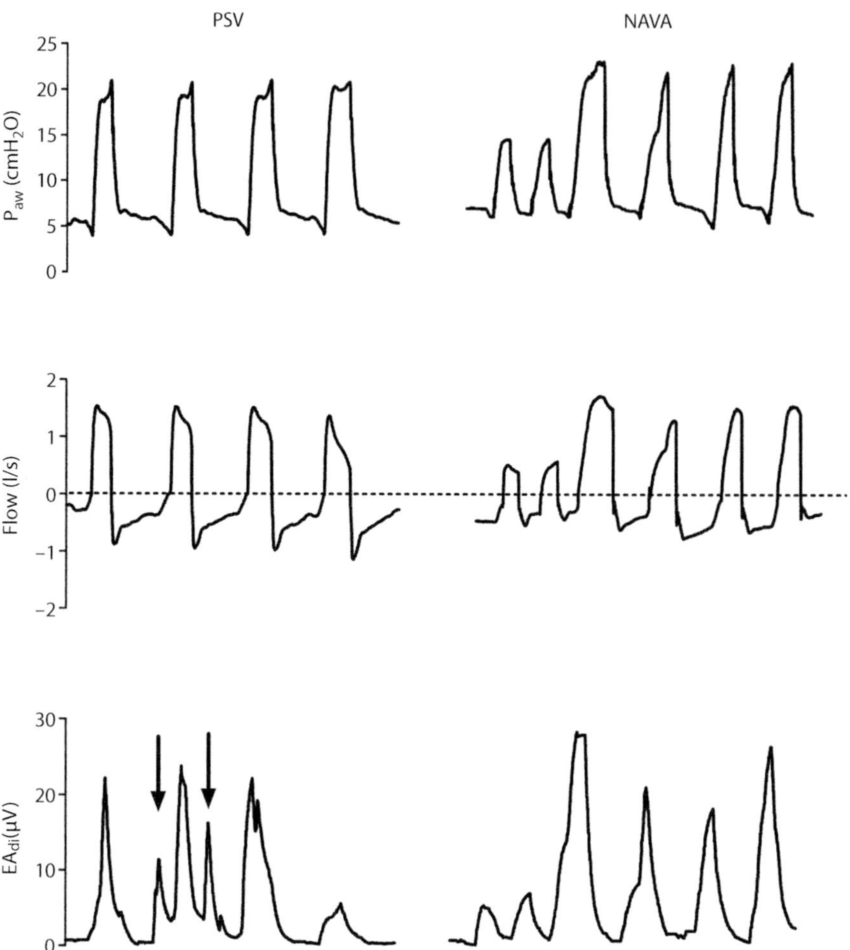

Figure 4.1 Examples of tracings from one patient receiving NIV in PSV (left panel) and NAVA (right panel) are displayed. Airway pressure (P_{aw}), flow and diaphragm electrical activity (EA_{di}) tracings are shown from top to bottom. The support delivered by the ventilator is proportional to EA_{di} in NAVA, while not in PSV. Also, the ineffective efforts occurring during PSV, as indicated by the mismatch between P_{aw} and EA_{di} (arrows), disappear with NAVA, despite the large air leaks.

of support provided instantaneously corresponds to the ventilatory demand (Figure 4.2).[27,28]

Several studies evaluated the use of NAVA to deliver NIV. Beck et al.[30] demonstrated in an animal model of acute lung injury that the application of NAVA through a leaky non-invasive interface was effective in unloading the respiratory muscles while guaranteeing good synchrony. The efficacy of NIV delivery was ensured also in the presence of large leaks.[30] Moerer et al.[31] compared the use of EA_{di} with a conventional pneumatic signal in healthy subjects for cycling on and off the ventilator during PSV via helmet. Subject–ventilator synchrony, triggering effort and breathing comfort were significantly less impaired at increasing levels of support and breathing frequency with EA_{di} as opposed to the conventional pneumatic signal.[31]

Cammarota et al.[32] compared the short-term effects of PSV and NAVA in delivering NIV through a helmet in patients with post-extubation hypoxaemic respiratory failure. There were no significant differences in gas exchange, respiratory rate and EA_{di} between the two modes, while patient–ventilator interaction and synchrony were significantly improved with NAVA as opposed to PSV.[32] These findings were then repeatedly confirmed when delivering non-invasive NAVA by mask.[33–35] Piquilloud et al.[33] compared PSV and NAVA, applied through a face mask in a series of patients with ARF or at risk of post-extubation respiratory failure. They also found EA_{di} and arterial blood gases no different between the two modes, and the trigger delays and asynchronies significantly improved with NAVA, compared to PSV.[33] Schmidt et al.[34] applied prophylactic NIV after extubation, with PSV and NAVA, both with and without automatic air-leak compensation. Breathing pattern and EA_{di} were no different among the four trials. Irrespective of air-leak compensation, NAVA reduced trigger delays and improved synchrony, compared to PSV.[34] Furthermore, the NIV algorithm significantly reduced the incidence of asynchronous events during PSV, but not in NAVA.[34] Similar results were obtained by Bertrand et al.[35] in a population of patients with ARF of varying aetiologies. Recently, Doorduin et al.[36] evaluated patient–ventilator interactions by means of an automated analysis in a group of 12 COPD patients receiving NIV in three different conditions: 1) PSV applied by a dedicated NIV turbine

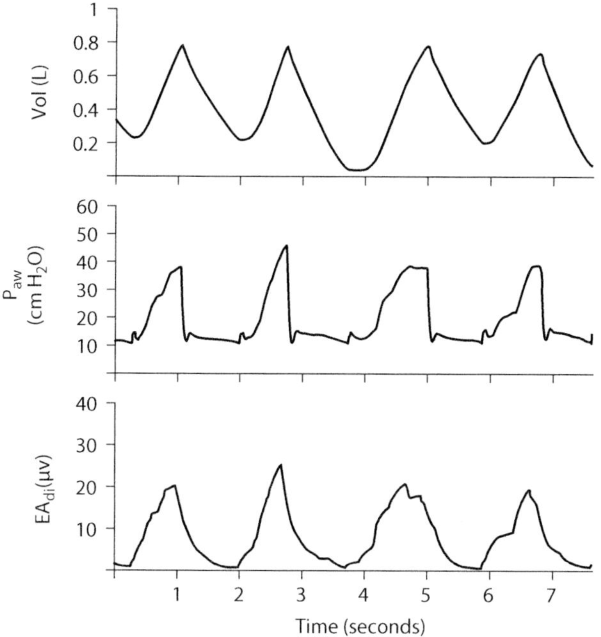

Figure 4.2 Volume, airway pressure (P_{aw}) and electrical activity of the diaphragm (EA_{di}) tracings are shown from a patient receiving NAVA. Note the precise synchronisation between patient effort (EA_{di}) and ventilator assistance (P_{aw}).

ventilator; 2) PSV with an ICU ventilator equipped with dedicated NIV software for air-leak compensation; and 3) NAVA using the same ICU ventilator. The automated analysis showed that NAVA improved patient–ventilator interaction compared to PSV, as delivered with both ventilators.[36]

NAVA improves patient–ventilator interaction during NIV. NAVA is air leaks insensitive and results in improved synchrony. As a nasogastric tube is necessary to apply NAVA, its use is limited to ICU patients. Assessing whether non-invasive NAVA can improve NIV success in the most severe and problematic patients requires further investigation.

VAPS MODES

VAPS modes combine PSV with a preset tidal volume by measuring or estimating the actual tidal volume and calculating the variations of inspiratory support necessary to achieve the target tidal volume. This can be achieved with a different algorithm. There are two VAPS algorithms applicable for NIV: average VAPS (AVAPS) and intelligent VAPS (iVAPS).

In AVAPS, the actual tidal volume is averaged over 1 min and IPAP accordingly adjusted breath-by-breath to maintain the target tidal volume.[3] Because the patient may increase his/her respiratory rate due to causes other than chemoreception, such as emotional (limbic), behavioural (cortical) and metabolic (fever) stimuli,[28] by delivering the same tidal volume at each breath, AVAPS may cause unwarranted high ventilation leading to excessive reduction of arterial carbon dioxide partial pressure ($PaCO_2$), sleep disruption and discomfort. To overcome this drawback, the iVAPS algorithm has been developed, which targets inspiratory assistance and backup respiratory rate to maintain constant minute alveolar ventilation, as estimated by an algorithm calculating the anatomic dead space according to the patient's height.[37]

The primary indications for the VAPS modes are the conditions leading to nocturnal alveolar hypoventilation, such as neuromuscular diseases, obesity hypoventilation syndrome (OHS) and overlap syndrome. VAPS modes should provide stable alveolar ventilation irrespective of variations of respiratory drive and effort during different sleep phases. In addition, they also adapt the amount of inspiratory pressure delivered in response to modifications in respiratory impedance, with the primary aim of improving the patient's safety by maintaining more stable gas exchanges. Moreover, by reducing the inspiratory assistance during wakefulness, they should also improve patient comfort and facilitate sleep onset.[38]

Using a crossover design, Storre et al.[4] studied 10 mildly hypercapnic patients with OHS who failed to respond to nocturnal CPAP (8.9 ± 1.0 mbar). Patients were randomised to undergo 6 weeks of nocturnal NIV either in conventional bi-level mode (IPAP 14.7 ± 2.4 mbar, EPAP 6.1 ± 1.1 mbar) or in AVAPS (IPAP 16.4 ± 3.9 mbar, EPAP 5.4 ± 1.2 mbar) and then switched to six further weeks of NIV with the complementary mode.[4] Compared with pre-treatment baseline, sleep quality and health-related quality of life were improved with both modes (CPAP not evaluated); furthermore, AVAPS, but not CPAP and bi-level ventilation, ameliorated transcutaneous carbon dioxide tension ($PtcCO_2$).[4] Janssens et al.[39] conducted a study with a crossover design including 12 OHS patients receiving in two consecutive nights NIV in bi-level mode and AVAPS. AVAPS significantly improved the control of nocturnal hypercapnia by increasing minute ventilation.[39] The polysomnography, however, showed more frequent awakenings with AVAPS, which was felt less comfortable by the patients, who reported the perception of receiving too much air and increased air leaks.[39] In a small population of nine COPD patients naive to NIV, PSV and AVAPS were randomly applied for two 5-day periods, with a crossover study design.[40] While compliance to treatment and arterial blood gases did not differ between the two modes, the sleep quality significantly improved with AVAPS, as opposed to PSV.[40] Another study comparing NIV delivered with PSV and AVAPS in 28 patients with CRF of varied aetiologies, however, found no difference regarding sleep efficiency between the two modes; AVAPS resulted in higher minute ventilation in the lateral decubitus, but not in the supine position.[3] More recently, a randomised controlled trial by Murphy et al.,[41] comparing PSV and AVAPS in 46 severely obese (BMI >40 kg/m^2) patients with OHS, found the two modes equally effective in reducing daytime hypercapnia even after 3 months of treatment.

The development of iVAPS is more recent and fewer studies are, therefore, presently available. A study including 27 COPD patients found high-intensity NIV and iVAPS equally effective in increasing in minute ventilation compared to spontaneous unassisted breathing, without significant differences between the two modes; subgroup analysis considering separately obese and non-obese patients also showed no difference between modes.[42] A small prospective single centre, randomised, parallel group trial comparing NIV by PSV and iVAPS reported no significant differences between the two groups in daytime arterial blood gas measurements, nocturnal oxygenation or compliance at 3 months follow-up. There were no significant differences between groups in the secondary outcomes of health-related quality of life assessment, dyspnoea, pulmonary function tests, exercise tolerance and nocturnal $PtcCO_2$ at 3 months.[43] Another recent study by Kelly et al.[44] randomised, with a crossover design, 18 patients with newly diagnosed nocturnal hypoventilation of varied aetiologies to receive NIV overnight by either PSV, initiated by a skilled healthcare professional, and iVAPS. There was no difference in outcome between the two modes for spirometry, respiratory muscle strength, sleep quality, arousals or oxygen desaturation index. However, iVAPS delivered a lower median inspiratory pressure, compared with standard PSV for the same ventilatory outcome, i.e. oxygen saturation and $PtcCO_2$, and resulted in better adherence to treatment.[44]

To date, only small studies enrolling relatively few patients are available for these two modes, with results either difficult to compare or lacking of consistency. In the absence of properly powered randomised controlled trials, it is presently impossible to draw a clear-cut conclusion in favour or against these modes in place of the conventional pressure-targeted NIV modes.

REFERENCES

1. Calderini E, Confalonieri M, Puccio PG et al. Patient–ventilator asynchrony during noninvasive ventilation: The role of expiratory trigger. *Intensive Care Med.* 1999;25(7):662–7.
2. Navalesi P, Costa R. New modes of mechanical ventilation: Proportional assist ventilation, neurally adjusted ventilatory assist, and fractal ventilation. *Curr Opin Crit Care.* 2003;9(1):51–8.
3. Ambrogio C, Lowman X, Kuo M et al. Sleep and non-invasive ventilation in patients with chronic respiratory insufficiency. *Intensive Care Med.* 2009;35(2):306–13.
4. Storre JH, Seuthe B, Fiechter R et al. Average volume-assured pressure support in obesity hypoventilation: A randomized crossover trial. *Chest.* 2006;130(3):815–21.
5. Miyoshi E, Fujino Y, Uchiyama A et al. Effects of gas leak on triggering function, humidification, and inspiratory oxygen fraction during noninvasive positive airway pressure ventilation. *Chest.* 2005;128(5):3691–8.
6. Carteaux G, Lyazidi A, Cordoba-Izquierdo A et al. Patient–ventilator asynchrony during noninvasive ventilation: A bench and clinical study. *Chest.* 2012;142(2):367–76.
7. Vignaux L, Vargas F, Roeseler J et al. Patient–ventilator asynchrony during non-invasive ventilation for acute respiratory failure: A multicenter study. *Intensive Care Med.* 2009;35(5):840–6.
8. Chiumello D, Pelosi P, Carlesso E et al. Noninvasive positive pressure ventilation delivered by helmet vs. standard face mask. *Intensive Care Med.* 2003;29(10):1671–9.
9. Tokioka H, Tanaka T, Ishizu T et al. The effect of breath termination criterion on breathing patterns and the work of breathing during pressure support ventilation. *Anesth Analg.* 2001;92(1):161–5.
10. Younes M, Kun J, Webster K, Roberts D. Response of ventilator-dependent patients to delayed opening of exhalation valve. *Am J Respir Crit Care Med.* 2002;166(1):21–30.
11. Tassaux D, Gainnier M, Battisti A, Jolliet P. Impact of expiratory trigger setting on delayed cycling and inspiratory muscle workload. *Am J Respir Crit Care Med.* 2005;172(10):1283–9.
12. Chiumello D, Polli F, Tallarini F et al. Effect of different cycling-off criteria and positive end-expiratory pressure during pressure support ventilation in patients with chronic obstructive pulmonary disease. *Crit Care Med.* 2007;35(11):2547–52.
13. Prinianakis G, Delmastro M, Carlucci A et al. Effect of varying the pressurisation rate during noninvasive pressure support ventilation. *Eur Respir J.* 2004;23(2):314–20.
14. Ambrosino N, Vitacca M, Polese G et al. Short-term effects of nasal proportional assist ventilation in patients with chronic hypercapnic respiratory insufficiency. *Eur Respir J.* 1997;10(12):2829–34.
15. Polese G, Vitacca M, Bianchi L et al. Nasal proportional assist ventilation unloads the inspiratory muscles of stable patients with hypercapnia due to COPD. *Eur Respir J.* 2000;16(3):491–8.
16. Porta R, Appendini L, Vitacca M et al. Mask proportional assist vs pressure support ventilation in patients in clinically stable condition with chronic ventilatory failure. *Chest.* 2002;122(2):479–88.
17. Serra A, Polese G, Braggion C, Rossi A. Non-invasive proportional assist and pressure support ventilation in patients with cystic fibrosis and chronic respiratory failure. *Thorax.* 2002;57(1):50–4.
18. Bianchi L, Foglio K, Pagani M et al. Effects of proportional assist ventilation on exercise tolerance in COPD patients with chronic hypercapnia. *Eur Respir J.* 1998;11(2):422–7.
19. Dolmage TE, Goldstein RS. Proportional assist ventilation and exercise tolerance in subjects with COPD. *Chest.* 1997;111(4):948–54.
20. Wysocki M, Richard JC, Meshaka P. Noninvasive proportional assist ventilation compared with noninvasive pressure support ventilation in hypercapnic acute respiratory failure. *Crit Care Med.* 2002;30(2):323–9.
21. Gay PC, Hess DR, Hill NS. Noninvasive proportional assist ventilation for acute respiratory insufficiency. Comparison with pressure support ventilation. *Am J Respir Crit Care Med.* 2001;164(9):1606–11.

22. Fernandez-Vivas M, Caturla-Such J, Gonzalez de la Rosa J et al. Noninvasive pressure support versus proportional assist ventilation in acute respiratory failure. *Intensive Care Med.* 2003;29(7):1126–33.
23. Rusterholtz T, Bollaert PE, Feissel M et al. Continuous positive airway pressure vs. proportional assist ventilation for noninvasive ventilation in acute cardiogenic pulmonary edema. *Intensive Care Med.* 2008;34(5):840–6.
24. Navalesi P, Hernandez P, Wongsa A et al. Proportional assist ventilation in acute respiratory failure: Effects on breathing pattern and inspiratory effort. *Am J Respir Crit Care Med.* 1996;154(5):1330–8.
25. Younes M, Kun J, Masiowski B et al. A method for noninvasive determination of inspiratory resistance during proportional assist ventilation. *Am J Respir Crit Care Med.* 2001;163(4):829–39.
26. Younes M, Webster K, Kun J, Roberts D et al. A method for measuring passive elastance during proportional assist ventilation. *Am J Respir Crit Care Med.* 2001;164(1):50–60.
27. Sinderby C, Navalesi P, Beck J et al. Neural control of mechanical ventilation in respiratory failure. *Nat Med.* 1999;5(12):1433–6.
28. Navalesi P, Longhini F. Neurally adjusted ventilatory assist. *Curr Opin Crit Care.* 2015;21(1):58–64.
29. Beck J, Gottfried SB, Navalesi P et al. Electrical activity of the diaphragm during pressure support ventilation in acute respiratory failure. *Am J Respir Crit Care Med.* 2001;164(3):419–24.
30. Beck J, Brander L, Slutsky AS et al. Non-invasive neurally adjusted ventilatory assist in rabbits with acute lung injury. *Intensive Care Med.* 2008;34(2):316–23.
31. Moerer O, Beck J, Brander L et al. Subject–ventilator synchrony during neural versus pneumatically triggered non-invasive helmet ventilation. *Intensive Care Med.* 2008;34(9):1615–23.
32. Cammarota G, Olivieri C, Costa R et al. Noninvasive ventilation through a helmet in postextubation hypoxemic patients: Physiologic comparison between neurally adjusted ventilatory assist and pressure support ventilation. *Intensive Care Med.* 2011;37(12):1943–50.
33. Piquilloud L, Tassaux D, Bialais E et al. Neurally adjusted ventilatory assist (NAVA) improves patient–ventilator interaction during non-invasive ventilation delivered by face mask. *Intensive Care Med.* 2012;38(10):1624–31.
34. Schmidt M, Dres M, Raux M et al. Neurally adjusted ventilatory assist improves patient–ventilator interaction during postextubation prophylactic noninvasive ventilation. *Crit Care Med.* 2012;40(6):1738–44.
35. Bertrand PM, Futier E, Coisel Y et al. Neurally adjusted ventilatory assist vs pressure support ventilation for noninvasive ventilation during acute respiratory failure: A crossover physiologic study. *Chest.* 2013;143(1):30–6.
36. Doorduin J, Sinderby CA, Beck J et al. Automated patient–ventilator interaction analysis during neurally adjusted non-invasive ventilation and pressure support ventilation in chronic obstructive pulmonary disease. *Crit Care.* 2014;18(5):550.
37. Hart M, Orzalesi M, Cook C. Relation between anatomic respiratory dead space and body size and lung volume. *J Appl Physiol.* 1963;18(3):519–22.
38. Oscroft NS, Ali M, Gulati A et al. A randomised crossover trial comparing volume assured and pressure preset noninvasive ventilation in stable hypercapnic COPD. *COPD.* 2010;7(6):398–403.
39. Janssens JP, Metzger M, Sforza E. Impact of volume targeting on efficacy of bi-level non-invasive ventilation and sleep in obesity-hypoventilation. *Respir Med.* 2009;103(2):165–72.
40. Crisafulli E, Manni G, Kidonias M et al. Subjective sleep quality during average volume assured pressure support (AVAPS) ventilation in patients with hypercapnic COPD: A physiological pilot study. *Lung.* 2009;187(5):299–305.
41. Murphy PB, Davidson C, Hind MD et al. Volume targeted versus pressure support non-invasive ventilation in patients with super obesity and chronic respiratory failure: A randomised controlled trial. *Thorax.* 2012;67(8):727–34.
42. Ekkernkamp E, Kabitz HJ, Walker DJ et al. Minute ventilation during spontaneous breathing, high-intensity noninvasive positive pressure ventilation and intelligent volume assured pressure support in hypercapnic COPD. *COPD.* 2014;11(1):52–8.
43. Oscroft NS, Chadwick R, Davies MG et al. Volume assured versus pressure preset non-invasive ventilation for compensated ventilatory failure in COPD. *Respir Med.* 2014;108(10):1508–15.
44. Kelly JL, Jaye J, Pickersgill RE et al. Randomized trial of 'intelligent' autotitrating ventilation versus standard pressure support non-invasive ventilation: Impact on adherence and physiological outcomes. *Respirology.* 2014;19(4):596–603.

5

Extracorporeal CO_2 removal

LARA PISANI AND V. MARCO RANIERI

KEY MESSAGES

- The extracorporeal carbon dioxide removal (ECCO2R) refers to a partial respiratory support in which an extracorporeal circuit is used for the primary purpose of removing CO_2 from the body.
- The topic is clinically relevant; the approach is innovative and takes advantage of the major technical improvements offered by industry in this field.
- Recently, the ECCO2R technique was implemented using a minimally invasive system based on a modified continuous veno-venous haemofiltration device. The main features of this system are a low extracorporeal blood flow and the use of small double-lumen catheters. However, full anticoagulation is required.
- By eliminating CO_2, ECCO2R has been proposed both in patients with ARDS and in patients with acute hypercapnic respiratory failure (AHRF) with different purpose. Mechanical ventilation may be supported by ECCO2R to remove the excessive CO_2 and therefore allow super-protective ventilatory strategies or to reverse life-threatening acidosis and hypercapnia, preventing the NIV failure and facilitating the weaning process as well.
- Future, well-planned studies are urgently warranted to further validate the efficacy and safety of this novel strategy.

The use of extracorporeal carbon dioxide removal (ECCO2R) for acute respiratory failure has markedly increased in recent years. Originally proposed for patients with acute respiratory distress syndrome (ARDS), more recently, a new generation of ECCO2R devices have been proposed as a therapeutic option in patients with chronic obstructive pulmonary disease (COPD) in addition to non-invasive mechanical ventilation (NIV) to avoid intubation and to facilitate weaning of patients who have been intubated and those who have been mechanically ventilated. This chapter addresses the physiological and technical aspects of this technique, as well as reviews the available clinical evidence, comparing and discussing studies in which ECCO2R was applied.

INTRODUCTION

Extracorporeal carbon dioxide removal (ECCO2R) refers to an extracorporeal circuit that is able to selectively extract carbon dioxide (CO_2) from blood by passing it through a membrane 'lung' (Figure 5.1). The concept of removing only CO_2, with little to no effect on oxygenation, is not new. It was originally proposed in 1997 by Dr Kolobow and Dr Gattinoni at the National Institutes of Health. By using a membrane 'lung' in seven unsedated lambs,[1] the authors found two important results:

1. CO_2 removal increased linearly with increase in blood flow and was dependent on $PaCO_2$ baseline level. A flow rate of 500 mL/min was able to remove approximately half of total body CO_2 production (about 100 L/min).[2]
2. As CO_2 removal increased, alveolar ventilation was reduced proportionately. When extracorporeal CO_2 removal reached 50% of CO_2 production, alveolar ventilation decreased by 50%. This is possible because blood oxygenation and CO_2 removal occur through different mechanisms.[3] It is essential to remember that only a small amount of oxygen is carried as a physical solution (0.31 mL per 100 mL) in venous blood. The rest is transported in combination with haemoglobin, which is normally 70% to 85% saturated. Therefore, the lungs can add just 40 to 60 mL of oxygen (O_2) per litre of venous blood. In addition, CO_2 is more soluble and diffuses more easily in blood than

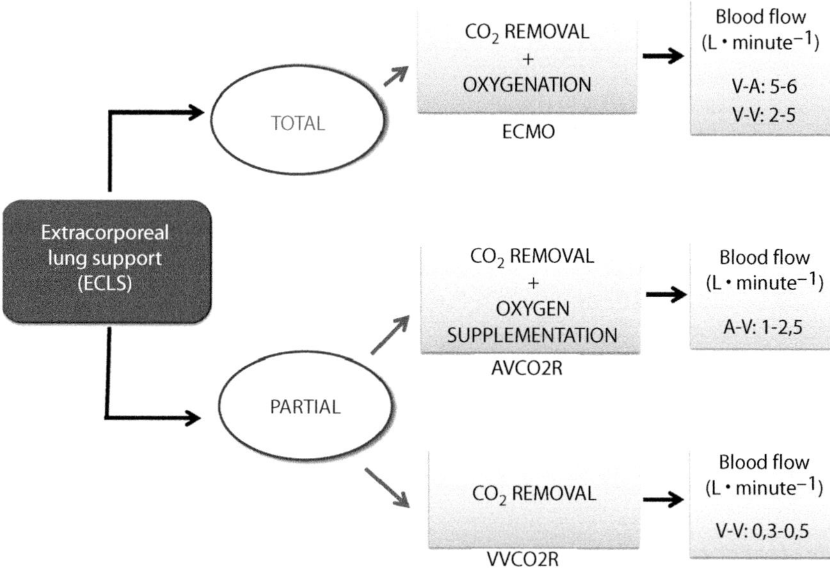

Figure 5.1 Extracorporeal lung support: a schematic view. ECMO: extracorporeal membrane oxygenation; AVCO2R: arteriovenous CO_2 removal; VVCO2R: veno-venous CO_2 removal.

the oxygen. Thus, oxygen uptake requires an amount of blood flow similar to the total cardiac output (4 to 7 L/min). In contrast, the quantity of blood flow needed to remove all metabolically produced CO_2 (normal resting CO_2 production averages 200 mL/min) through an efficient membrane 'lung' is only about 20% of the total cardiac output. As a consequence, ECCO2R devices have many advantages compared to conventional extracorporeal membrane oxygenation (ECMO) systems including a lower blood flow rate (range from 300 up 1500 mL/min) and smaller veno-venous catheters (12–14 French). Continuous infusion of heparin is still needed to 'prevent clotting' of the circuit.

CARBON DIOXIDE REMOVAL TECHNOLOGY: PRINCIPLES AND CIRCUITRY

The main features of ECCO2R devices include the following.[4]

Membrane 'lung'

This was not initially present but later introduced because of blood biochemical alterations caused by the air–fluid direct interface with blood. Different factors, including the diffusion gradient, the contact time with the blood and the membrane characteristics, determine the amount of CO_2 that can be exchanged. The modern membranes are generally made of hollow biocompatible material fibres (polymethylpentene or polypropylene) with a contact surface area that ranges from 1 to 3 m^2. In addition, the membranes are connected to a fresh gas flow source (i.e. oxygen flow of 6–8 L/min). In some cases, they are coated with heparin or other components designed to improve biocompatibility.

Pump

This is not required in an arteriovenous (AV) system, which takes advantage of the pressure gradient between arterial and venous blood. Pumpless systems result in less trauma to the blood and a lower risk of haemolysis, but require large arterial cannulas and an adequate cardiac output. Therefore, an AV device, depending on the AV shunt provided by the patient's haemodynamic status, can only be used if the left ventricular function is preserved and without severe peripheral vascular disease because limb ischaemia is a real risk.

In contrast, a venous-venous (VV) system is dependent on the work of a pump. The recent development of rotary pumps (centrifugal or diagonal) minimises blood trauma.[4,5] In addition, optimal control of gas exchange is possible by manipulating flow rates.

Catheters

Usually small double lumen catheters (13–17 French in calibre, similar to that used for haemodialysis) placed in either femoral or jugular veins, using the Seldinger technique and ultrasound guidance, are utilised for VV devices.[6] The use of single dual-lumen catheters and the percutaneous venous approach reduces the incidence of catheter placement-associated adverse events as well as the level of patient discomfort.

ECCO2R IN PATIENTS WITH ARDS

ARDS is characterised by damage to the lung parenchyma, caused by either indirect or direct insults. Consequently, a decrease in respiratory system compliance due to the presence of alveolar and interstitial fluid and the loss of surfactant occurs.[7] According to the recent Berlin definition, patients affected by ARDS are now categorised into three different categories (mild, moderate or severe), based on the PaO_2/FIO_2 ratio on 5 cmH_2O of CPAP/PEEP.[8]

The traditional approach to mechanical ventilation in patients with ARDS was completely changed when a clinical trial involving 10 different university centres in the Acute Respiratory Distress Syndrome Network (ARDSNet) was published.[9] This study compared an innovative lung protective strategy with low tidal volume (TV) (6 mL/kg/predicted body weight [PBW]) and a plateau pressure (Pplat) of 30 cmH_2O with the traditional ventilation, using a TV of 12 mL/kg/PBW and a Pplat of 50 cmH_2O or less. The trial showed mortality was lower in the group treated with the protective approach than in the control group (31.0% vs. 39.8%, $p = 0.007$).[9]

The rationale for this strategy was that smaller TVs are less likely to generate alveolar overdistension and cyclic alveolar recruitment/derecruitment during mechanical ventilation, which are the principal causes of ventilator-associated lung injury (VILI).

Although current guidelines for ARDS recommend a protective ventilation strategy, recent data have shown that ARDS patients may still be exposed to forces that can induce alveolar hyperinflation and stress, even using lower TVs.[10–12]

Thus, ECCO2R has been suggested in ARDS to allow very small TVs and manage the consequent permissive hypercapnia, in an attempt to minimise ventilator-induced lung injury.

To date, there is still a paucity of high-quality evidence in this area. In fact, only two randomised controlled trials (RCTs) on the use of ECCO2R in this setting have been conducted. In order to understand better the role and the efficacy of ECCO2R systems in patients with acute hypoxaemic respiratory failure due to ARDS, a recent review was published.[13] Fourteen studies with significant heterogeneity and a total of 495 patients were included (2 RCTs and 10 observational studies). No significant reduction in terms of mortality and organ failure free days or intensive care unit (ICU) length of stay was demonstrated. The incidence of ECCO2R-related adverse events ranged between 0% and 25%.

The study by Terragni et al.[14] provides for the first time clinical evidence that a low-flow extracorporeal device was able to remove the amount of carbon dioxide needed to avoid the respiratory acidosis consequent to VT reduction, allowing more protective ventilatory settings.

In addition, only two of the included studies evaluated the use of ECCO2 in increasing ventilator-free days. In the Xtravent study,[15] after a 'stabilisation period,' that means 24 hours with optimised therapy and high PEEP, 40 patients were randomly assigned to the treatment group (very low-TV strategy with 3 mL/kg/PBW associated with a pumpless extracorporeal lung assist system) and 39 patients to the control group (6 mL/kg/PBW without the extracorporeal device, according to the ARDSNet strategy).

This small trial showed that low-TV strategy with 3 mL/kg/PBW associated with a pumpless extracorporeal lung assist system did not result in significant difference in ventilator-free days between groups, the primary outcome, during 28 and 60 days after randomisation. However, a post-hoc analysis on cohorts based on PaO_2/FiO_2 showed that, in more hypoxaemic patients ($PaO_2/FiO_2 < 150$), a significant improvement of 60 ventilator-free days (VFD-60) in the treatment group compared to the control group occurred (VFD-60 = 40.9 ± 12.8 versus 28.2 ± 16.4, $p = 0.033$, respectively). A limitation of this study is the fact that only patients with stable haemodynamics were enrolled. As a result, the mortality rate was low (16.5%) and did not differ between groups, making it difficult to generalise the results to the overall ARDS population.

More recently, Fanelli et al.[16] evaluated the safety and feasibility of an 'ultra-protective' strategy consisting of very low TV (TV = 4 mL/kg/PBW) combined with extracorporeal CO_2 removal.

Fifteen patients with moderate ARDS ($100 < PaO_2/FiO_2 < 200$ with PEEP > 5 cm H_2O) were included. The use of ECCO2R ranged between 2 and 4 days. The gradual TV reduction (from 6.2 ± 0.7 to 4.8 ± 0.7 mL/kg) was associated with a significant decrease in Pplat and driving pressure (Pplat – PEEP). Minute ventilation was significantly decreased without respiratory acidosis by using ECCO2R. In addition, the incidence of ECCO2R-related adverse events was low. Only two patients experienced side effects such as intravascular haemolysis requiring transfusion and femoral central venous catheter malfunction. On the other hand, the authors reported severe hypoxaemia in six patients (40%): prone position and veno-venous ECMO were used as rescue therapies in four and two patients, respectively.

There are several possible mechanisms to explain this finding. As pointed out by Gattinoni,[17] worsening hypoxaemia during ECCO2R may be associated with the fact that the lung tends to collapse when the mean airway pressure decreases, thereby creating gravitational atelectasis. In fact, it is important to keep in mind that 30%–40% of recruitable lung remains closed when ARDS patients are ventilated with a Pplat target less than 25 cm H_2O. This implies that a sufficient pressure must be applied to reopen the newly formed atelectatic areas. In addition, by using lower ventilator settings, ventilation (VA)/perfusion (Q) ratio reaches more rapidly a critical level, accelerating the process of atelectasis reabsorption. Finally, during ECCO2R, the respiratory quotient (R) decreases when the CO_2 eliminated by the natural lungs decreases. Consequently, unrecognised alveolar hypoxia can occur.

Taking all this into account, the question arises: does a Pplat less than 25 cm H_2O really improve ARDS patient's outcomes?

The ongoing SUPERNOVA trial,[18] sponsored by the European Society of Intensive Care, will add important information to answer this question.

ECCO2R IN PATIENTS WITH COPD

COPD patients often experience acute hypercapnic respiratory failure (AHFR) during an episode of exacerbation. AHFR is considered an emergency situation, and its management has changed during the past decades.[19]

During an exacerbation, worsening expiratory flow limitation results in dynamic hyperinflation with increased end expiratory lung volume (EELV) and residual volume (RV).[20]

On the other hand, inspiratory capacity (IC) and inspiratory reserve volume (IRV) are significantly decreased as well. Consequently, because tidal breathing comes closer to total lung capacity (TLC), an increase in pressure generated by the respiratory muscles must be generated to maintain VT. In addition, a progressive reduction in expiratory time leading to the presence of positive intrapulmonary pressure at the end of expiration, intrinsic positive end expiratory pressure (PEEPi), increases the work of breathing (WOB).[21]

Therefore, the inability to sustain spontaneous breathing in COPD patients with an acute exacerbation (AECOPD) is the result of an imbalance between the load and the capacity of the respiratory muscles to generate pressure. This results in higher respiratory rates, leading to dynamic hyperinflation, elevated intrathoracic pressures, excessive WOB and finally CO_2 retention.

NIV is actually the first-line treatment in this setting.[19] Despite the positive results and the increasing experience with NIV, an important proportion of patients, especially those with severe acidosis, continue to fail and require intubation.[21] Additionally, COPD patients who require intubation have a poor prognosis and an increased risk of difficult weaning and prolonged ventilation.[22]

Recently, ECCO2R has been proposed as a new treatment in AECOPD patients. The rationale of this novel strategy is to combine ECCO2R with a 'conventional approach' that consists in the improvement of alveolar ventilation by using a mechanical ventilator working together with the respiratory pump, in order to avoid intubation in COPD patients refractory to NIV and to facilitate weaning in mechanically ventilated hypercapnic patients.

To date, no large RCTs have been published. As reported by a recent systematic review,[23] most of the evidence we have about the role of ECCO2R in patients with AECOPD comes from single centres and small studies. In fact, only 10 publications with a total of 85 patients were included in this analysis. Specifically, the larger ones were two case-control studies.[24,25] In addition, all papers differ in terms of patient characteristics, ECCO2R device used and study design.[23]

Despite these limitations, it was demonstrated that ECCO2R avoided intubation in 65/70 (93%) patients. Moreover, 9/17 (53%) patients were weaned successfully from invasive ventilation by using ECCO2R.[23] A large number of ECCO2R-related complications were the other side of the coin. In line with these results is a recent multicentre case-control study (ECLAIR study). Compared to the control group, intubation was avoided in 14 of 25 (56.0%) COPD patients at risk of NIV failure treated with venovenous ECCO2R. Again, the authors found that relevant complications occurred in over one-third of cases.[26]

Generally speaking, compared to ECMO, fewer complications have been described with new VV ECCO2R systems because they are less invasive. However, the procedure is not without adverse events. Potential adverse events during the procedure can be classified as mechanical (cannula problems, membrane 'lung' failure, clots in the circuit, air in the circuit, pump malfunction, tubing rupture, catheter displacement, system leaks) and patient-related (vein perforation, significant bleeding, haemodynamic instability, ischaemic/gangrenous bowel, pneumothorax, renal complications, infectious and thromboembolic complications). The incidence of these complications varies greatly across studies. Despite the two systematic reviews that assessed the efficacy and safety of ECCO2R not specifically focusing on the adverse effects of ECCO2R, a large number of patients included experienced ECCO2R-related adverse events.[13,23] Thus, the potential risks of ECCO2R need to be taken into account when considering patients for extracorporeal support.

Finally, we elucidated the physiologic effects of ECCO2R in COPD patients who failed at least two spontaneous breathing trials (SBTs), showing that ECCO2R may be indicated when WOB is increased, even in the absence of respiratory acidosis.[27]

In fact, the addition of ECCO2R to unsupported breathing is able to reduce the inspiratory effort, decreasing significantly the Pdi swing and the pressure–time products of the trans-diaphragmatic pressure, and improving the respiratory pattern. Moreover, ECCO2R prevents the increase in rapid shallow breathing index (f/VT) and $PaCO_2$ during a T-piece trial, thereby avoiding respiratory acidosis and accelerating the weaning process in those patients.[27]

In conclusion, these data provide the rationale for the application of ECCO2R in patients with AHRF. Future, well-planned RCTs are urgently warranted to further validate the efficacy and safety of this novel strategy.

OTHER APPLICATIONS

Low flow extracorporeal support can also be a bridge to lung transplantation (LT). Despite optimised ventilator settings, some patients listed for LT develop severe unresponsive respiratory acidosis. The only treatment option for these patients is extracorporeal life support (ECLS), such as ECMO. In recent years, the application of ECMO as a bridge to LT has progressively increased.[28] Although ECMO technology has advanced with better performance and an improved morbidity profile, several complications including bleeding, infection and renal failure remain.[28]

Fischer et al.[29] reported for the first time the use of the interventional lung assist NovaLung (iLA; NovaLung) as a bridge to LT in 30 patients with ventilation-refractory hypercapnia and respiratory acidosis.

Other studies have confirmed the usefulness of ECCO2R as a bridge to LT in adults with severe hypercapnic respiratory failure. The most common underlying diagnoses were emphysema, bronchiolitis obliterans syndrome, cystic fibrosis, idiopathic pulmonary fibrosis and chronic rejection of a previous double lung transplant, respectively.[30–36]

Several case reports describe other experiences of low-flow CO_2 removal devices intraoperatively during lung volume reduction surgery in patients with end-stage lung emphysema or during giant bullectomy.[37,38] To date, such uses are limited with insufficient clinical evidence.

FUTURE RESEARCH

Despite the promising results related to ECCO2R use, many questions remain to be answered. Major points of concern are as follows:

- *The lack of RCTs* with short-term and long-term clinical outcomes.
- *The need of technical skills and proper setting.* The most important skills that an ECCO2R technique requires include the ability to gain an accurate and valid vascular access and to maintain an adequate anticoagulation level, balancing the risks of haemorrhage and thrombosis. To date, heparin remains the most commonly used anticoagulant in these devices. In this respect, we look forward to technological progress that involves more simplified systems, making ECCO2R feasible outside a critical-care area.
- *A cost–benefit analysis.* Data are lacking on the cost-effectiveness of this treatment. The only study that has evaluated the economic implications of the use of this complex and expensive technology was a retrospective ancillary analysis[39] of data extracted from a multicentre case–control study.[25] This study compared the costs of an av-ECCO2R device to avoid intubation with costs for a conventional strategy of invasive mechanical ventilation after NIV failure in patients with acute or chronic hypercapnic respiratory failure. A lower median ICU length of stay (11.0 vs. 35.0 days), hospital length of stay (17.5 vs. 51.5 days) and treatment costs for the ECCO2R group (19.610 vs. 46.552 €, $p = 0.01$) were demonstrated.[39] However, this analysis has several biases including, especially, the study design, the different costs between a pumpless arterio-venous ECCO2R device applied in the original study and a veno-venous system as well as the consideration that the health-care provider's perspective on reimbursement plans varies greatly from country to country. Taking into account all these factors, the results from this study cannot be generalised.
- *The ethical implications.* A recent editorial[40] underlined the ethical controversy focuses on the use of ECCO2R especially in COPD patients.

In fact, subjects with ARDS and those who are admitted to the ICU after an episode of COPD exacerbation (AECOPD) are very different in terms of prognosis. Although survivors of ARDS can develop cognitive, psychological and physical impairments, their recovery process is often complete, albeit slow. In contrast, the 1 year mortality rate for patients with AECOPD requiring admission to ICU is 35%, particularly in those with major comorbidities.[41] In addition, as reported by Lynn et al.,[42] in this group, around 20% of patients spend the final 6 months in hospital with poor quality of life. Therefore, further studies are needed in order to understand better if the implementation of extracorporeal CO_2 removal with expensive devices can be ethically justified in patients with AECOPD.

CONCLUSION

ECCO2R is an appealing technique with an innovative approach that takes advantage of the major technical improvements offered by the industry in this field. To date, a few studies have shown the safety and efficacy of ECCOR devices in the acute care setting. Although indications for ECCO2R in both patients with ARDS and COPD patients with acute exacerbation are starting to be defined, further studies are needed before ECCO2R can become a routine treatment.

REFERENCES

1. Kolobow T, Gattinoni L, Tomlinson TA, Pierce JE. Control of breathing using an extracorporeal membrane lung. *Anesthesiology.* 1977;46(2):138–41.
2. Maclaren G, Combes A, Bartlett RH. Contemporary extracorporeal membrane oxygenation for adult respiratory failure: Life support in the new era. *Intensive Care Med.* 2011;38:210–20.
3. Pesenti A, Gattinoni L, Bombino M. Extracorporeal carbon dioxide removal. In: Tobin MJ, ed. *Principles and Practice of Mechanical Ventilation*, 3rd ed. New York: McGraw Hill; 2013.
4. Cove ME, MacLaren G, Federspiel WJ, Kellum JA. Bench to bedside review: Extracorporeal carbon dioxide removal, past present and future. *Crit Care.* 2012;16:232.
5. Reul HM, Akdis M. Blood pumps for circulatory support. *Perfusion.* 2000;15:295–311.
6. Wang D, Zhou X, Liu X et al. Wang–Zwische double lumen cannula—Toward a percutaneous and ambulatory paracorporeal artificial lung. *ASAIO J.* 2008;54:606–11.
7. Ware LB, Matthay MA. The acute respiratory distress syndrome. *N Engl J Med.* 2000;342:1334–7.
8. Ferguson ND, Fan E, Camporota L et al. The Berlin definition of ARDS: An expanded rationale, justification, and supplementary material. *Intensive Care Med.* 2012;38:1573–82.
9. ARDSnet. Ventilation with lower tidal volumes as compared with traditional tidal volumes for acute lung injury and the acute respiratory distress syndrome. The Acute Respiratory Distress Syndrome Network. *N Engl J Med.* 2000;342(18):1301–8.
10. Slutsky AS, Ranieri VM. Ventilator-induced lung injury. *N Engl J Med.* 2013;369(22):2126–36.
11. Bellani G, Guerra L, Musch G et al. Lung regional metabolic activity and gas volume changes induced by tidal ventilation in patients with acute lung injury. *Am J Respir Crit Care Med.* 2011;183(9):1193–9.

12. Grasso S, Strippoli T, De Michele M et al. ARDSnet ventilator protocol and alveolar hyperinflation: Role of positive end-expiratory pressure. *Am J Respir Crit Care Med.* 2007;176(8):761–7.
13. Fitzgerald M, Millar J, Blackwood B et al. Extracorporeal carbon dioxide removal for patients with acute respiratory failure secondary to the acute respiratory distress syndrome: A systematic review. *Crit Care.* 2014;18:222.
14. Terragni PP, Del Sorbo L, Mascia L et al. Tidal volume lower than 6 ml/kg enhances lung protection: Role of extracorporeal carbon dioxide removal. *Anesthesiology.* 2009;111:826–35.
15. Bein T, Weber-Carstens S, Goldmann A et al. Lower tidal volume strategy (≈3 ml/kg) combined with extracorporeal CO2 removal versus 'conventional' protective ventilation (6 ml/kg) in severe ARDS: The prospective randomized Xtravent-study. *Intensive Care Med.* 2013;39:847–856.
16. Fanelli V, Ranieri MV, Mancebo J et al. Feasibility and safety of low-flow extracorporeal carbon dioxide removal to facilitate ultra-protective ventilation in patients with moderate acute respiratory distress syndrome. *Crit Care.* 2016;20(1):36.
17. Gattinoni L. Ultra-protective ventilation and hypoxemia. *Crit Care.* 2016;20:130.
18. SUPERNOVA. SUPERNOVA: A strategy of ultra-protective lung ventilation with extracorporeal co2 removal for new-onset moderate to severe ARDS. http://www.esicm.org/research/trials-group/supernova.
19. Pisani L, Corcione N, Nava S. Management of acute hypercapnic respiratory failure. *Curr Opin Crit Care.* 2016 Feb;22(1):45–52.
20. O'Donnell DE, Parker CM. COPD exacerbations. 3: Pathophysiology. *Thorax.* 2006;61:354–61. Review.
21. Lindenauer PK, Stefan MS, Shieh MS et al. Outcomes associated with invasive and noninvasive ventilation among patients hospitalized with exacerbations of chronic obstructive pulmonary disease. *JAMA Intern Med.* 2014;174:1982–93.
22. Chandra D, Stamm JA, Taylor B et al. Outcomes of noninvasive ventilation for acute exacerbations of chronic obstructive pulmonary disease in the United States, 1998–2008. *Am J Respir Crit Care Med.* 2012;185:152–9.
23. Sklar MC, Beloncle F, Katsios CM et al. Extracorporeal carbon dioxide removal in patients with chronic obstructive pulmonary disease: A systematic review. *Intensive Care Med.* 2015;41:1752–62.
24. Del Sorbo L, Pisani L, Filippini C et al. Extracorporeal CO_2 removal in hypercapnic patients at risk of noninvasive ventilation failure: A matched cohort study with historical control. *Crit Care Med.* 2014;43:120–7.
25. Kluge S, Braune SA, Engel M et al. Avoiding invasive mechanical ventilation by extracorporeal carbon dioxide removal in patients failing noninvasive ventilation. *Intensive Care Med.* 2012;38:1632–9.
26. Braune S, Sieweke A, Brettner F et al. The feasibility and safety of extracorporeal carbon dioxide removal to avoid intubation in patients with COPD unresponsive to noninvasive ventilation for acute hypercapnic respiratory failure (ECLAIR study): Multicentre case-control study. *Intensive Care Med.* 2016;42:1437–44.
27. Pisani L, Fasano L, Corcione N et al. Effects of extracorporeal CO_2 removal on inspiratory effort and respiratory pattern in patients who fail weaning from mechanical ventilation. *Am J Respir Crit Care Med.* 2015 Dec 1;192(11):1392–4.
28. Del Sorbo L, Boffini M, Rinaldi M, Ranieri VM. Bridging to lung transplantation by extracorporeal support. *Minerva Anestesiol.* 2012;78:243–50.
29. Fischer S, Simon AR, Welte T et al. Bridge to lung transplantation with the novel pumpless interventional lung assist device NovaLung. *J Thorac Cardiovasc Surg.* 2006;131:719.
30. Ricci D, Boffini M, Del Sorbo L et al. The use of CO_2 removal devices in patients awaiting lung transplantation: An initial experience. *Transplant Proc.* 2010;42:1255.
31. Bartosik W, Egan JJ, Wood AE. The Novalung interventional lung assist as bridge to lung transplantation for self-ventilating patients – initial experience. *Interact Cardiovasc Thorac Surg.* 2011;13:198.
32. Haneya A, Philipp A, Mueller T et al. Extracorporeal circulatory systems as a bridge to lung transplantation at remote transplant centers. *Ann Thorac Surg.* 2011;91:250.
33. Ruberto F, Bergantino B, Testa MC et al. Low-flow veno-venous extracorporeal $C0_2$ removal: First clinical experience in lung transplant recipients. *Int J Artif Organs.* 2014 Dec;37(12):911–7.
34. Hermann A, Staudinger T, Bojic A et al. First experience with a new miniaturized pump-driven veno-venous extracorporeal CO2 removal system (iLA Activve): A retrospective data analysis. *ASAIO J.* 2014 May–Jun;60(3):342–7.
35. Schellongowski P, Riss K, Staudinger T et al. Extracorporeal CO_2 removal as bridge to lung transplantation in life-threatening hypercapnia. *Transpl Int.* 2015 Mar;28(3):297–304.
36. Redwan B, Ziegeler S, Semik M et al. Single-site cannulation veno-venous extracorporeal CO_2 removal as bridge to lung volume reduction surgery in end-stage lung emphysema. *ASAIO J.* 2016; 62(6):743–6.
37. Kim YR, Haam SJ, Park YG et al. Lung transplantation for bronchiolitis obliterans after allogeneic hematopoietic stem cell transplantation. *Yonsei Med J.* 2012;53:1054.

38. Dell'Amore A, D'Andrea R, Caroli G et al. Intraoperative management of hypercapnia with an extracorporeal carbon dioxide removal device during giant bullectomy. *Innovations (Phila).* 2016 Mar–Apr;11(2):142–5.
39. Braune S, Burchardi H, Engel M et al. The use of extracorporeal carbon dioxide removal to avoid intubation in patients failing non-invasive ventilation – a cost analysis. *BMC Anesthesiol.* 2015 4;15:160.
40. Nava S, Ranieri VM. Extracorporeal lung support for COPD reaches a crossroad. *Lancet Respir Med.* 2014;2(5):350–2.
41. Groenewegen KH, Schols AM, Wouters EF. Mortality and mortality related factors after hospitalization for acute exacerbation of COPD. *Chest.* 2003;124:459–67.
42. Lynn J, Ely EW, Zhong Z et al. Living and dying with chronic obstructive pulmonary disease. *J Am Geriatr Soc.* 2000;48:S91–100.

6

Interfaces

CESARE GREGORETTI, VINCENZO RUSSOTTO AND DAVIDE CHIUMELLO

INTRODUCTION

Patient comfort is crucial for non-invasive ventilation (NIV) success in both acute[1,2] and chronic[3] settings. It may be affected by the interface with respect to many factors, such as air leaks, claustrophobia, facial skin erythema, acneiform rash, eye irritation and skin breakdown.[4–19] In a survey of over 3000 home care patients ventilated with continuous positive airway pressure (CPAP), Meslier et al.[20] found that only about half of the patients classified their interface fit as 'good' or 'very good'. Although nasal masks are more comfortable for stable chronic patients undergoing long-term domiciliary NIV,[5] in patients with acute respiratory failure (ARF), who breathe through both the nose and the mouth, a face mask is preferred.[21] A review of studies using NIV showed that in ARF, the face mask is the most commonly used interface (63%) followed by nasal mask (31%), nasal pillow and mouthpiece.[5] Recent data[22] from a web-based survey of about 300 intensive care units (ICUs) and respiratory wards throughout Europe confirmed that oronasal masks are the most commonly used interfaces for ARF, followed by nasal masks, full face masks and helmets. In chronic respiratory failure, the most common interface used is the nasal mask (73%) followed by nasal pillow, face masks and mouthpieces.[15,23]

CHARACTERISTICS, ADVANTAGES AND DISADVANTAGES OF THE VARIOUS NIV INTERFACES

Box 6.1 summarises the characteristics of an ideal NIV interface.

Air-leak minimisation and comfort depend on the complex interplay between the patient (underlying disease, face contour and claustrophobia), the ventilator settings (mode of ventilation, inspiratory–expiratory applied pressures and inspiratory–expiratory trigger thresholds), the interface (type, size, material and shape) and the securing system (sites of attachment and tension).[15–22,24] NIV is now considered by most critical care physicians as an effective treatment for selected forms of ARF because of the continuous development of new materials and designs, which have increased the availability of interfaces and therefore enhanced the use of NIV.[24,25] The classes of NIV interface are shown in Box 6.2.

BOX 6.1: Characteristics of an ideal NIV interface and securing system

Interface and securing system

- Ideal interface
- Leak-free
- Good stability
- Non-traumatic
- Light-weight
- Long-lasting
- Non-deformable
- Non-allergenic material
- Low resistance to airflow
- Minimal dead space (when needed)
- Low cost
- Easy to manufacture (for the moulded interfaces)
- Available in various sizes

Ideal securing system

- Stable (to avoid interface movements or dislocation)
- Easy to put on or remove
- Non-traumatic
- Light and soft
- Breathable material
- Available in various sizes
- Washable, for home care
- Disposable, for hospital use

Modified from Nava S et al., *Respir Care*. 2009:54:71–84.

> **BOX 6.2: Classes of non-invasive ventilation interfaces**
>
> - Oral interfaces: mouthpiece placed between the patient's lips and held in place by lip seal or the teeth
> - Nasal mask: covers the nose but not the mouth
> - Nasal pillows: plugs inserted into the nostrils
> - Oronasal: covers the nose and mouth
> - Full face: covers the mouth, nose and eyes
> - Helmet: covers the whole head and all or part of the neck

Interfaces include standard commercially available ready-to-use models in various sizes (neonatal, paediatric and adult small, medium and large) or custom-fabricated, moulded directly on the patient or from a moulded cast previously obtained.[8–10] Many commercially available masks consist of two parts: a cushion of soft material (polyvinyl chloride, polypropylene, silicone, silicone elastomer or hydrogel), which forms the seal against the patient's face, and a frame of stiff material (polyvinyl chloride, polycarbonate or thermoplastic), which in many models is transparent. There are four types of face-seal cushion: transparent non-inflatable, transparent inflatable, full hydrogel and full foam. The mask frame has several attachment points (e.g. prongs) to anchor the headgear. The higher the number of attachment points, the higher the probability of obtaining the best fit and the ability to target the point of maximum pressure.[13] Many types of strap assemblies are available.[4] Straps secure the mask with hooks or Velcro. Some interfaces have one or more holes in the frame to prevent rebreathing (so-called 'vent system'; Figure 6.1). Such a mask should not be used with a circuit that has separate inspiratory and expiratory limbs or with an expiratory valve or other external device for carbon dioxide clearance (e.g. the Respironics Plateau valve).[15] A tube adapter allows insertion of a nasogastric tube and prevents the air leak and facial skin damage that could occur if the nasogastric tube was tucked under the seal of a conventional mask.[1–6] Chin straps, lips seals and mouth taping have also been proposed as means to prevent air leaks.[4] Reducing the risk of skin damage is one of the major goals (Box 6.3). Gregoretti et al.[6] performed a multicentre randomised study to evaluate patient comfort, skin breakdown and eye irritation in patients ventilated with different face masks in the acute setting. Interestingly, they found that 10 patients presented a certain amount of skin breakdown after only 24 hours. In a recent study aimed at surveying the effects of an oronasal interface for NIV, using a three-dimensional (3D) computational model with the

> **BOX 6.3: Reducing skin breakdown during NIV**
>
> - Rotate various types of interfaces
> - Proper harness and tightening
> - Skin and mask hygiene
> - Nasal-forehead spacer (to reduce the pressure on the bridge of the nose)
> - Forehead pads (to obtain the most comfortable position on the forehead)
> - Cushioning system between mask prong and forehead
> - Remove patient's dentures when making impression for a moulded mask
> - In home care, replace the mask according to the patient's daily use
> - Skin pad or woundcare dressing
>
> Modified from Nava S et al., *Respir Care*. 2009:54:71–84.

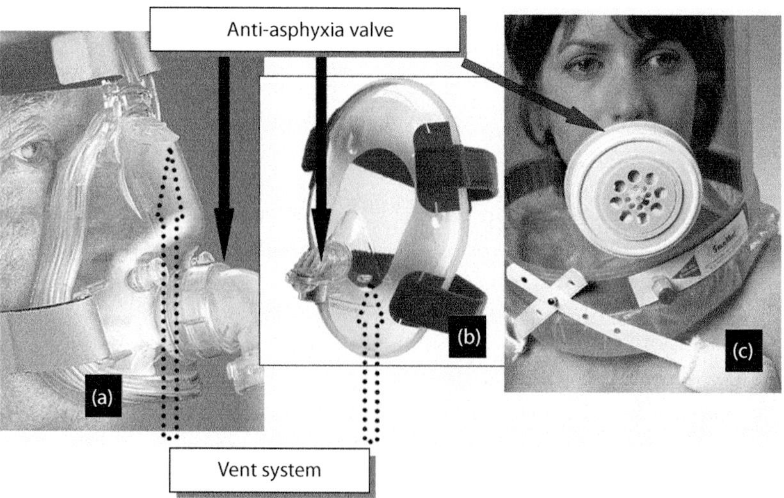

Figure 6.1 Anti-asphyxia and vent systems. **(a, b)** Vent system (dotted arrows) of a full face and of a total full face. **(c)** Anti-asphyxia valve (thick arrows) of a total full-face mask and of a helmet, respectively. (Courtesy of the manufacturers.)

ability to simulate and evaluate the main pressure zones of the interface on the human face, the authors found that a computer model identified several high-impact pressure zones in the nasal bridge and paranasal regions. The variation in soft tissue depth had a direct impact on the amount of applied pressure.[26] So far, the most important strategy to prevent skin damage is to avoid an excessively tight fit.[15] A simple method to avoid this risk is to leave enough space to allow two fingers to pass beneath the headgear.[13] A small amount of air leak is acceptable and should not strongly affect patient–ventilator interaction.[27] Woundcare dressing has also been used to limit or treat skin damage.[28] Long-term use of tight-fitting headgear retards facial skeletal development in children.[29,30]

Most of the interfaces are available in vented and non-vented versions. In the former configuration, there is a 'vented' system (some holes or slots on the frame or on the swivel elbow) that allows carbon dioxide diffusion during ventilation with 'intentional leak' circuit configuration.[31] The vented configuration of an oronasal and total-face mask is always equipped with an anti-asphyxia valve with automatic opening to prevent rebreathing in the case of a pressure failure or when airway pressure falls below 2–3 cmH_2O. The non-vented version fits only with a single or double respiratory circuit with valves.[32]

PHYSIOLOGICAL ASPECTS

Air leaks

Air leaks may reduce the efficiency of NIV and patient tolerance, increase patient–ventilator asynchrony (through loss of triggering sensitivity) and cause awakenings and fragmented sleep.[33,34] Several methods have been proposed to reduce air leaks (Box 6.4). During pressure support ventilation (PSV), leaks can hinder achievement of the inspiration termination criterion.[27,35] Vignaux et al.[36] conducted a prospective multicentre observational study to determine the prevalence of patient–ventilator asynchrony in patients receiving NIV for ARF. They found that ventilator asynchrony due to leaks is quite common in patients receiving NIV. Borel et al.[16] measured intentional leaks in seven different industrial masks to determine whether higher leaks could modify ventilator performance and quality of ventilation. The level of intentional leaks in the seven masks ranged from 30 to 45 L/min for an inspiratory pressure level of 14 cmH_2O. The capacity to achieve and maintain the set inspiratory pressure was significantly decreased with all ventilators and in all simulated lung conditions when intentional leaks increased.

BOX 6.4: Reducing air leaks in NIV

- Proper interface type and size
- Proper securing system
- Mask-support ring
- Comfort flaps
- Adapter for feeding tube
- Hydrogel or foam seals
- Chin strap
- Lips seal or mouth taping

Modified from Nava S et al., *Respir Care*. 2009:54:71–84.

In patients with neuromuscular disorders receiving nocturnal NIV, leaks are also associated with daytime hypercapnia.[37] Schettino et al.[38] evaluated air leaks and mask mechanics and estimated the pressure required to seal the mask to the skin and prevent leaks (mask–face seal pressure) as the difference between the airway pressure and the mask pressure against the face. Higher mask pressure against the face decreases air leaks, as does decreasing the airway pressure applied by the ventilator.

Dead space and carbon dioxide rebreathing

The dead space added by the interface is also recognised as a major problem, in particular, for the treatment of hypercapnic patients, because it may reduce NIV effectiveness in correcting respiratory acidosis.[39,40]

Bench studies have suggested that carbon dioxide rebreathing is significantly increased with masks having a large internal volume,[39] and conversely decreased with masks having a built-in exhalation port, as designed for use with single-circuit bi-level ventilators.[39,40] Navalesi et al.[7] measured the differences in apparatus dead space between a nasal mask and a full face mask. Although the in vitro difference was substantial (205 mL vs 120 mL with full face mask and nasal mask, respectively), the in vivo results (which took into account anatomical structures) were similar (118 mL vs 97 mL with full face mask and nasal mask, respectively). Nasal pillows add very little dead space and can be as effective as face masks in reducing arterial carbon dioxide and increasing pH, but are less tolerated by patients.[7] Different flow patterns and pressure waveforms may also influence the apparatus dead space. Saatci et al.[39] found that a face mask increased dynamic dead space from 32% to 42% of tidal volume above physiological dead space, during unsupported breathing. Other investigators have confirmed the importance of the site of the exhalation ports on carbon dioxide rebreathing.[41] Cuvelier et al.[19] conducted a randomised controlled study to compare the clinical efficacy of a cephalic mask versus an oronasal mask in 34 patients with acute hypercapnic respiratory failure. Compared with values at inclusion, pH, arterial carbon dioxide, encephalopathy score, respiratory distress score and respiratory frequency improved significantly and were similar with both masks.

Fraticelli et al.[18] evaluated the physiological effects of four interfaces with different internal volumes in patients with hypoxaemic or hypercapnic ARF receiving NIV through ICU ventilators. Three face masks with very high

(977 mL), high (163 mL) and moderate (84 mL) internal volume, and a mouthpiece having virtually no internal volume were tested. NIV decreased inspiratory effort and improved gas exchange with no significant difference between the four interfaces. An increased rate of air leaks and asynchrony, and reduced comfort were observed with the mouthpiece, as opposed to all three face masks. The leakage around the mask could act as a bias flow resulting in mask carbon dioxide washout, which could minimise the possible differences in dead space.[18] However, recently Fodil et al.[42] postulated that due to the streaming effects of the gas passing throughout the interface, the effective dead space of the interface could be different from the interface internal volume (labelled as interface gas region) delimited by the interface once fit to a mannequin face. They used numerical simulations with computational fluid dynamics (CFD) software to describe pressure, flow and gas composition in four types of interfaces (two oronasal masks with different internal volume, a cephalic mask and a helmet). CFD allowed this set of interfaces to be tested under strictly identical conditions. The authors found that effective dead space is not related to the internal gas volume included in the interface, suggesting that this internal volume should not be considered as a limiting factor for their efficacy during NIV. In patients undergoing NIV for ARF, the addition of a dead space through a heat and moisture exchanger was shown to reduce the efficacy of NIV, by increasing arterial carbon dioxide,[43] respiratory rate, minute ventilation[43,44] and the work of breathing.[44] The helmet has a much larger volume than any of the other NIV interfaces (always larger than tidal volume), and it behaves as a semi-closed environment, in which the increase in inspired partial pressure of carbon dioxide is an important issue. Similar to a pressurised aircraft,[45] the inspired partial pressure of carbon dioxide in a semi-closed environment depends on the amount of carbon dioxide produced by the subject(s) and the flow of fresh gas that flushes the environment (with a helmet this is called the 'helmet ventilation'). Taccone et al.[46] found in a bench study with a lung model and helmets of various sizes that a 33% reduction in helmet volume had no effect on the amount of carbon dioxide rebreathing at steady state. During either CPAP or NIV, the helmet affects carbon dioxide clearance. High gas flow (40–60 L/min) is required to maintain a low inspired partial pressure of carbon dioxide during helmet CPAP. In contrast, when they delivered CPAP with a ventilator, Taccone et al.[46] found considerable carbon dioxide rebreathing. The effect of a helmet on carbon dioxide during NIV was also evaluated in two physiological studies.[47,48] In both studies, the inspired partial pressure of carbon dioxide was significantly higher with helmet PSV than with mask PSV. However, a recent study[18] of two full-face masks found no significant negative effect of dead space on gas exchange or patient effort. In contrast, studies of masks versus helmets found a helmet less efficient in unloading the respiratory muscles,[49] especially in the presence of a resistive load[48] and higher likelihood of patient–ventilator asynchrony. This may be explained by the longer time required to reach the target pressure, because part of the gas delivered by the ventilator is used to pressurise the helmet.[47,48,50] Some portion of inspiratory effort is unassisted because of greater inspiratory-trigger and expiratory-trigger delay.[48,49,51] Vargas et al.[52] in a prospective crossover study evaluated the ventilatory setting (PSV plus PEEP and pressurisation rate) in 11 patients at risk for respiratory distress, undergoing in a random order face mask, helmet and helmet ventilation with specific setting (50% increases in both PSV and with the highest pressurisation rate). Compared with the face mask, the helmet with the same settings worsened patient–ventilator synchrony, as indicated by longer triggering-on and cycling-off delays.

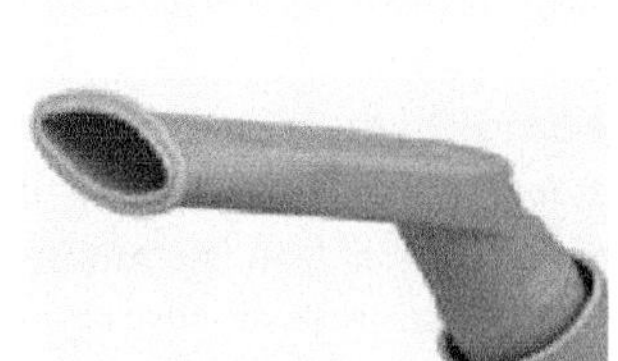
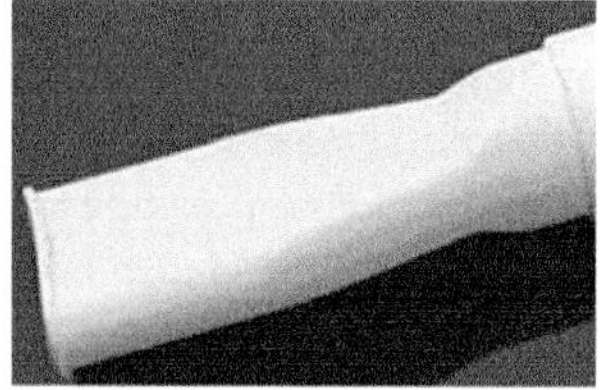

Figure 6.2 Oral interfaces from Respironics. (Courtesy of the manufacturer.)

ORAL INTERFACES

Figure 6.2 shows the oral NIV interfaces, and these are of two types: standard narrow mouthpieces with various degrees of flexion, which are held by the patient's teeth and lips; and custom-moulded bite plates. Oral interfaces are used for long-term ventilation of patients with severe chronic respiratory failure due to neuromuscular disease.[53,54]

In subjects who required several hours of ventilatory support, Bach et al.[53] reported the sequential use of a narrow flexed mouthpiece during the day time and a nasal mask overnight. They suggested the possible use of a standard mouthpiece with lip seal retention or custom-moulded orthodontic bites for overnight use.[53] One study used mouthpieces in patients with cystic fibrosis and acute or chronic respiratory failure.[55] A recent study suggested that a mouthpiece is as effective as a full-face mask in reducing inspiratory effort in patients receiving NIV for ARF.[18] Mouthpieces may elicit the gag reflex, salivation or vomiting. Long-term use can also cause tooth and jaw deformities. Vomit aspiration is another potential complication, though so far that risk has only been theoretical.[53] Mouth air leaks may be controlled with a tight-fitting lip seal. Nasal pledges or nose clips can be used to avoid air leak through the nares.[53]

NASAL MASKS AND PILLOWS

Although nasal masks are the first choice for long-term ventilation, they have also been used for acute hypercapnic[56–62] and hypoxaemic[60,63–69] respiratory failure. Nasal masks are shown in Figure 6.3, and Box 6.5 summarises the reported advantages of and contraindications to nasal masks.

Preliminary studies with normal adults suggested that nasal ventilation is of limited effectiveness when nasal resistance exceeds 5 cmH_2O.[70]

The two types of nasal mask are

- Full nasal mask: covers the whole nose
- External nostril mask (also called nasal slings): applied externally to the nares

Nasal pillows (Figure 6.4), like nasal slings, have less dead space than face masks, are less likely to produce claustrophobia and allow the patient to wear glasses.[4] They offer advantages similar to those of nasal masks; they allow expectoration, food intake and speech without removing the mask. Nasal pillows potentially also allow the user to wear glasses for reading.

With nasal pillows and masks, the presence of expiratory air leak makes tidal volume monitoring unreliable.[2] Nasal pillows can be alternated with oronasal and nasal masks to minimise friction and pressure on the skin, at least for a few hours, which could improve tolerance of NIV and therefore allow more hours of ventilation per day.

ORONASAL AND FULL-FACE MASKS

It is a common belief that oronasal masks are preferred for patients with ARF, because those patients generally breathe through the mouth to bypass nasal resistance.[57] Kwok et al.[21] studied a heterogeneous population of

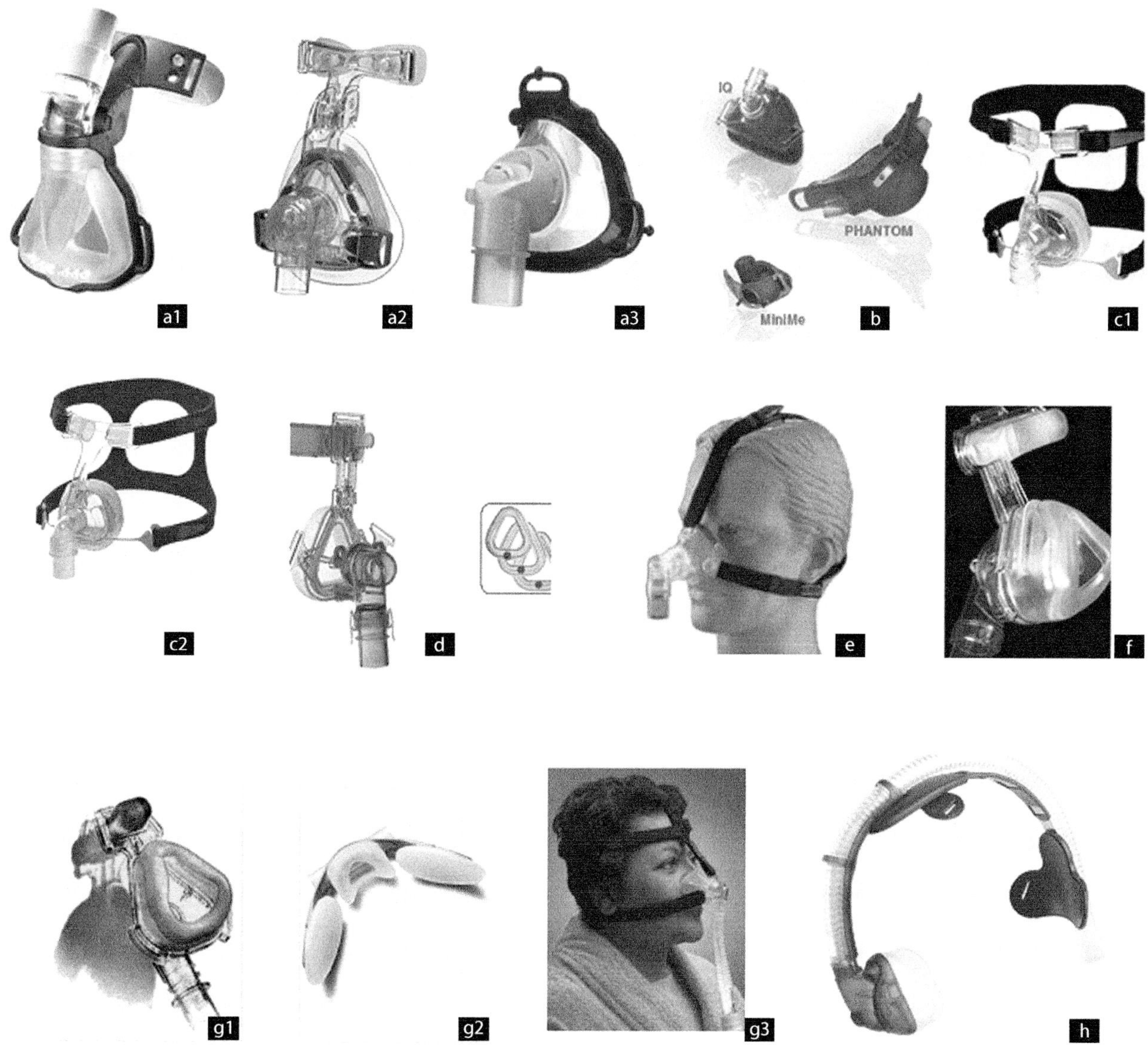

Figure 6.3 Nasal masks. ResMed: **(a1)** Papillon, **(a2)** Activa, **(a3)** Mirage Micro, **(b)** SleepNet IQ, Phantom, and MiniMe. Fisher and Paykel: **(c1)** HC407, **(c2)** Zest Clear Cut, **(d)** Koo Deluxe, **(e)** Hans Rudolph Nasal Alizes 7800, **(f)** CareFusion Standard Series Nasal Mask. Respironics: **(g1)** Comfort Classic, **(g2)** Comfort Curve, **(g3)** Simplicity, **(h)** Covidien Breeze DreamSeal. (Courtesy of the manufacturers.)

BOX 6.5: Advantages of and contraindications to nasal masks for non-invasive ventilation

Advantages

- Less interference with speech and eating
- Allows cough
- Less danger with vomiting
- Claustrophobia uncommon
- No risk of asphyxia in case of ventilator malfunction
- Less likely to cause gastric distension

Relative contraindications

- Edentulism
- Leaks from the mouth during sleep

Absolute contraindications

- Respiration from the mouth or unable to breathe through the nose
- Oronasal breathing in severe acute respiratory failure
- Surgery of the soft palate

Modified from Nava S et al., *Respir Care.* 2009:54:71–84.

35 patients with congestive heart failure, sepsis, acute lung injury, asthma, pneumonia and COPD. Although both masks performed similarly with regard to improving vital signs and gas exchange and avoiding intubation, the nasal mask was less tolerated than the oronasal mask in patients with ARF.

Girault et al.,[17] in patients with hypercapnic ARF due to acute COPD with mixed aetiology, compared the initial choice of face mask and nasal mask and its clinical effectiveness and tolerance. Patients randomised to nasal NIV had significant mask failure (75%), occurring within 6 hours of NIV therapy, mainly due to buccal air leak (94%), necessitating a switch to a face mask. None in the face NIV group needed mask change. In the nasal NIV group, no intubation was required among those who did not require a mask change, but in those who needed a change of mask, 18% needed intubation and mechanical ventilation. There were, however, no significant differences in intubation rate, ICU length of stay and ICU mortality. However, studies comparing two different interfaces cannot be blinded, and it is impossible to eliminate bias. The decision to change masks is based on subjective opinion by the attending physician and not based on objective criteria, and the use of different ventilators to deliver NIV could cause variations in outcome.[71] Figure 6.5 shows some types of oronasal masks.

One mask is a combination of a nasal pillow and an oral interface. Interestingly, it also skips the nasal bridge once fitted to the patient, thus avoiding nasal skin breakdown (Figure 6.5d1). A cephalic mask (total full-face mask or integral mask) has a soft cuff that seals around the perimeter of the face, so there is no pressure on areas that an oronasal mask contacts[9,18] (Figure 6.6). The frame of the total full-face mask may include an anti-asphyxia valve that automatically opens to room air in case of ventilator malfunction when airway pressure falls below 3 cmH_2O (Figure 6.1b). Compared with a full-face mask, a cephalic mask has a larger inner volume because it covers the entire anterior surface of the face. Its main advantage is that it limits the risk of deleterious cutaneous side effects during NIV.[6,9,18,19] This mask also is of potential interest as an alternative to conventional masks for patients with skin breakdown or morphologic characteristics hindering adaptation to other interfaces.[18] Fraticelli et al.[18] found that nose comfort was better with the mouthpiece and the cephalic mask. Cuvelier et al.[19] when comparing cephalic mask versus an oronasal mask, found that in spite of its larger inner volume, the cephalic mask had the same clinical efficacy and required the same ventilatory settings as the oronasal mask during ARF. Tolerance of the oronasal mask was improved at 24 hours and further. However, one patient with the cephalic mask had claustrophobia, but this did not lead to dropping

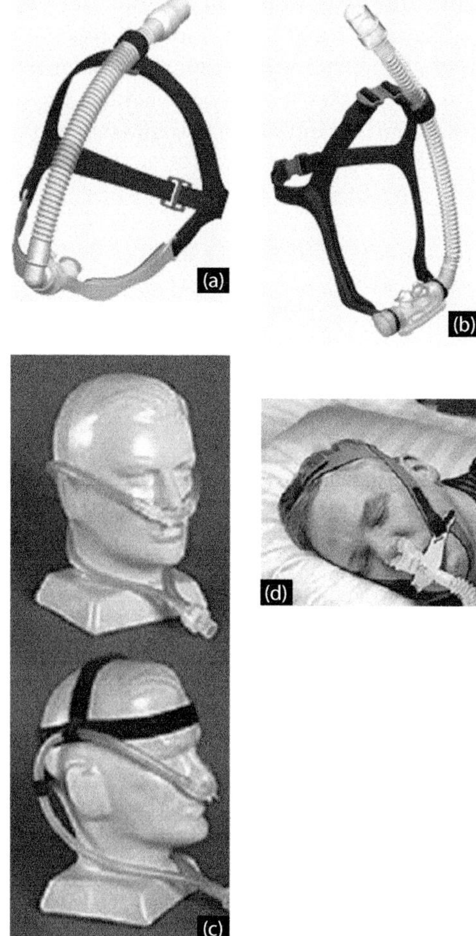

Figure 6.4 Nasal pillows. Fisher and Paykel: **(a)** New Opus; ResMed: **(b)** Mirage Swift II: **(c)** InnoMed Nasal-Airell. Respironics: **(d)** OptiLife. (Courtesy of the manufacturers.)

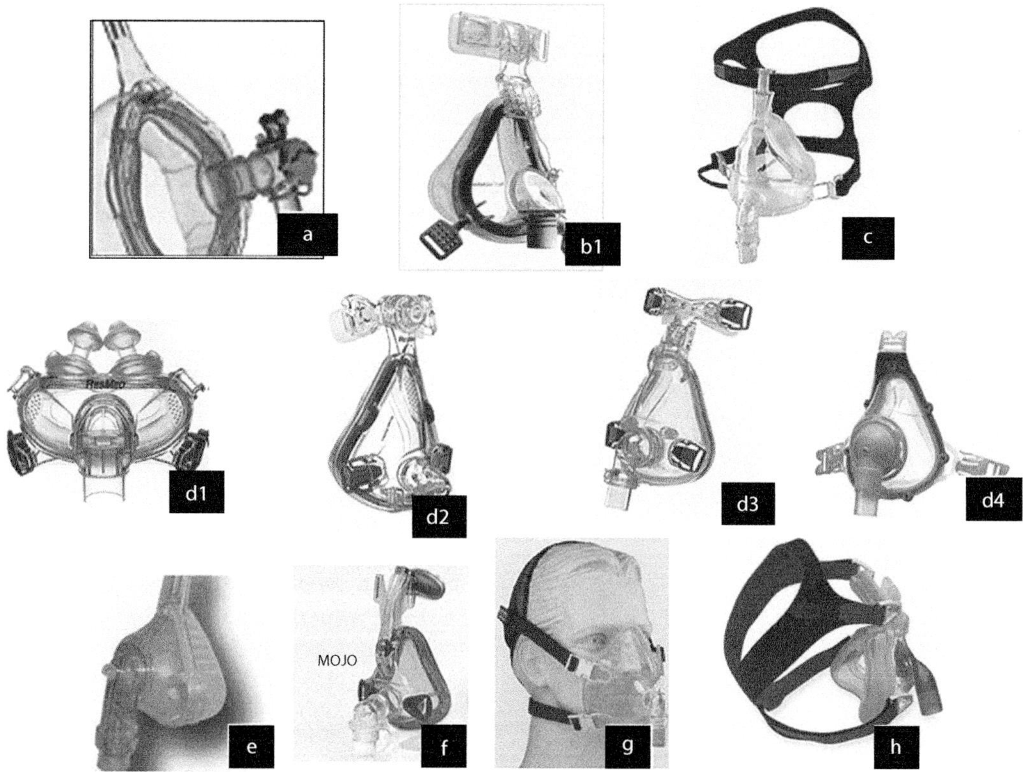

Figure 6.5 Full-face masks. Koo: **(a)** Blustar, **(b1)** Comfort Gel, **(c)** Fisher and Paykel HC431. ResMed: **(d1)** Mirage Quattro, **(d2)** Liberty, **(d3)** Mirage, **(d4)** Hospital Mirage, **(e)** Viasys, **(f)** SleepNet Mojo, **(g)** Hans Rudolph VIP 75/76, **(h)** Weinmann Joyce. (Courtesy of the manufacturers.)

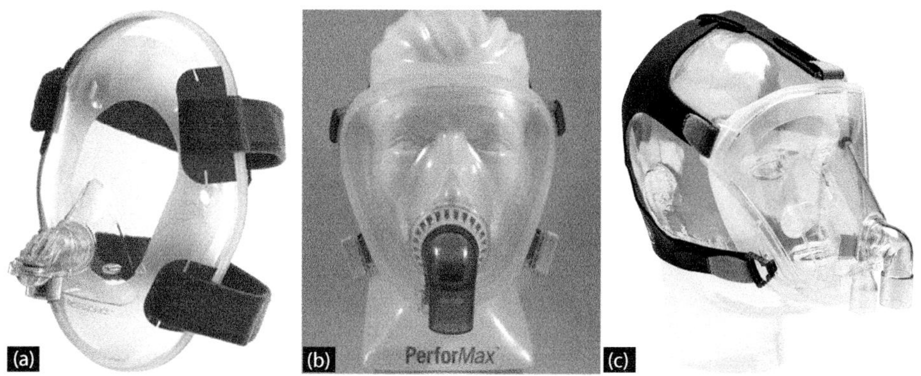

Figure 6.6 Total full face masks. Respironics: **(a)** Total, **(b)** PerforMax, and **(c)** Dimar DIMAX ZERO. (Courtesy of Respironics.)

out from the study. Cephalic mask has also been found to decrease patient–ventilator synchrony in turbine-driven ventilator equipped with an 'intentional leak' circuit.[72] Discussion is still also open if the cephalic mask would change the outcome.[73] In patients in hypercapnic ARF, for whom escalation to intubation is deemed inappropriate, switching to cephalic mask can be proposed as a last resort therapy when face mask-delivered non-invasive mechanical ventilation has already failed to reverse ARF. This strategy is particularly interesting because it can provide prolonged periods of continuous NIV while preventing facial pressure sore.[74] A new type of full-face mask, equipped with nasal and oral ports, is intended for use in endoscopic procedures both for elective ventilation and for emergencies. This is theoretically possible because this new interface is made of two symmetrical parts that can be joined even after the insertion of the endoscopic probe.[75]

Box 6.6 gives the advantages of and contraindications to oronasal and full-face masks.

HELMETS

A helmet has a transparent hood and soft (polyvinyl chloride or silicone) collar that contacts the body at the neck and/or shoulders (Figure 6.7). A helmet has at least two ports: one through which gas enters, and another from which gas

BOX 6.6: Advantages of and contraindications to oronasal and full face masks for NIV

Advantages (compared with nasal mask)

- Fewer air leaks with more stable mean airway pressure, especially during sleep
- Less patient cooperation required

Relative contraindications

- Tetraparetic patients with severe impairment in arm movement

Absolute contraindications

- Vomiting
- Claustrophobia

Modified from Nava S et al., *Respir Care.* 2009:54:71–84.

exits. The helmet is secured to the patient by armpit straps. All the available helmets are latex-free and available in multiple sizes. Helmets were originally used to deliver a precise oxygen concentration during hyperbaric oxygen therapy. The United States Food and Drug Administration has not approved any of the available helmets, but they have been approved in some other countries.[22,25,46,76,77] The helmet, which covers the head of the patient entirely, is particularly indicated in the presence of skin breakdown.[78] Costa et al.[79] comparing PSV delivered by a helmet, an oronasal interface or an endotracheal tube, found that patient–ventilator synchrony was significantly better with the last one. Helmet compared to the oronasal mask results in a worst synchrony due to a longer inspiratory trigger delay and a shorter time of synchrony between ventilator support and patient effort. However, recently helmets have been improved, with more comfortable seals against leak and a better ventilator interaction.[80–82] Box 6.7 lists the advantages of and contraindications to helmets.

BOX 6.7: Advantages of and contraindications to helmets

Advantages (compared with oronasal mask)

- Less resistance to flow
- Can be applied regardless of the facial contour, facial trauma or edentulism
- Allows coughing
- Less need for patient cooperation
- Better comfort
- Less interference with speech
- Less likelihood of causing skin damage

Relative contraindications

- Need for monitoring of volumes
- Likelihood of difficult humidification

Absolute contraindications

- Claustrophobia
- Tetraplegia

Modified from Nava S et al., *Respir Care.* 2009:54:71–84.

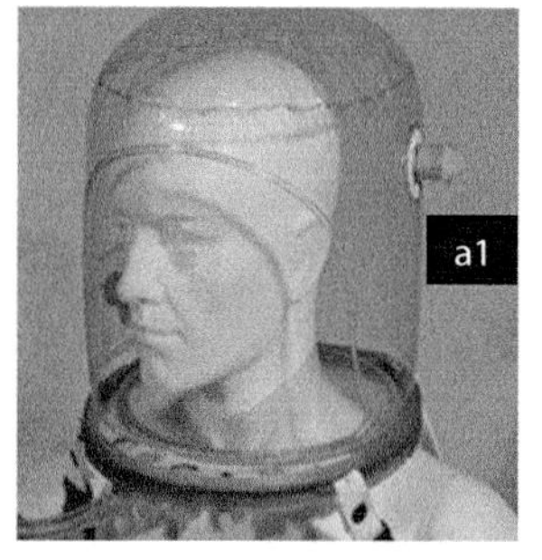

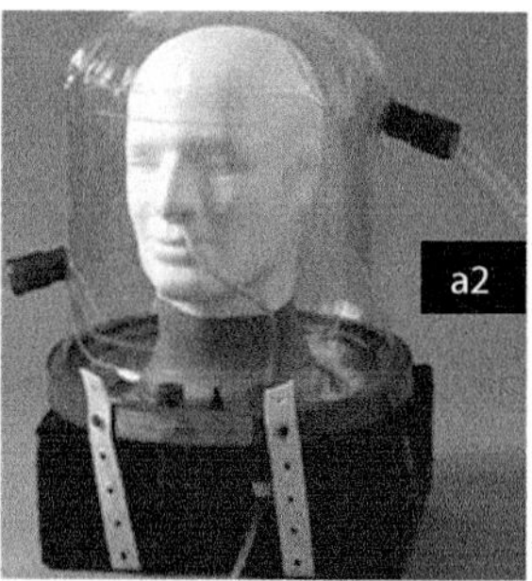

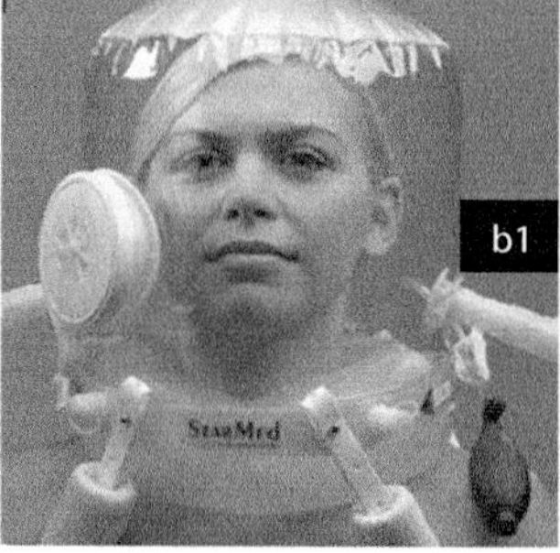

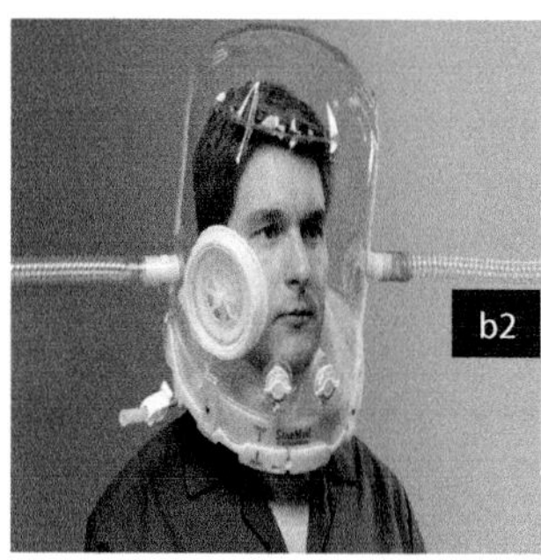

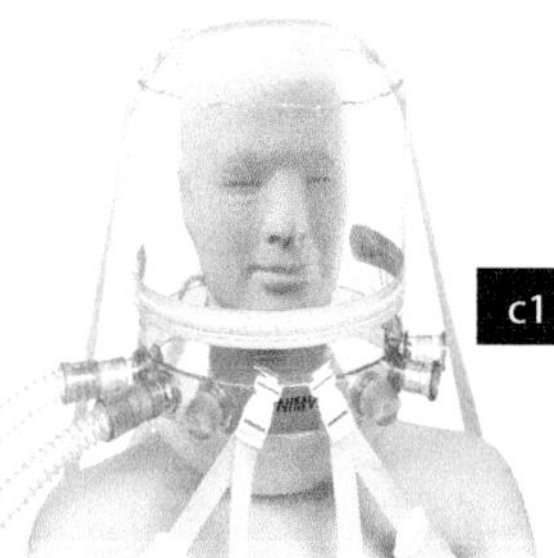

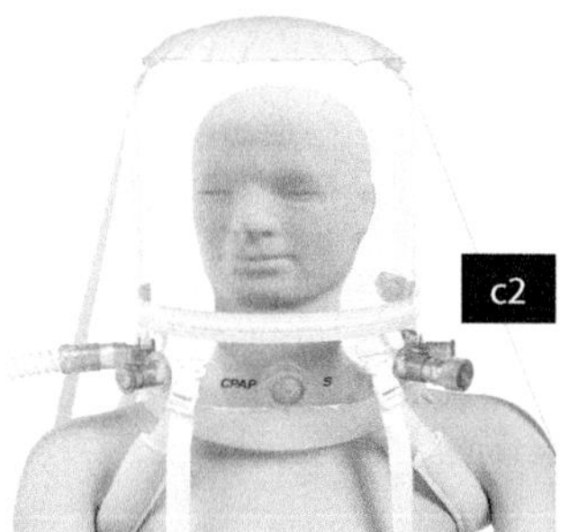

Figure 6.7 Helmets. Harol: **(a1)** NIV10201, **(a2)** NIV10301/X; **(b1)** Intersurgical Castar, **(b2)** Intersurgical Castar NIV Next, **(c1)** Dimar NIMV Comfort ZIP, **(c2)** Dimar CPAP Comfort ZIP. (Courtesy of the manufacturers.)

PAEDIATRIC INTERFACES

NIV is increasingly used in children.[83] Indeed, the choice of the optimal interface for NIV is mandatory for the success of NIV, especially in young children and those with facial deformity or asymmetry. The likelihood of skin injury, pain, discomfort or air leaks around the mask may result in poor children acceptance to NIV. Nasal masks are usually employed in neonates and in smaller children who are nose breathers. However, nasal prongs and facial masks may be also used in older individuals.[83] There is a paucity of literature regarding paediatric interfaces. In children, the choice of the interface is determined not only by the patient's age and the facial morphology but also by the ventilatory mode. According to the circuit configuration, as in the adult population, interfaces with manufactured leaks are used for 'vented' ventilation, and interfaces without manufactured leaks are used for 'non-vented' ventilation. The choice between these two ventilatory modes is mainly determined by the type of underlying disease with very small children probably better adapting to vented ventilation.[84–86] Long-term use of facial or nasal masks may cause facial hypoplasia, and for this reason, careful attention should be paid in smaller children. In the same way, nasal prongs may disrupt nostril anatomy.[28,30]

CONCLUSIONS

Practically, a full-face mask or a total full-face mask should be the first-line strategy in the initial management of hypercapnic acute respiratory failure with NIV. The internal volume of the mask seems not to be a major problem in terms of arterial blood gases and patient effort.[18] However, if NIV has to be prolonged, switching to a nasal mask may improve comfort by reducing face mask complications. In contrast, in mild ARF, we recommend trying a nasal mask first, which is better tolerated,[7,15] or nasal pillows, which are less likely to cause skin damage.[15] Helmet CPAP with continuous flow devices may also offer an appealing approach, taking into account the physical properties of the helmet and the problems related to carbon dioxide clearance.[76] However, physicians must bear in mind that, when switching from CPAP to intermittent positive ventilation, the mechanical properties of the helmet must be considered to achieve effective downloading of the patient's muscles.[52]

Nevertheless, a recent clinical study[87] shed interesting clues on helmet. Among patients with ARDS, treatment with helmet NIV resulted in a significant reduction of intubation rates. More multicentre studies are needed to replicate these findings.[87]

REFERENCES

1. Antonelli M, Conti G, Moro M et al. Predictors of failure of noninvasive positive pressure ventilation in patients with acute hypoxemic respiratory failure: A multi-center study. *Intensive Care Med.* 2001;27:1718–28.
2. Squadrone E, Frigerio P, Fogliati C et al. Noninvasive vs invasive ventilation in COPD patients with severe acute respiratory failure deemed to require ventilatory assistance. *Intensive Care Med.* 2004;30:1303–10.
3. Criner GJ, Brennan K, Travaline JM, Kreimer D. Efficacy and compliance with noninvasive positive pressure ventilation in patients with chronic respiratory failure. *CHEST J.* 1999;116:667–75.
4. Mehta S, Hill NS. Noninvasive ventilation. *Am J Respir Crit Care Med.* 2001;163:540–77.
5. Schönhofer B, Sortor-Leger S. Equipment needs for noninvasive mechanical ventilation. *Eur Respir J.* 2002;20:1029–36.
6. Gregoretti C, Confalonieri M, Navalesi P et al. Evaluation of patient skin breakdown and comfort with a new face mask for non-invasive ventilation: A multi-center study. *Intensive Care Med.* 2002;28:278–84.
7. Navalesi P, Fanfulla F, Frigerio P et al. Physiologic evaluation of noninvasive mechanical ventilation delivered with three types of masks in patients with chronic hypercapnic respiratory failure. *Crit. Care Med.* 2000;28:1785–90.
8. Tsuboi T, Ohi M, Kita H et al. The efficacy of a custom-fabricated nasal mask on gas exchange during nasal intermittent positive pressure ventilation. *Eur Respir. J.* 1999;13:152–6.
9. Criner GJ, Travaline JM, Brennan KJ, Kreimer DT. Efficacy of a new full face mask for noninvasive positive pressure ventilation. *CHEST J.* 1994;106:1109–15.
10. McDermott I, Bach JR, Parker C, Sorfor S. Custom-fabricated interfaces for intermittent positive pressure ventilation. *Int J Prosthodont.* 1989;2.
11. Bach J, Sortor S, Saporito L. Interfaces for non-invasive intermittent positive pressure ventilatory support in North America. *Eur Respir Rev.* 1993:254.
12. Cornette A, Mougel D. Ventilatory assistance via the nasal route: Masks and fittings. *Eur Respir Rev.* 1993:250.
13. Meduri G, Spencer S. Noninvasive mechanical ventilation in the acute setting. Technical aspects, monitoring and choice of interface. *Eur Respir Monogr.* 2001;6:106–24.
14. Navalesi P, Frigerio P, Gregoretti C. Interfaces and humidification in the home setting. In: Muir J-F, Ambrosino N, Simonds AK, eds. Noninvasive ventilation. *Eur Respir Monogr.* 2008;2:338–49.
15. Nava S, Navalesi P, Gregoretti C. Interfaces and humidification for noninvasive mechanical ventilation. *Respir Care.* 2009;54:71–84.
16. Borel JC, Sabil A, Janssens J-P et al. Intentional leaks in industrial masks have a significant impact on efficacy of bilevel noninvasive ventilation: A bench test study. *CHEST J.* 2009;135:669–77.

17. Girault C, Briel A, Benichou J et al. Interface strategy during noninvasive positive pressure ventilation for hypercapnic acute respiratory failure. *Crit Care Med.* 2009;37:124–31.
18. Fraticelli A, Lellouche F, L'her E et al. Physiological effects of different interfaces during noninvasive ventilation for acute respiratory failure. *Crit Care Med.* 2009;37:939–45.
19. Cuvelier A, Pujol W, Pramil S et al. Cephalic versus oronasal mask for noninvasive ventilation in acute hypercapnic respiratory failure. *Intensive Care Med.* 2009;35:519–26.
20. Meslier N, Lebrun T, Grillier-Lanoir V et al. A French survey of 3,225 patients treated with CPAP for obstructive sleep apnoea: Benefits, tolerance, compliance and quality of life. *Eur Respir J.* 1998;12:185–92.
21. Kwok H, McCormack J, Cece R et al. Controlled trial of oronasal versus nasal mask ventilation in the treatment of acute respiratory failure. *Crit Care Med* 2003;31:468–73.
22. Crimi C, Noto A, Esquinas A, Nava S. Non-invasive ventilation (NIV) practices: A European web-survey. *Eur Respir J.* 2008;32:1970.
23. Sferrazza Papa GF, Di Marco F, Akoumianaki E, Brochard L. Recent advances in interfaces for non-invasive ventilation: From bench studies to practical issues. *Minerva Anestesiol.* 2012;78:1146–53.
24. Navalesi P. Internal space of interfaces for noninvasive ventilation: Dead, but not deadly. *Crit Care Med.* 2009;37:1146–7.
25. Antonelli M, Conti G, Pelosi P et al. New treatment of acute hypoxemic respiratory failure: Noninvasive pressure support ventilation delivered by helmet—A pilot controlled trial. *Crit Care Med.* 2002;30:602–8.
26. Barros LS, Talaia P, Drummond M, Natal-Jorge R. Facial pressure zones of an oronasal interface for noninvasive ventilation: A computer model analysis. *J Bras Pneumol.* 2014;40:652–7.
27. Calderini E, Confalonieri M, Puccio P et al. Patient–ventilator asynchrony during noninvasive ventilation: The role of expiratory trigger. *Intensive Care Med.* 1999;25:662–7.
28. Li KK, Riley RW, Guilleminault C. An unreported risk in the use of home nasal continuous positive airway pressure and home nasal ventilation in children: Mid-face hypoplasia. *CHEST J.* 2000;117:916–8.
29. Callaghan S, Trapp M. Evaluating two dressings for the prevention of nasal bridge pressure sores. *Prof Nurse.* 1998;13:361–4.
30. Fauroux B, Lavis J-F, Nicot F et al. Facial side effects during noninvasive positive pressure ventilation in children. *Intensive Care Med.* 2005;31:965–9.
31. Szkulmowski Z, Belkhouja K, Le Q-H et al. Bilevel positive airway pressure ventilation: Factors influencing carbon dioxide rebreathing. *Intensive Care Med.* 2010;36:688–91.
32. Gregoretti C, Navalesi P, Ghannadian S et al. Choosing a ventilator for home mechanical ventilation. *Breathe.* 2013;9:394–409.
33. Meyer TJ, Pressman MR, Benditt J et al. Air leaking through the mouth during nocturnal nasal ventilation: Effect on sleep quality. *Sleep.* 1997;20:561–9.
34. Bach JR, Robert D, Leger P, Langevin B. Sleep fragmentation in kyphoscoliotic individuals with alveolar hypoventilation treated by NIPPV. *CHEST J.* 1995;107:1552–8.
35. Mehta S, McCool F, Hill N. Leak compensation in positive pressure ventilators: A lung model study. *Eur Respir J.* 2001;17:259–67.
36. Vignaux L, Vargas F, Roeseler J et al. Patient–ventilator asynchrony during non-invasive ventilation for acute respiratory failure: A multicenter study. *Intensive Care Med.* 2009;35:840–6.
37. Gonzalez J, Sharshar T, Hart N et al. Air leaks during mechanical ventilation as a cause of persistent hypercapnia in neuromuscular disorders. *Intensive Care Med.* 2003;29:596–602.
38. Schettino G, Tucci M, Sousa R et al. Mask mechanics and leak dynamics during noninvasive pressure support ventilation: A bench study. *Intensive Care Med.* 2001;27:1887–91.
39. Saatci E, Miller D, Stell I et al. Dynamic dead space in face masks used with noninvasive ventilators: A lung model study. *Eur Respir J.* 2004;23:129–35.
40. Schettino GP, Chatmongkolchart S, Hess DR, Kacmarek RM. Position of exhalation port and mask design affect CO_2 rebreathing during noninvasive positive pressure ventilation. *Crit Care Med.* 2003;31:2178–82.
41. Ferguson GT, Gilmartin M. CO_2 rebreathing during BiPAP ventilatory assistance. *Am J Respir Crit Care Med.* 1995;151:1126–35.
42. Fodil R, Lellouche F, Mancebo J et al. Comparison of patient–ventilator interfaces based on their computerized effective dead space. *Intensive Care Med.* 2011;37:257–62.
43. Jaber S, Chanques G, Matecki S et al. Comparison of the effects of heat and moisture exchangers and heated humidifiers on ventilation and gas exchange during non-invasive ventilation. *Intensive Care Med.* 2002;28:1590–4.
44. Lellouche F, Maggiore SM, Deye N et al. Effect of the humidification device on the work of breathing during noninvasive ventilation. *Intensive Care Med.* 2002;28:1582–9.
45. Lumb A. High altitude and flying. *Appl Respir Physiol.* 2000:357–74.

46. Taccone P, Hess D, Caironi P, Bigatello LM. Continuous positive airway pressure delivered with a "helmet": Effects on carbon dioxide rebreathing. *Crit Care Med.* 2004;32:2090–6.
47. Costa R, Navalesi P, Antonelli M et al. Physiologic evaluation of different levels of assistance during noninvasive ventilation delivered through a helmet. *Chest.* 2005;128:2984.
48. Racca F, Appendini L, Gregoretti C et al. Effectiveness of mask and helmet interfaces to deliver noninvasive ventilation in a human model of resistive breathing. *J Appl Physiol.* 2005;99:1262–71.
49. Navalesi P, Costa R, Ceriana P et al. Non-invasive ventilation in chronic obstructive pulmonary disease patients: Helmet versus facial mask. *Intensive Care Med.* 2007;33:74–81.
50. Chiumello D, Pelosi P, Severgnini P et al. Performance of a new" helmet" versus a standard face mask. *Intensive Care Med.* 2003;29:1671–9.
51. Moerer O, Fischer S, Hartelt M, Kuvaki B. Influence of two different interfaces for noninvasive ventilation compared to invasive ventilation on the mechanical properties and performance of a respiratory system: A lung model study. *Chest.* 2006;129:1424.
52. Vargas F, Thille A, Lyazidi A, Campo F, Brochard L. Helmet with specific settings versus facemask for noninvasive ventilation. *Critical Care Med.* 2009;37:1921.
53. Bach J, Alba A, Bohatiuk G et al. Mouth intermittent positive pressure ventilation in the management of postpolio respiratory insufficiency. *Chest.* 1987;91:859–64.
54. Bach J, Alba A, Saporito L. Intermittent positive pressure ventilation via the mouth as an alternative to tracheostomy for 257 ventilator users. *Chest.* 1993;103:174.
55. Madden B, Kariyawasam H, Siddiqi A et al. Noninvasive ventilation in cystic fibrosis patients with acute or chronic respiratory failure. *Eur Respir J.* 2002;19:310.
56. Benhamou D, Girault C, Faure C et al. Nasal mask ventilation in acute respiratory failure. Experience in elderly patients. *CHEST J.* 1992;102:912–7.
57. Hoo GWS, Santiago S, Williams AJ. Nasal mechanical ventilation for hypercapnic respiratory failure in chronic obstructive pulmonary disease: Determinants of success and failure. *Crit Care Med.* 1994;22:1253–61.
58. Confalonieri M, Aiolfi S, Gondola L et al. Severe exacerbations of chronic obstructive pulmonary disease treated with BiPAP® by nasal mask. *Respiration.* 1994;61:310–6.
59. Barbe F, Togores B, Rubi M et al. Noninvasive ventilatory support does not facilitate recovery from acute respiratory failure in chronic obstructive pulmonary disease. *Eur Respir J.* 1996;9:1240–5.
60. Alsous F, Amoateng-Adjepong Y, Manthous C. Noninvasive ventilation: Experience at a community teaching hospital. *Intensive Care Med.* 1999;25:458–63.
61. Bardi G, Pierotello R, Desideri M et al. Nasal ventilation in COPD exacerbations: Early and late results of a prospective, controlled study. *Eur Respir J.* 2000;15:98–104.
62. Carrey Z, Gottfried SB, Levy RD. Ventilatory muscle support in respiratory failure with nasal positive pressure ventilation. *CHEST J.* 1990;97:150–8.
63. Pennock B, Crawshaw L, Kaplan P. Noninvasive nasal mask ventilation for acute respiratory failure. Institution of a new therapeutic technology for routine use. *Chest.* 1994;105:441.
64. Tognet E, Mercatello A, Polo P et al. Treatment of acute respiratory failure with non-invasive intermittent positive pressure ventilation in haematological patients. *Clin Intensive Care.* 1994;5:282.
65. Sacchetti AD, Harris RH, Paston C, Hernandez Z. Bi-level positive airway pressure support system use in acute congestive heart failure: Preliminary case series. *Acad Emerg. Med.* 1995;2:714–8.
66. Mehta S, Jay GD, Woolard RH et al. Randomized, prospective trial of bilevel versus continuous positive airway pressure in acute pulmonary edema. *Crit Care Med.* 1997;25:620–8.
67. Conti G, Marino P, Cogliati A et al. Noninvasive ventilation for the treatment of acute respiratory failure in patients with hematologic malignancies: A pilot study. *Intensive Care Med.* 1998;24:1283–8.
68. Cuomo A, Delmastro M, Ceriana P et al. Noninvasive mechanical ventilation as a palliative treatment of acute respiratory failure in patients with end-stage solid cancer. *Palliat Med.* 2004;18:602–10.
69. Hillberg R, Johnson D. Noninvasive ventilation. *N Engl J Med.* 1997;337:1746.
70. Ohi M, Chin K, Tsuboi T. Effect of nasal resistance on the increase in ventilation during noninvasive ventilation. *Am J Respir Crit Care Med.* 1994;149:A643.
71. Martin TJ, Hovis JD, Costantino JP et al. A randomized, prospective evaluation of noninvasive ventilation for acute respiratory failure. *Am J Respir Crit Care Med.* 2000;161:807–13.
72. Nakamura MA, Costa EL, Carvalho CR, Tucci MR. Performance of ICU ventilators during noninvasive ventilation with large leaks in a total face mask: A bench study. *J Bras Pneumol.* 2014;40:294–303.
73. Chacur FH, Vilella Felipe LM, Fernandes CG, Lazzarini LC. The total face mask is more comfortable than the oronasal mask in noninvasive ventilation but is not associated with improved outcome. *Respiration.* 2011;82:426–30.

74. Lemyze M, Mallat J, Nigeon O et al. Rescue therapy by switching to total face mask after failure of face mask-delivered noninvasive ventilation in do-not-intubate patients in acute respiratory failure. *Crit Care Med.* 2013;41:481–8.
75. Scala R, Naldi M, Maccari U. Early fiberoptic bronchoscopy during non-invasive ventilation in patients with decompensated chronic obstructive pulmonary disease due to community-acquired-pneumonia. *Crit Care.* 2010;14:R80.
76. Patroniti N, Foti G, Manfio A et al. Head helmet versus face mask for non-invasive continuous positive airway pressure: A physiological study. *Intensive Care Med.* 2003;29:1680–7.
77. Cammarota G, Olivieri C, Costa R et al. Noninvasive ventilation through a helmet in postextubation hypoxemic patients: Physiologic comparison between neurally adjusted ventilatory assist and pressure support ventilation. *Intensive Care Med.* 2011;37:1943–50.
78. Racca F, Appendini L, Berta G et al. Helmet ventilation for acute respiratory failure and nasal skin breakdown in neuromuscular disorders. *Anesth Analg.* 2009;109:164–7.
79. Costa R, Navalesi P, Spinazzola G et al. Influence of ventilator settings on patient–ventilator synchrony during pressure support ventilation with different interfaces. *Intensive Care Med.* 2010;36:1363–70.
80. Vaschetto R, De Jong A, Conseil M et al. Comparative evaluation of three interfaces for non-invasive ventilation: A randomized cross-over design physiologic study on healthy volunteers. *Crit. Care.* 2014;18:R2.
81. Olivieri C, Costa R, Spinazzola G et al. Bench comparative evaluation of a new generation and standard helmet for delivering non-invasive ventilation. *Intensive Care Med.* 2013;39:734–8.
82. Pisani L, Carlucci A, Nava S. Interfaces for noninvasive mechanical ventilation: Technical aspects and efficiency. *Minerva Anestesiol.* 2012; 78:1154.
83. Ramirez A, Delord V, Khirani S et al. Interfaces for long-term noninvasive positive pressure ventilation in children. *Intensive Care Med.* 2012; 38:655–62.
84. Guilleminault C, Pelayo R, Clerk A et al. Home nasal continuous positive airway pressure in infants with sleep-disordered breathing. *J Pediatr.* 1995;127:905–12.
85. Marcus CL, Rosen G, Ward SLD et al. Adherence to and effectiveness of positive airway pressure therapy in children with obstructive sleep apnea. *Pediatrics.* 2006;117:e442–51.
86. Conti G, Gregoretti C, Spinazzola G et al. Influence of different interfaces on synchrony during pressure support ventilation in a pediatric setting: A bench study. *Respir Care.* 2015;60:498–507.
87. Patel BK, Wolfe KS, Pohlman AS et al. Effect of noninvasive ventilation delivered by helmet vs face mask on the rate of endotracheal intubation in patients with acute respiratory distress syndrome: A randomized clinical trial. *JAMA.* 2016 Jun 14;315:2435–41.

7

Quality control of non-invasive ventilation: Performance, service, maintenance and infection control of ventilators

JORDI RIGAU AND RAMON FARRÉ

INTRODUCTION

Treatment with non-invasive ventilation (NIV) is based on the use of sophisticated electromechanical equipment that is continually evolving because of the integration of the latest technological improvements.[1] The clinical outcome of NIV, like that of other medical treatments, depends not only on clinical aspects but also on technical issues.[2] Selection of the most suitable ventilator for each patient, appropriate adjustment of settings and correct maintenance of the equipment are all essential for ensuring adequate treatment, maximising its clinical outcome and minimising the occurrence of adverse events.[3–5] This is particularly important with respect to home mechanical ventilation (HMV) as there is no permanent supervision by specialised personnel. Accordingly, quality control procedures need to be implemented to ensure that patients receive the ventilatory support prescribed by the physician safely and precisely.[4,6]

Given that NIV is used in various scenarios (intensive care unit [ICU], general ward, home, emergency department, transportation),[7] the equipment employed is not the same in all applications, and therefore specific quality control, service and maintenance protocols are required. According to the current regulations for medical devices, it is the responsibility of the manufacturer to identify the applications for which a ventilator can be used.[8,9] Consequently, the manufacturer of the ventilator must analyse the potential risks that the technology poses to the patient or user based on its intended use. However, the equipment used during NIV comprises not only the ventilator device but also the patient interface (mask) and the tubing connecting the ventilator's outlet with the mask, as well as filters and valves. Each part plays a role in the correct functioning of the system and should be kept in good condition to ensure a correct application of the treatment.[3] These components must therefore also be taken into account in quality control procedures.

Some of the risks associated with NIV therapy are related to the ventilator and its accessories. Incidents such as device failure or malfunction, power cuts, misuse by the patient or user or incorrect maintenance of the equipment can generate adverse events of varying degrees of severity, such as incorrect treatment, infections, serious injuries or even the patient's death.[4] All these potential incidents should be identified and minimised, paying special attention to those with potentially life-threatening consequences. Thus, healthcare professionals – as well as patients and other agents involved in the application of NIV – should be trained in the basic principles of the treatment and maintenance of the equipment and be familiar with the characteristics and potential associated risks.[4]

This chapter focuses on the current situation with regard to quality control procedures for NIV. Several issues will be discussed: clinically relevant differences in the characteristics and performance of mechanical ventilators, current procedures for the service and maintenance of NIV equipment and the control of infections related to mechanical ventilation. Finally, the various phases and agents involved in the quality control of NIV will be addressed in the light of the regulations for medical devices.

CHARACTERISTICS AND PERFORMANCE OF MECHANICAL VENTILATORS

Like all other medical devices, mechanical ventilators are subjected to regulations issued by government authorities. These regulations vary in accordance with the country in which the medical device is commercially available, e.g. the European Directives 93/42/CEE on Medical Devices amended by Directive 2007/47/EC in Europe and the

Code of Federal Regulations Title 21 (CFR 21) of the Food and Drug Administration (FDA) in the US market.[8–10] The main aim of these regulations is to guarantee the safety of the patients, users and third parties by minimising the occurrence and effects of potential risks, and to ensure the device performs in accordance with the manufacturer's intentions.[8,9] To this end, the regulations define a number of essential requirements that medical devices have to satisfy before they can be put on the market or into service. These requirements are related to issues such as risk assessment and management, chemical, physical, electrical and biological properties, infection and microbiological contamination and protection against radiation.

To facilitate compliance with the regulations, a manufacturer can voluntarily adhere to harmonised standards that provide a presumption of conformity with the relevant essential requirements.[8] However, these essential requirements do not provide any rules or recommendations on how to design or manufacture a medical device, a strategy that allows for the development of new technical improvements. The current international standards for lung ventilators define basic requirements for some of the fundamental variables (tidal volume, inspiratory pressure, etc.), but other important issues such as inspiratory waveform and trigger sensitivity are not defined with full detail.[11–13] Consequently, the mechanical ventilation market offers a number of different modes for controlling artificial breathing, cycling from inspiration to expiration and starting inspiration, as well as a great variety of flow and pressure profiles and modes of ventilation.[14,15] Although these unrestricted technological developments have improved mechanical ventilation by overcoming specific problems or fulfilling needs for different pathologies and scenarios, the variability of the commercially available ventilators and their different characteristics sometimes makes it difficult to choose the correct ventilator for a specific patient.[16] Furthermore, the undemanding requirements imposed by harmonised standards make the level of device performance entirely dependent on the manufacturer. The regulations do not specify any minimum performance requirements or provide any indications on how to assess the correct functioning of devices.[8,9] Accordingly, the ventilators that are now available commercially offer a wide range of performance levels. In fact, several studies have analysed the functioning of mechanical ventilators from various viewpoints related to the main parameters of ventilatory support, revealing clinically relevant differences between devices.[17–23]

SERVICE AND MAINTENANCE OF HMV

The main advantages of mechanical ventilation in the home, as opposed to the hospital, are reductions in hospital-acquired infections, increased mobility, improved nutritional status, patient empowerment and lower healthcare costs.[3,24] However, since HMV is usually administered without the permanent supervision of specialised staff, there is an increased risk of adverse events or suboptimal treatment, which can be minimised with adequate service and maintenance procedures. The use of HMV has increased rapidly in recent decades, albeit in the absence of any standardised criteria and guidelines for implementing this therapy in clinical practice.[25,26] The lack of evidence about the best HMV procedures for the different patient groups, the complexity of HMV prescription, supply and follow-up logistics and the limited experience in the application of this relatively new therapy in many centres were some of the probable reasons for the application of many different non-standardised procedures for HMV, including the quality control of ventilators.[6] Between 2001 and 2002, a detailed survey of HMV use, called Eurovent, was carried out in Europe as part of a Concerted Action of the European Commission entitled 'The role of home respiratory ventilators in the management of chronic respiratory failure'.[26] This survey analysed HMV in 16 European countries to identify patterns of use in different countries and settings, on the basis of data from 329 HMV centres, representing around 21,500 HMV patients. Eurovent showed that quality control procedures varied considerably between the various HMV providers.[6] Indeed, although the servicing of home ventilators (including maintenance, repair and delivery of spare parts) was mainly undertaken by an external company, considerable differences were found between countries in the percentage of centres servicing HMV through an external company and in the mean regularity of routine servicing.

The variety of quality control procedures in different centres and countries may lead to inadequate treatment of patients in their homes. In effect, a survey of 300 patients using HMV reported that a non-negligible number of ventilators exhibited significant discrepancies between the actual measured main ventilator variables (minute ventilation or inspiratory pressure) and the corresponding values prescribed by the physician.[5] These differences were due in part to the inadequate performance of the ventilator and to inconsistencies between the values set in the ventilator control panel and the settings prescribed by the physician. It is important to note that the patient and the prescriber also have roles in equipment maintenance that are relevant in the quality control of HMV, as inadequate cleaning and maintenance of the ventilator at home has been associated with an increased risk of equipment contamination and patient colonisation.[27] The education of patients, families and caregivers is a key aspect of any homecare programme, as it helps them to use the equipment confidently and safely and to promptly identify simple problems, and encourages them to seek help or advice when necessary.[4]

Current data show that there is room for improvement in HMV quality control procedures. In contrast to the ICU setting, where professionals involved in NIV treatment work in a well-coordinated way in the same facility following protocols defined by the centre, the different partners involved in the treatment at home make HMV quality control a complex process (Figure 7.1). The role played by each agent (prescriber, patient/caregiver, home ventilation

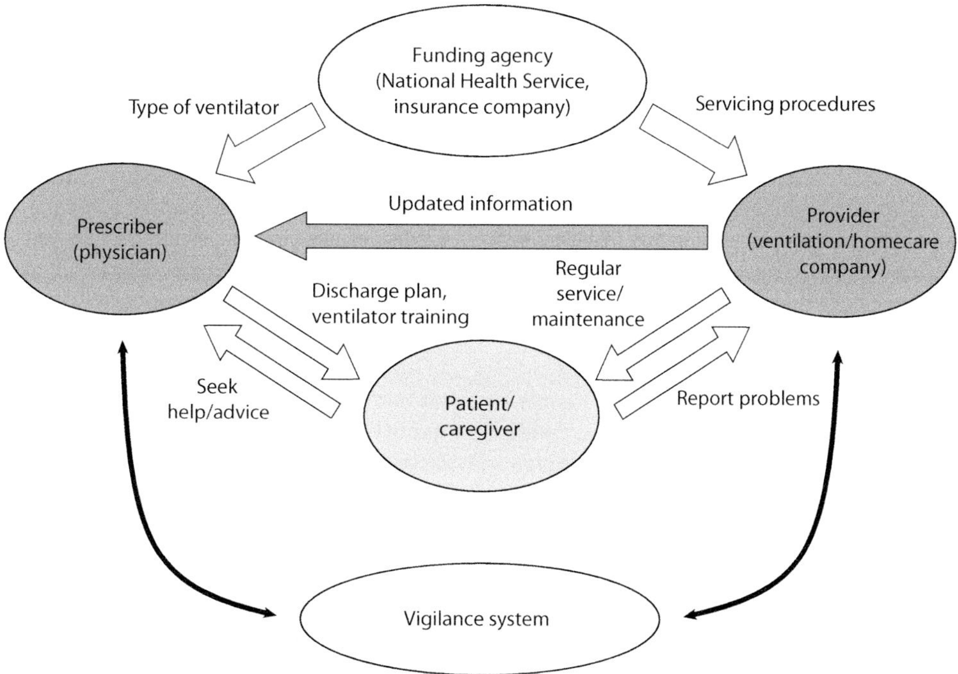

Figure 7.1 Roles of the different actors involved in the quality control process in home mechanical ventilation.

provider, funding agency and vigilance system) and their interaction are crucial in ensuring good treatment outcomes at home.[6] The agency funding HMV (a national health service or insurance company) regulates the kind of ventilator that can be prescribed to each patient and the procedures for servicing the equipment that the provider must follow. On the one hand, the prescriber should have a structured discharge plan adapted to the patient. The prescriber should provide adequate training to the patient/caregiver, including written instructions, to allow them to correctly operate and maintain the ventilator and solve basic technical problems.[4] It is also important to train caregivers in the recognition of early signs of clinical deterioration, basic life support procedures and the appropriate times to seek outside help. On the other hand, the provider is in charge of the regular servicing and planned preventive maintenance of the equipment in the patient's home. The provider should also provide regular training to the patient/caregiver on ventilator use and maintenance and facilitate easy communication channels for reporting problems (Figure 7.1). Moreover, the interaction between the provider and the prescriber should be optimised to ensure that the physician in charge of the patient is kept up to date as regards to the HMV application (e.g. incidents or change of equipment or settings). In this respect, the Eurovent survey showed that almost 30% of the prescribing centres were not regularly informed of any problems concerning the maintenance of the equipment. In addition, only 63% of centres were regularly updated on equipment servicing, and in some countries, the model of the ventilator could be changed without the agreement of the prescriber.[6]

One further aspect of the quality control procedure is that both the provider and the prescriber should be in contact with the corresponding vigilance system to report adverse events during treatment and receive updates on the current HMV quality control issues. Finally, since the patient is the centre of the HMV quality control procedure, all the partners involved should promote patient empowerment and encourage patients and caregivers to actively participate in consumer–patient associations aimed at improving the quality of HMV from their particular viewpoint (Figure 7.1).[28]

INFECTION CONTROL

Treatment with NIV is not exempt from potential risks of infection transmission, both when used in healthcare facilities and when used at home. The most common nosocomial infection in the ICU is ventilator-associated pneumonia (VAP), with an incidence ranging from 9% to 40%.[29] One of the main causes of VAP is endotracheal intubation,[29,30] which can be avoided by means of NIV in selected groups of patients with acute respiratory failure (ARF).[7,31] NIV may therefore reduce the risk of nosocomial pneumonia by maintaining the natural barriers provided by the glottis and the upper respiratory tract, by preserving the natural cough reflex and by reducing the duration of mechanical assistance and the need for sedation.[32,33] In fact, treatment with NIV in patients with ARF has been associated with a reduction in the total number of adverse events associated with mechanical ventilation, a reduction in the length of stay in the ICU, a lower rate of nosocomial pneumonia, reduced administration of antibiotics for nosocomial infections and reduced mortality.[32–34] Moreover, the early implementation of NIV in selected patients seems to be a promising alternative to standard weaning with controlled mechanical ventilation (CMV) and is associated with a lower risk of developing nosocomial pneumonia as well as reduced mortality at 2–3 months.[35,36]

There is a risk of nosocomial transmission of a wide range of respiratory pathogens as a result of the contamination of respiratory equipment.[29,37,38] Reusable equipment used in delivering NIV may be exposed to contamination during routine use through contact with the patient's skin, mucous membranes, respiratory secretions and blood.[37] Specially, if ventilator accessories, such as the mask, tubing and humidifiers, are not properly disinfected before use with a new patient, the risk of nosocomial transmission can be increased.[38] Furthermore, there is a potential risk of pathogen transmission to caregivers during the use of NIV in patients with ARF caused by infectious aetiologies, because of exposure to exhaled air from the ventilator.[39] In fact, the World Health Organization guideline on prevention and control of acute respiratory diseases in healthcare considers NIV as one of the aerosol-generating procedures in which the risk of pathogen transmission is 'controversial or possible', albeit undocumented.[40] Nevertheless, these risks can be easily minimised if appropriate precautions are taken: infected patients should be treated in an adequately ventilated single room, a bacterial/viral filter should be placed between the mask and the expiratory port of the ventilator and personal protective equipment should be worn by the caregivers.[40,41] Despite the above mentioned data, the risk of ventilator contamination is extremely low, since there is no airflow going back into the ventilator from the patient in most of the devices used for NIV.[37,42]

Non-invasive mechanical ventilators used at home are also at risk of becoming contaminated, although few studies have been published and the presence of potentially pathogenic microorganisms is controversial.[27,43,44] In the home setting, the main cause of infection is improper maintenance and cleaning of the respiratory equipment, particularly the mask and the humidifier (when used).[27,43,44] In recent years, various scientific societies and government agencies have published clinical guidelines for the management and control of healthcare-associated pneumonia, including VAP.[45–49] NIV is considered as a measure to minimise the risk of VAP in some patients with respiratory failure.[45,46,48] Other non-pharmacological measures for the prevention of VAP that are related to respiratory equipment are associated with the frequency of the changing of the ventilator circuits,[45,50] the use of heat and moist exchangers or heated humidifiers (although this is still controversial and depends on the duration of the mechanical ventilation),[45,47] the sterilisation or disinfection of reusable respiratory devices to avoid cross-contamination and the development of VAP,[42] and the hygienic measures taken by healthcare personnel when manipulating the respiratory equipment or when in contact with infected patients.[30,51] Despite the publication of these evidence-based guidelines, their implementation varies considerably, with poor adherence by physicians and nurses due to disagreement with the interpretation of the clinical trials analysed in the guidelines, unavailability of resources and patient discomfort.[45,52,53]

QUALITY CONTROL PROCEDURES

The current quality control procedures for NIV are not well standardised. Since the regulatory framework does not provide detailed indications on the performance of ventilators, the first step in the quality control of NIV is to select the most adequate device for each patient. This is currently undertaken on the basis of the experience of the prescribing physician or centre, the results of small observational trials, or the availability of ventilators, or on a trial-and-error basis.[15] Well-documented strategies based on both clinical evidence and technical issues are required to standardise quality control procedures. As with other medical devices, quality control procedures for NIV devices should focus not only on initial performance and safety but also on the whole lifecycle of the device, involving all the actors who have a role from the first idea of the device to its final elimination (Figure 7.2).

During the design and production of the device, the manufacturer is required to implement a quality assurance system and good manufacturing practices aimed at regulating the methods used for the design, manufacture, labelling, final inspection and servicing of medical devices (Figure 7.2).[8,9] Medical and scientific societies also have to specify the clinical conditions in which the device has been proved to be useful and effective, and the recommended minimal characteristics required for assuring the desired performance. Market approval is the second step in the lifecycle of a ventilator (Figure 7.2). According to the European Medical Devices directive, non-invasive ventilators are considered Class IIb devices (active therapeutic devices that can administer energy to the patient in a potentially hazardous way).[8] The FDA considers non-invasive ventilators as Class II devices (moderate risk for the patient/user) and require special controls to ensure the safety and effectiveness of the device.[9] Due to the classification level of ventilators, manufacturers of ventilators are required to obtain the approval of the health authorities for the commercialisation of their products by presenting a technical file on the product to the notified body in order to apply for a certification (CE mark in the EU market; premarket notification 510[k] or premarket approval for the US market).

Use and maintenance issues are crucial in quality control (Figure 7.2). From the quality assessment viewpoint, training of ventilator users (clinical staff and patients) is essential. Health professionals should be familiarised with the equipment that they will be using when attending to a patient requiring NIV. They should be aware of the technical characteristics of the range of ventilators currently available on the market and of the different performance levels of each device, depending on the clinical condition.[15,54] Furthermore, health professionals must know the potential risks posed to the patient during treatment with NIV and acquire the knowledge and skills to minimise them in the case of any adverse event. Clinical outcomes may be optimised with trained and experienced health professionals capable of carefully selecting patients eligible for NIV and

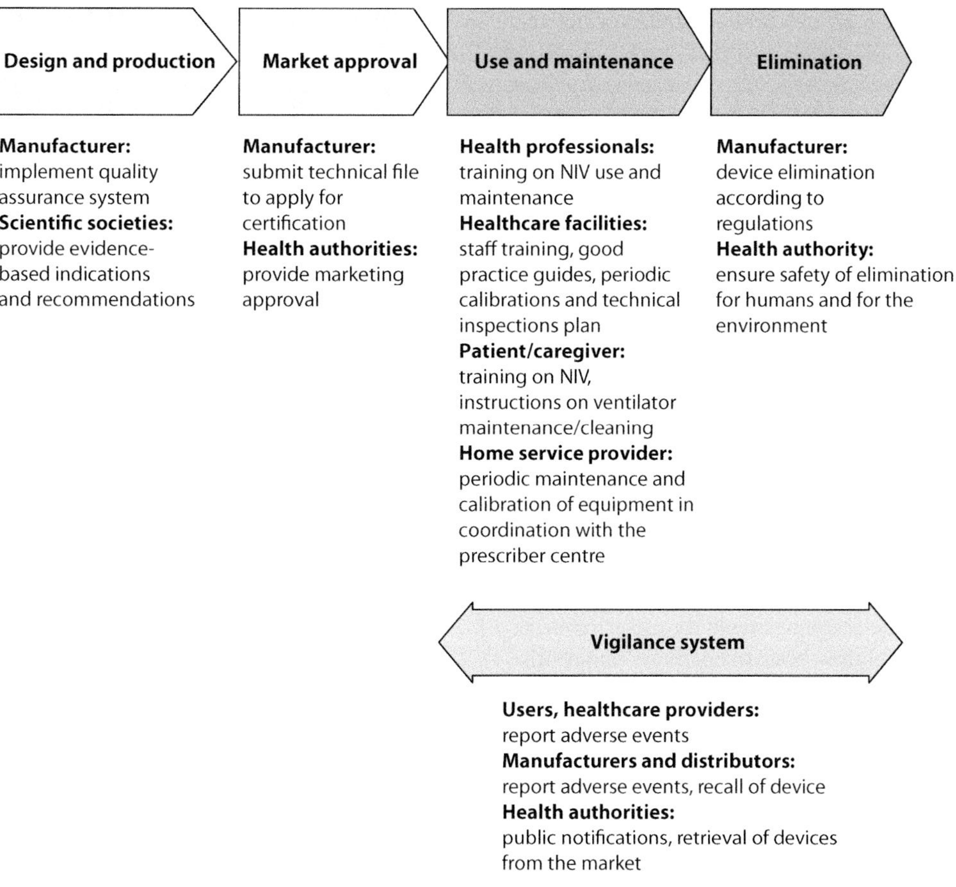

Figure 7.2 Quality control procedures during the lifecycle of a medical device. NIV, non-invasive ventilation.

the appropriate device, location and settings for the treatment.[31] It is also necessary that hospitals and other healthcare facilities provide regular training sessions to their staff and implement 'good practice' guidelines on the use and procedures of NIV,[55] including periodic calibrations, technical inspections and the prevention of infections in the hospital and home settings.

The maintenance of mechanical ventilators is also a key issue in quality control. According to the regulations, the manufacturer has to provide instructions and procedures for keeping the ventilator in good working order in the documentation accompanying the device. Since most European countries rely on external companies for servicing and maintenance of home ventilators,[6] coordination between home service providers and prescriber centres is essential to ensure good quality control of the respiratory equipment in patients' homes. Supplying the patient with more written information and education on the cleaning and maintenance of the equipment and assessing his or her abilities would enhance patient empowerment and also improve the quality control of HMV.[6] The final step in the use of a ventilator is the elimination of the device (Figure 7.2) at the end of its lifecycle, in accordance with the manufacturer's indications and applicable regulations.

The vigilance system is an extremely important element in the quality control of medical devices (Figure 7.2). Health authorities implement vigilance systems as a mechanism for identifying and monitoring significant adverse events involving medical devices. The goals of vigilance systems are the detection and correction of problems in a timely manner, to minimise their effects on the population and to take actions to prevent any reoccurrence of the problem.[8,9,56] When an adverse event is reported, the health authorities issue public notifications and, if required, take action to retrieve the device from the market. When a medical device is defective and/or could be a health risk, it must be recalled in order to address this problem. It is usually the company itself (manufacturer, distributor, etc.) that notifies the competent authority and recalls the device to correct the problem in the place where it is used or sold, or removes the device from the market, with the manufacturer being responsible for the adequate recall.[57] Health professionals have the responsibility to familiarise themselves with the guidelines in their facilities for reporting adverse events, but knowledge of these procedures is currently limited.[6]

CONCLUSIONS

There is a need for the standardisation of quality control procedures for NIV. These standards should be defined in accordance with the role of each agent in the various phases of the ventilator's lifecycle, and close interaction between the partners involved should be fostered, with the patient placed at the core of the process. The effectiveness of these procedures could be improved by the incorporation of new information technologies. The use of a telemedicine programme to provide ICUs with remote intensivist support showed improvements in clinical outcomes and reduced costs.[58] Weaning from HMV could also be successfully and safely completed in a patient's home with remote monitoring and call-centre response.[59] Moreover, a simple device connecting a ventilator to the Internet via the mobile phone network can be used to monitor HMV, making it possible to control the ventilator settings in real time to optimise patient ventilation.[60] Ventilator manufacturers are also promoting initiatives to improve patient–ventilator interaction in home treatment by including technological advances for collecting information from the device (usage time, pressure and flow waveforms, leaks, cycling, etc.) with the aim to increase both compliance with the treatment and patient comfort.[61] However, the strategies used by most manufacturers to protect their know-how from their competitors by means of patents favour the appearance on the market of 'black-box' devices, in which clinically relevant technical details are hidden from health professionals.[2,22,61,62] The future success of all these new technological developments will depend on the easy usability of the adopted solution, the prescriber's and the caregiver's learning curve for the technology, the evidence for their cost-effectiveness and a clearly defined legal framework.

REFERENCES

1. Kacmarek RM, Chipman D. Basic principles of ventilator machinery, In: Tobin MJ, ed. *Principles and Practice of Mechanical Ventilation*, 2nd ed. New York: McGraw-Hill; 2006:53–95.
2. Redline S, Sanders M. A quagmire for clinicians: When technological advances exceed clinical knowledge. *Thorax*. 1999;54:474–5.
3. Srinivasan S, Doty SM, White TR et al. Frequency, causes, and outcome of home ventilator failure. *Chest*. 1998;114:1363–7.
4. Simonds AK. Risk management of the home ventilator dependent patient. *Thorax*. 2006;61:369–71.
5. Farré R, Navajas D, Prats E et al. Performance of mechanical ventilators at the patient's home: A multicentre quality control study. *Thorax*. 2006;61:400–4.
6. Farré R, Lloyd-Owen SJ, Ambrosino N et al. Quality control of equipment in home mechanical ventilation: A European survey. *Eur Respir J*. 2005;26:86–94.
7. International consensus conferences in intensive care medicine: Noninvasive positive pressure ventilation in acute respiratory failure. *Am J Respir Crit Care Med*. 2001;163:283–91.
8. European Community Council. Council directive 93/42/CEE of 14 June 1993, concerning medical devices. OJ L169.
9. Code of Federal Regulations Title 21. Parts 800-1299. Available at http://www.accessdata.fda.gov/scripts/cdrh/cfdocs/cfcfr/cfrsearch.cfm (last update 1 April 2015) (accessed 1 May 2016).
10. Directive 2007/47/EC of the European Parliament and of the Council, of 5 September 2007, amending Council Directive 90/385/EEC on the approximation of the laws of the Member States relating to active implantable medical devices, Council Directive 93/42/EEC concerning medical devices and Directive 98/8/EC concerning the placing of biocidal products on the market. OJ L247.
11. International Organization for Standardization. ISO 10651:2004. Lung ventilators for medical use – particular requirements for basic safety and essential performance – Parts 2, 3, 5 and 6.
12. International Organization for Standardization. ISO 80601-2-12:2011. Medical electrical equipment – Part 2-12: Particular requirements for basic safety and essential performance of critical care ventilators.
13. International Organization for Standardization. ISO 80601-2-72:2015 Medical electrical equipment – Part 2-72: Particular requirements for basic safety and essential performance of home healthcare environment ventilators for ventilator-dependent patients.
14. Fink JB. Device and equipment evaluations. *Respir Care*. 2004;49:1157–64.
15. Branson RD, Johanningman JA. What is the evidence base for the newer ventilation modes? *Respir Care*. 2004;49:742–69.
16. Chatburn RL, Primiano FP. Decision analysis for large capital purchases: How to buy a ventilator. *Respir Care*. 2001;46:1038–53.
17. Lofaso F, Fodil R, Lorino H et al. Inaccuracy of tidal volume delivered by home mechanical ventilators. *Eur Respir J*. 2000;15:338–41.
18. Mehta S, McCool FD, Hill NS. Leak compensation in positive pressure ventilators: A lung model study. *Eur Respir J*. 2001;17:259–67.
19. Battisti A, Tassaux D, Janssens JP et al. Performance characteristics of 10 home mechanical ventilators in pressure-support mode. *Chest*. 2005;127:1784–92.
20. Stell IM, Paul G, Lee KC et al. Noninvasive ventilator triggering in chronic obstructive pulmonary disease. A test lung comparison. *Am J Respir Crit Care Med*. 2001;164:2092–7.
21. Rigau J, Montserrat JM, Holger W et al. Bench model to simulate upper airway obstruction for analyzing automatic continuous positive airway pressure devices. *Chest*. 2006;130:350–61.

22. Farre R, Navajas D, Montserrat JM. Technology for noninvasive mechanical ventilation: Looking into the black box. *ERJ Open Res.* 2016;2:00004.
23. Isetta V, Montserrat JM, Santano R et al. Novel approach to simulate sleep apnoea patients for evaluating positive pressure therapy devices. *PLoS ONE.* 2016;11(3):e0151530.
24. Windisch W, on behalf of the quality of life in home mechanical ventilation study group. Impact of home mechanical ventilation on health-related quality of life. *Eur Respir J.* 2008;32:1328–36.
25. Fauroux B, Howard P, Muir JF. Home treatment for chronic respiratory insufficiency: The situation in Europe in 1992. The European Working Group on home treatment for chronic respiratory insufficiency. *Eur Respir J.* 1994;7:1721–6.
26. Lloyd-Owen SJ, Donaldson GC, Ambrosino N et al. Patterns of home mechanical ventilation use in Europe: Results from the Eurovent survey. *Eur Respir J.* 2005;25:1025–31.
27. Rodríguez JM, Andrade G, de Miguel J et al. Bacterial colonization and home mechanical ventilation: Prevalence and risk factors. *Arch Bronconeumol.* 2004;40:392–6.
28. International Ventilator Users Network. Available at http://www.ventusers.org (last update 12 July 2009) (accessed 18 July 2009).
29. Safdar N, Crnich CJ, Maki DG. The pathogenesis of ventilator-associated pneumonia: Its relevance to developing effective strategies for prevention. *Respir Care.* 2005;50:725–41.
30. Girou E. Prevention of nosocomial infections in acute respiratory failure patients. *Eur Respir J.* 2003;22:72s–6.
31. Ambrosino N, Vagheggini G. Noninvasive positive pressure ventilation in the acute care setting: Where are we? *Eur Respir J.* 2008;31:874–86.
32. Brochard L, Mancebo J, Wysocki M et al. Noninvasive ventilation for acute exacerbations of chronic obstructive pulmonary disease. *N Engl J Med.* 1995;333:817–22.
33. Antonelli M, Conti G, Rocco M et al. A comparison of noninvasive positive-pressure ventilation and conventional mechanical ventilation in patients with acute respiratory failure. *N Engl J Med.* 1998;339:429–35.
34 Girou E, Schortgen F, Delclaux C et al. Association of noninvasive ventilation with nosocomial infections and survival in critically Ill patients. *JAMA.* 2000;284:2361–7.
35. Nava S, Ambrosino N, Clini E et al. Noninvasive mechanical ventilation in the weaning of patients with respiratory failure due to chronic obstructive pulmonary disease: A randomized, controlled trial. *Ann Intern Med.* 1998;128:721–8.
36. Ferrer M, Esquinas A, Arancibia F et al. Noninvasive ventilation during persistent weaning failure: A randomized controlled trial. *Am J Respir Crit Care Med.* 2003;168:70–6.
37. Singh A, Sterk PJ. Noninvasive ventilation and the potential risk of transmission of infection. *Eur Respir J.* 2008;32:816.
38. Gray J, George RH, Durbin GM et al. An outbreak of *Bacillus* cereus respiratory tract infections on a neonatal unit due to contaminated ventilator circuits. *J Hosp Infect.* 1999;41:19–22.
39. Hui DS, Hall SD, Chan MTV et al. Noninvasive positive-pressure ventilation. *Chest.* 2006;130:730–40.
40. WHO/CDS/EPR72007.6. Infection prevention and control of epidemic- and pandemic-prone acute respiratory diseases in health care. WHO interim guidelines. World Health Organization, Geneva; 2007.
41. Puro V, Fusco FM, Pittalis S et al. Noninvasive positive-pressure ventilation. *CMAJ.* 2008;178:597a.
42. Steinhauer K, Goroncy-Bermes P. Investigation of the hygienic safety of continuous positive airways pressure devices after reprocessing. *J Hosp Infect.* 2005;61:168–75.
43. Sanner BM, Fluerenbrock N, Kleiber-Imbeck A et al. Effect of continuous positive airway pressure therapy on infectious complications in patients with obstructive sleep apnea syndrome. *Respiration.* 2001;68:483–7.
44. Toussaint M, Steens M, Van Zeebroeck A et al. Is disinfection of mechanical ventilation tubing needed at home? *Int J Hyg Environ Health.* 2005;209:183–90.
45. Lorente L, Blot S, Rello J. Evidence on measures for the prevention of ventilator-associated pneumonia. *Eur Respir J.* 2007;30:1193–207.
46. Centers for Disease Control and Prevention. Guidelines for preventing health-care-associated pneumonia, 2003: Recommendations of CDC and the Healthcare Infection Control Practices Advisory Committee. *MMWR.* 2004;53:RR3.
47. Torres A, Carlet J, Members of the Task Force et al. Ventilator-associated pneumonia: European Task Force on ventilator-associated pneumonia. *Eur Respir J.* 2001;17:1034–45.
48. Guidelines for the management of adults with hospital-acquired, ventilator-associated, and healthcare-associated pneumonia. *Am J Respir Crit Care Med.* 2005;171:388–416.
49. Dodek P, Keenan S, Cook D et al. Evidence-based clinical practice guideline for the prevention of ventilator-associated pneumonia. *Ann Intern Med.* 2004;141:305–13.
50. Han JN, Liu YP, Ma S et al. Effects of decreasing the frequency of ventilator circuit changes to every 7 days on the rate of ventilator-associated pneumonia in a Beijing hospital. *Respir Care.* 2001;46:891–6.

51. Doebbeling BN, Stanley GL, Sheetz CT et al. Comparative efficacy of alternative hand-washing agents in reducing nosocomial infections in intensive care units. *N Engl J Med.* 1992;327:88–93.
52. Rello J, Lorente C, Bodí M et al. Why do physicians not follow evidence-based guidelines for preventing ventilator-associated pneumonia? *Chest.* 2002;122:656–61.
53. Ricart M, Lorente C, Diaz E et al. Nursing adherence with evidence-based guidelines for preventing ventilator-associated pneumonia. *Crit Care Med.* 2003;31:2693–96.
54. Gregoretti C, Navalesi P, Tosetti I et al. How to choose an intensive care unit ventilator. *The Buyer's Guide to Respiratory Care Products*; 2009; 94–118.
55. Girou E, Brun-Buisson C, Taille S et al. Secular trends in nosocomial infections and mortality associated with noninvasive ventilation in patients with exacerbation of COPD and pulmonary edema. *JAMA.* 2003;290:2985–91.
56. Food and Drug Administration. Medical device reporting for manufacturers. Department of Health and Human Services, Public Health Service. Rockville, MD; 1997.
57. Food and Drug Administration. Medical device recalls. Available at http://www.fda.gov/MedicalDevices/Safety/RecallsCorrectionsRemovals/default.htm (last update 19 June 2009) (accessed 7 July 2009).
58. Breslow MJ, Rosenfeld BA, Doerfler M et al. Effect of a multiple-site intensive care unit telemedicine program on clinical and economic outcomes: An alternative paradigm for intensivist staffing. *Crit Care Med.* 2004;32:31–8.
59. Vitacca M, Gerra A, Assoni G et al. Weaning from mechanical ventilation followed at home with the aid of a telemedicine program. *Telemed J E Health.* 2007;13:445–9.
60. Dellacá RL, Gobbi A, Govoni L et al. A novel simple Internet-based system for real time monitoring and optimizing home mechanical ventilation. *Int Conf E Health Telemed Soc Med.* 2009;209–15.
61. Evers G, Van Loey C. Monitoring patient/ventilator interactions: Manufacturer's perspective. *Open Respir Med J.* 2009;3:17–26.
62. Farré R, Montserrat JM, Rigau J et al. Response of automatic continuous positive airway pressure devices to different sleep breathing patterns: a bench study. *Am J Respir Crit Care Med.* 2002;166:469–73.

8

Humidifiers and drug delivery during non-invasive ventilation

ANTONIO M. ESQUINAS RODRIGUEZ AND MARIA VARGAS

The administration of gases in NIV requires an adequate level of humidification and heating. Humidity may be expressed in terms of absolute humidity (AH, $mgH_{(2)}O/L$) or relative humidity (RH, %). Humidity or hygrometric levels may extend over a wide range, thus giving rise to diverse consequences, all of which may be controlled by increasing the level of AH in the gas delivered to NIV.[1,2]

During normal breathing through an intact upper airway, inspired gas entering the trachea is warmed to 29°C–32°C and is fully saturated with water vapour. In the mid-trachea, temperature and AH reach approximately 34°C and AH is 34–38 $mgH_{(2)}O/L$. The point at which the gas reaches 37°C and 100% RH (which corresponds to an AH of 44 $mgH_{(2)}O/L$) is known as the 'isothermic saturation boundary', which is located below the carina during quiet breathing. During mechanical ventilation, the intensity of heat and moisture exchange increases with an increasing minute ventilation. Non-invasive ventilation (NIV) is a special condition in which patients are breathing high minute volume of dry and cool gases and then requires humidification.[3]

EFFECTS OF AN INADEQUATE AH

In acute NIV, a high respiratory rate causes the loss of internal AH. Mouth closure should prevent a decrease in AH.[4] Mouth or peripheral mask leak produces a constant loss in AH, which when combined with an inadequate AH level may cause a wide variety of potential problems, as has been described for acute or chronic NIV applications. The main alterations are summarised in Table 8.1.

INCREASE OF NASAL AIRWAY RESISTANCE

Nasal airway resistance (NAWR) is typically observed when the unidirectional airflow of low temperature and humidity induces a vasoconstriction response and therefore an increase of NAWR.[5,6] When this occurs in combination with an increased work of breathing (WOB), this effect may condition and/or perpetuate an acute respiratory failure (ARF) condition and therefore NIV failure (Figure 8.1).

ANATOMY AND FUNCTION OF NASAL MUCOSA

A decline in the anatomy and function of nasal mucosa (ciliary activity, mucus secretion) usually takes place when a patient breathes air with low or insufficient humidity.[7,8]

During NIV, the unidirectional and non-moistured inspiratory airflow dries the nasal mucosa that can lose the capacity to heat and humidify the inspired air and release inflammatory mediators.[9]

This aspect has been studied in detail in home-NIV patients, where the epithelium and the submucosa may suffer from metaplastic changes and keratinisation over time, when patients have been submitted to low or non-existent humidification during long periods of time.[7] This histopathological condition has also been observed during acute NIV applications by our Humivenis Group. Four patients with ARF without humidification had a nasal biopsy after 7 days of treatment and showed metaplastic changes and keratinisation in the respiratory nasal mucosa, similar to those observed by Hayes et al.[7] (Figure 8.2).

FUNCTIONAL LEVEL IN THE VENTILATORY PARAMETERS

Changes have been observed at a functional level in the ventilatory parameters (tidal volume, minute volume, gas exchange [hypercapnia increase] and WOB) in both acute and chronic NIV applications. Some of these effects may be associated with the selection of an active heat humidifier wire (HHW) or a heat and moisture exchanger filter (HMEF) as discussed below.

Although this condition has not been deeply studied, there have been some observations in patients, especially

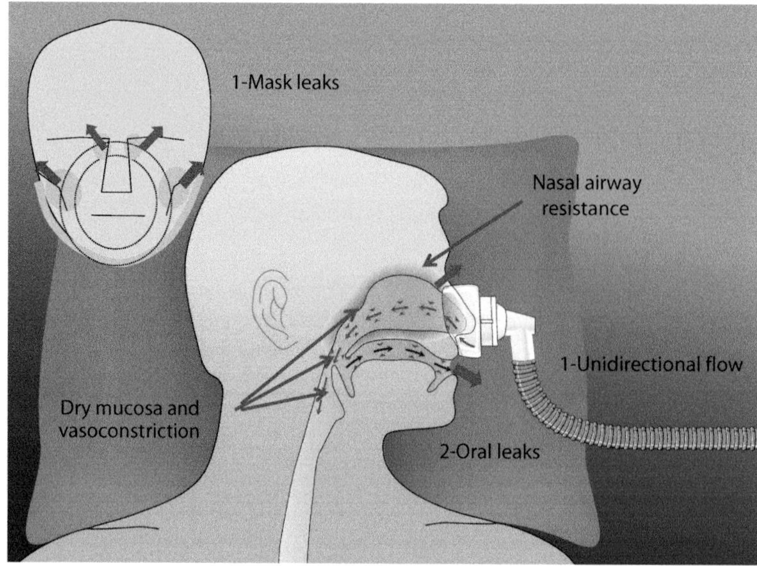

Figure 8.1 Pathophysiology and interaction leaks and humidification in upper airways related with NAWR and mucosae vasoconstriction.

Table 8.1 Effects of inefficient humidity during NIV

1. Increase of nasal resistance (NAWR)[5]
2. Function and anatomy decline of nasal mucosa[6,7]
3. Effects on ventilatory parameters, gas exchange and work of breathing (WOB)
4. Difficult intubation[8,9]
5. Intolerance, discomfort, low compliance and adherence in NIV

Sources: Tuggey JM et al. *Respir Med.* 2007 Sep;101(9):1874–9; Esquinas A et al. *Am J Respir Crit Care Med.* 2008 May;177:A 644; Hayes M et al. *Thorax.* 1995;50:1179–82; Esquinas A et al. *Am J Respir Crit Care Med.* 2002 April;165(8):A-385; Nava S et al. *Respir Care.* 2009 Jan;54(1):71–84.

those with bronchial secretions and a low humidification level. It has been observed that when NIV fails in those patients, a difficult endotracheal intubation (ETI) can result.[8,10] NIV has been associated with some risk factors associated with high airflow NIV-CPAP devices and high inspiratory oxygen fraction (FiO_2), especially in hypoxemic ARF (pneumonia, ARDS) conditions. Wood et al.[10] described a difficult ETI situation in this context, and our epidemiologic study *Humivenis* has also confirmed this observation.

INTOLERANCE, DISCOMFORT, LOW COMPLIANCE AND REDUCED ADHERENCE IN NIV

All these symptoms may improve after the optimisation of the AH level through the selected humidification system (HHW vs. HMEF) and are related to the NIV response.

Low levels of adherence may be affected by the control of respiratory mucosal dryness. This aspect has been observed in detail during home-NIV in patients with nasal SAOS-NIV where humidification delivery efficiently avoids dryness of respiratory mucosa, and improves comfort, adaptability and NIV compliance, when assessed using an analogue scale.[5] However, according to other authors, humidification does not have a significant effect on the final adherence to chronic NIV.[11] The discomfort level associated with NIV, defined as dryness at mouth and/or the thoracic level, was assessed by means of a scale (from 0 to 10), and a positive effect on discomfort could be observed with the application of HHW.[5,12]

The optimal AH level related to the symptoms in acute NIV applications is still unknown. In an experimental level, Wiest et al.[13] studied this condition and proved that the symptoms started to appear when the AH level was lower than 15 $mgH_{(2)}O/l$.

The most comprehensive compliance analysis was carried out by Nava et al. in home-NIV, when two humidification systems (HHW vs. HMEF) and the development of symptoms were compared. A greater compliance (75% of patients) was found in the HHW. However, in this same population, other symptoms such as thoracic dryness, amount of hospitalisations and development of complications caused by infections (mainly pneumonia) were similar with both systems (HHW vs. HMEF).[14] Massie et al.[15] published similar results, but they emphasise the concept of using humidification at the very onset of equipment use in order to reach the highest level of compliance in home-NIV.

Even if humidification can improve the quality of life in nasal NIV-CPAP, there is limited information in this respect. It may be inferred that, if the aforementioned symptoms associated with the inadequate humidification are controlled, the quality of life should be improved. Nevertheless, further studies are necessary to correlate both concepts.[11,15]

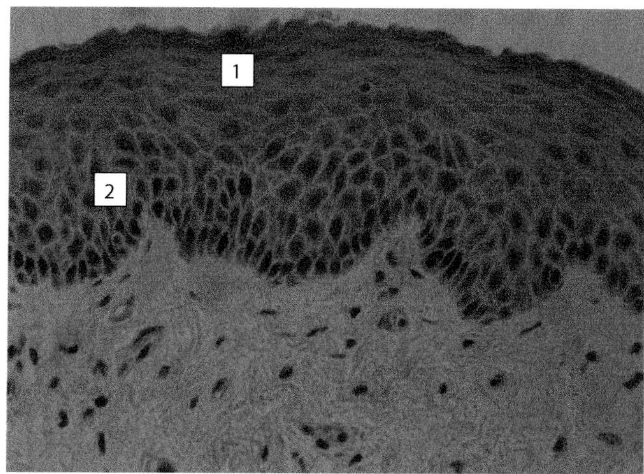

Figure 8.2 Biopsy nasal mucosa. Legend: Metaplastic and keratinisation changes in nasal respiratory mucosae in patients without humidification during NIV.[6] (1) Keratin and (2) metaplastic.

TECHNICAL CONSIDERATIONS

Hygrometric values in NIV

The recommended optimal hygrometric values of AH or RH in the different NIV applications are still unknown, since most information is provided by experimental studies from direct (nasal cavities) or indirect (thermometers) measurements.[16]

Hygrometric analysis during NIV is relevant to know temperature values at several critical points to achieve an accurate interpretation:(1) the temperature of the environment; (2) the temperature in the vaporisation chamber and the temperature of the inhaled gas[17]; (3) atmospheric pressure; (4) level and characteristics of airflow at the entrance of the selected humidification system (HHW vs. HMEF); and (5) typical characteristics of the selected NIV apparatus (ventilator type and interface).

Probably, the effects in NIV patients of the airflow entering the humidification chamber have been the most observed physical parameter, with special mention of the studies carried out by Wenzel et al., who compared the factors that determine the humidification capacity in a variable range of airflow at the entrance to the humidification chamber (20, 55 and 90 L/min).[18] The key aspects of this study are summarised in Figure 8.3.

On another level, we should mention those factors that are specific to the NIV technique. The main aspects are given next.

Interface

In recent years, the technological development provides different interfaces for NIV. The NIV interfaces may be divided in six classes: mouthpiece, nasal mask, nasal pillow, oronasal covers, full face and helmet.

The most commonly used interfaces to deliver NIV are nasal and facial mask. The nasal mask seems to have more air leaks and inadequate conditioning even if it avoids the change of RH related to mouth leaks.

Peripheral mask leaks and leaks from the expiratory connector in the respiratory circuit are the two constant points of inspiratory AH loss.[16] Mouth opening produces AH loss with nasal-NIV, although NIV with a face mask allows a better conservation since there is less mouth leakage. In both interface models, it becomes necessary to adjust the level of AH of the inhaled gas.

The use of helmet and gas conditioning should be carefully evaluated. The helmet has a much larger inner space, which may act as a 'reservoir' of humidity because of the amount of exhaled gas that remains there.[19]

Recently, Chiumello[20] compared hygrometric values in a helmet system using a mechanical ventilator without humidity to a helmet system with a continuous-flow NIV-CPAP for two flow rates (40 and 80 L/min). Patients with ARF were recruited and an HHW system used with both systems.[20] In this study, the HHW system increased the AH level, both with low flow (HA = 11.4 ± 4.8 to 33.9 ± 1.9 $mgH_{(2)}O/L$) and with high flow (HA = 6.4 ± 1.8 to 24.2 ± 5.4 $mgH_{(2)}O/L$). However, the AH values in the conventional mechanical ventilator without humidification were higher (HA = 18.4 ± 5.5 to 34.1 ± 2.8 $mgH_{(2)}O/L$). Neither of the groups showed significant differences in the level of patient comfort for these AH values. From this study, it should be inferred that (1) the effect of the flow applied to CPAP systems itself impacts as a limiting factor in the intra-helmet AH measured level, and (2) the early delivery of HHW in this case is recommended, unlike with helmet-NIV when applied by means of a conventional mechanical ventilator.

From these observations, it should be deduced that the type of interface and the leaks, together with the intra-interface airflow, will condition the AH values to be delivered.

Models of NIV ventilators

NIV mechanical ventilators (intensive care unit [ICU], bi-level positive airway pressure [BiPAP]), home care mechanical ventilators or high-flow CPAP systems operate by providing a very high inspiratory flow to compensate for the inspiratory demand of a patient with ARF. According to Poulton and Downs[21] this aspect is especially significant when high airflow CPAP systems are used in NIV.

ICU conventional mechanical ventilators provide a lower level of AH (5 $mgH_{(2)}O/L$) when compared to specific NIV turbine mechanical ventilators (13 $mgH_{(2)}O/L$), according to the studies carried out by Wiest et al.[22] The same author similarly determined the starting AH levels from which complications should be expected. AH levels lower than 5 $mgH_{(2)}O/L$ should be considered 'critical.[22]

In relation to specific mechanical ventilators, a broader study by Holland et al.[23] empirically compared RH values without humidification using a NIV-specific ventilator. They determined that the RH range in the respiratory

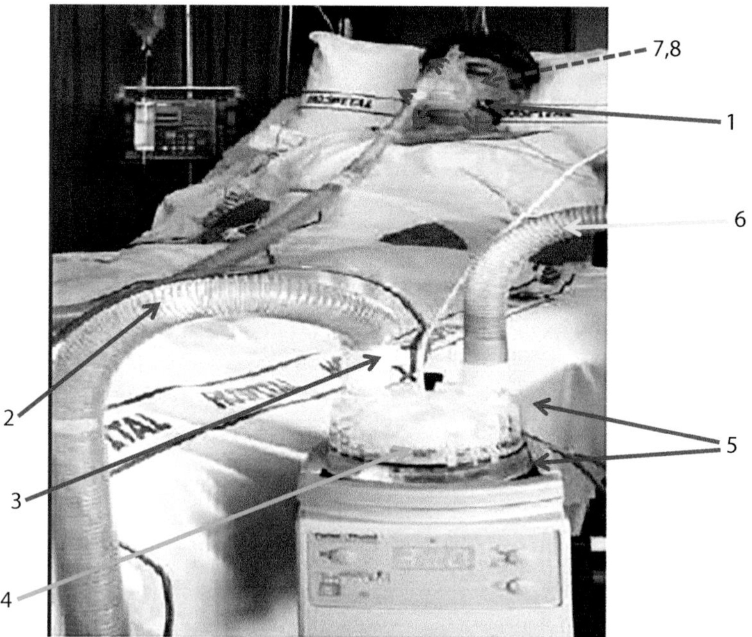

Figure 8.3 Key major physic element related with humidification. Legend: 1 = Interface; 2 = air velocity; 3 = water temperature in the chamber; 4 = air–water surface contact; 5 = physical characteristics of water chamber; 6 = air turbulence level; 7 = leaking level; 8 = humidity at the exit of the respiratory circuit.

circuit is lower than the environmental range (RH = 16.3%–26.5% vs. 27.6%–31.5%).[23]

The increase in the cmH_2O inspiratory positive airway pressure (IPAP) level led to a significant decrease in the RH, which turned back to normal parameters when an HHW was applied. This decreasing RH could be explained by an increase in the temperature (°C) at the entrance of the HHW system coming from the mechanical ventilator, probably due to an increase in the delivered flow and a faster rotation of the mechanical ventilator turbine. The HHW systems produce a small decrease in the selected IPAP level (0.5–1 cmH_2O), but the clinical consequences of this are yet to be determined. As this is an experimental model, the changes in the respiratory rate or in the inspiratory/expiratory ratio (i:e) did not affect the final RH measurement. As a key conclusion for this study, we should state that the incorporation of HHW systems in NIV increased the RH measured values.

Our group has analysed the AH values in 12 patients with NIV and hypoxemic ARF, with a BiPAP specific ventilator and a face mask, and observed the effects of a variable range of oxygen inspiratory fraction (FiO_2) in four different NIV environments: (1) without humidification; (2) with HHW-MR850; (3) with HHW-730; and (4) with an HME-Booster. The main observations showed that (1) FiO_2 increase led to a proportional AH decrease, being more evident in an environment without humidification, and more standard in the HHW and HME-Booster systems, and (2) the AH levels were 'critical' when FiO_2 was above 60%.[24]

Similarly, in the study by Holland et al., we could observe that the humidification application with HHW or HME-Booster systems increased AH (FiO_2 range value). However, when comparing both HHW and HME-Booster, the HA level was higher in the HME-Booster, but it was associated with a patient–ventilator asynchrony and an increase in pCO_2 values.[24]

ACTIVE (HHW) VS. PASSIVE (HMEF)

There is no uniform consensus to recommend one device over the other, and there is also limited epidemiological information to state what are the most adequate hospital practices and protocols in relation to humidification and the selected devices. Recently, our international group for the study of humidification (*Humivenis Working Group*) carried out a survey in 15 hospitals and determined that, in the usual practice, the HHW is used more in acute NIV applications compared to HME (53% vs. 6.6%). In fact, there is a lack of hospital protocols referring to humidification practices (55%).[9]

In general, HHW and HME technically produce similar AH levels (25–30 $mgH_{(2)}O/L$), which are adequate for the physiological functioning of the upper airway.

Using HHW or HME during NIV for ARF had also comparable effects on intubation rate and long-term outcome as length of stay and mortality.[32] In hypercapnic respiratory failure, HME leads to a small but significant increase in $PaCO_2$ despite the increased minute ventilation triggered by the added dead space of the HME.[33,34] However, humidification performance in each system may vary within a range of respiratory rate, especially the level of ventilator airflow that enters the system through the humidification chamber.[25] In NIV applications, significant disadvantages have been observed in the HME compared to the HHW, which are summarised in Tables 8.2 and 8.3.[25–30]

Table 8.2 HME in NIMV

Advantages	Disadvantages
1. Cost effective. 2. Extended use in the ICU. 3. Eliminates circuit condensation (hygroscopic models are recommended). 4. The application of a Booster system to a hydrophobic HME may preserve HA capacity when incoming gases are delivered within a temperature range (lower than 26°C) and a high flow.	1. Increases dead space (VD/VT). 2. Reduces efficacy in case of leaks. 3. Operation depends on the body temperature. 4. May lead to an increase in the AWR in patients with heavy secretions and respiratory tract bleeding.

Sources: Nava S et al. *Eur Respir J.* 2008 Aug;32(2):460–4; Carter BG et al. *J Aerosol Med.* 2002 Spring;15(1):7–13.

Table 8.3 HH in NIMV

Advantages	Disadvantages
1. Recommended in a dehydration condition with a temperature over 37°C. 4. Produces WOB improvement in the baseline values compared to HME systems. 5. Lower increase in $PaCO_2$ values. 6. Best humidification option, especially in patients with mild to severe hypercapnic ARF.	1. Reduces efficacy with elevated environmental temperature. 2. Produces an increase in mild resistance (6.7 ± 1.8 $cmH_{(2)}O \times L\ s^{-1}$) compared to no humidification system (5.7 ± 1.8 $cmH_{(2)}O \times L\ s^{-1}$). 3. Temperature of the gases coming through the ventilator may impact on the hygrometric levels.

Sources: Nava S et al. *Eur Respir J.* 2008 Aug;32(2):460–4; Jaber S et al. *Intensive Care Med.* 2002 Nov;28(11):1590–4; Lellouche F. *Intensive Care Med.* 2002 Nov;28(11):1582–9; Lellouche F. *Intensive Care Med.* 2009 Jun;35(6):987–95.

CONCLUSIONS

Most authors recommend that the technical limitations of the selected humidification systems, the environmental conditions, the NIV technique to be used and the characteristics of the airflow must always be clearly understood. We need to add to the above list, that it is important to understand the patients, underlying pathologies. It should not be construed that the presence of humidification in NIV shall always ensure accurate humidity delivery.[1,13] It is important to realise that no complete extrapolation should be attempted from the observations on humidity carried out in laboratory tests to the acute or chronic NIV environment, due to a wide range of variables and factors that impact in the final AH. A small provision of AH should always help to control the most common symptoms observed during acute or chronic NIV, even though more extensive studies should be conducted.[22]

However, there is no uniform consensus on the following: (1) when and what is the best role of humidification in acute and home-NIV; (2) what are the recommended hygrometric values; and (3) what is the efficacy of the current systems.[32]

AEROSOL THERAPY IN NIV

Aerosol therapy is a frequently used therapy during NIV in the exacerbation of COPD and bronchial asthma.[35] There is no extensive information on the aerosol behaviour due to the inner characteristics of NIV, as is developed in patients during invasive mechanical ventilation (IMV).[36–38]

Factors depending on the patient

According to the studies by Fink et al.,[39] during a spontaneous respiratory pattern, ventilation and its length (i:e ratio) will influence aerosolised drug deposition, largely ranging from 4.9% to 39.2% of the total amount of aerosolised particles.

A longer expiratory time should favour higher drug deposition in the lower airway,[39,40] as well as a low respiratory rate pattern[39] and a tidal volume increase. These correlated factors may cause higher aerosolised deposits in NIV patients.

A low respiratory rate allows a longer deposit time in the lower airway, and a high tidal volume is associated with a larger lung expansion and redistribution. Furthermore, as discussed below, the degree of airway obstruction, together with the auto-PEEP level, and the degree of lung restriction in NIV patients should be expected to interfere with the deposit of aerosolised particles.

Characteristic factors of the NIV technique

INTERFACE, LEAKS, GENERATOR POSITION

Aerosol loss may be generated at the expiratory port within the respiratory circuit, and by the level of peripheral mask leak as well. The optimisation of leaks and the type of interface should enhance the final aerosolised deposits getting into the respiratory airways.

It has been established that the efficacy of lung deposits is higher when the aerosol generator is positioned between the respiratory circuit and the interface.[39] Technically, it is important to know that the mask models with accessory expiratory ports included in the mask surface itself may cause additional loss of aerosols, as more aerosol leaks through them[41,42] (Figure 8.4).

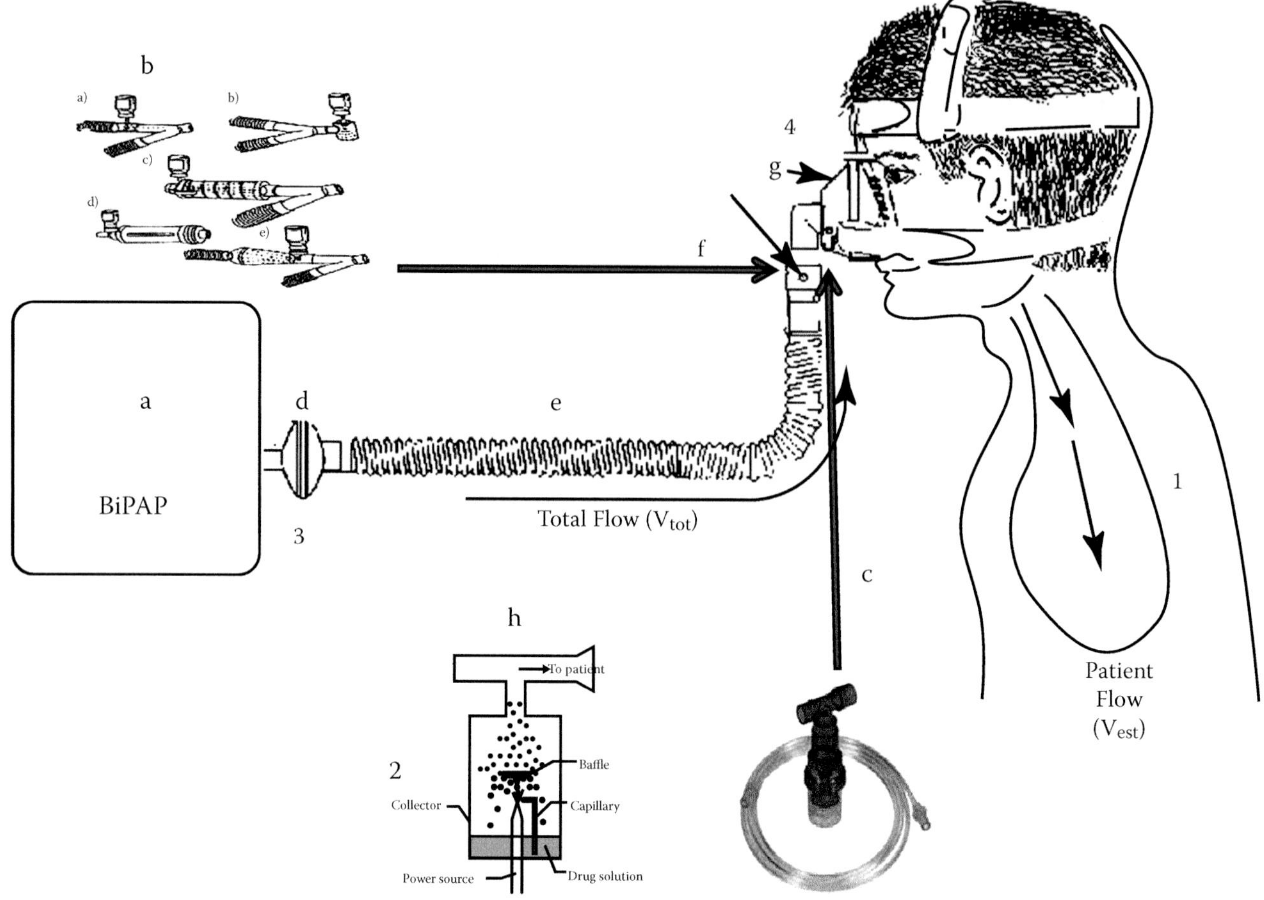

Figure 8.4 Aerosol therapy during NIV. Elements and factors related with airflow aerosolised. Legend: a = NIV ventilator; b = types MDI; c = nebuliser; d = bacterial filter; e = respiratory circuit; f = expiratory port; g = leaks with aerosols in expiratory port and inside mask (some models); h = generator nebuliser. Factor related airflow aerosolised: (1) = patient's inspiratory peak flow; (2) = generator airflow nebuliser; (3) = ventilator airflow (or positive pressure system).

VENTILATORY MODE

There is limited information relating to the effects of the different ventilatory modes selected in NIV. It is common to consider that, in all cases, the extent of lung expansion and a lower airway resistance should result in a higher distal deposit.[38]

CPAP MODE

The application of continued pressure (CPAP) may cause changes in the minute volume (MV) depending on the elasticity and lung resistance, therefore conditioning the final deposits.[43] However, this rule may not always apply due to some coincident factors:

1. The geometry of the respiratory airways (low calibre) caused by auto-PEEP-related condition.
2. The generation of large and heavy particles that impact on the interface and the higher airway.
3. A high inspiratory turbulent airflow from the positive pressure generation system selected (CPAP or NIV-mechanical ventilator).
4. Dynamic changes of the ventilatory pattern (respiratory rate/TV) during NIV.
5. It is known that some NIV-CPAP systems operate at a low temperature, which should reduce the final aerosol generation.[44]
6. Peripheral mask leaks.

Generally, the CPAP mode of NIV causes an improvement in the bronchodilator effect.

In a recent in vitro study by Ball et al.,[45] aerosol delivery during CPAP increased (1) while putting the nebuliser as close to the patient as possible, (2) as CPAP level increased and (3) connecting CPAP to high-flow Venturi generator. At present, these observations are still limited, and it should be carefully extrapolated to acute patients, as mentioned by Newhouse et al.[46]

BiPAP MODE

NIV with BiPAP mode has potential effects in aerosol therapy, and its bi-level features are obtained by means of direct observation of the beneficial effects associated with an improvement of NIV in the BiPAP mode. As mentioned above, it enhances the ventilatory pattern (low respiratory rate, increase of tidal volume and WOB). The experiences of Pollack et al.[47] and Brandao et al.[48] in patients with exacerbations of asthma undergoing aerosol therapy and NIV should be noted.

Type of device, level of positive pressure and drug dose

The type of NIV ventilator (volumetric, pressure-metric, CPAP systems), the range of selected pressure and the drug dose apparently do not directly interfere with the amount of aerosol deposited. Similarly, no significant alteration has been observed during the ventilator's operation.[37,47,49]

AIRWAY FLOW

Airway flow constitutes a 'critical' factor that may be modified and affect the final amount of aerosol deposited.

The main factors related to the inspiratory airflow generation during aerosol therapy are (1) age, (2) level of bronchoconstriction, (3) type of generator (nebuliser/metered dose inhalator [MDI]) and (4) ventilator airflow (or CPAP system).

The total flow delivered carrying aerosol particles is the result of a final balance obtained after eliminating the proportion of aerosol lost by peripheral mask leaks and by the expiratory connector during aerosol therapy, as summarised in the following text box and in Figure 8.4:

$$\text{Total flow} = \{(\text{patient's inspiratory peak flow} + \text{generator flow} + \text{ventilator flow (or positive pressure system)}\} - (\text{flow loosed by leaks})$$

A high inspiratory flow leads to a limited bronchodilator effect mainly due to (1) lower deposition, (2) higher aerosol loss caused by peripheral mask leaks, (3) turbulent airflow with higher particle impact in proximal airway and (4) generation of large-size particles.[39,50]

TWO FACTORS DERIVED FROM AEROSOL THERAPY TECHNIQUE

Type of generator: Nebuliser vs. MDI

There is not enough information on whether nebulisation is superior in terms of efficacy to inhalation (MDI) systems in NIV. The most extensive information available has been obtained from some studies carried out in patients undergoing IMV[35,36] (Figure 8.4).

NIV-nebulisers: Nebulisation is the most widespread method to generate aerosols, according to Dhan et al.[35] The most favourable position to achieve an optimal deposit is to put the nebulisation device between the interface and the respiratory circuit.[37,51] Pollack et al.[47] and Brandao et al.[48] used nebulisers during NIV in patients with exacerbations of asthma, and favourable effects were observed in clinical terms.

As regards NIV-MDIs, Nava et al. compared NIV with and without space chambers in patients with COPD. They could not find significant differences between the options, though favourable clinical and ventilatory effects were observed.[52]

Position of generator

The positioning of the generator during nebulisation between the interface and the expiratory port influences the amount of aerosol deposits.[40] If an MDI system is used, efficacy should be similar for the same position, but it should be noted that this system requires synchronicity during the inspiratory phase.[49] However, with a high-flow generator system, the highest aerosol delivery may be obtained capping one outlet of the T-piece and positioning the nebuliser between the capped outlet and the patients.[45]

Type of drug and dose

Most studies have been carried out using bronchodilator drugs for aerosol therapy in NIV.[37] There is no standard rule from the published studies as to the selection of a bronchodilator drug, its corresponding dose and whether the option of one of them may cause a higher or lower deposit performance.[37,47] Similarly, there is limited information on the efficacy of final drug deposits, which could be estimated at about 25% of the total delivered amount.[37] Other drugs such as the deposition of antibiotics have also been studied. We should mention a study by Reychler[53] that compared the deposits of nebulised amikacin with a NIV-CPAP-Boussignac in healthy subjects. A lower deposit rate was found in the NIV procedure vs. conventional nebulisation.[53]

In the paediatric population, aerosol therapy and NIV are also an open subject with the same conditioning issues, and limited information is available due to the lack of comprehensive studies. Other aerosol drugs such as corticoids, antibiotics, prostaglandins, surfactants and mucolytics have been studied with quite different results.[37,38]

Effects of aerosolised bronchodilators during NIV

COPD-NIV

Nava et al.[49] observed an increase in the obstruction ventilatory parameters measured by a FEV_1/FVC quotient independently of the application mode with MDI in NIV. However, no changes were seen during gas exchange. Subsequently, two further studies observed similar results when comparing aerosol therapy in NIV to a placebo.

ASTHMA-NIV

Pollack et al.[47] and Brandao et al.[48] compared NIV-nebulisation in BiPAP mode to a placebo. Improvements were found in some aspects (respiratory rate, heart rate, O_2 saturation, peak expiratory flow, forced expiratory volume at 1 s, forced vital capacity and forced expiratory flow between 25% and 75%).

CONCLUSIONS

In both NIV aerosol therapy options, nebulisation vs. MDI, the results should be carefully extrapolated, since in the real-world practice, there are many variables that have not been studied and that could impact the selection and the final outcome.[35,38,54]

It should be concluded that aerosol therapy in NIV must be considered, taking into account that there are still a few studies in this area, and all the physical variables that may impact in the generation and final deposits of bronchodilator drugs must be taken into account. During an acute phase, the ventilatory pattern, the high flow as well as peripheral mask leaks shall condition the selection of the nebulisation vs. an MDI device.

ABBREVIATIONS

AH	absolute humidity ($mgH_{(2)}O/L$)
ARDS	acute respiratory distress syndrome
ARF	acute respiratory failure
Auto-PEEP	intrinsic positive end expiratory pressure
BiPAP	bi-level positive airway pressure
COPD	chronic obstructive pulmonary disease
CPAP	continuous positive airway pressure
ET	expiratory time
ETI	endotracheal intubation
FiO_2	oxygen inspiratory fraction
HHW	heated humidifier wire
HMEF	heat and moisture exchanger/filter
i:e	inspiratory/expiratory ratio
ICU	intensive care unit
IMV	invasive mechanical ventilation
IPAP	inspiratory positive airway pressure
MDI	metered dose inhalator
MV	minute volume
NAWR	nasal airway resistance
NIV	non-invasive ventilation
RAW	respiratory airways
RH	relative humidity
SAOS	sleep apnoea obstructive syndrome
TV	tidal volume time
TE	expiratory volume
WOB	work of breathing

REFERENCES

1. Miyoshi E. Effects of gas leak on triggering function, humidification, and inspiratory oxygen fraction during noninvasive positive airway pressure ventilation. *Chest.* 2005 Nov;128(5):3691–8.
2. Duong M. Jayaram L, Camfferman D et al. Use of heated humidification during nasal CPAP titration in obstructive sleep apnoea syndrome. *Eur Respir J.* 2005 Oct;26(4):679–85.
3. Branson RD, Gentile MA. Is humidification always necessary during non invasive ventilation in the hospital? *Respir Care.* 2010 Feb;55(2):209–16.
4. Martins De Araújo MT, Vieira SB, Vasquez EC, Fleury B. Heated humidification or face mask to prevent upper airway dryness during continuous positive airway pressure therapy vivo efficacy. *Chest.* 2000 Jan;117(1):142–7.
5. Tuggey JM, Delmastro M, Elliott MW. The effect of mouth leak and humidification during nasal non-invasive ventilation. *Respir Med.* 2007 Sep; 101(9):1874–9.
6. Esquinas A, Nava S, Scala R et al. Humidification and difficult endotraqueal intubation in failure of noninvasive mechanical ventilation (NIV). Preliminary results. *Am J Respir Crit Care Med.* 2008 May;177:A 644.
7. Hayes M, McGregor F, Roberts D et al. Continuous nasal positive airway pressure with a mouth leak: Effect on nasal mucosal blood flux and geometry. *Thorax.* 1995;50:1179–82.
8. Esquinas A, Escobar C, Chavez A, Picazos C. Noninvasive mechanical ventilation and humidification in acute respiratory failure. A morpho histological and clinical study of side effects. *Am J Respir Crit Care Med.* 2002 Apr;165(8):A-385.
9. Nava S, Navalesi P, Gregoretti C. Interfaces and humidification for noninvasive mechanical ventilation. *Respir Care.* 2009 Jan;54(1):71–84.
10. Wood KE, Flaten AL, Backes WJ. Inspissated secretions: A life threatening complication of prolonged noninvasive ventilation. *Respir Care.* 2000;45(5):491–3.
11. Mador MJ, Krauza M, Pervez A et al. Effect of heated humidification on compliance and quality of life in patients with sleep apnea using nasal continuous positive airway pressure. *Chest.* 2005 Oct;128(4):2151–8.
12. Chanques G, Constantin JM, Sauter M et al. Discomfort associated with underhumidified high-flow oxygen therapy in critically ill patients. *Intensive Care Med.* 2009 Jun;35(6):996–1003.

13. Wiest GH, Foerst J, Fuchs FS et al. Heated humidifiers used during CPAP-therapy for obstructive sleep apnea under various environmental conditions. *Sleep*. 2001 Jun 15;24(4):435–40.
14. Nava S, Cirio S, Fanfulla F et al. Comparison of two humidification systems for long-term noninvasive mechanical ventilation. *Eur Respir J*. 2008 Aug;32(2):460–4.
15. Massie CA, Hart RW, Peralez K, Richards GN. Effects of humidification on nasal symptoms and compliance in sleep apnea patients using continuous positive airway pressure. *Chest*. 1999 Aug;116(2):403–8.
16. Fischer Y, Keck T. Measurements were taken in a climatic chamber and relative humidity. *Sleep Breath*. 2008 Nov;12(4):353–7.
17. Severgnini P, D'Onofrio D, Frigerio A et al. A rationale basis for airways conditioning: Too wet or not too wet?. *Minerva Anestesiol*. 2003 Apr;69(4):297–301.
18. Wenzel M, Wenzel G, Klauke M et al. Characteristics of several humidifiers for CPAP-therapy invasive and non-invasive ventilation and oxygen therapy under standardised climatic conditions in a climatic chamber. *Pneumologie*. 2008 Jun;62(6):324–9.
19. Crimi C, Noto A, Princi P, Nava S. Survey of noninvasive ventilation practices: A snapshot of Italian practice. *Minerva Anestesiol*. 2010;77:971–8.
20. Chiumello D. Effect of a heated humidifier during continuous positive airway pressure delivered by a helmet. *Crit Care*. 2008;12(2):R55.
21. Poulton TJ, Downs JB. Humidification of rapidly flowing gas. *Crit Care Med*. 1981 Jan;9(1):59–63.
22. Wiest GH, Fuchs FS, Brueckl WM et al. In vivo efficacy of heated and non-heated humidifiers during nasal continuous positive airway pressure (nCPAP) – therapy for obstructive sleep apnoea. *Respir Med*. 2000 Apr;94(4):364–8.
23. Holland AE, Denehy L, Buchan CA, Wilson JW. Efficacy of a heated passover humidifier during noninvasive ventilation: A bench study. *Respir Care*. 2007 Jan;52(1):38–44.
24. Esquinas A, Carrillo, A González, G Humivenis Working Group. Absolute humidity variations with a variable inspiratory oxygenation fraction in noninvasive mechanical ventilation (NIV). A pilot study. *Am J Respir Crit Care Med*. 2008 May;177:A 644.
25. Schumann S, Stahl CA, Möller K et al. Moisturizing and mechanical characteristics of a new counterflow type heated humidifier. *Br J Anaesthesiol*. 2007 Apr;98(4):531–8.
26. Randerath WJ, Meier J, Genger H et al. Efficiency of cold passover and heated humidification under continuous positive airway pressure. *Eur Respir J*. 2002 Jul;20(1):183–6.
27. Jaber S, Chanques G, Matecki S et al. Comparison of the effects of heat and moisture exchangers and heated humidifiers on ventilation and gas exchange during non-invasive ventilation. *Intensive Care Med*. 2002 Nov;28(11):1590–4.
28. Carter BG, Whittington N, Hochmann M, Osborne A. The effect of inlet gas temperatures on heated humidifier performance. *J Aerosol Med*. 2002 Spring;15(1):7–13.
29. Campbell RS, Davis K Jr, Johannigman JA, Branson RD. The effects of passive humidifier dead space on respiratory variables in paralyzed and spontaneously breathing patients. *Respir Care*. 2000 Mar;45(3):306–12.
30. Lellouche F. Effect of the humidification device on the work of breathing during noninvasive ventilation. *Intensive Care Med*. 2002 Nov;28(11):1582–9.
31. Lellouche F. Water content of delivered gases during non-invasive ventilation in healthy subjects. *Intensive Care Med*. 2009 Jun;35(6):987–95.
32. Lellouche F, L'Her E, Abroug F et al. Impact of humidification device on intubation rate during noninvasive ventilation with ICU ventilators: Results of a multicentre randomized controlled trial. *Intensive Care Med*. 2014 Feb;40(2):211–9.
33. Lellouche F. Pignataro C, Maggiore SM et al. Short-term effects of humidification devices on respiratory pattern and arterial blood gases during non invasive ventilation. *Respir Care*. 2012 Nov;57(11):1879–86.
34. Lellouche F, Taille S, Lefancois F et al. Humidification performance of 48 passive airway humidifiers: Comparison with manufacturer data. *Chest*. 2009 Feb;135(2):276–86.
35. Dhand Rajiv MD. Aerosol bronchodilator therapy during noninvasive positive-pressure ventilation. *Respir Care*. 2005;50(12):1621–2.
36. Hess D. The mask for noninvasive ventilation: Principles of design and effects on aerosol delivery. *J Aerosol Med*. 2007:20(Suppl 1):S85–98.
37. Chatmongkolchart S, Schettino GP, Dillman C et al. In vitro evaluation of aerosol bronchodilator delivery during noninvasive positive pressure ventilation: Effect of ventilator settings and nebulizer position. *Crit Care Med*. 2003:30(11):2515–9.
38. Dhand R, Tobin MJ. Inhaled bronchodilator therapy in mechanically ventilated patients. *Am J Respir Crit Care Med*. 1997;156(1):3–10.
39. Fink JB. Aerosol delivery from a metered-dose inhaler during mechanical ventilation. An in vitro model. *Am J Respir Crit Care Med*. 1996 Aug;154 (2 Pt 1):382–7.

40. Dolovich M. Influence of inspiratory flow rate, particle size, and airway caliber on aerosolized drug delivery to the lung. *Respir Care.* 2000:45(6):597–608.
41. Branconnier MP, Hess DR. Albuterol delivery during noninvasive ventilation. *Respir Care.* 2005 Dec;50(12):1649–53.
42. Branconnier MP, Hess DR. Albuterol delivery during noninvasive ventilation. *Respir Care.* 2005;50(12):1649–53.
43. Parkes SN, Bersten AD. Aerosol kinetics and bronchodilator efficacy during continuous positive airway pressure delivered by face mask. *Thorax.* 1997;52(2):171–5.
44. Parkes SN, Bersten AD. Aerosol kinetics and bronchodilator efficacy during continuous positive airway pressure delivered by face mask. *Thorax.* 1997;52:171–5.
45. Ball L, Sutherasan Y, Caratto V et al. Effects of nebulizer position, gas flow, and CPAP on aerosol bronchodilator delivery: An in vitro study. *Respir Care.* 2016 Mar;39(61):263–8.
46. Newhouse MT, Dolovich MB. Control of asthma by aerodilator. *N Engl J Med.* 1986;315:870–3.
47. Pollack CV Jr, Fleisch KB, Dowsey K. Treatment of acute bronchospasm with beta-adrenergic agonist aerosols delivered by a nasal bilevel positive airway pressure circuit. *Annals Emerg Med.* 1995;26(5):552–7.
48. Brandao DC, Lima VM, Filho VG et al. Reversal of bronchial obstruction with bi-level positive airway pressure and nebulization in patients with acute asthma. *J Asthma.* 2009 May;46(4):356–61.
49. Nava S, Karakurt S, Rampulla C et al. Salbutamol delivery during non-invasive mechanical ventilation in patients with chronic obstructive pulmonary disease: A randomized controlled study. *Intensive Care Med.* 2001:27(10):1627–35.
50. Laube BL, Links JM, LaFrance ND et al. Homogeneity of bronchopulmonary distribution of 99mTc aerosol in normal subjects and in cystic fibrosis patients. *Chest.* 1989:95(4):822–30.
51. Miller DD, Amin MM, Palmer LB et al. Aerosol delivery and modern mechanical ventilation: In vitro/in vivo evaluation. *Am J Respir Crit Care Med.* 2003;168(10):1205–9.
52. Diot P, Morra L, Smaldone GC. Albuterol delivery in a model of mechanical ventilation: Comparison of metered-dose inhaler and nebulizer efficiency. *Am J Respir Crit Care Med.* 1995 Oct;152(4 Pt 1): 1391–4.
53. Reychler G. Effect of continuous positive airway pressure combined to nebulization on lung deposition measured by urinary excretion of amikacin. *Respir Med.* 2007 Oct;101(10):2051–5.
54. Mercer TT. Production of therapeutic aerosols. Principles and techniques. *Chest.* 1981;80(S):813–8.

9

How to start a patient on non-invasive ventilation

RAFFAELE SCALA AND MARTIN LATHAM

INTRODUCTION

The use of non-invasive ventilation (NIV) to treat both acute respiratory failure (ARF) and chronic respiratory failure (CRF) has tremendously expanded in the last two decades in terms of spectrum of successfully managed diseases,[1,2] locations of application[3–5] and achievable goals.[6,7] Despite the huge amount of literature, a 'clear recipe' for starting NIV in clinical practice is lacking. Results of RCTs obtained by expert centres cannot be translated into a 'real-world scenario' where skills, standardisation and expertise may not be adequate.[8–10] This is not surprisingly since NIV, like other medical treatments, has to be considered as a rational 'art' and not just as application of 'science'; in other words, NIV requires the ability to choose the best 'ingredients' (i.e. patient selection, interface, ventilator, interface, methodology, etc.) to calibrate specific protocols for each case.[11]

This chapter focuses on the 'key ingredients' for 'how to start NIV' in ARF and CRF.

ACUTE RESPIRATORY FAILURE

Personnel

Reasons for low use of NIV are inappropriate equipment, poor experience and inadequately trained staff (Figure 9.1).[12,13] Success is achieved by good education and communication within the multidisciplinary team where everyone fully understands indications, benefits and concerns associated with NIV.[1,11]

Medical doctors have to be experts in pathophysiology and practice of mechanical ventilation, including endotracheal intubation (ETI), and management of cardiorespiratory emergencies[4,13]; familiarity with analgo-sedation, ability on bronchoscopy and sensibility to ethics issues are also required.[7,14–16] When starting NIV, doctors have to select patients according to the achievable goals (resolution of acute decompensation or palliation) with a careful balance between environment and ARF severity.[1,6,7,16]

The role in NIV application of nurses and respiratory therapists (RTs) differs from country to country. In Europe, nurses are usually the main staff group dealing with NIV,[4,17] while RTs are mainly involved in chest physiotherapy.[18] Conversely, in North America, even though nurses are familiar with NIV, RTs assume the leadership in implementing ventilation.[10,19] Practical skills and theoretical knowledge of nurses and RTs should be periodically refreshed and protocols updated with staff turnover and introduction of new equipment.[10,11]

Experience in NIV is the most important factor predicting success and workload. Established practice with NIV in an Italian Respiratory high-dependency care unit (RHDCU) allowed treatment of more severely ill patients with the same success rate keeping staff, equipment and environment constant.[8] These data are negatively mirrored by a Spanish study[9] showing that the greater rate of NIV failure reported in a general versus a respiratory ward was due to poorer staff training.

Concerning workload in RHDCU, nurses, RTs and MD time consumption to manage chronic obstructive pulmonary disease (COPD) exacerbations was similar for NIV versus both medical therapy and invasive mechanical ventilation (IMV), with a significant reduction of NIV workload after the first hours of ventilation.[17,20] In two ward-based RCTs in the United Kingdom,[21,22] nursing NIV patients was not different from the controls despite the inclusion of a supernumerary NIV research staff in one study.[21] However, there were no data regarding either the care of other non-ventilated patients or whether the outcome would have been better if nurses had spent more time with ventilated patients.[3]

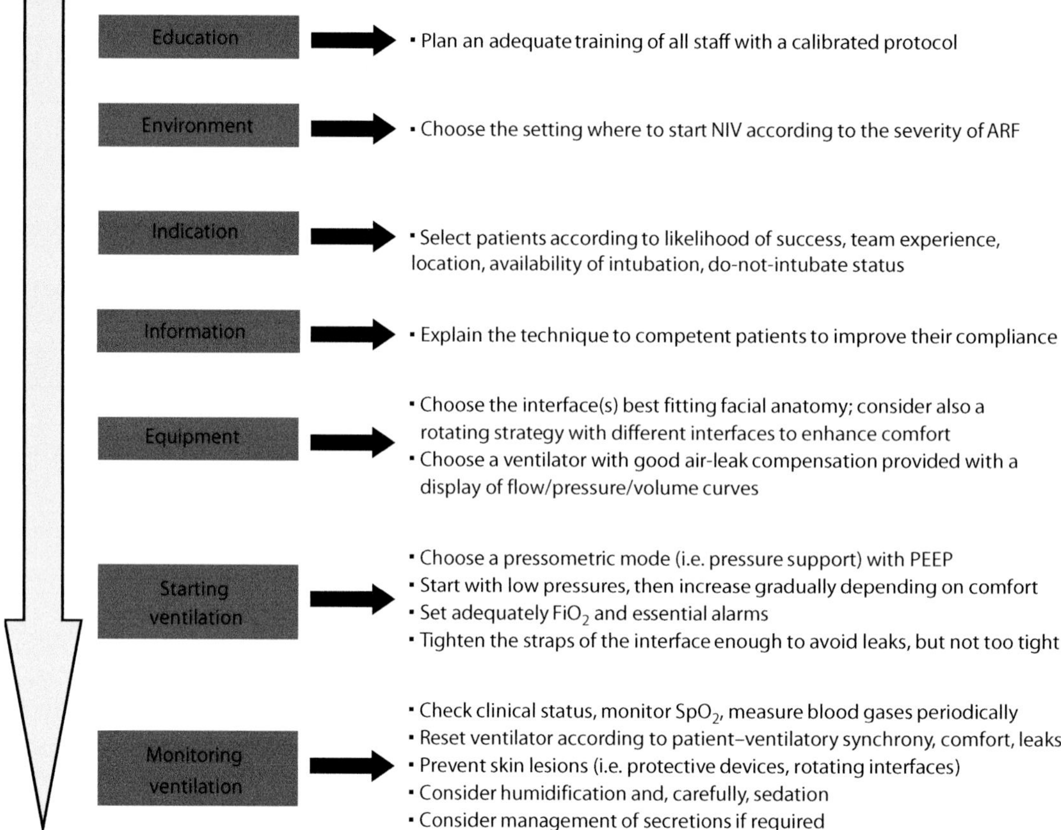

Figure 9.1 Sequential pathway for starting non-invasive ventilation (NIV) in patients with acute respiratory failure (ARF). PEEP, positive end-expiratory pressure.

Location

The 'ideal environment' for starting NIV[3] should have expert staff in adequate numbers for 24-h cover, facilities for monitoring, rapid access to IMV and reasonable cost (Table 9.1). Since ICU offers the highest care level at the higher costs, this is the appropriate location for starting NIV in sickest patients for whom ventilatory support is mandatory.[23] The existence of an RHDCU in a hospital is likely to reduce ICU admission for NIV.[4,24] In this context, 'respiratory patients' is the category of subjects that are more likely to be refused in ICU because they are either 'too ill' or 'too well'.[25] One of the most innovative aspects of acute NIV is the possibility of initiating ventilation outside ICU[1,3,4,21,23,26] with the advantage of treating less severe patients with similar success but at lower costs.[24] However, lower levels of care provided in some areas might increase the risk that deterioration will not be promptly recognised.

The question of where to start NIV is still debated for the heterogeneity of settings capable of delivering NIV even within the same hospital.[3,10,12] Choice of where to start NIV is based on the patient's need for monitoring, the unit's monitoring capabilities, staff experience and time response to NIV.[1,3] Patients with ARF poorly responsive to NIV, such as pneumonia, ARDS and asthma, should be treated in ICU, where immediate ETI is available.[16] One exception is when NIV is applied in 'do-not-intubate'/'do-not-resuscitate'(DNI)/DNR) context to palliate symptoms.[7] Fast-responding diseases (i.e. acute cardiogenic pulmonary oedema) may be appropriately ventilated in short-stay settings, such as pre-hospital transport and emergency department (ED).[3] This is more feasible for CPAP than for NIV as the former is easier to be applied and cheaper.[26,27]

The strategy[28] based on medical emergency teams to provide and monitor NIV outside ICU is feasible, but concerns on the safety of this model still remain.

Starting NIV in ED may be advantageous in 'rapid-solving' diseases to avoid delay in initiating ventilation and DNR/DNI status,[3,7] as well as to 'buy time' for patients to make end-of-life choices.[3] However, findings of RCTs[13,29] dealing with NIV in ED are inconsistent for several reasons: unsuitable environment for 'slow-solving' disorders (i.e. COPD exacerbations, pneumonia, ARDS), quick improvement of several patients after optimised oxygen therapy[30] and inadequate experience of ED staff in NIV. Conversely, starting NIV in ED and then continuing ventilation in RHDCU could reduce in-hospital mortality and length of stay in ICU/RHDCU for most acute patients.[31]

RHDCU are specialised units providing an intermediate care between ICU and ward.[4] RHDCU may work as a

Table 9.1 Advantages and disadvantages of starting NIV in different settings

Location	Advantages	Disadvantages
Pre-hospital	Rapid application (CPAP) (feasible in ACPE)	Limited equipment and monitoring Difficulty in corrected diagnosis Low level of evidence
Emergency department	Rapid application (more feasible in ACPE) Close monitoring in high-intensity room	Temporary location In many units, staff without NIV skill and experience Low level of evidence
General ICU	Highest nurse/patient ratio	Resource-intensive and too costly for low-risk patients
	Usually dedicated RT Maximal monitoring capabilities Suitable for high-risk patients	Beds in short supply
RHDCUs	Central monitoring available Specialised NIV skills	Not present in many hospitals Variable nurse/patient ratio (from 1:2 to <1:4)
	Often dedicated RT Cost-effective for ARF in chronic diseases	MD not available 24/24 h in all units Heterogeneity in levels of care
General ward	Higher availability of beds	Lowest monitoring capabilities and nurse/patient ratio
	Lower costs for NIV therapy	In many units, staff without NIV skill and experience
	Suitable for low-risk patients	Usually, lack of dedicated RT Risk of unduly delay in ETI for NIV failures

Abbreviations: ACPE = Acute cardiogenic pulmonary oedema; ETI = endotracheal intubation.

'step-down unit' for stabilised patients transferred from ICU and as a 'step-up unit' for cases failing medical therapy in EDs or wards. As well as having experience in NIV, some RHDCUs are capable of managing IMV and prolonged weaning.[4] Starting NIV in RHDCU gives the chance of successfully treating ARF in chronic respiratory disorders with similar efficacy[32] and lower costs than in ICU.[24] Opening of a RHDCU may be advantageous to reduce in-hospital mortality, need for ICU admission and hospital stay as compared to ward and ED settings.[33] Unfortunately, in several countries, the number of RHDCUs is insufficient,[3] as shown by an Italian survey.[34]

General/respiratory wards vary considerably in the ability to manage patients on NIV. Wards having nursing staff experienced with NIV, readily available skilled RTs and central telemetry may deliver NIV safely to selected acute patients. Conversely, NIV is unlikely to be successful on wards with few nurses and other non-ventilated unstable patients.[3,22]

Selection of patients

Several points should be considered when starting NIV (Figure 9.2).

First, aims of NIV should be considered[1,6]: (1) to prevent an impending ARF or post-extubation failure; (2) to prevent ETI when ARF is already established but ventilation not mandatory; (3) as an alternative to IMV when ventilation is mandatory or to facilitate weaning from IMV; and (4) as a palliative care in DNI/DNR patients with end-stage respiratory or neoplastic diseases.[7] NIV should be started early because a delay increases the likelihood of failure (Table 9.2).[1] However, there is no point in starting NIV too early in patients with mild ARF.[20]

Second, clinicians should identify the type of ARF to be treated with NIV. Hypercapnic ARF – mostly occurring in patients with pre-existent respiratory disorders (i.e. COPD, chest-wall deformities, neuromyopathies) – are more responsive to NIV than hypoxemic or 'de novo' ARF, occurring in patients without pre-existent cardiorespiratory diseases (i.e. ARDS).[1,16]

Third, care should be taken to exclude patients with contraindications for NIV (Table 9.3). With the exception of cardiorespiratory arrest, other contraindications have not been proved but are derived from exclusion criteria of RCTs.[1] For instance, moderate hypercapnic encephalopathy may be 'safely' treated with NIV,[32,35] which has been found to be associated with a similar short- and long-term survival and fewer infections than IMV.[32] Moreover, NIV

Likelihood of NIV success	Stage of ARF: Not established	Stage of ARF: Mild-moderate (early)	Stage of ARF: Severe (late)
High	• Extubation failure in high risk hypercapnic patients (i.e. COPD)	• COPD exacerbations • Immunocompromised patients • ACPE	• Weaning from invasive ventilation (only COPD)
Moderate	• Post-abdominal surgery	• Post-operative after lung resection • Fiberoptic bronchoscopy • Do not intubate order • Chest trauma • CAP	• COPD exacerbations • Pre-intubation oxygenation
Low	• COPD exacerbations	• Extubation failure • Hypoxaemic (ARDS) • Asthma exacerbations	• Hypoxaemic (ARDS/CAP) • Do not intubate order
Goals of NIV	To prevent ARF	To prevent Intubation	Alternative to invasive ventilation

Figure 9.2 Flowchart showing steps in selection of patients for non-invasive ventilation (NIV) according to the level of literature evidence, the severity of acute respiratory failure (ARF) and the goals to be achieved with NIV. ACPE, acute cardiogenic pulmonary oedema; ARDS, acute respiratory distress syndrome; CAP, community-acquired pneumonia. (Modified from Nava S et al., *Intensive Care Med.* 2006;32:361–70.)

Table 9.2 When to Start NIV in acute patients?

- Clinical signs
  - Rest dyspnoea (from moderate to severe)
  - Tachypnoea (RR >25 breaths/min)
  - Increased respiratory work (accessory muscles use, paradoxical breathing)
- Blood gases
  - Respiratory acidosis (pH <7.35 with $PaCO_2$ > 45 mmHg)
  - Hypoxemia (PaO_2/FiO_2 <300)

Abbreviation: RR = respiratory rate.

Table 9.3 When to not start NIV in acute patients?

Cardiac or respiratory arrest

- Non-hypercapnic encephalopathy
- Severe hypercapnic encephalopathy (i.e. Kelly–Matthay score > 4)
- Psychomotor agitation not controlled with sedation
- Severe gastrointestinal bleeding
- Bowel obstruction
- Multiple comorbidities
- Severe haemodynamic instability with or without unstable cardiac angina
- Fixed upper airway obstruction
- Inability to protect the airway and/or high risk of aspiration
- Inability to clear secretions despite cough assist techniques
- Untreated pneumothorax

may successfully treat ARF patients with depressed cough thanks to an integrated management of secretions.[36,37]

Finally, risk factors and timing of NIV failure should be evaluated (Table 9.4).[38]

Equipment

This topic is covered elsewhere in this book. Here, some issues dealing with choice of interface and ventilator will be discussed.

INTERFACES

The interface used to start acute NIV is crucial as excessive air leaks, poor tolerance and skin lesions are predictors of failure.[38,39] The NIV team should have a variety of interfaces, with different types and sizes, to ensure the best fit to the patient's facial anatomy.[39]

Full-face mask should be the first-line strategy in starting acutely NIV, while in stabilised patients requiring prolonged NIV, switch to nasal mask may improve comfort.[40] Switching to total face mask may be a successful rescue option when full-face mask has failed, especially for preventing facial damages.[41] Although a helmet is well tolerated, NIV delivered with helmet is associated with worse patient–ventilator interaction, unloading of respiratory muscles and CO_2 clearance compared with full-face mask ventilation.[42] Ventilation with a new helmet shows better patient–ventilator interaction and capability of reducing $PaCO_2$ in COPD exacerbations.[43,44]

The other interfaces (i.e. nasal pillows, mouthpiece) show limited application in acute NIV.[38] Open-mouthpiece ventilation may be an effective alternative to nasal NIV in preventing deterioration of gas exchange in mild-to-moderate acidotic COPD exacerbations.[45]

Table 9.4 How to decide to start NIV in acute patients?

Predictors of NIV failure in Hypercapnic ARF

- Before starting ventilation
  - Low BMI
  - Poor pre-morbid condition (i.e. ADL score <2)
  - Community acquired pneumonia
  - Excessive secretions
  - Colonisation with non-fermenting gram-negative bacilli (e.g. *Pseudomonas aeruginosa*)
  - RR > 35 breaths/min
  - Severe respiratory acidosis (i.e. pH <7.25)
  - Severe altered level of consciousness (i.e. Kelly–Matthay score >3, GCS <12)
  - Severe acute illness (i.e. high APACHE II scores >29)
- After starting ventilation
  - No improvement within 2 h of NIV in pH, RR, $PaCO_2$, APACHE II score, sensorium
  - Late clinical–physiological worsening after initial successful response to NIV
  - Inability to minimise leak
  - Inability to co-ordinate with NIV
  - Burden of secretion not manageable with both non-invasive and invasive techniques
  - Poor compliance to NIV and/or agitation not manageable with cautious sedation

Predictors of NIV failure in Hypoxemic ARF

- Before starting ventilation
  - Moderate–severe ARDS (i.e. <200)
  - Age >40 year
  - Shock (i.e. systolic blood pressure <90 mmHg despite vasopressors)
  - Multiple acute organ insufficiency
  - Metabolic acidosis (i.e. pH <7.25)
  - Severe acute illness (i.e. SAPS II score >34)
- After starting ventilation
  - Failure to improve oxygenation within first hour of NIV (PaO_2/FiO_2 <175 mm Hg)

Abbreviation: RR = respiratory rate
Note: Consider clinical and physiological variables predicting NIV failure in ARF.

'Rotational' strategy of different interfaces is associated with greater efficacy and comfort.[40]

VENTILATORS

NIV-dedicated ventilators demonstrated better performance than several ICU ventilators.[46,47] Some features should be considered when choosing a ventilator to start acute NIV: (1) capability to air-leak compensate; (2) availability of flow–volume–pressure waveforms and chance of setting trigger sensitivity, pressurisation speed and expiratory cycling to detect and correct patient–ventilator asynchronies; (3) high-pressure oxygen source to set a reliable FiO_2;[48] (4) staff experience; and (5) costs.[1,46,47]

Practical issues

Pressure support ventilation (PSV) is mostly used in ARF because, despite similar clinical–physiological improvement, it is better tolerated than volume-target modes.[39,46,47] Newer hybrid presso-volumetric modes of NIV, such as average volume-assured pressure support (VAPS), have been largely used in clinical practice despite the lack of benefits over PSV in both ARF and CRF.[49]

Levels of pressure support and positive end-expiratory pressure (PEEP) are not standardised but should be titrated depending on interface fitting, tolerance and clinical–physiological response. It is advisable to start with low pressures while the mask is held to the face once patients realise that NIV improves dyspnoea.[11] Then, the mask may be fixed and pressure support increased (usually 8–20 cmH_2O/hPa) according to expiratory tidal volume (6–10 mL/kg), respiratory rate (RR) (<25 breaths/min), leaks, comfort and blood gases.[39] Peak pressures above lower oesophageal sphincter opening pressure (25–30 cmH_2O) should be avoided to prevent gastro-distension.

Masks should be neither too tight nor too loose; too tight can cause skin breakdown, while too loose causes air leaks and patient–ventilator asynchronies.[1,50]

Monitoring patients during NIV is mandatory to verify its clinical–physiological efficacy.[11,43,50] Even if positive response after 1–2 h of NIV is a predictor of success, 'late failures' occur in 20% of cases.[38]

Air leaks are detected by monitoring the difference between inspired and expired tidal volumes and flow–pressure–volume waveforms.[39,48,50] The most common dyssynchronies are inspiratory 'hung-up', auto-triggering and ineffective efforts.[50]

Adherence to NIV may be improved by providing humidification in patients with dry throat and/or thick secretions. Heated humidifiers (HH) show clinical–physiological advantages versus heat-moisture exchangers.[51] The integrated use of high-flow nasal oxygen may improve compliance and effectiveness of NIV in hypoxemic patients.[52] Early management of accumulated secretion may be considered when starting NIV in high-risk COPD patients with depressed cough.[14]

Finally, 'safe' sedation may reduce NIV failure due to the patient's discomfort, but careful selection of candidates, close monitoring, expertise of team and prompt availability of ETI are required.[15]

CHRONIC RESPIRATORY FAILURE

Education

Many of the issues reported for starting NIV in ARF are applicable to CRF. Some long-term conditions (Table 9.5) expose patients to the risk of developing CRF, and the

Table 9.5 Long-term conditions that cause CRF leading to NIV

Type of condition	Examples
Muscular-skeletal	Scoliosis Kyphoscoliosis Thoracoplasty
Neuro-muscular	Duchenne and other dystrophies Amylotrophic lateral sclerosis Myotonic dystrophy Spinal muscular atrophy Post-polio syndrome Myopathies Charcot–Marie–Tooth syndrome Diaphragmatic paralysis Cervical–spinal cord injury Myasthenia gravis Multiple sclerosis Polyneuropathies
Neurological	Congenital central hypoventilation syndrome Brain-stem stroke
Obesity	Obesity–hypoventilation syndrome Severe obstructive sleep apnoea syndrome Prader–Willi syndrome
Pulmonary parenchymal or vascular	COPD Cystic fibrosis Fibrosing alveolitis Primary pulmonary hypertension Cheynes–Stokes ventilation with heart failure Bridge to lung transplantation
Idiopathic	Idiopathic non-obstructive alveolar hypoventilation

progression into hypercapnic ventilatory failure is often predictable.[2,53–55] This predictability of the progression into CRF offers the opportunity of preparing patients, familiars and caregivers in advance for the eventuality of NIV.[56] Several patient organisations produce excellent leaflets[56,57] detailing signs and symptoms of CRF, as well as treatment options. Some specifically discuss the need for NIV, explaining what is involved and giving advice on troubleshooting. It is useful to signpost patients to these available resources.

In certain life-limiting and progressive illnesses such as ALS, when starting NIV, it is also important if appropriate to ask the patient to consider at which point he or she may want to stop NIV. The patient may wish to discuss an advanced directive to refuse treatment in the event of the benefits of NIV being outweighed by the symptoms of advancing disease and disability.[55] The discussion may include advice about involving palliative care and withdrawal of ventilation.[58,59]

Table 9.6 Signs and symptoms related to CRF

Group	Sign and symptom
Sleep	Sleep fragmentation Frequent arousals Nightmares or vivid dreams Excessive daytime sleepiness Nocturnal hypoventilation
Respiratory	Severe orthopnoea Vital capacity <50% of predicted value Daytime hypercapnoea Repeated chest infections Paradoxical abdominal breathing pattern Use of accessory muscles of respiration
Neurological	Excessive fatigue Impaired cognitive function Morning headaches
Muscular	Respiratory muscular weakness Reduced exercise tolerance Weak cough
Metabolic	Failure to thrive Poor appetite

Timing

NIV is usually started once the patient begins to develop signs and symptoms of diurnal ventilatory failure or has symptomatic nocturnal hypoventilation (Table 9.6).[2,60–62] When to assess and monitor patients at risk of developing CRF is covered in another chapter.

The question of timing of NIV needs to be considered in the light of the natural history of the underlying disease. Patients with rapidly progressive diseases should be educated in the signs and symptoms of CRF and monitored closely so that CRF is identified rapidly and acted upon.[2,63] When starting this group on NIV, there is the need to rapidly titrate patients onto treatment against a background of progressive deterioration.

Patients with a chronically stable condition such as a kyphoscoliosis will deteriorate more gradually, so the clinical evolution is more subtle and often missed by the patient.[2] Often the patients will ascribe the excessive daytime fatigue to the ageing process rather than to sleep fragmentation. Depending on the severity of the presenting CRF, the imperative to rapidly achieve effective treatment is not so great in this group. Where the CRF is mild, then titration to effective treatment may take several weeks or months. There is, however, evidence[64] that, in the absence of signs and symptoms of CRF or nocturnal hypoventilation, commencing NIV too early may be counterproductive.

Location

The location for initiating NIV in CRF will depend on the individual circumstances of the providing organisation, but

Table 9.7 Locations for starting NIV in CRF

Location	Advantages	Disadvantages
Home	Familiar environment especially for patients with complex needs Using NIV in situ Remote monitoring allows accurate titration	Clinical staff should operate away from hospital Portable equipment
Outpatient department (1–2 h)	Shorter appointment for patient All equipment available Remote monitoring allows accurate titration	Time constraints May require repeat visits to problem-solve Large volume of information for patient/carers to assimilate in a short time
Day-case (up to 8 h)	More time to acclimatise to ventilation than outpatient Patient can use a bed Carers can stay	May require repeat visits to problem solve No overnight titration
Overnight stay (up to 30 h)	Able to titrate ventilation overnight More time to acclimatise to ventilation and problem solve	Unfamiliar environment Equipment patient normally uses not available Problems may only become apparent once home Carers may not be able to stay
Inpatient stay (several days and nights)	Able to titrate ventilation accurately Plenty of time to acclimatise to ventilation Problems more likely to become apparent and be solved	Unfamiliar environment Equipment patient normally uses not available Time-consuming for patient and provider Carers may not be able to stay

there are a wide variety of options that can be tailored to suit the needs of patients, family and caregivers (Table 9.7).

Where a rapid acclimatisation to NIV is required, then an inpatient stay may be more appropriate. However, if they have complex care needs provided for by caregivers in a specially adapted home environment, then it may be easier for the patient to be started on NIV there than in a hospital.

Patients with a chronically stable condition may prefer outpatient or daycase initiation as this has less impact on work and home life. A study[5] suggests that there is an equivalent outcome whether patients were initiated as outpatients compared with inpatients in terms of improvement in ventilatory failure and compliance. What is key to success irrespective of the location chosen to initiate NIV is the need to have staff who are fully competent in NIV.[3]

Equipment

INTERFACE

Like in ARF, there is currently a wide range of interfaces available for a chronic setting. A good selection of masks is the key for achieving success in starting NIV in CRF.[65] All the available options should be discussed and shared with the patient. There are many components to choosing the right interface, as each particular mask has its own advantages and disadvantages. For example, a patient who likes to read in bed may prefer an interface that allows the wearing of spectacles, such as nasal pillows. Another patient may prefer the stability that a mask with a forehead support offers as they are a restless sleeper. Similar to ARF, giving the chronic patient as much choice as possible can improve NIV compliance. Acclimatisation to mask wearing may take a considerable time.

VENTILATOR

The choice of a ventilator in CRF depends on several factors. Conditions where respiratory drive is good (i.e. COPD) could use a simple ventilator that works in a spontaneous mode, whereas those in whom the respiratory drive is absent must have a mandatory back-up rate. For patients with neuromuscular disorders who may progress to more than 12 h a day, ventilator use will need battery back-up and possibly wheelchair mounting.[2,61] Some individuals, especially those with neuromuscular disease, may find it difficult to cope with PEEP at first as they cannot speak easily or keep their mouth closed when wearing nasal masks and may benefit from intermittent positive pressure ventilation (IPPV) during the acclimatisation period; this can be easier to cope with compared with bi-level ventilation. Some ventilators have the ability to set low PEEP levels or reduce PEEP during exhalation, which may be useful. Conditions where the patient generates intrinsic PEEP, such as in COPD, may benefit from bi-level ventilation as the addition of PEEP can reduce the work of breathing.[2,60]

Generally at the start, the pressures can be kept low, which will help with compliance, and then increased to achieve a therapeutic effect.[66] The duration of titration depends on the underlying condition and location where NIV is started; titration may be done overnight or over several weeks. Modern ventilators also offer the possibility of auto-titration of pressures using novel modes such as VAPS, where a range of pressure support can be programmed into the device. This has the advantage of offering less support when the patient is awake and does not need it, only increasing support once the patient is asleep.[66] This can be set low and then revised upwards as the patient adjusts to ventilation. The latest versions of ventilators using mobile phone technology allow remote access by the clinician so the settings can be changed on a daily basis if required to allow a rapid titration even at home. In those individuals with obstructive sleep apnoea overlap then the addition of auto-titrating PEEP can be useful, and again this can be capped and then reviewed as patient acclimatisation occurs.

Where time constrains allow patients, they may prefer to acclimatise to NIV during the day, gradually increasing use until they are able to cope with NIV for at least an hour, then switching to night-time use. Ventilators that have a ramp facility to build up the pressures may also be useful where the patient is having difficulty coping with ventilation. There are a couple of considerations when starting with low pressures: the work of breathing could be increased if IPAP is too low; and CO_2 rebreathing may occur depending on the mask if PEEP is below 4 cmH_2O.[46]

Practical issues

Starting NIV in CRF is a complex process with many subtle factors at play, so preparing individuals fully and giving them as much choice as possible are key factors in ensuring success. Early and timely problem solving is key to maintaining NIV once it has been started. By far, the most common problems are related to the interface and to the drying effects of NIV, which can be rectified with the addition of adequate humidification. HHs are efficient at delivering warm moist air with manufacturers producing ventilators with integral humidifiers.

Another issue that has to be dealt is the noise which may occur during ventilation. Careful positioning of the exhaust port on the mask may help reduce noise; for example, running the tube over the top of the bed may direct the exhaust flow away from the ears. Noise disturbance affects partners too, and they may need to use earplugs. Care must also be taken when setting the alarms on the ventilator to ensure that they will only function when a genuine need arises, as frequent spurious alarms can significantly disturb sleep. With remote monitoring, spurious alarms can be identified and dealt with easily.

Getting the patient involved in their care is crucial to success of NIV; manufacturers have and are developing ways to engage patients with their NIV through information technology. Apps allow patients to review the efficiency of their treatment and mask fit, gaining positive feedback and tips on how to improve.

CHAPTER SUMMARY

The 'ingredients' to start a successful 'NIV recipe' both in ARF and CRF are as follows: education and staff training; location adequately matched with the patient's clinical status; selection of patients according to the presentation of acute/chronic symptoms and 'shared goals' of the treatment; and identification of a suitable caregiver for home treatment. Clinicians should also choose carefully interface, ventilator and mode of ventilation, including suitable humidification; consider the patient's needs for information, care and 'human support'; monitor for excessive mask leaks and patient–ventilator synchrony; and ensure comfortable breathing.

CASE STUDY IN CHRONIC VENTILATORY FAILURE

June Long* is a 73-year-old lady with compensated hypercapnic ventilatory failure secondary to chronic obstructive pulmonary disease. Arterial blood gases: pH 7.36, pCO_2 8.1 kPa, pO_2 7.2 kPa, HCO_3 37 mmol. She attended an outpatient appointment to have an oxygen trial but became acidotic on a flow rate of 1.0 L/min, so it was suggested that she should start NIV. June became quite distressed at the suggestion that she would have to wear a mask. The clinician discussed with June why she should be so fearful of the mask and she explained why: 'During the second world war I was issued with a gas mask and I hated it because it was smelly. When I was naughty my parents would make me wear the gas mask as punishment, so I don't like anything on my head or face'.

The clinician was able to reassure June that masks were different and showed her the range of masks available, inviting her to choose one. Obviously the full-face masks were too much like the gas mask, but the nasal pillows were similar to the nasal cannulae that she had tolerated for the oxygen trial. With support June tried the nasal pillows on but did not like them. June suggested that she needed more time, so a plan was made to bring her back to outpatients in 3 weeks to start NIV; she would take the nasal pillows home and wear them during the day, gradually increasing the length of time she would wear them.

* The patient's name has been changed.

The clinician removed the tube from the nasal pillows to minimise the dead space and suggested that June wear them when she was doing something such as reading or watching television, as this would distract her from the presence of the mask. No minimum time limit for wearing the mask was set for June so as not to set her up to fail.

Three weeks later, June returned to start NIV, and she had managed to wear the mask building up from 2 to 45 min with no problems; she thought it was less trouble than she had anticipated. June was started on a pressure support ventilator, which has a ramp to allow the pressures to build slowly over 10 min. Starting with an IPAP pressure of 6 hPa and an EPAP pressure of 2 hPa allowed June to get used to the sensation of ventilation while still being gentle; the ramp allowed the pressure to build to IPAP 8 hPa and EPAP 4 hPa, then the clinician gently increased the IPAP from 8 to 12 hPa; the EPAP remained at 4 hPa. June coped well with this, keeping the mask on for 30 min. Having a transcutaneous CO_2 monitor in situ, she could also see the benefits as her tCO_2 fell by 1 kPa, and her SpO_2 improved significantly. June returned home with the ventilator and a plan to use it during the day as she had used the mask and when she was ready to try using overnight.

REFERENCES

1. Nava S, Hill N. Non-invasive ventilation in acute respiratory failure. *Lancet*. 2009;374:250–9.
2. Ozsancak A, D'Ambrosio C, Hill NS. Nocturnal non-invasive ventilation. *Chest*. 2008;133:1275–86.
3. Hill NS. Where should noninvasive ventilation be delivered? *Respir Care*. 2009;54:62–70.
4. Corrado A, Roussos C, Ambrosino N et al. Respiratory intermediate care units: A European survey. *Eur Respir J*. 2002;20:1343–50.
5. Chatwin M, Nickol AH, Morrell MJ et al. Randomised trial of inpatient versus outpatient initiation of home mechanical ventilation in patients with nocturnal hypoventilation. *Respir Med*. 2008;102:1528–35.
6. Nava S, Navalesi P, Conti G. Time of non-invasive ventilation. *Intensive Care Med*. 2006;32:361–70.
7. Scala R, Nava S. NIV and palliative care. *Eur Respir Mon*. 2008;41:287–306.
8. Carlucci A, Delmastro M, Rubini F et al. Changes in the practice of non-invasive ventilation in treating COPD patients over 8 years. *Intensive Care Med*. 2003;29:419–25.
9. Lopez-Campos JL, Garcia Polo C, Leon Jimenez A et al. Staff training influence on non-invasive ventilation outcome for acute hypercapnic respiratory failure. *Monaldi Arch Chest Dis*. 2006;65:145–51.
10. Schettino G, Altobelli N, Kacmarek RM. Noninvasive positive-pressure ventilation in acute respiratory failure outside clinical trials: Experience at the Massachusetts General Hospital. *Crit Care Med*. 2008;36:441–7.
11. Kacmarek RM. Noninvasive positive-pressure ventilation: The little things do make the difference! *Respir Care*. 2003;48:919–21.
12. Maheshwari V, Paioli D, Rothaar R et al. Utilization of noninvasive ventilation in acute care hospitals: A regional survey. *Chest*. 2006;129:1226–33.
13. Wood KA, Lewis L, Von Harz B et al. The use of noninvasive positive pressure ventilation in the emergency department: Results of a randomized clinical trial. *Chest*. 1998;113:1339–46.
14. Scala R. Flexible bronchoscopy during noninvasive positive pressure mechanical ventilation: Two are better than one? *Panminerva Med*. 2016 [Epub ahead of print].
15. Scala R. Sedation during non-invasive ventilation to treat acute respiratory failure. *Shortness Breath*. 2013;2:35–43.
16. Demoule A, Girou E, Richard JC et al. Benefits and risks of success or failure of noninvasive ventilation. *Intensive Care Med*. 2006;32:1756–65.
17. Nava S, Evangelisti I, Rampulla C et al. Human and financial costs of noninvasive mechanical ventilation in patients affected by COPD and acute respiratory failure. *Chest*. 1997;111:1631–8.
18. Norrenberg M, Vincent JL. A profile of European intensive care unit physiotherapists. *Intensive Care Med*. 2000;26:988–94.
19. Keenan SP, Powers CE, McCormack DG. Noninvasive positive-pressure ventilation in patients with milder chronic obstructive pulmonary disease exacerbations: A randomized controlled trial. *Respir Care*. 2005;50:610–16.
20. Kramer N, Meyer TJ, Meharg J et al. Randomized, prospective trial of noninvasive positive pressure ventilation in acute respiratory failure. *Am J Respir Crit Care Med*. 1995;151:1799–806.
21. Bott J, Carroll MP, Conway JH et al. Randomised controlled trial of nasal ventilation in acute ventilatory failure due to chronic obstructive airways disease. *Lancet*. 1993;341:1555–7.
22. Plant PK, Owen JL, Elliott MW. Early use of non-invasive ventilation for acute exacerbations of chronic obstructive pulmonary disease on general respiratory wards: A multicentre randomised controlled trial. *Lancet*. 2000;355:1931–5.
23. Conti G, Antonelli M, Navalesi P et al. Noninvasive vs. conventional mechanical ventilation in patients with chronic obstructive pulmonary disease after failure of medical treatment in the ward: A randomized trial. *Intensive Care Med*. 2002;28:1701–7.
24. Bertolini G, Confalonieri M, Rossi C et al. Costs of the COPD. Differences between intensive care unit and respiratory intermediate care unit. *Respir Med*. 2005;99:894–900.

25. Iapichino G, Corbella D, Minelli C et al. Reasons for refusal of admission to intensive care and impact on mortality. *Intensive Care Med.* 2010;36:1772–9.
26. Bolton R, Bleetman A. Non-invasive ventilation and continuous positive pressure ventilation in emergency departments: Where are we now? *Emerg Med J.* 2008;25:190–4.
27. Plaisance P, Pirracchio R, Berton C et al. A randomized study of out-of-hospital continuous positive airway pressure for acute cardiogenic pulmonary oedema: Physiological and clinical effects. *Eur Heart J.* 2007;28:2895–901.
28. Cabrini L, Idone C, Colombo S et al. Medical emergency team and non-invasive ventilation outside ICU for acute respiratory failure. *Intensive Care Med.* 2009;35:339–43.
29. Barbé F, Togores B, Rubí M et al. Noninvasive ventilatory support does not facilitate recovery from acute respiratory failure in chronic obstructive pulmonary disease. *Eur Respir J.* 1996;9:1240–5.
30. Plant PK, Owen JL, Elliott MW. One year period prevalence study of respiratory acidosis in acute exacerbations of COPD: Implications for the provision of non-invasive ventilation and oxygen administration. *Thorax.* 2000;55:550–4.
31. Tomii K, Seo R, Tachikawa R et al. Impact of non-invasive ventilation trial for various types of acute respiratory failure in the emergency department; decreased mortality and use of the ICU. *Respir Med.* 2009;103:67–73.
32. Scala R, Nava S, Conti G et al. Noninvasive versus conventional ventilation to treat hypercapnic encephalopathy in chronic obstructive pulmonary disease. *Intensive Care Med.* 2007;33:2101–8.
33. Confalonieri M, Trevisan R, Demsar M et al. Opening of a respiratory intermediate care unit in a general hospital: Impact on mortality and other outcomes. *Respiration.* 2015;90:235–42.
34. Scala R, Corrado A, Confalonieri M et al. Increased number and expertise of Italian Respiratory High-Dependency Care Units: The second national survey. *Respir Care.* 2011;56:1100–7.
35. Scala R, Naldi M, Archinucci I et al. Noninvasive positive pressure ventilation in patients with acute exacerbations of COPD and varying levels of consciousness. *Chest.* 2005;128:1657–66.
36. Vianello A, Corrado A, Arcaro G et al. Mechanical insufflation-exsufflation improves outcomes for neuromuscular disease patients with respiratory tract infections. *Am J Phys Med Rehabil.* 2005;84:83–8.
37. Vargas F, Bui HN, Boyer A et al. Intrapulmonary percussive ventilation in acute exacerbations of COPD patients with mild respiratory acidosis: A randomized controlled trial. *Crit Care.* 2005;9:R382–9.
38. Ozyilmaz E, Ugurlu AO, Nava S. Timing of non-invasive ventilation failure: Causes, risk factors, and potential remedies. *BMC Pulm Med.* 2014;14:19.
39. Maggiore SM, Mercurio G, Volpe C. NIV in the acute setting: Technical aspects, initiation, monitoring and choice of interface. *Eur Respir Mon.* 2008;41:173–88.
40. Girault C, Briel A, Benichou J et al. Interface strategy during noninvasive positive pressure ventilation for hypercapnic acute respiratory failure. *Crit Care Med.* 2009;37:124–31.
41. Lemyze M, Mallat J, Nigeon et al. Rescue therapy by switching to total-face mask after failure of face mask-delivered noninvasive ventilation in do-not-intubate patients in acute respiratory failure. *Crit Care Med.* 2013;41:481–8.
42. Navalesi P, Costa R, Ceriana P et al. Non-invasive ventilation in chronic obstructive pulmonary disease patients: Helmet versus facial mask. *Intensive Care Med.* 2007;33:74–81.
43. Pisani P, Mega C, Vaschetto R et al. Oronasal mask versus helmet in acute hypercapnic respiratory failure. *Eur Respir J.* 2015;45:691–9.
44. Olivieri C, Longhini F, Cena T et al. New versus conventional helmet for delivering noninvasive ventilation: A physiologic, crossover randomized study in critically ill patients. *Anesthesiology.* 2016;124:101–8.
45. Nicolini A, Santo M, Ferrari-Bravo M et al. Open-mouthpiece ventilation versus nasal mask ventilation in subjects with COPD exacerbation and mild to moderate acidosis: A randomized trial. *Respir Care.* 2014;59:1825–31.
46. Scala R, Naldi M. Ventilators for noninvasive ventilation to treat acute respiratory failure. *Respir Care.* 2008;53:1054–80.
47. Vignaux L, Tassaux D, Jolliet P. Performance of non-invasive ventilation modes on ICU ventilators during pressure support: A bench model study. *Intensive Care Med.* 2007;33:1444–51.
48. Marco F, Centanni S, Bellone A et al. Optimization of ventilator setting by flow and pressure waveforms analysis during noninvasive ventilation for acute exacerbations of COPD: A multicentric randomized controlled trial. *Crit Care.* 2011;24;15:R283.
49. Pluym M, Kabir AW, Gohar A. The use of volume-assured pressure support noninvasive ventilation in acute and chronic respiratory failure: A practical guide and literature review. *Hosp Pract (1995).* 2015;43:299–307.
50. Scala R. Monitoring choices in acute NIV. In: Simonds AK, ed. *ERS Practical Handbook of Noninvasive Ventilation.* Sheffield, ERS, 2015;pp. 93–101.
51. Jaber S, Chanques G, Matecki S et al. Comparison of the effects of heat and moisture exchangers and heated humidifiers on ventilation and gas exchange during non-invasive ventilation. *Intensive Care Med.* 2002;28:1590–4.

52. Frat JP, Brugiere B, Ragot S et al. Sequential application of oxygen-therapy via high-flow nasal cannula and noninvasive ventilation in acute respiratory failure: An observational pilot study. *Respir Care.* 2015;60:170–8.
53. Casey KR, Cantillo KO, Brown LK. Sleep-related hypoventilation/hypoxemic syndromes. *Curr Opinion Pulm Med.* 2007;131:1936–48.
54. Dhand UK, Dhand R. Sleep disorders in neuromuscular diseases. *Curr Opinion Pulm Med.* 2006;12:402–8.
55. Motor neurone disease: Assessment and management. NICE guidelines (NG 42). London: NICE, 2016. Available at http://www.nice.org.uk/guidance/ng42 (accessed 29 May 2016).
56. Motor Neurone Disease Association. Information sheet 8A. Support for breathing problems. Northampton: MNDA, 2015. Available at http://www.mndassociation.org/wp-content/uploads/2015/07/08A-Support-for-breathing-problems.pdf (accessed 30 May 2016).
57. Simonds AK. Making breathing easier. London: Muscular Dystrophy Campaign, 2015. Available at http://cdn5.musculardystrophyuk.org/app/uploads/2015/02/Making-Breathing-Easier-2016.pdf (accessed 30 May 2016).
58. Davidson C, Banham S, Elliott M et al. BTS/ICS Guidelines for the ventilator management of acute hypercapnic respiratory failure in adults. *Thorax.* 2016;71(supplement 2).
59. Association of Palliative Medicine of Great Britain and Ireland. Withdrawal of Assisted Ventilation at the request of a patient with Motor neurone disease. Southampton: APM, 2015. Available at apmonline.org/wp-content/uploads/2016/03/Guidance-with-logos-updated-210316.pdf (accessed 29 May 2016).
60. Turkington PM, Elliott MW. The rationale for the use of non-invasive ventilation in chronic ventilatory failure. *Thorax.* 2000;55:417–23.
61. ATS Consensus Conference. Respiratory care of the patient with Duchenne muscular dystrophy. *Am J Respir Crit Care Med.* 2004;170:456–65.
62. Ward S, Chatwin M, Heather S et al. Randomised controlled trial of non-invasive ventilation for nocturnal hypoventilation in neuromuscular and chest wall disease patients with daytime normocapnia. *Thorax.* 2005;60:1019–24.
63. Bourke SC, Bullock RE, Williams TL et al. Noninvasive ventilation in ALS, indications and effect on quality of life. *Neurology.* 2003;61:171–7.
64. Raphael JC, Chevret S, Chastang C et al. Randomised trial of preventive nasal ventilation in Duchenne muscular dystrophy. *Lancet.* 1994;343:1600–4.
65. Elliott MW. The interface: Crucial for successful non-invasive ventilation. *Eur Respir J.* 2004;23:7–8.
66. Murphy PB, Davidson C, Hind MD et al. Volume targeted versus pressure support non-invasive ventilation in patients with super obesity and chronic respiratory failure: A randomised controlled trial. *Thorax.* 2012:67:727–34.

PART 2

The practice – acute NIV

10	How to set up an acute non-invasive ventilation service *Paul K. Plant and Gregory A. Schmidt*	85
11	Education programmes/assessment of staff competencies *Alanna Hare*	95
12	Monitoring during acute non-invasive ventilation *Eumorfia Kondili, Nektaria Xirouchaki and Dimitris Georgopoulos*	101
13	Troubleshooting non-invasive ventilation *Nicholas S. Hill, Mayanka Tickoo and Najia Indress*	111
14	Sedation and delirium *Lara Pisani, Maria Laura Vega and Cesare Gregoretti*	122
15	Timing of non-invasive ventilation *Stefano Nava and Paolo Navalesi*	131
16	Why non-invasive ventilation works in acute respiratory failure? *Miguel Ferrer and Antoni Torres*	139
17	Predicting outcome in patients with acute hypercapnic respiratory failure *Tom Hartley and Stephen C. Bourke*	149
18	Use of NIV in the real world *Mihaela Stefan, Peter Lindenauer, Najia Indress, Faisal Tamimi and Nicholas S. Hill*	157

10

How to set up an acute non-invasive ventilation service

PAUL K. PLANT AND GREGORY A. SCHMIDT

KEY POINTS

- NIV is a highly effective intervention that is often underutilised or started later than recommended. The main barriers to service provision are usually the lack of a structured service and the inexperience of clinicians.
- Hospitals should have a NIV multi-disciplinary team who champion the service, develop local guidelines and standards, select locations to offer NIV and ensure staff in those locations are trained.
- All relevant clinical staff should be educated in the indications for NIV, monitoring, the identification of NIV failure and escalation plans.
- Staff applying NIV require competency in achieving adaptation to NIV (mask fitting and initial ventilator set-up), ensuring effective ventilation (adjustment of pressures/equipment in response to monitoring) and be able to respond to the patient's perceptions and behaviours (e.g. maximising concordance, time on NIV).
- NIV services benefit from regular audit and ongoing service improvement.

INTRODUCTION

The indications for the use of non-invasive ventilation (NIV) have increased, based on improved outcomes (compared with invasive ventilation) and reduced risks (such as fewer nosocomial infections). At the same time, NIV has made it possible to support or palliate patients who have elected to forego more invasive life-sustaining measures, such as endotracheal intubation. Despite evidence that NIV can prevent intubations and improve mortality, especially in chronic obstructive pulmonary disease (COPD) exacerbations, cardiogenic pulmonary oedema and immunocompromised patients with hypoxaemic respiratory failure, underutilisation is common. Some hospitals miss opportunities to provide NIV because they lack expertise, fail to invest the necessary resources, have no champions or resist change. Although NIV is becoming more common, it could be used more extensively and often at an earlier stage in the evolution of a patient's respiratory failure. Therefore, we emphasise a multidisciplinary team approach to building the competencies necessary for an institution to succeed at providing NIV safely to those most likely to benefit.

Starting a NIV service is a complex process that relies on multiple factors for its success, related to both the clinicians and the organisational structure of the healthcare setting. These factors include the practice, educational programmes, beliefs and attitudes of clinicians, expectations of the patients, clinicians or administrators, the organisational context of the hospital including resources and current care processes and public policy or legislation that can influence practice.[1,2] Each of these factors is vital to a successful new paradigm and must be addressed. In this chapter, we present methods and suggestions on how to set up an acute NIV unit in the hospital setting. Issues include identification of appropriate use opportunities, the setting of use, training and types of personnel, necessary infrastructure and barriers to acceptance (Box 10.1). Although a comprehensive approach to implementing and maintaining a NIV service is presented, marked differences in healthcare settings and practices across regions and the world contribute to the challenge of change.

BOX 10.1: Key ingredients in starting a non-invasive ventilation programme

- Identify a 'champion' to lead the process
- Assemble a multidisciplinary team with training and experience in NIV
- Incorporate hospital administration, departmental leaders, and clinical providers into initial set-up decision-making
- Decide on a location for NIV and/or mobile service
- Establish monitoring methods and assemble equipment
- Create protocols including initiation, training and maintenance of NIV
- Establish quality management strategies and outcomes monitoring
- Anticipate resistance to change and establish strategies to overcome barriers

WHY A NIV SERVICE?

Current data suggest that NIV is underutilised despite growing evidence of its success in decreasing the need for initiation of mechanical ventilation, preventing failure of extubation, decreasing nosocomial pneumonias and improving short- and long-term mortality.[3]

For instance, in one utilisation study, two thirds of intensive care unit (ICU) patients who had a diagnosis of COPD or cardiogenic pulmonary oedema at admission and fulfilled criteria for use of NIV were intubated without a trial.[4] Maheshwari et al.[5] studied utilisation practices in northeastern United States and found marked variation in utilisation rates (0% to greater than 50%), noting that the two main perceived barriers to utilisation were lack of physician knowledge and inadequate equipment. Undoubtedly, the reasons behind this variability are more complex. However, this study highlights the necessity for increased education and visibility of this technique to aid in widespread safe and effective use.

Cabrini et al.[3] in their meta-analysis also concluded that NIV should be used early in a patient's decline and that switching to NIV after clinical deterioration was less effective. Hence, underutilisation can be both the failure to offer NIV and also the administration of it late in a patient's decline.

A UK study explored the prevalence of respiratory acidosis in 983 consecutive patients admitted with acute exacerbations of COPD (AECOPD).[6] After initial therapy, 16% of patients had a respiratory acidosis. The pH was below 7.25 in 22%; 78% had a pH between 7.25 and 7.35. The British Thoracic Society NIV Audit of 2013 explored the use of NIV in 2693 patients admitted to 148 UK hospitals in a 2 month period.[7] UK guidelines recommend NIV for COPD patients with a pH < 7.35 and a $PaCO_2$ > 6 kPa. The median pH at initiation of NIV was 7.24, suggesting that milder acidosis was not being treated promptly. The mortality rate in the audit was high at 34% compared to published series. The authors concluded that this was due to underutilisation in milder disease.

Next, lack of a structured service and inexperience with the technique can also lead to misuse of NIV and suboptimal care. For instance, in a review of 91 patients in whom NIV was initiated, physician orders were missing for 15% of the NIV trials, cardiorespiratory monitoring was not explicitly ordered in any patient and documentation of equipment was lacking.[8] Further, experience of operators is particularly important in severely ill patients. A review of the outcomes of patients on NIV over a 7 year period of time found that increased experience with NIV may allow increasingly severely ill patients to be treated without compromising the rate of success.[9]

A MULTIDISCIPLINARY TEAM

It is important to have one clinician or a small group of clinicians who serve as 'champions' or leaders of the process (Figure 10.1).[2] The champion should be available to answer questions, troubleshoot and maintain momentum of the process. This person must remain flexible to problems and suggestions, implementing changes in protocols and processes where needed. To be the most effective, leaders also need to maintain knowledge of the latest technologies and evidence regarding NIV, and maintain collaborations with other institutions for advice and consultation. Having a champion increases awareness and knowledge, and promotes an evidence-based culture, thereby increasing appropriate utilisation.

The champion should be integrally involved in both the planning and implementation phases of the acute NIV service, serving to bridge this gap. Planning will involve a different group of team members than the actual

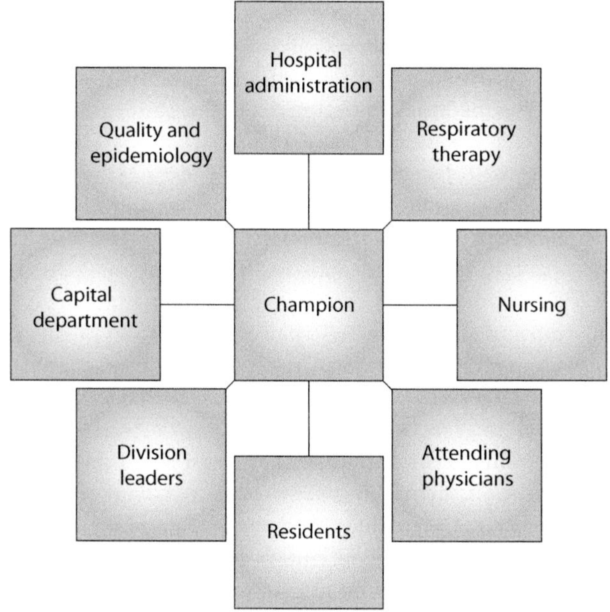

Figure 10.1 Role of the champion.

implementation team. In planning, hospital administration, a member of the capital department and division leaders should be involved in cost analyses, resource allocation, logistics and public relations.

The exact location and design of the NIV service will depend on the local setting. However, successful NIV depends on having an understanding of the demand on the service, a clear pathway of care to ensure access to NIV, a highly trained team able to provide NIV plus educators to ensure sustainability of the service as new members join and quality control to ensure high-quality NIV.

The specific professional groups offering NIV vary in different healthcare settings. In the United States, NIV is often initiated by respiratory therapists, but it can also be by doctors, nurses, respiratory physiologists, physicians' assistants or nurse practitioners.[10] The prevalence of each of these caregivers varies regionally and internationally, and the make-up of the implementation team depends on local availability. Overall, it is important to involve different types of caregivers as each brings a different expertise to the forefront of care, all inherent to patient success.

THE LOCATION FOR NIV

An acute NIV service can be located in a particular ward or unit in a hospital, or can be defined more broadly to include a team that administers NIV in various locations within the hospital.[10] Currently, NIV is used in a variety of places. One study showed that the primary site of initiation of NIV in the hospital was the emergency department, although the ICU and the clinical teaching unit incorporated the most total hours of NIV.[8] Other reviews confirm that the emergency department, ICU and general wards are the most common sites of initiation.[5,12] Clinical teaching units that use NIV most frequently are internal medicine, pulmonology and cardiology. More recently, successful use of NIV has been shown in the post-operative care units,[13] particularly in treating acute respiratory failure after lung resection.[14] Outside of the hospital, NIV started in-home and upon transport has been shown to be a feasible and effective method to improve the emergency management of patients with pulmonary oedema[15] and may become increasingly used for other causes.[16,17]

Factors influencing the location of NIV use include monitoring capabilities of the unit, ICU bed capacity, convenience if intubation is required, nurse-to-patient ratio, respiratory therapy availability, cost-effectiveness and clinician experience.[18] While it is often recommended that candidates for NIV be treated in an ICU for reasons of safety (especially in North America), this is not always possible because such beds are often in short supply. At the same time, costly ICU beds may not be necessary for appropriately selected patients. Experience is critically important in judging which patients can be managed safely outside the ICU. Key factors include the type and severity of illness, respiratory parameters, mental status and ability to clear secretions, in combination with the type of equipment needed and ward infrastructure, when deciding on a location for NIV initiation (Box 10.2). Level of consciousness should be taken into account as decreased levels have been associated with worse outcomes in some studies.[8,19] Nevertheless, obtundation is not a contraindication to NIV. Finally, the decision on where to monitor should take into account the experienced clinician's subjective judgement regarding the severity of illness and potential for deterioration.

BOX 10.2: Patients who can be managed outside an ICU

The ideal candidate

- COPD exacerbation
- Haemodynamically stable
- Alert, cooperative and able to remove the mask themselves when appropriate
- Capable of tolerating brief periods off NIV
- Adequate cough with no excessive secretions
- Shows improvement of pH and respiratory rate during first 1–2 hours of therapy
- Staff are experienced in NIV use

Higher risk of NIV failure

- Acute respiratory failure of undetermined aetiology
- Hypoxaemic respiratory failure not due to cardiogenic pulmonary oedema
- Agitation or poor mask tolerance
- Greater overall illness severity
- Tolerance off NIV unproved
- Excessive or tenacious secretions or poor cough
- Not clearly improving after initial trial of therapy
- Staff less experienced in recognising respiratory deterioration, troubleshooting NIV or facilitating endotracheal intubation

EMERGENCY WARD

The emergency department is an important venue as it is one of the earliest opportunities to institute NIV to prevent intubation, with the impetus that NIV has a higher success rate if started early.[20] Initiating NIV in the emergency department may also decrease the need for ICU admission,[21,22] and thereby reduce ICU costs.[23] Administration of NIV in the emergency department also mitigates against delays in transferring patients to busy respiratory wards where NIV is routinely performed.

Careful application in the emergency department setting is imperative, as use for inappropriate indications or lack of appropriate monitoring can delay life-saving care in some cases.[24] Challenges in the emergency department include the tentative nature of the respiratory failure diagnosis, high risk of intubation need in the first hours of NIV, staff inexperience in the longitudinal management of NIV and lack of continuity with the team that will manage the subsequent hospital care. Moreover, NIV success benefits from time taken to engage the patient, troubleshoot the equipment, titrate the settings and judge the impact – an approach that sometimes contradicts a goal of securing the airway and transferring to a ward. A NIV service can provide education for emergency department physicians and staff with regard to how to maximise success. Guidelines regarding use should be enforced to prevent adverse events in a hectic emergency department where monitoring and communication may be difficult. Posted protocols, e.g. attached to the ventilator, can help provide an easy reference regarding selection of patients, instructions on who to call for placement of NIV, monitoring requirements and how to recognise a failing patient.[11] Often, a separate consult service can help alleviate strain on the emergency department personnel.

Success and ease of use in the emergency department setting are important, as many potential patients are seen. However, perceived failures or lack of ease of use can lead to frustration and scepticism on the part of emergency department staff. Failure rates can also appear higher in this setting given the heterogeneity of patients and potential for inappropriate use. Last, it should be emphasised that NIV is most often a bridge to admission and continuation of NIV, as a majority of patients require more than a few hours of use. Nevertheless, there is some experience with using NIV to improve vital signs and acid/base parameters, followed by an assessment for immediate discharge to an unmonitored general ward. For example, following an initial 90 min period of NIV for acute cardiogenic pulmonary oedema, 43 of 58 patients who tolerated 15 min of NIV removal without dyspnoea or haemodynamic instability were treated on a general ward.[21] None of these patients subsequently died, was intubated or required ICU transfer. Overall, in light of these complexities, a NIV service can be of particular importance to the emergency department environment in order to capture patients who would benefit, alleviate a considerable time and effort, burden off emergency department personnel and potentially improve outcomes in a cost-effective process.

GENERAL WARD

Similarly, NIV can be used on general wards in certain patients depending on severity of illness. Intense monitoring standards must be applied, as well as proper education and training of nurses, as NIV cannot be applied universally on wards without these factors in place. Furthermore, high concern for patient selection based on current evidence should be implemented. For example, one study shows that early use of NIV in COPD patients with mild or moderate acidaemia on general wards resulted in fewer intubations and decreased in-hospital mortality.[25] Therefore, NIV may be reasonable in these cases. Also, institutions highly experienced with NIV have treated an increasing fraction of moderately ill patients (COPD exacerbation and pH > 7.28) on a general medical ward without compromising safety.[9] Alternatively, studies have shown that patients in hypercapnic coma can be treated with NIV.[26,27] However, these studies were performed in controlled, well-monitored ICUs or respiratory monitoring units, and therefore, these patients should not be placed on a regular ward. Patients on the ward should be awake enough to take off the mask in case of vomiting or able to press a call button for a nurse. It has been suggested that patients should be capable of breathing spontaneously for 1 h without NIV.[12] In addition, documentation of monitoring and checks is essential to ensure identification of a failing patient in need of more specialised care. We believe that use of NIV on general wards in non-COPD respiratory failure (such as hypoxaemic failure or pulmonary oedema) is rarely appropriate, unless there has been a clear decision to limit life-sustaining treatments.

RESPIRATORY INTERMEDIATE CARE UNIT

In those patients with more potential for failure, a specialised NIV ward can be utilised with similar monitoring to an ICU. These wards may be less stressful for patients than the ICU atmosphere and contribute to increased sleep, comfort and improved experience for the patient. A number of studies have suggested that these units can be cost-effective and successful.[18,28–31] Elpern et al.[28] found that using a non-invasive ventilatory unit for specialty care of mechanically ventilated patients was a cost-saving measure primarily due to savings from ICU time. Use of an intermediate respiratory unit can free up vital ICU resources and decrease nursing requirements. The number of beds can vary according to the needs and resources of different institutions, and therefore, assessment of patient population, bed utilisation and overall need is necessary prior to setting up this type of ward. The size often ranges from 4 to 10 beds.[32] It is also important that the institution have at least a minimum number of patients, not only for cost structuring but also to maintain the experience of the teams involved in patient care. This type of ward can often be the most efficient place for NIV and offer high-quality care, given the specialisation.

The Intensive Care Assembly of the European Respiratory Society Task Force has adopted criteria defining a respiratory intermediate care unit, which includes criteria for admission, type of intervention and equipment and staffing.[32] Criteria for admission are single organ failure, acute respiratory failure requiring monitoring (but not mechanical ventilation) or tracheostomy-ventilated patients coming from the ICU. The unit should have NIV, availability of conventional ventilators and monitoring equipment. Staffing should be a ratio of four or fewer patients to every one nurse, a respiratory physiotherapist and a doctor with the same profile as the senior doctor (training in pneumology and NIV) immediately available 24 h per day.

INTENSIVE CARE UNIT

The ICU provides the highest standard of monitoring, with high ratios of nurses and dedicated respiratory therapists.

It is important to note that a majority of the evidence regarding NIV efficacy and safety is derived from ICU environments. If NIV is used only in the ICU, however, there is likely to be underutilisation of NIV. On the other hand, if NIV is used anywhere, there may be overutilisation, sacrificing patient safety. We believe it is prudent to treat most respiratory failure patients who are candidates for NIV in an ICU or dedicated NIV unit, whenever such beds are readily available. One of the functions of a NIV service should be to balance these issues of utilisation and patient safety, taking into account the capabilities of the individual institution.

MONITORING

Monitoring is essential to the successful use of NIV and should be available (for further details, see Chapter 12). Experienced personnel, preferably including a physician, should be available on a 24 h basis. Monitoring the patient in the first hours after initiation is particularly intensive and vital to patient safety (Box 10.3).

Utilisation reviews show that intubation rate and death are higher in hospital settings outside of clinical trials, and this may be partially due to a lack of systematic monitoring.[8] Communication between the ICU teams, wards and during shift changes can also be standardised to improve patient safety. Correct interpretation of monitoring data to guide decision-making is crucial, and therefore, training in this area is important.

SET-UP AND EQUIPMENT

Obtaining and maintaining equipment needed for the NIV service requires the efforts of hospital administration, the capital department, champion physicians and the respiratory therapists and nurses who administer the equipment. This is important, as one of the main barriers to usage has been lack of adequate equipment.[5] Further, having more ventilators available has been associated with increased NIV usage.[33] Therefore, an assessment of projected usage is important to ensure cost-effectiveness, balanced by adequate resources for all patients in whom a trial of NIV is indicated.

BOX 10.3: Tasks in the first hours of NIV

- Educate and reassure the patient
- Assess mask fit, comfort and tolerance
- Seek and correct leaks
- Determine synchrony of patient and ventilator
- Titrate inspiratory positive airway pressure (IPAP) and expiratory positive airway pressure (EPAP)
- Monitor heart rate, respiratory rate, accessory muscle use and level of consciousness
- Judge cough adequacy and secretions
- Consider the role for judicious sedation
- Analyse arterial blood gas values at 1 hour
- Actively estimate the probability of failure and reevaluate the level of monitoring
- Diagnose and treat the underlying cause of respiratory failure

TRAINING

Protocols for training can be implemented across a variety of healthcare professionals to ensure safe and effective utilisation of NIV (Box 10.4). In a survey of NIV use in the United Kingdom, the two primary reasons for lack of utilisation were lack of senior physician and of other staff training.[34] The best practices on how to train physicians and healthcare professionals on NIV are currently unclear. However, it is likely that a combination of methods is effective. The training also depends on the type of practitioner involved. A survey of 242 physicians who used NIV revealed that the most common method of learning about NIV was from physician and respiratory therapy colleagues, rather than from educational conferences or direct examination of the evidence.[33] Elliott et al.[18] support this premise of preceptorship when they found that clinician experience, and not necessarily training, led to increased use of NIV on the wards.

In general, physicians, nurses and other ward personnel should be educated on the indications for NIV, because

BOX 10.4: Training goals for the NIV programme*

Theory

- Practical theory of mechanical ventilation
- Evidence base supporting NIV

Equipment

- How to initiate NIV
- Mask fit, headgear, comfort and leak detection
- Machines and modes
- Titration of pressures and settings
- Troubleshooting alarms
- Standards of monitoring
- Maintaining and stocking equipment

Patient care

- Identification of appropriate candidates for NIV
- Coaching the patient
- Interpreting arterial blood gases during NIV
- Symptoms and signs of NIV failure
- Indications for intubation

*The ideal programme includes simulation, case-based learning and preceptorship during real patient care. Programmes that reinforce learning at regular intervals, such as twice yearly, are more likely to effect long-lasting change.

any of these groups can help identify appropriate candidates and initiate NIV. This includes residents and physicians in all areas of the hospital. For the same reason, signs and symptoms of failure of NIV should be taught to all of those involved in order to maintain safe use. This can be accomplished through conferences, didactic sessions or direct teaching by champions and leaders during rounds and patient care. Furthermore, training and education directed towards the entire healthcare team may be necessary to improve guideline awareness and increase comfort with recommended practices.[35]

More targeted training should be directed to those healthcare professionals directly involved in initiating and placing NIV on a patient. This mainly includes respiratory therapists, but can also be nurses or physicians, particularly in regions where respiratory therapists do not exist. The failure to educate staff fully can lead to the failure of the service.[36] Sorensen et al.,[37] in a qualitative study of expert NIV nurse practitioners, identified three key skills required by staff to deliver NIV successfully. The first was 'achieving NIV adaptation', the second was 'ensuring effective ventilation' and the third was 'responding attentively to patient's perceptions'.

'Achieving adaptation' included not only the technical aspects of machine specifics and mask application but also the ability to problem-solve around mask fit, air leakage and asynchronous ventilation. In essence, this is the earliest phase of NIV. The training material of those directly involved in initiating the ventilator and monitoring the patient should include how to put on equipment, provide facial care, titrate pressures, troubleshoot alarms and monitor. The complexity of the technical training is often based on the type of the ventilator utilised. At a minimum, this education includes basic ventilatory mechanics and theory.

'Ensuring effective ventilation' includes how to monitor the patient with both clinical and technical assessments and then ensure optimum ventilator settings. The participants emphasised the need to look at the patient for chest movement and respiratory rate and understand technical measures, e.g. arterial blood gases. This assessment needed to be accompanied by the confidence and competence to amend ventilator settings as required. This secondary phase to delivering NIV was considered important not least in ensuring that initial starting pressures were escalated to target pressures.

The third step was 'responding attentively to the patient's perception of NIV'. Helping the patient achieve a sense of well-being on the ventilator is a complex process but essential in ensuring concordance with NIV. The nurse participants reported complex responses including physical, social, psychological and ethical support. The importance and complexity is captured in the following transcript extract:

'On a workday when my patient feels that the NIV doesn't relieve his shortness of breath and he even feels that the mask is unpleasant to wear, I have to use all my persuasive skills to make him give it another chance. On days like this, I explain the same things to the patient over and over again. I tell him why it's important, I explain that it will get better if he can stand the mask a little bit longer each time, e.g. I make deals with him about when to have a break, I coax him into holding on, I try to do everything to entice him to endure it a little longer. For example, I wet his lips, position him, encourage and comfort him and make sure the ventilation is appropriate. Sometimes I use a firm voice and tell him to do this and that. And very important I never leave him alone. We do not force or coerce patients on NIV, but sometimes I help stimulate and persuade the patient so much that it borders on making me feel uncomfortable. On the other hand, maybe I know more about the consequences of failed treatment than the patient does? I feel the responsibility heavily; it's a human life! A day like this is extremely tiring, because I use myself in a certain way'.

The training is best done with hands-on workshops with demonstrations of masks, tubing and ventilators, but also can include some lectures or didactics. Simulation sessions can also be very helpful, such as mask applications practised on classmates. However, Sorensen also concluded that some of the skills are only obtained with experience over time, which she described as 'practical wisdom'. This is probably why units are able to manage sicker patients over time with similar levels of success.[9] Hence, shadowing and preceptorship with clinical rotations accompanying those who place the masks and initiate ventilation should be incorporated to train healthcare professionals with actual patients. Problem solving and case-based learning can simulate true ward situations. These training objectives should be documented, and ongoing routine training on a biannual or annual basis should be enforced. This ongoing training requirement is particularly important in units where resident and practitioner turnover is high.

One university teaching hospital accounted its success to training and orientation of caretakers.[12] They incorporated a 4 h training session for respiratory therapy on application of NIV to patients, while nurses received classroom orientation and bedside instruction by respiratory therapy. Certification may also be helpful for a variety of reasons. First, certifications can help to assure standardised training amongst different groups. Second, certifications can be useful to track outcomes as they relate to training, which can reveal a cause or contributory factor to increased failure rate.

QUALITY MANAGEMENT

NIV services should undertake audit regularly and benchmark to other organisations and national standards. The British Thoracic Society National NIV audits of 2010 and 2013 are examples that showed that outcomes varied significantly between centres with overall outcomes worse than published trials.[7,38] Local audit/quality assurance should look at access to the service, how NIV is delivered and outcomes. Access can include the percentage of eligible patients treated and timeliness to the initiation of NIV, e.g. door to nose time. Delivery can be assessed by hours of use, pressures achieved and correction of arterial blood gases. Outcomes should include failure rate, intubation rate and mortality. It is important to share these results with colleagues, hospital administration and the community in order to increase buy-in and support for NIV. Deficits in the service should be approached with continuous service improvement.

However, there is an inherent failure rate of NIV even when used strictly according to the evidence. Review of one's own care practices, as well as others, can help implement important quality and safety measures to ensure ongoing success.

INSTITUTING CHANGE

Mechanical ventilation practices are changing internationally, based on evolving evidence.[39] Instituting organisational change can be a challenge, and knowledge of organisational change models can be helpful. In one study assessing change-avid respiratory therapy departments, it was found that the main differences between change-avid and non-change-avid departments was the presence of a vision for change, effective leadership, engaging employees in the change effort, celebrating wins and assuring the sustainability of the change.[40] Conversely, the least desirable traits included an authoritative culture, passive leadership and limited communication with respiratory therapy staff. These concepts highlight the important role of having a champion of the effort, leading change and promoting a clear vision and effective plan.

Involvement of those personnel on the 'front lines' is imperative to successful change. This involves communication with respiratory therapists or nurses who will be responsible for implementing the service. The champion should be open and available to listen to suggestions and input. Furthermore, empowering this group to take responsibility is often desirable for both the physicians and the respiratory therapists, and may even translate to improved care of the patient. Multiple studies have shown that implementation of respiratory care protocols by non-physician healthcare professionals can improve outcomes for critically ill patients.[41–43] Increasing the roles and involvement of the therapists encourages internal change and ownership of the plan. Empowerment has been effective in other realms and is accomplished by appropriate delegation of work, guidelines and protocols.

Implementing a change is the first battle – however, sustaining change is equally important. First, success should be acknowledged in a global sense. Second, the champions should commend individuals for efforts and successes. It is important to recognise the programme and individuals on a continuing basis in order to maintain motivation and ongoing positive change. This is also where it is important to be conservative at the beginning of the service, as to decrease the likelihood of an early failure, which can be a considerable setback to the morale of the programme. For instance, it may be prudent to focus initial implementation in one or two key locations in the hospital. Growth to other venues can then occur as the service becomes more accepted and successes become obvious to all stakeholders. Recognition of efforts sets the stage for forward growth and continuous improvement.

When instituting change, resistance should always be expected. In one evaluation assessing the difficulties in instituting infection control practices, active resistance was present in 14/14 sites, primarily by attending physicians or competing authorities. Mid- to high-level administration also created barriers with ambivalence, passive resistance or active blocking of an initiative.[44] This leads to poor morale and frustration at an organisational level. Suggested solutions to overcome the 'active resister' and 'organisational constipator' include regular feedback, effective champions, participation in collaborative efforts, improving communication with executives and working around or excluding individuals who are barriers to change.[44]

'SELLING YOUR SERVICE': NEEDS ASSESSMENT AND HOSPITAL BUY-IN

The implementation of a NIV service will involve 'buy in' by a number of groups, including hospital administration, physician colleagues in multiple specialties and ward personnel who care for the patient. Often, this involves education on the evidence behind the benefits of a successful programme such as patient safety, improved outcomes and increased patient satisfaction. Furthermore, financial justification is becoming an increasingly important problem that the champion will encounter.

In the planning phase, the champion must argue that the NIV service is worth the input of resources by the hospital, personnel and colleagues. A careful assessment of the projected need based on patient admissions and missed opportunity for NIV is necessary. Resources must be allocated towards purchase of equipment and training of the staff. Importantly, time and effort of the team must not be overlooked. For instance, Kramer et al.[45] found that respiratory therapy may spend up to an hour of time in the first 8 h of initiation of NIV, and the time involved by staff in care of NIV may be similar to invasive ventilation. Overall, these resources must be enacted in entirety, as a programme lacking in any one of the components, whether it is time, equipment or enthusiasm, is increasingly likely to fail.

Improved outcome and patient safety should be the primary reasons to implement a NIV service. This is supported by multiple reports of decreased mortality and improved outcomes.

Cost-effectiveness of NIV will be an important argument for overall buy-in. Multiple studies have demonstrated that, if implemented correctly, NIV can be a cost-saving measure. Keenan et al.[29] found that using NIV in COPD exacerbations is not only more effective, but less expensive. A similar analysis in the UK hospital system indicated that providing a NIV service will avoid six deaths and three to nine admissions to ICUs per year, with an associated cost reduction of £12,000–£53,000 per year.[30] Furthermore, the use of NIV for COPD and acute respiratory failure of other causes doubled from 1998 to 2004, coinciding with a 50%

reduction in the overall numbers of patients in the ICU with a primary diagnosis of COPD or cardiogenic pulmonary oedema.[39] This aspect is important when considering the investment in equipment and personnel, which may initially seem prohibitive.

PROBLEMS AND OBSTACLES

In any institution, problems and obstacles to implementation are expected to occur as with introduction of many new devices or protocols. First, the effects on other departments or services should not be minimised. A NIV service may be perceived as an effort to limit another service's privileges or infringement upon their independence to provide care. This is where the champion can make a concerted effort to educate all services on the known benefits and confer support, rather than dominance, with the technique. At times, finding collaborators in different departments to relay information to his or her colleagues or subordinates can be useful. It is also important to circulate success rates and 'advertising' to build support and visibility among the departments.

Logistics can be an issue, particularly if the service is not confined to one ward.[6] Skills are retained more easily if patients are managed regularly in one location for the full duration of their NIV treatment. A similar volume of work distributed over several wards naturally means less experience per location but also increases the probability of protracted time without needing to use NIV, during which skills erode. Being aware of the need for the service therefore informs the model.

The skills include not only the ability of the NIV team physically to reach a patient but also the ability to monitor, the availability of emergency response, and proximity to more intensive care. Placing a patient in a room closer to a nursing station, incorporating emergency carts in each location and having immediate availability of personnel to help in emergency situations (such as a 'rapid response team') can help to alleviate some of these concerns.

Staffing will also be an important issue that should be first addressed in the planning phase. A 24 h service staffed with trained and experienced personnel requires availability and cooperation of the team. Hospital administration should be involved in the investment of resources towards this goal, and team members must be willing to provide care for patients, including night coverage. Furthermore, nursing coverage, particularly on a specialised NIV ward service, should include a group of experienced and trained nurses who can provide continuity of care. Large numbers of 'floating' nurses through this area should be avoided to ensure that appropriate specialised care is provided. A mobile team could be formed to provide NIV and aid in the care of patients on general wards.

USE OF PROTOCOLS

Protocols can improve practice, help implement evidence-based strategies, reduce errors and ensure uniformity and quality of care. Essential to adherence to guidelines in the intensive care setting are effective leadership and positive interprofessional team dynamics, education tailored to the learning preferences of different groups, repeated education and feedback.[46] Using guidelines and protocols can lead to an increase in NIV utilisation, although the question of whether this equates to improved mortality outcomes is still unproven.[47] However, evidence on the use of non-physician-implemented protocols is gaining momentum in the care of critically ill patients, improving outcomes and allocation of respiratory care services.[42]

The creation of new protocols or modification of existing ones should involve multidisciplinary input from physicians, respiratory therapy and nursing. This collaboration can serve to decrease obstacles and problems in implementation and increase confidence towards usage. Pre-printed orders or computerised order entry order sets can be useful for fast, uniform implementation, as are pocket cards for care personnel with algorithms, guidelines and troubleshooting (Figure 10.2). Protocols must be concrete, explicit and easy to follow. Complicated algorithms will lead to lack of acceptance by hospital caregivers.

Due to the complexity of care of a patient with NIV, multiple protocols or guidelines may be necessary (Box 10.5). For example, protocols may be necessary for initiation of NIV and maintenance and assessment of the patient currently on NIV. These may also differ or include information based on the type of respiratory failure or unit (ICU, step-down unit or ward). Protocols may be written or implemented for titration of NIV or how to identify and treat the

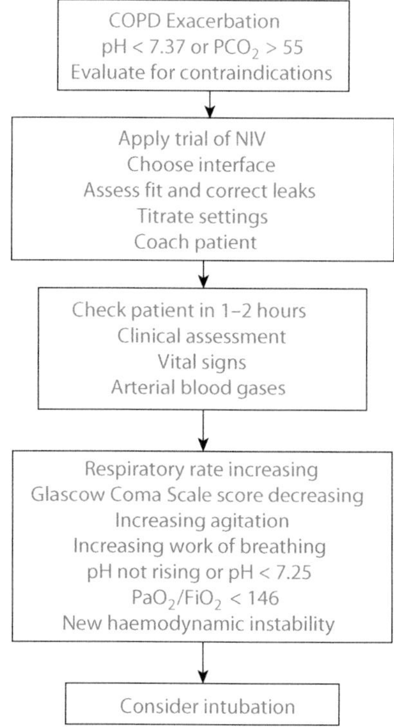

Figure 10.2 Example guideline for care of a COPD patient. NIV: non-invasive ventilation.

BOX 10.5: Types of protocols for NIV

- Indications for NIV
- Applying NIV
- Monitoring
- Titrating NIV
- Identifying the failing patient
- Intubation

failing patient. All protocols must be reassessed regularly to ensure their effectiveness and use. Published protocols may be used, but often need modification depending on institutional infrastructure and personnel.

Implementation of protocols can also meet resistance, particularly from physicians who may feel a lack of control over patients. In this respect, attention to education on the evidence supporting protocols, monitoring of compliance and maintaining feedback can help to facilitate the process.[42] Furthermore, it should be reinforced that protocols are second to a clinician's judgement, and should serve as guidelines rather than strict rules to a decision-making process.

CONCLUSIONS

With increased use of NIV and the emergence of new indications, there is now an increasing need for acute NIV services in hospitals. Creation of a service requires intense planning and the cooperation of physicians, hospital administration, nursing and respiratory therapists. Problems such as generalised acceptance, logistics and resource allocation must be expected. Of utmost importance to a programme's success is the training and education of the caregivers. Despite these complexities, a successful acute NIV service can provide better outcomes, improved patient experience and a cost-effective system.

REFERENCES

1. Grol R, Grimshaw J. Evidence-based implementation of evidence-based medicine. *Joint Comm J Q Improve*. 1999;25:503–13.
2. Hess DR. How to initiate a noninvasive ventilation program: Bringing the evidence to the bedside. *Respir Care*. 2009;54:232–43; discussion 43–5.
3. Cabrini L, Landoni G, Oriani A et al. Noninvasive ventilation and survival In acute care settings: A comprehensive systematic review and meta-analysis of randomised controlled trials. *Crit Care Med*. 2015;43(4):880–8.
4. Sweet DD, Naismith A, Keenan SP et al. Missed opportunities for noninvasive positive pressure ventilation: A utilization review. *J Crit Care*. 2008;23:111–7.
5. Maheshwari V, Paioli D, Rothaar R et al. Utilization of noninvasive ventilation in acute care hospitals: A regional survey. *Chest*. 2006;129:1226–33.
6. Plant PK, Owen JL, Elliott MW. One year period prevalence study of respiratory acidosis in acute exacerbations of COPD: Implications for the provision of non-invasive ventilation and oxygen administration. *Thorax*. 2000;55:550–4.
7. British Thoracic Society NIV audit 2013. http://britthoracic.org.uk/audit.aspx
8. Sinuff T, Cook D, Randall J et al. Noninvasive positive-pressure ventilation: A utilization review of use in a teaching hospital. *CMAJ*. 2000;163:969–73.
9. Carlucci A, Delmastro M, Rubini F et al. Changes in the practice of non-invasive ventilation in treating COPD patients over 8 years. *Intensive Care Med*. 2003;29:419–25.
10. Topple M, Ryan B, Baldwin I et al. Tasks completed by nursing members of a teaching hospital medical emergency team. *Int Crit Care Nursing*. 2016;32:12–9.
11. Ward K, Horobin H. Does the application of an algorithm for non-invasive ventilation in COPD improve the initiation process and patient outcomes. *Physiotherapy*. 2012;98(2):151–9.
12 Schettino G, Altobelli N, Kacmarek RM. Noninvasive positive-pressure ventilation in acute respiratory failure outside clinical trials: Experience at the Massachusetts General Hospital. *Crit Care Med*. 2008;36:441–7.
13. Jhanji S, Pearse RM. The use of early intervention to prevent postoperative complications. *Curr Opin Crit Care*. 2009;15:349–54.
14. Auriant I, Jallot A, Herve P et al. Noninvasive ventilation reduces mortality in acute respiratory failure following lung resection. *Am J Respir Crit Care Med*. 2001;164:1231–5.
15. Weitz G, Struck J, Zonak A et al. Prehospital noninvasive pressure support ventilation for acute cardiogenic pulmonary edema. *Eur J Emerg Med*. 2007;14:276–9.
16. Bruge P, Jabre P, Dru M et al. An observational study of noninvasive positive pressure ventilation in an out-of-hospital setting. *Am J Emerg Med*. 2008;26:165–9.
17. Duchateau FX, Beaune S, Ricard-Hibon A et al. Prehospital noninvasive ventilation can help in management of patients with limitations of life-sustaining treatments. *Eur J Emerg Med*. 2010;17:7–9.
18. Elliott MW, Confalonieri M, Nava S. Where to perform noninvasive ventilation? *Eur Respir J*. 2002;19:1159–66.
19. Ambrosino N, Foglio K, Rubini F et al. Non-invasive mechanical ventilation in acute respiratory failure due to chronic obstructive pulmonary disease: Correlates for success. *Thorax*. 1995;50:755–7.
20. Celikel T, Sungur M, Ceyhan B et al. Comparison of noninvasive positive pressure ventilation with standard medical therapy in hypercapnic acute respiratory failure. *Chest*. 1998;114:1636–42.

21. Giacomini M, Iapichino G, Cigada M et al. Short-term noninvasive pressure support ventilation prevents ICU admittance in patients with acute cardiogenic pulmonary edema. *Chest.* 2003;123:2057–61.
22. Soroksky A, Stav D, Shpirer I. A pilot prospective, randomized, placebo-controlled trial of bilevel positive airway pressure in acute asthmatic attack. *Chest.* 2003;123:1018–25.
23. Huang DT. Clinical review: Impact of emergency department care on intensive care unit costs. *Crit Care.* 2004;8:498–502.
24. Wood KA, Lewis L, Von Harz B et al. The use of noninvasive positive pressure ventilation in the emergency department: Results of a randomized clinical trial. *Chest.* 1998;113:1339–46.
25. Plant PK, Owen JL, Elliott MW. Early use of non-invasive ventilation for acute exacerbations of chronic obstructive pulmonary disease on general respiratory wards: A multicentre randomised controlled trial. *Lancet.* 2000;355:1931–5.
26. Diaz GG, Alcaraz AC, Talavera JC et al. Noninvasive positive-pressure ventilation to treat hypercapnic coma secondary to respiratory failure. *Chest.* 2005;127:952–60.
27. Scala R, Naldi M, Archinucci I et al. Noninvasive positive pressure ventilation in patients with acute exacerbations of COPD and varying levels of consciousness. *Chest.* 2005;128:1657–66.
28. Elpern EH, Silver MR, Rosen RL et al. The noninvasive respiratory care unit. Patterns of use and financial implications. *Chest.* 1991;99:205–8.
29. Keenan SP, Gregor J, Sibbald WJ et al. Noninvasive positive pressure ventilation in the setting of severe, acute exacerbations of chronic obstructive pulmonary disease: More effective and less expensive. *Crit Care Med.* 2000;28:2094–102.
30. Plant PK, Owen JL, Parrott S et al. Cost effectiveness of ward based non-invasive ventilation for acute exacerbations of chronic obstructive pulmonary disease: Economic analysis of randomised controlled trial. *BMJ.* 2003;326:956.
31. Carrera M, Marin JM, Anton A et al. A controlled trial of noninvasive ventilation for chronic obstructive pulmonary disease exacerbations. *Am J Respir Crit Care Med.* 2009;179:533–41.
32. Corrado A, Roussos C, Ambrosino N et al. Respiratory intermediate care units: A European survey. *Eur Respir J.* 2002;20:1343–50.
33. Burns KE, Sinuff T, Adhikari NK et al. Bilevel noninvasive positive pressure ventilation for acute respiratory failure: Survey of Ontario practice. *Crit Care Med.* 2005;33:1477–83.
34. Doherty MJ, Greenstone MA. Survey of non-invasive ventilation (NIPPV) in patients with acute exacerbations of chronic obstructive pulmonary disease (COPD) in the UK. *Thorax.* 1998;53:863–6.
35. Sinuff T, Kahnamoui K, Cook DJ et al. Practice guidelines as multipurpose tools: A qualitative study of noninvasive ventilation. *Crit Care Med.* 2007;35:776–82.
36. Lopez-Campos JL, Garcia Polo C, Leon Jimenez A et al. Staff training influence on non-invasive ventilation outcome for acute hypercapnic respiratory failure. *Monaldi Arch Chest Dis.* 2006;3:145–51.
37. Sorensen D, Frederiksen K, Grofte T et al. Practical wisdom: A qualitative study of the care and management of non-invasive ventilation patients by experienced Intensive care nurses. *Intensive Crit Care Nursing.* 2013;29(3);174–81.
38. British Thoracic Society NIV audit 2010. http://britthoracic.org.uk/audit.aspx
39. Esteban A, Ferguson ND, Meade MO et al. Evolution of mechanical ventilation in response to clinical research. *Am J Respir Crit Care Med.* 2008;177:170–7.
40. Stoller JK, Kester L, Roberts VT et al. An analysis of features of respiratory therapy departments that are avid for change. *Respir Care.* 2008;53:871–84.
41. Kollef MH, Shapiro SD, Silver P et al. A randomized, controlled trial of protocol-directed versus physician-directed weaning from mechanical ventilation. *Crit Care Med.* 1997;25:567–74.
42. Ely EW, Meade MO, Haponik EF et al. Mechanical ventilator weaning protocols driven by nonphysician health-care professionals: Evidence-based clinical practice guidelines. *Chest.* 2001;120:454S–63S.
43. Marelich GP, Murin S, Battistella F et al. Protocol weaning of mechanical ventilation in medical and surgical patients by respiratory care practitioners and nurses: Effect on weaning time and incidence of ventilator-associated pneumonia. *Chest.* 2000;118:459–67.
44. Saint S, Kowalski CP, Banaszak-Holl J et al. How active resisters and organizational constipators affect health care-acquired infection prevention efforts. *Joint Comm J Q Patient Safety/Joint Comm Resour.* 2009;35:239–46.
45. Kramer N, Meyer TJ, Meharg J et al. Randomized, prospective trial of noninvasive positive pressure ventilation in acute respiratory failure. *Am J Respir Crit Care Med* 1995;151:1799–806.
46. Sinuff T, Cook D, Giacomini M et al. Facilitating clinician adherence to guidelines in the intensive care unit: A multicenter, qualitative study. *Crit Care Med.* 2007;35:2083–9.
47. Sinuff T, Cook DJ, Randall J et al. Evaluation of a practice guideline for noninvasive positive-pressure ventilation for acute respiratory failure. *Chest.* 2003;123:2062–73.

11

Education programmes/assessment of staff competencies

ALANNA HARE

KEY MESSAGES

- Developing effective educational programmes and ensuring the acquisition and maintenance of professional competence in non-invasive ventilation (NIV) delivery are vital if we wish to increase NIV utilisation rates and enhance the success of NIV therapy.
- One single method of training and assessment will never be adequate if we want a multiprofessional team that is skilled and competent to carry out NIV. Instead, a portfolio of educational tools and assessment methods should be utilised to build an educational programme that brings together professional groups in an integrated fashion, which is reflective of how the service is delivered.
- Key competencies should be identified at the outset, both to ensure transparency and accountability, and to inform the development of the curriculum for training.
- The 'spiral curriculum' is a useful concept in which new clinical skills are related to, and build on, existing skills and knowledge.
- Assessment of competence is key, and skills and knowledge should be evaluated in contextualised, clinical settings to ensure learners are able to integrate their skills and knowledge and wider personal and interpersonal attributes, and can adapt and develop these in different clinical situations.
- Simulation-based education has a great deal to offer in terms of both delivering the curriculum and undertaking assessments. Furthermore, it offers learners a safe and controlled environment to practice and develop skills using the principles of deliberate practice.
- Didactic teaching also has a place in curriculum delivery, and learning can and indeed should, continue at the bedside in daily clinical practice.
- A holistic approach to education and competency assessment for NIV should therefore be adopted, utilising a variety of training and assessment approaches, and thereby laying the foundation for the development of a clinically competent practitioner with the requisite physical and cognitive skills to impact the care of patients requiring NIV in a positive and significant way.

INTRODUCTION

In many areas, despite robust evidence supporting the use of non-invasive ventilation (NIV) across a broad spectrum of respiratory conditions, uptake and use of NIV remains poor.[1–3] There is extensive evidence that medical and nursing team members lack key skills in NIV and feel ill-prepared and unsafe to deliver NIV in accordance with guidelines.[4] The main reasons given for lower utilisation rates of NIV in surveys across the United States and Europe are lack of clinician knowledge and training. Furthermore, clinical experience with NIV seems to be an important factor in its success. A systematic review of the predictors of NIV failure found that patient tolerance of and compliance with NIV therapy is closely related to clinician expertise.[5] Girou et al.,[6] in a study of French intensive care departments, demonstrated a significant reduction in mortality and in the incidence of nosocomial pneumonia as the rate of NIV utilisation increased, changes which the authors attributed to a 'learning effect'. Carlucci et al.[7] also found that increasing clinical experience with the use of NIV meant that more severely ill patients could be treated, whilst maintaining a constant NIV success rate.[7] We know that NIV used in appropriately selected patient groups saves lives and reduces utilisation of resources, and that the way in which NIV is used affects patient outcomes; furthermore, the evidence would suggest that the gap between best evidence and real world practice is, at least in part, driven by a lack of adequate training and education. It seems clear, then, that developing effective educational programmes and ensuring the acquisition and maintenance of professional competence in NIV delivery, are vital if we wish to increase NIV utilisation rates and enhance the success of NIV therapy.

Currently, training in NIV is often neither systematic nor structured. Well-validated educational tools are not used and proven adjunctive methods for procedural teaching are not being translated into clinical practice. This chapter will describe how to build an outcomes-focused curriculum of competencies, utilise evidence-based educational techniques and enhance interprofessional learning to effectively train the multiprofessional team in NIV, in order to ensure high-quality care delivery.

DEVELOPING OUTCOMES FOR LEARNING

The first step in improving education and training in NIV is to develop specific and clear evidence-based learning objectives or competencies. This involves defining and standardising educational outcomes and key competencies for training in NIV at the outset. Explicit standards guide trainees' learning and trainers' instruction. Outcomes should be clinically relevant and emphasise current best practice. In addition to medical knowledge and skills, clinical competence is defined by skill level in multiple functional domains such as interprofessional communication, ethics, attitudes and values, motivation and reflection.[8,9] Competency in NIV requires skills in all of these domains.

In a competency-based approach, it is not knowledge per se that is most important, but rather how this knowledge can be successfully applied.[10] Skills in the practice of NIV should be separated into specific behavioural objectives (competencies) that can be assessed and measured against predetermined standards.[11] This is vital in the healthcare professions in an era of greater public accountability[12] where it is not appropriate for skills in one domain (for example, communication) to compensate for lack of skills in another (for example, procedural skill).[13] It may be appropriate to develop a series of professional competencies, which are appropriate for different professional groups and reflect each group's differing roles and responsibilities in the provision of NIV.

DESIGNING A CURRICULUM FOR LEARNING IN NIV

A competency-based approach to curriculum design ensures that not only are the outcomes of the educational programme clearly defined at the outset, but that they are also taught, learned and assessed during the training programme. Learning should be integrated across the NIV curriculum, so that curricular elements build upon one another, with the predefined competencies as the organising framework.[14] The content of the curriculum should be focused on the qualities and attributes required of competent NIV practitioners.

As shown in Figure 11.1, a spiral curriculum approach[15] is useful and is appropriate to training in clinical skills such as NIV. In this approach, there is consistent revision of core clinical skills throughout the curriculum. Clinical skills are revisited at multiple levels of difficulty and new clinical skills are related to existing skills. The competence of learners thereby increases with each visit to the clinical skill.

Curriculum delivery should ideally utilise a combination of pedagogic approaches. Didactic lectures and written materials may be appropriate to deliver training on patient selection, the physiologic rationale for NIV and the evidence base for practice. Practical, hands-on sessions, by contrast, may focus on interface selection and fitting, and the initial choice and subsequent titration of ventilator settings. Self-directed learning, including online learning, should be encouraged. The use of 'professional' patient educators or carers, who have experience in receiving NIV therapy, can also prove invaluable for training. Training should include practical problem-solving, which may include review of clinical cases that have a number of key learning points that illustrate curricular items. Groups of trainees may also work together, undertaking case-based discussions and presenting their findings and conclusions to other learners for further review. Simulation-based education does not have to involve a large initial financial outlay, since even simple, inexpensive techniques can add value and interest to an educational programme: this will be discussed in more detail later in the chapter.

When developing a new educational programme, trainers would be well-advised to seek out colleagues who already run well-established training programmes for NIV, to gain their advice on what is successful, and what is less so, and to share educational materials. Longer-running training programmes should also be continuously assessed and

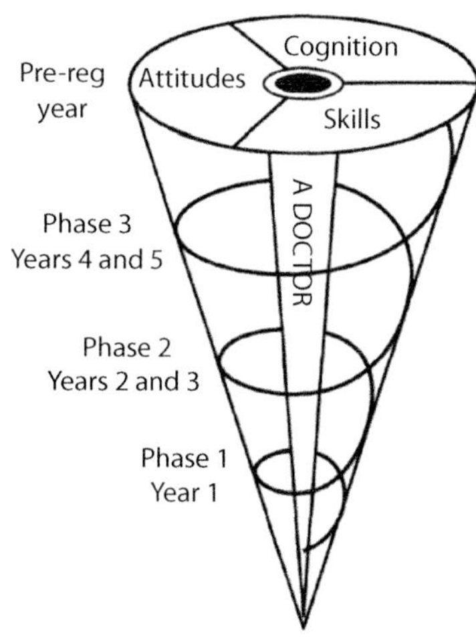

Figure 11.1 Spiral curriculum. (Reproduced from Harden RM, *Med Teach*. 1999;21(2):141–3. With permission.)

reviewed, to ensure the material remains relevant, and the educational programme is delivering the desired outcomes.

A key component of a competency-based curriculum is a reduced emphasis on the time spent training in a particular skill, and a focus instead on progression of skills and attributes.[13] Since different learners will progress at different rates, the amount of time spent in achieving key competencies in NIV will vary and should be tailored to their needs. This kind of training programme therefore needs to be individualised and flexible,[16] and is then more likely to be efficient and engaging.[14] Learners should be encouraged to take responsibility for their own progress through the curriculum, aided by transparent standards, so that they can plan and map their own progression through the training programme.[17] Finally, the importance of ongoing learning and training 'on the job' should not be ignored or underestimated. In a survey by Burns et al.,[18] physicians reported learning more commonly about NIV from colleagues in the workplace than in conferences and hospital education settings. Training and education should therefore continue at the bedside, even once the formal period of instruction in an educational programme has ended.

ASSESSING COMPETENCE IN NIV

Assessment of competence is a key component for ensuring standards in NIV delivery. Once key competencies have been determined, and the curriculum designed to ensure acquisition of these key competencies, learners' progress must be assessed on the basis of demonstrated performance.[16]

In some cases, it may be appropriate for assessments of competence to focus on the demonstration of mastery of some components of practice separately, for example, the understanding of the physiologic rationale for NIV, the evidence base for NIV and appropriate patient selection. For these training outcomes, it may be appropriate for assessments to take place outside of the 'real world' of clinical practice, and a short written examination or verbal assessment (such as a viva) may suffice. The written examination may include the use of multiple choice question formats, and this is particularly advisable if a large number of learners are being tested. Pre- and post-training course assessments are particularly valuable in ensuring the quality of the training programme itself, since they provide a form of quality assurance, ensuring that the programme is fit for purpose in developing NIV competence.

Learners' performance in particular skills may be assessed at the bedside using pre-coded checklists and/or rating scales, which break down the encounter into a series of predetermined performance criteria, aimed at identifying whether the learner has acquired particular competencies. This type of assessment is particularly well suited to, for example, selection and fitting of NIV interfaces, and choice of appropriate initial settings. There are numerous examples of the use of checklists and scoring tools in the evaluation of clinical skills competence in the literature, and it is suggested that educators and trainers review these well-validated tools and use them as a basis for developing their own assessments for NIV competency (see, for example, Schroedl et al.[21] and Wayne et al.[19,20]).

Finally, it is worth commenting that assessment is also a tool for learning, and can provide guidance to the learner, enabling critical self-reflection and effective formative feedback for development.[9]

SIMULATION-BASED EDUCATION FOR NIV

Of course, it is inherently difficult to articulate a complex clinical practice, such as the practical application of NIV, into individual components, and some argue that breaking down a professional clinical role into discrete tasks risks ignoring the links between those tasks, and thereby fails to represent adequately the complexities of real-world clinical practice.[16] There is also a risk that this approach may lead to fragmented learning, and a failure to acquire a coherent understanding of the body of disciplinary knowledge required for the practice of NIV, so that scientific knowledge is shifted into the background at the expense of 'problem-solving'. One potential solution to this problem is the use of simulation-based education.

Simulation-based education is defined as follows:

> 'a person, device or set of conditions which attempts to present [education and] evaluation problems authentically. The student or trainee is required to respond to the problem as he or she would under natural circumstances'[22]

Simulation can take many forms: from static anatomical models for task training such as mannequins for mask-fitting, to computer-based automated simulations, to full-body high-fidelity computer-driven simulators that accurately replicate physiological responses to stimuli. Simulation-based education is based on the principles of Deliberate Practice,[23,24] which involves

> '(a) repetitive performance of psychomotor skills in a focused domain coupled with (b) rigorous skills assessment that provides learners with (c) specific, informative feedback, which results in increasingly (d) betters skills performance in a controlled setting'.[20]

Research in instructional science demonstrates that the acquisition and maintenance of skills expertise in a wide range of skills, including performance in sports, music and chess, but also in clinical medicine, depend on a learner's engagement in deliberate practice of desired educational outcomes.[23] Progress depends on sustained efforts to enhance particular aspects of performance, and repetition alone is not sufficient. Deliberate practice involves learners engaging in repetitive practice with gradually increasing levels of difficulty until the desired standard is achieved.

A key feature of simulation-based education is that learners develop knowledge and skills in clinical practice by engaging in activities that are representative of the real clinical context in which those skills will be used. The focus is on training in accurately reproduced clinical environments, so that learners develop and use their skills in an authentic domain. Individualised learning is encouraged, since the goal is to ensure all learners achieve all educational objectives with little or no variation in outcome.[24]

A growing body of research demonstrates that simulation-based education is effective in terms of skills acquisition[25–28] and that clinical skills acquired during simulation-based training translate directly into improved patient care and better clinical outcomes.[29–31] Simulation provides a safe and controlled environment where learners at all levels, and from across the multiprofessional team, have the opportunity to practice and refine their clinical skills whilst protecting patients from harm.

Simulation-based education therefore offers a number of opportunities for educational programmes in NIV: the practice of selection and fitting of an interface could be performed on a static mannequin, or even on a fellow learner, in a 'low fidelity' environment; selection and titration of settings could be taught through the use of a 'high fidelity' simulated emergency department, or through the use of a computer-driven simulator that accurately models physiologic outcomes of changes in ventilator settings, as in the European Respiratory Society's web-based NIV simulator programme shown in Figure 11.2 (available at http://www.ers-education.org/e-learning/simulators.aspx). There is growing evidence that simulation-based training programmes for NIV are effective in improving knowledge and confidence in NIV.[32,33]

Simulation also enables the assessment of integrated professional performance, enabling evaluation of the complex combination of knowledge, skills and attitudes that are required for the professional practice of NIV in context and in practice. In this form of assessment, there is an inherent recognition that competence in practice requires more than individual domains of knowledge and skill, but also the ability to integrate those skills into professional performance.

INTERPROFESSIONAL EDUCATION

Patients receiving NIV are treated by hospital doctors, general or community doctors, physiotherapists, nurses, technicians, respiratory therapists and many others, and the success of their treatment involves the performance of that group as an effective team.[34,35] Like the other professional competencies described earlier in this chapter, interprofessional learning is a key part of medical education and should be integrated into all clinical training programmes. Lack of knowledge about the work and skills of other professionals, and lack of competence in interprofessional communication, create barriers to achieving effective and safe patient care.[36] McPherson et al., argues that

> 'If interprofessional working is central to good patient care, then being able to work in a team and collaborate with other professionals can no longer be an "optional extra" but must become a core competency'.[34]

There is therefore a powerful argument for bringing the care team together in training for NIV. One way to achieve this might be to create a 'virtual practice' and teach based on the timeline a patient actually experiences: the patient arrives in the emergency room; they are seen and assessed by a nurse, then reviewed by a respiratory therapist or physiotherapist, then admitted to the ward by a doctor. Many mistakes are made at times of care transition; these can and should be addressed in this kind of educational

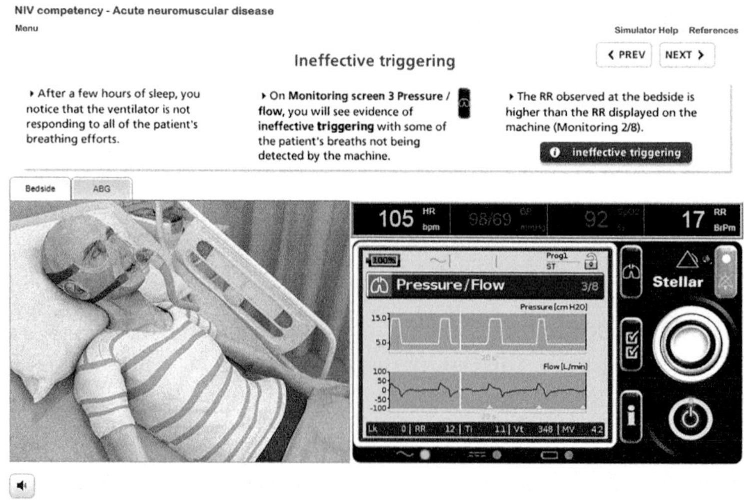

Figure 11.2 European Respiratory Society web-based NIV simulator programme.

approach: teaching the whole team together so they treat the patient together; in this way, learners can discover how to manage the patient, not just set up the ventilator. It is also worth considering whether aspects of the curriculum could be delivered by different members of the multiprofessional team, to further break down professional barriers and engender respect and communication.

REFERENCES

1. Maheshwari V, Paioli D, Rothaar R, Hill NS. VNI – Utilization of noninvasive ventilation in acute care hospitals: A regional survey. *Chest.* 2006;129:1226–33.
2. Vanpee D, Delaunois L, Lheureux P et al. Survey of non-invasive ventilation for acute exacerbation of chronic obstructive pulmonary disease patients in emergency departments in Belgium. *Eur J Emerg Med.* 2002 Sep;9(3):217–24.
3. Carlucci A, Richard JC, Wysocki M et al. Noninvasive versus conventional mechanical ventilation. An epidemiologic survey. *Am J Respir Crit Care Med.* 2001 Mar;163(4):874–80.
4. Plumb JOM, Juszczyszyn M, Mabeza G. Non-invasive ventilation (NIV) a study of junior doctor competence. *Open Med Educ J.* 2010;3:11–7.
5. Nava S, Ceriana P. Causes of failure of noninvasive mechanical ventilation. *Respir Care.* 2004 Mar;49(3):295–303.
6. Girou E, Brun-Buisson C, Taillé S et al. Secular trends in nosocomial infections and mortality associated with noninvasive ventilation in patients with exacerbation of COPD and pulmonary edema. *JAMA.* 2003 Dec 10;290(22):2985–91.
7. Carlucci A, Delmastro M, Rubini F et al. Changes in the practice of non-invasive ventilation in treating COPD patients over 8 years. *Intensive Care Med.* 2003 Mar;29(3):419–25.
8. Kouwenhoven W. Competence based curriculum development in Higher Education: A globalised concept! In: Lazinica A, Calafte C, eds. *Technology, Education and Development.* Vukovar, Croatia: In-Tech; 2009.
9. Epstein RM, Hundert EM. Defining and assessing professional competence. *JAMA.* 2002;287(2): 226–35.
10. Everwijn SEM, Bomers GBJ, Knubben JA. Ability- or competence-based education: Bridging the gap between knowledge acquisition and ability to apply. *High Educ.* 1993;25(4):425–38.
11. Schilling JF, Koetting JR, Lac F Du. Underpinnings of competency-based education. *Athl Train Educ J.* 2010;5(4):165–9.
12. Frank JR, Jabbour M, Fréchette D et al. The CanMEDS 2005 Physician Competency Framework. Better standards. Better physicians. Better care. *Framework.* 2005:1–40 pp.
13. Frank JR, Snell LS, Cate O Ten et al. Competency-based medical education: Theory to practice. *Med Teach.* 2010;32(8):638–45.
14. Carraccio C, Wolfsthal SD, Englander R et al. Shifting paradigms: From Flexner to competencies. *Acad Med.* 2002;77(5):361–7.
15. Harden RM. What is a spiral curriculum? *Med Teach.* 1999;21(2):141–3.
16. Leung W-C. Learning in practice competency based medical training: Review. *BMJ.* 2002;325: 693–6.
17. Harris P, Snell L, Talbot M, Harden RM. Competency-based medical education: Implications for undergraduate programs. *Med Teach.* 2010;32(8):646–50.
18. Burns KE, Sinuff T, Adhikari NKJ et al. Bilevel noninvasive positive pressure ventilation for acute respiratory failure: Survey of Ontario practice. *Crit Care Med.* 2005;33(7):1477–83.
19. Wayne DB, Butter J, Siddall VJ et al. Simulation-based training of internal medicine residents in advanced cardiac life support protocols: A randomized trial. *Teach Learn Med.* 2005;17(3):202–8.
20. Wayne DB, Butter J, Siddall VJ et al. Mastery learning of advanced cardiac life support skills by internal medicine residents using simulation technology and deliberate practice. *J Gen Intern Med.* 2006;21(3):251–6.
21. Schroedl CJ, Corbridge TC, Cohen ER et al. Use of simulation-based education to improve resident learning and patient care in the medical intensive care unit: A randomized trial. *J Crit Care.* 2012;27(2).
22. McGaghie W. Simulation in professional competence assessment: Basic considerations. In: Tekian A, McGuire CH, McGaghie WC, eds. *Innovative Simulations for Assessing Professional Competence.* Chicago: University of Illinois at Chicago, Department of Medical Education; 1999.
23. Ericsson KA. Deliberate practice and the acquisition and maintenance of expert performance in medicine and related domains. *Acad Med.* 2004;79(10 Suppl):S70–81.
24. McGaghie WC, Siddall VJ, Mazmanian PE, Myers J. Lessons for continuing medical education from simulation research in undergraduate and graduate medical education: Effectiveness of continuing medical education: American College of Chest Physicians Evidence-Based Educational Guidelines. *Chest.* 2009;135(3 Suppl):62S–8S.
25. Barsuk JH, Cohen ER, Feinglass J et al. Use of simulation-based education to reduce catheter-related bloodstream infections. *Arch Intern Med.* 2009;169(15):1420–3.
26. Kim J, Park J-H, Shin S. Effectiveness of simulation-based nursing education depending on fidelity: A meta-analysis. *BMC Med Educ.* 2016;16(1):152.

27. McGraw R, Chaplin T, McKaigney C et al. Development and evaluation of a simulation-based curriculum for ultrasound-guided central venous catheterization. *CJEM*. 2016 May 16;1–9.
28. Reed T, Pirotte M, McHugh M et al. Simulation-based mastery learning improves medical student performance and retention of core clinical skills. *Simul Healthc*. 2016 Jun;11(3):173–80.
29. Blum MG, Powers TW, Sundaresan S. Bronchoscopy simulator effectively prepares junior residents to competently perform basic clinical bronchoscopy. *Ann Thorac Surg*. 2004;78(1):287–91.
30. Draycott TJ, Crofts JF, Ash JP et al. Improving neonatal outcome through practical shoulder dystocia training. *Obstet Gynecol*. 2008;112(1):14–20.
31. Seymour NE, Gallagher AG, Roman SA et al. Virtual reality training improves operating room performance: Results of a randomized, double-blinded study. *Ann Surg*. 2002;236(4):458–63; discussion 463–4.
32. Chatwin M, Hare A, Kurosinski P et al. Evaluation of the educational outcomes of simulation-based training (SBT) for NIV: Table 1. *Eur Respir J*. 2015 Sep 30;46(suppl 59):OA4778.
33. McQueen S, Dickinson M, Pimblett M. Human patient simulation can aid staff training in non-invasive ventilation. *Nurs Times*. 106(26):20.
34. McPherson K, Headrick L, Moss F. Working and learning together: Good quality care depends on it, but how can we achieve it? *Qual Health Care*. 2001 Dec;10(Suppl 2):ii46–53.
35. Thistlethwaite J. Interprofessional education: A review of context, learning and the research agenda. *Med Educ*. 2012 Jan;46(1):58–70.
36. Kohn LT, Corrigan JM, Donaldson MS. *To Err Is Human: Building a Safer Health System*. Vol. 21, Annales francaises d'anesthesie et de reanimation; 2000:453–4.

12

Monitoring during acute non-invasive ventilation

EUMORFIA KONDILI, NEKTARIA XIROUCHAKI AND DIMITRIS GEORGOPOULOS

KEY POINTS

- Monitoring is essential to evaluate the efficacy of NIV.
- Significant information is provided by thoughtful clinical observation.
- Continuous recording of heart rate, breathing frequency and pulse oximetry is critical.
- Measurement of expired tidal volume and evaluation of patient–ventilator synchrony may influence the decision-making process.
- For proper monitoring, accurate estimation of leakage is fundamental.
- Non-invasive ventilators do not measure tidal, volume or leak directly, but provide estimates; this should be borne in mind when interpreting the results.

INTRODUCTION

Several studies have shown that non-invasive mechanical ventilation (NIV) represents an effective treatment for acute respiratory failure. This technique has been applied in patients with acute exacerbation of chronic obstructive pulmonary disease (COPD), cardiogenic pulmonary oedema and hypoxaemic respiratory failure due to various causes.[1–4] In addition, NIV has been also used in post-extubation respiratory failure and as a weaning tool mainly in patients with COPD.[5–7] Monitoring is essential to evaluate the efficacy of NIV and to identify patients who will fail on this technique. During the first few hours of NIV, monitoring is mainly performed by a continuous evaluation of the patient's clinical status and arterial blood gases to assess the initial response to this treatment.[8–10] More advanced monitoring is important in order to optimise the efficacy of therapy. This should include monitoring of air leakage, expired tidal volume, patient–ventilator synchrony and sleep quality. Box 12.1 summarises the monitoring requirements during NIV.

The intensive care unit (ICU) or high-dependency unit (HDU) is the best environment of applying NIV.[11,12] These locations offer many capabilities, and close monitoring of the patients is feasible. Nevertheless, due to shortage of ICU or HDU beds, many patients receive NIV in wards.[13] In this case, the intensity of monitoring should be determined by the severity of the respiratory failure and particularly by the risk of NIV failure. The latter is probably the most important determinant of the intensity of monitoring. Therefore, risk factors for NIV failure should be carefully sought and identified[14–16] (see Box 12.1). A patient with multiple risk factors should be closely monitored in the ICU or HDU.[11,12]

CLINICAL EVALUATION

Bedside clinical evaluation is essential, particularly during the first few hours of treatment where the majority of failures occur. Clinical evaluation should include monitoring of patient comfort, work of breathing and neurological and mental status.

Patient comfort

Several studies have shown that poor tolerance to this technique and thus discomfort is an independent risk factor of NIV failure.[8,17] It follows that patient comfort should be closely monitored. Of the various scales that quantify the patient's comfort, the most common is the visual analogue

BOX 12.1: Monitoring during acute NIV

Essential

Regular clinical evaluation

- Comfort (mask and ventilator settings)
- Breathing effort: accessory muscle use; paradoxical breathing
- Synchrony: triggering; expiratory asynchrony
- Air leaks
- Agitation
- Delirium
- Secretion clearance

Complications: nasal erythema, ulceration; conjunctivitis; gastric distention

Continuous recording of heart rate and breathing frequency

Continuous pulse oximetry

Arterial blood gases 1–4 h NPPV and after 1 h of any change in ventilator settings or FiO_2

Desirable

Electrocardiogram

Objective quantification of leaks

Monitoring of expired tidal volume

Graphical display to monitor patient–ventilator synchrony

Invasive monitoring for patients with hemodynamic instability

Sleep evaluation

scale (VAS), which has been validated in mechanically ventilated patients.[18] In addition to patient comfort, attention should be paid to the mask. It is important to make sure that the mask is of an appropriate size with the correct headgear and correctly positioned. Also, attention should be paid to the mask pressures.[19,20] Excessive mask pressures lead to discomfort and skin damage, whereas a weak mask sealing may facilitate air leakage.[10,20]

Work of breathing

One of the main goals of NIV is to minimise the patient's work of breathing. Although precise estimation of work of breathing necessitates the placement of an oesophageal balloon, there are clinical signs that may serve as indirect indices of increased work of breathing. The use of accessory muscles during inspiration, paradoxical abdominal motion and active expiratory efforts are reliable sign of excessive work of breathing. Other signs are tachycardia, increased respiratory rate and diaphoresis.[9,12,21] All these signs should be recorded and carefully monitored. Increased work of breathing is also associated with dyspnoea, which, however, is a highly subjective symptom. It is important for patient monitoring to quantify the dyspnoea sensation, as quantitative measurements of dyspnoea provide a baseline to assess the efficacy of NIV. There are several dyspnoea scales that can be easily used in clinical practice and permit the quantification of dyspnoea and monitor change.[22,23] Ultrasonography allows direct visualisation of the diaphragm and might represent a reliable monitoring technique in evaluating diaphragmatic function during NIV. Indeed, it has been shown that ultrasonographic measurement of the thickening fraction of the diaphragm, calculated as (thickness at inspiration – thickness at expiration)/thickness at expiration, shows a good correlation with diaphragmatic pressure time product – an indirect index of work of breathing (Figure 12.1)[24] (see also Chapter 20).

Evaluation of mental and neurological status

This task is essential especially in patients with acute hypercapnic respiratory failure. Several scales can be used to evaluate the neurological impairment.[25,26] Although in the past, coma has been considered a contraindication for NIV, studies have shown a high success rate of NIV in patients with hypercapnic coma.[27,28] In addition to neurological status, another important aspect that should be monitored is delirium. Several studies have now confirmed that delirium occurs in 60%–80% of mechanically ventilated patients and in up to 50% of non-intubated critically ill patients.[29] Delirium is an independent risk factor for increased morbidity and mortality.[30,31] Although data are lacking regarding the incidence of delirium in patients during NIV, these patients are theoretically prone to this complication since risk factors of delirium are usually present in this population.[32] The occurrence of delirium may significantly affect the patient's tolerance to this treatment. In this regard, we suggest that patients on NIV should be carefully monitored for delirium and treated accordingly.[33] The delirium status can be assessed several times during the day using a well-validated and highly reliable instrument: the Confusion Assessment Method for the ICU (CAM-ICU).[29]

Conventional vital signs

Heart rate and breathing frequency should be monitored, preferably continuously.[34] A decrease in breathing frequency and heart rate within 1 h of NIV is a sign of success.[34,35] In patients without haemodynamic instability, arterial blood pressure may be recorded non-invasively. Urine output should be also measured. Patients with acute hypoxaemia and/or persistent respiratory acidosis, or whose condition is deteriorating, require a higher level of monitoring, which includes central venous access, arterial line and urine catheter.[35] This is particularly true in patients with haemodynamic instability in whom the rate of failure on NIV is very high.[35]

Gas exchange

Improving the gas exchange defects (hypoxaemia and/or hypercapnia) is a priority during NIV. The most commonly

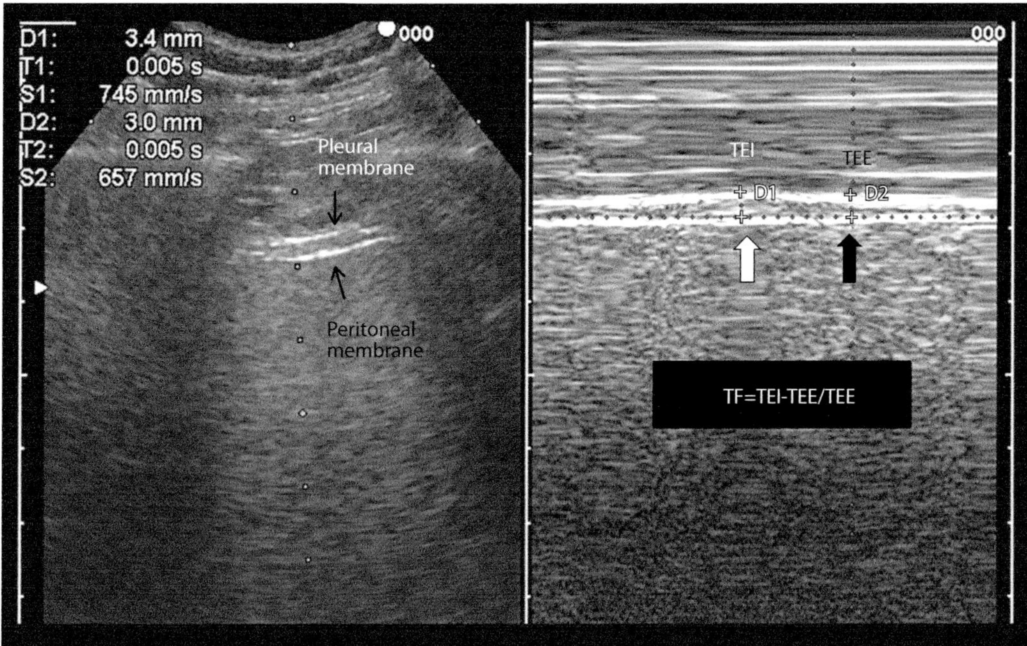

Figure 12.1 Ultrasonographic view of the diaphragm and method of measurement of diaphragmatic thickness at end inspiration and end expiration in time motion mode in one of our patients receiving NIV. TEI, thickness at end inspiration; TEE, thickness at end expiration. In this patient, the work of breathing is relatively low as indicated by the low thickening fraction (TF 13%), thus confirming the ability of NIV to unload the diaphragm.

used method to access oxygenation is the continuous arterial oxygen saturation (SaO_2), which is feasible by continuous pulse oximetry at the bedside (SpO_2).[34,35] All patients should be monitored with pulse oximetry. It should be noted that the addition of oxygen during NIV may occasionally worsen the hypercapnia, particularly in patients with high $PaCO_2$ and rapid shallow breathing pattern.[36,37] If patients have COPD or other risk factors for hypercapnic respiratory failure, a saturation of 88%–92% is recommended, but this can be adjusted to 94%–98% if the $PaCO_2$ is normal (unless there is a history of respiratory failure requiring NIV or invasive positive pressure ventilation).[37] Blood gases should be rechecked after 30–60 min.[37]

Assessment of the $PaCO_2$ remains the gold standard for the evaluation of alveolar ventilation. The opportunity to assess $PaCO_2$ continuously and non-invasively is desirable particularly in patients receiving NIV on a ward. There are two different techniques for non-invasive $PaCO_2$ monitoring: the end-tidal carbon dioxide and the transcutaneous PCO_2 measurements.[38–40] End tidal CO_2 is not accurate in patients with lung disease particularly during NIV and should not be used even as a trend monitor. See Chapter 19.

Blood gases should be obtained on admission and after 1–4 h.[12,35] Several studies have shown that changes in arterial blood gases and acid–base status after a short period of NIV application predict the successful outcome.[41–43] Arterialised capillary or venous blood gases are an alternative (see Chapter 19). Ventilator settings should be adjusted based on results of blood gases obtained within 1 h and as necessary at 2–4 h intervals.[35,44]

MONITORING OF LEAKS

NIV is a semi-open system, and thus air leaks are inherent to its design. Leaks commonly occur through the mouth (with nasal masks) or around the interface. These are termed non-intentional leaks. Leaks may also occur through expiratory ports or valves that are placed in the circuit close to or directly on the mask (intentional leaks). An important characteristic of a ventilator delivering NIV is its ability to recognise and compensate for leaks in the system. Ideally, leak compensation should automatically affect the triggering and cycling-off functions to maintain optimum ventilator performance. Even though most of the modern ICU ventilators and bi-level devices may compensate for leakage, this ability is significantly compromised in the presence of excessive leaks.[45] In addition, marked differences have been observed between ventilators as far as the ability to compensate for leaks is concerned.[45–47]

Excessive non-intentional leaks have a detrimental effect on the efficiency of NIV. With all modes of mechanical ventilation, air leaks reduce the efficiency of NIV by altering the actual tidal volume that the patient receives and impairing the triggering and cycling-off functions of the ventilator (see below).[45–47] Furthermore, excessive leaks may cause the patient discomfort, arousal and sleep fragmentation.[45,48] In addition to non-intentional leaks, intentional leaks may also affect ventilator performance and the quality of ventilation.[45] In this regard, independently of their origin, air leaks should be monitored. Gross air leaks can be easily assessed at the bedside. Vibration of lips or other structures around

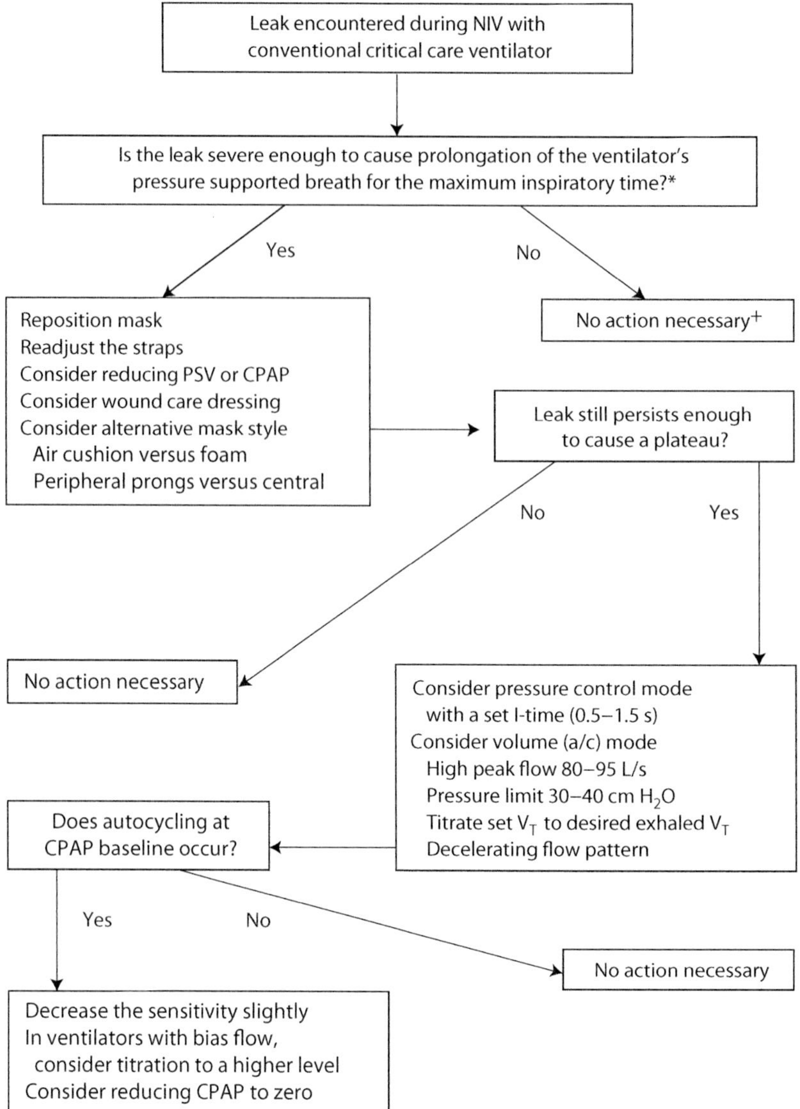

Figure 12.2 Approach in patients with significant air leakage while receiving continuous positive airway pressure and pressure support. *: this can reduce respiratory rate, cause air trapping and increase work of breathing. +: tidal volume (V_T) remains constant as long as the leak does not cause an inspiration plateau. (From Meduri GU, *Clin Chest Med.* 1996;17(3):513–53. With permission.)

the airway is indicative of air leaks. Less obvious leaks can be detected by tactile means, i.e. by placing hands near the mouth or seal and feeling for air; however, this method has low sensitivity, and it does not allow for quantification of the amount of air leakage. In some ventilators, the expired volume is continuously monitored, and leaks can be calculated by subtracting expired volume from the corresponding inspiratory volume. In some new-generation bi-level positive airway pressure (BiPAP) devices, leaks are automatically estimated with sophisticated algorithms and are displayed on the screen of the ventilator breath by breath. Even with these systems, estimates of the quantity of leakage may be inaccurate. Inspection of the pressure volume and flow waveform provided by the new-generation ventilators on a breath-by-breath basis may be helpful for identifying leakage. Greater area under the inspiratory flow curve than that under the expiratory flow is indicative of air leaks. In addition, identification of leak-associated asynchronies such as auto-triggering and prolonged inspiration (see below) allows the detection of air leaks. Since leaks may affect both the function of the ventilator and patient comfort, every effort should be made to minimise these (Figure 12.2).

MONITORING TIDAL VOLUME

During NIV, the tidal volume results from both the airway pressure delivered by the ventilator and the respiratory muscle pressure generated by the patient's respiratory drive. A recent study performed by Carteaux et al.[49] examined the relationships between tidal volume and NIV failure in patients with acute de novo hypoxaemic respiratory failure.

A tidal volume target of 6–8 mL/kg PBW was impossible to achieve in the majority of patients receiving NIV. Additionally, a tidal volume higher than 9.5 mL/kg PBW over the first 4 h of NIV application accurately predicts NIV failure in patients with moderate to severe hypoxaemia.[49]

MONITORING PATIENT–VENTILATOR ASYNCHRONY

Asynchrony is defined as the uncoupling of ventilator-delivered inspiratory flow from the patient's ventilatory demands in terms of either timing or drive.[50,51] In intubated patients, the mode of ventilation, ventilator settings and respiratory system mechanics are the main factors that determine both the incidence and the severity of asynchrony.[50,51] During NIV, there are two additional factors that modify the patient–ventilator asynchrony. These are the presence of air leaks and the type of interface. These factors complicate the issue of patient–ventilator synchrony during NIV. The prevalence of patient–ventilator asynchrony during NIV was recently evaluated in a multicentre study by Vignaux et al.[52] who studied a group of 60 patients receiving NIV for acute respiratory failure and found that 43% of the patients exhibited severe asynchrony. The most frequent asynchrony was prolonged insufflation, which was present in 23% of the patients. This was followed by double triggering (15%), auto-triggering (13%), ineffective efforts (13%) and premature cycling (12%).[52]

Patient–ventilator asynchrony can be assessed at the bedside by the interpretation of ventilator waveforms.[51,53] In most of the new-generation ICU and portable ventilators, pressure, flow and volume waveforms are continuously displayed on the screen on a breath-by-breath basis. This non-invasive approach is a valuable tool that allows the physician to recognise patient–ventilator asynchrony and take the appropriate action.[51,53] However, it should be noted that significant information can be provided by clinical observation. The physician should focus on the expansion of both the rib cage and the abdomen while listening for the timing and coordinated triggering of the ventilator.

Non-invasive methods such as impedance plethysmography and magnetometry may also be helpful for identifying patient–ventilator asynchrony; however, currently both methods are mainly used for research proposes and not for everyday clinical practice. More detailed monitoring, such as estimation of various indices of respiratory neural and motor output, requires complex methods such as evaluation of diaphragmatic EMG and calculation of transdiaphragmatic pressure and instantaneous pressure output of the respiratory muscles. These approaches, however, necessitate the placement of oesophageal electrodes and oesophageal and gastric catheters.

Recently, new technologies for automatic detection of patient–ventilator asynchrony have been introduced aiming to monitor and improve patient–ventilator interaction.[54–57] These systems use the airway pressure, volume and flow waveforms as a tool to identify patient effort. The effectiveness of these systems in intubated patients in terms of recognising triggering delay, ineffective effort and expiratory asynchrony has been clinically evaluated and recently reported.[54–57] It should be noted, however, that data are lacking regarding the accuracy of these systems during NIV, in which the occurrence of leaks is a common phenomenon.

Identifying patient–ventilator asynchrony during the triggering phase

AUTO-TRIGGERING

Auto-triggering occurs when the ventilator is triggered in the absence of inspiratory muscle contraction.[51,53] It may be caused by a low triggering threshold, excessive leaks, the presence of water in the circuit and/or cardiogenic oscillation.[51,53] During NIV, air leaks represent by far the most significant factor leading to auto-triggering. It has been shown that the use of a ventilator with good leak compensation system practically eliminates this type of dyssynchrony.[49] With pressure triggering, an absence of the initial pressure drop below the end-expiratory pressure is indicative of auto-triggering.[51,53] A short cycle during PSV with different flow-time waveform than previous breaths is also indicative of auto-triggering (Figure 12.3). Cycles triggered by signals that do not come from the patient may cause, among other complications, discomfort and should be corrected.[51,53]

EXCESSIVE TRIGGERING DELAY AND INEFFECTIVE EFFORT

During NIV, air leaks and excessive ventilator support are the most important causes of triggering delay and ineffective effort. A recent clinical study showed a significant correlation between the magnitude of leaks and the number of ineffective efforts.[52] Although most of the modern ventilators compensate for air leaks by automatically adjusting the triggering threshold, this capability is significantly affected by the presence of large intentional or non-intentional leaks.[43,46,47] Furthermore, clinical studies have demonstrated that the type of interface may also affect patient–ventilator asynchrony during the triggering phase.[58,59] Ineffective efforts and triggering delays can be detected with accuracy through the inspection of flow-time and/or airway pressure–time waveforms (Figure 12.3).[51,53]

Identifying patient–ventilator asynchrony during the pressure delivery phases

Ineffective efforts during the pressure delivery phase represent a common form of asynchrony during NIV.[52] It is mainly promoted by high ventilator assistance, which, during pressure support, is associated with prolonged inspiration due to increased air leaks.[52] Ineffective efforts during insufflation can be identified using the flow or P_{aw} (airways pressure) waveform depending on the mode of support.[51,53] With assist volume control, ineffective efforts are mainly presented as a transient P_{aw} distortion, although this distortion is not

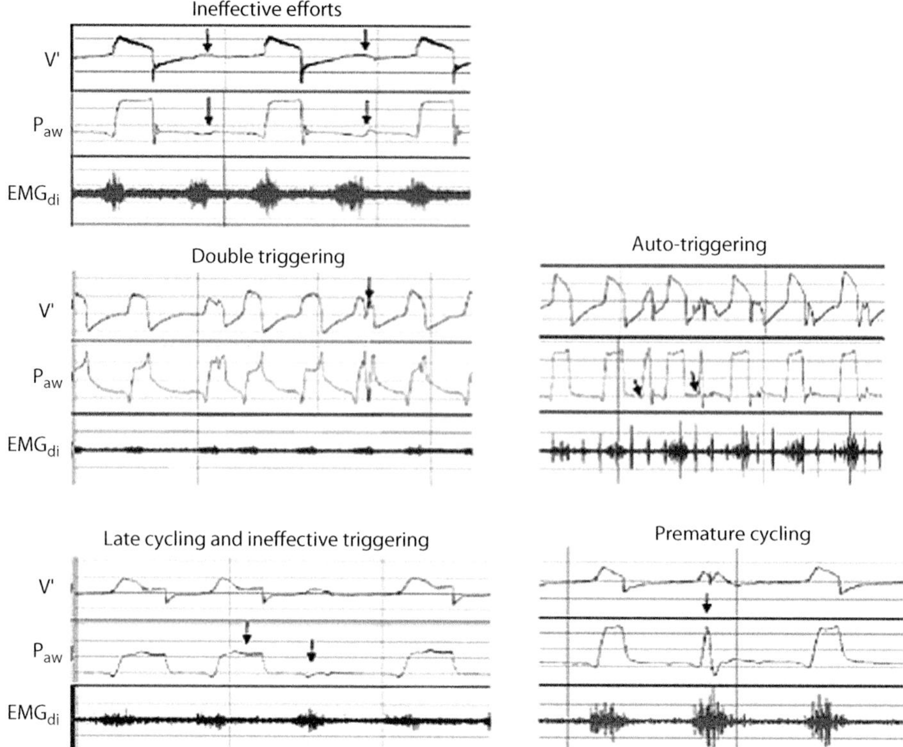

Figure 12.3 Flow (V'), airway pressure (P_{aw}) and diaphragmatic electromyography (EMGdi), in a patient ventilated on pressure support during NIV. *Ineffective efforts:* Observe the flow distortion during expiration (arrows), which is not followed by a mechanical breath, signifying the presence of ineffective efforts. Note also that the signal of flow distortion is much clearer than the corresponding P_{aw} change. *Double triggering:* Note that in the sixth breath (arrow), one inspiratory effort triggered the ventilator twice. *Auto-triggering:* Observe that the third and fifth breaths (arrows) are triggered in the absence of the patient's inspiratory effort (no EMG activity). Note also that auto-triggering results in a distortion in flow waveform (arrows). *Premature cycling:* Note that in the second breath, EMGdi activity continues far beyond the end of the ventilatory inspiratory time. Also note that in this breath the premature opening of the exhalation valve is indicated by an abrupt drop in P_{aw} from peak pressure to baseline (arrow). *Late cycling and ineffective triggering:* Note that in all breaths due to the presence of leaks, the ventilator continues to insufflate far beyond the end of EMGdi activity (arrow). Under this circumstance, the time available for expiration is reduced, resulting in the presence of an ineffective effort. (Modified from Vigneaux L et al., *Intensive Care Med.* 2009;35(5): 840–846. With permission.)

always easy to recognise. With pressure support, ineffective efforts are mainly observed during prolonged insufflations as an abrupt increase in inspiratory flow.[51,53]

In some of the new-generation ventilators, the pressurisation rate with PS (defined as the incremental increase in P_{aw} per time unit) is adjustable in order to optimise patient–ventilator synchrony. Prinianakis et al.[60] observed that a rapid pressurisation rate was associated with a reduction in the pressure–time product, an index of oxygen consumption of the diaphragm. However, this resulted in increased air leakage[60] (Figure 12.4). Since both leaks and patient discomfort may modify the effectiveness of NIV, the pressurisation rate should not be set to very high.[60] Finally, the caregiver should check whether the demands of the patient are being met by the ventilator-delivered flow.[53] By observing the contour of P_{aw} during assist volume control and that of flow during PS, the caregiver may have an estimate of the patient respiratory effort.[53] Nevertheless, we should note that the presence of leaks may interfere with this technique, and monitoring this type of asynchrony is not always easy.

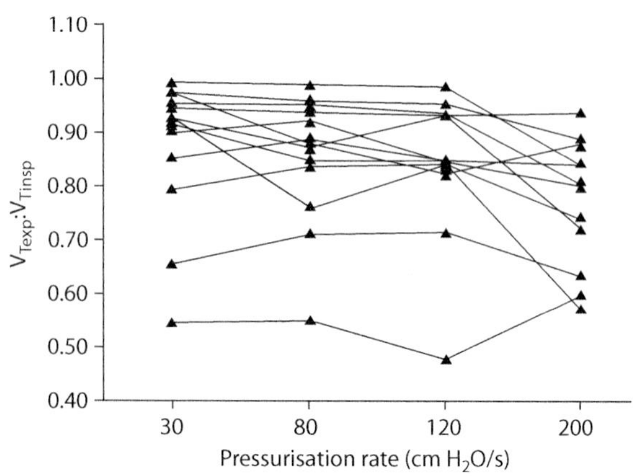

Figure 12.4 Amount of air leaks through the mask, as assessed by the ratio between expiratory (VTexp) and inspiratory tidal volume (VTinsp) for the different values of pressurisation rate for each patient. (From Prinianakis G et al., *Eur Respir J.* 2004;23(2):314–320. With permission.)

Identifying patient–ventilator asynchrony during the cycling-off phase (expiratory asynchrony)

Two types of expiratory asynchrony have been recognised: premature opening of the expiratory valve, in which the end of mechanical inflation precedes the end of neural inspiration; and delayed opening of the expiratory valve, in which the end of mechanical inflation follows the end of neural inspiration.[51,53]

PREMATURE OPENING OF THE EXHALATION VALVE

During assisted modes of support, premature opening of the exhalation valve is evidenced by the presence of zero or small inspiratory flow for some time immediately after P_{aw} decreases to the positive end-expiratory pressure (PEEP) level,[51,53] and a sharp decline in the peak expiratory flow that lasts a few milliseconds and is followed by an increase and then a gradual decrease to zero at the end of expiration (Figure 12.3).[51,53] In the P_{aw} waveform, premature expiratory opening is indicated by an abrupt drop from peak pressure to baseline rather than the expected gradual decay because of the finite resistance of the expiratory ventilator circuit.[51,53]

In some breaths, inspiratory effort after opening of the exhalation valve reverses the expiratory flow to an inspiratory flow (in-flow triggering system); in addition, inspiratory effort can reduce P_{aw} to below the PEEP and thereby initiate the triggering process. In this case, one inspiratory effort triggers the ventilator twice (or even more; see Figure 12.3).[51,53] Expiratory asynchrony due to premature opening of the valve may be minimised by actions that increase the mechanical inflation time or decrease the neural inspiratory time. The latter is particularly important in patients with prolonged inspiratory efforts due to excessive administration of opioids. On the other hand, in order to increase the mechanical inflation time, the mode of support should be taken into consideration. In patients ventilated with pressure mode, mechanical inflation time may be increased by decreasing the flow threshold for cycling off, increasing the pressure support level or decreasing the rising time. With pressure or volume control modes, the increase in mechanical inflation may be easily achieved by proper adjustment of ventilator setting (i.e. inspiratory time, pause time, inspiratory flow).

DELAYED OPENING OF THE EXHALATION VALVE

The ventilator permits transition from inspiration to expiration according to a predetermined cycling-off criterion. The most commonly used criterion is the decrease in inspiratory flow to a predetermined percentage of peak inspiratory flow. During NIV, the presence of leaks may lead to a prolonged mechanical inspiration because the delivered flow remains above the flow threshold for cycling off. Under this circumstance, the time available for expiration is reduced and the patient is at risk of triggering delay and ineffective efforts (Figure 12.3). The frequency of delayed cycling and ineffective efforts correlates with the magnitude of the leaks.[52] Prolonged mechanical inspiration can be eliminated by reducing either the leaks or the ventilator inspiratory time.[52,60,61] Calderini et al.[61] demonstrated that patient–ventilator synchrony is improved and patient effort is reduced with time cycling compared to flow cycling (Figure 12.5). In

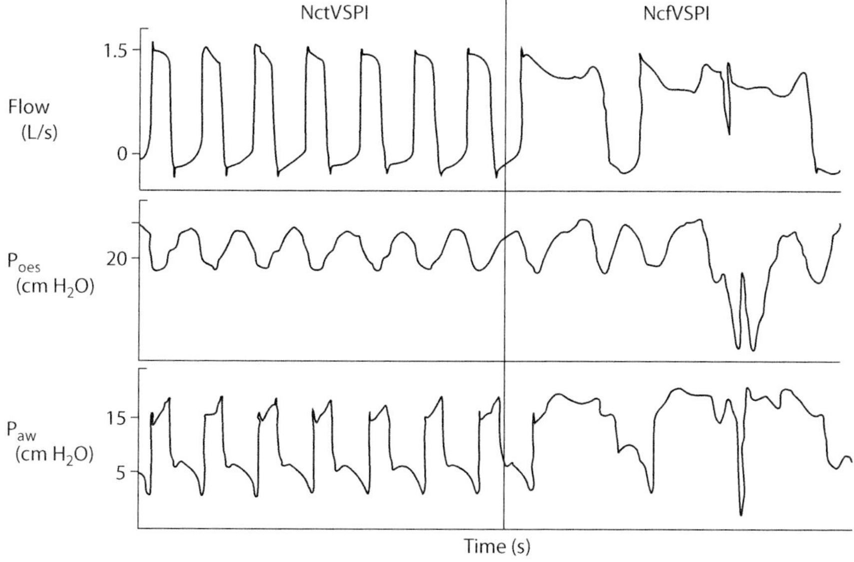

Figure 12.5 Representative experimental record in a patient treated with NIV using time and conventional flow percentage as cycling-off criterion. Notice the perfect synchronisation between patient and machine during time cycling-off criterion. With flow cycling-off criterion, the prolonged mechanical assist into the neural expiratory time results into wasted next inspiratory effort, as evident by the following negative deflections on the Poes curve. (From Calderini E et al., *Intensive Care Med.* 1999;25(7):662–667. With permission.)

patients ventilated with PS, the continuation of mechanical inflation into neural expiration is evidenced by a rapid decrease in inspiratory flow followed by an exponential decline toward the end of mechanical inspiration, and a small spike (increase) in airway pressure (P_{aw}) near the end of the breath.[51,53]

SLEEP EVALUATION

Clinical studies using both polysomnographic data and patients' perceptions have shown a poor quality of sleep among mechanically ventilated patients.[62–66] Although data are lacking regarding the sleep quality of patients during NIV, it is unlikely to be better than those on invasive mechanical ventilation in acute settings, considering the significant sleep disruptions that are caused by the frequent mask readjustments required to prevent air leakage, the air leak per se and the significant sleep deprivation.[63,67,68] Detailed sleep evaluation is only feasible through overnight polysomnography studies. Considering the difficulty of performing polysomnography studies in acute settings and the absence of data supporting the necessity of routine sleep evaluation, we do not recommend sleep studies in this population. Evaluation of sleep might be done using clinical criteria, which, however, are not accurate.

MONITORING OF COMPLICATIONS

Complications that should be monitored during NIV are skin necrosis particularly over the bridge of the nose (with masks), carbon dioxide retention (with helmet), retention of secretions, abdominal distension and upper airway obstruction.[69]

CONCLUSIONS

During NIV, close monitoring is important in order to optimise therapy and minimise complications as well as the risk of treatment failure. The intensity of monitoring depends on the patient's condition and the location where NIV is applied. Essential monitoring should include regular clinical evaluation and continuous pulse oximetry. In the last two decades, significant technical advances in ventilators and interfaces have allowed detailed monitoring, which may guide the caregiver to take actions to reduce leaks and improve the patient–ventilator synchrony, crucial obstacles during this modality of ventilatory support. It should, however, be emphasised that advanced monitoring is not a substitute for detailed clinical evaluation. In addition, advanced monitoring effectiveness depends on adequate data interpretation, a task that is not always easy, necessitating background knowledge and skills.

REFERENCES

1. Brochard L, Mancebo J, Wysocki M et al. Noninvasive ventilation for acute exacerbations of chronic obstructive pulmonary disease. *N Engl J Med.* 1995;333(13):817–22.
2. Confalonieri M, Potena A, Carbone G et al. Acute respiratory failure in patients with severe community-acquired pneumonia. A prospective randomized evaluation of noninvasive ventilation. *Am J Respir Crit Care Med.* 1999;160(5 Pt 1):1585–91.
3. Ferrer M, Esquinas A, Leon M et al. Noninvasive ventilation in severe hypoxemic respiratory failure: A randomized clinical trial. *Am J Respir Crit Care Med.* 2003;168(12):1438–44.
4. Lightowler JV, Wedzicha JA, Elliott MW, Ram FS et al. Non-invasive positive pressure ventilation to treat respiratory failure resulting from exacerbations of chronic obstructive pulmonary disease: Cochrane systematic review and meta-analysis. *BMJ.* 2003;326(7382):185.
5. Keenan SP, Powers C, McCormack DG, Block G. et al. Noninvasive positive-pressure ventilation for postextubation respiratory distress: A randomized controlled trial. *JAMA.* 2002;287(24):3238–44.
6. Ferrer M, Valencia M, Nicolas JM et al. Early non-invasive ventilation averts extubation failure in patients at risk: A randomized trial. *Am J Respir Crit Care Med.* 2006;173(2):164–70.
7. Nava S, Gregoretti C, Fanfulla F et al. Noninvasive ventilation to prevent respiratory failure after extubation in high-risk patients. *Crit Care Med.* 2005;33(11):2465–70.
8. Demoule A, Girou E, Richard JC et al. Increased use of noninvasive ventilation in French intensive care units. *Intensive Care Med.* 2006;32(11):1747–55.
9. Nava S, Hill, N. Non-invasive ventilation in acute respiratory failure. *Lancet.* 2009; 374(9685): p. 250–9.
10. Kelly CR, Higgins AR, Chandra S. Noninvasive positive-pressure ventilation. *N Engl J Med.* 2015;373(13):1279.
11. Hill NS. Where should noninvasive ventilation be delivered? *Respir Care.* 2009;54(1):62–70.
12. Elliott MW, Confalonieri M, Nava S. Where to perform noninvasive ventilation? *Eur Respir J.* 2002;19(6):1159–66.
13. Plant PK, Owen JL, Elliott MW. Early use of non-invasive ventilation for acute exacerbations of chronic obstructive pulmonary disease on general respiratory wards: A multicentre randomised controlled trial. *Lancet.* 2000;355(9219):1931–5.
14. Confalonieri M, Garuti G, Cattaruzza MS et al. A chart of failure risk for noninvasive ventilation in patients with COPD exacerbation. *Eur Respir J.* 2005;25(2):348–55.

15. Thille AW, Boissier F, Ben-Ghezala H et al. Easily identified at-risk patients for extubation failure may benefit from noninvasive ventilation: A prospective before-after study. *Crit Care*. 2016;20:48.
16. Lightowler JV, Elliott MW. Predicting the outcome from NIV for acute exacerbations of COPD. *Thorax*. 2000;55(10):815–6.
17. Demoule A, Girou E, Richard JC et al. Benefits and risks of success or failure of noninvasive ventilation. *Intensive Care Med*. 2006;32(11):1756–65.
18. Mahler DA. Dyspnea: Diagnosis and management. *Clin Chest Med*. 1987;8(2):215–30.
19. Fraticelli AT, Lellouche F, L'her E et al. Physiological effects of different interfaces during noninvasive ventilation for acute respiratory failure. *Crit Care Med*. 2009;37(3):939–45.
20. Kwok H, McCormack J, Cece R et al. Controlled trial of oronasal versus nasal mask ventilation in the treatment of acute respiratory failure. *Crit Care Med*. 2003;31(2):468–73.
21. Garpestad E, Brennan J, Hill NS. Noninvasive ventilation for critical care. *Chest*. 2007;132(2):711–20.
22. Borg GA. Psychophysical bases of perceived exertion. *Med Sci Sports Exerc*. 1982;14(5):377–81.
23. Mahler DA, Weinberg DH, Wells CK, Feinstein AR et al. The measurement of dyspnea. Contents, interobserver agreement, and physiologic correlates of two new clinical indexes. *Chest*. 1984;85(6):751–8.
24. Vivier E, Mekontso Dessap A, Dimassi S et al. Diaphragm ultrasonography to estimate the work of breathing during non-invasive ventilation. *Intensive Care Med*. 2012;38(5):796–803.
25. Pape TL, Senno RG, Guernon A, Kelly JP. A measure of neurobehavioral functioning after coma. Part II: Clinical and scientific implementation. *J Rehabil Res Dev*. 2005;42(1):19–27.
26. Jagger J, Jane JA, Rimel R. The Glasgow coma scale: To sum or not to sum? *Lancet*. 1983;2(8341):97.
27. Diaz GG, Alcaraz AC, Talavera JC et al. Noninvasive positive-pressure ventilation to treat hypercapnic coma secondary to respiratory failure. *Chest*. 2005;127(3):952–60.
28. Scala R, Naldi M, Archinucci I et al. Noninvasive positive pressure ventilation in patients with acute exacerbations of COPD and varying levels of consciousness. *Chest*. 2005;128(3):1657–66.
29. Ely EW, Inouye SK, Bernard GR et al. Delirium in mechanically ventilated patients: Validity and reliability of the confusion assessment method for the intensive care unit (CAM-ICU). *JAMA*. 2001;286(21):2703–10.
30. Ely EW, Shintani A, Truman B et al. Delirium as a predictor of mortality in mechanically ventilated patients in the intensive care unit. *JAMA*. 2004;291(14):1753–62.
31. Thomason JW, Shintani A, Peterson JF et al. Intensive care unit delirium is an independent predictor of longer hospital stay: A prospective analysis of 261 non-ventilated patients. *Crit Care*. 2005;9(4):R375–81.
32. Girard TD, Pandharipande PP, Ely EW. Delirium in the intensive care unit. *Crit Care*. 2008;12(Suppl 3):S3.
33. Charlesworth M, Elliott MW, Holmes JD. Noninvasive positive pressure ventilation for acute respiratory failure in delirious patients: Understudied, under-reported, or underappreciated? A systematic review and meta-analysis. *Lung*. 2012;190(6):597–603.
34. Organized jointly by the American Thoracic Society, the European Respiratory Society, the European Society of Intensive Care Medicine, and the Société de Réanimation de Langue Française, and approved by ATS Board of Directors. International Consensus Conferences in Intensive Care Medicine: Noninvasive positive pressure ventilation in acute Respiratory failure. *Am J Respir Crit Care Med*. 2001;163(1):283–91.
35. Hill NS, Brennan J, Garpestad E, Nava S et al. Noninvasive ventilation in acute respiratory failure. *Crit Care Med*. 2007;35(10):2402–7.
36. Stradling JR. Hypercapnia during oxygen therapy in airways obstruction: A reappraisal. *Thorax*. 1986;41(12):897–902.
37. O'Driscoll BR, Howard LS, Davison AG; British Thoracic Society. et al. BTS guideline for emergency oxygen use in adult patients. *Thorax*. 2008;63(Suppl 6):vi1–68.
38. Cox M, Kemp R, Anwar S et al. Non-invasive monitoring of CO2 levels in patients using NIV for AECOPD. *Thorax*. 2006;61(4):363–4.
39. Storre JH, Steurer B, Kilobits HJ et al. Transcutaneous PCO2 monitoring during initiation of noninvasive ventilation. *Chest*. 2007;132(6):1810–6.
40. Lermuzeaux M, Meric H, Sauneuf B et al. Superiority of transcutaneous CO2 over end-tidal CO2 measurement for monitoring respiratory failure in nonintubated patients: A pilot study. *J Crit Care*. 2016;31(1):150–6.
41. Meduri GU, Abou-Shala N, Fox RC et al. Noninvasive face mask mechanical ventilation in patients with acute hypercapnic respiratory failure. *Chest*. 1991;100(2):445–54.
42. Meduri GU. Noninvasive positive-pressure ventilation in patients with acute respiratory failure. *Clin Chest Med*. 1996;17(3):513–53.
43. Mehta S, Hill NS. Noninvasive ventilation. *Am J Respir Crit Care Med*. 2001;163(2):540–77.
44. Elliott MW. Noninvasive ventilation in chronic ventilatory failure due to chronic obstructive pulmonary disease. *Eur Respir J*. 2002;20(3):511–4.
45. Borel JC, Sabil A, Janssens JP et al. Intentional leaks in industrial masks have a significant impact on efficacy of bilevel noninvasive ventilation: A bench test study. *Chest*. 2009;135(3):669–77.

46. Ferreira JC, Chipman DW, Hill NS, Kacmarek RM. Bilevel vs ICU ventilators providing noninvasive ventilation: Effect of system leaks: A COPD lung model comparison. *Chest*. 2009;136(2):448–56.
47. Vignaux L, Tassaux D, Jolliet P. Performance of noninvasive ventilation modes on ICU ventilators during pressure support: A bench model study. *Intensive Care Med*. 2007;33(8):1444–51.
48. Wysocki M, Richard JC, Meshaka P. Noninvasive proportional assist ventilation compared with noninvasive pressure support ventilation in hypercapnic acute respiratory failure. *Crit Care Med*. 2002;30(2):323–9.
49. Carteaux G, Lyazidi A, Cordoba-Izquierdo A et al. Patient–ventilator asynchrony during noninvasive ventilation: A bench and clinical study. *Chest*. 2012;142(2):367–76.
50. Kondili E, Prinianakis G, Georgopoulos D. Patient–ventilator interaction. *Br J Anaesth*. 2003;91(1):106–19.
51. Kondili E, Xirouchaki N, Georgopoulos D. Modulation and treatment of patient-ventilator dyssynchrony. *Curr Opin Crit Care*. 2007;13(1):84–9.
52. Vignaux L, Vargas F, Roeseler J et al. Patient-ventilator asynchrony during non-invasive ventilation for acute respiratory failure: A multicenter study. *Intensive Care Med*. 2009;35(5):840–6.
53. Georgopoulos D, Prinianakis G, Kondili E. Bedside waveforms interpretation as a tool to identify patient-ventilator asynchronies. *Intensive Care Med*. 2006;32(1):34–47.
54. Chen CW, Lin WC, Hsu CH et al. Detecting ineffective triggering in the expiratory phase in mechanically ventilated patients based on airway flow and pressure deflection: Feasibility of using a computer algorithm. *Crit Care Med*. 2008;36(2):455–61.
55. Mulqueeny Q, Ceriana P, Carlucci A et al. Automatic detection of ineffective triggering and double triggering during mechanical ventilation. *Intensive Care Med*. 2007;33(11):2014–8.
56. Younes M, Brochard L, Grasso S et al. A method for monitoring and improving patient–ventilator interaction. *Intensive Care Med*. 2007;33(8):1337–46.
57. Blanch L, Sales B, Montanya J et al. Validation of the Better Care(R) system to detect ineffective efforts during expiration in mechanically ventilated patients: A pilot study. *Intensive Care Med*. 2012;38(5):772–80.
58. Vargas F, Thille A, Lyazidi A et al. Helmet with specific settings versus facemask for noninvasive ventilation. *Crit Care Med*. 2009;37(6):1921–8.
59. Miyoshi E, Fujino Y, Uchiyama A et al. Effects of gas leak on triggering function, humidification, and inspiratory oxygen fraction during noninvasive positive airway pressure ventilation. *Chest*. 2005;128(5):3691–8.
60. Prinianakis G, Delmastro M, Carlucci A et al. Effect of varying the pressurisation rate during noninvasive pressure support ventilation. *Eur Respir J*. 2004;23(2):314–20.
61. Calderini E, Confalonieri M, Puccio PG et al. Patient–ventilator asynchrony during noninvasive ventilation: The role of expiratory trigger. *Intensive Care Med*. 1999;25(7):662–7.
62. Cooper AB, Thornley KS, Young GB et al. Sleep in critically ill patients requiring mechanical ventilation. *Chest*. 2000;117(3):809–18.
63. Gonzalez MM, Parreira VF, Rodenstein DO. Noninvasive ventilation and sleep. *Sleep Med Rev*. 2002;6(1):29–44.
64. Parthasarathy S. Sleep during mechanical ventilation. *Curr Opin Pulm Med*. 2004;10(6):489–94.
65. Parthasarathy S, Tobin MJ. Effect of ventilator mode on sleep quality in critically ill patients. *Am J Respir Crit Care Med*. 2002;166(11):1423–9.
66. Parthasarathy S, Tobin MJ. Sleep in the intensive care unit. *Intensive Care Med*. 2004;30(2):197–206.
67. Gonzalez J, Sharshar T, Hart N et al. Air leaks during mechanical ventilation as a cause of persistent hypercapnia in neuromuscular disorders. *Intensive Care Med*. 2003;29(4):596–602.
68. Meyer TJ, Pressman MR, Benditt J et al. Air leaking through the mouth during nocturnal nasal ventilation: Effect on sleep quality. *Sleep*. 1997;20(7):561–9.
69. Gregoretti C, Confalonieri M, Navalesi P et al. Evaluation of patient skin breakdown and comfort with a new face mask for non-invasive ventilation: A multi-center study. *Intensive Care Med*. 2002;28(3):278–84.

13

Troubleshooting non-invasive ventilation

NICHOLAS S. HILL, MAYANKA TICKOO AND NAJIA INDRESS

KEY MESSAGES

- NIV failure is common, ranging from less than 10% to more than 50% depending on the patient population and other factors.
- Risk for NIV failure can be assessed a priori based on known risk factors, and should be considered when deciding whether or not to initiate NIV.
- Once initiated, NIV should be closely monitored in an appropriate setting.
- Common problems applying NIV such as mask discomfort and suboptimal ventilator settings should be handled proactively by adjusting masks and settings, and trying alternative masks.
- Other common problems include excessive unintentional air leaks, patient–ventilator asynchrony and inability to ventilate or oxygenate.
- Appropriate measures should be undertaken to stabilize and reverse these problems, but it can't be overemphasized that if these have failed, delaying a needed intubation is dangerous and to be avoided.

INTRODUCTION

Non-invasive ventilation (NIV) has assumed an important role in the management of respiratory failure, with surveys indicating that it comprises 20%–40% of initial ventilator starts in acute care hospitals in Europe and North America.[1,2] Strong evidence now supports the use of NIV as the ventilator modality of first choice to treat respiratory failure due to chronic obstructive pulmonary disease (COPD) exacerbations[3] and acute cardiogenic pulmonary oedema[4] with numerous other potential applications.[5] Yet, NIV can be very challenging to administer, with failure rates (need for intubation or death, mainly in do-not-intubate patients) exceeding 40% in some studies.[6,7] This high failure rate underlines the importance of troubleshooting for reversible contributing factors and strategies for managing them. The following presents a systematic approach to management of problems frequently encountered during use of NIV that predisposes to failure and is meant to serve as a troubleshooting guide for clinicians aiming to optimise success rates. The focus will be on the acute care setting, but some principles discussed will be relevant to the long-term setting as well.

PREDICTORS OF NIV FAILURE (SEE ALSO CHAPTER 17)

A number of investigations have identified factors associated with NIV success or failure, as summarised in Boxes 13.1[8–10] and 13.2.[11,12] These can be useful in informing clinicians on identifying potentially modifiable factors as well as avoiding patients at high risk of failing NIV so that success rates can be improved.

A fairly consistent picture emerges from these studies to assess the risk of NIV failure. Patients with an inability to cooperate with the technique or coordinating their breathing with the ventilator, unable to handle their secretions, excessive air leaking or a high severity of acute illness, especially with multi-organ system failure, fare poorly with NIV. Greater severity of the oxygenation defect is also a risk factor for failure, but not so for greater carbon dioxide retention, which correlates with success in some studies.

BOX 13.1: Predictors of failure: NIV for hypercapnic respiratory failure

- Advanced age
- Higher acuity of illness (APACHE score)
- Uncooperative
- Poor neurological score
- Unable to coordinate breathing with ventilator
- Large air leaks
- Edentulous
- Tachypnoea (>35/min)
- Acidaemia (pH <7.18)
- Failure to improve pH, heart and respiratory rates or Glasgow Coma Score within the first 2 hours*

*Most powerful predictor.

Adapted from Soo Hoo GW et al., *Crit Care Med* 1994; 22: 1253–61; Ambrosino N et al., *Thorax* 1995; 50: 755–7; Confalonieri M et al., *Eur Respir J* 2005; 25: 348–55.

BOX 13.2: Predictors of failure: NIV for hypoxaemic respiratory failure

- Diagnosis of acute respiratory distress syndrome (ARDS) or pneumonia
- Simplified Acute Physiology Score (SAPS) ≥35
- Lower PaO_2/FIO_2 (low 100s or below)
- Low pH
- Age >40 years
- Septic shock
- Multiorgan system failure
- Failure to improve PaO_2/FIO_2 >146 within first hour

Adapted from Antonelli M et al., *Intensive Care Med* 2001; 27: 1718–28; Rana S et al., *Crit Care* 2006; 10: R79.

Furthermore, the failure to manifest an early (within an hour or two) favourable response to NIV is a strong predictor of a poor outcome.

REASONS FOR NIV FAILURE

Predictors of NIV failure permit clinicians to estimate the risk of failure in a given candidate being considered for NIV, but specific reasons for failure can be identified only after failure has occurred. Thus, a major goal of NIV management is to anticipate problems likely to arise during NIV use and address them before they lead to NIV failure. Common specific reasons for NIV failure are listed in Box 13.3.[13] Considerable overlap exists between the categories, so it is difficult to accurately determine the occurrence of the specific reasons for failure. For example, patients who fail to improve their ventilation on NIV may be unable to tolerate adequate inspiratory pressure or to synchronise with the ventilator, or have excessive air leaking or airway secretions or some combination of these factors. Investigators analysing reasons for failure attempt to categorise patients according to primary reasons for failure, but these categorisations are open to interpretation. Nonetheless, these categories assist clinicians in identifying situations that may lead to failure and lead to strategies for dealing with them. The following will address each of these reasons commonly cited for NIV failure and discuss possible approaches to alleviating them.

BOX 13.3: Common reasons for NIV failure

Environmental/caregiver team factors
- Lack of skilled, experienced caregiver team
- Poor patient selection
- Lack of adequate monitoring

Patient-related factors
- Intolerance
- Mask problems: discomfort; poor fit; skin ulceration; claustrophobia
- Agitation
- Excessive secretions, inability to protect airway
- Progression of underlying disease

Technical factors
- Inadequate equipment
- Failure to ventilate
- Failure to oxygenate
- Patient–ventilator asynchrony
- Air leaks

Environmental/caregiver team factors in NIV failure

In order to avoid problems with NIV and promptly deal with those that arise, NIV must be administered in an appropriate environment by a knowledgeable, skilled team in well-selected patients. The importance of developing a skilled, experienced team to optimise the delivery of mechanical ventilation is discussed in more detail in Chapter 10.

Selection of appropriate patients for NIV

Regardless of the specific reason for NIV failure, selection of patients at very high risk of NIV failure will lead to high failure rates. Thus, one of the most important ways to avoid problems with the administration of NIV is to select appropriate recipients and avoid those at very high risk. Patient selection is a key responsibility of the physician and should be based on evidence from the medical literature, available guidelines and knowledge of risk factors for NIV failure (as discussed above) and clinical judgement.

As evidence regarding the use of NIV has accumulated,[14] it has become clear that certain forms of respiratory failure, such as that due to COPD exacerbations or cardiogenic pulmonary oedema, are well suited for it.[3,15] These entities are usually characterised by intact upper airway function and prompt reversibility with medical therapy, usually within hours for cardiogenic pulmonary oedema and within days for COPD. Other forms of acute respiratory failure that may benefit from NIV include that occurring in immunocompromised patients, who are at very high risk of healthcare-acquired pneumonias and other infections that are avoided by NIV.[16,17] NIV may be tried in many other forms of acute respiratory failure, but the evidence to support these applications is weaker, and such patients should be monitored closely to optimise success.

An assessment of risk factors for NIV failure is also important when deciding on whether a patient should receive NIV. The risk factors listed in Boxes 13.1 and 13.2 are helpful in stratifying risk for patients with hypercapnic and hypoxaemic respiratory failure, respectively, and should be considered before initiating NIV. Patients deemed at excessively high risk for NIV failure should forego a trial entirely, and those at high risk might undergo a cautious trial in a closely monitored ICU setting with plans to intubate if there is no clear evidence of improvement within the first hour or two.

The decision to initiate NIV, though, must often be made quickly at the bedside with little information other than that gleaned from direct observation of the patient. Thus, it must be based on simple observations and measurements, often before arterial blood gas results are known, because loss of valuable time initially can predispose to failure later. The first step in selection is to assess the need for ventilatory assistance (Box 13.4) based on the presence of at least moderate dyspnoea, evidence of increased work of breathing and an appropriate cause of respiratory failure. Such patients are at risk of needing intubation if NIV is not initiated promptly.

The second step is to ascertain that there are no contraindications to NIV that would render its use excessively risky (Box 13.5). Some of these are absolute, such as a respiratory arrest, but most are relative, such as excessive agitation or secretions, and require assessment based on experience.

BOX 13.4: Selection guidelines for NIV in the acute setting

- Appropriate diagnosis with potential reversibility (i.e. COPD or congestive heart failure [CHF])
- Establish need for ventilatory assistance
  - Moderate to severe respiratory distress

and

  - Tachypnoea (>24 for COPD, >30 for CHF)
  - Accessory muscle use or abdominal paradox
  - Blood gas derangement: pH <7.35, $PaCO_2$ >45, or PaO_2/FiO_2 <300*

*Awaiting return of blood gas results is discouraged in very dyspnoeic patients to avoid delays in initiation.

BOX 13.5: Contraindications to NIV

- Respiratory or cardiac arrest
- Too unstable (e.g. hypotensive shock, myocardial infarction requiring intervention, uncontrolled ischaemia or arrhythmias, uncontrolled upper gastrointestinal bleed, unevacuated pneumothorax)
- Unable to protect airway*
  - Excessive secretions
  - Poor cough
  - Impaired swallowing
- Aspiration risk*
  - Distended bowel; obstruction or ileus
  - Frequent vomiting
- Uncooperative or agitated*
- Unable to fit mask
- Recent upper airway or oesophageal surgery
- Multiorgan system failure (more than 2)

*Relative contraindications.

Once again, when in doubt, the clinician can either intubate upfront or initiate a trial of NIV in a closely monitored setting and proceed to intubation if there is no improvement.

Proper monitoring of NIV

Effective troubleshooting of NIV is impossible without adequate monitoring. Unless detected and addressed promptly, problems arising with the administration of NIV can precipitate NIV failure. Selection of a proper location for administration of NIV is important, based on the patient's need for monitoring and the capabilities of the unit.[18] Patients deemed at higher risk of NIV failure, such as those with greater gas exchange derangement, increased airway secretions, impaired cough, severe respiratory distress, marginal vital signs or altered mental status, should be monitored in a more closely observed setting such as an ICU or respiratory step-down unit. One potentially useful method for establishing the patient's need for monitoring is to temporarily remove the NIV mask and determine the length of time before deterioration occurs and NIV must be reinitiated. If this occurs within minutes, a closely monitored setting would be mandatory. Alternatively, if the patient can tolerate more than 20 or 30 min without needing NIV and is capable of calling for help if necessary, location on a regular hospital ward might be appropriate. Erring on the side of caution is prudent, however, with patients placed in a higher intensity setting until it is clear that they have stabilised.

Potential complications should be anticipated and prevented, if possible, such as by routinely using artificial skin or other protective coverings at the first sign of skin redness over the bridge of the nose. The value of monitoring by a skilled and experienced team cannot be overestimated. For further information about monitoring during NIV, see Chapter 11.

PATIENT-RELATED FACTORS CONTRIBUTING TO NIV FAILURE

Problems may arise during NIV because of patient-related factors such as inability to tolerate NIV or agitation that often precipitate NIV failure unless promptly addressed. Sometimes these occur in a particularly anxious patient or are related to progression of the underlying process rendering NIV failure inevitable, but these may be reversible if recognised and managed early enough. A strategy to deal with intolerance/agitation is depicted in Figure 13.1.

Intolerance of NIV

Intolerance is one of the most commonly cited reasons for NIV failure but is not precisely defined. In a general sense, it describes a patient who becomes uncomfortable or agitated and demands that the mask be removed or removes it themselves. Specific reasons for intolerance include mask discomfort, the sensation of claustrophobia and discomfort related to excessive pressure from the ventilator. Respiratory distress and associated anxiety causing agitation also contribute to the problem. While most patients with intolerance to NIV essentially 'declare' themselves at the initiation of therapy, late failure (after >48 h of initial improvement) has also been reported in patients with acute hypercapnic respiratory failure, underlining the importance of continued monitoring.[19]

Mask discomfort

Many patients find the interfaces used for NIV uncomfortable, and this is one of the most common reasons for intolerance of NIV. Some discomfort occurs in most patients using NIV, and the aim should be to make the mask tolerable. Patients with respiratory distress initially may feel a sense of suffocation when the mask is first strapped on and need reassurance. Giving cooperative patients a sense of control by having them hold the mask in place may facilitate initiation.

An ill-fitting mask, a mask type that is unacceptable to the patient, or excessively tightened straps may also contribute to mask intolerance. A properly fitting mask is essential to NIV tolerance. Some masks come with gauges to assist with fitting. Usually, the smallest mask that just accommodates the nose and mouth is the best choice; excessively large masks can contribute to air leaking and may necessitate more tightening of the straps to control the leaks.

Patients also differ markedly in their preferences for mask types. In the acute setting, oronasal masks that cover both the nose and mouth are better tolerated than nasal masks as the initial mask choice, largely because of better control of mouth leaks.[20] In the long-term setting, however, nasal masks are rated by patients as more comfortable than oronasal.[21] Thus, switching to a nasal mask after initial oronasal mask use may be desirable for some patients who are to be continued on NIV after the first days or so of use. Also, patients who are claustrophobic or are expectorating

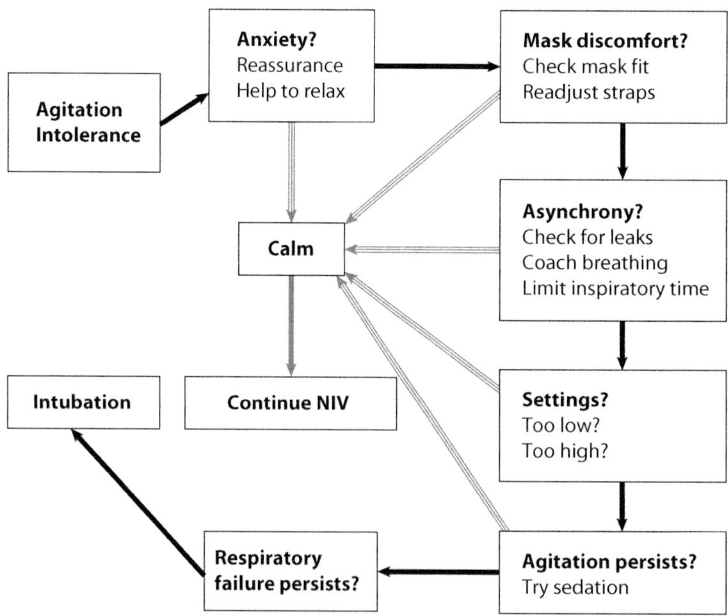

Figure 13.1 Schematic suggesting an approach to the agitated/intolerant patient using NIV. Black solid arrows indicate persisting agitation despite intervention, and striped arrows indicate that the patient is becalmed so that NIV can continue. According to the schema, the first step is to see if anxiety responds to reassurance. Failing that, readjust the mask, eliminate asynchrony and check the ventilator settings. If those fail, try chemical sedation. If the patient remains agitated and in respiratory failure, perform intubation.

frequently may fare better with the nasal mask for initiation. If a nasal mask is used, however, the patency of the nasal passages should be assured.

Many mask types besides the typical nasal or oronasal ones are now available that may be more comfortable for some patients because they are larger and seal around the perimeter of the face, avoiding the nose and mouth. Nasal prongs may be useful in patients developing nasal ulcers because they seal in the nares and not on the bridge of the nose. These and 'hybrid' masks that combine nasal prongs with a mask that fits over the mouth are more often used in the long-term setting. The 'helmet', used mainly in certain European centres,[22] seals over the neck and shoulders using straps secured under the axillae and may offer a more comfortable alternative for some patients. A recent single center study randomised ARDS patients to receive NIV via a helmet as opposed to a facemask and showed significant reductions in intubation rate as well as 90 day mortality in those using the helmet.[23] However, cost and noise (related to the high gas flow rates needed to minimise rebreathing) may be barriers to more widespread helmet use.[24] As mentioned above, the capability of quickly trying different mask types may enhance tolerance in the acute setting, so having a 'mask bag' containing a number of different choices attached to the non-invasive ventilator can be advantageous (see also Chapter 6).

Other mask-related problems

In the past, ulceration on the bridge of the nose has been reported to occur in up to 40% of patients using certain kinds of masks,[25] but should be an infrequent occurrence today because of advances in mask technology and heightened awareness of the problem. Newer masks have soft silicone seals that are less apt to traumatise the face, and some have forehead spacers that help to relieve tension on the nose. In addition, artificial skin should be applied over the bridge of the nose either routinely or at the first sign of nasal skin irritation as indicated by redness over the bridge of the nose.

Claustrophobia

Claustrophobic reactions commonly lead to NIV intolerance. Many patients feel panic when a mask is tightly strapped over their nose or nose and mouth, especially when they are sensing respiratory distress. Self-reported patient dyssynchrony in the form of increased sensation of pressure and subjective dyspnea has been reported to be an independent predictor of NIV failure.[26] These patients have a natural desire to remove the mask, but may respond to verbal reassurance. Giving them control over the mask during initiation by having them hold it in place may also help. Using a mask that covers less of the face such as a nasal mask or nasal prongs instead of an oronasal mask may help, but many patients require sedation (see below). Sometimes, though, the claustrophobic reaction and aversion to the mask are so intense that NIV failure is unavoidable.

Intolerance of ventilator settings

Suboptimal adjustment of ventilator settings may also contribute to intolerance. Excessively high pressures contribute to discomfort, not only via direct effects on the ears and sinuses causing burning and pain, but also because they promote air leaks and necessitate greater tightening of the mask straps. Insufficient pressures may contribute to intolerance because of inadequate alleviation of respiratory distress. An excessively high backup rate or increase in inspiratory pressure 'rise time' may also contribute to ventilator asynchrony and intolerance. (See later the section 'Patient–Ventilator Asynchrony' for a more extensive discussion.)

Agitation

Agitation is another commonly cited reason for NIV intolerance and failure. It refers to a state of high anxiety, usually associated with uncooperativeness, with the patient grabbing at and removing the mask, and unable to coordinate breathing with the ventilator. The term is non-specific and may be precipitated by claustrophobia or mask discomfort. It may also be associated with underlying delirium, referring to a state of inattention and disorientation, which becomes manifest when the patient is stressed by having to use NIV. Agitation contributes to NIV failure because the patient is unable to relax and let the ventilator assist with the breathing load.

Strategies to deal with agitation should first focus on non-pharmacological measures such as verbal reassurance, efforts to enhance comfort, giving the patient control over the mask or, if the respiratory insufficiency is not too severe, frequent 'vacations' from NIV (Figure 13.1). Sometimes, however, sedation is necessary to calm the patient. Most pulmonary and critical care physicians in North America and Europe are reluctant to use sedation because of the perceived risks of interfering with ability to protect the airway or depressing respiratory drive.[27,28] (See Chapter 14 for a detailed review of the use of sedation during NIV.)

Excessive secretions

Excessive secretions or the inability to adequately cough or swallow are listed as contraindications to NIV. However, these are relative, because many patients succeed with NIV despite the presence of secretions or cough or swallowing impairment. Thus, a clinical judgement must be made in these patients as to whether the problems are so severe as to preclude the use of NIV. Sometimes, patients with mild or moderate impairment of airway protection undergo a trial of NIV under close observation and preparedness to intubate if they fail to respond favourably.

While these patients are under observation, some interventions may be helpful. Clinicians should ascertain that hydration is adequate and provide humidification of inhaled gas to avoid desiccation of mucus. Mucolytics such as acetylcysteine should also be considered, although this may provoke bronchospasm in patients with airway hyperreactivity. In some patients, chest physiotherapy sometimes coupled with postural drainage can help. Vest-like devices that vibrate the chest can also help to dislodge mucus, although they appear to be of greatest help in patients with bronchiectasis or cystic fibrosis.[29] For patients with weakened cough muscles, cough in-exsufflators can be sufficiently effective in facilitating cough to avoid intubation.[30] They are used most often in outpatients with neuromuscular disease,[31] but may have applications in the acute setting as well. Recently, interest has been mounting in high flow nasal therapy (HFNT) as a means to facilitate secretion removal by virtue of humidifying gas at high flows, avoiding dessication of mucus and preserving mucociliary function.[9]

Progression of the underlying process

NIV may succeed initially yet fail after the first 24 or 48 h because of progression of the underlying disease.[32] This is a particular concern in patients with severe hypoxaemic respiratory failure and underlying pneumonia or ARDS who may succumb to excessive secretions, progressive hypoxaemia or multiorgan system failure, conditions that overwhelm the capabilities of NIV and necessitate intubation. Antonelli et al.[13] found that in a cohort of 354 patients with hypoxaemic respiratory failure treated with NIV, inability to correct hypoxaemia was the most common cause of NIV failure between 24 and 48 h after initiation of therapy, while inability to manage secretions or to correct dyspnoea were distant second and third causes. Higher severity of illness scores including septic shock,[9] APACHE II[33] or SAPS II[34] scores, low PaO_2:FiO_2 ratio in ARDS[35] as well as higher lactate[7] at presentation (markers of severity of critical illness) have all been found to predict increased NIV failure. While hypercarbic respiratory failure usually responds well to NIV, the presence of bronchiectasis and pneumonia, low GCS and cough strength at initiation as well as failure of improvement in PaO_2:FiO_2 ratio between hours 1 and 3 of therapy predict late failure for these patients.[36] Other comorbidities at presentation such as severe hyperglycaemia or significant functional impairment also predict late NIV failure.[36] Considering that unanticipated emergency intubations add to the morbidity and mortality of these patients and are to be avoided, patients deemed to be at risk of NIV failure due to progression of the underlying disease must be monitored closely in a general or respiratory ICU and intubated promptly when deemed necessary to avoid a respiratory arrest and its attendant morbidity and mortality.

TECHNICAL FACTORS CONTRIBUTING TO NIV FAILURE

NIV failure may sometimes be related to inadequate equipment, inability to reverse hypoventilation or hypoxaemia, asynchrony or inadequately controlled air leaks.

Proper equipment for NIV

The skill to properly apply equipment is probably more important than the equipment itself. But proper equipment can make a difference, particularly masks. As discussed in the section 'Intolerance of NIV', having familiarity with the many mask choices available and a mask bag containing a variety of types and sizes of masks attached to the ventilator is strongly recommended.

No studies have convincingly demonstrated the superiority of one ventilator type over another. For acute applications of NIV, newer 'bi-level positive pressure devices' have advantages over older bi-level devices in that they have much improved monitoring and alarm systems, better graphic displays, oxygen blenders, sophisticated algorithms to limit inspiratory time and enhance synchrony and an internal battery to facilitate transport. These factors, especially the oxygen blender, can make the difference between success and failure in patients with hypoxaemic respiratory failure. Most other 'bi-level ventilators' were designed to deliver NIV at home and not to ventilate challenging hypoxaemic patients. They lack an oxygen blender, and even when oxygen is supplemented into a 'T' connector in the ventilator tubing or directly into the mask, maximal fraction of inhaled oxygen concentration (FiO_2) reaches only 45%–50%.[37]

On most 'critical care ventilators', 'NIV' modes are now available that enhance leak compensation, silence 'nuisance' alarms and limit inspiratory time. Few have been tested clinically, but bench studies indicate that these do not all function the same.[38,39] In the face of air leaks, caregivers must be prepared to make additional adjustments on most of these ventilators,[39] but they appear to function better at delivering NIV than traditional pressure support modes that were used in the past. Despite the advantages of the newer ventilators, it is important to keep in mind that many ventilator types, including both 'bi-level' and 'critical care', can be adjusted to deliver NIV successfully. The lack of newer, sophisticated ventilators is no reason to avoid using NIV unless a patient with hypoxaemic respiratory failure cannot be adequately oxygenated.

Failure to ventilate

A commonly cited reason for NIV failure, failure to adequately assist ventilation, is encountered most often in patients with acute hypercapnic respiratory failure, most of whom have COPD. Reported NIV success rates among patients with acute hypercapnic respiratory failure are high, usually above 70%[13,17] and sometimes even exceeding 90%.[40]

Nonetheless, failures to improve ventilation do occur, often associated with other factors that interfere with the effectiveness of NIV, including intolerance or agitation, patient–ventilator asynchrony or excessive air leaks.

Obviously, a major aim in treating acute or acute-on-chronic respiratory acidosis is to lower $PaCO_2$ and raise pH. For this reason, clinicians are encouraged to obtain baseline arterial blood gases for comparison with a repeat test after the first hour or two of therapy. If $PaCO_2$ rises substantially during this interim (>10 mm Hg, for example), intubation should be contemplated. However, the drop in $PaCO_2$ is often gradual,[17] and as long as other aims are being achieved (decreased respiratory rate and dyspnoea in a haemodynamically stable patient), a rise in $PaCO_2$ might be tolerated initially without resorting to intubation.

Nonetheless, reasons for lack of improvement in $PaCO_2$ should be sought, even if intubation is not deemed urgent, to reduce the eventual need. Intolerance, refusal to wear the mask and asynchrony with the ventilator can be addressed as discussed above, and air leaks are discussed in more detail below. Failure to adequately ventilate can also be caused if the ventilator is set inappropriately and the driving pressure or 'pressure support' that assists each patient breath is too small. Low inspiratory (8–10 cm H_2O) and expiratory (4–5 cm H_2O) pressures are often used to facilitate patient tolerance initially, but unless the difference between inspiratory and expiratory pressure – the 'driving' pressure or pressure support – is promptly increased, many patients will derive too little ventilatory assistance to improve ventilation. As with the use of pressure support in an intubated patient, the pressure support level should be increased until the patient's tidal volume reaches 6–7 mL/kg and respiratory rate decreases, ideally, to the low 20s.[41] These targets may not be achievable if the increase in inspiratory pressure causes too much discomfort, but the highest tolerable inspiratory pressure should be used. Arterial blood gases, vital signs and subjective adaptation should be monitored closely in an ICU or intermediate care environment until stability is assured.

Failure to oxygenate

With the exception of cardiogenic pulmonary oedema, failure rates for NIV are higher for hypoxaemic than for hypercapnic failure, approaching or even exceeding 50% in some studies.[42,43] Also, most non-cardiogenic oedema patients with hypoxaemic respiratory failure are poor candidates for NIV, and selection of appropriate candidates with hypoxaemic respiratory failure is challenging. Nonetheless, there may be subgroups of patients with hypoxaemic respiratory failure whose outcomes would be improved by use of NIV (see above).[44] Although multiple reasons contribute to the higher NIV failure rate, including mask intolerance and failure to correct dyspnoea, the most commonly cited reason in these patients is failure to oxygenate.[13]

Strategies to deal with persistent hypoxaemia during NIV include assurance that a mask that covers the nose and mouth is being used. In a prospective, randomised trial, Kwok et al.[23] found that the oronasal mask was better tolerated initially than nasal masks because of fewer mouth leaks and associated desaturation episodes. In addition, hypoxaemic patients must be watched closely in an intensive care unit (ICU) until stabilised because mask dislodgement can precipitate severe desaturations that lead to NIV failure unless detected and corrected promptly. Furthermore, as discussed above, the ventilator must be capable of delivering high FiO_2s, generally by means of an oxygen blender, and sufficient FiO_2 must be delivered to maintain a target O_2 saturation, usually greater than 90%. Also, as mentioned above, different interfaces such as the helmet may offer benefit for patients with ARDS.[2]

Once the appropriateness of the mask and ventilator to treat hypoxaemic patients is assured, ventilator adjustments may be helpful to enhance oxygenation. Just as positive end-expiratory pressure (PEEP) is helpful to maintain oxygenation in invasively ventilated patients, so increases in expiratory pressure are helpful in oxygenating patients on NIV. However, increases are limited because of patient intolerance and the tendency of high mask pressures to increase air leaks. Also, to maintain the pressure support level, the inspiratory pressure must be raised in tandem with the expiratory pressure, something that can heighten intolerance. Thus, during acute applications of NIV to treat oxygenation failure, the maximum tolerated expiratory pressure is usually in the range of 8–10 cm H_2O. As is true in invasive mechanical ventilation, excessive tidal volumes may be harmful in patients with de novo acute hypoxic respiratory failure treated with NIV; Carteaux et al.[45] found that patients with higher mean tidal volumes (VT_e) had a higher rate of NIV failure than those with lower tidal volumes. In another group of patients with hypoxaemic respiratory failure, L'Her et al.[46] found that, as might be anticipated, increases in pressure support to as high as 15 cm H_2O improved ventilation and reduced dyspnoea. On the other hand, increases in PEEP to 10 cm H_2O improved oxygenation, but at the expense of reduced patient comfort. They recommended titration to arrive at a compromise, enhancing oxygenation without sacrificing too much comfort.

Patients with respiratory failure due to pneumonia or ARDS are at risk for progression of the underlying process over a period of hours or days after initiation of NIV. For this reason, NIV for oxygenation failure may still fail even after 24–48 h of ventilation.[13] The need to watch these patients in a closely monitored setting and to avoid delays in needed intubation cannot be overemphasised. Also, a chest radiograph should be obtained routinely in patients with failure to ventilate or oxygenate because progression of pneumonia, worsening CHF and pneumothoraces are possible contributors.

Unanticipated respiratory arrests and the need for emergency intubation in these patients greatly add to morbidity and mortality and should be avoided by anticipating the need for intubation before it arises. Also, if PEEP levels of

10 cm H_2O or below are insufficient to adequately oxygenate patients with hypoxaemic respiratory failure or if sophisticated ventilatory techniques such as pressure release ventilation or high-frequency oscillation are needed, then intubation and invasive ventilator management should be performed without delay.

Patient–ventilator asynchrony

In the ideal situation, the ventilator should precisely follow the patient's neural output from the respiratory centre, as signified by neural activity of the phrenic nerves, assisting or replacing the action of the diaphragm. Patients breathing asynchronously with the ventilator cannot take full advantage of the pressure increase meant to be delivered in time with diaphragmatic activity and thus do not realise the benefits of reduced inspiratory work of breathing or improved gas exchange. Furthermore, the asynchrony contributes to discomfort and agitation as the patient exhales against the higher inspiratory pressure or inhales when the ventilator is providing insufficient airflow. Thus, patient–ventilator asynchrony is a significant cause of NIV failure.

Intermittent patient–ventilator asynchrony is virtually universal among patients receiving NIV and need not be cause for concern as long as the large majority of breaths are synchronous and the patient is reasonably comfortable. But as more breaths become asynchronous, the efficacy of NIV becomes more compromised and NIV failure more likely. Vignaux et al.[47] found that 43% of patients receiving NIV for ARF had severe asynchrony that contributed to discomfort. Thus, prompt attention to the problem of patient–ventilator synchrony is a key to NIV success.

Asynchrony can be related to many potentially reversible factors during NIV use. Patients must learn how to adjust their breathing pattern to benefit from NIV when first starting, and coaching from an experienced caregiver with instructions like 'try to breathe slower and let the respirator breathe for you' can be very helpful. Many patients become anxious and uncomfortable during initiation of NIV, causing them to breathe asynchronously, and may respond to reassurance or, if these non-pharmacological interventions fail, judicious doses of anxiolytics and/or analgesics. Mask discomfort or inappropriate ventilator settings (too high contributing to discomfort or too low failing to relieve respiratory distress) may also contribute to agitation and thereby asynchrony.

Pressure support modes commonly have problems synchronising with the breathing pattern of COPD patients, whether ventilated invasively or non-invasively. Auto-PEEP occurs commonly during exacerbations, increasing the inspiratory effort required to initiate the next breath and leading to failure to trigger (initiate the next ventilator breath). Also, inspiratory flow may not drop rapidly at the end of inspiration related to lack of lung recoil causing the ventilator to continue inspiratory pressure in the face of the patient's attempt to exhale, referred to as failure to cycle or 'expiratory asynchrony'.[48] The inspiration can be quite prolonged, as some ventilator algorithms permit a maximal inspiratory phase of up to 3 s.[39]

Excessive expiratory asynchrony contributes to patient discomfort and loss of ventilator efficacy.[39,44] Strategies to alleviate these types of asynchrony include reducing the level of pressure support to lower tidal volume and thereby auto-PEEP, and raising the cycling threshold so that it triggers at higher inspiratory flow.[49] Limiting inspiratory time[50] and minimising air leaks that can also contribute to these forms of asynchrony (see below) are also effective strategies.

Other avenues for improving the matching of ventilator output and patient effort include adjustments in inspiratory flow or 'rise time' (found on some 'bi-level' ventilators to permit adjustments in the time to reach target inspiratory pressure),[45] adaptive servoventilation, proportional-assist ventilation (PAV) and neurally adjusted ventilatory assistance (NAVA). COPD patients tend to prefer relatively rapid inspiratory flow rates (in the range of 60 L/min).[51] Such flow rates reduce inspiratory work compared with lower flow rates, but excessively rapid rates can add to patient discomfort.[52]

Air leaks

Air leaks are virtually universal during NIV because the system is open. 'Bi-level' positive pressure ventilators have intentional leaks in the mask or ventilator tubing, of course, because they use single circuit tubing and must have a fixed exhalation port to minimise CO_2 rebreathing. Although some earlier studies raised concern about the possibility of rebreathing contributing to NIV failure during use of 'bi-level' devices,[53] this has never been demonstrated in a clinical setting and seems unlikely as long as expiratory pressure is kept at 4 cm H_2O or higher to maintain a sufficiently high bias flow. Interfaces like the helmet may be more susceptible to rebreathing and require high airflows that are associated with loud noise levels.[54–56]

Other contributors to leak include nasal as opposed to oronasal masks because of leakage through the mouth.[23] Yet, even when properly fitted masks are applied using 'critical care ventilators' with dual limb circuits that do not require fixed intentional leaks, some leakage occurs under the mask seal, because of the irregularity of the facial contour and the laxity of the mandible. Air leaking is intensified by poorly fitted masks and high ventilator pressures.

The consequences of air leaks depend on the severity of the leak. Smaller leaks, in the range of 30 L/min or less, are generally well compensated by the ventilators and do not interfere with ventilator function. Large leaks (>60 L/min) wreak havoc, contributing to patient discomfort and agitation, patient–ventilator asynchrony, diminished tidal volumes and NIV failure. Leaks in between these limits cause problems depending on the location of the leak, the capability of the ventilator to compensate and synchronise and the patient's level of tolerance.[57]

Air leaks under the mask seal can be noisy and frightening to patients. Leaks not uncommonly occur along the sides of the nose, sometimes flowing into the eyes and causing conjunctivitis. With the use of nasal masks, leaks through the mouth cause increased airflow through the nose as the ventilator compensates by increasing and prolonging inspiratory flow. This can cause nasal dryness or congestion as well as nasal mucosal cooling, which can increase nasal resistance.[58] Some air can leak into the oesophagus, causing gastric insufflation and distension, which can occasionally interfere with ventilation. But the most concerning consequences of leak are patient–ventilator asynchrony and NIV failure.

As mentioned in the section 'Patient–Ventilator Asynchrony', the high airflow rates associated with leak make it difficult for ventilators to sense the onset of inspiration and exhalation, leading to delayed and sometimes totally asynchronous ventilator inspiratory triggering as well as cycling.[46] Some ventilators respond to excessive leak by auto-cycling as their triggering function mistakes the leak for the patient's inspiratory flow.[53] Others delay cycling into expiration for more than 2 s. At the extreme, excessively large leaks interfere with delivery of target pressure or volume leading to NIV failure.

The first step in managing air leaks is to monitor for them with the aim of detecting and managing them before adverse consequences occur. Some ventilators provide digital displays of leak flow rate that can be early indicators. Others have graphic displays of inspiratory flow that show the increases associated with leak. Most will alarm when target pressure or volume is not being reached. Once a leak is detected and is deemed large enough to cause problems, it should be located. Often the patient is aware of the leak, but the fingers can be used to detect leaks as well, moving them around the perimeter of the mask seal, keeping in mind that, during bi-level ventilation, some of the leaks are intentional.

Once detected, attempts are made to eliminate the leak or at least minimise it. Often, the initial reflex is to tighten the mask straps, sometimes intensifying discomfort and raising the risk of facial ulcers. Rather, the first step should be to pull the mask away from the face to reposition the mask and reseat the seal, which sometimes eliminates the problem. Next, straps should be adjusted, always attempting to use the lowest tension necessary to control the leak. When patients are using nasal masks, verbal instructions to close the mouth may help and chin straps may be helpful. But more often, switching to an oronasal or other larger mask may be necessary. When leaks are happening repeatedly, humidification of air may be helpful to avoid desiccation of mucosa and to enhance comfort. Gastric insufflation may be treated with agents such as simethicone or, in the unusual circumstance that it interferes with ventilation, nasogastric suction. Lowering inspiratory pressure or tidal volume is also an effective strategy to reduce air leaking, but may also intensify respiratory distress if lowered too much. Humidification of inspired gas may also help to alleviate mucosal drying, enhance comfort and alleviate work of breathing.[59]

SUMMARY AND CONCLUSIONS

Over the past 20 years, NIV has occupied a growing role in the treatment of acute respiratory failure due to COPD exacerbations and acute cardiogenic pulmonary oedema and early in association with immunocompromised states. It is also the ventilatory modality of first choice for chronic respiratory failure associated with neuromuscular disease or obesity and possibly stable COPD. Although it is generally well tolerated, adverse effects are not uncommon and it suffers from a failure rate approaching 40% in some series in the acute setting. Problems arising with NIV use are best avoided or dealt with promptly by selecting appropriate patients and monitoring them closely as long as they are acutely ill. Intolerance is a common problem related to mask discomfort, agitation or inappropriate ventilator settings. Using the right equipment delivered by skilled, experienced staff helps to optimise outcomes. When there is a failure to ventilate or oxygenate, clinicians should rapidly assess the situation for reversible contributing factors, but be prepared to intubate without undue delay if rapid reversal cannot be achieved. A systematic approach to troubleshooting can help assure the best possible NIV outcomes.

REFERENCES

1. Demoule A, Girou E, Richard JC et al. Increased use of noninvasive ventilation in French intensive care units. *Intensive Care Med.* 2006;32:1747–55.
2. Ozsancak Ugurlu A, Sidhom SS, Khodabandeh A et al. Use and outcomes of noninvasive positive pressure ventilation in acute care hospitals in Massachusetts. *Chest.* 2014;145:964–71.
3. Lightowler JV, Wedjicha JA, Elliot MW et al. Non-invasive positive pressure ventilation to treat respiratory failure resulting from exacerbations of chronic obstructive pulmonary disease: Cochrane systematic review and meta-analysis. *BMJ.* 2003;326:185–9.
4. Masip J, Roque M, Sanchez B et al. Noninvasive ventilation in acute cardiogenic pulmonary edema. *JAMA.* 2005;294:3124–30.
5. Nava S, Hill N. Non-invasive ventilation in acute respiratory failure. *Lancet.* 2009;374:250–9.
6. Schettino G, Altobelli N, Kacmarek RM. Noninvasive positive pressure ventilation reverses acute respiratory failure in selected 'do-not-intubate' patients. *Crit Care Med.* 2005;33:1976–82.
7. Levy M, Tanios MA, Nelson D et al. Outcomes of patients with do-not-intubate orders treated with noninvasive ventilation. *Crit Care Med.* 2004;32:2002–7.
8. Soo Hoo GW, Santiago S, Williams AJ. Nasal mechanical ventilation for hypercapnic respiratory failure in chronic obstructive pulmonary disease: Determinants of success and failure. *Crit Care Med.* 1994;22:1253–61.

9. Ambrosino N, Foglio K, Rubini F et al. Non-invasive mechanical ventilation in acute respiratory failure due to chronic obstructive pulmonary disease: Correlates for success. *Thorax*. 1995;50:755–7.
10. Confalonieri M, Garuti G, Cattaruzza MS et al. Italian noninvasive positive pressure ventilation (NPPV) study group. A chart of failure risk for noninvasive ventilation in patients with COPD exacerbation. *Eur Respir J*. 2005;25:348–55.
11. Antonelli M, Conti G, Moro ML et al. Predictors of failures of noninvasive positive pressure ventilation in patients with acute hypoxemic respiratory failure: A multi-center study. *Intensive Care Med*. 2001;27:1718–28.
12. Rana S, Hussam J, Gay P et al. Failure of non-invasive ventilation in patients with acute lung injury: Observational cohort study. *Crit Care*. 2006;10:R79.
13. Nava S, Ceriana P. Causes of failure of noninvasive mechanical ventilation. Respir Care. 2004;49: 295–303.
14. Carlucci A, Delmastro M, Rubini F et al. Changes in the practice of non-invasive ventilation in treating COPD patients over 8 years. *Intensive Care Med*. 2003;29:419–25.
15. Keenan SP, Sinuff T, Cook DJ et al. Which patients with acute exacerbation of chronic obstructive pulmonary disease benefit from noninvasive positive-pressure ventilation? A systematic review of the literature. *Ann Intern Med*. 2003;138:861–70.
16. Rocco M, Dell'Utri D, Morelli A et al. Noninvasive ventilation by helmet or face mask in immunocompromised patients: A case-control study. *Chest*. 2004;126:1508–15.
17. Nourdine K, Combes P, Carton MJ et al. Does noninvasive ventilation reduce the ICU nosocomial infection risk? A prospective clinical survey. *Intensive Care Med*. 1999;25:567–73.
18. Hill NS. Where should noninvasive ventilation be delivered? *Respir Care*. 2009;54:62–70.
19. Çiledağ A, Kaya A, Erçen Diken Ö et al. The risk factors for late failure of non-invasive mechanical ventilation in acute hypercapnic respiratory failure. *Tuberk Toraks*. 2014;62:177–82.
20. Kwok H, McCormack J, Cece R et al. Controlled trial of oronasal versus nasal mask ventilation in the treatment of acute respiratory failure. *Crit Care Med*. 2003;31:468–73.
21. Navalesi P, Fanfulla F, Frigerio P et al. Physiologic evaluation of noninvasive mechanical ventilation delivered by three types of masks in patients with chronic hypercapnic respiratory failure. *Crit Care Med*. 2000;28:1785–90.
22. Navalesi P, Costa R, Ceriana P et al. Non-invasive ventilation in chronic obstructive pulmonary disease patients: Helmet versus facial mask. *Intensive Care Med*. 2007;33:74–81.
23. Patel BK, Wolfe KS, Pohlman AS, Hall JB, Kress JP. Effect of noninvasive ventilation delivered by helmet vs face mask on the rate of endotracheal intubation in patients with acute respiratory distress syndrome: A randomized clinical trial. *JAMA*. 2016;315:2435–41.
24. Cavaliere F, Conti G, Costa R et al. Noise exposure during noninvasive ventilation with a helmet, a nasal mask, and a facial mask. *Intensive Care Med*. 2004;30:1755–60.
25. Gregoretti C, Confalonieri M, Navalesi P et al. Evaluation of patient skin breakdown and comfort with a new face mask for non-invasive ventilation: A multi-center study. *Intensive Care Med*. 2002;28:278–84.
26. Liu J, Duan J, Bai L, Zhou. Noninvasive ventilation intolerance: Characteristics, predictors, and outcomes. *Respir Care*. 2016;61(3):277–84.
27. Devlin JW, Nava S, Fong JJ et al. Survey of sedation practices during noninvasive positive-pressure ventilation to treat acute respiratory failure. *Crit Care Med*. 2007;35:2298–302.
28. Salluh JI, Dal-Pizzol F, Mello PV et al. Delirium recognition and sedation practices in critically ill patients: A survey on the attitudes of 1015 Brazilian critical care physicians. *J Crit Care*. 2009;24:556–62.
29. Arens R, Gozal D, Omlin KJ. Comparison of high frequency chest compression and conventional chest physiotherapy in hospitalized patients with cystic fibrosis. *Am J Respir Crit Care Med*. 1994;150:1154–7.
30. Tzeng AC, Bach JR. Prevention of pulmonary morbidity for patients with neuromuscular disease. *Chest*. 2000;118:1390–6.
31. Simonds AK. Recent advances in respiratory care for neuromuscular disease. *Chest*. 2006;130:1879–86.
32. Moretti M, Cilione C, Tampieri A et al. Incidence and causes of non-invasive mechanical ventilation failure after initial success. *Thorax*. 2000;55:819–25.
33. Corrêa TD, Sanches PR, de Morais LC et al. Performance of noninvasive ventilation in acute respiratory failure in critically ill patients: A prospective, observational, cohort study. *BMC Pulm Med*. 2015;15:144.
34. Thille AW, Contou D, Fragnoli C et al. Non-invasive ventilation for acute hypoxemic respiratory failure: Intubation rate and risk factors. *Crit Care*. 2013;17(6):R269.
35. Chawla R, Mansuriya J, Modi N et al. Acute respiratory distress syndrome: Predictors of noninvasive ventilation failure and intensive care unit mortality in clinical practice. *J Crit Care*. 2016 31:26–30.
36. Çiledağ A, Kaya A, Erçen Diken Ö et al. The risk factors for late failure of non-invasive mechanical ventilation in acute hypercapnic respiratory failure. *Tuberk Toraks*. 2014;62:177–82.

37. Schwartz AR, Kacmarek RM, Hess DR. Factors affecting oxygen delivery with bi-level positive airway pressure. *Respir Care.* 2004;49:270–5.
38. Brochard L, Mancebo J, Wysocki M et al. Noninvasive ventilation for acute exacerbations of chronic obstructive pulmonary disease. *N Engl J Med.* 1995;333:817–22.
39. Mehta S, McCool FD, Hill NS. Leak compensation in positive pressure ventilators: A lung model study. *Eur Respir J.* 2001;17:259–67.
40. Iwama H, Suzuki M. Combined local-propofol anesthesia with noninvasive positive pressure ventilation in a vasectomy patient with sleep apnea syndrome. *J Clin Anesth.* 2003;15:375–7.
41. Abou-Shala N, Meduri U. Noninvasive mechanical ventilation in patients with acute respiratory failure. *Crit Care Med.* 1996;24:705–15.
42. Schettino G, Altobelli N, Kacmarek RM. Noninvasive positive-pressure ventilation in acute respiratory failure outside clinical trials: Experience at the Massachusetts General Hospital. *Crit Care Med.* 2008;36:441–7.
43. Jolliet P, Abajo B, Pasquina P et al. Non-invasive pressure support ventilation in severe community-acquired pneumonia. *Intensive Care Med.* 2001; 27:812–21.
44. Antonelli M, Conti G, Esquinas A et al. A multiple-center survey on the use in clinical practice of noninvasive ventilation as a first-line intervention for acute respiratory distress syndrome. *Crit Care Med.* 2007;35:18–25.
45. Carteaux G, Millán-Guilarte T, De Prost N et al. Failure of noninvasive ventilation for de novo acute hypoxemic respiratory failure: Role of tidal volume. *Crit Care Med.* 2016; 44:282–90.
46. L'Her E, Deye N, Lellouche F et al. Physiologic effects of noninvasive ventilation during acute lung injury. *Am J Respir Crit Care Med.* 2005;172:1112–8.
47. Vignaux L, Vargas F, Roeseler J et al. Patient-ventilator asynchrony during non-invasive ventilation for acute respiratory failure: A multicenter study. *Intensive Care Med.* 2009;35:840–6.
48. Parthasarathy S, Jubran A, Tobin MJ. Cycling of inspiratory and expiratory muscle groups with the ventilator in airflow limitation. *Am J Respir Crit Care Med.* 1998;158:1471–8.
49. Hess DR. Ventilator waveforms and the physiology of pressure support ventilation. *Respir Care.* 2005;50:166–86.
50. Calderini E, Confalonieri M, Puccio PG et al. Patient–ventilator asynchrony during noninvasive ventilation: The role of expiratory trigger. *Intensive Care Med.* 1999;25:662–7.
51. Bonmarchand G, Chevron V, Chopin C et al. Increased initial flow rate reduces inspiratory work of breathing during pressure support ventilation in patients with exacerbation of chronic obstructive pulmonary disease. *Intensive Care Med.* 1996;22:1147–54.
52. Prinianakis G, Delmastro M, Carlucci A. Effect of varying the pressurization rate during noninvasive pressure support ventilation. *Eur Respir J.* 2004;23:314–20.
53. Vignaux L, Tassaux D, Jolliet P. Performance of noninvasive ventilation modes on ICU ventilators during pressure support: A bench model study. *Intensive Care Med.* 2007;33:1444–51.
54. Ferguson GT, Gilmartin M. CO_2 rebreathing during BiPAP ventilatory assistance. *Am J Respir Crit Care Med.* 1995;151:1126–35.
55. Lofaso F, Brochard L, Touchard D et al. Evaluation of carbon dioxide rebreathing during pressure support ventilation with BiPAP devices. *Chest.* 1995;108:772–8.
56. Schettino GPP, Chatmongkolchart S, Hess D et al. Position of exhalation port and mask design affect CO2 rebreathing during noninvasive positive pressure ventilation. *Crit Care Med.* 2003;31:2178–82.
57. Cavaliere F, Conti G, Costa R et al. Noise exposure during noninvasive ventilation with a helmet, a nasal mask, and a facial mask. *Intensive Care Med.* 2004;30:1755–60.
58. Richards GN, Cistulli PA, Ungar RG et al. Mouth leak with nasal continuous positive airway pressure increases nasal airway resistance. *Am J Respir Crit Care Med.* 1996;154:182–6.
59. Lellouche F, Maggiore SM, Deye N et al. Effect of the humidification device on the work of breathing during noninvasive ventilation. *Intensive Care Med.* 2002;28:1582–9.

14

Sedation and delirium

LARA PISANI, MARIA LAURA VEGA AND CESARE GREGORETTI

KEY MESSAGES

- Sedation has been used during non-invasive ventilation (NIV) to reduce agitation, often related to mask intolerance.
- However, it should only be used after a non-pharmacological approach has been attempted.
- There are currently no guidelines on the use of sedation during NIV.
- Opioids and hypnotic agents can be used taking into account their pharmacokinetic and pharmacodynamics properties, the patient's age and comorbidities.
- Sedation should be titrated against a sedation scale.
- Delirium should be monitored with appropriate scales and should be prevented, favouring circadian sleep cycles and avoiding sleep disruption.

INTRODUCTION

The use of non-invasive ventilation (NIV) has increased significantly in recent years reducing the rate of intubation and its complications in selected patients affected by acute respiratory failure (ARF).[1,2] NIV is considered to be the 'gold standard' in ARF due to exacerbations of chronic obstructive pulmonary disease (COPD), with success rates of 80%–85%. Other indications with solid scientific evidence include acute cardiogenic pulmonary oedema, pneumonia in immunocompromised patients and weaning from invasive ventilation in COPD patients. However, NIV is not suitable for all patients with ARF, and the patient's cooperation and tolerance are crucial factors for NIV success.[3] Mask intolerance due to pain, discomfort or claustrophobia is the main reason for early discontinuation of NIV.[4] In addition, if delirium and agitation are observed during NIV, these represent relative contraindications to continuation with this treatment.[5] Although sedative drugs may reduce the risk of NIV failure, and consequently the rate of intubation, in patients with interface-related issues and discomfort, sedation during NIV is still debated.[6] This chapter will give a comprehensive and practical overview of sedation and analgesia during NIV, based on the limited available evidence-based medicine data and expert opinion. The pharmacokinetic and pharmacodynamic properties of the most frequently used agents will be also discussed.

NIV AND SEDATION IN REAL LIFE

A recent Cochrane review[7] on the role of NIV as a weaning strategy from invasive mechanical ventilation found only one study[8] that used a standardised sedation protocol before or after initiation of NIV. Only eight small clinical studies have investigated the use of sedation during NIV.[9–16] A survey published in 2007[17] found that sedation and analgesia were infrequently used to treat acute respiratory failure in patients undergoing NIV. In addition, a number of different factors including geography and specialties conditioned the attitudes of respondents towards sedation. Benzodiazepines alone were the preferred used drugs in North America; on the other hand, only 29% of respondents, mostly European physicians, chose opioids alone as the sedation regimen of choice. Moreover, sedation was usually administered as an intermittent intravenous bolus according to clinical experience, outside of an institutional sedation protocol. More recently, Matsumoto et al.[18] evaluated retrospectively the role of sedation in agitated patients treated with

NIV after an episode of acute respiratory failure. Of 3506 patients who received NIV, 120 subjects (81 patients with non-intubation code [DNI] and 39 non-DNI) were sedated in order to control mask intolerance, pressure discomfort or the combination of the two; 72 (60%) patients received sedation intermittently, 37 (31%) patients switched from intermittent to continuous administration and sedation was applied continuously from the outset only in 11 (9%) patients. Risperidone or haloperidol was used for intermittent use and dexmedetomidine, midazolam or propofol for continuous infusion. All sedatives were titrated against the Richmond Agitation Sedation Scale (RASS).[19] Although 48% of the patients had weak indications for NIV, such as acute respiratory distress syndrome (ARDS), severe pneumonia and acute exacerbation of interstitial lung disease, the authors concluded that sedation is potentially useful to avoid NIV failure in both groups of patients (DNI and non-DNI). Very recently, an international prospective, observational multicentre study has been published that evaluated the effects of sedative-analgesic therapy in NIV failure.[20] The study involved 322 ICUs in 30 countries, including more than 840 patients in the analysis who had received, as initial treatment, at least 2 h of NIV after admission to the ICU. Muriel et al.[20] found that analgesia and sedation were used only in 19.6% of patients, confirming the data of the previous investigation.[17] Analgosedation did not bring any benefits in terms of reduction of NIV failure, defined as the need to intubate the patient. Indeed, using a rigorous statistical method, based on marginal structural models, an increase in risk of NIV failure and increased mortality in patients who were treated with both analgesic and sedative agents were seen.

RATIONALE FOR USING SEDATION DURING NIV

In intubated and critically ill patients, sedation and analgesia are essential to increase tolerance of the endotracheal tube and suction procedures, reduce anxiety, modify the sleep–wake cycle, allowing a better adaptation of the patient to the hospital environment, facilitate patient–ventilator interaction and finally make invasive procedures tolerable.[21] NIV is usually applied only in spontaneously breathing patients, able to trigger the ventilator and to protect the airway. Sedation in patients undergoing NIV should guarantee good control of agitation, anxiety and dyspnoea, as well as improve patient–ventilator interaction and sleep.[22,23] Moreover, sedation during NIV should reduce respiratory rate and inspiratory effort while avoiding abolition of respiratory drive and preserving upper airway patency.[24,25] Sedation may reduce the risks associated with ventilation at high volumes and thus reduce transpulmonary pressure and the incidence of ventilator-induced lung injury.[26] Bellani et al.[27] recently found that the use of NIV in moderate to severe ARDS may be associated with a worse ICU outcome than invasive mechanical ventilation. While mortality rate was low for patients who were successfully managed with NIV, patients who failed NIV had a high mortality. The main hypothesis to explain these results is that patients who are dyspnoeic and anxious generate high transpulmonary pressures.[28] Theoretically, this points to the importance of identifying and evaluating the anxiety component of dyspnoea with an appropriate scale. Therefore, sedation to reduce anxiety could be indicated when dyspnoea has a high affective component.

BOX 14.1

- Reducing dyspnoea
- Reducing anxiety
- Reducing respiratory drive
- Reducing respiratory rate
- Improving patient–ventilator synchrony

BOX 14.2

- Anxiolytic and analgesic properties
- Not abolish respiratory drive
- Rapid on-set and off-set
- A constant half-life time
- No accumulation in case of renal or liver failure
- No impairment of circulatory function

During NIV, only a hypnotic/sedative agent or opioid should be used so as to limit the risk of oversedation that could lead to a risk of orotracheal intubation. In fact, regardless of its effect on intolerance and patient agitation, there are a number of potential beneficial effects of analgesia and sedation when using NIV (Box 14.1).

Using the appropriate agent, each of these effects can be achieved separately, i.e. opioids can reduce respiratory rate but not respiratory drive; propofol reduces respiratory drive but may cause upper airway obstruction; and dexmedetomidine causes sedation, but does not decrease respiratory rate and drive.[29,30]

Therefore, the ideal drug for sedation during NIV should include all of the items mentioned in Box 14.2.

Although new drugs have most of these characteristics, so far, no drug fully meets all these requirements.

CHOOSING THE RIGHT DRUG FOR THE RIGHT PATIENT

Analgesic agents

Opioid drugs, such as morphine and semisynthetic–synthetic compounds, are used in a wide variety of clinical situations, producing different biological responses in the body. In particular, their μ and κ receptor activation contributes to analgesia and control of pain. In contrast, stimulation of other receptors determines adverse events such as respiratory depression and modulation of cardiorespiratory function. For example, opioid-induced hypotension typically depends on different factor combinations that include sympatholysis, vagal stimulation and release of histamine. Other important side effects include depression of the level of consciousness and intestinal transit. All these aspects should be taken into account when opioids are administered during NIV. Promoting pharyngeal collapse and inhibiting rapid eye movement (REM) sleep (with consequent 'REM rebound' when the drug is stopped) opioids are particularly risky in patients with obstructive sleep apnoea (OSA) and in patients with central apnoea.[31] Given its very rapid onset of action, naloxone is the drug of choice in acute opioid intoxication.

MORPHINE

Morphine metabolism takes place primarily in the liver, and almost 87% of a dose of morphine appears in the urine within 72 h of administration. Thus, dose adjustment is recommended in patients with hepatic and/or renal impairment in order to decrease the accumulation of active metabolites that result in a prolonged opioid effect. In a pilot study published in 1999,[10] the authors reported the outcome of 10 patients with acute lung injury who underwent a trial of NIV on 12 occasions. Morphine was used in 9 of the 12 NIV trials. Success, defined as a withdrawal of face-mask ventilation without the need for further assisted ventilation for the following 72 h, was achieved on six of nine occasions (66%). There are no guidelines for the use of morphine during NIV. In our clinical experience, morphine can be administered as a bolus of 0.03 mg/kg or as a continuous infusion at 0.01 to 0.02 mg/kg/h. Doses of morphine necessarily require continuous titration of the effective dose to prevent the risk of accumulation, especially in acute or chronic renal failure.

Theoretical pros/cons of morphine are listed in Table 14.1.

REMIFENTANIL

Remifentanil is a 4-anilidopiperidine short-acting opioid with selectivity for μ receptor and pharmacodynamic properties similar to those of other opioids but with a unique pharmacokinetic profile. Its metabolism is not influenced by hepatic or renal dysfunction, being metabolised by blood and tissue nonspecific esterases into a pharmacologically inactive metabolite.[32,33]

Table 14.1 Pros/cons of morphine use

Pro
- ↓ Pain
- ↓ Respiratory rate
- Hydrophilic agents (ideal in obese patients)
- Rapid onset
- Synergic effect with α2 agonist
- Cheap

Con
- Requires continuous titration
- Increase central apnoea and possibly OSA

This drug has an onset time of approximately 1 min, reaches 70% of the plasma concentration in about 3 min and equilibrates rapidly between the brain and the blood after approximately 20 min; and it has a reduced distribution volume. The elimination half-life of remifentanil is less than 10 min and is independent of infusion duration.[34] The pKa of remifentanil (i.e. the pH at which the opioid is 50% ionised) is lower than the physiological pH, allowing the drug to cross the blood–brain barrier and rapidly reach a good sedation level. Remifentanil is, therefore, an ideal drug for analgesia and sedation because of its easy titration and organ-independent metabolism. Low doses of remifentanil (0.05 μg/kg/min) have been shown to provide analgesia and sedation in critically ill patients without decreasing respiratory drive.[35] Compared with sedative-hypnotic approaches, remifentanil-based treatments were associated with shorter duration of mechanical ventilation, faster weaning and shorter ICU stay. Analgosedation was well tolerated, with no significant differences in haemodynamic stability compared to sedative-hypnotic treatments.[36] These characteristics make remifentanil very easy to titrate and allow the administration of opiates without concerns about accumulation and unpredictable and/or delayed recovery.

There are limited data regarding the use of remifentanil during NIV. In a prospective preliminary study, Constantin et al.[12] evaluated the efficacy and safety of the use of remifentanil in 13 patients (10 with acute hypoxaemic respiratory failure and 3 with acute hypercapnic respiratory failure) at risk of failing NIV. Continuous infusion of remifentanil (mean remifentanil dose 0.1 ± 0.03 μg/kg/min) to obtain a conscious sedation (equal to a value of 2–3 of the Ramsay scale) led to a decrease in respiratory rate and improvement in arterial blood gases after 1 h, avoiding intubation in 9 of 13 patients (69%). However, the dose of remifentanil used in this study was quite high, and three patients also required propofol, with a possible risk of oversedation.[34]

The efficacy and safety of remifentanil was evaluated in 36 patients with persistent acute respiratory failure[36] ($PaO_2/FiO_2 < 200$ after a first-line trial of NIV to avoid intubation) who refused to continue treatment because of intolerance of two different interfaces (helmet and total face mask). The initial dose of the drug was 0.025 μg/kg/min increased by 0.010 μg/kg/min every minute until reaching a level of sedation equal to 2–3 of the Ramsay scale and in any case up to a dose not higher than 0.12 μg/kg/min; 61% of patients continued NIV after the initiation of remifentanil infusion. Although the dose administrated was even higher than the recommended safety dose, patients did not require propofol.[34] No patient showed haemodynamic changes or reduction in respiratory drive during the study period. Fourteen patients were intubated: 12 for persisting discomfort and 2 for haemodynamic instability due to septic shock. In addition, the analgosedation with remifentanil leads to a decrease in respiratory rate and an improvement in blood gas values, both in mask or helmet ventilated patients.

Despite these promising results, the use of sedation with remifentanil during NIV is still very limited, and there

Table 14.2 Pros/cons of remifentanil use

Pro
– Fast elimination (very short half-life time) with no accumulation
– ↓ Pain
– ↓ Respiratory rate in a dose-dependent way (Te increases at the expense of an RR reduction)
– Optimal delivery in total controlled infusion (TCI) mode
– Synergic effect with α2 agonist
Con
– Hyperalgesia
– Increase central apnoea and possibly OSA
– IV bolus not indicated
– More expensive compared to the other opioids

are no guidelines for its use in this situation. Remifentanil should not be used outside the ICU. It must not be administered as a bolus due to the risk of muscle and chest wall stiffness.[37] In our clinical experience, it should be titrated in a continuous intravenous infusion at 0.05–0.08 μg/kg/min (ideal body weight).[34] Higher doses can cause apnoea and muscle stiffness.[37] A dedicated intravenous line is needed.

Theoretical pros/cons of remifentanil are listed in Table 14.2.

Drugs for sedation

DEXMEDETOMIDINE

It is a selective agonist of α2-adrenergic receptors and inhibits the release of norepinephrine from sympathetic nerve endings. Its sedative and analgesic activity is mediated by α2-adrenoceptor in the locus coeruleus. Dexmedetomidine has eight times greater affinity for α2 receptors than clonidine and a shorter half-life. Also, dexmedetomidine has the lowest risk of depressing the respiratory centres among all sedative drugs. It is protein bound, and 94% of the drug is metabolised in the liver.[30]

Dexmedetomidine may result in a reduction of heart rate and blood pressure through central sympathetic action, but at higher concentrations, it causes peripheral vasoconstriction leading to hypertension. A recent meta-analysis,[38] which included 1994 patients from 16 randomised controlled trials, found that compared to lorazepam, midazolam or propofol, dexmedetomidine was associated with a reduction in ICU length of stay (WMD = −0.304; 95% CI [−0.477, −0.132]; $p = 0.001$), days of mechanical ventilation (WMD = −0.313, 95% CI [−0.523, −0.104]; $p = 0.003$) and incidence of delirium (RR = 0.812, 95% CI [0.680, 0.968]; $p = 0.020$). Dexmedetomidine is also associated with a higher incidence of bradycardia (RR = 1.947, 95% CI [1.387, 2.733]; $p = 0.001$) and hypotension (RR = 1.264; 95% CI [1.013, 1.576]; $p = 0.038$). The first experience of its use during NIV appears in a Japanese pilot study[14] in which the drug was administered by continuous infusion in 10 patients undergoing NIV. After 1 h of infusion, the authors recorded an improvement in gas exchange and respiratory rate. Subsequently, Senoglu et al.[15] compared the profile of sedation and adverse effects of dexmedetomidine with midazolam in patients who underwent NIV in intensive care for an episode of acute respiratory failure secondary to COPD exacerbation. Patients were randomised to receive dexmedetomidine (group D, $n = 20$) or midazolam (group M, $n = 20$). The first group was administered a loading dose of 1 mg/kg followed by a maintenance dose of 0.5 mg/kg/h. The patients in group M, however, were treated with a loading dose of 0.05 mg/kg followed by a continuous infusion of 0.1 mg/kg/h of midazolam. In both groups, however, the dosage was titrated to maintain a mild-to-moderate sedation target (score of 2–3 according to the RSS; score of 3–4 according to the Riker Sedation Agitation Scale [RSAS] or a level Bispectral Index [BIS] > 85). The monitoring in terms of level of sedation and vital parameters were maintained for 24 h. Both groups manifested an adequate level of sedation. Only one patient in the midazolam group showed excessive sedation (RSS > 4 and RSAS < 2), so the infusion of midazolam was suspended at the eighth hour. In addition, no difference was found in terms of respiratory rate and blood gases between the two groups. By contrast, heart rate and blood pressure were significantly lower in the group treated with dexmedetomidine during the period after the administration of the loading dose (incidence of bradycardia: 18.2% vs. 0, $p = 0.016$). However, no patient manifested clinically significant adverse cardiovascular events. Similar results are derived from another randomised trial[16] involving 62 patients with hypoxaemic respiratory failure secondary to acute pulmonary oedema and unable to continue treatment with NIV because of excessive discomfort, claustrophobia and marked agitation. The authors concluded that, despite similar levels of sedation and safety profile of dexmedetomidine and midazolam, it was possible to awaken patients more rapidly with dexmetomidine and there were reduced healthcare-associated infections (possibly because of less suppression of the cough reflex) and decreased length of stay in intensive care. Despite these encouraging findings, a recently published study[39] showed that early administration of intravenous dexmedetomidine soon after the start of NIV in patients with acute respiratory failure does not improve the tolerance of NIV. In this study, 33 patients were randomised within 8 h from the beginning of NIV to receive dexmedetomidine (from 0.2 up to 0.7 μg/kg/h) to maintain a sedation level corresponding to a 3–4 Sedation–Agitation Scale (SAS) score or placebo for up to a maximum of 72 h of treatment or up to 2 h after the suspension of NIV if the patient was stable or if the patient was intubated. In both groups, patients who did not reach a level of sedation or optimal pain control could receive an additional dose of midazolam or fentanyl intravenously with a minimum 3 h interval; moreover, in case of delirium, repeated bolus of haloperidol (0.5 to 1 mg every 6 h) could be administered. The authors showed that in a population of subjects in which only one third presented at baseline signs of

Table 14.3 Pros/cons of dexmedetomidine

Pro
– Selective alpha-2 receptor agonist
– Short distribution $T_{1/2\alpha}$ 6 min
– Short elimination $T_{1/2\beta}$ 2 h
– Opioid and sedative sparing effect
– Could help to reduce delirium in critically ill patients
Con
– Bradycardia
– Hypotension
– IV bolus not indicated

intolerance to NIV, the routine and early administration of dexmedetomidine presents no benefit when compared with the intermittent use of midazolam and fentanyl, in terms of prevention of agitation and delirium, reduction in failure rate of NIV or improvement of patient/nursing staff comfort. As for most of the drugs, there are no guidelines on the use of dexmedetomidine during NIV. Dexmedetomidine can be used outside the ICU in some countries where the drug is registered. Boluses should be discouraged because of an adverse effect on haemodynamics. In our experience, it can be titrated in continuous intravenous infusion from 0.2 to 1.4 μg/kg/h (ideal body weight), but higher doses (i.e. 1–1.4 μg/kg/h for 30 min) are suggested at the beginning of treatment to reach a suitable blood concentration. Doses should be reduced in elderly patients.

Theoretical pros/cons of dexmedetomidine during NIV are listed in Table 14.3.

PROPOFOL

It is a phenolic derivative, highly lipophilic and insoluble in water. It is formulated with an oil solution of glycerol and egg lecithin for intravenous administration. Its minimally active metabolites are excreted by the kidney. It has no analgesic effects, a rapid onset (about 90 s) and an equally rapid offset (about 20 min). Propofol produces dose-dependent respiratory depression and decreases blood pressure. There is no antagonistic for this drug. It should only be used by clinicians who have airway management skills. In both adults and paediatric patients, a severe syndrome because of the infusion of propofol (propofol infusion syndrome [PRIS]) at high doses (>4 mg/kg/h) and for prolonged periods has been described. It is characterised by metabolic acidosis, renal failure and rhabdomyolysis.[40,41] In a pilot study, Clouzeau et al.[42] evaluated the safety use of the infusion of propofol with target-controlled infusion (TCI) technique for the sedation of 10 patients at risk of NIV failure due to poor tolerance. The TCI technique uses devices that achieve a specific plasma drug concentration by selecting a set of pharmacokinetic parameters with built-in computer technology included in an infusion pump.

Interestingly, Vaschetto et al.[43] found that during invasive mechanical ventilation in pressure support mode, deep propofol sedation increased asynchronies, while light sedation did not. Propofol reduced the respiratory drive, while breathing timing was not significantly affected. Gas exchange and breathing pattern were also influenced by propofol infusion to an extent that varied with the level of sedation and the ventilation mode. In our clinical experience, propofol can be used for light sedation (i.e. 0.3–0.8 mg/kg/h) as the only agent when the target is to reduce respiratory drive and transpulmonary pressure. Nevertheless, there are no guidelines on the use of propofol during NIV.

Theoretical pros/cons of propofol during NIV are listed in Table 14.4.

Table 14.4 Pros/cons of propofol use

Pro
– Rapid onset time
– Reduce respiratory drive
– ⇓Cerebral metabolic rate of oxygen (CMRO2) and anticonvulsant effect
– Intra- and also extra-hepatic metabolism
Con
– Dose-dependent cardio-circulatory effects
– Plasma concentration may increase for prolonged infusion
– Respiratory depression and loss of upper airway patency
– Can increase plasma lipids because of the phospholipid carrier

BENZODIAZEPINE

Midazolam and lorazepam are more commonly used benzodiazepines for sedation in intensive care because they can be used both intermittently and by continuous infusion. They bind to a specific receptor of gamma aminobutyric acid complex (GABA) in the central nervous system. Anxiolysis is achieved at low doses. High doses are associated with sedation, muscle relaxation, including of the muscles of the upper airways, anterograde amnesia and respiratory and cardiovascular depression.

However, the pharmacokinetic and pharmacodynamics of benzodiazepines are often unpredictable; the effects can vary from patient to patient, causing side effects even at low doses. Benzodiazepine may worsen upper airway collapse in patients with OSA syndrome.[44] Benzodiazepines and opioids may accumulate after repeated doses,[21,45] and their effects on the cardiorespiratory system are amplified when they are administered both at the same time. In addition, prolonged sedation with benzodiazepines is often associated with a longer hospital stay and a higher incidence of delirium. Currently, guidelines agree in suggesting operational protocols that use drugs other than benzodiazepines (propofol and dexmedetomidine) to reduce the duration of invasive mechanical ventilation, ICU stay and the incidence of delirium.[21] Nevertheless, benzodiazepines are especially useful in cases of anxiety, epileptic fits or amnesia, and are also useful during procedures such as bronchoscopy.

As for all the above-mentioned drugs, there are no guidelines for the use of midazolam (the most used

Table 14.5 Pros/cons of midazolam

Pro
– Rapid onset time (120–300 s)
– Synergic effect with alpha2 agonist
Con
– Paradoxical agitation
– Great individual variability – half-life (2–24 h)
– Active metabolite (alfa-idrossimetazolam) with risk of accumulation
– Causes selective inhibition of upper airway activity

benzodiazepine) during NIV. In our clinical experience, a regimen of intermittent boluses of 0.015 to 0.03 mg/kg (ideal body weight) should be encouraged because of the risk of accumulation during continuous infusion. Again, according to our clinical experience, if intravenous continuous infusion is needed, it should be titrated against a sedation scale (i.e. RASS).[19]

Theoretical pros/cons of midazolam during NIV are listed in Table 14.5.

DELIRIUM

Several publications have addressed its diagnostic criteria, risk factors, prevention and treatment strategies and outcomes.[46,47] Delirium is present in as many as 60%–80% of mechanically ventilated patients and 20%–50% of non-mechanically ventilated patients.[21,46] It is characterised by the acute to sub-acute onset of altered consciousness and cognition, frequently with a reduced awareness of the environment, impaired attention and/or disorganised thinking.[48,49] Delirium presents as three major subtypes: hyperactive (agitated), hypoactive (quiet) and mixed (features of both), with hypoactive and mixed the most common presentations in critically ill patients.[50,51] Screening for a diagnosis of delirium in mechanically ventilated patients has been reported using the Intensive Care Delirium Screening Checklist (ICDSC) and the Confusion Assessment Method for the Intensive Care Unit (CAM-ICU), with both now being recommended for routine use in the ICU.[21] However, there is still an inability to accurately identify delirium in the ICU.[47] So far, no pharmacologic treatment has been found to alter the course of delirium. A placebo-controlled trial (HOPE-ICU) found that intravenous haloperidol, the most commonly prescribed antipsychotic in critical care, had no impact on the duration of delirium or coma or other relevant outcomes.[52] Reade et al.[53] found in a preliminary pilot study that dexmedetomidine was a promising agent for the treatment of ICU-associated delirious agitation. These data were confirmed by a recent meta-analysis suggesting that dexmedetomidine could help to reduce delirium in critically ill patients.[54,55] The awakening and breathing coordination, choice of sedative, delirium monitoring and management and early mobility (ABCDE) bundle was specially designed to minimise sedation, encourage early liberation from the ventilator, improve assessment of and management of delirium and facilitate early mobilisation in the ICU.[56]

Critically ill patients treated with this bundle have been found to spend three more days breathing without assistance. However, this bundle only partially fits with patients receiving NIV.

An important issue is also the environment in which the patient is admitted. Zaal et al.[57] found that ICU environment may influence the course of delirium. Data regarding delirium in patients undergoing NIV including the prognostic impact of delirium in NIV failure are scarce. Tanaka et al.[58] conducted a multinational survey of ICU professionals to determine the practices of the assessment and management of delirium and their perceptions and attitudes towards its evaluation and impact in patients requiring NIV. An electronic questionnaire was created and distributed to evaluate the profiles of the respondents and their related ICUs. Approximately 61% of the respondents reported no delirium assessment in the ICU, and 31% evaluated delirium in patients receiving NIV. CAM-ICU was the most reported validated diagnostic tool (66.9%). Concerning the indication of NIV in patients already presenting with delirium, 16.3% of respondents never allowed the use of NIV in this clinical context. The authors concluded that their survey provides data that strongly reemphasise poor assessment and management of delirium in the ICU setting, especially regarding patients requiring NIV. NIV failure may be associated with the development of agitation and deterioration of mental status, as in delirious patients, and the ability to cooperate with and tolerate NIV decreases (Table 14.6).

In mechanically ventilated patients, ventilator asynchrony may adversely affect sleep.[22,59] Late NIV failure in elderly patients with acute hypercapnic respiratory failure was associated with early sleep disturbances including an abnormal electroencephalographic pattern, disruption of the circadian sleep cycle and decreased REM sleep.[23] These data suggest that sleep disturbances may promote delirium. Charlesworth et al.[60] performed a systematic review and meta-analysis of the literature to determine the prevalence of delirium in patients receiving NIV for acute respiratory failure and to quantify the prognostic impact of delirium with respect to NIV failure; 239 patients receiving NIV who were assessed for delirium were included. The prevalence of delirium was recorded at between 33% and 38% with a pooled prevalence of 37%. Two studies reported prognostic data, and the risk ratios for NIV failure in delirium were calculated as 1.79 (95% CI 1.09–2.94) and 3.28 (95% CI 1.60–6.73). A meta-analysis was performed and the pooled risk ratio was found to be 2.12 (95% CI 1.41–3.18). Smith et al.[65] described the subjective experiences of individuals treated with NIV for acute hypercapnic respiratory failure in qualitative face-to-face interviews analysed using thematic analysis. Participants described balancing the benefits and burdens of NIV, with the goal of achieving another chance at life. Gaps in recall of their treatment with NIV were frequent, potentially suggesting underlying delirium. The findings of this study inform patient-centred care and have implications for the care of patients requiring NIV and for advance care planning discussions.

Table 14.6 Suggestions indications for the most commonly used analgosedation drugs

	Consider if	Avoid if
Morphine	Relief of dyspnoea Management of refractory Symptoms at the end of life	Nausea Occlusion or paralytic ileus Caution in severe chronic kidney disease
Remifentanil*	Need for sedation and for decreasing respiratory rate and dyspnoea Renal impairment Severe liver disease	Nausea Occlusion or paralytic ileus Bradycardia
Dexmedetomidine	Need for sedation without affecting respiratory drive Delirium Severe respiratory disease (minimal respiratory depression)	Bradycardia Hypotension
Propofol	Need for decreasing respiratory drive Bronchospasm	Obstructive/central sleep apnoea Bradycardia Hyperlipidaemia Prolonged use and/or high doses
Midazolam	Need for decreasing respiratory drive Management of refractory Symptoms at the end of life	Obstructive sleep apnoea Psychosis or delirium Caution in severe chronic kidney disease Severe liver disease Acute narrow-angle glaucoma

*Use restricted in ICU with a dedicated line.

CONCLUSIONS

The literature shows that there is still much debate on these topics. Although preliminary results are encouraging regarding the use of analgosedation in patients intolerant of NIV, the lack of randomised controlled trials with sufficient numbers of patients makes it impossible to draw a conclusion on the real benefit in clinical practice. As mentioned above, sedative medications with the exception of dexmedetomidine may produce respiratory depression. Most of the agents may increase upper airways collapsibility in a dose-dependent way even in normal subjects.[25,61,62]

However, patients who are already predisposed to the collapse of the upper airway or have central apnoeas are more sensitive to the effects of opioids and sedatives. Analgosedation is not routinely required in patients receiving NIV, but it can help in specific situations only after a non-pharmacological approach (i.e. mask fitting/tolerance; a leak compensated software/ventilator; reassuring the patients; proper environment minimizing noise and disturbance) has been attempted first, so as to enhance the patient's adaptation to ventilation. For this purpose, the use of an interface rotation strategy in cases of patients with little autonomy in NIV, as well as the use of manoeuvres to improve patient–ventilator synchrony, may play an important role. Implementation of effective delirium screening is feasible but requires careful attention to implementation methods. This would include a change in the current ICU culture and behaviour that believes delirium is inevitable, to a future culture that views delirium as a dangerous syndrome that may also lead to NIV failure.

REFERENCES

1. Walkey AJ, Wiener RS. Use of noninvasive ventilation in patients with acute respiratory failure, 2000–2009: A population based study. *Ann Am Thorac Soc.* 2013;10 (1):10–7.
2. Nava S, Hill N. Non-invasive ventilation in acute respiratory failure. *Lancet.* 200918;374:250–9.
3. Demoule A, Chevret S, Carlucci A et al. Changing use of noninvasive ventilation in critically ill patients: Trends over 15 years in francophone countries. *Intensive Care Med.* 2016;42:82–92.
4. Carlucci A, Richard JC, Wysocki M et al. SRLF Collaborative Group on Mechanical Ventilation. Noninvasive versus conventional mechanical ventilation. An epidemiologic survey. *Am J Respir Crit Care Med.* 2001;163:874–80.
5. Smith TA, Agar M, Jenkins CR et al. Experience of acute noninvasive ventilation-insights from 'Behind the Mask': A qualitative study. *BMJ Support Palliat Care.* Published Online First: 26 August 2016. doi: 10.1136/bmjspcare-2015-000908.
6. Longrois D, Conti G, Mantz J et al. Sedation in non-invasive ventilation: Do we know what to do (and why)? *Multidiscipl Respir Med.* 2014; 9:56.
7. Burns KE, Meade MO, Premji A et al. Noninvasive ventilation as a weaning strategy for mechanical ventilation in adults with respiratory failure: A Cochrane systematic review. *CMAJ.* 2014; 186:E112–22.

8. Hill NS, Lin D, Levy M et al. Noninvasive positive pressure ventilation (NPPV) to facilitate extubation after acute respiratory failure: A feasibility study [abstract]. *Am J Respir Crit Care Med.* 2000;161:B18.
9. Takasaki Y, Kido T, Samba K. Dexmedetomidine facilitates induction of noninvasive positive pressure ventilation for acute respiratory failure in patients with severe asthma. *J Anesth.* 2009;23:147–50.
10. Rocker GM, Mackenzie MG, Williams B et al. Non invasive positive pressure ventilation: Successful outcome in patients with acute lung injury/ARDS. *Chest.* 1999;115:173–7.
11. Scala R. Sedation during non-invasive ventilation to treat acute respiratory failure. *Shortness Breath.* 2013;2(1):35–43.
12. Constantin JM, Schneider E, Cayot-Constantin S et al. Remifentanil-based sedation to treat noninvasive ventilation failure: A preliminary study. *Intensive Care Med.* 2007;33(1):82–7.
13. Rocco M, Conti G, Alessandri E et al. Rescue treatment for noninvasive ventilation failure due to interface intolerance with remifentanil analgosedation: A pilot study. *Intensive Care Med.* 2010;36(12):2060–5.
14. Akada S, Takeda S, Yoshida Y et al. The efficacy of dexmedetomidine in patients with noninvasive ventilation: A preliminary study. *Anesth Analg.* 2008;107:167–70.
15. Senoglu N, Oksuz H, Dogan Z et al. Sedation during noninvasive mechanical ventilation with dexmedetomidine or midazolam: A randomized, double-blind, prospective study. *Curr Ther Res Clin Exp.* 2010;71:141–53.
16. Huang Z, Chen YS, Yang ZL et al. Dexmedetomidine versus midazolam for the sedation of patients with non-invasive ventilation failure. *Intern Med.* 2012;51:2299–305.
17. Devlin JW, Nava S, Fong JJ et al. Survey of sedation practices during noninvasive positive-pressure ventilation to treat acute respiratory failure. *Crit Care Med.* 2007;35(10):2298–302.
18. Matsumoto T, Tomii K, Tachikawa R et al. Role of sedation for agitated patients undergoing noninvasive ventilation: Clinical practice in a tertiary referral hospital. *BMC Pulm Med.* 2015 Jul 13;15:71.
19. Sessler CN, Gosnell MS, Grap MJ et al. The Richmond Agitation-Sedation Scale: Validity and reliability in adult intensive care unit patients. *Am J Respir Crit Care Med.* 2002 Nov 15;166(10):1338–44.
20. Muriel A, Peñuelas O, Frutos-Vivar F et al. Impact of sedation and analgesia during noninvasive positive pressure ventilation on outcome: A marginal structural model causal analysis. *Intensive Care Med.* 2015 Sep;41(9):1586–600.
21. Barr J, Fraser GL, Puntillo K et al. Clinical practice guidelines for the management of pain, agitation, and delirium in adult patients in the intensive care unit. *Crit Care Med.* 2013;41:263–306.
22. Fanfulla F, Taurino AE, Lupo ND et al. Effect of sleep on patient/ventilator asynchrony in patients undergoing chronic non-invasive mechanical ventilation. *Respir Med.* 2007;101:1702–7.
23. Roche Campo F, Drouot X, Thille AW et al. Poor sleep quality is associated with late noninvasive ventilation failure in patients with acute hypercapnic respiratory failure. *Crit Care Med.* 2010;38:477–85.
24. Zhuang PJ, Wang X, Zhang XF et al. Postoperative respiratory and analgesic effects of dexmedetomidine or morphine for adenotonsillectomy in children with obstructive sleep apnoea. *Anaesthesia.* 2011;66:989–993.
25. Olofsen E, Boom M, Nieuwenhuijs D et al. Modeling the non-steady state respiratory effects of remifentanil in awake and propofol-sedated healthy volunteers. *Anesthesiology.* 2010;112:1382–95.
26. Demoule A, Hill N, Navalesi P. Can we prevent intubation in patients with ARDS? *Intensive Care Med.* 2016;42:768–71.
27. Bellani G, Laffey JC, Pham T et al. Non-invasive ventilation of patients with ARDS: Insights from the LUNG SAFE Study. *Am J Respir Crit Care Med.* 2017 1;195:67–77.
28. Parshall MB, Schwartzstein RM, Adams L et al. An official American Thoracic Society statement: Update on the mechanisms, assessment, and management of dyspnea. *Am J Respir Crit Care Med.* 2012;185:435–52.
29. Eastwood PR, Platt PR, Shepherd K et al. Collapsibility of the upper airway at different concentrations of propofol anesthesia. *Anesthesiology.* 2005;103:470–7.
30. Bhana N, Goa KL, McClellan KJ. Dexmedetomidine. *Drugs.* 2000;59:263–8 [discussion 269–70].
31. Filiatrault ML, Chauny JM, Daust R et al. Medium increased risk for central sleep apnea but not obstructive sleep apnea in long-term opioid users: A systematic review and meta-analysis. *J Clin Sleep Med.* 2016;12(4):617–25.
32. Conti G, Costa R, Pellegrini A et al. Analgesia in PACU: Intravenous opioids. *Curr Drug Targets.* 2005;6:767–71.
33. Hoke JF, Shlugman D, Dershwitz M et al. Pharmacokinetics and pharmacodynamics of remifentanil in persons with renal failure compared with healthy volunteers. *Anesthesiology.* 1997;87:533–41.
34. Cavaliere F, Antonelli M, Arcangeli A et al. A low-dose remifentanil infusion is well tolerated for sedation in mechanically ventilated, critically-ill patients. *Can J Anaesth.* 2002;49:1088–94.
35. Devabhakthuni S, Armahizer MJ, Dasta JF et al. Analgosedation: A paradigm shift in intensive care unit sedation practice. *Ann Pharmacother.* 2012;46:530–40.
36. Rocco M, Conti G, Alessandri E et al. Rescue treatment for noninvasive ventilation failure due to interface intolerance with remifentanil analgosedation: A pilot study. *Intensive Care Med.* 2010;36(12):2060–5.

37. Afshan G. Are we anesthesiologists, aware about the incidence of muscle stiffness associated with remifentanil? *Anesth Pain Med.* 2012;1(3):218.
38. Constantin JM, Momon A, Mantz J et al. Efficacy and safety of sedation with dexmedetomidine in critical care patients: A meta-analysis of randomized controlled trials. *Anaesth Crit Care Pain Med.* 2016;35:7–15.
39. Devlin JW, Al-Qadheeb NS, Chi A et al. Efficacy and safety of early dexmedetomidine during noninvasive ventilation for patients with acute respiratory failure: A randomized, double-blind, placebo-controlled pilot study. *Chest.* 2014;145(6):1204–12.
40. Bray RJ. Propofol infusion syndrome in children. *Pediatr Anaesth.* 1998;8:491–9.
41. Cremer OL, Moons KG, Bouman EA et al. Long term propofol infusion and cardiac failure in adult head-injured patients. *Lancet.* 2001;357:606–7.
42. Clouzeau B, Bui HN, Vargas F et al. Target controlled infusion of propofol for sedation in patients with non-invasive ventilation failure due to low tolerance: A preliminary study. *Intensive Care Med.* 2010;36:1675–80.
43. Vaschetto R, Cammarota G, Colombo D et al. Effects of propofol on patient-ventilator synchrony and interaction during pressure support ventilation and neurally adjusted ventilatory assist. *Crit Care Med.* 2014 Jan;42(1):74–82.
44. Dhonneur G, Combes X, Leroux B et al. Postoperative obstructive apnea. *Anesth Analg.* 1999;89:762–7.
45. Devlin JW, Roberts RJ. Pharmacology of commonly used analgesics and sedatives in the ICU: Benzodiazepines, propofol, and opioids. *Anesthesiol Clin.* 2011;29(4):567–85.
46. Brummel NE, Vasilevskis EE, Han JH et al. Implementing delirium screening in the ICU: Secrets to success. *Crit Care Med.* 2013;41:2196–208.
47. Devlin J et al. The accurate recognition of delirium in the ICU: The emperor's new clothes? *Intensive Care Med.* 2013;39:2196–9.
48. American Psychiatric Association. *Diagnostic and Statistical Manual of Mental Disorders: DSM-IV-TR.* 4th ed. Washington, DC: American Psychiatric Association; 2000.
49. Meagher DJ, Moran M, Raju B et al. Motor symptoms in 100 patients with delirium versus control subjects: Comparison of subtyping methods. *Psychosomatics.* 2008;49:300–8.
50. Peterson JF, Pun BT, Dittus RS et al. Delirium and its motoric subtypes: A study of 614 critically ill patients. *J Am Geriatr Soc.* 2006;54:479–84.
51. Pandharipande P, Cotton BA, Shintani A et al. Motoric subtypes of delirium in mechanically ventilated surgical and trauma intensive care unit patients. *Intensive Care Med.* 2007;33:1726–31.
52. Page VJ, Ely EW, Gates S et al. Effect of intravenous haloperidol on the duration of delirium and coma in critically ill patients (Hope-ICU): A randomised, double-blind, placebo controlled trial. *Lancet Respir Med.* 2013;1:515–23.
53. Reade MC, O'Sullivan K, Bates S et al. Dexmedetomidine vs. haloperidol in delirious, agitated, intubated patients: A randomised open-label trial. *Crit Care.* 2009;13:R75.
54. Pasin L, Landoni G, Nardelli P et al. Dexmedetomidine reduces the risk of delirium, agitation and confusion in critically Ill patients: A meta-analysis of randomized controlled trials. *J Cardiothorac Vasc Anesth.* 2014 Dec;28(6):1459–66.
55. Zhang H, Lu Y, Liu M et al. Strategies for prevention of postoperative delirium: A systematic review and meta-analysis of randomized trials. *Crit Care.* 2013 Mar 18;17(2):R47.
56. Balas MC, Vasilevskis EE, Olsen KM et al. Effectiveness and safety of the awakening and breathing coordination, delirium monitoring/management, and early exercise/mobility bundle. *Crit Care Med.* 2014;42:1024–36.
57. Zaal IJ, Spruyt CF, Peelen LM et al. Intensive care unit environment may affect the course of delirium. *Intensive Care Med.* 2013;39:481–8.
58. Tanaka LM, Salluh JI, Dal-Pizzol F et al. Delirium in intensive care unit patients under noninvasive ventilation: A multinational survey. *Rev Bras Ter Intensiva.* 2015;27:360–8.
59. Bosma K, Ferreyra G, Ambrogio C et al. Patient–ventilator interaction and sleep in mechanically ventilated patients: Pressure support versus proportional assist ventilation. *Crit Care Med.* 2007;35:1048–54.
60. Charlesworth M, Elliott MW, Holmes JD. Noninvasive positive pressure ventilation for acute respiratory failure in delirious patients: Understudied, under-reported, or underappreciated? A systematic review and meta-analysis. *Lung.* 2012;190:597–603.
61. Ankichetty S, Wong J, Chung F. A systematic review of the effects of sedatives and anesthetics in patients with obstructive sleep apnea. *J Anaesthesiol Clin Pharmacol.* 2011;27:447–58.
62. Eastwood PR, Platt PR, Shepherd K et al. Collapsibility of the upper airway at different concentrations of propofol anesthesia. *Anesthesiology.* 2005;103:470–7.

15

Timing of non-invasive ventilation

STEFANO NAVA AND PAOLO NAVALESI

INTRODUCTION

The timing of non-invasive ventilation (NIV) application is important.[1] If, on the one hand, the chances of successful application of NIV are increased when it is initiated early to avert excessive progression of the underlying disorder, or, on the other hand, if it is started too early, when the patients' condition is such that ventilatory assistance is not truly needed, the patient is more likely to develop mask intolerance.

As summarised in Figure 15.1, NIV may therefore be used at different times.

NIV TO PREVENT ACUTE RESPIRATORY FAILURE

Exacerbation of chronic obstructive pulmonary disease and hypercapnic respiratory failure

Very few studies have assessed the efficacy of NIV in preventing the occurrence of ARF, and all of those that have done this have included patients with only a mild exacerbation of chronic obstructive pulmonary disease (COPD). Bardi et al.[2] randomised 30 patients, the large majority of whom had a pH > 7.35, to early NIV or medical therapy alone. No significant reduction was found in mortality, or improvement in need for endotracheal intubation or time spent in the hospital. In a similar population, Keenan et al.[3] reported no difference in any clinical outcome, but a significant reduction in dyspnoea with NIV, although mask ventilation was found to be very poorly tolerated. Conversely, Pastaka et al.[4] found that patients with a pH > 7.35 receiving NIV demonstrated good tolerance to the technique and, in contrast to those in the control group who received only standard medical treatment, had faster improvement in arterial blood gases and shorter length of hospital stay. A large Chinese study[5] started NIV between 24 and 48 h of admission; the mean pH at randomisation was 7.35 for NIV versus 7.34 for standard therapy group; there was a decrease in the number of patients meeting the criteria for intubation with NIV, but no difference in mortality. Subgroup analysis of patients with a normal pH showed a beneficial effect of NIV for patients meeting the criteria for intubation versus those that did not, but not for mortality. However, NIV was started much later than in other studies, and the number of patients deteriorating to the point at which ETI was considered appropriate was surprisingly high, considering the mild acidosis. Furthermore, oxygen levels were high, suggesting that, in these patients, ventilatory failure was precipitated by inappropriate oxygen administration.

According to these studies, anticipating the use of NIV in patients with an exacerbation of COPD to prevent, rather than to treat, respiratory distress may be futile and would therefore be an unnecessary waste of resources. Official ERS/ATS clinical practice guidelines: noninvasive ventilation for acute respiratory failure.[6]

Cardiogenic pulmonary oedema

Some studies performed on cardiogenic pulmonary oedema (CPO) did not include as a primary enrolment criterion the presence of ARF. For example, Park et al.[7] studied those patients with acute onset of respiratory distress (breathing rate > 25 breaths/min), associated tachycardia and diaphoresis, and findings of pulmonary congestion on physical examination, and similar criteria were used by Crane et al.[8] All these investigations showed overall a more rapid improvement of gas exchange, dyspnoea and, in one study,[5] reduction in intubation rate, using either continuous positive airway pressure (CPAP) or pressure support with the addition of CPAP versus oxygen therapy alone.

These results suggest a possible role of NIV to prevent the occurrence of ARF during an episode of CPO with respiratory distress.

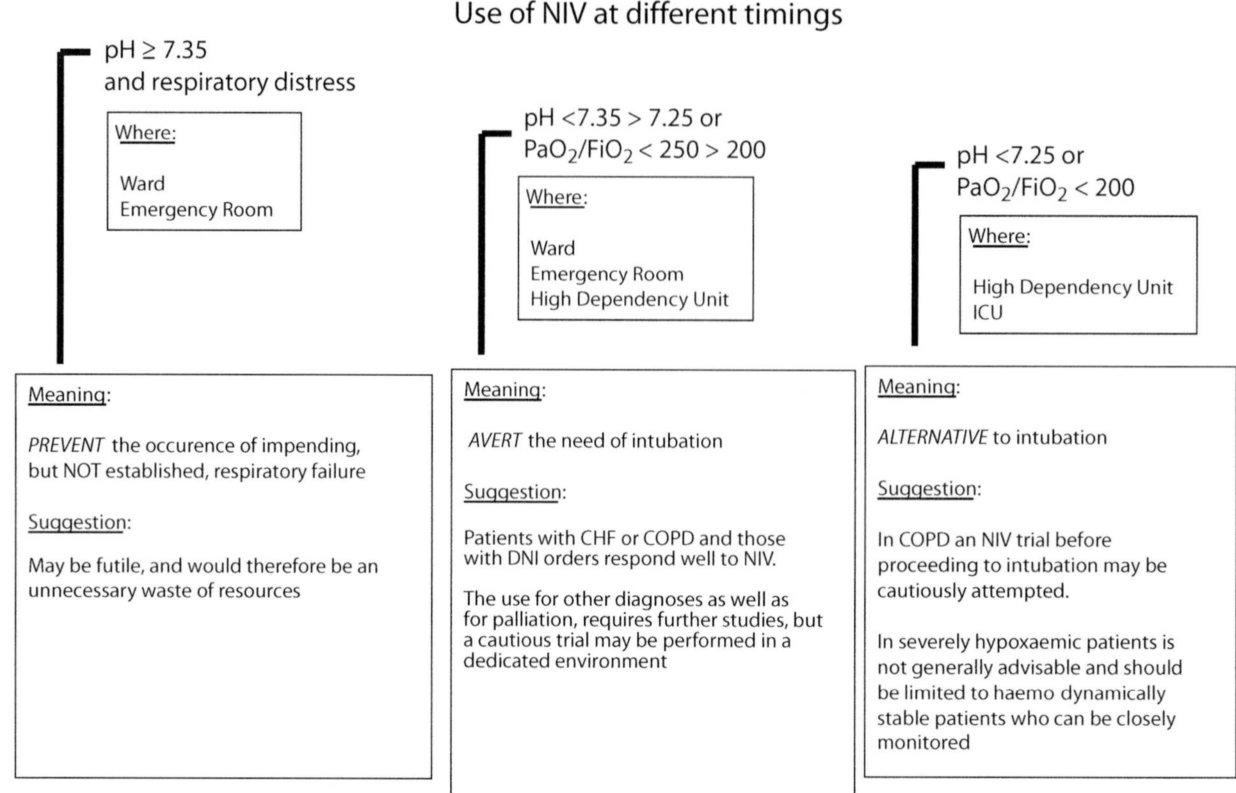

Figure 15.1 Use of NIV at different times in the patient journey.

De novo hypoxic respiratory failure

There are no studies on the use of NIV to prevent an episode of ARF in this condition.

NIV TO AVERT THE NEED FOR ENDOTRACHEAL INTUBATION AND REINTUBATION

COPD exacerbation and hypercapnic respiratory failure

The patients who benefit most from NIV are those with acute respiratory acidosis caused by an exacerbation of COPD.[8,9] In the past decade, several randomised controlled trials (RCTs) have shown that the addition of NIV to medical treatment relieves dyspnoea, improves vital signs and gas exchange, prevents endotracheal intubation, reduces complications, lowers mortality and shortens the time spent in the hospital.[10] Brochard et al.,[11] however, found that the benefits of NIV over standard treatment vanished when only those patients in whom treatment failed and those who required intubation were considered.

Notwithstanding a general consensus on the value of NIV, resulting from this large body of evidence, some aspects still deserve consideration. For example, one randomised trial[12] found that adding NIV to standard treatment in hypercapnic COPD patients admitted to a respiratory ward with very mild ARF did not produce further advantages; the success rate, however, was 100% for both NIV and standard treatment. In a large multicentre trial, Plant et al.[13] found that the rate of intubation and mortality were overall reduced when NIV was added to standard medical therapy; a subgroup analysis, however, indicated that the improvement was limited to those patients who had a pH ≥ 7.30. The authors surmised that the patients with pH < 7.30 might have fared better in the intensive care unit (ICU) rather than in the ward, despite that in experienced wards, sicker patients may be treated successfully.[14] Last, it has been shown in two US studies that the use of NIV for COPD exacerbations has increased steadily, whereas invasive ventilation use has declined, and this was associated with decreased intubation and mortality rates; however, there was a rising mortality rate in the small group of patients failing NIV and therefore requiring intubation.[15,16]

In conclusion, considering the strong evidence of efficacy and the relatively low risk of failure, in COPD patients with mild to moderate ARF, NIV is considered the ventilatory therapy of first choice and can be safely administered in appropriately monitored and staffed areas outside the ICU.

Cardiogenic pulmonary oedema

NIV has been used to avoid intubation during an episode of ARF in patients with CPO.[17,18] Indeed, helmet CPAP was shown to be feasible, efficient and safe in pre-hospital treatment of presumed CPO in an observational study.[19] Meta-analyses[17,18] have concluded that the addition to the standard medical therapy of non-invasive CPAP (n-CPAP) or NIV reduces the rate of intubation. These conclusions have been challenged by the results of a large multicentre trial comparing oxygen therapy alone, n-CPAP and NIV.[20] This trial found no difference in intubation rate or mortality at 7 and 30 days. However, interpretation of the results is limited by the high crossover rate and by the potential different aetiology of heart failure, with different responses haemodynamically in patients with an ischaemic or hypertensive cardiomyopathy and those with a dilated left ventricle. One potential explanation for the low intubation rate may be that the appropriate use of nitrates, compared to most of the other studies, was a more important factor in survival.

In conclusion, based on systematic reviews[21,22] that have incorporated the data from Gray et al., it may be concluded that (1) NIV decreases the need for intubation, (2) NIV is associated with a reduction in hospital mortality, (3) NIV is not associated with increased myocardial infarction and (4) CPAP and NIV have similar effects on these outcomes.

De novo hypoxic respiratory failure

Several clinical trials have evaluated NIV as a means to prevent intubation in patients with mild to moderate hypoxaemic ARF (i.e. $PaO_2/FiO_2 \geq 200$) of varied aetiology.

Wysocki et al.[23] showed that, compared with standard therapy, NIV reduced the need for endotracheal intubation, shortened the duration of ICU stay and decreased the mortality rate only in the subgroup of patients with associated hypercapnia. In contrast, in a similar group of patients, Martin et al.[24] found that NIV reduced the rate of intubation. Ferrer et al.[25] randomised a group of 105 patients with hypoxaemic ARF to receive either NIV or high oxygen concentration alone. NIV reduced the need for endotracheal intubation, incidence of septic shock, ICU mortality and 90 day mortality.

One of the major confounders in these studies was the marked variability of the case mix; patients with different underlying disorders and pathophysiological pathways were included under the same generic definition of having hypoxaemia. Confalonieri et al.[26] evaluated NIV in patients with ARF consequent to community acquired pneumonia (CAP). Compared with standard treatment alone, NIV produced a significant reduction in respiratory rate, need for endotracheal intubation and ICU stay. However, a subgroup analysis showed that the benefits of NIV occurred only in the subgroup of COPD patients. In a later study,[27] enrolling patients with more severe hypoxia and excluding COPD patients, it was shown that helmet CPAP reduces the risk of meeting intubation criteria compared to oxygen therapy. Until recently, almost all studies with NIV compared it to oxygen delivered with high concentration masks, like Venturi masks or reservoir masks. Recently, the technique of high flow nasal cannula oxygen (HOF) delivery has been proposed and seems an attractive alternative.[28] In a multicentre study, Frat et al.[29] included 313 patients, the large majority with CAP, assigned to HOF, oxygen continuously via a non-rebreather face mask and NIV. The treatments did not result in significantly different cumulative incidence of endotracheal intubation during the 28 days after randomisation. However, a post hoc analysis on cohorts based on PaO_2/FiO_2 showed that in more hypoxaemic patients ($PaO_2/FiO_2 < 200$), the intubation rate was significantly lower in the HOF group than in the other two groups. This probably helps to explain why there was a significant difference in favour of high-flow oxygen in 90 day mortality.

Major surgery is sometimes complicated by the occurrence of atelectasis and pneumonia, which lead to hypoxaemia and respiratory distress during the early post-operative period. A randomised study[30] showed that n-CPAP delivered through a helmet decreases atelectasis and prevents pneumonia more effectively than standard therapy alone during an episode of mild respiratory failure after upper abdominal surgery.

More recently, those previous data were confirmed even in patients with severe hypoxaemic respiratory failure following abdominal surgery, where the use of NIV compared with standard oxygen therapy reduced the risk of tracheal reintubation within 7 days.[31]

NIV may be used in the early treatment of ARF secondary to lung resection, a fatal complication in up to 80% of cases. Auriant et al.[32] showed that NIV is safe and effective in reducing the need for intubation and improving survival. Early NIV application may be extremely helpful in immunocompromised patients, in whom intubation greatly increases the risk of pneumonia, infections and ICU mortality.

Antonelli et al.[33] compared NIV with standard therapy in solid organ transplant recipients with hypoxaemic ARF. Within the first hour of treatment, PaO_2/FiO_2 improved in 70% of patients in the NIV group and in only 25% of patients receiving medical therapy alone. NIV was associated with a significant reduction in the rate of intubation, complications, mortality and duration of ICU stay among survivors. In patients with immunosuppression, Hilbert et al.[34] compared early NIV with standard treatment. All patients had fever, bilateral pulmonary infiltrates and hypoxaemia. Fewer patients in the NIV group required intubation, had serious complications or died in the ICU or in the hospital.

In a multicentre randomised trial including 374 immunocompromised subjects,[35] early NIV, compared with standard oxygen therapy, did not cause any harm, but was not associated with clinical advantage in terms of mortality, ICU-acquired infections, duration of mechanical ventilation or length of ICU stay. The generalisation of the results of this study was, however, limited by the fact that high-flow nasal oxygen was used in about two-fifths of these patients and may have served to decrease the intubation and mortality rates.

Concerning the use of NIV to prevent intubation in ARF due to ARDS, there is to our knowledge only one RTC[36] that demonstrated that NIV versus standard oxygen treatment may reduce intubation and mortality rate. However, these patients had mild ARDS,[37] while in general, NIV is more likely to fail in moderate to severe ARDS patients,[38,39] particularly in the presence of shock, metabolic acidosis and high severity scores of illness.

Patients with severe irreversible chronic medical diseases often eschew invasive mechanical ventilation when they present with ARF and/or distress, and it may even be medically inappropriate when they are in the terminal stages of their disease. NIV may be seen as an intermediate step for relieving symptoms as well as for achieving hospital survival in some cases. Two large US-based studies[40,41] on patients with ARF and do not intubate (DNI) orders observed that about half of the patients treated with NIV survived and were discharged from the hospital. The underlying disease was an important determinant of survival; patients with congestive heart failure (CHF) and COPD had better survival rates than those with pneumonia or cancer. The only two RCTs were performed in patients with advanced cancer with the sole aim of reducing dyspnoea, comparing NIV either versus 'regular' oxygen therapy or humidified high oxygen flow (HOF). The study of Hui et al.[42] showed a similar improvement in dyspnoea score, between NIV and HOF, while the larger multicentre study[43] demonstrated a significantly greater reduction in breathlessness using NIV, especially in the hypercapnic subgroup of patients.

In conclusion, the outcome of NIV in patients with hypoxaemic ARF for whom endotracheal intubation is not mandatory yet depends primarily on the type and evolution of the underlying disorder. The high rate of failure of NIV in community-acquired pneumonia and acute respiratory distress syndrome suggests for these patients a cautious approach consisting of early treatment and avoidance of delay of needed intubation. A trial of NIV is advisable in immunosuppressed patients, after lung resection and major abdominal surgery. Patients with DNI orders and COPD or CHF respond well to NIV, but use for other diagnoses as well as for palliation requires further study.

NIV AS AN ALTERNATIVE TO INVASIVE VENTILATION

Exacerbations of COPD

Two RCTs have compared NIV with invasive ventilation in COPD patients with severe ARF.[44,45] The average pH in those studies entry was about 7.20 for both groups, indicating that these patients had more severe ARF than those enrolled in the clinical trials in which NIV was used at an earlier stage. In the Italian study,[44] NIV group, treatment failed in 52% of patients who were thus intubated. The patients in the NIV group had a lower rate of sepsis and septic shock and showed a trend toward a lower incidence of nosocomial pneumonia during their time in the ICU. In addition, at a 12 month follow-up, the rate of hospital readmissions and the number of patients on long-term oxygen therapy were lower in the NIV group. The study of Jurjevic et al.[45] found that invasive ventilation brought about a more rapid improvement in physiological abnormalities in the first few hours but was associated with a longer total duration of ventilation and ICU length of stay. Mortality was similar in the two groups. Patients receiving NIV had less ventilator-associated pneumonia and requirement for tracheostomy.

These results were confirmed by a subsequent case–control clinical trial[46] including 64 consecutive COPD patients with severe ARF caused by exacerbation or community-acquired pneumonia. The average pH in the patients and controls on entry into the study was 7.18. The mortality rate, duration of mechanical ventilation, time spent in the ICU and duration of post-ICU hospitalisation were similar in the two groups; however, patients in the NIV group had fewer complications and showed a trend toward a lower probability of remaining on mechanical ventilation after 30 days.

In all the aforementioned studies, NIV was used in an ICU, and the study protocols had predefined criteria for NIV failure, which led in all cases to a prompt intubation, when required.

In conclusion, in patients with COPD deemed severe enough to require ventilatory support, the use of NIV at a more advanced stage of ARF is more likely to fail. A NIV trial before proceeding to intubation does not, however, harm the patient and may be cautiously attempted, avoiding excessive delay of the required intubation.

Cardiogenic pulmonary oedema

There are no studies formally assessing the use of NIV as a real alternative to intubation for CPO, despite the only randomised trial[47] that has so far evaluated the use of NIV in hypoxaemic patients considered sufficiently ill to require mandatory ventilatory assistance, which enrolled about 20% of patients with this pathology. Interestingly, four of seven patients in the NIV group did not require intubation, so that it may be suggested that a cautious NIV trial may be performed even in the presence of severe ARF due to CPO.

De novo hypoxic respiratory failure

Antonelli et al.[47] compared NIV with conventional ventilation through an endotracheal tube in selected patients with hypoxaemic ARF. Sixty-four consecutive patients were enrolled. After 1 h of mechanical ventilation, the PaO_2/FiO_2 ratio had improved in both groups. Ten patients in the NIV group required intubation. Patients randomised to conventional ventilation more frequently developed serious complications and, in particular, infections secondary to endotracheal intubation. Among survivors, the duration of mechanical ventilation and ICU stay was shorter in patients randomised to NIV. It should, however, be kept in mind that this single study was conducted in selected patients in one well-experienced centre.

A study performed in three European ICUs having expertise with NIV clarifies the issue of the 'real life' use of NIV in these conditions.[48] It was shown that 'only' 16.5% of the patients admitted with acute respiratory distress syndrome may be successfully treated with this technique. Over 2 years, 479 patients were admitted; the majority of these patients (69%) were already intubated at admission, so only 147 were eligible for this study. NIV improved gas exchange and avoided intubation in 54% of this subset of patients, leading to an overall success rate of <20%. This was associated with less ventilator-associated pneumonia and lower ICU mortality rate (6% versus 53%).

In summary, the use of NIV as an alternative to invasive ventilation in severely hypoxaemic patients is not generally advisable and should be limited to haemodynamically stable patients who can be closely monitored in an ICU.

NIV TO PREVENT EXTUBATION FAILURE IN THOSE PATIENTS PREVIOUSLY INTUBATED

Post-extubation failure is a major clinical problem in ICUs.[49]

Two randomised trials have been performed to assess whether NIV is effective in preventing the occurrence of post-extubation failure in patients at risk.[50,51] Both studies, which adopted similar criteria to define patients at risk and had comparable study designs, showed that the groups treated with NIV had a lower rate of reintubation than the groups in which standard therapy was used; furthermore, in one of the two studies, a post hoc analysis showed that ICU mortality was also reduced in the subgroup of hypercapnic patients treated with NIV.[51] A subsequent RCT performed in this specific condition has confirmed this important result.[52] Two smaller single-centre trials also randomised patients to receive NIV or standard treatment after planned extubation.[53,54] In the first one, Khilnani et al. enrolled only COPD patients and found no differences regarding intubation rate and ICU and hospital lengths of stay. The second one was performed in a group of patients for whom the only inclusion criterion was the use of invasive mechanical ventilation for more than 72 h, predominantly patients with COPD exacerbation, and, despite the small number of patients, found a reduction of the rates of reintubation and death in the NIV group.

In conclusion, promptly initiated NIV for at least 48 h in selected patients 'at risk' may prevent post-extubation respiratory failure, especially in those patients with persistent hypercapnia.

NIV TO TREAT ESTABLISHED POST-EXTUBATION RESPIRATORY FAILURE OR DISTRESS

The use of NIV has been suggested in an attempt to avoid reintubation in patients who show signs of 'incipient' or even overt respiratory failure following extubation.[55] In one RCT, NIV was applied to patients who developed ARF within 48 h after extubation and compared with standard medical therapy.[56] The patients were randomised to standard therapy alone or to NIV. The authors did not find any difference in reintubation rate, hospital mortality rate and ICU and hospital stay, despite there being a trend to a shorter duration of hospital stay in the NIV group.

Esteban et al.[57] conducted a large multicentre, randomised trial to evaluate the effect of NIV on mortality in this clinical setting. Patients who had respiratory failure were randomly assigned within the subsequent 48 h to either NIV (114 patients) or standard medical therapy (107 patients). There was no difference between the two groups in the need for reintubation, but ICU mortality was higher in the NIV group (25% versus 14%; relative risk = 1.78); the median time from respiratory failure to reintubation was longer in the NIV group, raising the doubt that this delay in reintubation may have influenced the negative results. The authors concluded that NIV does not prevent the need for reintubation or reduce mortality in unselected patients who have respiratory failure after extubation. It is noteworthy that NIV was used as a 'rescue' therapy in the patients who failed standard therapy, and the rate of success was much higher than in the NIV group.

In summary, NIV does not prevent the need for reintubation or reduce mortality in unselected patients with established post-extubation respiratory failure.

NIV TO FACILITATE THE PROCESS OF WEANING FROM INVASIVE VENTILATION

In the majority of cases, withdrawal of mechanical ventilation is possible immediately after resolution of the underlying problems responsible for ARF. However, there is a group of ventilated patients who require more gradual and longer withdrawal of mechanical ventilation. In ventilator-dependent COPD patients, NIV has been shown to be as effective as invasive ventilation in reducing inspiratory effort and improving arterial blood gases.[58] The first RCT of this strategy was performed in severely ill COPD patients ventilated through an endotracheal tube.[59] Patients who failed the T-piece trial were randomised to either extubation, with immediate application of NIV, or continued weaning with the endotracheal tube in place. Overall, this study showed that when NIV is used as a weaning technique, the likelihood of weaning success is increased, whereas the duration of mechanical ventilation and ICU stay is decreased.

A second RCT was conducted on patients with chronic respiratory disorders, intubated for an episode of ARF.[60] This study also found a shorter duration of invasive mechanical ventilation in the groups weaned non-invasively, although no differences were found in ICU or hospital stay or 3 month survival.

Several studies were performed on this topic in the following years. Burns et al.[61] identified 16 RCTs enrolling 994 participants overall, mostly with COPD (9/16). Compared with conventional weaning through the ETT, NIV was associated with a significant decrease in mortality, ventilator-associated pneumonia, ICU and hospital length of stay and total duration of mechanical ventilation.

The only pilot study aimed to assess the feasibility of early extubation, in patients with resolving hypoxaemic ARF, demonstrated a non-inferiority of the NIV approach to weaning.[62]

In conclusion, NIV may be safely and successfully used in ICU to shorten the process of liberation from mechanical ventilation in stable patients recovering from an episode of hypercapnic ARF who had previously failed a weaning trial.

CONCLUSIONS

Following on from a 'pioneering era', NIV is currently a therapeutic strategy that belongs to the real world of clinical practice. It should primarily be used for the early treatment of established episodes of ARF, in order to avoid further deterioration and intubation, and eventually to shorten the duration of invasive mechanical ventilation in COPD patients. Depending on the type and severity of the episode of ARF, on the prognosis of the underlying disease, on the setting where it is applied and on the level of expertise of the team involved, NIV may be profitably applied at different timings. To paraphrase from a famous song, 'time is on NIV's side'.[63]

REFERENCES

1. Nava S, Navalesi P, Conti G. Time of non-invasive ventilation. *Intensive Care Med.* 2006;32:361–70.
2. Bardi G, Pierotello R, Desideri M et al. Nasal ventilation in COPD exacerbations: Early and late results of a prospective, controlled study. *Eur Respir J.* 2000;15:98–104.
3. Keenan SP, Powers CE, McCormack DG. Noninvasive positive-pressure ventilation in patients with milder chronic obstructive pulmonary disease exacerbations: A randomized controlled trial. *Respir Care.* 2005;50:610–6.
4. Pastaka C, Kostikas K, Karetsi E et al. Non-invasive ventilation in chronic hypercapnic COPD patients with exacerbation and a pH of 7.35. *Eur J Intern Med.* 2007;18:524–30.
5. Collaborative Research Group of Noninvasive Mechanical Ventilation for Chronic Obstructive Pulmonary Disease. Early use of non-invasive positive pressure ventilation for acute exacerbations of chronic obstructive pulmonary disease: A multicentre randomized controlled trial. *Chin Med J (Engl).* 2005;118:2034–40.
6. Rochwerg B, Brochard L, Elliott MW et al. Official ERS/ATS clinical practice guidelines: noninvasive ventilation for acute respiratory failure. *Eur Respir J.* 2017 Aug 31;50(2).
7. Park M, Sangean MC, Volpe MS et al. Randomized, prospective trial of oxygen, continuous positive airway pressure, and bilevel positive airway pressure by face mask in acute cardiogenic pulmonary edema. *Crit Care Med.* 2004;32:2407–15.
8. Crane SD, Elliott MW, Gilligan P et al. Randomised controlled comparison of continuous positive airways pressure, bilevel non-invasive ventilation, and standard treatment in emergency department patients with acute cardiogenic pulmonary edema. *Emerg Med J.* 2004;21:155–61.
9. Lightowler JV, Wedzicha JA, Elliott MW et al. Non-invasive positive pressure ventilation to treat respiratory failure resulting from exacerbations of chronic obstructive pulmonary disease: Cochrane systematic review and meta-analysis. *BMJ.* 2003;326:185.
10. Quon BS, GanWQ, Sin DD. Contemporary management of acute exacerbations of COPD: A systematic review and meta-analysis. *Chest.* 2008;133:756–66.
11. Brochard L, Mancebo J, Wysochi M et al. Noninvasive ventilation for acute exacerbation of chronic obstructive pulmonary disease. *N Engl J Med.* 1995;333:817–22.
12. Barbè F, Togores B, Rubi M et al. Noninvasive ventilatory support does not facilitate recovery from acute respiratory failure in chronic obstructive pulmonary disease. *Eur Respir J.* 1996;9:1240–5.
13. Plant PK, Owen JL, Elliot MW. A multicentre randomised controlled trial of the early use of non-invasive ventilation in acute exacerbation of chronic obstructive pulmonary disease on general respiratory wards. *Lancet.* 2000;335:1931–5.
14. Fiorino S, Bacchi-Reggiani L, Detotto E et al. Efficacy of non-invasive mechanical ventilation in the general ward in patients with chronic obstructive pulmonary disease admitted for hypercapnic acute respiratory failure and pH < 7.35: A feasibility pilot study. *Intern Med J.* 2015;45:527–37.
15. Chandra D, Stamm JA, Taylor B et al. Outcomes of noninvasive ventilation for acute exacerbations of chronic obstructive pulmonary disease in the United States, 1998–2008. *Am J Respir Crit Care Med.* 2012;185:152–9.
16. Lindenauer PK, Stefan MS, Shieh MS et al. Outcomes associated with invasive and noninvasive ventilation among patients hospitalized with exacerbations of chronic obstructive pulmonary disease. *JAMA Intern Med.* 201;174:1982–93.
17. Masip J, Rocha M, Sanchez B et al. Non invasive ventilation in acute pulmonary edema. Systematic review and meta-analysis. *JAMA.* 2005;294:3124–30.
18. Peter JV, Moran JL, Phillips-Hughes J et al. Effect of non-invasive positive pressure ventilation on mortality in patients with acute cardiogenic pulmonary oedema: A meta-analysis. *Lancet.* 2006;367:1155–63.

19. Foti G, Sangalli F, Berra L et al. Is helmet CPAP first line pre-hospital treatment of presumed severe acute pulmonary edema? *Intensive Care Med.* 2009;35:656–62.
20. Gray A, Goodacre S, Newby DE et al. Noninvasive ventilation in acute cardiogenic pulmonary edema. *N Engl J Med.* 2008;359:142–51.
21. Vital FM, Ladeira MT, Atallah AN. Non-invasive positive pressure ventilation (CPAP or bilevel NPPV) for cardiogenic pulmonary oedema. *Cochrane Database Syst Rev.* 2013;5:CD005351.
22. Cabrini L, Landoni G, Oriani A et al. Noninvasive ventilation and survival in acute care settings: A comprehensive systematic review and metaanalysis of randomized controlled trials. *Crit Care Med.* 2015;43:880–8.
23. Wysocki M, Tric L, Wolff MA et al. Noninvasive pressure support ventilation in patients with acute respiratory failure. A randomized comparison with conventional therapy. *Chest.* 1995;107:761–8.
24. Martin TJ, Hovis JD, Costantino JP et al. A randomized, prospective evaluation of noninvasive ventilation for acute respiratory failure. *Am J Respir Crit Care Med.* 2000;161:807–13.
25. Ferrer M, Esquinas A, Leon M et al. Noninvasive ventilation in severe hypoxemic respiratory failure: A randomised clinical trial. *Am J Respir Crit Care Med.* 2003;168:1438–44.
26. Confalonieri M, Della Porta R, Potena A et al. Acute respiratory failure in patients with severe community-acquired pneumonia: A prospective randomized evaluation of noninvasive ventilation. *Am J Respir Crit Care Med.* 1999;160:1585–91.
27. Brambilla AM, Aliberti S, Prina E et al. Helmet CPAP vs. oxygen therapy in severe hypoxemic respiratory failure due to pneumonia. *Intensive Care Med.* 2014;40:942–9.
28. Spoletini G, Alotaibi M, Blasi F et al. Heated humidified high-flow nasal oxygen in adults: Mechanisms of action and clinical implications. *Chest.* 2015;148:253–61.
29. Frat JP, Thille AW, Mercat A et al. High-flow oxygen through nasal cannula in acute hypoxemic respiratory failure. *N Engl J Med.* 2015;372:2185–96.
30. Squadrone V, Coha M, Cerutti E et al. Continuous positive airway pressure for treatment of postoperative hypoxemia. *JAMA.* 2005;293:589–95.
31. Jaber S, Lescot T, Futier E et al. Effect of noninvasive ventilation on tracheal reintubation among patients with hypoxemic respiratory failure following abdominal surgery: A randomized clinical trial. *JAMA.* 2016;315:1345–53.
32. Auriant I, Jallot A, Herve P et al. Noninvasive ventilation reduces mortality in acute respiratory failure following lung resection. *Am J Respir Crit Care Med.* 2001;164:1231–5.
33. Antonelli M, Conti G, Bufi M et al. Noninvasive ventilation for treatment of acute respiratory failure in patients undergoing solid organ transplantation: A randomized trial. *JAMA.* 2000;283:235–41.
34. Hilbert G, Gruson D, Vargas F et al. Noninvasive ventilation in immunosuppressed patients with pulmonary infiltrates, fever, and acute respiratory failure. *N Engl J Med.* 2001;344:481–7.
35. Lemiale V, Mokart D, Resche-Rigon M et al. Effect of noninvasive ventilation vs oxygen therapy on mortality among immunocompromised patients with acute respiratory failure a randomized clinical trial. *JAMA.* 2015;314:1711–9.
36. Zhan Q, Sun B, Liang L et al. Early use of noninvasive positive pressure ventilation for acute lung injury: A multicenter randomized controlled trial. *Crit Care Med.* 2012;402:455–60.
37. ARDS Definition Task Force, Ranieri VM, Rubenfeld GD, Thompson BT et al. Acute respiratory distress syndrome: The Berlin definition. *AMA.* 2012;307:2526–33.
38. Antonelli M, Conti G, Moro ML et al. Predictors of failure of noninvasive positive pressure ventilation in patients with acute hypoxemic respiratory failure: A multi-center study. *Intensive Care Med.* 2001;27:1718–28.
39. Rana S, Jenad H, Gay PC et al. Failure of non-invasive ventilation in patients with acute lung injury: Observational cohort study. *Crit Care.* 2006;10, R79–1619.
40. Levy M, Tanios MA, Nelson D et al. Outcomes of patients with do-not-intubate orders treated with noninvasive ventilation. *Crit Care Med.* 2004;32:2002–7.
41. Schettino G, Altobelli N, Kacmarek RM. Noninvasive positive pressure ventilation reverses acute respiratory failure in selected 'do-not-intubate' patients. *Crit Care Med.* 2005;33:1976–82.
42. Hui D, Morgado M, Chisholm G et al. High-flow oxygen and bilevel positive airway pressure for persistent dyspnea in patients with advanced cancer: A phase II randomized trial. *J Pain Symptom Manage.* 2013;46:463–73.
43. Nava S, Ferrer M, Esquinas A et al. Palliative use of non-invasive ventilation in end-of-life patients with solid tumours: A randomised feasibility trial. *Lancet Oncol.* 2013;14:219–27.
44. Conti G, Antonelli M, Navalesi P et al. Noninvasive vs. conventional mechanical ventilation in patients with chronic obstructive pulmonary disease after failure of medical treatment in the ward: A randomized trial. *Intensive Care Med.* 2002;28:1701–7.
45. Jurjevic M, Matic I, Sakic-Zdravcevic K et al. Mechanical ventilation in chronic obstructive pulmonary disease patients, noninvasive vs. invasive method (randomized prospective study). *Collegium Antropol.* 2009;33:791–7.

46. Squadrone E, Frigerio P, Fogliati C et al. Noninvasive vs invasive ventilation in COPD patients with severe acute respiratory failure deemed to require ventilatory assistance. *Intensive Care Med.* 2004;30:1303–10.
47. Antonelli M, Conti G, Rocco M et al. A comparison of noninvasive positive-pressure ventilation and conventional mechanical ventilation in patients with acute respiratory failure. *N Engl J Med.* 1998;339:429–35.
48. Antonelli M, Conti G, Esquinas A et al. A multiple-center survey on the use in clinical practice of noninvasive ventilation as a first-line intervention for acute respiratory distress syndrome. *Crit Care Med.* 2007;35:18–25.
49. Epstein SK, Ciubataru RL, Wong JB. Effect of failed extubation on the outcome of mechanical ventilation. *Chest.* 1997;112:186–92.
50. Nava S, Gregoretti C, Fanfulla F et al. Noninvasive ventilation to prevent respiratory failure after extubation in high risk patients. *Crit Care Med.* 2005;33:2465–70.
51. Ferrer M, Valencia M, Nicolas JM et al. Early non-invasive ventilation averts extubation failure in patients at risk: A randomized trial. *Am J Respir Crit Care Med.* 2006;173:164–70.
52. Ferrer M, Sellarés J, Valencia M et al. Non-invasive ventilation after extubation in hypercapnic patients with chronic respiratory disorders: Randomised controlled trial. *Lancet.* 2009;374:1082–8.
53. Khilnani GC, Galle AD, Hadda V et al. Non-invasive ventilation after extubation in patients with chronic obstructive airways disease: A randomised controlled trial. *Anaesth Intensive Care.* 2011;39(2):217–23.
54. Ornico SR, Lobo SM, Sanches HS et al. Noninvasive ventilation immediately after extubation improves weaning outcome after acute respiratory failure: A randomized controlled trial. *Crit Care.* 2013;17(2):R39.
55. Espstein SK, Ciubotaru RL. Independent effects of etiology of failure and time of reintubation on outcome for patients failing extubation. *Am J Respir Crit Care Med.* 1998;158:489–93.
56. Keenan SP, Powers C, McCormack DG et al. Noninvasive positive-pressure ventilation for postextubation respiratory distress. *JAMA.* 2002;287:3238–44.
57. Esteban A, Frutos-Vivar F, Ferguson ND et al. Non-invasive positive pressure ventilation for respiratory failure after extubation. *N Engl J Med.* 2004;350:2452–60.
58. Vitacca M, Ambrosino N, Clini E et al. Physiological response to pressure support ventilation delivered before and after extubation in patients not capable of totally spontaneous autonomous breathing. *Am J Respir Crit Care Med.* 2001;164:638–41.
59. Nava S, Ambrosino N, Clini E et al. Noninvasive mechanical ventilation in the weaning of patients with respiratory failure due to chronic obstructive pulmonary disease. A randomized, controlled trial. *Ann Intern Med.* 1998;128:721–8.
60. Girault C, Daudenthun I, Chevron V et al. Noninvasive ventilation as a systematic extubation and weaning technique in acute-on-chronic respiratory failure. A prospective, randomized controlled study. *Am J Respir Crit Care Med.* 1999;160:86–92.
61. Burns KE, Meade MO, Premji A et al. Noninvasive ventilation as a weaning strategy for mechanical ventilation in adults with respiratory failure: A Cochrane systematic review. *CMAJ.* 2014;186:E112–22.
62. Vaschetto R, Turucz E, Dellapiazza F et al. Noninvasive ventilation after early extubation in patients recovering from hypoxemic acute respiratory failure: A single-centre feasibility study. *Intensive Care Med.* 2012;38:1599–606.
63. Winding K and his orchestra. *Time Is on My Side.* Verve Records, 1963.

16

Why non-invasive ventilation works in acute respiratory failure?

MIGUEL FERRER AND ANTONI TORRES

KEY MESSAGES

- Non-invasive ventilation (NIV) decreases the work of breathing in obstructive lung disease by the addition of inspiratory pressure support and counterbalancing intrinsic positive end-expiratory pressure (PEEPi).
- Similar mechanisms may help in facilitating extubation of ventilator-dependent patients with chronic respiratory disorders.
- In cardiogenic pulmonary oedema, positive airway pressure results in reduced cardiac preload and afterload, and recruitment of collapsed alveolar units.
- In hypoxaemic patients, appropriate levels of inspiratory positive pressure and PEEP are needed to unload the respiratory muscles and relieve dyspnoea.
- The benefits of high-flow nasal cannula oxygenation appear related to delivery of heated and humidified gas through comfortable interfaces.

INTRODUCTION

Non-invasive ventilation (NIV) has been used in various clinical settings for patients with severe acute respiratory failure (ARF). The clearest evidence for benefit has been shown in severe exacerbations of chronic obstructive pulmonary disease (COPD),[1] to facilitate weaning and extubation in COPD patients,[2] cardiogenic pulmonary oedema[3] and immunosuppressed patients.[4] Recently, high-flow nasal cannula oxygenation (HFNCO) has been introduced in different clinical settings with promising results.[5]

This chapter will revise the physiological effects of NIV, including spontaneous breathing with continuous positive airway pressure (CPAP) and HFNCO, and the mechanisms of action in the different conditions leading to ARF.

SEVERE COPD EXACERBATION

The derangements in ventilatory mechanics, muscle function and gas exchange that characterise severe acute exacerbations of COPD (AECOPD) with respiratory failure have been extensively investigated.[6,7] Critical expiratory flow limitation and the consequent dynamic lung hyperinflation and decreased inspiratory capacity appear to be the predominant deleterious factors. It results in tachypnoea, increased ventilatory drive, worsening gas exchange with increased dead space, neuromechanical uncoupling and worsening cardiovascular function, with increased pulmonary artery pressure, decreased right ventricle preload and increased left ventricle afterload.

Dynamic hyperinflation results in increased intrinsic positive end-expiratory pressure (PEEPi).[8] The increased PEEPi and decreased lung compliance increase the work of breathing (WOB). Dynamic hyperinflation and air trapping result in diaphragm flattening and shortened respiratory muscle fibres, both of which reduce the effective power output of the respiratory muscle pump. In response to an adverse change in the load/capacity balance of the respiratory system, patients develop a rapid, shallow breathing pattern to protect against respiratory muscle fatigue, but this leads to reduced alveolar ventilation and hypercapnia and respiratory acidosis. Respiratory muscle function is then further compromised by acidosis.[9] NIV may partially reverse these abnormalities by unloading the respiratory muscles and improving gas exchange[6] (Figure 16.1). By using external PEEP or CPAP, the elastic workload due to dynamic hyperinflation may decrease

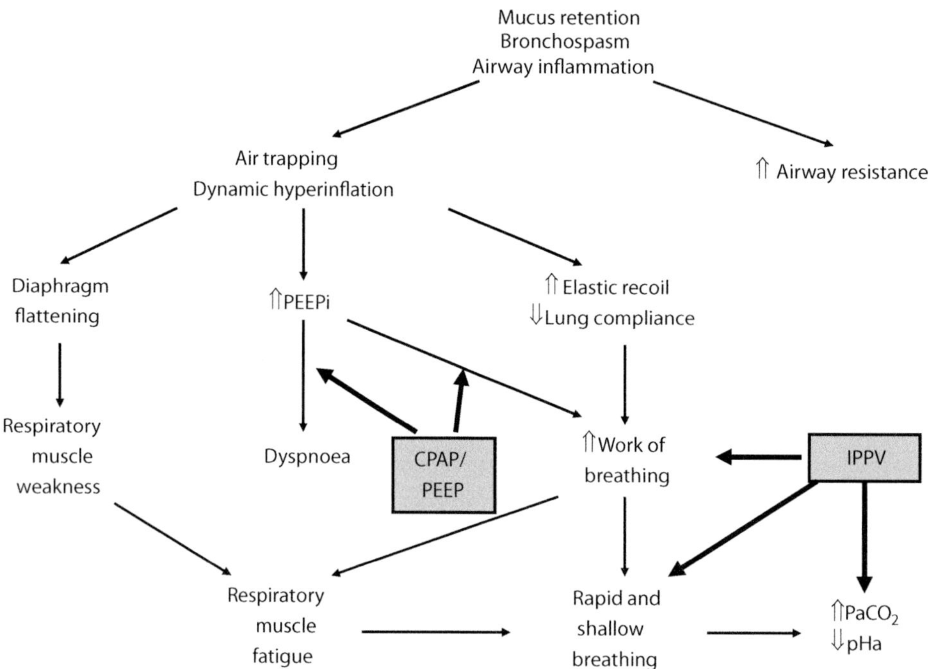

Figure 16.1 Schematic physiological effects of NIV in COPD exacerbation. When $PaCO_2$ is increased, the respiratory muscles are failing to generate sufficient alveolar ventilation to eliminate CO_2. Means of correcting this pathophysiology include increasing alveolar ventilation by increasing tidal volume and reducing CO_2 production by decreasing the WOB. Respiratory muscle failure can occur when the WOB is normal (e.g. neuromuscular problems) or increased (e.g. COPD, asthma, obesity hypoventilation syndrome), and presumably because of inadequate oxygen delivery to the respiratory muscles (e.g. some patients with cardiogenic pulmonary oedema). CPAP/PEEP decreases the elastic WOB because it supplies all or part of the driving pressure required to overcome PEEPi and initiate inspiratory flow. Adding inspiratory positive pressure ventilation (IPPV) further unloads the inspiratory muscles, reduces the WOB, corrects the rapid and shallow breathing pattern and decreases the increased $PaCO_2$ and decreased arterial pH (pHa). (Adapted in part from *Am J Respir Crit Care Med* 2001;163:283–91.)

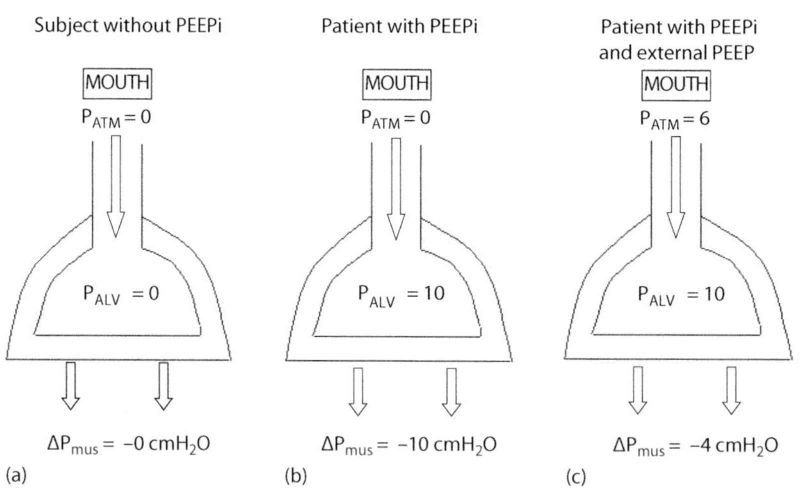

Figure 16.2 Intrinsic PEEP as superimposed inspiratory effort. **(a)** Healthy subject without PEEPi. At end expiration, alveolar pressure (P_{ALV}) is equal to the mouth atmospheric pressure (P_{ATM}); therefore, inspiratory flow begins as the inspiratory muscles start contraction. **(b)** Patient with PEEPi 10 cm H_2O. At end expiration, P_{ALV} is 10 cm H_2O higher than P_{ATM}; therefore, the inspiratory muscles first generate 10 cm H_2O negative pressure (P_{mus}) in order to decrease P_{ALV} to the level of P_{ATM} before inspiratory flow begins. **(c)** Patient with PEEPi 10 cm H_2O and external PEEP 6 cm H_2O. The inspiratory muscles generate a negative pressure of only 4 cm H_2O, since P_{ALV} should decrease to the levels of external PEEP.

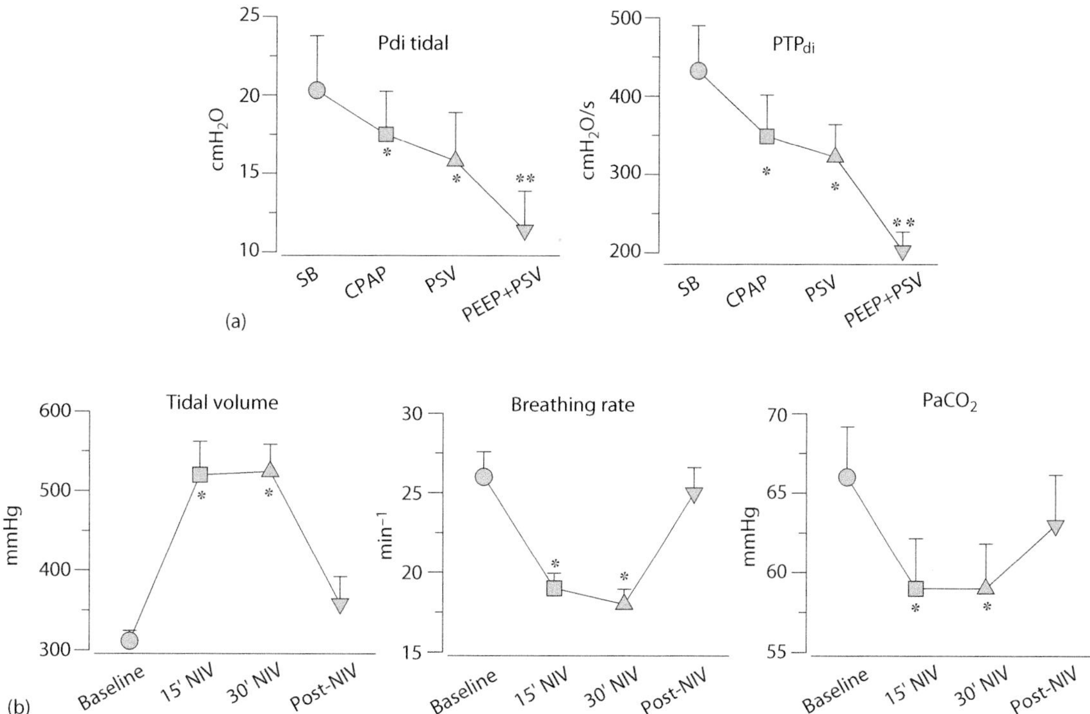

Figure 16.3 **(a)** Mean±SEM values of tidal transdiaphragmatic pressure (Pdi tidal) and pressure–time product of the diaphragm (PTP_{di}) during spontaneous breathing (SB), CPAP, PSV and PSV with positive end expiratory pressure (PEEP) of patients with COPD exacerbation. Single asterisks denote differences compared with SB. Double asterisks denote differences with CPAP and PSV alone. **(b)** Mean±SEM values of tidal volume, breathing frequency and arterial CO_2 tension ($PaCO_2$) during baseline in spontaneous breathing, after 15 and 30 min of NIV, and again in spontaneous breathing 15 min after withdrawal of NIV. Asterisks denote differences compared with baseline. ([a] Adapted from Appendini L et al., *Am J Respir Crit Care Med* 1994;149:1069–76; [b] Adapted from Diaz O et al., *Am J Respir Crit Care Med* 1997; 156: 1840–5.)

because part of the pressure required to overcome PEEPi and initiate inspiratory flow or trigger the ventilator is supplied (Figure 16.2).[10] The addition of pressure support ventilation (PSV) further unloads the inspiratory muscles and decreases the WOB, increases tidal volume and minute ventilation and improves gas exchange in these patients (Figure 16.3).[10]

Using NIV in patients with AECOPD and hypercapnic respiratory failure helps correct the rapid, shallow breathing pattern. The V_A/Q indices improve due to the combined increased minute ventilation and decreased lung perfusion, without major changes in V_A/Q mismatching.[11] These mechanisms result in increased PaO_2 and arterial pH, and decreased $PaCO_2$ (Figure 16.3).

DISCONTINUATION OF INVASIVE MECHANICAL VENTILATION

Discontinuation of invasive mechanical ventilation (IMV) is a challenging period that may represent 40%–50% of the total duration of ventilation.[12] Discontinuation of IMV may be particularly difficult in patients with chronic respiratory disorders.[13] As longer IMV is associated with increased mortality,[14] reducing the weaning period to an optimal duration is advisable.

Pathophysiology of weaning failure (Table 16.1)

Patients who cannot be weaned immediately from IMV often develop a rapid and shallow breathing pattern during the spontaneous breathing trial (SBT).[15,16]

Table 16.1 Pathophysiologic bases of weaning failure during transition from positive pressure ventilation to spontaneous breathing

- Rapid and shallow breathing pattern
- Increased workload for the respiratory muscles due to
  - Increased intrinsic positive end-expiratory pressure
  - Increased elastance and resistance of the respiratory system
  - Increased WOB
  - Increased effective inspiratory impedance
  - Increased load/capacity balance
- Inappropriate cardiovascular response
  - Increased venous return to right ventricle
  - Increased negative deflections in intrathoracic pressure
  - Increased left ventricular afterload
  - Fall of mixed venous oxygen pressure and saturation
- Impaired neurological status

The cardiovascular response to the switch from positive pressure ventilation to spontaneous breathing is also important to achieve successful weaning. An increase in the venous return to the right ventricle and, consequently, a leftward shift of the ventricular septum caused by ventricular interdependence and the large negative deflections in intrathoracic pressure due to the inspiratory threshold load, increases left ventricular afterload.[17] An inappropriate cardiovascular response to these changes with left ventricular dysfunction and increased pulmonary artery occlusion pressure occurs during weaning failure.[17,18] Weaning failure is also associated with decreased mixed venous oxygenation during spontaneous breathing,[19] which remains unchanged or increased during a successful SBT.[19–21]

Table 16.2 Physiologic effects of non-invasive positive pressure ventilation

- Effect on respiratory mechanics
  - Decrease negative deflections of intrathoracic pressure
  - Decrease WOB
  - Additive effects of positive pressure ventilation and external positive end-expiratory pressure in reducing the WOB
- Effects on gas exchange
  - Improvement of hypoxaemia and hypercapnia secondary to slower and deeper breathing pattern
  - No effects on ventilation–perfusion mismatch

Effects of NIV during unsuccessful weaning (Table 16.2)

The rationale for using NIV to facilitate weaning is based on its ability to offset several pathophysiological mechanisms associated with unsuccessful weaning. The effects of NIV on respiratory mechanics and gas exchange in non-intubated COPD patients with acute hypercapnia also apply in intubated patients.[10,11] Intubated ventilator-dependent patients with chronic respiratory disorders have been studied after recovery from the acute episode.[22] Invasive and non-invasive PSV were equally effective in reducing the WOB and improving arterial blood gases, compared to spontaneous breathing. In addition,

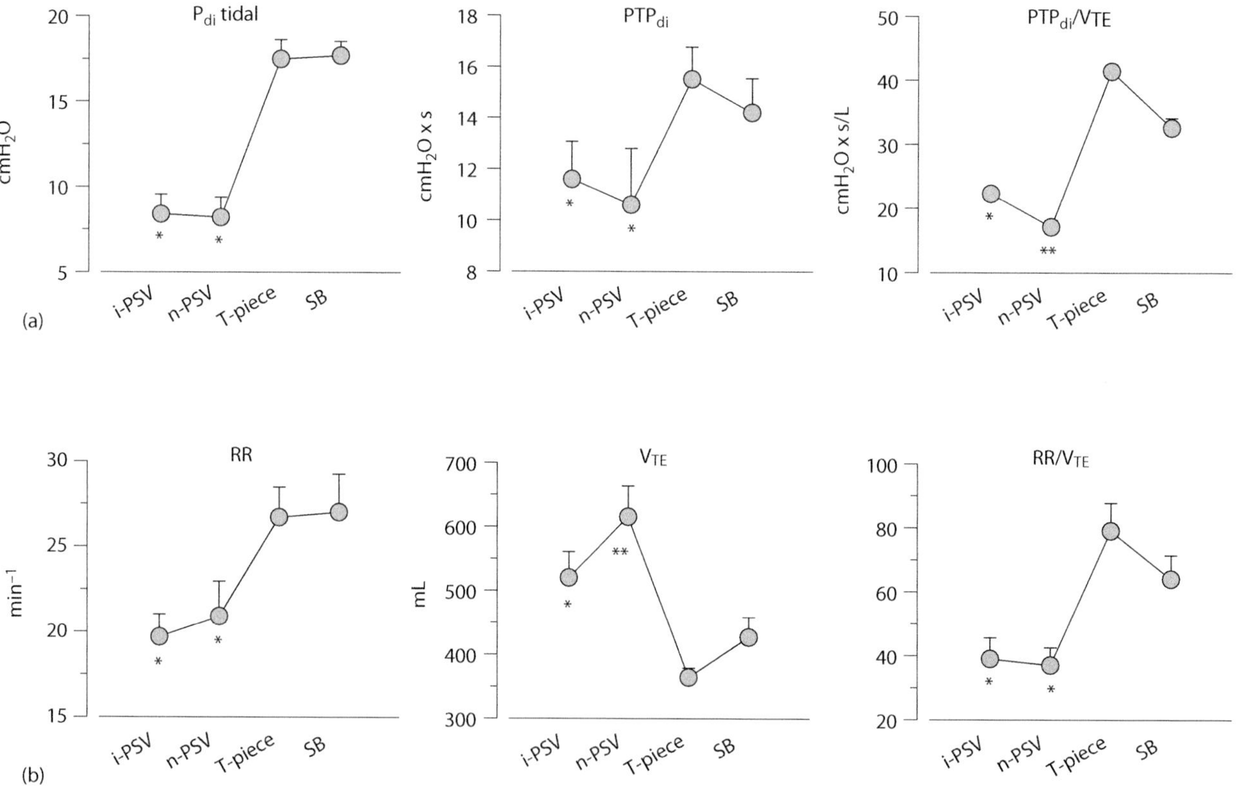

Figure 16.4 Physiologic effects of NIV in the weaning from IMV in ventilator-dependent patients with chronic respiratory disorders. Sequential measurements were done, prior to extubation, during a T-piece trial (T-piece) and invasive PSV (i-PSV), and later after extubation, in spontaneous breathing (SB) with oxygen mask and non-invasive PSV (n-PSV). **(a)** Mean±SEM values of tidal transdiaphragmatic pressure (P_{di} tidal), pressure–time product of the diaphragm (PTP_{di}) and the efficacy of the respiratory pump, assessed by the ratio of PTP_{di} and the expired tidal volume (V_{TE}). **(b)** Mean±SEM values of respiratory rate (RR), V_{TE} and rapid shallow breathing index (RR/V_{TE}). Single asterisks denote differences of i-PSV and n-PSV versus T-piece and SB. Double asterisks denote differences of n-PVS versus i-PSV. (Adapted from Vitacca M et al., *Am J Respir Crit Care Med* 2001;164:638–41.)

NIV improved the breathing pattern, the respiratory pump efficacy and tolerance better than invasive PSV (Figure 16.4). Therefore, the physiological effects of NIV observed in non-intubated COPD patients are present during the weaning period.

ACUTE CARDIAC FAILURE

The effects of NIV in heart failure are extensively discussed in Chapters 35 and 36. Changes in intrathoracic pressure during the respiratory cycle are transmitted to the heart, with changes in the pressure gradients for both systemic venous return (right ventricle preload) and systemic arterial outflow (left ventricular afterload).[23]

The decrease in pleural pressure during inspiratory efforts can become extremely negative in patients with heart failure.[24,25] When positive inspiratory pressure is applied and the respiratory muscles are unloaded, the negative swings of pleural pressure during inspiration decrease. Furthermore, PEEP or CPAP increases pleural pressure during expiration.[24,26]

Hypercapnia is common in patients with severe acute cardiac failure and may be associated with respiratory co-morbidities such as COPD or the obesity-hypoventilation syndrome. However, up to 50% of patients with severe acute cardiac failure, without chronic lung disease, are hypercapnic at admission.[27] Hypercapnia in these patients is associated with older age, obesity and systemic muscle weakness.

The most relevant physiologic effects of CPAP or NIV in patients with heart failure are as follows: (1) decreased venous return and ventricular preload as a consequence of increased right atrial pressure[28,29]; (2) decreased left ventricle afterload as a consequence of attenuation of negative pleural pressure swings during inspiration (Figure 16.5)[25,28–30]; (3) decreased WOB and oxygen consumption by unloading the respiratory muscles,[24] with higher systemic and mixed venous oxygenation and decreasing lactic acidosis[31]; and (4) variable effects on right ventricle afterload due to the combination of reversing hypoxic pulmonary vasoconstriction by recruiting collapsed lung areas with positive pressure, and development of pulmonary hyperinflation due to the positive airway pressure.

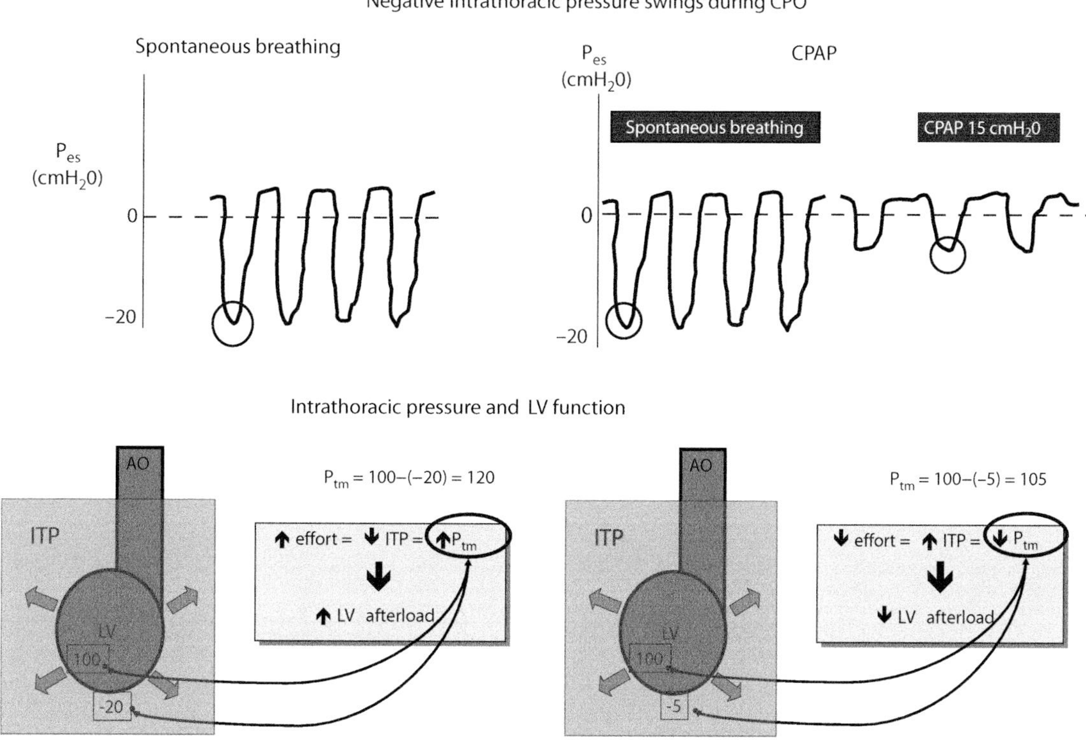

Figure 16.5 Schematic representation of the effects of CPAP on the negative inspiratory deflections of pleural pressure and left ventricle (LV) afterload in a patient with cardiogenic pulmonary oedema (CPO). Left upper panel: Pleural pressure during spontaneous breathing. The exaggerated negative swings of pleural pressure, assessed by oesophageal pressure (P_{es}), may reach up to −20 cm H_2O. Left lower panel: The transmural pressure (P_{tm}) represents the pressure needed by the LV to overcome both the aortic (AO) and the negative intrathoracic pressure (ITP). Due to the highly negative ITP, the increased P_{tm} of the LV results in increased LV afterload. Right upper panel: Pleural pressure while breathing with CPAP. The negative swings of pleural pressure are attenuated by the increase in pleural pressure induced by CPAP. Right lower panel: As a result of the decreased negative deflection of ITP, P_{tm} of the LV decreases, which results in decreased LV afterload. (Courtesy of Dr Stefano Nava, Bologna, Italy.)

ACUTE HYPOXAEMIC RESPIRATORY FAILURE

In selected patients with acute hypoxaemic respiratory failure, early institution of NIV may help in reversing the acute episode and reduce the need for endotracheal intubation.[32] However, the efficacy of NIV in these patients is far from optimal, and switching to invasive ventilation is often required.

Applying PEEP to the airway may increase alveolar recruitment and functional residual capacity (FRC), and improve respiratory mechanics and gas exchange.[33] CPAP has been used in order to prevent subsequent clinical deterioration and reduce the need for endotracheal intubation.[34,35]

The inspiratory effort expended by patients with acute hypoxaemic respiratory failure is approximately four to six times the normal value and can be brought down near to the normal range by careful selection of ventilator settings.[36] Non-invasive CPAP, which is the simplest way to apply positive airway pressure, raises intrathoracic pressure and reduces the transpulmonary WOB in intubated patients, indicating an improvement in respiratory mechanics, decreases intrapulmonary shunting, and may improve oxygenation and dyspnoea.[34]

The short-term physiologic effects of two combinations of PSV above PEEP and CPAP alone were studied in patients with acute hypoxaemic respiratory failure treated with NIV.[37] This study showed that PSV at two different levels reduced neuromuscular drive, unloaded the inspiratory muscles and improved dyspnoea. When used alone in this setting, CPAP was unable to reduce inspiratory effort. The greatest improvement in arterial oxygenation was achieved at a PEEP level of 10 cm H_2O, either with CPAP or PSV; the greatest improvement in dyspnoea was obtained with the highest level of PSV.[37] Figure 16.6 shows the most relevant findings of this study.[37] The absence of an effect of CPAP on respiratory effort may explain the failure of non-invasive CPAP to provide clinical benefits in these hypoxaemic patients.[38] These results also emphasise that improving oxygenation, as with CPAP alone, should not be the sole objective, because it is not always associated with a decrease in respiratory effort. Indeed, signs of exhaustion were the most frequent feature at the time of intubation in a controlled clinical trial on the efficacy of NIV in patients with acute hypoxaemic respiratory failure.[39]

The lack of beneficial effects of CPAP in patients with acute hypoxaemic respiratory failure observed in this study[37] does not rule out potential clinical benefits for CPAP in other populations. In the post-operative period, loss of lung volume, atelectasis and oxygenation impairment are frequent and may be the main pathophysiologic pathways of respiratory complications.[40–43] CPAP initiated during the post-operative period might reduce post-operative atelectasis, pneumonia and need for reintubation.[44]

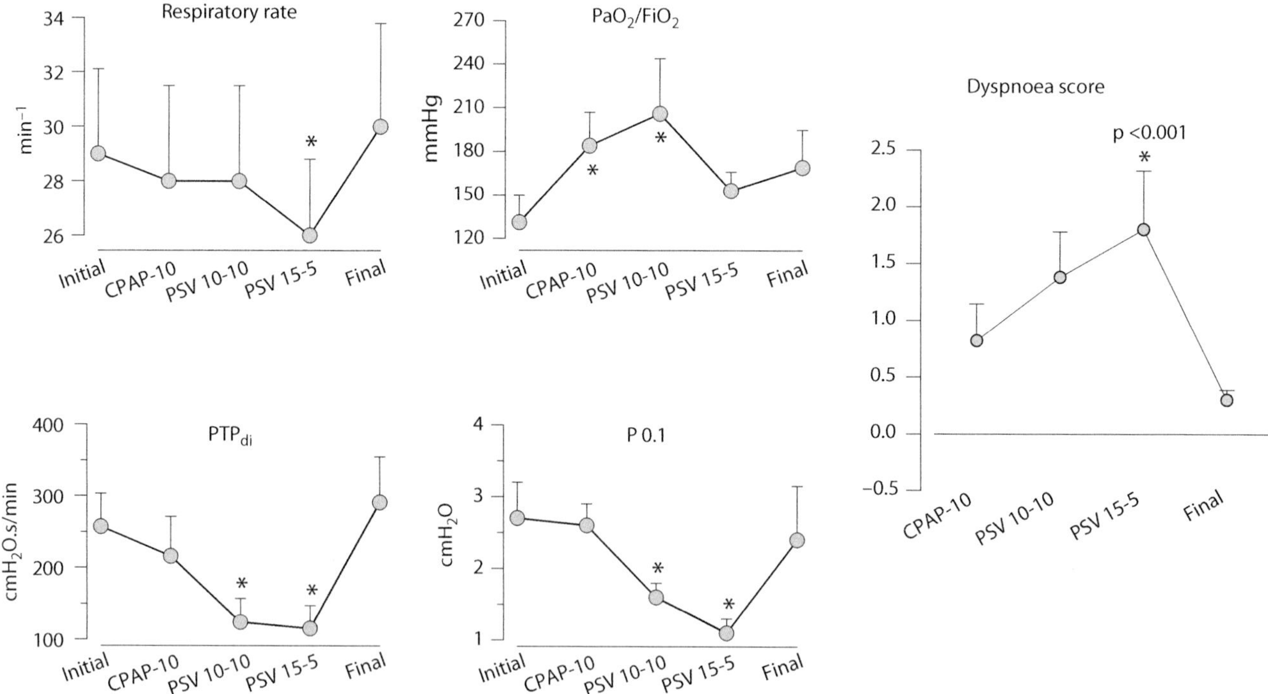

Figure 16.6 Summary of the most relevant physiologic effects of NIV in patients with acute hypoxaemic respiratory failure under spontaneous breathing (initial and final part of the study), during CPAP 10 cm H_2O, and during two combinations of PSV and PEEP 10–10 and 15–5 cm H_2O. PTP_{di} = pressure–time product of the diaphragm; P0.1 = neuromuscular drive, assessed by the oesophageal pressure decrease after 0.1 s. Changes in dyspnoea were assessed on the following scale: +2, marked improvement; +1, slight improvement; 0, no change; -1, slight deterioration; and -2, marked deterioration. (Adapted from L'Her E et al., *Am J Respir Crit Care Med* 2005;172:1112–8.)

HIGH-FLOW NASAL CANNULA OXYGENATION

In patients breathing at high inspiratory flow, conventional oxygen sources result in additional air entraining around the mask, thereby diluting the oxygen and lowering the FiO_2. In addition, conventional delivery devices have other drawbacks that reduce their efficacy and tolerance such as insufficient humidification and warming of the inspired gas at high flows that cause patient discomfort.[45]

HFNCO delivers oxygen flows of up to 60 L/min. The gas source is connected through an active heated humidifier to a nasal cannula and allows FiO_2 adjustment independently from the flow (Figure 16.7).[5]

Recent studies have suggested that HFNCO is effective in enhancing patients' comfort and oxygenation,[46,47] and it could be associated with better outcomes.[5] HFNCO maintains a good control of the actual FiO_2 by delivering flows higher than the spontaneous inspiratory demand, thereby diminishing room-air entrainment. As the difference between the patients' inspiratory flow and the delivered flow is small with HFNCO, the FiO_2 remains relatively stable. However, the flow rate must be set to match the patients' inspiratory demand and/or the severity of respiratory distress.

The clinical benefits of HFNCO are also related to an optimal conditioning of the delivered gas because the nasal air/oxygen mixtures are warmed and humidified closely to physiological conditions.[45,48] Thus, oxygen flow is better tolerated and provides greater comfort especially with flows up to 60 L/min.

Another mechanism is related to high-flow delivery. HFNCO therapy generates a flow-dependent positive airway pressure; the higher the flow delivered, the higher the positive airway pressure generated,[48,49] with consistently higher levels of airway pressure with the mouth closed as compared to open.[48,50] This issue is relevant when HFNCO is used in critically ill patients with acute hypoxaemic respiratory failure, who often breathe through an open mouth rather than through the nose.

The use of HFNCO is also associated with increased end-expiratory lung impedance in post-cardiac surgery patients, suggestive of increased FRC.[51] In obese post-cardiac surgery patients, the increase in FRC was significantly greater when HFNCO was used as compared to low-flow oxygen therapy, and may be the result of alveolar recruitment and prevention of further alveolar collapse due to the low level of positive pressure generated by HFNCO.[51] The higher PaO_2/FiO_2 reported in patients using HFNCO could be attributed in part to an increase in alveolar units available for ventilation. The clearance of CO_2 from the anatomical dead space also contributed to the improvement in subjective dyspnoea and decrease in respiratory rate.[47,52,53] Although the positive airway pressure generated by HFNCO is modest,[48–50] it could partially counteract PEEPi leading to decreased WOB and improved comfort in patients with dynamic hyperinflation. The continuous CO_2 flush out from the upper airway is another potential benefit of HFNCO, resulting in increased alveolar ventilation.

Thoracic-abdominal synchrony can also be improved with HFNCO as compared with face mask oxygen therapy.[54] Furthermore, HFNCO was associated with a lower respiratory rate while tidal volume was maintained, indicating a decrease in minute ventilation.[51,54]

All the currently available data suggest that HFNCO is an effective method for delivering oxygen therapy.

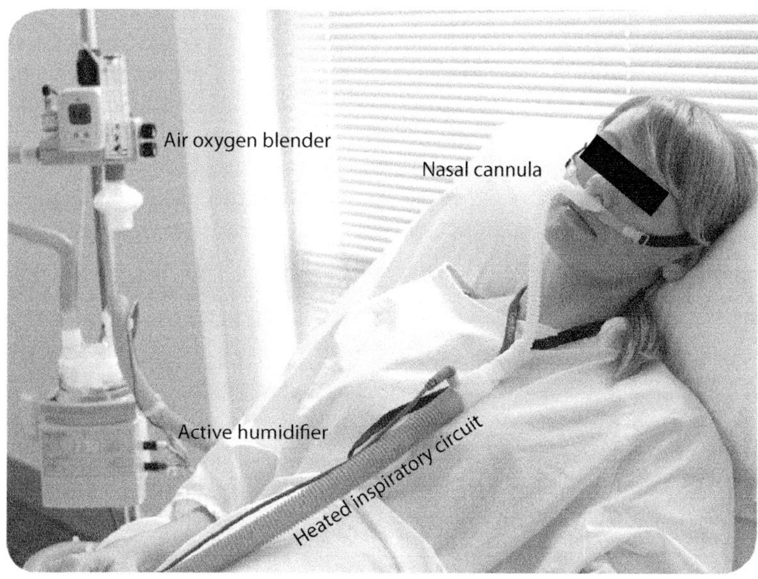

Figure 16.7 High-flow nasal cannula oxygenation device. An air/oxygen blender, allowing FiO_2 ranging from 0.21 to 1.0, generates flows of up to 60 L/min. The gas is heated and humidified by an active heated humidifier and delivered via a single limb.

Table 16.3 Potential physiological benefits of high-flow nasal cannula oxygenation compared to conventional oxygen therapy

Higher and stable FiO_2 values
Delivered gas flow higher than the spontaneous inspiratory demand
Smaller difference between the delivered flow rate and the patient's inspiratory flow rate
Flow set to match the patient's inspiratory demand and/or the severity of the respiratory distress
Improved ventilation/perfusion ratio and oxygenation
Decreased effect of the anatomical dead space by washout of the nasopharyngeal space
Participation of a larger fraction of minute ventilation in gas exchange
Decreased WOB
HFNCO mechanically stents the airway
Flow rates provided match the patient's inspiratory flow
Markedly attenuates the inspiratory resistance associated with the nasopharynx
More efficient respiratory efforts
Improved thoracic–abdominal synchrony
Heated and humidified gas delivered
Reduced WOB and improved mucociliary function by warm humid gas
Facilitated secretion clearance
Decreased risk of atelectasis
Less energy spent to warm and humidify the inspired gas
Better conductance and pulmonary compliance associated with warm humid gas, compared to dry, cooler gas
Adequately warmed and humidified gas only when flow is >40 L/min
Increased positive airway pressures
Continuous positive pressures in the pharynx (up to 8 cm H_2O)
Depends on flow and mouth opening
Lung distension by positive pressure
Lung recruitment
Decreased pulmonary ventilation–perfusion mismatch
Greater end-expiratory lung volume compared with low-flow oxygen therapy

Source: Papazian L et al., *Intensive Care Med* 2016.

Compared to conventional low-flow oxygen devices, HFNCO improves gas exchange, respiratory rate and comfort. HFNCO seems safer than a face mask, with less interface displacement and less episodes of oxygen desaturation.[47] The unique features of HFNCO lie in the simplicity of use,[55] the enhanced tolerance and comfort[47] in comparison with other forms of oxygen delivery, including NIV,[56,57] and its practicality in terms of oxygen and ventilation equipment management. The potential physiological benefits of HFNCO compared to conventional oxygen therapy are summarised in Table 16.3.

CONCLUSION

Increased knowledge of the pathophysiology of different clinical conditions causing ARF and the effects of NIV may contribute to improve the clinical application of this support measure in these patients. HFNCO, a most novel technique recently introduced in clinical practice, still needs studies to better understand the mechanisms of action.

REFERENCES

1. Ram FS, Picot J, Lightowler J et al. Non-invasive positive pressure ventilation for treatment of respiratory failure due to exacerbations of chronic obstructive pulmonary disease. *Cochrane Database Syst Rev.* 2004;CD004104.
2. Burns KE, Meade MO, Premji A et al. Noninvasive ventilation as a weaning strategy for mechanical ventilation in adults with respiratory failure: A Cochrane systematic review. *CMAJ.* 2014;186:E112–22.
3. Vital FM, Ladeira MT, Atallah AN. Non-invasive positive pressure ventilation (CPAP or bilevel NPPV) for cardiogenic pulmonary oedema. *Cochrane Database Syst Rev.* 2013;CD005351.
4. Nava S, Hill N. Non-invasive ventilation in acute respiratory failure. *Lancet.* 2009;374:250–9.
5. Papazian L, Corley A, Hess D et al. Use of high-flow nasal cannula oxygenation in ICU adults: A narrative review. *Intensive Care Med.* 2016;42:1336–49.
6. O'Donnell DE, Parker CM. COPD exacerbations. 3: Pathophysiology. *Thorax.* 2006;61:354–61.

7. Barbera JA, Roca J, Ferrer A et al. Mechanisms of worsening gas exchange during acute exacerbations of chronic obstructive pulmonary disease. *Eur Respir J.* 1997;10:1285–91.
8. Rossi A, Polese G, Brandi G et al. Intrinsic positive end-expiratory pressure (PEEPi). *Intensive Care Med.* 1995;21:522–36.
9. Yanos J, Wood LD, Davis K et al. The effect of respiratory and lactic acidosis on diaphragm function. *Am Rev Respir Dis.* 1993;147:616–9.
10. Appendini L, Patessio A, Zanaboni S et al. Physiologic effects of positive end-expiratory pressure and mask pressure support during exacerbations of chronic obstructive pulmonary disease. *Am J Respir Crit Care Med.* 1994;149:1069–76.
11. Diaz O, Iglesia R, Ferrer M et al. Effects of noninvasive ventilation on pulmonary gas exchange and hemodynamics during acute hypercapnic exacerbations of chronic obstructive pulmonary disease. *Am J Respir Crit Care Med.* 1997;156:1840–5.
12. Esteban A, Ferguson ND, Meade MO et al. Evolution of mechanical ventilation in response to clinical research. *Am J Respir Crit Care Med.* 2008;177:170–7.
13. Boles JM, Bion J, Connors A et al. Weaning from mechanical ventilation. *Eur Respir J.* 2007; 29:1033–56.
14. Esteban A, Anzueto A, Frutos F et al. Characteristics and outcomes in adult patients receiving mechanical ventilation: A 28-day international study. *JAMA.* 2002;287:345–55.
15. Tobin MJ, Perez W, Guenther SM et al. The pattern of breathing during successful and unsuccessful trials of weaning from mechanical ventilation. *Am Rev Respir Dis.* 1986;134:1111–8.
16. Jubran A, Tobin MJ. Pathophysiologic basis of acute respiratory distress in patients who fail a trial of weaning from mechanical ventilation. *Am J Respir Crit Care Med.* 1997;155:906–15.
17. Lemaire F, Teboul J, Cinotti L et al. Acute left ventricular dysfunction during unsuccessful weaning from mechanical ventilation. *Anesthesiology.* 1988;69:171–9.
18. Richard Ch, Teboul JL, Archambaud F et al. Left ventricular function during weaning of patients with chronic obstructive pulmonary disease. *Intensive Care Med.* 1994;20:181–6.
19. Jubran A, Mathru M, Dries D et al. Continuous recordings of mixed venous oxygen saturation during weaning from mechanical ventilation and the ramifications thereof. *Am J Respir Crit Care Med.* 1998;158:1763–9.
20. Torres A, Reyes A, Roca J et al. Ventilation-perfusion mismatching in chronic obstructive pulmonary disease during ventilator weaning. *Am Rev Respir Dis.* 1989;140:1246–50.
21. Ferrer M, Iglesia R, Roca J et al. Pulmonary gas exchange response to weaning with pressure-support ventilation in exacerbated COPD patients. *Intensive Care Med.* 2002;28:1595–9.
22. Vitacca M, Ambrosino N, Clini E et al. Physiological response to pressure support ventilation delivered before and after extubation in patients not capable of totally spontaneous autonomous breathing. *Am J Respir Crit Care Med.* 2001;164:638–41.
23. Bradley TD, Hall MJ, Ando S et al. Hemodynamic effects of simulated obstructive apneas in humans with and without heart failure. *Chest.* 2001;119:1827–35.
24. Lenique F, Habis M, Lofaso F et al. Ventilatory and hemodynamic effects of continuous positive airway pressure in left heart failure. *Am J Respir Crit Care Med.* 1997;155:500–5.
25. Naughton MT, Rahman MA, Hara K et al. Effect of continuous positive airway pressure on intrathoracic and left ventricular transmural pressures in patients with congestive heart failure. *Circulation.* 1995;91:1725–31.
26. Monnet X, Teboul JL, Richard C. Cardiopulmonary interactions in patients with heart failure. *Curr Opin Crit Care.* 2007;13:6–11.
27. Contou D, Fragnoli C, Cordoba-Izquierdo A et al. Severe but not mild hypercapnia affects the outcome in patients with severe cardiogenic pulmonary edema treated by non-invasive ventilation. *Ann Intensive Care.* 2015;5:55.
28. Bradley TD, Holloway RM, McLaughlin PR et al. Cardiac output response to continuous positive airway pressure in congestive heart failure. *Am Rev Respir Dis.* 1992;145:377–82.
29. Baratz DM, Westbrook PR, Shah PK et al. Effect of nasal continuous positive airway pressure on cardiac output and oxygen delivery in patients with congestive heart failure. *Chest.* 1992;102:1397–401.
30. De HA, Liu PP, Benard DC et al. Haemodynamic effects of continuous positive airway pressure in humans with normal and impaired left ventricular function. *Clin Sci (Lond).* 1995;88:173–8.
31. Pinsky MR. Cardiovascular issues in respiratory care. *Chest.* 2005;128:592S–7S.
32. Keenan SP, Sinuff T, Cook DJ et al. Does noninvasive positive pressure ventilation improve outcome in acute hypoxemic respiratory failure? A systematic review. *Crit Care Med.* 2004;32:2516–23.
33. Mehta S, Hill NS. Noninvasive ventilation (state of the art). *Am J Respir Crit Care Med.* 2001;163:540–77.
34. Katz JA, Marks JD. Inspiratory work with and without continuous positive airway pressure in patients with acute respiratory failure. *Anesthesiology.* 1985;63:598–607.

35. Hilbert G, Gruson D, Vargas F et al. Noninvasive continuous positive airway pressure in neutropenic patients with acute respiratory failure requiring intensive care unit admission. *Crit Care Med.* 2000;28:3185–90.
36. Tobin MJ. Advances in mechanical ventilation. *N Engl J Med.* 2001;344:1986–96.
37. L'Her E, Deye N, Lellouche F et al. Physiologic effects of noninvasive ventilation during acute lung injury. *Am J Respir Crit Care Med.* 2005;172:1112–8.
38. Delclaux C, L'Her E, Alberti C et al. Treatment of acute hypoxemic nonhypercapnic respiratory insufficiency with continuous positive airway pressure delivered by a face mask: A randomized controlled trial. *JAMA.* 2000;284:2352–60.
39. Ferrer M, Esquinas A, Leon M et al. Noninvasive ventilation in severe hypoxemic respiratory failure: A randomized clinical trial. *Am J Respir Crit Care Med.* 2003;168:1438–44.
40. Dureuil B, Cantineau JP, Desmonts JM. Effects of upper or lower abdominal surgery on diaphragmatic function. *Br J Anaesth.* 1987;59:1230–5.
41. Simonneau G, Vivien A, Sartene R et al. Diaphragm dysfunction induced by upper abdominal surgery. Role of postoperative pain. *Am Rev Respir Dis.* 1983;128:899–903.
42. Magnusson L, Spahn DR. New concepts of atelectasis during general anaesthesia. *Br J Anaesth.* 2003;91:61–72.
43. Eichenberger A, Proietti S, Wicky S et al. Morbid obesity and postoperative pulmonary atelectasis: An underestimated problem. *Anesth Analg.* 2002;95:1788–92.
44. Ireland CJ, Chapman TM, Mathew SF et al. Continuous positive airway pressure (CPAP) during the postoperative period for prevention of postoperative morbidity and mortality following major abdominal surgery. *Cochrane Database Syst Rev.* 2014;8:CD008930.
45. Chanques G, Constantin JM, Sauter M et al. Discomfort associated with underhumidified high-flow oxygen therapy in critically ill patients. *Intensive Care Med.* 2009;35:996–1003.
46. Cuquemelle E, Pham T, Papon JF et al. Heated and humidified high-flow oxygen therapy reduces discomfort during hypoxemic respiratory failure. *Respir Care.* 2012;57:1571–7.
47. Roca O, Riera J, Torres F et al. High-flow oxygen therapy in acute respiratory failure. *Respir Care.* 2010;55:408–13.
48. Chanques G, Riboulet F, Molinari N et al. Comparison of three high flow oxygen therapy delivery devices: A clinical physiological cross-over study. *Minerva Anestesiol.* 2013;79:1344–55.
49. Parke RL, McGuinness SP. Pressures delivered by nasal high flow oxygen during all phases of the respiratory cycle. *Respir Care.* 2013;58:1621–4.
50. Parke RL, Eccleston ML, McGuinness SP. The effects of flow on airway pressure during nasal high-flow oxygen therapy. *Respir Care.* 2011;56:1151–5.
51. Corley A, Caruana LR, Barnett AG et al. Oxygen delivery through high-flow nasal cannulae increase end-expiratory lung volume and reduce respiratory rate in post-cardiac surgical patients. *Br J Anaesth.* 2011;107:998–1004.
52. Schmidt M, Banzett RB, Raux M et al. Unrecognized suffering in the ICU: Addressing dyspnea in mechanically ventilated patients. *Intensive Care Med.* 2014;40:1–10.
53. Moller W, Celik G, Feng S et al. Nasal high flow clears anatomical dead space in upper airway models. *J Appl Physiol.* 2015;118:1525–32.
54. Itagaki T, Okuda N, Tsunano Y et al. Effect of high-flow nasal cannula on thoraco-abdominal synchrony in adult critically ill patients. *Respir Care.* 2014;59:70–4.
55. Lenglet H, Sztrymf B, Leroy C et al. Humidified high flow nasal oxygen during respiratory failure in the emergency department: Feasibility and efficacy. *Respir Care.* 2012;57:1873–8.
56. Frat JP, Brugiere B, Ragot S et al. Sequential application of oxygen therapy via high-flow nasal cannula and noninvasive ventilation in acute respiratory failure: An observational pilot study. *Respir Care.* 2015;60:170–8.
57. Frat JP, Thille AW, Mercat A et al. High-flow oxygen through nasal cannula in acute hypoxemic respiratory failure. *N Engl J Med.* 2015;372:2185–96.

17

Predicting outcome in patients with acute hypercapnic respiratory failure

TOM HARTLEY AND STEPHEN C. BOURKE

KEY POINTS

- Clinicians overestimate mortality and underutilise NIV. Clinical intuition is unreliable. Risk assessment should be based on objective criteria, ensuring patients make a truly informed choice.
- The index condition is of key importance. Outcomes are particularly favourable in COPD, OHS and NMD without severe bulbar impairment.
- In favourable conditions, coexistent pneumonia, hypercapnic coma or severe acidaemia are indications for closer monitoring, not contraindications to NIV.
- Other important predictors of poor outcome include poor stable state performance status and AHRF occurring 24 h or more after admission.
- NIV should not be a default treatment of AHRF; use should be based on objective risk assessment, and patients appropriately informed.

INTRODUCTION

In selected patients with acute hypercapnic respiratory failure (AHRF), non-invasive ventilation (NIV) is highly effective and offers advantages over invasive mechanical ventilation (IMV). Outcomes are particularly favourable in acute exacerbations of COPD (AECOPD), obesity hypoventilation syndrome (OHS) and neuromuscular disease (NMD) without severe bulbar impairment. However, decisions about escalation to NIV can be difficult, especially in multi-morbid individuals with poor performance status. There is troubling evidence that clinician estimates of outcome tend to be overly pessimistic (see below).[1] Consequently, patients likely to have a favourable outcome may not be offered, or be dissuaded from accepting, NIV. Conversely, in certain cases, immediate intubation or alternative palliation may be more appropriate. NIV is an intrusive therapy, and identification of patients with a poor prognosis should improve the appropriate provision of palliative care, which is poor in chronic respiratory illness. Objective and accurate estimation of outcome should guide selection of patients suitable for NIV and inform discussions with patients about treatment options. Risk assessment may also influence service design, facilitating timely initiation of NIV when a favourable outcome is likely whilst ensuring careful senior review in other cases and identification of patients who may benefit from closer monitoring during NIV. Within this process, it is essential that predictors of outcome are dispassionately assessed.[2] Both the condition being treated and individual patient factors strongly influence outcome. This chapter seeks to evaluate current knowledge of prognosis prediction.

CURRENT PRACTICE

Despite the marked increase in NIV use over recent decades,[3] under-utilisation remains a concern. The 2014 UK National COPD Audit showed that only 50.4% of patients with respiratory acidaemia on the first arterial blood gas (ABG), and 65.9% with persistent or new acidaemia on serial ABG, received ventilation.[4] US and Scandinavian studies show significant variation in ventilation rates.[3,5] NIV is now provided in various locations including emergency departments, admission and respiratory wards, respiratory support units/high dependency units and ICU, and a range of clinicians may be involved in the decision to initiate treatment, with significant variation between healthcare systems. Ward-based NIV is effective,[6] but, at least in high risk patients, higher levels of care offer better outcomes.[6,7]

HOW GOOD ARE CLINICIANS AT PREDICTING OUTCOME?

The COPD and asthma outcomes study (CAOS) assessed clinician-predicted mortality and actual mortality at 180 days in 92 ICUs and 3 respiratory HDUs in the United Kingdom[1,8]; 80% of predictions were unduly pessimistic. Better-than-expected survival was not achieved at an unacceptably high morbidity cost; 96% of survivors would choose to be ventilated again, and 73% reported equivalent or improved quality of life compared to a stable period prior to their index event. Within units, practice was fairly consistent, but between units, important patient characteristics such as age and baseline functional status varied markedly. Outside of specialist units, a wider variety of clinicians make similar clinical predictions; performance is unlikely to be better. Well-designed prognostic tools outperform expert judgement in various clinical settings; the same is true of simple statistical models in other walks of life. However, it is important to recognise the limitations of prognostic models. In patients requiring assisted ventilation, current purpose designed tools offer modest performance. This may reflect over-reliance on routinely captured physiological indices, whilst other important predictors of outcome, such as recent performance status when stable, were not assessed during development.[9–11] Additional objective criteria should be considered.

One reason for poor prediction of outcome as exemplified in the CAOS study is inherent bias. There are over 100 established types of cognitive bias that may influence clinical decision making, unless consciously avoided. This chapter does not aspire to provide a review of cognitive bias in medicine, but its effects, especially when considering such a fundamental decision as provision (or denial) of ventilatory support, should be borne in mind. Important biases are shown in Box 17.1.

In respect to assisted ventilation, a decision not to treat is usually a self-fulfilling prophecy, potentially reinforcing bias. Clinicians and teams are typically reasonably consistent within their own units, further limiting the opportunity for feedback on the accuracy of such judgements.

BOX 17.1: Examples of cognitive bias in medical practice

1. Bandwagon effect/herd mentality: the tendency to do what others do.
2. Confirmation bias: the tendency to select and interpret information to confirm our preconception.
3. Framing: differing conclusions can be drawn from the same information depending on how it is presented.
4. Anchoring: the tendency to rely too heavily or anchor to a particular piece of information.
5. Super-additivity and sub-additivity: the tendency to over- or underestimate the probability of the whole as compared to its component parts. Complicating this, clinicians struggle to recognise indices that confer true independent risk.

BASE MORTALITY RATE OF THE PRESENTING CONDITION

The most important prognostic information in any field is the base rate of an event's occurrence. In this setting, it is the mortality rate associated with provision of NIV for the presenting condition. Randomised controlled trials typically have a lower mortality than real-life audit data; this is likely to primarily reflect selection criteria, and perhaps closer monitoring, within clinical trials. In AECOPD requiring ventilation, real-life inpatient mortality is 25%–35%.[3,4,8] Among those who survive to discharge, 1 year mortality is 23.2%–49.1%.[12–15] In OHS, both outcomes tend to be more favourable. In NMD, most patients survive episodes of acute decompensation without escalation to invasive ventilation, provided bulbar function is not severely impaired. In contrast, outcomes with isolated pneumonia (not complicating the conditions listed above) and, in particular, idiopathic pulmonary fibrosis (IPF), are much less favourable.

COPD

Several of the prognostic indices in this section may be applicable to other conditions, but the populations in which they were derived were in whole or in the most part patients with AECOPD; care must be taken in cross-interpretation. Care must also be taken to differentiate between markers of inpatient mortality and predictors of NIV failure. The former is arguably the more clinically relevant. The definition of NIV failure is not standardised and inevitably subjective indices are included introducing a potential source of bias. Unless otherwise stated, inpatient mortality is being discussed.

Steady-state variables

Age has an uncertain effect on outcome: In a randomised controlled trial (RCT) of NIV vs. standard medical therapy in patients aged over 75 with AHRF predominantly secondary to COPD, rates of endotracheal intubation and mortality were lower in the NIV group.[16] In Confalonieri et al.'s work,[11] age was associated with NIV failure on univariate analysis but not after logistic regression. Age has been identified as an adverse factor in national audits, but it is uncertain whether this represents an independent risk or an association with other factors such as increasing disability, comorbidities or aggressiveness of treatment.[4] Age alone should not be used as the basis for treatment denial.[17]

Performance status: In AECOPD, stable state exercise capacity, most commonly assessed by the Medical Research Council dyspnoea scale (MRCD: 1–5), is a strong predictor of in-hospital mortality. The extended version (eMRCD) further improves prediction of outcome,[18,19] including in patients requiring ventilation.[20] Patients who are unable to leave their home unassisted are subdivided into levels 5a and 5b, depending on whether they need assistance washing and dressing (a measure of frailty). The Dyspnoea (eMRCD), Eosinopenia, Consolidation, Acidaemia and atrial Fibrillation (DECAF) prognostic score estimates risk of inpatient death in AECOPD, is easy to apply in the acute setting and offers excellent performance in unselected cohorts (AUROC = 0.82–0.86). It was developed in 2645 patients across six UK hospitals, with capture of consecutive unique admissions at each site. Outcomes in those receiving NIV stratified by the eMRCD scale are shown in Figure 17.1. Similarly, requiring limited or total assistance in activities of daily living is a predictor of late failure of NIV.[18,21] Stable state exercise capacity and independence in ADLs should be assessed routinely.

Low body mass index (BMI) is associated with both inpatient[22] and post-discharge mortality.[12,14] In a large cohort including non-ventilated patients, BMI < 18.5 and unintentional weight loss were associated with in-hospital mortality, but only the former was an independent predictor.[18]

Cough effectiveness has shown promise[23] but is inherently subjective. Nevertheless, it is intuitive that patients who are unable to clear secretions may have worse outcome, as is the case in other conditions such as amyotrophic lateral sclerosis (ALS) and bronchiectasis.

Of note, *FEV1* is a poor correlate with outcome. *Long-term oxygen* use may be linked to increased mortality (it is post discharge[12,24]), but further evaluation is necessary. On the basis of the available evidence, neither should be used as a sole reason for treatment denial.

Severity and timing of respiratory acidaemia

A *lower pH* is associated with higher mortality risk,[11,25] with a threshold of <7.25 most commonly cited. In a large UK audit of NIV in AECOPD (n = 9716),[26] inpatient mortality by admission pH was pH = 7.26–7.34 = 17%; pH ≤ 7.25 = 26%. Inpatient mortality is also related to the *timing of acidaemia*: (1) lowest pH on admission = 12%; (2) acidaemia on admission but lower pH later recorded = 21%; (3) normal pH on admission with subsequent acidaemia = 33%. Similar findings have been seen in UK annual audits[27] and were confirmed in a later study, which also showed that the adverse effects of severe acidaemia, late development of acidaemia and poor stable state performance status and frailty (eMRCD5b) are additive, and in combination confer a very poor prognosis.[20]

Investigations

Biochemical indices have been extensively studied due to their routine capture in clinical databases and are included in composite scores such as APACHE II and CAPS. *Neutrophil count,*[20] *Eosinopenia,*[18] *CRP,*[28] *creatinine,*[28] *urea,*[25] *bilirubin,*[23] *albumin*[29] and *glucose*[30] are associated with mortality, but with variation between studies. No one blood marker should be relied on in isolation. In AECOPD complicated by *pneumonia*, NIV is associated with a lower risk of intubation acutely and lower mortality at 2 months. Co-existent pneumonia should not exclude patients with AECOPD from NIV.[31]

Observations

Multiple physiological indices show relation to mortality and are included within composite scores. Evidence of other organ failure, including *low blood pressure* unresponsive to fluid resuscitation, raises concern. An elevated *respiratory rate* (RR) is a consistent independent predictor of mortality,

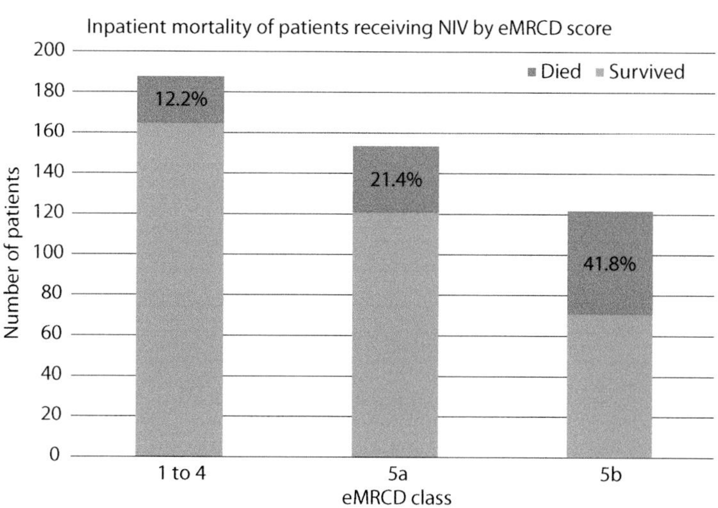

Figure 17.1 In-hospital mortality of patients with an exacerbation of COPD treated with NIV for AHRF, stratified by eMRCD score. Data from DECAF programme of research (n = 464; overall mortality 23.1%). (Unpublished data.)

particularly RR > 30.[30] A low *Glasgow Coma Scale* (GCS) is also associated with adverse outcome in some studies,[11,23] but this is not a consistent finding. Of importance, in a case mixed, dual centre series of 958 patients receiving NIV on ICU, in-hospital mortality was: GCS ≤ 8 = 26.3%; GCS > 8 = 33.2%.[32] Patients with GCS < 8 were managed with nasogastric tubes to reduce risk of aspiration. Low GCS presumed due to hypercapnia should not be regarded as a contraindication to NIV, but rather it identifies patients who should be considered higher risk and managed in an environment allowing close monitoring. In patients deteriorating despite optimal NIV, or in those with another cause for low GCS, IMV or alternative palliation may be appropriate.

Predictive tools

Several prognostic tools have been specifically developed, or at least assessed, in AECOPD requiring assisted ventilation. APACHE II, COPD and Asthma Physiology score (CAPS) and the simplified acute physiology score (SAPS)[10,11,32,33] are mainly composed of physiological indices, are complex to score and offer only modest performance. The largest study developed a tool to predict NIV failure (Figure 17.2). It offers modest prediction (AUROC 0.71) prior to initiation, but better performance when rescored after 2 hours (AUROC 0.83). The score is based on a GCS, pH, RR and APACHE II score; adoption outside of the ICU setting may have been hampered by the need to calculate a full APACHE II score.[11] DECAF offers simple scoring and excellent performance in general AECOPD. Whilst it has not been validated in this subgroup, mortality is very low in those who are otherwise low risk by DECAF. The highest scores are associated with both high mortality and a short time to death.[21]

Post initiation

Markers of poor outcome after NIV has been commenced are both intuitive (i.e. patients who do not improve following instigation of treatment do worse) and less useful than markers present prior to initiation as they do not aid patient selection. NIV failure is associated with higher APACHE II scores.[33] Failing to improve (or falling) pH is probably the strongest determinant of failure.[11,15,25] Varying time cut-offs (1–4 hours) have been mooted. Similarly, failure to improve physiological indices such as GCS, RR or heart rate may indicate worse prognosis.

Late failure of NIV, following initial correction of respiratory acidaemia, is associated with mortality and is more common in patients who require limited or complete assistance with ADLs (frailty). Moretti et al. used the following definition: "a sudden or progressive worsening of arterial blood gas tensions (pH < 7.34 with an increase in $PaCO_2$ of >15%–20% compared with previous arterial blood gas tensions), dyspnoea and/or sensory deterioration while still on mechanical ventilation for at least 6 hours/day." Mortality was high in both arms, but continuing NIV in lieu of invasive ventilation conferred an extremely poor prognosis (mortality: NIV group 92%, Intubated group 53%). Of note, group selection was based on patient preference, pH at the time of late failure was much lower in the NIV group and patient numbers were low.[34] In a similar ICU cohort, late failure of NIV was associated with 80% mortality.[35] Cardiac complications and nosocomial infection were important contributors to deterioration and death; however, the definition of late failure included non-objective criteria, limiting wider generalisabilty. In contrast, in a small cohort from our institution (n = 14) in whom late failure was managed with high-pressure NIV, we found that in-hospital mortality was substantially lower (32%).[36] Further study of late failure is warranted to draw definitive conclusion. A binary choice between intubation or palliation should late failure develop as advocated by some is questionable; a trial of intensification of NIV with close monitoring, and careful clinical review to ensure the underlying condition is optimally managed, may be beneficial.

OTHER CONDITIONS

Some or even all of the individual prognostic factors identified in COPD populations may apply to other conditions, but this is not definitively known. As previously highlighted, a key predictor outcome is the condition being treated. The following section will overview other key situations in which NIV may be used.

		pH admission < 7.25		pH admission 7.25–7.29		pH admission > 7.30	
	RR	APACHE > 29	APACHE < 29	APACHE ≥ 29	APACHE < 29	APACHE ≥ 29	APACHE < 29
GCS 15	<30	29	11	18	6	17	6
	30–34	42	18	29	11	27	10
	≥35	42	24	37	15	35	14
GCS 12–14	<30	48	22	33	13	33	12
	30–34	63	34	48	22	46	21
	≥35	71	42	57	29	55	27
GCS ≤11	<30	64	35	49	23	47	21
	30–34	76	49	64	35	62	33
	≥35	82	59	72	44	70	42

Figure 17.2 Chart of failure risk for NIV in patients with COPD exacerbation. NIV failure was defined as intubation or death. (From Confalonieri M et al., *Eur Respir J.* 2005;25(2):348–55.)

Obesity hypoventilation syndrome

In AHRF due to OHS, RCTs comparing NIV to IMV or no ventilation have not been conducted. However, compared to real-world studies in AECOPD, cohort studies show lower rates of in-hospital mortality[26,37,38] and late failure, with a trend towards better survival at 1 year.[37] NIV outcomes are also better than those receiving IMV, either primarily or after an initial trial of NIV.[39] The presenting diagnosis remains the best predictor of outcome, and a trial of NIV should generally be offered. However, recognition that AHRF is due to OHS is essential. Of concern, in a cohort of 61 such patients, pre-admission 75% were inappropriately treated for COPD or asthma (none had obstructive spirometry), and only three had a diagnosis of OHS, whilst the admitting diagnosis in all was AECOPD and/or heart failure.[40] Vigilance is required. Higher BMI predicts late failure[39]; whilst the risk is not sufficient to justify immediate intubation or withholding NIV, closer monitoring should be considered in the super-obese (BMI > 50). In patients with AECOPD, coexistent obesity is associated with lower rates of late failure and 1 year readmission; the latter may in part be explained by more frequent use of domiciliary NIV.[37]

Neuromuscular disease

In NMD, ventilation decisions are most challenging in patients not previously established on home ventilation, and particularly if AHRF is the first presentation of a previously undiagnosed condition. The rate of progression of the underlying condition and bulbar function are of particular importance. In rapidly progressive conditions such as ALS and Duchenne muscular dystrophy, almost all patients will require long-term ventilation if they survive, even if acute decompensation was triggered by a reversible event. Consequently, it is important to clarify the patient's views on home ventilation. Although the same is true in most patients with a slowly progressive condition such as myotonic dystrophy, there is a better chance of weaning from ventilation; thus, in those who do not wish long-term ventilation, it is more reasonable to still consider NIV acutely. Severe bulbar impairment is the strongest predictor of NIV failure[41]; either immediate IMV or alternative palliation may be more appropriate. In patients without severe bulbar impairment, NIV improves survival and reduces ITU length of stay and complications (including ventilator-associated pneumonia) compared to match controls receiving IMV.[42] In addition to NIV, non-invasive sputum clearance techniques are important. Mechanical insufflation–exsufflation offers better results than alternatives, but it is also less effective in patients with severe bulbar impairment.

Asthma

There is currently insufficient evidence to recommend routine use of NIV in patients with asthma. However, reported outcomes tend to be favourable, and this may be particularly true of patients with a substantial degree of airways remodelling.[17] If NIV is used, this should be in an area with close monitoring and rapid access to IMV if required.

Pneumonia

Pneumonia has consistently been shown to be a strong predictor of NIV failure and in-hospital mortality.[23,27,33] Nevertheless, the difference between pneumonia complicating a NIV-responsive underlying condition and isolated pneumonia should be noted. Complicating pneumonia should not be considered a contraindication to NIV, but rather a marker of increased risk and need for closer monitoring. Indeed, in pneumonic exacerbations of COPD, NIV is associated with better outcomes compared to IMV, including 2 month survival.[31] Similarly, in pneumonia complicating OHS or NMD without severe bulbar impairment, a trial of NIV is usually justified. In contrast, in isolated pneumonia, persisting with NIV may worsen outcomes.

IPF

Patients with IPF are often slightly younger, with a rapid progression from good health. Outcomes following NIV or IMV for exacerbations of IPF are poor; mortality is typically 80%–90% overall and tends to be higher with IMV than NIV.[43–45] Of those who survive to discharge, most die within 6 months. Limited data suggest that an elevated BNP level is a marker of exceptionally poor outcome. These factors should emphasise to all those caring for patients with IPF the importance of advanced care planning with particular consideration paid to shared, informed, future ventilation decisions. More recent data from the US National Inpatient Sample (2006–2012) showed much better outcomes: IMV (n = 1703) mortality = 51.9%; NIV (n = 778) mortality = 30.9%[46]; this is probably related to inclusion of patients in whom IPF was simply a comorbidity rather than the primary reason for AHRF. Of note, other (potentially more reversible) forms of interstitial lung disease such as drug-induced pneumonitis may benefit from NIV or IMV in the acute setting and should be identified on a case-by-case basis.

Pulmonary oedema

Mortality in acute pulmonary oedema is of the order 10%–12%.[47,48] The relative merits of CPAP vs. NIV will not be discussed here, although CPAP is usually sufficient even if acidaemia is present. CPAP/NIV is associated with more rapid relief of breathless and physiological improvement, and probably improves survival, particularly in patients not showing an early improvement with medical therapy alone. Of note, acidaemia is a poor predictor of mortality in pulmonary oedema and should not be used to determine treatment.[48,49] Using regression modelling of data from the 3CPO trial, the study group identified a prediction model

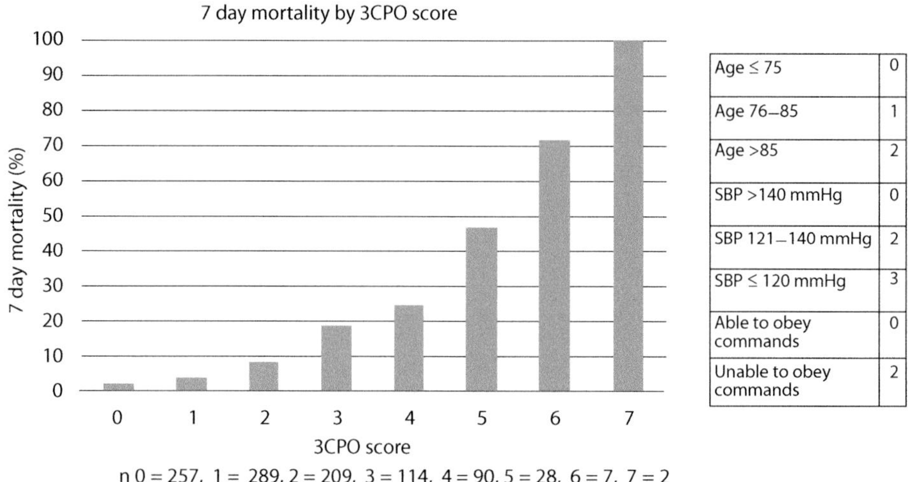

Age ≤ 75	0
Age 76–85	1
Age >85	2
SBP >140 mmHg	0
SBP 121–140 mmHg	2
SBP ≤ 120 mmHg	3
Able to obey commands	0
Unable to obey commands	2

Figure 17.3 Seven day mortality risk by 3CPO score in pulmonary oedema. (From Gray A et al., *Circ Heart Failure.* 2010;3(1):111–7.)

of 7 day mortality that includes age, systolic blood pressure and inability to obey commands.[50] The adverse scores across all three indices conferred a particularly poor outcome (Figure 17.3).

CONCLUSIONS AND SUGGESTED APPROACH

NIV is among the most effective clinical interventions; in favourable conditions, the NNT is substantially lower than PCI for acute coronary syndromes or thrombolysis in stroke. Despite this, it is underutilised. Reliance on clinical intuition alone is unreliable. Unduly pessimistic estimates of survival may lead to well-intended clinicians either withholding or dissuading patients from accepting NIV in favour of palliative care. In the latter situation, the patient's choice is not an (appropriately) informed choice. Risk assessment should be based on objective criteria, which in turn will drive improvements in patient-centred decision-making, clinical care and outcomes. A better understanding of NIV outcomes should also drive improvements in structures of care.

The presenting diagnosis strongly influences outcome; this should be rapidly confirmed bearing in mind that AHRF may be the first presentation of a previously undiagnosed condition. OHS is often unrecognised both prior to and during episodes of acute decompensation. Previously unrecognised NMD can present a diagnostic challenge. Outcomes are particularly favourable in AECOPD, OHS and NMD without severe bulbar impairment; NIV should be offered by default. Adverse factors such as hypercapnic coma or co-existent consolidation are indications for closer monitoring, not contraindications to NIV. Occasionally, in those with a combination of highly adverse factors, immediate intubation or alternative palliation may be appropriate. Outcomes from assisted ventilation for exacerbations of IPF are poor; CPAP or NIV may be considered in fully informed patients, but if they continue to deteriorate, palliation rather than IMV is generally appropriate. In other conditions, such as acute asthma, isolated pneumonia and NMD with severe bulbar impairment, IMV probably offers better outcomes than NIV and should not be delayed if appropriate. In patients deemed 'not for intubation', NIV should not be used as a default ceiling of care, but rather such decisions should be informed by objective risk assessment, taking account of the patients' appropriately informed views.

Performance status on a good day in the last 3 months, and independence in activities of daily living, should be assessed. The timing of respiratory academia should be considered. Clinical deterioration after admission despite primary treatment, with the late development of respiratory acidaemia, is associated with worse outcomes. Important co-morbidities and other adverse prognostic markers should be reviewed. Age, and specifically in COPD, FEV1 and LTOT, should not be the basis for treatment denial. Physiological and blood markers such as a higher RR, pH < 7.25 or elevated urea have frequently been associated with poorer outcome but should be afforded little individual weighting.

Services should be established to rapidly assess patients and minimise unnecessary delays in instigating treatment when a favourable outcome is likely. Shorter door to mask time reduces mortality. Whilst, particularly in COPD, a proportion of patients correct with medical therapy alone, this is likely to have fallen with the reduction in the inappropriate use of excess oxygen. During such trials, patients should remain closely monitored and NIV commenced if improvement is not seen within 1 h.

REFERENCES

1. Wildman MJ, Sanderson C, Groves J et al. Implications of prognostic pessimism in patients with chronic obstructive pulmonary disease (COPD) or asthma admitted to intensive care in the UK within the COPD and asthma outcome study (CAOS): Multicentre observational cohort study. *BMJ*. 2007;335(7630):1132.
2. Meehl PE. *Clinical versus Statistical Prediction: A Theoretical Analysis and a Review of the Evidence*. Minneapolis, MN, US: University of Minnesota Press; 1954. x, 149 p.
3. Chandra D, Stamm JA, Taylor B et al. Outcomes of noninvasive ventilation for acute exacerbations of chronic obstructive pulmonary disease in the United States, 1998–2008. *Am J Respir Crit Care Med*. 2012;185(2):152–9.
4. Stone R, Holzhauer-Barrie J, Lowe D et al. COPD: Who cares matters. National Chronic Obstructive Pulmonary Disease (COPD) Audit Programme: Clinical audit of COPD exacerbations admitted to acute units in England and Wales. 2014;2015.
5. Liaaen ED, Henriksen AH, Stenfors N. A Scandinavian audit of hospitalizations for chronic obstructive pulmonary disease. *Respir Med*. 2010; 104(9):1304–9.
6. Plant PK, Owen JL, Elliott MW. Early use of non-invasive ventilation for acute exacerbations of chronic obstructive pulmonary disease on general respiratory wards: A multicentre randomised controlled trial. *Lancet*. 2000;355(9219):1931–5.
7. Brochard L, Mancebo J, Wysocki M et al. Noninvasive ventilation for acute exacerbations of chronic obstructive pulmonary disease. *N Engl J Med*. 1995;333(13):817–22.
8. Wildman MJ, Sanderson CF, Groves J et al. Survival and quality of life for patients with COPD or asthma admitted to intensive care in a UK multicentre cohort: The COPD and Asthma Outcome Study (CAOS). *Thorax*. 2009;64(2):128–32.
9. Knaus WA, Draper EA, Wagner DP et al. APACHE II: A severity of disease classification system. *Crit Care Med*. 1985;13(10):818–29.
10. Wildman MJ, Harrison DA, Welch CA et al. A new measure of acute physiological derangement for patients with exacerbations of obstructive airways disease: The COPD and Asthma Physiology Score. *Respir Med*. 2007;101(9):1994–2002.
11. Confalonieri M, Garuti G, Cattaruzza MS et al. A chart of failure risk for noninvasive ventilation in patients with COPD exacerbation. *Eur Respir J*. 2005;25(2):348–55.
12. Chung LP, Winship P, Phung S et al. Five-year outcome in COPD patients after their first episode of acute exacerbation treated with non-invasive ventilation. *Respirology*. 2010;15(7):1084–91.
13. Steer J, Gibson GJ, Bourke SC. Longitudinal change in quality of life following hospitalisation for acute exacerbations of COPD. *BMJ Open Respir Res*. 2015;2(1):e000069.
14. Chu CM, Chan VL, Lin AW et al. Readmission rates and life threatening events in COPD survivors treated with non-invasive ventilation for acute hypercapnic respiratory failure. *Thorax*. 2004; 59(12):1020–5.
15. Plant PK, Owen JL, Elliott MW. Non-invasive ventilation in acute exacerbations of chronic obstructive pulmonary disease: long term survival and predictors of in-hospital outcome. *Thorax*. 2001;56(9):708–12.
16. Nava S, Grassi M, Fanfulla F et al. Non-invasive ventilation in elderly patients with acute hypercapnic respiratory failure: A randomised controlled trial. *Age Ageing*. 2011;40(4):444–50.
17. Davidson AC, Banham S, Elliott M et al. BTS/ICS guideline for the ventilatory management of acute hypercapnic respiratory failure in adults. *Thorax*. 2016;71(Suppl 2):ii1–ii35.
18. Steer J, Gibson J, Bourke SC. The DECAF Score: Predicting hospital mortality in exacerbations of chronic obstructive pulmonary disease. *Thorax*. 2012;67(11):970–6.
19. Steer J, Norman EM, Afolabi OA et al. Dyspnoea severity and pneumonia as predictors of in-hospital mortality and early readmission in acute exacerbations of COPD. *Thorax*. 2012;67(2):117–21.
20. Steer J, Gibson J, Bourke S. Predicting mortality in patients hospitalised with acute exacerbations of COPD (AECOPD) requiring assisted ventilation. *Eur Respir J*. 2012;40(Suppl 56).
21. Echevarria C, Steer J, Heslop-Marshall K et al. Validation of the DECAF score to predict hospital mortality in acute exacerbations of COPD. *Thorax*. 2016;71(2):133–40.
22. Ambrosino N, Foglio K, Rubini F et al. Non-invasive mechanical ventilation in acute respiratory failure due to chronic obstructive pulmonary disease: Correlates for success. *Thorax*. 1995;50(7):755–7.
23. Sidhom S, Ugurlu A, Khodabandeh A et al. Predictors of noninvasive ventilation failure in acute respiratory failure. D104 Mechanical ventilation. American Thoracic Society International Conference Abstracts: American Thoracic Society. 2011;83:A6238.
24. Hajizadeh N, Goldfeld K, Crothers K. What happens to patients with COPD with long-term oxygen treatment who receive mechanical ventilation for COPD exacerbation? A 1-year retrospective follow-up study. *Thorax*. 2015;70(3):294–6.
25. Miller D, Fraser K, Murray I et al. Predicting survival following non-invasive ventilation for hypercapnic exacerbations of chronic obstructive pulmonary disease. *Int J Clin Pract*. 2012;66(5):434–7.

26. Roberts CM, Stone RA, Buckingham RJ et al. Acidosis, non-invasive ventilation and mortality in hospitalised COPD exacerbations. *Thorax*. 2010.
27. Davies M. Report British Thoracic Society NIV Audit. British Thoracic Society; 2013.
28. Ucgun I, Metintas M, Moral H et al. Predictors of hospital outcome and intubation in COPD patients admitted to the respiratory ICU for acute hypercapnic respiratory failure. *Respir Med*. 2006; 100(1):66–74.
29. Connors AF, Jr., Dawson NV, Thomas C et al. Outcomes following acute exacerbation of severe chronic obstructive lung disease. The SUPPORT investigators (Study to Understand Prognoses and Preferences for Outcomes and Risks of Treatments). *Am J Respir Crit Care Med*. 1996;154(4 Pt 1):959–67.
30. Chakrabarti B, Angus RM, Agarwal S et al. Hyperglycaemia as a predictor of outcome during non invasive ventilation in decompensated COPD. *Thorax*. 2009;64:857–86.
31. Confalonieri M, Potena A, Carbone G et al. Acute respiratory failure in patients with severe community-acquired pneumonia. A prospective randomized evaluation of noninvasive ventilation. *Am J Respir Crit Care Med*. 1999;160(5 Pt 1): 1585–91.
32. Diaz GG, Alcaraz AC, Talavera JC et al. Noninvasive positive-pressure ventilation to treat hypercapnic coma secondary to respiratory failure. *Chest*. 2005;127(3):952–60.
33. Phua J, Kong K, Lee KH et al. Noninvasive ventilation in hypercapnic acute respiratory failure due to chronic obstructive pulmonary disease vs. other conditions: effectiveness and predictors of failure. *Intensive Care Med*. 2005;31(4):533–9.
34. Moretti M, Cilione C, Tampieri A et al. Incidence and causes of non-invasive mechanical ventilation failure after initial success. *Thorax*. 2000;55(10): 819–25.
35. Carratù P, Bonfitto P, Dragonieri S et al. Early and late failure of noninvasive ventilation in chronic obstructive pulmonary disease with acute exacerbation. *Eur J Clin Investig*. 2005;35(6):404–9.
36. Palmer E, Burns H, Bourke SC. Late failure of non-invasive ventilation in COPD. European Respiratory Society International Congress, Abstract. 2014.
37. Carrillo A, Ferrer M, Gonzalez-Diaz G et al. Noninvasive ventilation in acute hypercapnic respiratory failure caused by obesity hypoventilation syndrome and chronic obstructive pulmonary disease. *Am J Respir Crit Care Med*. 2012;186(12):1279–85.
38. Rabec C, Merati M, Baudouin N et al. Management of obesity and respiratory insufficiency. The value of dual-level pressure nasal ventilation. *Rev Mal Respir*. 1998;15(3):269–78.
39. Duarte AG, Justino E, Bigler T et al. Outcomes of morbidly obese patients requiring mechanical ventilation for acute respiratory failure. *Crit Care Med*. 2007;35(3):732–7.
40. Marik PE, Desai H. Characteristics of patients with the "malignant obesity hypoventilation syndrome" admitted to an ICU. *J Intensive Care Med*. 2013;28(2):124–30.
41. Servera E, Sancho J, Zafra MJ et al. Alternatives to endotracheal intubation for patients with neuromuscular diseases. *Am J Phys Med Rehabi/Assoc Acad Physiatr*. 2005;84(11):851–7.
42. Vianello A, Bevilacqua M, Arcaro G et al. Non-invasive ventilatory approach to treatment of acute respiratory failure in neuromuscular disorders. A comparison with endotracheal intubation. *Intensive Care Med*. 2000;26(4):384–90.
43. Mollica C, Paone G, Conti V et al. Mechanical ventilation in patients with end-stage idiopathic pulmonary fibrosis. *Respiration*. 2010;79(3):209–15.
44. Vianello A, Arcaro G, Battistella L et al. Noninvasive ventilation in the event of acute respiratory failure in patients with idiopathic pulmonary fibrosis. *J Crit Care*. 2014;29(4):562–7.
45. Fumeaux T, Rothmeier C, Jolliet P. Outcome of mechanical ventilation for acute respiratory failure in patients with pulmonary fibrosis. *Intensive Care Med*. 2001;27(12):1868–74.
46. Rush B, Wiskar K, Berger L et al. The use of mechanical ventilation in patients with idiopathic pulmonary fibrosis in the United States: A nationwide retrospective cohort analysis. *Respir Med*. 2016;111:72–6.
47. Roguin A, Behar D, Ben Ami H et al. Long-term prognosis of acute pulmonary oedema—An ominous outcome. *Eur J Heart Failure*. 2000;2(2):137–44.
48. Gray A, Goodacre S, Newby DE et al. Noninvasive ventilation in acute cardiogenic pulmonary edema. *N Engl J Med*. 2008;359(2):142–51.
49. Aliberti S, Piffer F, Brambilla AM et al. Acidemia does not affect outcomes of patients with acute cardiogenic pulmonary edema treated with continuous positive airway pressure. *Crit Care (Lond)*. 2010;14(6):R196.
50. Gray A, Goodacre S, Nicholl J et al. The development of a simple risk score to predict early outcome in severe acute acidotic cardiogenic pulmonary edema: The 3CPO score. *Circ Heart Fail*. 2010;3(1):111–7.

18

Use of NIV in the real world

MIHAELA STEFAN, PETER LINDENAUER, NAJIA INDRESS,
FAISAL TAMIMI AND NICHOLAS S. HILL

INTRODUCTION

In the past 20 years, use of non-invasive ventilation (NIV) has increased from rare to highly prevalent in many intensive care units (ICUs) around the world.[1] This increase in use has been driven by accumulating evidence from randomised controlled trials (RCTs) and meta-analyses that have led to wide agreement that acute hypercapnic respiratory failure (AHcRF), mainly due to chronic obstructive pulmonary disease (COPD), and acute cardiogenic pulmonary oedema (CPE) are the main indications for NIV. As important as RCTs are for establishing the safety and efficacy of an intervention, though, they do not inform us as to how an intervention is actually being used in 'real life' – at hospitals or other settings in the community.

Approaches to obtaining data on 'real-life' applications have been evolving including surveys of caregivers[2] and of patient management at different institutions, but such approaches have limitations. Surveys of providers reveal what the respondents think they do, not necessarily what they do, and large multi-institutional surveys reflect what is done at institutions that are willing to participate, but not at those unwilling, and they are limited in what can be done to validate data. Recently, analyses of 'big data' using pooled data from large multi-institutional databases, usually based on diagnostic codes and billing data, have provided information on up to millions of admissions for a particular diagnosis and thus are useful in tracking global trends in resource utilisation and doing analyses of patient characteristic- or hospital-related outcomes. Although they provide large numbers, 'big data' approaches are limited by the accuracy of diagnostic coding as well as lack of granularity.

In the following, we describe and analyse studies from around the world including caregiver surveys, patient records and 'big data' approaches in order to assess current use of NIV worldwide, and understand trends in utilisation.

INSIGHTS FROM SURVEYS

Epidemiologic data on use of NIV for ARF are entirely lacking from most countries in the world. However, available data suggest that NIV use began increasing during the 1990s and has continued through the 2010s. In a single 26 bed French ICU, NIV use for patients with acute respiratory failure (ARF) due to COPD and CPE increased from 20% of ventilator starts in 1994 to nearly 90% in 2001, associated with reductions in healthcare acquired pneumonias and ICU mortality from 20% to 8% and 21% to 7%, respectively.[3] In a multicentre survey performed in French ICUs in 1997 and again in 2002, NIV use increased from 16% to 24% of the total ventilated patients and from 35% to 52% of the patients starting ventilation in the ICU.[4]

However, NIV use may vary greatly depending on the geographical location and even between institutions within the same region.[2] Providing an international view of NIV utilisation, a serial survey conducted in more than 40 countries enrolling more than 18,000 ventilated patients, overall NIV use increased from 4.4% to 11.1% and to 14% in 1998, 2004 and 2010, respectively.[5,6] Between 1998 and 2004, use in patients with ARF due to COPD and ACPE increased from 48% to 78% and from 35% to 65% of ventilator starts, respectively, and between 1998 and 2010, mortality fell significantly from 31% to 28%.

Some surveys in other countries have suggested low utilisation rates related to lack of education, knowledge and proper equipment.[2] A 2003 national audit found that 39% of ICUs in the United Kingdom were not applying NIV to COPD patients at all.[7] In German ICUs, NIV use was estimated at less than 10% of ventilator starts in most of the units.[8] Another survey from Korea found that only 2 of 24 university ICUs were using NIV, constituting only 4% of total ventilator starts.[9] Despite these challenges, NIV use has also increased outside the ICU setting, including high-dependency units, respiratory wards, emergency rooms and post-surgical recovery rooms.[10,11]

Another older survey of Directors of Respiratory Care in the United States demonstrated large variability in use between institutions, suggesting that adoption of NIV has been inconsistent.[2] The hospitals using less NIV (<15% of ventilator starts) identified lack of knowledge or experience concerning the technique, insufficient technical equipment such as specific ventilators and ad hoc interfaces and lack of funding.[12]

The increasing awareness of the effectiveness of NIV along with the shortage of available ICU beds has led to increasing use of NIV outside the ICU setting. An international web-based survey focusing on NIV use for ARF on general wards was conducted in 51 countries. In 66% of the hospitals, NIV was applied in general wards without monitoring.[13]

In a more recent epidemiologic survey performed between 2005 and 2007 at eight institutions in Massachusetts, USA, NIV use as a percentage of ventilator starts was up to 40% overall, and for respiratory failure due to COPD or CPE, it was 82% and 69%, respectively.[14] This survey's accuracy was assured by identification of actual cases of NIV use and did not rely on opinions of caregivers. Success rate was 76% for respiratory failure due to COPD and 79% for CPE, and mortality rates were 12% and 18%, respectively. Raising concern about possible overzealous use of NIV, 41% of patients with hypoxemic respiratory failure due to pneumonia were put on NIV initially, with a success rate of only 47% and mortality of 25%. This study also showed that full face, nasal and total masks were used in 86.7%, 7.1% and 0.5% of NIV starts, respectively (5.7% unknown). Bi-level-type pressure-limited ventilators were used in 91.4% of applications and an ICU-type ventilator in 4.3% (4.3% unknown). Mean initial IPAP and EPAP/CPAP settings were 12.5 and 5.6 cm H_2O, respectively. A pressure support-like ventilator mode with a backup rate was selected in 87.7% of NIV patients; CPAP was utilised in 12.3% of patients, mainly with CPE.

Presently, it is difficult to conclude much about worldwide use based on survey data alone. The serial surveys indicate that NIV use has increased substantially throughout the world over the past 20 years, while evidence has accumulated to support a variety of applications, mainly COPD and CPE. There is also the suggestion that NIV use varies enormously from country to country and even between institutions within countries. But these surveys also have a number of inherent limitations. Unless the survey is repeated at fairly frequent intervals, the information rapidly becomes obsolete and may poorly reflect current use. The information in them generally is not validated in any way and reflects the experience (often as estimated by caregivers working there) of selected institutions that may not be generalisable to institutions or individuals declining to participate in the survey, which may constitute the large majority of individuals polled. This accumulating evidence suggests that NIV is being used too little in some circumstances, too much in others, and raises the question of how to optimise the use of NIV. Clearly, there is no one optimal rate of NIV use that is applicable to all institutions at all times. Different hospitals serve different patient populations with quite variable prevalences of COPD and CPE.

So the question is how to avoid underuse or overuse of NIV and achieve the optimal level of use for a given institution. At the global level, international societies play an important role by providing educational sessions at their meetings, publishing high-quality clinical studies in their journals and formulating guidelines. At the level of individual countries, professional societies again play an important role in disseminating information and guidelines. Resources also have to be made available by policymakers so that appropriate equipment can be purchased and practitioners adequately trained. But the most important level is institutional, where individual practitioners can become 'champions' and help others learn the new techniques and gain relevant experience. They can make sure that other practitioners are appropriately educated, becoming aware of the evidence and guidelines and gaining valuable experience. Other strategies for using NIV well include giving respiratory therapists autonomy and functioning as a team, starting early with the right equipment on appropriate patients, monitoring closely in the right setting.[15] This is how the use of a technique like NIV, proven to improve outcomes for patients with ARF due to aetiologies like COPD and CPE, has been spreading worldwide. However, it is important that the spread continues to institutions and countries currently underutilising NIV, and that, by the same token, overzealous use be avoided in situations where prompt intubation would be safer, with the goal of optimising patient outcomes.

As discussed above, surveys of clinicians have limitations when trying to track actual use and outcomes. Another approach is to use large databases that rely on codes and resource utilisation. These databases track actual transactions and not estimates and beliefs as do most surveys. On the other hand, large databases have limitations too. They depend on accurate coding and reliable data entry, and are hindered by changes in coding practices and systems over time. Nonetheless, 'big data' provide valuable information, largely by virtue of the enormous number of data points that enables use of sophisticated statistical analyses to control for patient and hospital characteristics and allow for identification of secular trends and predictors of use and outcomes. In the following, we review results from studies using large databases to gain insights on trends of NIV use as well as factors associated with outcomes. These databases have been accrued in the United States so global generalisability is limited, but some of the observations likely reflect global trends and outcomes.

OBSERVATIONS USING LARGE DATABASES

NIV for COPD exacerbations

One of the earliest studies to understand trends in utilisation of NIV for COPD used the National Inpatient Sample, a database receiving input from hundreds of hospitals across the United States. Chandra et al.[16] analysed over 7.5 million hospital admissions for COPD exacerbations in this database between 1998 and 2008. They found a steady increase in NIV starts from 1% to 4.5% (462% increase) with a concomitant decrease in invasive mechanical ventilation (IMV) from 6% to 3.5% (42% decrease) (Figure 18.1). They also noted that the group of patients that transitioned from NIV to IMV, indicative of NIV failure, had a 61% higher risk of death compared to those begun on IMV initially. They raised the concern that NIV failures may have been inappropriate candidates for NIV or were kept on NIV too long, contributing to the relatively greater mortality.

In another analysis of the Nationwide Inpatient Sample based on ICD-9 codes and consisting of almost 2.4 million admissions for ARF between 2000 and 2009, Walkey and Wiener[17] found similar trends with respect to COPD, with use of NIV increasing from 3.5% to 12% (250% increase). But more remarkably, use of NIV for ARF due to non-COPD diagnoses increased from 1.2% to 6% (400% increase). Patients without COPD had higher NIV failure rates than those with COPD, and similar to the Chandra et al. study,[16] patients with NIV failure in the Walkey study had higher mortality rates than those begun on IMV.[17] This worse outcome may reflect the sicker population of patients prone

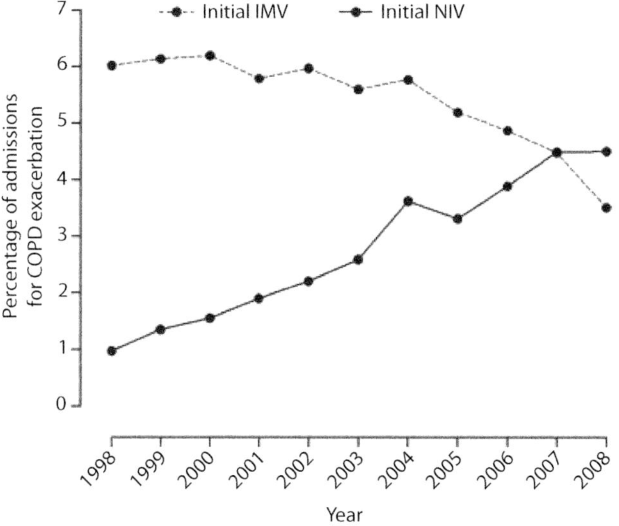

Figure 18.1 Temporal trends in the use of non-invasive positive pressure ventilation (NIV) and IMV as the initial form of respiratory support in patients hospitalised with acute exacerbations of COPD in the United States, 1998–2008. (From Chandra D et al., *Am J Respir Crit Care Med.* 2012 Jan 15;185(2):152–9. With permission.)

to NIV failure, but could also be due to excessive delay of needed intubation in patients begun on NIV.

Stefan et al.,[18] using the large, US-based, retrospective Premier database, examined a span of 10 years (2001 to 2011) including more than 700,000 hospitalisations for an exacerbation of COPD at 475 hospitals and identified patient factors that predicted use of NIV and outcomes. Similar to previous 'big data' studies, NIV use increased by 15.1% annually (from 5.9% to 14.8%), while IMV use declined by 3.2% annually (from 8.7% to 5.9%). By 2004, the rate of initial NIV use had surpassed that of initial IMV use. In all, 59% of patients who received ventilator support were treated with NIV (79% in 2011), and 16.6% of the admissions initially started on NIV were subsequently intubated (i.e. NIV failure). The annual rate of NIV failure declined slightly from 17.9% to 16.7%, probably reflecting an improvement in patient selection and accumulating experience of clinicians. Elderly patients (>85 years) had a 22% higher likelihood of receiving NIV compared to those aged <65 years, while blacks (OR 0.86) and Hispanics (OR 0.91) were less likely to receive NIV than whites. Over the 10 years of the study, the use of NIV increased more and the use of IMV decreased more in older patients relative to the youngest patients, suggesting that the intensity of treatment decreases with advancing age. Patients hospitalised with COPD with a high burden of comorbidities and those with concomitant pneumonia had higher rates of NIV failure and were more likely to receive initial IMV, which is in line with reports of the relatively low effectiveness of NIV in patients with pneumonia.[17] Although IMV use in patients with COPD had a substantial decline, there was an overall increase in the use of mechanical ventilation, suggesting that NIV was used in patients who might not in the past have received any ventilation.

Multiple randomised studies and meta-analyses have demonstrated the efficacy of NIV in exacerbations of COPD to improve dyspnoea, vital signs and gas exchange; avoid intubation; and reduce mortality compared to use of conventional supplemental oxygen therapy,[19] and guidelines including the recent ERS/ATS NIV guidelines[20] give a strong recommendation for NIV as the first ventilator modality in patients with an exacerbation of COPD. However, these results were obtained in the context of controlled trials using protocols at skilled centres and may not reflect what happens in actual 'real-life' practice situations. In a retrospective cohort study using the Premier database, Lindenauer et al.[21] compared the outcomes of patients with COPD treated with NIV to those treated with IMV. The study population consisted of 25,628 patients hospitalised for an exacerbation of COPD at 420 US hospitals. A total of 17,978 (70%) were initially treated with NIV on hospital day 1 or 2. In a propensity-adjusted analysis, NIV was associated with a lower risk of hospital-acquired pneumonia (OR 0.53) and mortality (OR 0.54), a shorter length of stay (OR 0.81) and lower costs (ratio 0.68), but no difference in 30 day all-cause readmission (OR 1.04) or COPD-specific readmission (OR 1.05) compared to IMV. The relative advantage of

NIV was attenuated in the face of higher comorbidity burden and among those with pneumonia present on admission. These findings indicate that the same benefits seen in controlled trials are discernible in comparative effective analyses using databases reflecting real-life experience.

Similar findings were derived from data accrued from 38 hospitals participating in the APACHE database from 2008 through 2012.[22] Of a total of 3520 patients with acute COPD exacerbations treated in the ICU, 27.7% received NIV and 45.5% received IMV. NIV failure occurred in 13.7% of the patients initiated on NIV. Hospital mortality was 7.4% for patients who succeeded with NIV, 16.1% for those treated initially with IMV and 22.5% for those who failed NIV. In the propensity-matched analysis, patients initially treated with NIV had a 41% lower risk of death than those treated with IMV (RR: 0.59). These results provide further support for the use of NIV as a first-line therapy in appropriately selected critically ill patients with COPD while also highlighting the risks associated with NIV failure and the need to be cautious with NIV in the face of severe disease. The rate of NIV relative to IMV use was lower than in some prior studies, but this may reflect the location of the patients exclusively in ICUs.

Rate of hospital use of NIV in COPD patients is also a factor in patient outcomes. Lindenauer et al.[23] found that the median NIV rate of use for ventilated COPD patients was 75.1% with a range of 9.2% to 94.1%. In a risk-stratified analysis, they reported that hospitals with a higher rate of NIV use had lower risk-standardised rates of IMV, modestly higher risk-standardised total rates of ventilation, lower risk-standardised mortality and marginally lower mortality rates among all patients compared with hospitals utilising less NIV. Higher NIV use was also associated with lower hospital costs, shorter length of stay and lower NIV failure rates.[23] In a more recent analysis of the effect of hospital rate of NIV use on outcomes, Stefan et al.[24] used the California State Inpatient Database and found that, overall, NIV use for strong evidence conditions like COPD exacerbations and heart failure constituted only 30% of NIV applications. Hospitals with greater use of NIV for strong evidence conditions had lower rates of NIV failure for both strong evidence conditions as well as non-strong evidence conditions. Based on two studies that have found that outcomes are no better at higher as opposed to lower NIV volume hospitals,[24,25] the better outcomes described above are apparently not related just to volume of NIV use. One of the studies even found that greater volume of NIV use was associated with higher rates of NIV failure, perhaps related to selection of higher risk patients at higher volume centres.

In summary, multiple lines of evidence from 'big data' studies demonstrate steadily increasing use of NIV in the United States from the early 2000s through 2011, especially in the elderly, associated with decreasing rates of IMV. The use of NIV as first-line ventilatory therapy for COPD exacerbations varies considerably between different hospitals, with hospitals that are having higher rates of initial use having better success rates. Overall NIV failure rates are in the range of 17%, with mortality in NIV failures exceeding that even of patients intubated initially, raising concerns about overzealous use of NIV in higher risk COPD patients or inadequate monitoring or management. Patient selection for NIV appears to be important in achieving success, and delay of needed intubation may be a contributor to mortality among NIV failures.

NIV FOR ASTHMA EXACERBATIONS

Very few studies on use of NIV for asthma exacerbations have been published, and the recent ERS/ATS guideline determined that evidence was insufficient to make a recommendation on use of NIV for acute asthma. Large databases at hundreds of hospitals provide an opportunity to track use of NIV for asthma in 'real-life' situations and gain insights into associated outcomes. In a retrospective cohort study using data from 97 US hospitals, almost 14,000 patients were hospitalised with an acute asthma exacerbation.[26] The median age was 53 years, 73% were women and 54% were white. NIV was used in 4% of these patients amounting to 44% of patients requiring ventilator support. The use of NIV increased from 2.3% in 2009 to 4.7% in 2012. Compared with patients treated with IMV, those treated with NIV were older, more likely to have a prior hospitalisation requiring NIV, less likely to have associated pneumonia and had lower severity of illness at admission. On the other hand, patients with status asthmaticus, prior IMV use, weight loss and neurological disorders were less likely to receive NIV. In a propensity-matched analysis, patients treated with NIV had lower mortality (1.0% vs. 8.1%) and shorter hospital lengths of stay (5.6 vs. 10.0 days) than those receiving IMV. Only 5% of patients treated with NIV had to be intubated (NIV failure) suggesting that NIV was being used selectively for lower risk patients. Patients who failed NIV had mortality comparable to those treated with IMV initially (15.4 vs. 14.7%, $p = 0.92$) and longer median hospital lengths of stay (10.9 vs. 6.7 days, $p = 0.007$). Independent predictors of NIV failure were prior admission for asthma in the previous year, and pneumonia and diabetes mellitus as comorbidities.

In a follow-up study using the same patient cohort,[27] the same authors characterised hospital patterns of NIV use in patients with asthma and evaluated the association between the rate of use of IMV and mortality. NIV was not used at all for asthma exacerbations at 38% of the hospitals. At hospitals using NIV, hospital-level adjusted NIV usage rates varied considerably (range, 0.4%–33.1%; median, 5.2%). Higher hospital rates of NIV use were not associated with lower IMV rates (5.4% vs. 5.7%), but they were associated with a small but significantly shorter hospital length of stay.

These results are in line with a study by Nanchal et al.[28] that used the Healthcare Cost and Utilization Project Nationwide Inpatient Sample to identify patients discharged with a principal diagnosis of asthma exacerbation. They found a substantial increase in the use of mechanical ventilation accompanied by a shift from IMV to NIV. However, despite the increased use of NIV, the adjusted mortality rate for asthma exacerbations treated with NIV or IMV was unchanged from 2000 to 2008.

These studies document the infrequent but gradually rising use of NIV to treat asthma exacerbations in recent years in the United States, but there is great variability between hospitals. Although it likely reflects the selection of less ill patients, those treated with NIV had lower mortality rates and hospital lengths of stay than those treated with IMV, and this finding could be used to justify a trial of NIV in carefully selected patients under close monitoring who do not respond to standard treatment. The steady increase in the use of NIV in patients with asthma seems to be the result of a 'spill-over' effect of a technology from one indication to another without necessarily improving outcomes. In contrast to COPD exacerbations, failure of NIV in patients with asthma exacerbations was not associated with higher mortality than in IMV patients, but it would still be prudent to observe these patients closely and be ready for prompt intubation because of the risk for rapid deterioration in patients with status asthmaticus.

NIV FOR PNEUMONIA

Using the HealthFacts multihospital electronic medical record database, Stefan et al.[29] examined outcomes of NIV and IMV in 3971 ventilated patients with pneumonia, 1109 (27.9%) of whom were initially treated with NIV. NIV patients had lower acuity of illness scores and were more likely to have congestive heart failure and chronic pulmonary disease than IMV patients. Mortality was 15.8%, 29.8% and 25.9.0% among patients treated with initial NIV, initial IMV and those with NIV failure, respectively. NIV patients had a lower risk of death than IMV patients in the propensity-matched analysis (relative risk: 0.71, 95% CI: 0.59–0.85). Mortality was less among NIV patients with cardiopulmonary comorbidities (relative risk 0.59, 95% CI: 0.47–0.75) but not in those without (relative risk 0.96, 95% CI: 0.74–0.1.25). Also, NIV failure was significantly (p = 0.002) less common in patients with cardiopulmonary conditions (13.8%) compared to those without these conditions (21.3%).

A retrospective cohort study[30] using a database composed of Medicare beneficiaries aged >64 years examined outcomes in patients with pneumonia admitted to acute-care hospitals in the United States from 2010 to 2011 and receiving mechanical ventilation. Among 65,747 Medicare beneficiaries with pneumonia who required mechanical ventilation, 12,480 (19%) received NIV. Patients receiving NIV were more likely to be older, male, white and rural-dwelling; have fewer comorbidities; and were less likely to be acutely ill as measured by organ failures. Overall, 30 day mortality rate was greater in the NIV than the IMV group (57.6% vs. 54.2%, respectively). However, in an instrumental variable analysis on 'marginal' patients defined as those who received initial NIV because of their proximity to high NIV user hospitals, NIV use was not significantly associated with differences in 30 day mortality when compared with IMV (54% vs. 55%; p = 0.92; 95% CI of absolute difference, −13.8 to 12.4) but was associated with significantly lower Medicare spending ($18,433 vs. $27,051; p = 0.02).

These findings demonstrate that NIV is commonly used to treat patients with pneumonia (varying from 1/5 to 1/3 in the two studies) in real-life situations in the United States. They also suggest that initial NIV is associated with variable outcomes compared to initial IMV to treat pneumonia, with one of the studies reporting better mortality and the other worse mortality overall. This difference may reflect the selection of patients in the two studies, with the inclusion of more patients with sepsis in the study with higher mortality associated with initial NIV, as well as the differing methods used to adjust for confounders. This also reflects the differing outcomes of RCTs on NIV.[31,32] The authors concluded that NIV should be used with caution in patients with pneumonia. If it is to be tried, careful consideration should be given to selection, keeping in mind that outcomes were better in the subgroup of patients hospitalised with pneumonia who had underlying COPD or heart failure. Also, the fact that NIV failures had high in-hospital mortality emphasises the importance of careful monitoring and being prepared to switch promptly to IMV when managing pneumonia patients with NIV.

NIV FOR POST-OPERATIVE USE

NIV use has increased in the post-operative period to prevent or treat acute hypoxic respiratory failure. Patients undergoing bariatric, abdominal and thoracic surgery are at higher risk for post-operative hypoxemic respiratory failure especially if they have obstructive sleep apnoea (OSA). Anaesthesia, analgesics for post-operative pain and the location of the surgery predispose to respiratory complications including restriction of lung volumes, atelectasis and diaphragm dysfunction, all exacerbating hypoventilation and hypoxaemia.[33]

Prior studies have shown that patient factors such as COPD, age over 60, obesity, CHF and American Society of Anesthesiologist (ASA) class III or higher increase the risk for post-operative complications.[34] Post-operative NIV may improve gas exchange, decrease work of breathing and reduce atelectasis (improving alveolar recruitment), and may be an important tool to prevent or treat post-operative respiratory complications including ARF and avoid intubation.

Although several RCTs have evaluated the impact of NIV in the post-operative period after abdominal[35] and cardiac surgery,[36] very few observational studies have characterised NIV use in the perioperative period, and little is known about the patterns of use in routine 'real-life' clinical practice.

In a study of more than 5000 patients with OSA undergoing bariatric surgery at 161 hospitals in the United States, Stefan et al.[37] examined the relationship of early initiation of NIV with post-operative outcomes. They found that 18.9% of the patients received post-operative NIV in the first 48 h post-surgery, and 3.8% received IMV within 3 days post-surgery. There was a large variability between hospitals in the use of early NIV among these bariatric surgical patients with known OSA; the median rate of use was 8.6%, but it ranged from 0.6% at the 10th percentile to 66.7% at the 90th percentile. When compared to patients who did not receive early NIV, those who were treated with NIV were slightly older, were more likely to have chronic pulmonary disease (34.2% vs. 27.7%) and received a higher dose of narcotics on the day of surgery. Patients who received early NIV were also more likely to be admitted to hospitals with high rates of OSA among bariatric patients and higher rates of NIV use among all surgical patients with OSA. Reintubation rate (4.5% vs. 3.8%), prolonged mechanical ventilation, arrhythmias, mortality and length of stay were similar between NIV-treated vs. untreated patients.

These findings may reflect a lack of effectiveness of early use of NIV to prevent post-operative adverse outcomes, but it should be borne in mind that this was a retrospective study using an administrative database, and it was challenging to differentiate prophylactic NIV from NIV treatment for a patient experiencing respiratory deterioration.

CONCLUSIONS

Real-world data can provide us with insights that RCTs cannot such as trends in NIV usage and global outcomes in large populations. Survey approaches may be limited by reporter biases and lack of validation, but they indicate that NIV use is increasing in multiple countries worldwide. Large databases avoid the potential biases of surveys, but they are limited by the need for accurate coding and possible changes in coding practices and systems over time. The large US databases tell us that NIV is being used much more in the United States since the turn of the millennium, especially for COPD, but there remains wide variability in usage rates between different hospitals. Somewhere around 2004, NIV became more often used for COPD exacerbations than IMV, and these large observational studies indicate that the advantages of NIV over oxygen plus, if needed, IMV that have been reported in multiple RCTs hold up in real life settings. For other indications like asthma exacerbations, NIV use has been gradually climbing but is still being used much less frequently than for COPD. Patients with asthma had lower mortality and hospital lengths of stay than those treated with IMV, but this was likely related to lower severity of illness. For post-bariatric surgical patients with OSA, NIV is used often at some hospitals and infrequently at others, and it has been difficult to discern any effect in preventing complications. Overall, use of NIV for non-COPD patients has increased almost as much as in COPD patients, raising concerns about overzealous use of NIV for patients with ARF due to diagnoses such as pneumonia that are not as well supported by evidence. Evidence from large databases on real-life use of NIV permits assessment of practice patterns, outcomes and adherence with guidelines that can help to inform efforts to improve practices and optimise application of NIV.

REFERENCES

1. Esteban A, Frutos-Vivar F, Muriel A et al. Evolution of mortality over time in patients receiving mechanical ventilation. *Am J Respir Crit Care Med.* 2013; 188(2):220–30.
2. Maheshwari V, Paioli D, Rothaar R et al. Utilization of noninvasive ventilation in acute care hospitals: A regional survey. *Chest.* 2006;129:1226–33.
3. Girou E, Brun-Buisson C, Taillé S et al. Secular trends in nosocomial infections and mortality associated with noninvasive ventilation in patients with exacerbation of COPD and pulmonary edema. *JAMA.* 2003;290(22):2985–91.
4. Demoule A, Girou E, Richard JC et al. Increased use of noninvasive ventilation in French intensive care units. *Intensive Care Med.* 2006;32(11):1747–55.
5. Esteban A, Ferguson ND, Meade MO et al. Evolution of mechanical ventilation in response to clinical research. *Am J Respir Crit Care Med.* 2008;177(2):170–7.
6. Esteban A, Frutos-Vivar F, Muriel A et al. Evolution of mortality over time in patients receiving mechanical ventilation. *Am J Respir Crit Care Med.* 2013 15;188(2):220–30.
7. Kaul S, Pearson M, Coutts I et al. Non-invasive ventilation (NIV) in the clinical management of acute COPD in 233 UK hospitals: Results from the RCP/BTS 2003 National COPD Audit. *COPD.* 2009;6(3):171–6.
8. Kumle B, Haisch G, Suttner SW. Current status of non-invasive ventilation in German ICU's: A postal survey. *Anasthesiol Intensivmed Notfallmed Schmerzther.* 2003;38:32–7.
9. Hong SB, Oh BJ, Kim YS et al. Characteristics of mechanical ventilation employed in intensive care units: A multicenter survey of hospitals. *J Korean Med Sci.* 2008;23(6):948–53.
10. Plant PK, Owen JL, Elliott MW. Early use of non-invasive ventilation for acute exacerbations of chronic obstructive pulmonary disease on general respiratory wards: A multicentre randomised controlled trial. *Lancet.* 2000;355:1931–5.
11. Poponick JM, Renston JP, Bennett RP. Use of a ventilatory support system (BiPAP) for acute respiratory failure in the emergency department. *Chest.* 1999;116:166–71.
12. Hess DR, Pang JM, Camargo CA. A survey of the use of noninvasive ventilation in academic emergency departments in the United States. *Respir Care.* 2009;54:1306–12.
13. Cabrini L, Esquinas A, Pasin L et al. An international survey on noninvasive ventilation use for acute respiratory failure in general non-monitored wards. *Respir Care.* 2015;60:586–92.
14. Ozsancak Ugurlu A, Sidhom SS, Khodabandeh A et al. Use and outcomes of noninvasive positive pressure ventilation in acute care hospitals in Massachusetts. *Chest.* 2014 May;145(5):964–71.

15. Fisher KA, Mazor KM, Goff S et al. Successful use of noninvasive ventilation in chronic obstructive pulmonary disease. How do high-performing hospitals do it? *Ann Am Thorac Soc.* 2017;14(11):1674–81.
16. Chandra D, Stamm JA, Taylor B et al. Outcomes of non-invasive ventilation for acute exacerbations of COPD in the United States, 1998–2008. *Am J Respir Crit Care Med.* 2012 Jan 15;185(2):152–9.
17. Walkey AJ, Wiener R. Use of noninvasive ventilation in patients with acute respiratory failure, 2000–2009: A population-based study. *Ann Am Thor Soc.* 2013;1:10–7.
18. Stefan MS, Shieh MS, Pekow PS et al. Trends in mechanical ventilation among patients hospitalized with acute exacerbation of COPD in the United States, 2001 to 2011. *Chest.* 2015 Apr;147(4):959–68.
19. Ram FS, Picot J, Lightowler J, Wedzicha JA. Non-invasive positive pressure ventilation for treatment of respiratory failure due to exacerbations of chronic obstructive pulmonary disease. *Cochrane Database Syst Rev.* 2004;(3):CD004104.
20. Rochwerg B, Brochard L, Elliott MW et al. Official ERS/ATS clinical practice guidelines: Noninvasive ventilation for acute respiratory failure. *Eur Respir J.* 2017 Aug 31;50(2):1–20.
21. Lindenauer PK, Stefan MS, Shieh MS et al. Outcomes associated with invasive and noninvasive ventilation among patients hospitalized with exacerbations of chronic obstructive pulmonary disease. *JAMA Intern Med.* 2014 Dec 1:174(12):1982–93L.
22. Stefan MS, Nathanson BH, Higgins TL et al. Comparative effectiveness of noninvasive and invasive ventilation in critically ill patients with acute exacerbation of COPD. *Crit Care Med.* 2015;43(7):1386–94.
23. Lindenauer PK, Stefan MS, Shieh MS et al. Hospital patterns of mechanical ventilation for patients with exacerbations of COPD. *Ann Am Thorac Soc.* 2015;12(3):402–9.
24. Stefan MS, Pekow PS, Shieh MS et al. Hospital volume and outcomes of noninvasive ventilation in patients hospitalized with an acute exacerbation of chronic obstructive pulmonary disease. *Crit Care Med.* 2017 Jan;45(1):20–7.
25. Mehta AB, Douglas IS, Walkey AJ et al. Hospital noninvasive ventilation case volume and outcomes of acute exacerbations of chronic obstructive pulmonary disease. *Ann Am Thorac Soc.* 2016;13(10):1752–9.
26. Stefan MS, Nathanson BH, Lagu T et al. Outcomes of noninvasive and invasive ventilation in patients hospitalized with asthma exacerbation. *Ann Am Thorac Soc.* 2016;13(7):1096–104.
27. Stefan MS, Nathanson BH, Priya A et al. Hospitals' patterns of use of noninvasive ventilation in patients with asthma exacerbation. *Chest.* 2016 Mar;149(3):729–36.
28. Nanchal R, Kumar G, Majumdar T et al. Utilization of mechanical ventilation for asthma exacerbations: Analysis of a national database. *Respir Care.* 2014 May;59(5):644–53.
29. Stefan MS, Priya A, Pekow PS et al. The comparative effectiveness of noninvasive and invasive ventilation in patients with pneumonia. *J Crit Care.* 2017 23;43:190–6.
30. Valley TS, Walkey AJ, Lindenauer PK et al. Association between noninvasive ventilation and mortality among older patients with pneumonia. *Crit Care Med.* 2017 Mar;45(3):e246–54.
31. Frat JP, Thille AW, Mercat A et al. High-flow oxygen through nasal cannula in acute hypoxemic respiratory failure. *N Engl J Med.* 2015;372:2185–96.
32. Patel BK, Wolfe KS, Pohlman AS et al. Effect of noninvasive ventilation delivered by helmet vs face mask on the rate of endotracheal intubation in patients with acute respiratory distress syndrome: A randomized clinical trial. *JAMA.* 2016 Jun 14;315(22):2435–41.
33. Lindberg P, Gunnarsson L, Tokics L et al. Atelectasis and lung function in the postoperative period. *Acta Anaesthesiol Scand.* 1992;36:546–53.
34. Daabiss M. American Society of Anaesthesiologists physical status classification. *Indian J Anaesth.* 2011;55(2):111–5.
35. Jaber S, Lescot T, Futier E et al. NIVAS Study Group effect of noninvasive ventilation on tracheal reintubation among patients with hypoxemic respiratory failure following abdominal surgery: A randomized clinical trial. *JAMA.* 2016 Apr 5;315(13):1345–53.
36. Stéphan F, Barrucand B, Petit P et al. High-flow nasal oxygen vs noninvasive positive airway pressure in hypoxemic patients after cardiothoracic surgery: A randomized clinical trial. *JAMA.* 2015;313:331–9.
37. Stefan MS, Hill NS, Raghunathan K et al. Outcomes associated with early postoperative noninvasive ventilation in bariatric surgical patients with sleep apnea. *J Clin Sleep Med.* 2016;12(11):1507–16.

PART 3

The practice – chronic NIV

19 Chronic ventilator service 165
Maxime Patout, Antoine Cuvelier, Jean-François Muir and Peter Wijkstra

20 Diagnostic tests in the assessment of patients for home mechanical ventilation 175
Michael Polkey, Patrick B. Murphy and Nicholas Hart

21 Ultrasound 190
Daniel A. Lichtenstein

22 Patient and caregiver education 200
Ole Norregaard

23 Discharging the patient on home ventilation 207
Joan Escarrabill and Ole Norregaard

24 Monitoring during sleep during chronic non-invasive ventilation 216
Jean-Paul Janssens, Jean-Christian Borel, Dan Adler and Jean-Louis Pépin

25 Continuity of care and telemonitoring 223
Michele Vitacca

19

Chronic ventilation service

MAXIME PATOUT, ANTOINE CUVELIER, JEAN-FRANÇOIS MUIR AND PETER WIJKSTRA

KEY MESSAGES

- Patients with chronic respiratory failure are best initiated on home mechanical ventilation, and their treatment regularly assessed, in a specialist chronic ventilation service (CVS).
- The care of these patients requires a sometimes very large, multi-disciplinary team; all the necessary components must be in place.
- The provision of home ventilation is complex and involves much more than just the purchase of a machine and ancillary equipment; home mechanical ventilation should not be delivered on an occasional basis by general pulmonology units.
- The CVS may be hospital-based or delivered at home by a mobile team.
- Training, and expertise, of medical, nursing and physiotherapy staff are key to the success of a CVS.
- The CVS must provide a 24 h service, either itself or through a home care service – there must be access to clinical advice and technical support, in case of equipment malfunction.

INTRODUCTION

Home mechanical ventilation (HMV) delivered either non-invasively or via a tracheostomy is the key treatment for patients with chronic respiratory failure and hypercapnia. Non-invasive ventilation (NIV) has progressively replaced tracheotomy ventilation, although this last modality still has some specific indications, especially during difficult weaning.

The overall prevalence of HMV in Europe is around 6.6/100,000, but this varies greatly between countries.[1] The increasing prevalence of severe COPD and severe obesity, better identification of adult neuromuscular diseases and the increasing lifespan of the general population point to a major increase in the disease burden associated with chronic respiratory failure in the next 20 years. The development of NIV by chest physicians during the early 1990s has led to the growth of centres delivering NIV to patients with chronic or acute-on-chronic respiratory failure. The wide variations between local organisations, from the technical, administrative and economic points of view, including the variable investment of chest physicians in the field of chronic respiratory failure and the relationships with the local intensive care units, have led to heterogeneous management. The need to rationalise healthcare costs and the development of more sophisticated technological tools imposes the obligation for better structures for the management of patients receiving HMV, beginning with titration and long-term monitoring and including rehabilitation and the management of acute episodes.[2] Clinical research in chronic respiratory failure patients is difficult to perform, but we can take advantage of the experience acquired in sleep laboratories. In a slightly different setting, clinicians in these units have developed a rational management structure and have produced quality research on ventilator assistance, titration and monitoring.

In this chapter, we describe a chronic ventilation service (CVS) that was set up in a university hospital in the early 1990s in France. This structured network manages around 200 new chronic respiratory failure patients each year, in connection with a non-profit provider for domiciliary management. This way of working is probably not valid for all healthcare organisations but is an example of how to organise the management of such patients. This chapter will describe the two components of a CVS: the specific activities provided in the hospital and the support provided at home. At the end of this chapter, the unique organisation of a CVS in the Netherlands will be described to illustrate an alternative model.

CVS IN THE HOSPITAL

Creation of a CVS first requires a sustained collaboration between physicians and the hospital administration, beginning with the identification of the number of NIV or tracheostomy-ventilated patients who may enter the CVS. This calculation clearly influences the subsequent choices about location, the medical and nursing staffing requirements and the technical equipment required to run the CVS. Our experience is that offering such a CVS immediately leads to an increase in the number of patients utilising such a service compared with the predicted needs. The different components of a CVS may be schematised as shown in Figure 19.1.

It is still not known if a CVS in the hospital improves the management of patients as compared with conventional management in the ward or with domiciliary-based management. Its impact should be assessed through objective endpoints, such as waiting time for initiation of HMV and the length of stay in the facility to initiate HMV, the number or unplanned hospitalisations or hospital-based assessments, the number of acute hypercapnic respiratory failure episodes, long-term ventilatory compliance and the effect on symptoms and quality of life. It is plausible that a CVS has some economic justifications because of longer-term savings, by reducing future healthcare costs despite the numbers of medical and nursing staff required to run it and the complexity of the technologies involved.

Organisation

The CVS is integrated into a network of departments of different competencies (Figure 19.2). The heart of the CVS is the place where patients are received and routinely assessed in the hospital. New patients enter the CVS through the titration unit, where planned HMV may be started and settings chosen and adjusted. The titration unit organises planned hospitalisations, usually after a chest physician consultation or after referral from a sleep laboratory. The relationship with the sleep laboratory is crucial since many chronic respiratory failure patients are diagnosed during investigations for sleep respiratory disturbances, particularly sleep apnoea. NIV is initiated over 3 to 5 days. Beds from the intermediate respiratory care unit or the pulmonary ward may be used to initiate HMV; our approach has the advantage that admissions are not delayed by the constant pressure to get available beds for unplanned pulmonary patients. In most centres, the expertise in invasive ventilation and NIV is available in intensive care units, and one of the challenges for the CVS is to take advantage of this expertise for patients with chronic respiratory failure on a long-term basis.

The second part of a CVS is the monitoring unit. This unit is dedicated to scheduled and sometimes unplanned assessments of long-term chronic respiratory failure patients having NIV or tracheostomy ventilation at home. These assessments are performed at regular intervals that vary according to the aetiology of the chronic respiratory failure; in some situations, the assessments may also be performed irregularly, owing to an unpredicted change, for instance, if HMV becomes less tolerated or is less efficient. It is probably better if the monitoring unit is localised in the same place as the titration unit, and both units may be under one administrative structure. However, both units are very different in their operational functioning, especially regarding the duration of patient stay. In our department, the titration unit accepts patients from 2 to 5 days, and the monitoring unit accepts patients for only 8 h long daytime assessments. If a patient requires more than this, he or she has to be transferred to the titration unit for one to several nights in order to modify the ventilator settings. Respiratory events have been reported in a significant proportion of patients treated by domiciliary NIV,[3] and night-time ventilatory

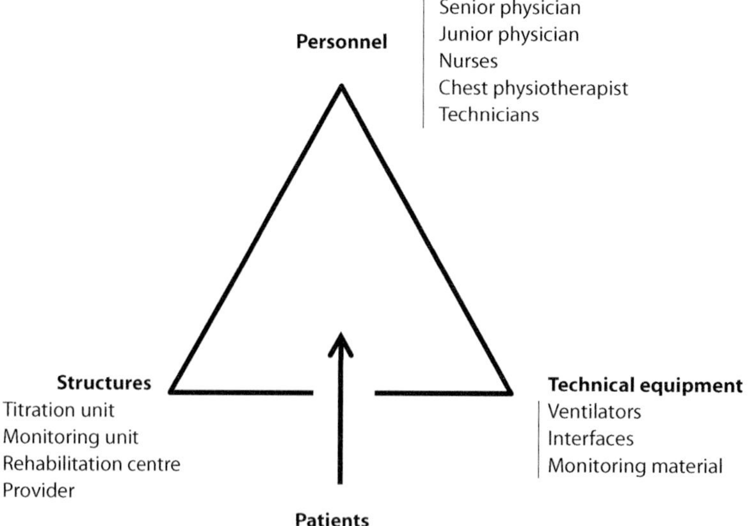

Figure 19.1 Organisation of a CVS.

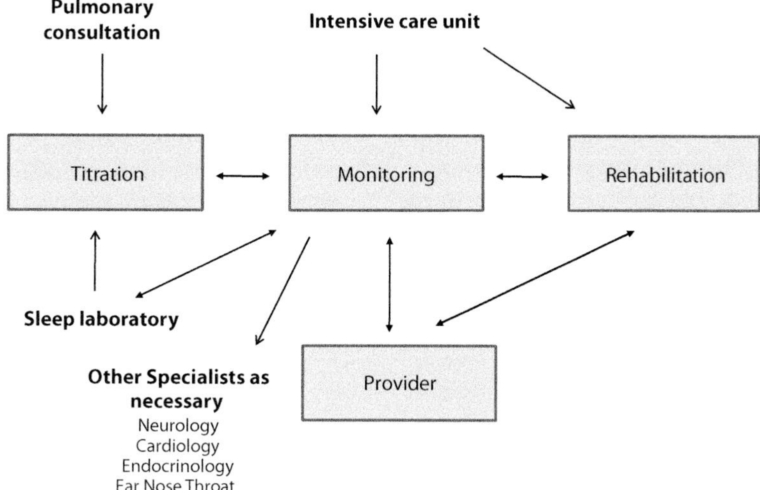

Figure 19.2 Network organisation of the clinical management of patients with chronic respiratory failure requiring HMV. The network is organized around the chronic ventilator service (in grey) and its correspondents.

assessments may be then justified in chronically ventilated patients. Such assessments may be performed at home through the provider, but their consequences on the treatment and the course of the disease still need to be evaluated on an immediate and a long-term basis. The recent characterisation of polysomnography during NIV[4,5] will perhaps modify the nature of these assessments and may lead to a larger number of one-night hospitalisations in selected patients. A high proportion of patients treated with NIV or tracheostomy ventilation are introduced to their ventilatory treatment during an episode of acute hypercapnic respiratory failure, managed in an intensive care or an intermediate care unit. Therefore, these patients enter the CVS via the monitoring unit and are subsequently managed like all other chronic respiratory failure patients. This unit should be accessible to patients with reduced mobility. It should also be organised to receive input from various professionals such as non-respiratory physicians, dieticians, occupational therapists, social services, etc. The multidisciplinary approach is key to the success of such a program. Regular reports from the monitoring unit should be sent to the patients' general practitioners (GPs), nurses and chest physiotherapists in the community.

The third component of a CVS organisation is the rehabilitation unit. Pulmonary rehabilitation is a major component of the management of chronic obstructive pulmonary disease (COPD), even in those severe patients requiring domiciliary NIV[6] and is now used in domiciliary ventilated patients with other diseases.[7] Pulmonary rehabilitation improves clinical symptoms and quality of life in patients with chronic respiratory failure[6] and may be performed in the hospital or in the home. It should always be delivered by dedicated staff, usually a chest physiotherapist, who can visit the patients in their homes.

Finally, the last component of the CVS is the equipment provider, which should be integrated in the activities of the centre, in order to provide and manage the ventilatory equipment at home. The importance of a high-quality coordination between the CVS and the provider will be described later.

Dedicated staff

The success of a CVS largely depends on the availability of dedicated medical, nursing and physiotherapy staff. The ratio of patients to staff varies greatly between centres and between different healthcare organisations. The nursing staff should be distinct from the staff in the pulmonary ward and should have competencies in NIV initiation and monitoring, not only during the day but also during sleep. Medical staff and the physiotherapists should be trained in the management of these patients, but there is no need that they are exclusively dedicated to the CVS. Technical support from the provider, which should be able to establish the link between the CVS and the home, is also very important. The role of the provider's technicians begins as soon as the titration is finished and is followed by an iterative supervision/renewal of the ventilator and ancillary equipment, as well as all notifications and alerts about these devices.[8]

STAFF TRAINING (SEE ALSO CHAPTER 11)

Undoubtedly, the success of a CVS largely depends on its medical, nursing and physiotherapist staff competence. In our view, the best training is based on regular caregiver teaching at bedside and is therefore largely dependent on the number of patients managed and experience from encountering and resolving various problems. This competence is also improved by regular teaching about the basis of mechanical ventilation and also through ventilator workshops using domiciliary devices and/or simulators. This is particularly true for learning how to set a ventilator and manipulate the interfaces, to install the ventilator circuits and the humidification devices. A low level of training will decrease the efficiency of the whole healthcare team and probably affect the short- and long-term benefits for the patient. Also, every component of training should be regularly reinforced, probably twice a year, but there is no consensus at present regarding the schedule of learning. Training for physicians should be organised in a similar way, but they should also keep abreast of the medical literature, current technological advances and availability and the various guidelines that may be published by health agencies. These guidelines should be adopted after being suitably adapted for the local needs by all the members of the CVS. Finally, it is recommended that the physicians involved in a CVS should have basic knowledge about intensive care and should be able to perform an endotracheal intubation as quickly as possible.

Training, which has to be tailored to all the different caregivers in the CVS team, should also include a good level of theoretical knowledge about ventilation physiology, ventilatory modes and the indications and contraindications for domiciliary ventilation. It should also include bedside practice, including examination of the patient and also the technical skills necessary to set the ventilator and interpret the effects of different modes and settings, especially during sleep. These competencies should be complemented by the appropriate skills for communicating with the patient and their family, in order to make treatment acceptable to them and to achieve high compliance. Training should also aim to develop the capacity for clinical reasoning and problem solving, for instance, intolerance of long-term NIV, patient–ventilator asynchronies, persistent nocturnal hypoxaemia or diurnal hypercapnia.

Equipment

The third component of a CVS is a stock of up-to-date equipment.

VENTILATORS

An active CVS inventory should consist of most domiciliary ventilators available on the market, and the staff should be trained to use them. Bench tests have shown great performance variability between different domiciliary ventilators, especially about triggering response,[9] battery duration,[9] tidal volumes, cycling off and airways pressurisation.[10] A ventilator may behave differently when applied to patients with different conditions,[11] in the presence of leaks,[12,13] and the comfort during ventilation may also vary greatly according to the machine.[14] Today, such discrepancies between ventilators are rarely due to hardware differences, but rather to software algorithm differences.[10] Moreover, large variations about ventilator characteristics and software navigation may also be perceived as a barrier to the training of physicians, nurses and physiotherapists. This is not the case in our experience, especially for people who are already familiar with one type of ventilator and if theoretical knowledge about triggering, cycling and pressurisation has been acquired. Therefore, careful attention should be paid to the teaching of ventilatory modes and the associated nomenclature, which is unfortunately very heterogeneous and confusing from one machine to another. Specific teaching should be provided to new staff, and regular courses should be aimed at strengthening the knowledge and skills of younger healthcare workers.

In order to titrate the patients with their domiciliary ventilators, the CVS should have the capacity to collect and interpret a substantial amount of monitoring data like clinical tolerance and compliance, evolution of signs of respiratory failure and the secondary effects due to pressure delivery or the effect of the interface (see Chapter 6). Dedicated ventilators are no longer needed for the titration step, because most bi-level domiciliary ventilators can now display nightly reports about flow/pressure variations, cycle rates, leaks and even an integrated SpO_2 curve. Regarding batteries, French legislation obliges the physician to prescribe a domiciliary ventilator with an internal or an external battery, once the prescribed ventilation is ≥12 h/day.

INTERFACES (SEE CHAPTER 6)

Interfaces are another factor influencing the efficacy and compliance with treatment. Their management by the CVS is largely the same as for the ventilators, as discussed in the previous section. The large number of available masks (nasal, facial or nasal plugs) allows management of most (if not all) adult patients. Custom-moulded interfaces still have a place in very specific situations such as older children with facial deformities. Seventy-five per cent of all our domiciliary ventilated patients are treated with only two models of nasal or facial interface. The difficulty therefore arises in the case of the minority of patients in whom several interfaces should be tested to get a balance between tolerance and efficacy. This phenomenon is still poorly understood because of the various related factors such as the amount of intentional leaks according to the delivered pressure, the configuration of intentional leaks on the mask or the circuit and the gas trajectory into the interface.[15,16] Also, an additional psychological factor cannot be excluded, including claustrophobia or treatment reluctance that may be expressed as interface intolerance. Any attempt by a hospital administration to provide only one standardised interface in their centres will compromise the care for around 25% of patients. Accordingly, a large variety of interfaces should be available in an expert CVS, both in the titration and the monitoring units. In France, the home care providers are not allowed to modify the ventilator model, the ventilator settings nor the interface. Finally, caregivers should be able to detect any complication and intolerance related to an interface and should be able to suggest a solution to the patients and their family: counselling about interface utilisation, trying out another interface, optimisation of humidification devices, etc. This approach is different for tracheostomised ventilation patients since tracheostomy cannulas have roughly similar technical characteristics, and their clinical performance is less influenced by the ventilatory mode.

Monitoring

The third technical component of a CVS is its monitoring capacity, including regular clinical monitoring of the underlying respiratory disease, regular identification of secondary effects of flow/pressure delivery or NIV interfaces and also patient–ventilator adaptation that is best evaluated at night, since most domiciliary ventilatory treatments are used during sleep. This topic is detailed in another part of this book, especially in Chapters 23–25.

CVS IN THE COMMUNITY

Definition and goals

The role of the respiratory home care service (RHCS) is to provide health services to patients and caregivers at home (Figure 19.3), to restore and maintain an acceptable clinical status and to minimise the consequences of chronic hypoventilation and disability and to reduce the number of episodes of acute respiratory events or failure. When they are discharged from the in-hospital CVS, and thus are considered as clinically stable, patients on long-term mechanical ventilation need an adequate environment to continue their treatment. They may be orientated towards either a long-term in-hospital facility or more often stay at home. At home, they need a structure to get adequate monitoring and maintenance of their equipment. As chronic respiratory failure patients are becoming older and more and more frail, with frequent comorbidities, they must be under the charge of not only respiratory technicians for their equipment but also other home care services as they are frequently dependent of them.

Thus, RHCS organisations represent a complex set of medical, ethical and social issues that involve multiple interest groups[17]: ventilator-assisted individuals, those who are completely dependent upon assisted ventilation for life support, those needing tracheostomy (generally neurological or neuromuscular patients, or severe end-of-life COPD patients) and partially dependent patients with varying degrees of severity and different aetiologies for respiratory failure treated by NIV.

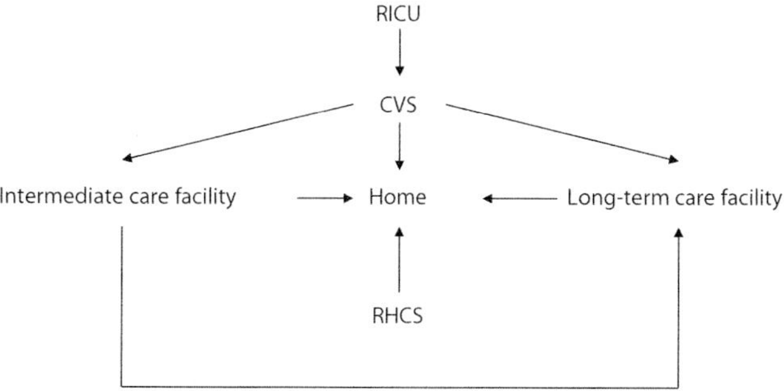

Figure 19.3 Place of the RHCS among other in- and out-hospital facilities. RICU: Respiratory intermediate care unit.

Transition to home (see also Chapters 22 and 23)

The transition between the CVS and home is a crucial period. It is important that the first days at home are successful as they will impact on the long-term acceptance of HMV by the patient. The keys for success are discussed below.

CONTINUUM OF THE IN-HOSPITAL EDUCATION PROGRAM FOR THE PATIENT AND THEIR FAMILY

Discharge from the CVS to home must be anticipated by in-hospital education involving a dedicated team consisting of physicians, nurses, respiratory therapists and social workers on one hand, and technicians and nurses of the RHCS who made contact with the patient in the hospital, on the other hand.[18] According to the aetiology of chronic respiratory failure, other professionals should be consulted, such as psychologists, dieticians and speech therapists. Prior to discharge, the RHCS team should meet the patient and their family, perform a home visit to plan the installation of the equipment and discuss potential improvement of the home setting in order to optimise the transfer and settling in of the patient.[19]

The training of patient and his or her family has to start as soon as possible during the stay in the hospital and is continued after the patient has returned home.[20] The home nursing staff who are directly involved in the day-to-day care of the patient have the task to demonstrate and repeat, as needed, the instructions to the patient and their caregivers on medication and nasal/face mask use.[21] Another important item is to ask the RHCS technician to check, at home, the level of knowledge of the patient and their family with regard not only to the equipment for its 'chronic' use but also the equipment and procedures to be used at home in case of an emergency (self-inflating manual resuscitator) for the most severe.[21]

The follow-up scheme and the 24 h free telephone line must be explained, as well as the therapeutic protocol indicating the timing and duration of night ventilation, and daytime oxygen therapy, sometimes interrupted by NIV sessions. The follow-up scheme must be planned with adequate frequency of follow-up. It is also important to ensure a 24 h free helpline for emergency telephone calls. A physician should be contactable concerning any information about treatment or other management problems. This same arrangement should also be in place for contacting the device manufacturing companies and technicians.

Finally, the patient should be made aware that the main goals of RHCS are to enhance their quality of life, to reduce hospital admissions and to be cost-effective, and also to supervise compliance with therapy. These goals are achieved by ensuring that the clinical and physiological functions (mainly adequate ventilation) and the patient's safety are maintained (see also Chapter 24).

SOCIAL CONSIDERATIONS

An important factor for success is to coordinate the social assistance that will be available at home. The spectrum ranges from the simplest case where the patient has numerous, motivated, available family members to no relatives in proximity. If the patient wants to go back home and if his or her clinical status permits it, collaboration with social workers must be organised according to the financial possibilities of the society and the social network. In France, for instance, patients with established chronic respiratory failure benefit from 100% reimbursement for their healthcare costs. Social services have budgets that are supported by the social charges (*cotisations*; like the National Insurance in the United Kingdom) paid by workers and their employers. These services are available in France for the most ventilator-dependent patients.

HOME CARE SETTING

The home equipment for ventilator-assisted individuals depends on the aetiology of the chronic respiratory failure, the degree of impairment, the upper airway function and the mode of ventilatory support. If clinically stable, a middle-aged patient requiring nocturnal NIV does not require a large amount of equipment (i.e. just a ventilator with the circuit and filters, and a mask). This type of patient does not need any humidifier device or additional oxygen in the circuit and no internal or external battery. Additional elements are needed for patients on long-term oxygen therapy or those requiring mechanical cough assistance. Ventilator-dependent individuals should always have a backup ventilator, an emergency power source and a manual resuscitation bag. The electricity supplier and the regional emergency medical assistance service should be aware of these individuals.

RHCSs: Obligations, organisation and costs

OBLIGATIONS

A RHCS must provide a 24 h service with facilities for on-call intervention at home by skilled technicians, nurses or other qualified employees. The availability of a physician who is a part- or full-time employee of the organisation ensures superior quality of home care.

In parallel, the RHCS also works with technicians who get involved either at home to ensure optimal maintenance of the equipment as well as education and motivation of the patient and their family, or in the maintenance workshop, generally located in the headquarters of the RHCS. Such technicians provide a regular daytime service and are also on-call during the night or at weekends. The frequency of the daytime visits varies according to the patient's needs. In France, the reimbursements to the RHCS are also different, depending on the type of respiratory home care provided to the patients. Specific contracts stating a precise frequency of visits and the obligations of the RHCS may be submitted for reimbursement.

Respiratory physiotherapists also have a role in managing patients with bronchial hypersecretion and decreased cough efficacy and those patients who will benefit from pulmonary rehabilitation. The availability of on-call respiratory technicians is crucial to provide answers to patients who require information about emergency situations or technical problems, especially with ventilator-dependent patients. A RHCS also needs a well-planned administrative structure to manage the financial budget, which is important in terms of deciding future investments and purchase of equipment. Criteria, procedures and quality standards to be certified by health services or quality control commissions widely vary between different countries.

ORGANISATION

The early national public health services that historically initiated home care services have largely been replaced by the trend towards cooperation between public and private organisations. In some countries, home care is supplied entirely by private companies; in others, the public health service still has a monopoly.

In France, the Association Nationale pour les Traitements à Domicile, l'Innovation et la Recherche (ANTADIR) initiated a large public network in the beginning of the 1980s that created a federation of 33 regional associations, devoted to home respiratory care.[22] At the beginning, these non-profit associations were intended to treat chronic respiratory failure patients at home by providing oxygen therapy and/or ventilatory assistance. They were funded by French Social Security to ensure delivery and maintenance of the equipment. This system largely developed alone nearly without any challenge from the private sector during the first 10 years; however, private health services became more and more interested in the business opportunities afforded by this model of care. Nowadays in France, RHCS (including treatments by continuous positive airway pressure [CPAP] for sleep apnoea syndrome) is shared between several regional associations (35%) and private national or international companies (65%). Generally, the most severe patients (i.e. those who are discharged by the public hospitals) are managed by the associative network, and patients who are less severe are managed by the private sector.

With the increasing demand, RHCS is looking to manage not only respiratory care but also the whole package for health maintenance at home (e.g. provision and installation of complex 'medical' beds, artificial feeding, home perfusion treatments, subcutaneous insulin, wheelchairs, etc.) and social worker management.

COSTS OF HOME CARE

Several studies have proven that home care is less expensive than in-hospital treatment, either in acute-care hospitals or in long-term facilities.[22] NIV is effective in maintaining the clinical stability of patients with chronic respiratory failure and reducing the need for further hospitalisations. In case of slowly progressive diseases with favourable long-term prognosis, such as post-polio syndrome or thoracic deformities, the costs of the ventilatory equipment, maintenance and the possible requirement for additional oxygen constitute a major economic burden. The decision whether to purchase or rent a ventilator should be made in the light of the prognosis of the disease and economic considerations in the contract with the local dealer (accessories, maintenance, other services) and varies from one country to another. In most European countries, a national policy regarding prescription modalities, reimbursement, assistance and medical supervision (if it exists) does not provide complete coverage, even if the costs of long-term oxygen therapy and the ventilator are usually reimbursed by the national health service or an insurance company. In France, social security covers the costs of installation, maintenance, medical and technical supervision of patients with chronic respiratory failure receiving domiciliary respiratory support through specific contracts according to the modality of the prescribed respiratory assistance. Patients are reimbursed at a 100% rate for all their specific costs related to the respiratory disease (pharmacological treatments, chest physiotherapy, etc.), but indirect costs must also be considered (Table 19.1). French social security is increasingly supported by private insurance funds through the associative network mainly regulated by ANTADIR with its public service philosophy,[22] and also through private networks that have strongly increased their presence in this field during the past 10 years. When the severity of the disease increases, the cost of respiratory assistance cannot be separated from the cost of chronic care, especially in progressive neuromuscular diseases or severe COPD, leading sometimes to ventilatory dependence. Caregivers in Europe are usually family members who face progressively increasing socio-medical requirements for cooking, bathing and toileting. A home care program that includes these specific needs is obviously desirable, but funding is presently lacking in most developed countries in the world and patients must pay themselves for this part of the care.

Table 19.1 Components of home care costs

Direct costs
Physician fees
Formal services purchased by family
Hospital and skilled nursing facility inpatient days
Medication
Equipment rental
Oxygen
Ambulance
Medical supplies
Extra-utility charges
Major one-time purchases or remodelling
Indirect costs
Alterations in employment
Lost wages resulting from caregiving

Monitoring the patient treated by HMV (Table 19.2)

Patients on long-term mechanical ventilation require regular follow-up on a clinical basis by their GP, in collaboration with the chest physician and the CVS. The frequency of visits is greater during the first year of follow-up, or if the disease is rapidly progressive or unstable. It is more convenient for the patient to come for a daytime consultation where the clinical status and the equipment are controlled, in collaboration with the RHCS. Moreover, it allows routine investigations (chest x-rays, electrocardiogram, arterial blood gases breathing room air or oxygen and during mechanical ventilation as needed) to be performed. However, such assessments do not provide any evaluation of patient–ventilator adaptation during the night and do not verify the correction of respiratory disturbances during sleep. Rabec et al.[3] have demonstrated that about half of patients considered as correctly ventilated at home still have desaturation during night-time or other respiratory events that are not identified by daytime assessments. Remote monitoring is now a new field for clinical, technological and research developments. See also Chapters 23 and 24.

HMV IN THE NETHERLANDS

HMV has a long history in the Netherlands. It started in the 1960s as a spin-off after the poliomyelitis epidemic, as a large group of patients became dependent on long-term mechanical ventilation.[23] In 1965, the first patient from Groningen was sent home with a ventilator.

Organisation of HMV in the Netherlands

While in the beginning different hospitals in our country were involved in HMV, the Dutch government decided in 2004 that only four centres, geographically spread over the country and associated with a university hospital, could initiate HMV. If patients need HMV, they have to be referred to one of these centres. To be even more precise, the postal code of the place where the patient lives determines to which centre the patient should be referred. This is the only way in which reimbursement of HMV is guaranteed. All HMV centres in the Netherlands work in more or less the same way, and the teams consist of physicians, specialised nurses and technicians. In contrast to many other HMV centres in the world, the Dutch teams work both inside and outside the hospital. This means that the centres are responsible both for the start of the HMV and for the follow-up. As more and more patients needed HMV and safety issues became more important, the government forced us in 2012 to develop a Dutch guideline. It was developed with all societies who are involved in this process, including GPs, intensive care physicians, physiatrists, neurologists and of course patients. In this guideline, a Dutch HMV centre is clearly defined: (1) it initiates HMV in at least 50 patients per year, (2) it is

Table 19.2 Monitoring the patient treated by HMV

ITEM	M1	M3	M6	M9	M12	M18	M24
Clinical evaluation	X	X	X	X	X	X	X
Chest x-ray	X				X		X
EKG	X				X		X
Biology	X				X		X
Diurnal arterial blood gases	X	X	X	X	X	X	X
Compliance recording	X	X	X	X	X	X	X
Pulmonary function tests	X				X		X
Ventilator software analysis	X	X	X	X	X	X	X
Equipment maintenance	X	X	X	X	X	X	X

responsible for follow-up of at least 200 patients yearly and (3) all patients are regularly monitored according to the disease leading to CRF.

Indication for HMV

The number of patients on HMV shows linear growth over time in all patient groups (Figure 19.4). The group including patients with a neuromuscular, central or peripheral nervous system disorder is the largest group in our country. Examples are patients with various muscular disorders, amyotrophic lateral sclerosis, spinal cord injury or diaphragm paralysis.

The second group entails patients with a thoracic cage problem, for example, congenital kyphoscoliosis. The obesity–hypoventilation syndrome belongs also to this group, as the obesity has a negative effect on the mobility of the thoracic cage. The latter diagnosis is valid if patients fulfil all the following criteria: a BMI > 30 kg/m^2, an arterial PCO_2 > 6.0 kPa (45 mmHg) and hypercapnia that cannot be explained by a disease other than the obesity.

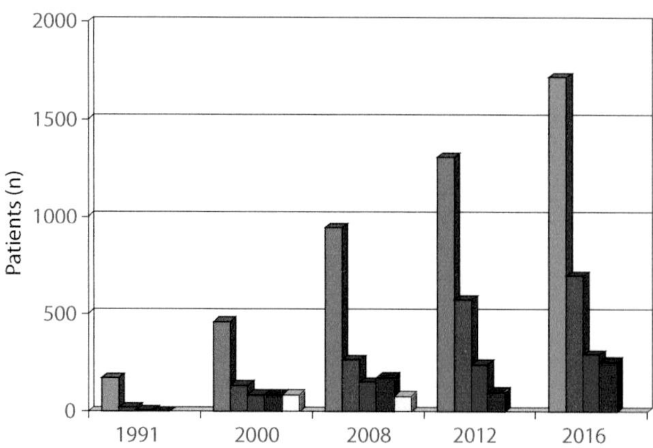

Figure 19.4 Different patient groups on HMV in the Netherlands from 1991 to 2016. Green: neuromuscular; red: thoracic cage problems; blue: lung; purple: sleep related; grey: miscellaneous.

The third group entails patients with lung diseases, and as shown in Figure 19.4, this is a small group in the Netherlands. The reason for this is that a recent meta-analysis did not show beneficial effects of HMV in COPD patients with stable hypercapnic failure.[24] However, this group will show a significant growth in the future, as a recent German study showed both an improved survival and improved quality of life due to chronic HMV.[25]

The fourth group contains patients with sleep-related breathing disorders, like obstructive sleep apnoea syndrome and central sleep apnoea syndrome. HMV might be an option in these patients if CPAP is not effective.

Referral and outpatient clinic

As mentioned previously, HMV can only be started after the patients have been referred to one of the four centres. After referral, patients will first be seen at the outpatient clinic by both a physician and specialised nurse. The task of the physician is to assess whether there is an indication for starting HMV, while the nurse will provide information about HMV and evaluates whether the social circumstances are sufficient for HMV. Spirometry, daytime arterial blood gases, nocturnal oximetry and transcutaneous capnography are the usual baseline assessments. In addition to information about chronic ventilatory support, the specialised nurse will also check the effectiveness of the patient's cough and will teach air stacking if needed. At the end of the visit, a decision will be made whether HMV should be started or not.

Start of HMV

If the patient fulfils the criteria for HMV, he/she will be admitted to the hospital. The four centres all have different settings in the hospital where HMV should be started. Some admit the patients to the ICU; some initiate HMV on the pulmonary ward. Despite the difference in settings, all wards must have specific knowledge of chronic ventilatory support and adequate monitoring, and safety must be guaranteed, being requested by the Dutch guideline. Regular nocturnal oximetry and transcutaneous capnography and readings from the ventilator give us insight into how the patient is ventilated. During this process, training of the patient and family/partner is started to teach them how to handle the mask and the machine. After the patient is adjusted to the ventilator and the settings are correct, the patient is ready to go home.

As we believe that the way we set up chronic ventilatory support is too expensive and less comfortable for the patient, we recently carried out a local study showing that initiation of HNV at home is equally effective, safe and cheaper compared to inpatient initiation.[26] To implement this nationally, we are currently conducting a study with all four centres in patients with a neuromuscular disorder or a thoracic cage.

Discharge and follow-up

Discharge can only take place at the time that safety issues around HMV are guaranteed. The patient and all healthcare providers get instruction on how to use the equipment and are informed about the possible alarms and the actions to be taken if problems occur. On the day of discharge, the patient is visited at home by our specialised nurse and the equipment installed. The department of HMV can be contacted 24/7 and is therefore always available in case of problems. Once a year, both oxygen saturation and carbon dioxide during the night will be checked while the patient is being ventilated, and if needed, this can be done more frequently. At least once a year, the patient will visit the outpatient clinic of the HMV centre.

The GP is the physician with primary responsibility for patients on HMV and the first to contact in case of problems. The activities and the role of the GP depend on the degree of disability of the patient and the severity of the underlying disease. In the final stages of the disease, the family, caregivers and healthcare professionals are coordinated by the GP to provide effective palliative care.

CONCLUSIONS

The provision of home ventilation is complex and involves much more than just the purchase of a machine and ancillary equipment. It is best delivered by a specialist service looking after a large number of patients, with a well-trained, and experienced, multidisciplinary team. It should not be delivered on an occasional basis by a general pulmonology service.

REFERENCES

1. Lloyd-Owen SJ, Donaldson GC, Ambrosino N et al. Patterns of home mechanical ventilation use in Europe: Results from the Eurovent survey. *Eur Respir J.* 2005;25:1025–31.
2. Haute Autorité de Santé. Practical aspects of long-term noninvasive positive pressure ventilation at home in neuromuscular disease. Clinical practice guidelines. 2006: Available at www.has-sante.fr/portail/jcms/c_334439 (accessed 22 July 2009).
3. Rabec C, Georges M, Kabeya NK et al. Evaluating noninvasive ventilation using a monitoring system coupled to a ventilator: A bench-to-bedside study. *Eur Respir J.* 2009;34:902–13.
4. Falsaperla R, Wenzel A, Pavone P et al. Polysomnographic evaluation of non-invasive ventilation in children with neuromuscular disease. *Respirology.* 2014;19:80–4.
5. Gonzalez-Bermejo J, Perrin C, Janssens JP et al. Proposal for a systematic analysis of polygraphy or polysomnography for identifying and scoring abnormal events occurring during non-invasive ventilation. *Thorax.* 2012;67:546–52.
6. Duiverman ML, Wempe JB, Bladder G et al. Two-year home-based nocturnal noninvasive ventilation added to rehabilitation in chronic obstructive pulmonary disease patients: A randomized controlled trial. *Respir Res.* 2011;12:112.
7. Dreher M, Ekkernkamp E, Schmoor C et al. Pulmonary rehabilitation and noninvasive ventilation in patients with hypercapnic interstitial lung disease. *Respiration.* 2015;89:208–13.
8. Chatwin M, Heather S, Hanak A et al. Analysis of home support and ventilator malfunction in 1,211 ventilator-dependent patients. *Eur Respir J.* 2010;35:310–6.
9. Blakeman TC, Rodriquez D, Jr., Hanseman D, Branson RD. Bench evaluation of 7 home-care ventilators. *Respir Care.* 2011;56:1791–8.
10. Chen Y, Cheng K, Zhou X. Performance characteristics of seven bilevel mechanical ventilators in pressure-support mode with different cycling criteria: A comparative bench study. *Med Sci Monit.* 2015;21:310–7.
11. Fauroux B, Leroux K, Desmarais G et al. Performance of ventilators for noninvasive positive-pressure ventilation in children. *Eur Respir J.* 2008;31:1300–7.
12. Ueno Y, Nakanishi N, Oto J, Imanaka H, Nishimura M. A bench study of the effects of leak on ventilator performance during noninvasive ventilation. *Respir Care.* 2011;56:1758–64.
13. Fauroux B, Leroux K, Pepin JL et al. Are home ventilators able to guarantee a minimal tidal volume? *Intensive Care Med.* 2010;36:1008–14.
14. Vitacca M, Barbano L, D'Anna S et al. Comparison of five bilevel pressure ventilators in patients with chronic ventilatory failure: A physiologic study. *Chest.* 2002;122:2105–14.
15. Schettino GP, Chatmongkolchart S, Hess DR, Kacmarek RM. Position of exhalation port and mask design affect CO2 rebreathing during noninvasive positive pressure ventilation. *Crit Care Med.* 2003;31:2178–82.

16. Schettino GP, Tucci MR, Sousa R et al. Mask mechanics and leak dynamics during noninvasive pressure support ventilation: A bench study. *Intensive Care Med.* 2001;27:1887–91.
17. Gilmartin M. Transition from the intensive care unit to home: Patient selection and discharge planning. *Respir Care.* 1994;39:456–77.
18. Huang TT, Peng JM. Role adaptation of family caregivers for ventilator-dependent patients: Transition from respiratory care ward to home. *J Clin Nurs.* 2010;19:1686–94.
19. Muir JF. *Architecture intérieure et handicap respiratoire.* Paris: Margaux Orange; 2007.
20. Fischer DA, Prentice WS. Feasibility of home care for certain respiratory-dependent restrictive or obstructive lung disease patients. *Chest.* 1982;82:739–43.
21. Swedberg L, Michelsen H, Chiriac EH, Hylander I. On-the-job training makes the difference: Healthcare assistants' perceived competence and responsibility in the care of patients with home mechanical ventilation. *Scand J Caring Sci.* 2015;29:369–78.
22. Stuart M, Weinrich M. Integrated health system for chronic disease management: Lessons learned from France. *Chest.* 2004;125:695–703.
23. Hazenberg A, Cobben NA, Kampelmacher MJ et al. HomeNed Tijdschr Geneeskd. *Ned Tijdschr Geneeskd.* 2012;156:A3609.
24. Struik FM, Lacasse Y, Goldstein R, Kerstjens HM, Wijkstra PJ. Nocturnal non-invasive positive pressure ventilation for stable chronic obstructive pulmonary disease. *Cochrane Database Syst Rev.* 2013;6:CD002878.
25. Kohnlein T, Windisch W, Kohler D et al. Non-invasive positive pressure ventilation for the treatment of severe stable chronic obstructive pulmonary disease: A prospective, multicentre, randomised, controlled clinical trial. *Lancet Respir Med.* 2014;2:698–705.
26. Hazenberg A, Kerstjens HA, Prins SC et al. Initiation of home mechanical ventilation at home: A randomised controlled trial of efficacy, feasibility and costs. *Respir Med.* 2014;108:1387–95.

20

Diagnostic tests in the assessment of patients for home mechanical ventilation

MICHAEL POLKEY, PATRICK B. MURPHY AND NICHOLAS HART

KEY MESSAGES

- The range of testing employed to assess patients undergoing home mechanical ventilation (HMV) should be tailored to the individual patient and, in addition to measurements of carbon dioxide level, the test used should reflect underlying disease pathology and as a minimum should include
  - Neuromuscular disease – forced vital capacity (FVC), inspiratory muscle strength and expiratory muscle strength
  - Obesity – weight and FVC
  - Obstructive airways diseases – forced expiratory volume in 1 s (FEV1) and FEV1/FVC ratio
- A stepwise approach for monitoring should be adopted with inpatient assessment and overnight polygraphy reserved for patients failing to respond to HMV therapy and refractory to manipulation in the outpatient setting.
- When assessment of carbon dioxide levels is required, consideration should be given to less painful and invasive techniques, such as transcutaneous capnometry over traditional arterial blood gas sampling.
- In patients with respiratory muscle weakness, both inspiratory and expiratory muscle testing should be performed with careful clinical assessment of cough function.

INTRODUCTION

The respiratory system maintains oxygen and carbon dioxide homeostasis, which requires repetitive cyclical neural activation (neural respiratory drive [NRD]) of the respiratory (principally inspiratory) muscles. Activation of the inspiratory muscles results in an increase in intrathoracic volume, and consequent decrease in intrathoracic pressure, which generates a pressure gradient causing airflow into the lungs. The efficiency of the respiratory muscle system is dependent on the strength and endurance of the respiratory muscles (respiratory muscle capacity) working against the resistance and compliance of the airways, lung and chest wall (respiratory muscle load). Respiratory failure arises due to an imbalance in the relationship between NRD, respiratory muscle capacity and respiratory muscle load (Figure 20.1). Non-invasive ventilation (NIV) is commonly used to augment alveolar ventilation during acute and chronic ventilatory failure.

While superficially it could be imagined that the evaluation of patients with chronic respiratory failure (CRF) necessitating home mechanical ventilation (HMV) requires no more than measurement of arterial blood gas (ABG) tension of oxygen and carbon dioxide, in practice, detailed physiological assessment of these key areas is often appropriate. This not only ensures that the correct diagnosis for the cause of CRF is made but also can enhance patient adherence by maximising the therapeutic benefit and optimising comfort. As with all patient care, history and clinical examination should be used to direct further investigations. Evaluation has been divided into

- Basic clinical assessment
- Gas exchange
- Pulmonary mechanics
- Respiratory muscle function
- Patient–ventilator interaction
- Overnight physiological monitoring

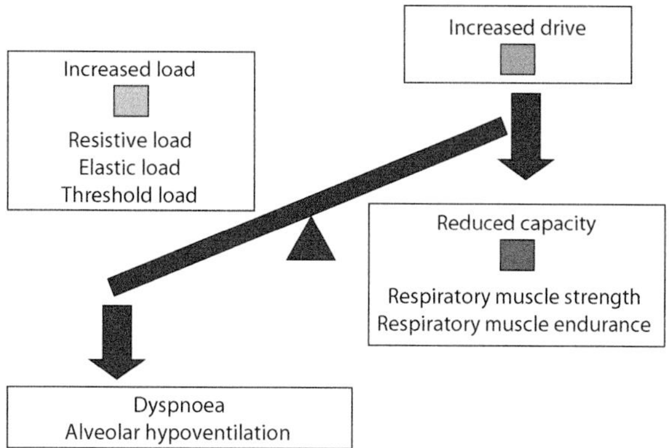

Figure 20.1 Illustrates the interaction between load capacity and drive essential to produce ventilation.

BASIC CLINICAL ASSESSMENT

The specific assessments undertaken during clinic consultations will depend on the underlying aetiology of CRF (where known), but a variety of issues are common across diagnoses regarding domiciliary ventilation and should be focused on to ensure that adequate patient–ventilator interaction and effective ventilation are achieved. The primary goal of the consultation should be for the clinician to demonstrate that the overall effect of HMV is both beneficial and acceptable to the patient, and this can be judged by the adherence of the patient to the nocturnal prescription of NIV and by the effect with sustained use on arterial carbon dioxide tensions. The majority of home ventilators now have internal monitoring clocks that measure and record the total 'blower' hours with data cards that can be used for the measurement of adherence. These data should be compared against the patient reported adherence and any discrepancies discussed with the patient. Poor adherence should prompt further questioning to identify areas to improve compliance. Failure to follow this approach may result in inappropriate investigation of persistent hypercapnia when the reason for treatment failure is actually sub-optimal treatment adherence. A range of clinical investigations are available to assist with the assessments of patients for HMV. These cover simple bedside tests to more complicated invasive testing used in research. The investigations are summarised in Table 20.1a and b, indicating those 'basic' tests used in routine clinical practice (Table 20.1a) and 'advanced' procedures used in research (Table 20.1b).

GAS EXCHANGE

ABG analysis is an important tool in the assessment of patients receiving HMV. The test is simple to perform by skilled operators, and the results are rapidly available allowing prompt clinical decisions. Many units now use arterialised ear lobe blood gas (ELBG) as an alternative to ABGs. These have been shown to reflect $PaCO_2$ accurately and can be less painful than the arterial equivalent.[1] However, ELBGs can be a less faithful reflection of PaO_2, since wide limits of agreement may underestimate PaO_2 in the normal range and therefore ELBG-derived PaO_2 should be interpreted in this light or used in conjunction with pulse oximetry.[2] The use of lidocaine to reduce pain associated with arterial puncture is advocated in some guidelines but is frequently not used in routine clinical practice.[3] Pre-procedure anxiety contributes to pain perception of the procedure and may dissuade patients from consenting to this important test and thus affect the ability to manage them appropriately.[4] Transcutaneous measures of CO_2 (discussed in more detail later in this chapter) have now been shown reliable for 'spot' readings of CO_2 and offers a pain-free method of assessment.[5] A range of parameters can be measured by the modern blood gas analysis machines, but those of most interest are the partial pressures of oxygen and carbon dioxide dissolved in the liquid component of blood (PaO_2 and $PaCO_2$, respectively) and the bicarbonate $\left(HCO_3^-\right)$ concentration. These parameters are used to define respiratory failure, which is divided into type 1, hypoxic respiratory failure (PaO_2 < 8 kPa or <60 mmHg), and type 2, hypercapnic respiratory failure ($PaCO_2$ > 6 kPa or >45 mmHg).

Oxygen

Oxygen delivery to the tissues is dependent on cardiac output and oxygen content of blood. While the contribution of dissolved oxygen in blood to total oxygen content is small, it is linked to haemoglobin saturation level and that contributes predominantly to oxygen content ($CaO_2 = 1.34 \times SaO_2 \times (Hb) + 0.003 \times PaO_2$). The correction of hypoxia with HMV is via a combination of improving hypoventilation,

Table 20.1a Basic investigations used in the assessment of HMV

Basic Investigation	Unit	Assessment
SNIP	cmH_2O	Global inspiratory muscle strength
MIP	cmH_2O	Global inspiratory muscle strength
MEP	cmH_2O	Global expiratory muscle strength
Spirometry (FEV_1/FVC)	L	Lung volume and airflow obstruction
Cough expiratory flow	L/min	Global expiratory muscle strength
Arterial blood gases	Various	Gas exchange and acid–base status

Table 20.1b Advanced investigations used in the assessment of HMV

Advanced Investigation	Unit	Assessment
Sniff oesophageal pressure	cmH_2O	Global inspiratory muscle strength
Cough gastric pressure	cmH_2O	Global expiratory muscle strength
Sniff trans-diaphragmatic pressure (P_{di})	cmH_2O	Volitional diaphragm strength
Twitch P_{di}	cmH_2O	Non-volitional diaphragm strength
PEEPi	cmH_2O	Threshold load
Pulmonary compliance	L/cmH_2O	Elastic load
Diaphragm $EMG_{\%max}$	%	Neural respiratory drive

abolishing upper airways obstruction and, in part, alveolar recruitment. If there is additional intrinsic lung disease, the addition of supplementary oxygen may be required to maintain adequate oxygenation. Although correction of daytime hypoxia has been shown to be beneficial in chronic obstructive pulmonary disease (COPD),[6] there is no clear randomised controlled trial evidence for the use of long-term oxygen therapy (LTOT) in other diseases causing respiratory failure. Therefore, in clinical practice, the same degree of hypoxia is used for non-COPD disease with LTOT prescribed when the $PaO_2 < 7.3$ kPa (<55 mmHg) or with a $PaO_2 < 8$ kPa (<60 mmHg) if there is evidence of sleep-disordered breathing, cor pulmonale, right heart strain on the electrocardiogram and/or a haematocrit level greater than 50%.

Carbon dioxide

The main function of HMV is to correct nocturnal hypoventilation; it is therefore given in the context of hypercapnic respiratory failure. In contrast to oxygen, the majority of carbon dioxide in arterial blood is dissolved in the liquid component rather than being protein bound. Due to the intrinsic properties of carbon dioxide, it rapidly crosses and equilibrates across the alveolar–capillary membrane and thus is inversely proportional to alveolar ventilation. Alveolar ventilation (V_A) is a product of respiratory rate (RR) and the difference between tidal volume (V_T) and the dead space (V_{DS}) ($V_A = (V_T - V_{DS}) \times RR$). Thus, hypoventilation can occur through increased dead space, decreased tidal volume or decreased respiratory rate. It is therefore possible to manipulate these variables using NIV, although one must appreciate that the ventilator circuit will produce a small increase in dead space. However, this is far outweighed by the significant improvements in tidal volume to enhance alveolar ventilation.

Acid–base balance

Acid–base balance is integrally linked to $PaCO_2$ homeostasis and the control of ventilation. Unlike hypoxia, which directly stimulates ventilation via action of the carotid sinus, CO_2 mediates its effects on ventilation via alteration in intracellular pH detected by peripheral and central chemoreceptors. Chronic (via renal bicarbonate retention) and acute (via the Henderson–Hasselbach equation) hypoventilations cause a rise in HCO_3^- levels that aim to buffer the effect on pH of rising $PaCO_2$. The presence of respiratory acidosis (pH < 7.35) on blood gas analysis indicates an acute deterioration in respiratory failure that is yet to be compensated for and indicates the need for prompt treatment.

PULMONARY MECHANICS

A clear understanding of pulmonary mechanics is useful for the physician to enable optimal individualised ventilator settings to be prescribed for the patient. Assessment of pulmonary mechanics ranges from basic spirometry, which can be routinely used in bedside testing and in clinics with portable meters, to full lung function testing with measurements of static and dynamic compliance. The interpretation of respiratory function abnormalities is the subject of a number of previous publications, and thus, an overview with particular relevance to HMV will be provided. Common patterns of spirometry are found in patients requiring HMV, with the typical lung function abnormalities found in COPD, obesity and neuromuscular disease summarised in Table 20.2 and Figure 20.2.

Lung volumes

The pattern of change of lung volumes depends on the underlying disease with lung hyperinflation occurring in COPD and reduced lung volumes in obesity and restrictive thoracic disorders, such as chest wall disease and neuromuscular disease. Functional residual capacity (FRC) is the point at which outward elastic recoil of the chest wall balances inward recoil of the lungs. A change in FRC may move the patient to an inefficient position on the pressure–volume curve, increasing work of breathing; this may be at higher lung volume (as is the case with COPD[7]) or lower (as is the case in obesity[8]). A number of techniques can be used to measure FRC, including helium dilution and nitrogen washout, and arithmetically from whole body plethysmography. Each technique has potential advantages and disadvantages, but, in clinical practice, the methods produce similar results except when there are large areas of unventilated

Table 20.2 Typical trends in lung function testing in HMV population

	COPD	NMD	Obesity
FEV_1	–	N/–	N/–
FVC	–	N/–	N/–
FEV_1/FVC	–	N/+	N/+
TLC	+	N/–	N/–
RV	+	–	N/+
RV/TLC	+	N/+	N/+
DL_{co}	–	–	–
PI_{max}	N/–	–	N

Legend: COPD, chronic obstructive pulmonary disease; NMD, neuromuscular disease; FEV_1, forced expiratory volume in 1 s; FVC, forced vital capacity; TLC, total lung volume; RV, residual volume; DL_{co}, diffusing capacity of the lung; PI_{max}, maximum static inspiratory pressure; N, normal; –, decreased; +, increased.

lung as is the case in patients with bullous emphysema but may occur in any patient with significant airflow obstruction. Usually the differences are only important when conducting research or considering highly specialised therapies such as lung volume reduction surgery. It is important to recognise that a truly accurate FRC measurement can only be measured with the respiratory muscles relaxed.

Basic spirometry, used to measure forced expiratory volume in 1 s (FEV_1) and forced vital capacity (FVC), is the most commonly encountered measure of pulmonary mechanics and is used to monitor progression of a range of diseases including COPD; it is also of some value in predicting survival in neuromuscular disease, including amyotrophic lateral sclerosis.[9] In the obese patient with obstructive sleep apnoea, FVC can predict CRF with a cut-off of 3.5L and 2.3L in men and women, respectively.[10] A fall in FVC of greater than 20% from sitting to supine is abnormal and may indicate significant diaphragmatic weakness.[11] A detailed review of the compartmentalisation of the lung volumes, in particular review of the residual volume (RV) measurement, can allow the clinician to separate those patients with combined inspiratory and expiratory muscle weakness and those with predominantly inspiratory muscle weakness.[12] However, because of the non-linear relationship between volume and pressure, tests of respiratory muscle strength (RMS) that measure the pressure generated by the respiratory muscles are a more sensitive marker of declining respiratory function than the measurement of lung volumes.[13] In clinical practice, this will include sniff nasal inspiratory pressure (SNIP) and maximal inspiratory pressures (MIPs) measured at the mouth, which are discussed in the section 'Respiratory Muscle Testing'.

Advanced physiological measurements

The detailed measurement of pulmonary mechanics requires the use of specialist equipment and skills, but it is increasingly feasible in the clinical arena (Figure 20.3). The basic mechanics of the respiratory system involve the action of respiratory muscles to produce negative intrathoracic pressure changes that result in airflow. To study this phenomenon requires the measurement of pressure changes throughout the system and the flow generated. This is most commonly achieved with the use of differential pressure transducers and a pneumotachograph; the signals from these devices are amplified and converted from analogue to digital signals and presented by commercially available software packages. Once digitised, the signals can be later manipulated and studied to measure

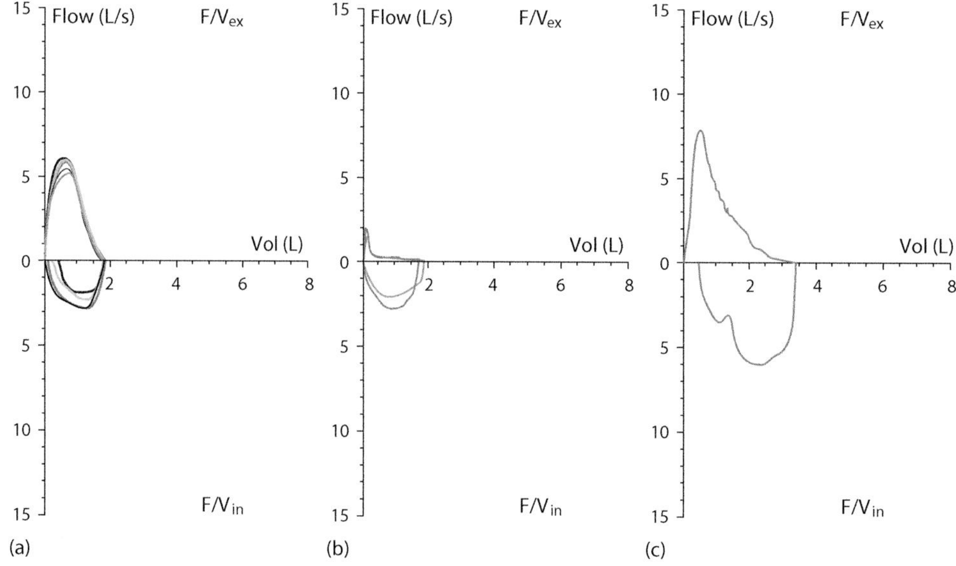

Figure 20.2 Flow volume loops from patients with **(a)** Neuromuscular disease (myotonic dystrophy) showing reduced lung volumes and without airway obstruction. **(b)** Chronic obstructive pulmonary disease showing a typical concave expiratory loop indicating airways obstruction. **(c)** Obesity revealing mildly reduced lung volumes with some concavity of the expiratory loop consistent with early airway closure.

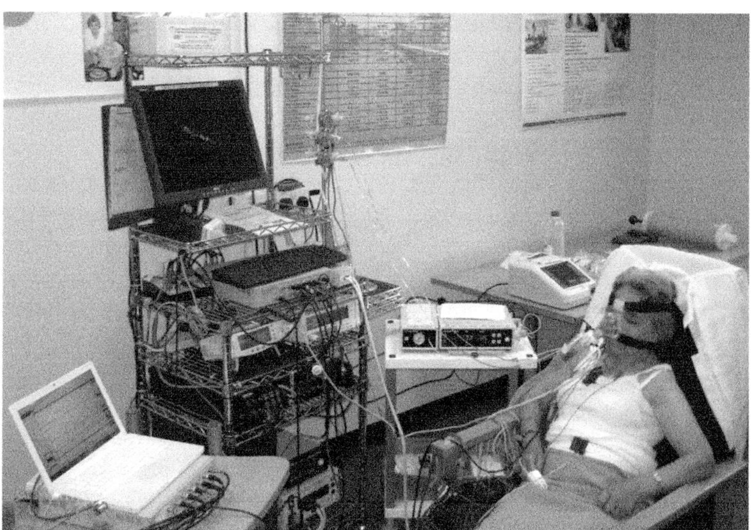

Figure 20.3 Patient attending for physiological evaluation including measurement of RMS, NRD and pulmonary mechanics on and off NIV. Illustrates the range of equipment needed for specialist invasive testing.

pulmonary mechanics. As pleural pressure cannot be measured directly, mid-oesophageal pressure (P_{oes}) is used as a surrogate marker and is measured with a balloon pressure monitoring catheter inserted pernasally.[14] Pressure measurements are also acquired from balloon catheters situated in the stomach (P_{ga}), to determine transdiaphragmatic pressure (P_{di}), and at the mouth (P_{mo}), in order to calculate pressures across the system as a whole (transpulmonary pressure). Combined balloon-electrode catheters allow the measurement of the diaphragm electromyogram (EMG_{di}) without the disadvantages of poor signals acquired from surface electrodes.[15] Despite initial concern with regard to changes in EMG_{di} signal with changes in lung volume, studies have shown the reliability and reproducibility of this technique using multipair recording electrodes during wake and sleep.[16]

Compliance

Compliance of the respiratory system (C_{rs}) reflects the ease at which pressure changes produced by the respiratory muscles change the volume of the lung. It is defined as the change in lung volume per unit change in pressure across the respiratory system. Importantly, compliance for a given individual varies with lung volume. In obese patients, for example, the C_{rs} can be reduced, meaning the lungs are more difficult to inflate, and such patients require higher levels of pressure support to ensure adequate ventilation.[17] Patients with neuromuscular disease often have a normal or slightly reduced lung and chest wall compliance[12] due to the loss of muscle mass, and thus the overall compliance of the respiratory system is preserved, meaning that these patients can usually be ventilated at lower pressures.

Compliance may be measured as a static or dynamic measure, each providing useful physiological data and both having advantages and disadvantages. The measurement of static compliance (C_{Lstat}) requires the use of specialised equipment, including a body box for plethysmography, and relies on the ability of the patient to completely relax their respiratory muscles and make no respiratory effort as the measurements are taken at zero flow to exclude airway resistance. This is, in practice, very difficult to achieve in spontaneously breathing, as opposed to paralysed and ventilated critically ill patients. Although modified techniques exist to measure C_{Lstat}, such as rapid airway occlusion, these are still limited in the clinical setting.[18] However, dynamic compliance (C_{Ldyn}) can be achieved easily in spontaneously breathing patients, although like C_{Lstat} measurements, it does require the insertion of a balloon catheter to measure P_{oes} and rests on the assumption that the respiratory muscles are inactive at the point of zero flow. The patient simply performs resting breathing through a pneumotachograph with an oesophageal balloon in situ. The integration of the flow from the pneumotachograph provides a value for V_T, and this is divided by the pressure change between end inspiration to end expiration (ΔP_{oes}). Values are averaged over 5 to 10 stable breaths. During inspiration, a proportion of the pressure produced by the respiratory muscles is to overcome surface tension and airways resistance, and thus C_{Ldyn} is measured in the relaxed expiratory phase. The main limitation of C_{Ldyn} is that it can be inaccurate in obstructive lung disease as there remains intrapulmonary airflow at the end of inspiration. Furthermore, those using the measurement should be aware that C_{Ldyn} is rate-dependent especially in patients with COPD.[19]

Positive end-expiratory pressure

Intrinsic positive end-expiratory pressure (PEEPi) occurs due to airflow limitation resulting from the narrowing of airways thus creating residual positive pressure in the alveolus (and so also the pleura) at the end of expiration. This results in an increase in the work of breathing by preventing a return to FRC and has a negative impact on ventilator triggering. Although it is not often measured in the HMV population and is more pertinent in acute ventilation in critical care, knowledge of the concept can enhance patient set-up for HMV. The presence of PEEPi can occur due to a range of processes including

- Insufficient expiratory time to allow pressure equalisation across lung units due to airway obstruction, e.g. COPD
- Dynamic airway collapse causing flow limitation, e.g. emphysema or obesity
- Pulmonary oedema resulting in airways oedema and airway obstruction, e.g. cardiac failure

Both static and dynamic PEEPi can be measured and requires the use of an oesophageal pressure catheter and a pneumotachograph, similar to the measurement of compliance. For the measurement of static PEEPi, airway occlusion is required at the end of passive expiration with complete relaxation of the respiratory muscles. The resultant plateau pressure represents the average PEEPi across the whole lung and may vary considerably between lung units in disease processes associated with profound heterogeneity, e.g. emphysema. Active expiration will cause a falsely high value, and patients should be coached to avoid this phenomenon.[20] Dynamic PEEPi can be measured in the spontaneously breathing patient without the need for airway occlusion. The ΔP_{oes} from the onset of respiratory effort to the point of inspiratory flow represents the lowest level of PEEPi within the lung that is required to be overcome in order to instigate flow. This can therefore be substantially lower than static PEEPi, most notably in those with airflow obstruction. If active expiration occurs, this can be partly compensated for by subtracting the ΔP_{ga} from the value of PEEPi calculated.[21] In the clinical setting, failure to correctly titrate expiratory positive airway pressure (EPAP) to a high-enough level to match the patient's intrinsic PEEP can lead to increased work of breathing, discomfort and triggering problems, especially in the acute setting. Equally, an EPAP set too high can worsen gas trapping and again lead to patient–ventilator asynchrony. PEEPi depends on underlying disease and, in general, it is usually absent in neuromuscular disease, but can be a significant problem in patients with both obstructive airways disease and obesity. Significant PEEP occurs in obese patients in the supine position due to the pressure exerted by the abdominal contents, and therefore, the position of the patient during measurements must be taken into consideration when interpreting measured PEEP values and setting EPAP.[22] It must also be noted that during HMV, EPAP is also used to abolish upper airway obstruction and maintain airway patency if there is coexistent obstructive sleep apnoea, which can be achieved with a manual titration technique or indeed using an automated ventilator with a specialised algorithm.[23]

Work of breathing

In the normal state, the respiratory system consumes a small proportion of the total oxygen consumption, typically less than 5%, but in illness this can rapidly escalate to more than 30% of the total. Although rarely measured in a clinical setting, unloading the respiratory muscles and reducing work of breathing have been shown to be associated with improved ventilator comfort and can be used to compare the effectiveness of modes of ventilation.[24] Again, measurements are taken during spontaneous breathing using a catheter to measure P_{oes} and a pneumotachograph with the integration ΔP_{oes} between points of zero flow generating the pressure–time product, which correlates with oxygen consumption and metabolic work of breathing.[25] This technique can show changes in work of breathing against changes in respiratory load, but with the addition of assisted ventilation, it can be difficult to interpret as the changes in P_{oes} represent, in part, the work performed by the ventilator rather than respiratory muscles.[24] To accurately measure changes in work of the respiratory muscles during ventilation, either change in oxygen consumption from spontaneous breathing to assisted breathing can be measured or the respiratory muscle activity can be measured using the EMG_{di}. These methods allow the physiological effects of modes of ventilation to be compared in detail as well as providing insights into the pathological processes involved in patients requiring HMV. Patients with high work of breathing during spontaneous respiration include those with COPD and obesity due to the high load on the respiratory system imposed by either airflow obstruction and hyperinflation or low chest wall and abdominal compliance.

RESPIRATORY MUSCLE TESTING

Respiratory muscle weakness can be a cause of unexplained breathlessness with classical symptoms of diaphragm paralysis including orthopnoea, breathlessness in water and breathlessness on exercise.[26,27] Although routine imaging techniques may raise the suspicion of diaphragm paralysis, the sensitivity and specificity of these tests are poor and should not be relied upon to make a diagnosis.[28] Profound respiratory muscle weakness initially leads to nocturnal hypoventilation prior to diurnal hypercapnia becoming established, and this may be used as an early detector of need for nocturnal ventilatory support in at-risk populations.[13,29] Tests of RMS are used in the diagnosis of unexplained hypercapnic respiratory failure, and abnormalities require further testing to ascertain whether there is a generalised systemic neuromuscular problem or whether it is isolated to the diaphragm. The latter can often be a consequence of neuralgic amyotrophy. Although either isolated unilateral or bilateral diaphragm weakness may produce sleep-disordered breathing, a further pathological process is usually required to cause respiratory failure necessitating treatment with NIV.[30,31]

Non-invasive tests

The change in vital capacity from sitting to supine is a simple test of RMS. However, other more specific tests, including SNIP and MIP, are available that better predict the presence of sleep-disordered breathing and need for NIV, particularly in patients with neuromuscular disorders.[32] Both these pressure measurements can be performed using handheld devices with a nasal bung or mouth piece, respectively. SNIP and MIP reflect overall RMS and are generally performed from FRC. Although the early literature reported that MIP testing should be performed from RV, more recent work has shown that it is reasonable to simplify the procedure by measuring peak pressure from FRC.[33,34] Previous work has shown good correlation between airway pressure and P_{oes} during sniff manoeuvres in patients without significant airway obstruction.[35] Due to a wide normal range of MIP values and technical difficulty some patients have with performing the procedure, particularly those with bulbar dysfunction, SNIP may provide a better method of excluding significant respiratory muscle weakness without the need for invasive testing.[36] However, it is also the case that MIP values may be higher than the SNIP,[37] and therefore multiple tests to assess RMS are required to exclude weakness in symptomatic patients.[38] Details on the test protocols can be found in the European Respiratory Society and American Thoracic Society statement on respiratory muscle testing.[33]

Expiration at rest is passive in upright humans; however, expiratory muscle function may be assessed non-invasively using maximum expiratory pressure (MEP) with pressure measured at the mouth in an analogous fashion to MIP during a forced expiration (from total lung capacity [TLC]) manoeuvre. It is important to prevent the subject from using buccal manoeuvres to increase the mouth pressure. As with MIPs, MEPs have a wide normal range, meaning low readings should be interpreted within a clinical evaluation. Cough peak expiratory flow (cough PEF) is another simple and commonly used test of expiratory muscle function.[39] This can be performed using a standard peak flow meter attached to a face mask and usually requires little or no coaching to produce acceptable technique. It must be appreciated that although this test reflects expiratory muscle strength at high lung volumes, the test is lung volume-dependent and also requires coordinated bulbar function to open and close the glottis rapidly during cough pressure generation and release. Therefore, values obtained will be reduced in patients with inspiratory muscle weakness due to inability to perform deep inspiration prior to cough initiation, and in those patients with bulbar dysfunction as well as those with true expiratory muscle weakness.[40] Patients with a cough PEF < 180 L/min have been shown to be unable to clear secretions independently.[39] These patients can augment cough response with manual physiotherapy and using insufflation–exsufflation devices,[41] and this augmented cough level is associated with improved prognosis independent of vital capacity or breathing pattern.

Table 20.3 Normal ranges for voluntary respiratory muscle manoeuvres

	Male	Female
$Sniff_{Pdi}$	148 (24)	122 (25)
$Sniff_{na}$	105 (24.5)	94 (21)
PI_{max} (FRC)	106 (22)	87 (21)
PI_{max} (RV)	114 (27)	88 (18)

Source: Miller JM et al. *Clin Sci (Lond).* 1985 Jul;69(1):91–6; Uldry C, Fitting J-W, *Thorax.* 1995;50:371–5.

Legend: $Sniff_{Pdi}$, transdiaphragmatic sniff pressure; $Sniff_{na}$, sniff nasal pressure; PI_{max}, maximum static inspiratory pressure; FRC, functional residual capacity; RV, residual volume. Units given as cmH_2O and are mean (SD).

The normal ranges for voluntary respiratory manoeuvres are provided in Table 20.3.[42]

Invasive tests

As both SNIP and MIP are volitional tests, a low value does not necessarily indicate inspiratory muscle weakness but could represent inadequate effort in performing the test. Therefore, if the non-invasive testing value is equivocal or a more accurate assessment is needed, invasive respiratory muscle testing can be performed. These require both a technically skilled operator as well as more specialised, but commercially available, equipment. For these reasons, these tests are usually performed in tertiary specialist units. They require measurement of P_{oes}, P_{ga} and EMG_{di}.

Voluntary manoeuvres are performed – maximal sniff efforts ($Sniff_{Poes}$ and $Sniff_{Pdi}$; Figure 20.4) and maximal cough effort ($Cough_{Pga}$). The pressures generated will, in part, be affected by lung volumes, and this should be taken into account when analysing the results. These tests produce a measure of global RMS, but to assess diaphragm function in isolation, phrenic nerve stimulation must be performed. Currently, this is performed using magnetic rather than electrical phrenic nerve stimulation as it is better tolerated and easier to perform.[43] The measurement of P_{di} following supramaximal phrenic nerve stimulation (twitch P_{di}; TwP_{di}) is the gold standard for demonstrating unilateral or bilateral diaphragm weakness; normal ranges for phrenic nerve stimulation are provided in Table 20.4.[44,45] Furthermore, diaphragm activation can be stimulated centrally via transcranial magnetic stimulation.[46–48] This allows accurate measurement of nerve conduction time, central and peripheral diaphragm fatigue, EMG_{di} latency and amplitude as either compound muscle action potential or motor evoked potential. These measurements are generally used as research tools, although these detailed assessments are required when evaluating patients for intramuscular diaphragmatic pacer insertion.[49]

The use of an oesophageal electrode to measure EMG_{di} during tidal breathing can be normalised to the maximum EMG_{di} produced during voluntary manoeuvres.[50] This can provide an index of NRD, which is the proportion of

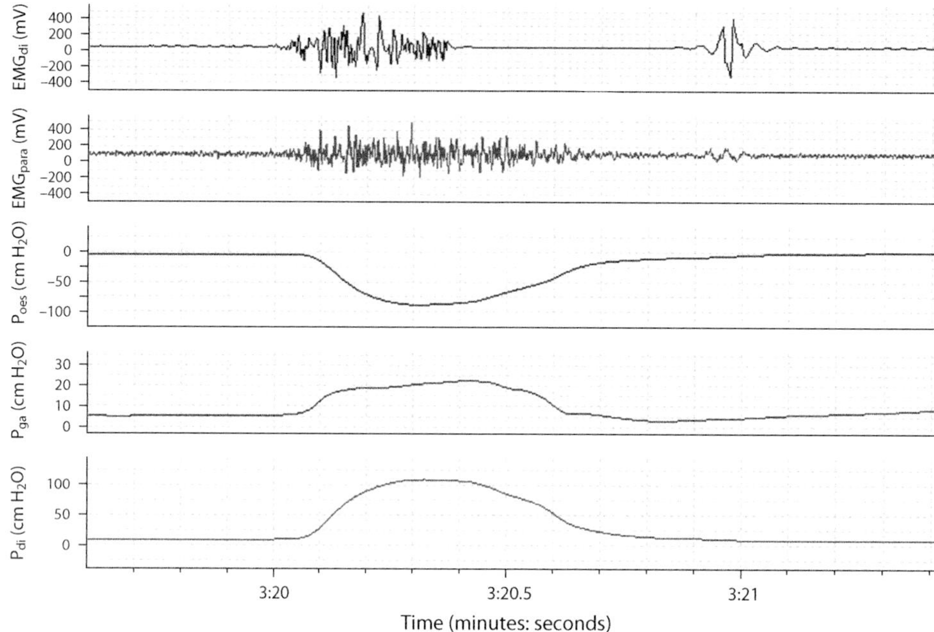

Figure 20.4 Trace showing a maximum sniff manoeuvre in a healthy volunteer with coordinated activity of diaphragm and parasternal muscles preceding respiratory system pressure changes. Figure shows diaphragm EMG (EMG_{di}), parasternal EMG (EMG_{para}), oesophageal pressure (P_{oes}), gastric pressure (P_{gas}) and transdiaphragmatic pressure (P_{di}). All pressure traces are shown in cmH_2O and EMG traces in mV after amplification (×1000).

maximum muscle activation required to perform tidal breathing. This provides insights into the physiological reserve in the respiratory system to cope with increased demand, e.g. during pulmonary infection; NRD can now be performed non-invasively using the electrical activity of the second intercostal space parasternal muscles, and may become a useful clinical tool in the future.[51] This technique may also have utility in the future for assessing patient–ventilator interaction by allowing investigation of unloading of the respiratory muscles and neuroventilator coupling (Figure 20.5); preliminary data suggest that patient–ventilator asynchrony is common in NIV users, although its significance remains unclear.[52] Respiratory drive can also be assessed using $P_{0.1}$, representing the pressure developed during the first 100 ms of inspiration as this is believed to be relatively free of voluntary control.[53] While initially thought to reflect respiratory motor output accurately and be unaffected by pulmonary mechanics

Table 20.4 Normal ranges for twPdi performed by magnetic stimulation

	Pressure
Bilateral TwP_{di}	31 (6)
Left TwP_{di}	16 (3)
Right TwP_{di}	12 (4)

Source: Hamnegard C-H et al., *Thorax*. 1996;51:1239–42; Mills GH et al., *Thorax*. 1995/11;50(11):1162–72.
Legend: TwP_{di}, twitch transdiaphragmatic pressure. Units given as cmH_2O and are mean (SD).

or respiratory pattern, it is now appreciated that it can be affected by altering the force–length relationship of the diaphragm, such as in lung hyperinflation.[54] It is therefore sometimes expressed using a ratio of the $P_{0.1}$ during tidal breathing to that produced during a maximum inspiratory manoeuvre ($P_{0.1}$:$P_{0.1\ max}$). The gradient of the P_{oes} curve during spontaneous breathing may serve a similar function.[55]

PATIENT–VENTILATOR INTERACTION

The principal areas that should be addressed during the consultation include

- *Interface* including mask leak, mouth leak, mask seal, head gear, mask and head gear age and skin pressure areas
- *Trigger efficiency* including inspiratory and expiratory synchronisation, frequency of auto-cycling, frequency of prolonged inspiratory support
- *Airway pressurization* including symptoms of excessive daytime hypersomnolence and morning headache, worsening breathlessness, continued snoring with symptoms and signs of cor pulmonale as well as excessive or inadequate pressure delivered

Sufficient time must be allowed during the initial HMV set-up to individualise the ventilator settings. Furthermore, regular follow-up must be undertaken to assess adherence to, and efficacy of, HMV, as a failure to improve and stabilise gas exchange and poor adherence may represent patient–ventilator

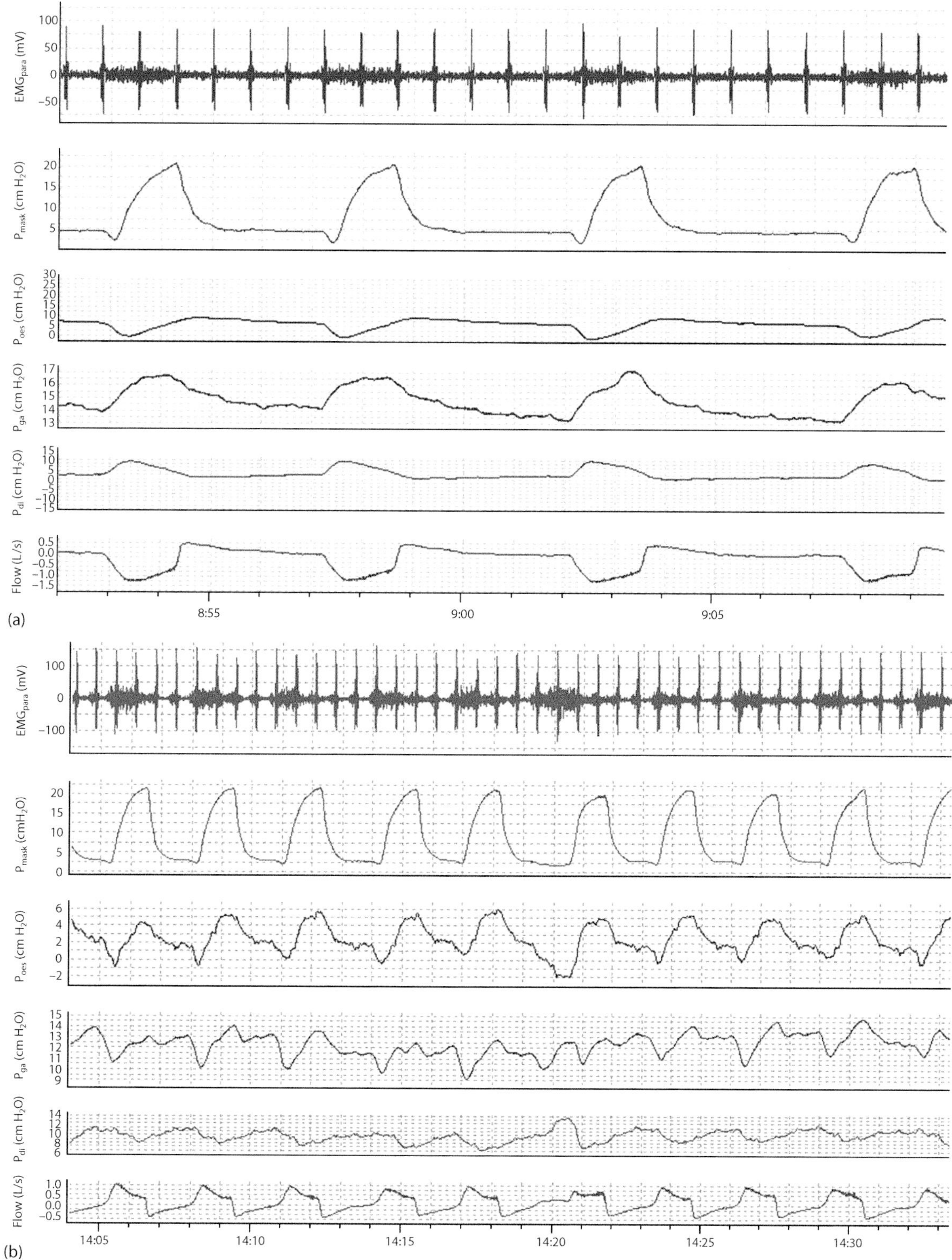

Figure 20.5 Section of physiological monitoring during a patient study examining patient–ventilator interaction showing parasternal EMG (EMG$_{para}$), mask pressure, oesophageal pressure, gastric pressure, transdiaphragmatic pressure and flow. The use of EMG$_{para}$ allows neuro-ventilator coupling to be investigated. **(a)** Figure shows a period of ventilation with pressure control ventilation and adequate trigger with inspiratory activity (indicated by EMG$_{para}$) resulting in ventilator activation and augmented ventilation. **(b)** Figure shows poor patient–ventilator interaction with inspiratory activity (indicated by EMG$_{para}$) failing to cause ventilator activation and resulting in wasted patient effort.

asynchrony, progression of the underlying disease or ventilator malfunction. The use of physiological targeted set-up has been reported by some investigators to improve patient comfort and enhances patient–ventilator interaction.[24,56] Although some patient–ventilator interactions can be assessed clinically, others require the use of more extensive testing to assess the problem (Figures 20.6 and 20.7). For a detailed report on monitoring patient–ventilator asynchrony and methods to manage the problems, see Chapters 12 and 24.

OVERNIGHT PHYSIOLOGICAL MONITORING

The investigations discussed so far in this chapter allow the physician to understand the interaction between respiratory muscle load, respiratory muscle capacity and NRD. However, this is directed to daytime measurements in the awake state for diagnosis of the clinical problem. The assessment of the respiratory physiological changes occurring during sleep that alter the load, capacity and drive relationship are required to assess for nocturnal ventilatory support. There are a range of home and hospital systems, from simple to advanced, and these are used to

- Diagnose sleep-disordered breathing
- Assess the severity of the problem
- Monitor efficacy of treatment

Oximetry

Overnight oximetry offers a simple, non-invasive and robust measure of nocturnal oxygenation and is a useful screening test in patients for the presence of sleep-disordered breathing. Due to its ease and low cost, it has been used extensively in obstructive sleep apnoea but is insufficiently sensitive to exclude a diagnosis in that condition.[57] The use of oximetry in the assessment of HMV can provide the clinician with valuable insights into the severity of disease and efficacy of treatment without requiring the patient to be admitted into the hospital for full physiological monitoring studies, and an experienced analyst can use these simple studies to diagnose a range of more complex sleep-disordered breathing (Figure 20.8). Computerised scoring systems provide automated analysis producing oxygen desaturation index, time spent with oxygen saturations <90% and heart rate variability allowing objective measures of sleep-disordered breathing. There is limited evidence available to set a standard lower level of nocturnal oxygenation, although clinical practice would aim for oxygen saturation levels greater than 88%. Although these devices have widespread availability, the user should appreciate their limitations. This is most noticeable when patients are receiving nocturnal oxygen therapy, resulting in a relatively normal oximetry trace as the hypoventilation and/or upper airways obstruction may result in minimal changes in oxygen saturations.

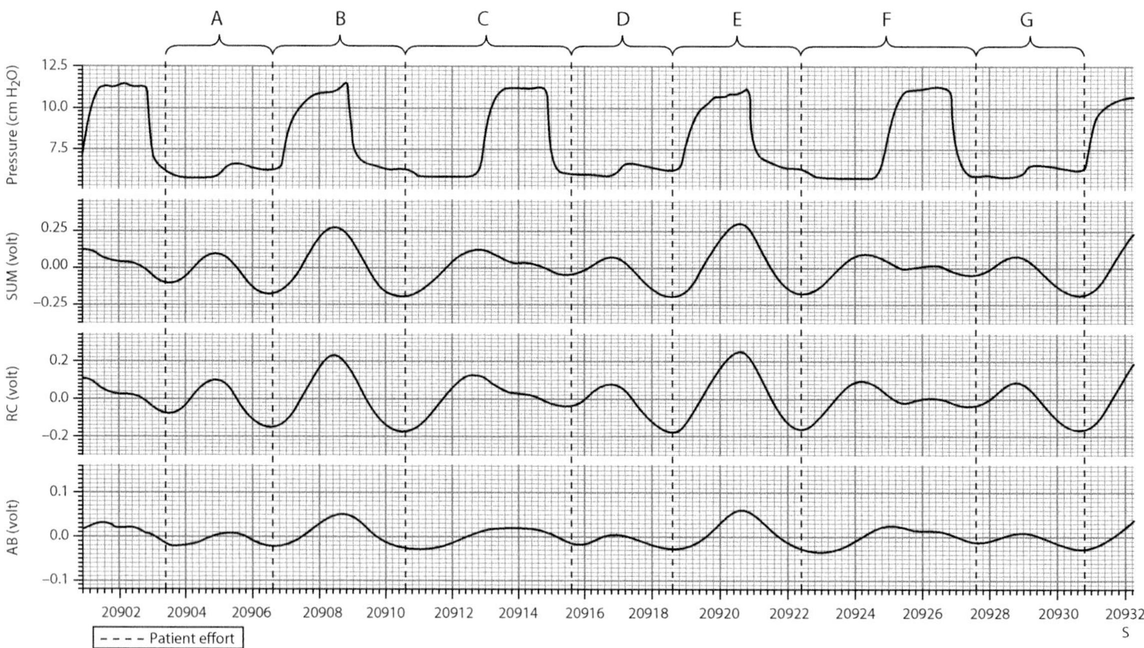

Figure 20.6 Section of respiratory monitoring on a patient initiating NIV showing, from the top trace, mask pressure, respiratory inductance plethysmography total (RIP sum), thoracic component (RIP RC) and abdominal component (RIP AB). The tracing shows poor synchronisation with ventilator pressurisation not responding to patient effort. Breaths B and E are synchronised with patient effort and ventilator pressurisation occurring together. Breaths A, E and G show patient effort without ventilator response with a small rise in mask pressure during expiration. Breaths C and F show respiratory effort unrewarded by pressure support with auto-cycling during expiration.

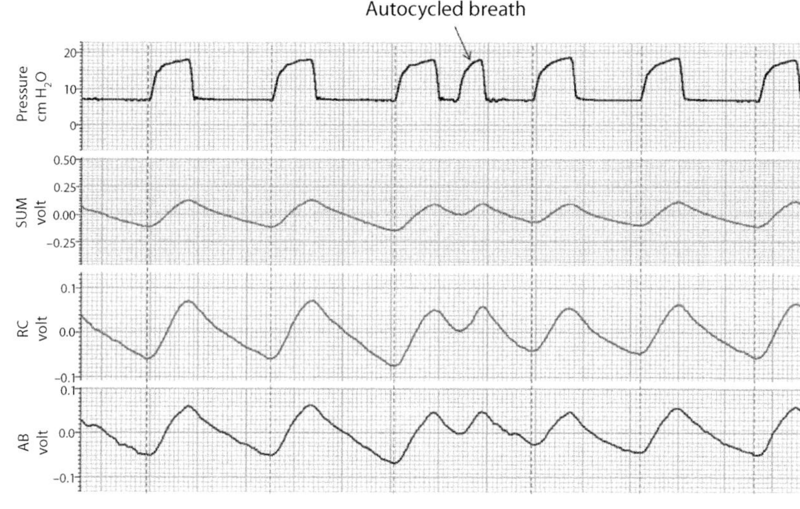

Figure 20.7 Section of respiratory monitoring on a patient initiating pressure control ventilation showing, from the top trace, mask pressure, respiratory inductance plethysmography total (RIP sum), thoracic component (RIP RC) and abdominal component (RIP AB). The trace shows an auto-cycled breath occurring during patient expiration.

Transcutaneous capnography

The hallmark of hypoventilation is an increase in $PaCO_2$. Previously, monitoring changes in CO_2 used either intermittent arterial sampling or end tidal monitoring; the former is invasive and the latter unreliable in obstructive airways disease and during HMV. The advent of robust and reliable transcutaneous CO_2 (T_cCO_2) monitoring has allowed for improved analysis of nocturnal breathing disorders. T_cCO_2 is measured electrochemically using a Severinghaus pH electrode to quantify the potentiometric difference between a reference and a measuring electrode. The resultant potential difference is proportional to the negative logarithm of $PaCO_2$. The technical constraints of the technique must be realised along with the appreciation that it is transcutaneous and not arterial values that are being measured. The measurements are taken using a heated electrode, allowing increased permeability of the skin to carbon dioxide facilitating measurement. The temperature settings will vary between systems but are usually in the order of 40°C–42°C. This elevation in temperature causes an increase in the local $PaCO_2$, and combined with the fact that the skin is a metabolically active tissue, consuming oxygen and producing carbon dioxide, further increases the recorded value. The commercially available systems correct for this with an automated algorithm that incorporates these factors and produces a value that should reflect $PaCO_2$. Clinical studies have shown T_cCO_2 to reflect $PaCO_2$ reliably and reproducibly in a range of clinical situations and conditions including critical care and acute NIV, as well as in sleep-disordered breathing and obesity.[58]

The introduction of combined pulse oximeter and T_cCO_2 sensors has further increased the usefulness of these devices simplifying the amount of monitoring equipment necessary to study respiratory disorders during sleep. The sensors need to be calibrated at the beginning and end of use to ensure accuracy.

Advanced sleep studies

Full polysomnography with electroencephalogram monitoring is rarely required in HMV management, although it can be useful if it is desired to elucidate the cause of persistent sleepiness despite therapy.[59] The use of limited respiratory polygraphy including transcutaneous carbon dioxide, nasal flow and respiratory inductance plethysmography (RIP) allows full assessment of patients prior to initiation and during follow-up. These modalities allow full assessment and the appropriate identification of complex sleep-disordered breathing, differentiating obstructive from central apnoeas, documenting hypoventilation as well as diagnosing periodic breathing abnormalities, such as Cheyne–Stokes respiration. Differentiation of obstructive from central events is made by the absence of respiratory effort in the latter, which is measured using RIP to measure abdominal and thoracic excursion (Figure 20.9). The technique is widely accepted, well tolerated by patients and easy to perform; however, it may overdiagnose central events.[60] Respiratory sleep studies can also be used in initial titration of HMV settings and diagnosing synchronisation issues between the patient and the ventilator.

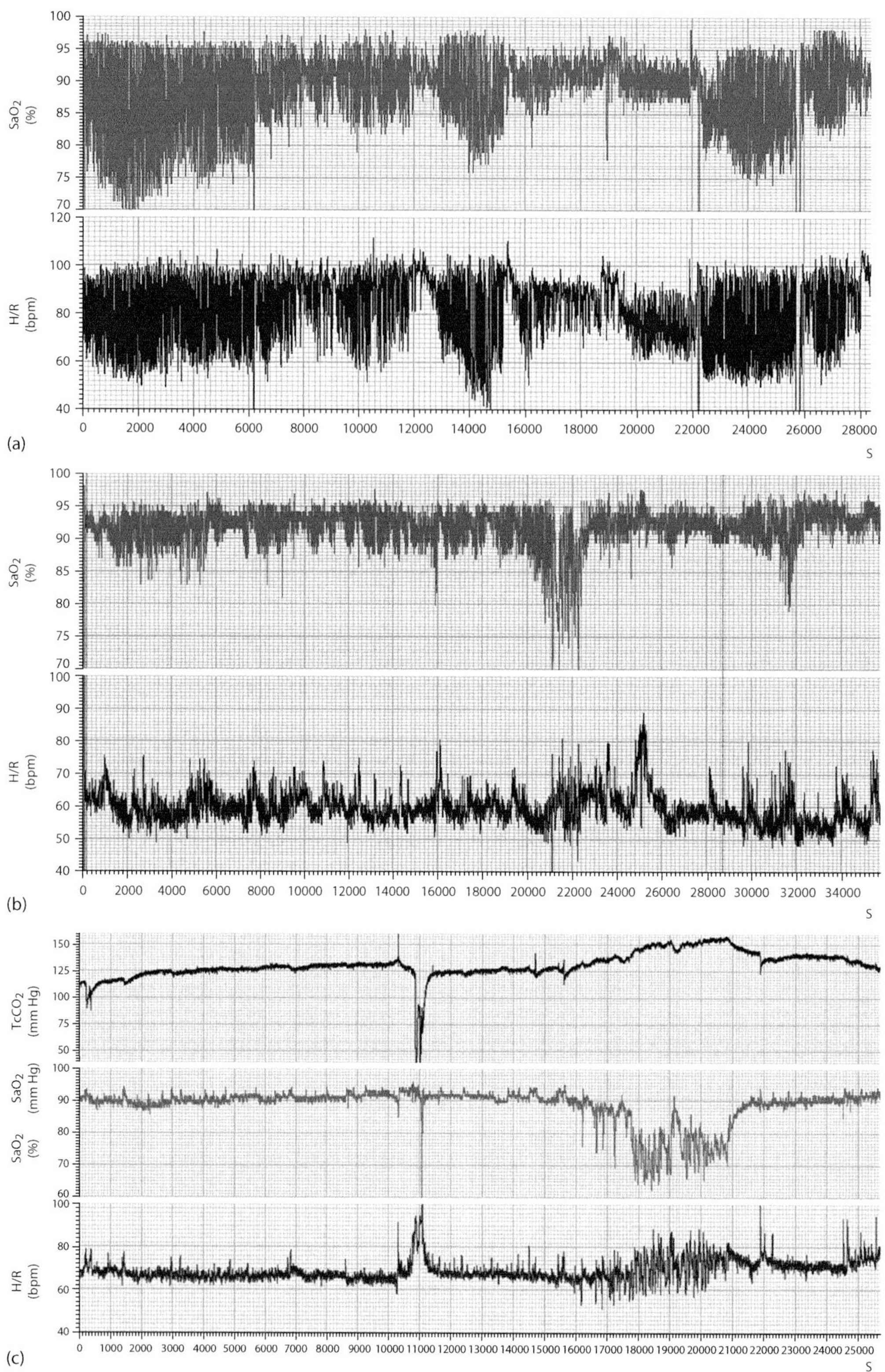

Figure 20.8 Examples of overnight oximetries (SpO_2 = red, heart rate = blue and T_cCO_2 = black) demonstrating patterns of common sleep-disordered breathing. **(a)** Oximetry tight repetitive desaturations with heart rate variability consistent with obstructive sleep apnoea. **(b)** This trace shows features of both hypoventilation and obstructive apnoeas with prolonged deep desaturations superimposed on rapid repetitive desaturations. Additionally there is transcutaneous CO_2 monitoring confirming hypoventilation. This pattern is classical of obesity hypoventilation syndrome with obstructive sleep apnoea. **(c)** Trace shows periods of sleep state or positional prolonged deep desaturation suggestive of hypoventilation.

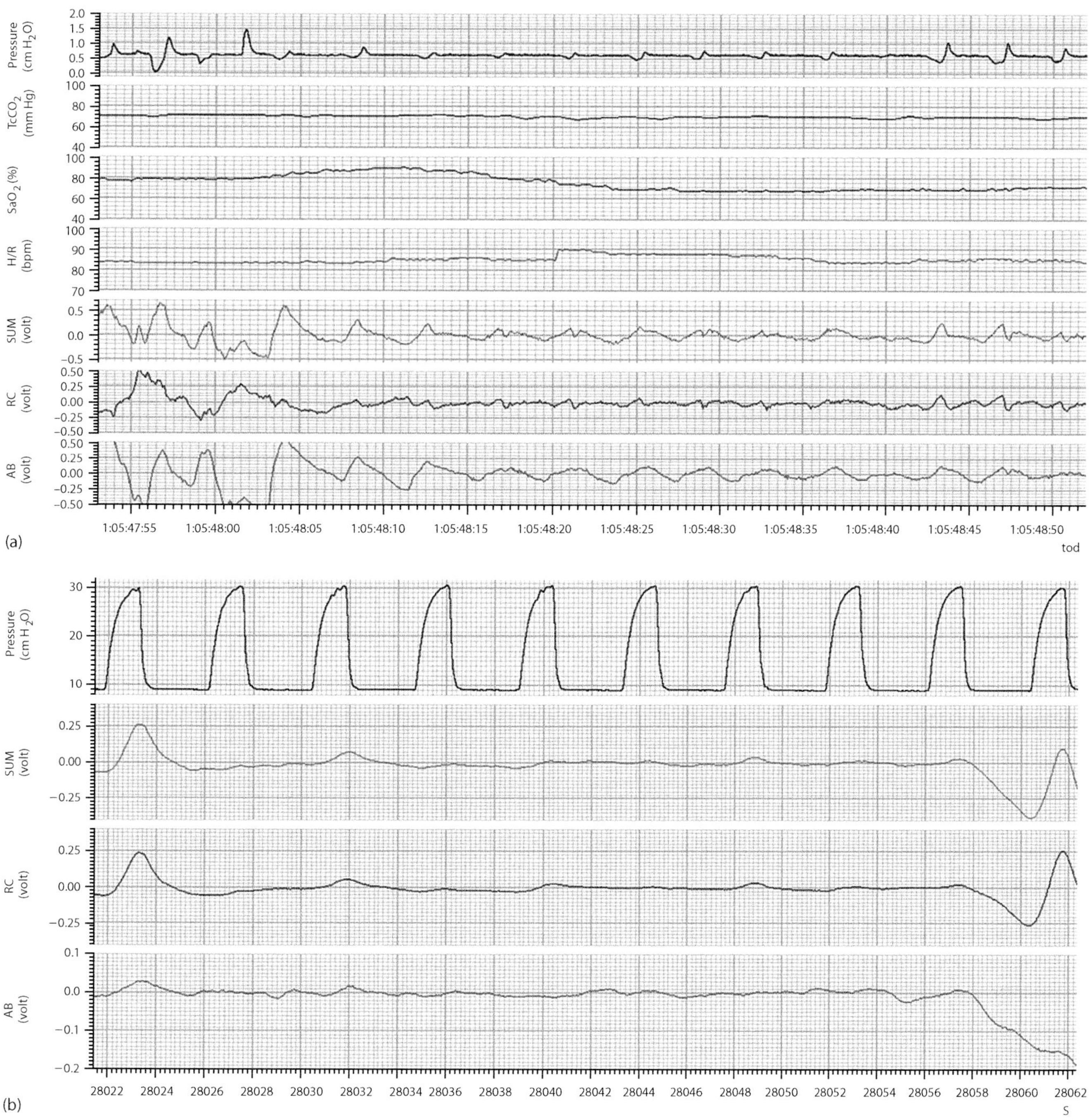

Figure 20.9 **(a)** Section of a diagnostic sleep study with recording of nasal pressure, transcutaneous CO_2, heart rate, oxygen saturations, RIP sum, RIP thorax and RIP abdomen. Shows obstructive hypopnea with chest wall paradox. **(b)** Section of respiratory sleep study on patient initiating ventilation for obesity hypoventilation syndrome. Shows central apnoea/hypopnea with absent/reduced respiratory effort and cycling of the ventilator at the back-up rate without respiratory movement suggesting upper airways obstruction preventing transmission of pressure.

CONCLUSION

The management of patients receiving HMV requires a detailed working knowledge of respiratory physiology and pathophysiology with a clear understanding of the relationship between respiratory muscle load, respiratory muscle capacity and NRD. In addition to the respiratory physiological changes that occur during sleep, the assessment of patients receiving HMV requires the clinician to have an integrated advanced knowledge of ventilator technology and the issues that are common to specific underlying disease processes. In order to achieve this, a coordinated team approach involving physicians, physiological technicians and specialist nurses is required.

REFERENCES

1. Dar K, Williams T, Aitken R et al. Arterial versus capillary sampling for analysing blood gas pressures. *BMJ*. 1995 Jan 7;310(6971):24–5.
2. Sauty A, Uldry C, Debetaz LF et al. Differences in PO2 and PCO2 between arterial and arterialized earlobe samples. *Eur Respir J*. 1996 Feb;9(2):186–9.
3. Lightowler JV, Elliott MW. Local anaesthetic infiltration prior to arterial puncture for blood gas analysis: A survey of current practice and a randomised double blind placebo controlled trial. *J R Coll Phys Lond*. 1997 Nov–Dec;31(6):645–6.
4. Patout M, Lamia B, Lhuillier E et al. A randomized controlled trial on the effect of needle gauge on the pain and anxiety experienced during radial arterial puncture. *PLoS One*. 2015;10(9):e0139432.
5. Aarrestad S, Tollefsen E, Kleiven AL et al. Validity of transcutaneous PCO2 in monitoring chronic hypoventilation treated with non-invasive ventilation. *Respir Med*. 2016 Mar;112:112–8.
6. Nocturnal Oxygen Therapy Trial Group. Continuous or nocturnal oxygen therapy in hypoxaemic chronic obstructive lung disease. *Ann Intern Med*. 1980;93:391–8.
7. Sciurba FC, Rogers RM, Keenan RJ et al. Improvement in pulmonary function and elastic recoil after lung-reduction surgery for diffuse emphysema. *N Engl J Med*. 1996;334:1095–9.
8. Steier J, Lunt A, Hart N et al. Observational study of the effect of obesity on lung volumes. *Thorax*. 2014 Aug;69(8):752–9.
9. Baumann F, Henderson RD, Morrison SC et al. Use of respiratory function tests to predict survival in amyotrophic lateral sclerosis. *Amyotroph Lateral Scler*. 2010;11(1–2):194–202.
10. Mandal S, Suh ES, Boleat E et al. A cohort study to identify simple clinical tests for chronic respiratory failure in obese patients with sleep-disordered breathing. *BMJ Open Respir Res*. 2014;1(1):e000022.
11. Allen SM, Hunt B, Green M. Fall in vital capacity with posture. *Br J Dis Chest*. 1985;79:267–71.
12. Hart N, Cramer D, Ward SP et al. Effect of pattern and severity of respiratory muscle weakness on carbon monoxide gas transfer and lung volumes. *Eur Respir J*. 2002 Oct;20(4):996–1002.
13. Lyall RA, Donaldson N, Polkey MI et al. Respiratory muscle strength and ventilatory failure in amyotrophic lateral sclerosis. *Brain*. 2001;124(Pt 10):2000–13.
14. Mead J, McIlroy MB, Selverstone NJ, Kriete BC. Measurement of intraesophageal pressure. *J Appl Physiol*. 1955;7:491–5.
15. Luo YM, Moxham J, Polkey MI. Diaphragm electromyography using an oesophageal catheter: Current concepts. *Clin Sci (Lond)*. 2008 Oct;115(8):233–44.
16. Xiao SC, He BT, Steier J et al. Neural respiratory drive and arousal in patients with obstructive sleep apnea hypopnea. *Sleep*. 2015;38(6):941–9.
17. Parameswaran K, Todd DC, Soth M. Altered respiratory physiology in obesity. *Can Respir J*. 2006 May–Jun;13(4):203–10.
18. D'Angelo E, Robatto FM, Calderini E et al. Pulmonary and chest wall mechanics in anesthetized paralyzed humans. *J Appl Physiol*. 1991 Jun;70(6):2602–10.
19. Guerin C, Coussa ML, Eissa NT et al. Lung and chest wall mechanics in mechanically ventilated COPD patients. *J Appl Physiol*. 1993;74:1570–80.
20. Purro A, Appendini L, Patessio A et al. Static intrinsic PEEP in COPD patients during spontaneous breathing. *Am J Respir Crit Care Med*. 1998 Apr;157(4 Pt 1): 1044–50.
21. Appendini L, Patessio A, Zanaboni S et al. Physiologic effects of positive end-expiratory pressure and mask pressure support during exacerbations of chronic obstructive pulmonary disease. *Am J Respir Crit Care Med*. 1994;149:1069–76.
22. Steier J, Jolley CJ, Seymour J et al. Neural respiratory drive in obesity. *Thorax*. 2009 Aug;64(8):719–25.
23. Murphy PB, Arbane G, Ramsay M et al. Safety and efficacy of auto-titrating noninvasive ventilation in COPD and obstructive sleep apnoea overlap syndrome. *Eur Respir J*. 2015 Aug;46(2):548–51.
24. Fauroux B, Pigeot J, Polkey MI et al. In vivo physiologic comparison of two ventilators used for domiciliary ventilation in children with cystic fibrosis. *Crit Care Med*. 2001;29(11):2097–105.
25. Thomas AM, Turner RE, Tenholder MF. Esophageal pressure measurements in cardiopulmonary exercise testing. *Chest*. 1997 Sep;112(3):829–32.
26. Hart N, Nickol AH, Cramer D et al. Effect of severe isolated unilateral and bilateral diaphragm weakness on exercise performance. *Am J Respir Crit Care Med*. 2002 May 1;165(9):1265–70.
27. Schoenhofer B, Koehler D, Polkey MI. Influence of immersion in water on muscle function and breathing pattern in patients with severe diaphragm weakness. *Chest*. 2004 Jun;125(6):2069–74.
28. Chetta A, Rehman AK, Moxham J et al. Chest radiography cannot predict diaphragm function. *Respir Med*. 2005 Jan;99(1):39–44.
29. Ward S, Chatwin M, Heather S, Simonds AK. Randomised controlled trial of non-invasive ventilation (NIV) for nocturnal hypoventilation in neuromuscular and chest wall disease patients with daytime normocapnia. *Thorax*. 2005 Dec;60(12):1019–24.
30. Steier J, Jolley CJ, Seymour J et al. Sleep-disordered breathing in unilateral diaphragm paralysis or severe weakness. *Eur Respir J*. 2008 Dec;32(6):1479–87.
31. Bennett JR, Dunroy HM, Corfield DR et al. Respiratory muscle activity during REM sleep in patients with diaphragm paralysis. *Neurology*. 2004 Jan 13;62(1):134–7.

32. Hughes PD, Polkey MI, Kyroussis D et al. Measurement of sniff nasal and diaphragm twitch mouth pressure in patients. *Thorax*. 1998;53:96–100.
33. American Thoracic Society/European Respiratory S. ATS/ERS Statement on respiratory muscle testing. *Am J Respir Crit Care Med*. 2002 Aug 15;166(4):518–624.
34. Fanfulla F, Delmastro M, Berardinelli A et al. Effects of different ventilator settings on sleep and inspiratory effort in patients with neuromuscular disease. *Am J Respir Crit Care Med*. 2005 Sep 1;172(5):619–24.
35. Koulouris N, Vianna LG, Mulvey DA et al. Maximal relaxation rates of esophageal, nose, and mouth pressures during a sniff reflect inspiratory muscle fatigue. *Am Rev Respir Dis*. 1989;139(5):1213–7.
36. Miller JM, Moxham J, Green M. The maximal sniff in the assessment of diaphragm function in man. *Clin Scie (Lond)*. 1985 Jul;69(1):91–6.
37. Hart N, Polkey MI, Sharshar T et al. Limitations of sniff nasal pressure in patients with severe neuromuscular weakness. *J Neurol Neurosurg Psychiatr*. 2003 Dec;74(12):1685–7.
38. Steier J, Kaul S, Seymour J et al. The value of multiple tests of respiratory muscle strength. *Thorax*. 2007 Nov;62(11):975–80.
39. Bach JR, Saporito LR. Criteria for extubation and tracheostomy tube removal for patients with ventilatory failure. A different approach to weaning. *Chest*. 1996;110:1566–71.
40. Polkey MI, Lyall RA, Green M et al. Expiratory muscle function in amyotrophic lateral sclerosis. *Am J Respir Crit Care Med*. 1998;158:734–41.
41. Mustfa N, Aiello M, Lyall RA et al. Cough augmentation in amyotrophic lateral sclerosis. *Neurology*. 2003 Nov 11;61(9):1285–7.
42. Storre JH, Steurer B, Kabitz HJ et al. Transcutaneous PCO2 monitoring during initiation of noninvasive ventilation. *Chest*. 2007 Dec;132(6):1810–6.
43. Man WDC, Moxham J, Polkey MI. Magnetic stimulation for the measurement of respiratory and skeletal muscle function. *Eur Respir J*. 2004 Nov 1, 2004;24(5):846–60.
44. Meyer TJ, Pressman MR, Benditt J et al. Air leaking through the mouth during nocturnal nasal ventilation: Effect on sleep quality. *Sleep*. 1997;20:561–9.
45. Luo YM, Tang J, Steier J et al. Distinguishing obstructive from central sleep apnea events: Diaphragm electromyogram and esophageal pressure compared. *Chest*. 2008 Dec 31.
46. Murphy K, Mier A, Adams L, Guz A. Putative cerebral cortical involvement in the ventilatory response to inhaled CO2 in conscious man. *J Physiol*. 1990 Jan;420:1–18.
47. Sharshar T, Hopkinson NS, Jonville S et al. Demonstration of a second rapidly conducting cortico-diaphragmatic pathway in humans. *J Physiol*. 2004 Nov 1;560(Pt 3):897–908.
48. Similowski T, Straus C, Coic L, Derenne JP. Facilitation-independent response of the diaphragm to cortical magnetic stimulation. *Am J Respir Crit Care Med*. 1996;154:1771–7.
49. Similowski T, Straus C, Attali V et al. Assessment of the motor pathway to the diaphragm using cortical and cervical magnetic stimulation in the decision making process of phrenic pacing. *Chest*. 1996;110:1551–7.
50. Jolley CJ, Luo YM, Steier J et al. Neural respiratory drive in healthy subjects and in COPD. *Eur Respir J*. 2009 Feb;33(2):289–97.
51. Murphy PB, Kumar A, Reilly C et al. Neural respiratory drive as a physiological biomarker to monitor change during acute exacerbations of COPD. *Thorax*. 2011 May 19.
52. Ramsay M, Mandal S, Suh ES et al. Parasternal electromyography to determine the relationship between patient-ventilator asynchrony and nocturnal gas exchange during home mechanical ventilation set-up. *Thorax*. 2015 Oct;70(10):946–52.
53. Whitelaw WA, Derenne JP, Milic-Emili J. Occlusion pressure as a measure of respiratory center output in conscious man. *Respir Physiol*. 1975;23:181–99.
54. Polkey MI, Kyroussis D, Hamnegard CH et al. Diaphragm strength in chronic obstructive pulmonary disease. *Am J Respir Crit Care Med*. 1996 Nov;154(5):1310–7.
55. Hamnegard CH, Polkey MI, Kyroussis D et al. Maximum rate of change in oesophageal pressure assessed from unoccluded breaths: An option where mouth occlusion pressure is impractical. *Eur Respir J*. 1998 Sep;12(3):693–7.
56. Fanfulla F, Taurino AE, Lupo ND et al. Effect of sleep on patient/ventilator asynchrony in patients undergoing chronic non-invasive mechanical ventilation. *Respir Med*. 2007 Aug;101(8):1702–7.
57. Williams AJ, Yu G, Santiago S, Stein M. Screening for sleep apnea using pulse oximetry and a clinical score. *Chest*. 1991 Sep;100(3):631–5.
58. Maniscalco M, Zedda A, Faraone S et al. Evaluation of a transcutaneous carbon dioxide monitor in severe obesity. *Intensive Care Med*. 2008 Jul;34(7):1340–4.
59. Senn O, Clarenbach CF, Kaplan V et al. Monitoring carbon dioxide tension and arterial oxygen saturation by a single earlobe sensor in patients with critical illness or sleep apnea. *Chest*. 2005 Sep;128(3):1291–6.
60. Storre JH, Magnet FS, Dreher M, Windisch W. Transcutaneous monitoring as a replacement for arterial PCO(2) monitoring during nocturnal non-invasive ventilation. *Respir Med*. 2011 Jan;105(1):143–50.

21

Ultrasound

DANIEL A. LICHTENSTEIN

Lung function has always been assessed using physical examination,[1] radiography[2,3] or computed tomography (CT).[4] None of these tools is perfect, because of limited accuracies for some and dangers of irradiation or transportation, among others.[5–9] Since the advent of intensive care units (ICUs), the community succeeded to live with this dilemma, but today, after long and confidential debuts, critical ultrasound, centered on the lung, is now becoming routine in the critically ill. Although paradoxical for a discipline not supposed to exist,[10] lung ultrasound in the critically ill (LUCI) has however shown to be superior in almost all instances to bedside chest radiographs. Compared to CT, it shows usually slightly inferior results, but also slightly superior results. The use of LUCI in ventilated patients is therefore of prime importance.

A REMINDER OF THE TECHNICAL APPROACH TO LUCI

Here are the seven principles of LUCI. Basic points regard the equipments and the signs, which aim to decrease a lot of confusion in this 'young' domain.

1. *LUCI requires simple machines.* Laptop units are popular in our ICUs and emergency rooms today, and they are good machines. However, we still use for LUCI and whole-body critical ultrasound our 1992 technology (last update, 2008), for features which we do not find in new generations. Mainly, the size favours bedside use, with a 32-cm width (no matter the height, it is not a useful parameter in a hospital, provided the unit is on a cart with *wheels*). The 7-s start-on time makes the machine suitable for cardiac arrest, as well as iterative daily uses. Its 5-MHz, high-resolution microconvex probe allows a whole-body assessment, a critical detail, and is perfect for the lung, veins, and all structures from 0.6 to 17 cm. For cardiac arrest, this is of prime importance (see SESAME-protocol below). Its flat, easy-to-clean keyboard begins to inspire some manufacturers. A flat keyboard and the use of a single probe are, to our opinion, the best warrant for efficient cleaning, that is, minimal *asepsis*.

   Its simple technology uses three useful buttons, has an instant response image, and mainly respects the lung artefacts (often destroyed by modern filters). Its intelligent cart is narrow and prevents any drop. Last, the resolution is fully suitable (see figures). Its low cost allows one to consider that ICUs already equipped with sophisticated units for echocardiographic assessment should have, besides, this simple equipment for hundred daily tasks (including simple cardiac assessments).

   Note that modern machines can be used; they just make LUCI more difficult and require more skill, more time and more costs mainly.
2. *The earth–sky axis must be respected.* The disorders are located according to the gravity rules.
3. *The lung is the most voluminous organ.* Where to apply the probe may be a challenge, but standardised points of analysis were defined, the BLUE-points[11] (Figure 21.1). We prefer longitudinal, rib short-axis scans which allow the detection of the bat sign, giving permanent location of the pleural line, regardless of whether the patient is dyspnoeic, bariatric, agitated, emphysematous and so on.
4. *The pleural line must be carefully detected.* In a longitudinal scan, two ribs are visible. The pleural line is located ½ cm below the rib line in adults. The pleural line and ribs generate the bat sign (Figure 21.2).
5. *Below the pleural line, artefacts are under special focus.* The space between the pleural line, the shadow of the ribs and the bottom of the screen has been called Merlin's space (Figure 21.2). The A-lines, equidistant repetitions of the pleural line, indicate gas (alveolar or dead) below the pleural line (Figure 21.2). Vascular probes are often not deep enough for exploiting this artefact.

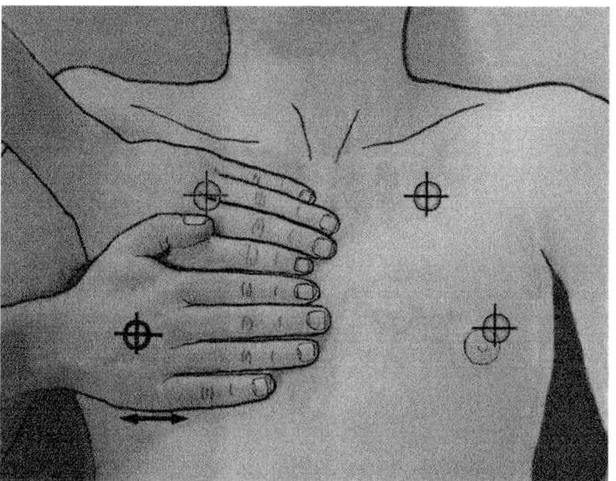

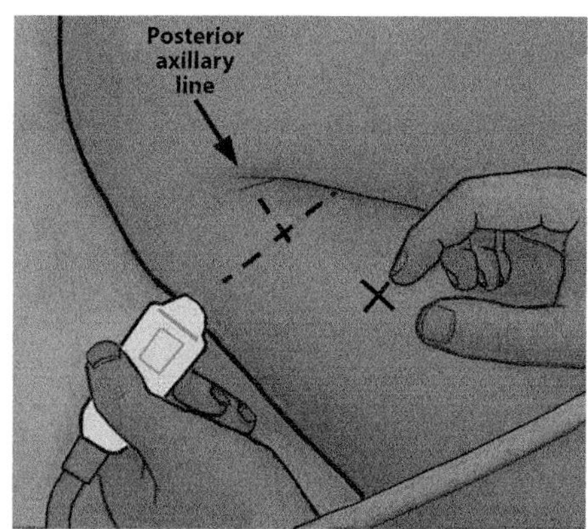

Figure 21.1 The BLUE-points. The standardised BLUE-points for performing a BLUE-protocol. Left: upper BLUE-point and lower BLUE-point. The hands are joined together, from the upper hand touching the podal border of the clavicle (hence oblique) to the lower hand, without thumbs for both, the lowest finger being therefore transversal. The tips of the hands touch the midline. The doctor's hand must be roughly the patient's size, unless adaptations are done (neonates, etc). The middle of the upper hand defines the upper BLUE-point, and the middle of the lower palm defines the lower BLUE-point. This definition has the advantage of avoiding the heart and making a roughly geometrical landmark of the lungs. The lower finger determines the lower limit of the lung (phrenic line). Right: the PLAPS-point is obtained by continuing laterally the lower BLUE-point up to the posterior axillar line, but ideally as far as possible near the rachis. The probe must be perpendicular to the chest wall, pointing to the sky as far as possible since the probe is jammed between the patient's back and the bed. One understands why a short (microconvex) probe is a critical advantage. Slightly turning the patient offers some degrees of vision. If the PLAPS-point shows no PLAPS, one or two podal extensions are done for detecting small or very small PLAPS, until the probe shows abdominal structures (liver, spleen). Anterior points inform mainly on pneumothorax and pulmonary oedema. PLAPS-point informs on most pleural or alveolar disorders. In the Pink-protocol, the examination is more comprehensive, is not limited to three points and includes the apex and others.

6. *Lung signatures are dynamic.* Lung sliding is the main dynamic sign. Associated with A-lines, it defines a normal lung surface[12] (Figure 21.2).
7. *Almost all life-threatening disorders reach the chest wall and are usually extensive.* This allows the elaboration of fast protocols.

A REMINDER OF THE SIGNS (WITH UPDATES)

Lung sliding in the critically ill

We define lung sliding as a twinkling of the whole of Merlin's space, that is, beginning at the very pleural line and spreading homogeneously below (generating the seashore sign in M-mode).

Easy to detect in healthy subjects, lung sliding can be difficult in the critically ill. In very dyspnoeic patients, muscular contractions contaminate the dynamic above the pleural line (the hectic variant of lung sliding); this requires experience or the simple use of the M-mode. In much sedated patients, lung sliding can be subtle (the quiet variant); here, again, M-mode can help.

Pleural effusions

They generate one constant sign, regardless of echogenicity (from anechoic to echoic) and volume: the quad sign, indicating this quad between the pleural line, shadow of ribs and a regular line roughly parallel to the pleural line: the lung line, indicating the visceral pleura (Figure 21.3). Another sign is dynamic in free cases, the sinusoid sign, indicating that the lung line moves toward the pleural line: this means that a fine needle is suitable for withdrawing fluid.[13]

Lung consolidations

The nontranslobar cases generate a structural image from he pleural line with a shredded deep border (the fractal sign), with air artefacts below (Figure 21.3). In translobar cases, this sign disappears, and the lung looks like an anatomical lung (the lung sign). It is useless to specify that a consolidation is 'subpleural', since all visible consolidations are subpleural. The air bronchograms, dynamic or static, are not needed for the definition of lung consolidation.[14]

PLAPS

Considering together posterolateral alveolar and/or pleural syndromes (PLAPS) allows one to deeply simplify the BLUE-protocol, since the distinction between both disorders does not change its accuracy (Figure 21.3).

Interstitial syndrome

Its definition still generates confusions in the literature. Our definition avoids most confusions.[15] Interstitial

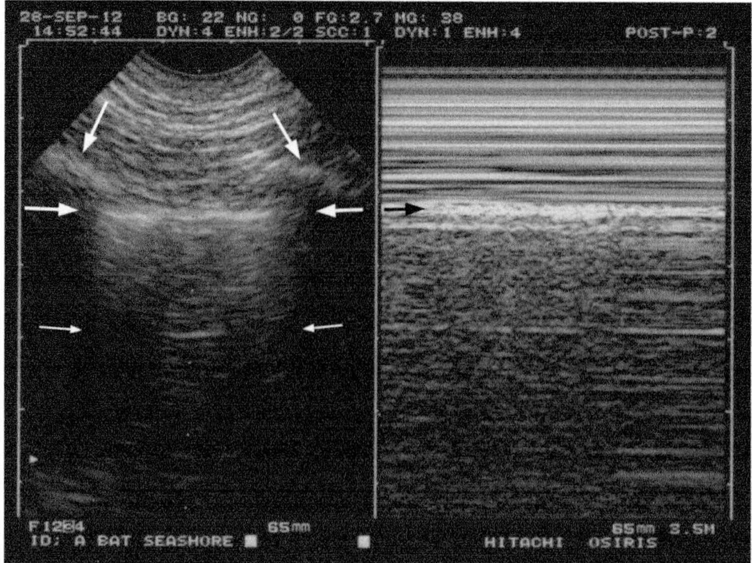

Figure 21.2 Normal lung surface. Left (real time): longitudinal scan of an intercostal space. Ribs (oblique arrows) cast frank acoustic shadows. The pleural line, a horizontal hyperechoic line, is located (upper horizontal arrows) between two ribs, 1/2 cm lower in the adult. The pleural line always indicates the parietal pleura. The upper rib, pleural line and lower rib outline the *bat sign*, a useful landmark. The space located between the pleural line, shadow of ribs and lower limit of screen has been called *Merlin's space*. Inside Merlin's space, the pleural line is repeated at the skin–pleural line distance, here discreetly; this repetition generates the *A-line* (lower horizontal arrow). A-lines indicate gas: pure air (pneumothorax) or quasi-pure air (normal lung surface). In the newborn, the same bat sign is visible. Right (M-mode): it makes the *seashore sign* appear (sandy pattern below the pleural line, wave pattern above), which indicates *lung sliding* on this frozen image (arrow, pleural line). Lung sliding indicates the presence of the lung against the wall (no pneumothorax) and correct lung expansion (no obstructive atelectasis). The reader can see here a rare pattern nowadays: both images are exactly aligned, making the detection of the pleural line easy on M-mode, even in stressful conditions. Left and right: at the anterior wall in supine patients, the combination of A-lines with lung sliding defines the *A-profile.*

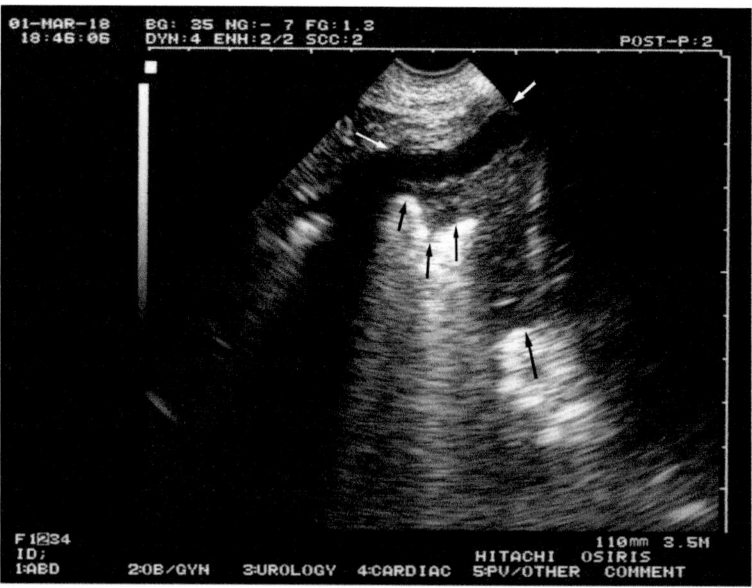

Figure 21.3 PLAPS. Small but typical PLAPS. At the PLAPS-point (more precisely at the second podal extension), from the pleural line (horizontal white arrows), a 6-mm echoic pleural effusion is described, with a regular lung line (and a sinusoid sign, not visible in a frozen real-time image). Then, a roughly 1 to 4-cm nontranslobar lower lobe consolidation follows, with the fractal sign shown by the vertical arrows arising from different parts, making a shredded line. Below the fractal line, air artefacts from aerated lung are visible (here called sub-B-lines). This PLAPS is just above the diaphragm, well seen here, i.e., is seen below the theoretical PLAPS-point, which indicates if needed a small PLAPS (larger mensurations indicate larger disorders).

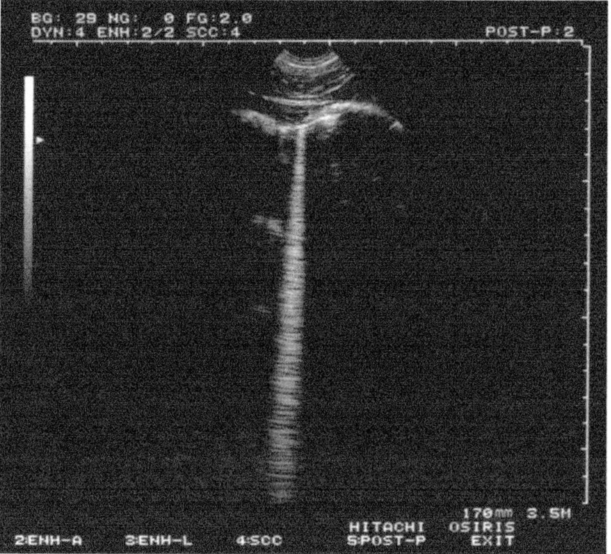

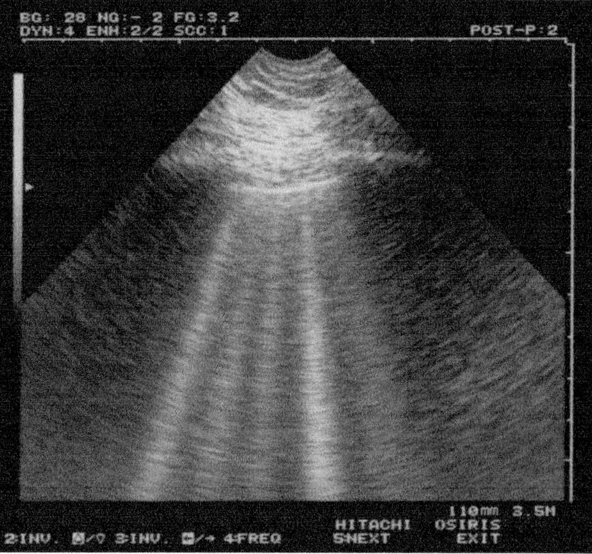

Figure 21.4 Lung rockets. The B-line is generated by a kind of chain reaction resulting from a 1% fluid mingling in an air medium. Left: We take the opportunity of one isolated B-line (labelled b-line) for reminding its main peculiarities. Three are constant. This is, always, a comet-tail artefact. It arises, always, from the pleural line. It always follows lung sliding (when there is lung sliding). Four criteria are quite constant (95% roughly). The B-line is long and does not fade. The B-line is well defined and laser-like (here narrow, but it can be broader). The B-line obliterates the A-lines. The B-line is hyper-echoic, as echoic as the pleural line. Normal subject, right lower BLUE-point likely indicating the horizontal fissure. Right: Four or five B-lines are seen here between two ribs. More than two B-lines visible between two ribs are labelled 'lung rockets'. Lung rockets indicate interstitial syndrome. Patient with acute haemodynamic pulmonary oedema.

syndrome is defined by a given concentration of B-lines. B-lines are a certain kind of comet-tail artefacts. The B-line has seven criteria, of which three are constant: comet-tail artefact, arising from the pleural line and moving in concert with lung sliding. Four are *quite* constant: long, well defined, erasing A-lines and hyperechoic. This definition is universal (works all the time). Lung rockets are defined by *more than two* B-lines between two ribs. Lung rockets define interstitial syndrome (Figure 21.4).

Pneumothorax

It generates other confusions. Our definition includes two *sequential* signs.[15] The first sign is the A′-profile (Figure 21.5). This profile combines, anteriorly in a supine patient, abolished lung sliding with exclusive A-lines. This profile combines in the M-mode the stratosphere sign in quiet ventilation and the Avicenne sign in hectic dyspnoea. The Keyes sign is a label indicating that parasite movements are seen superficial to the pleural line, because of muscular recruitment. This makes the assessment of lung sliding more difficult; in this case, the analysis of the M-mode is of prime importance. The A′-profile is constant in pneumothorax. The second sign should be sought for *only* when an A′-profile has been detected: the lung point (Figure 21.6). This is a fleeting visualisation of thoracic activity replacing an A′-profile at a given point, probe motionless; this sign is specific.[16] It also indicates the volume of the pneumothorax (anterior, it is usually radioccult; lateral, it is moderate; at the PLAPS-point or more posteriorly, it is substantial; not found, massive, or not a pneumothorax).

LUCI IN THE EMERGENCY ROOM: THE BLUE-PROTOCOL

The BLUE-protocol provides in a few minutes the diagnoses of the six most frequent causes of acute respiratory failure: pneumonia, haemodynamic pulmonary oedema, pulmonary embolism, asthma, exacerbated chronic obstructive pulmonary disease (COPD) and pneumothorax.[17] The hectic variant of lung sliding is usually present. Schematically, the anterior association of lung sliding with lung rockets (the B-profile, see Question 4) favours the diagnosis of haemodynamic pulmonary oedema. The anterior association of lung sliding with A-lines is seen in most cases of massive pulmonary embolism (and is also the usual profile in severe asthma or exacerbated COPD). The association of this A-profile with deep vein thrombosis (DVT) is 99% specific to pulmonary embolism.[17] Lung sliding abolished with lung rockets (B′-profile) favours the diagnosis of pneumonia, as well as the C-profile (anterior consolidation), the A/B-profile (unilateral anterior lung rockets), and the A-V-PLAPS-profile: A-profile, no DVT, and PLAPS.

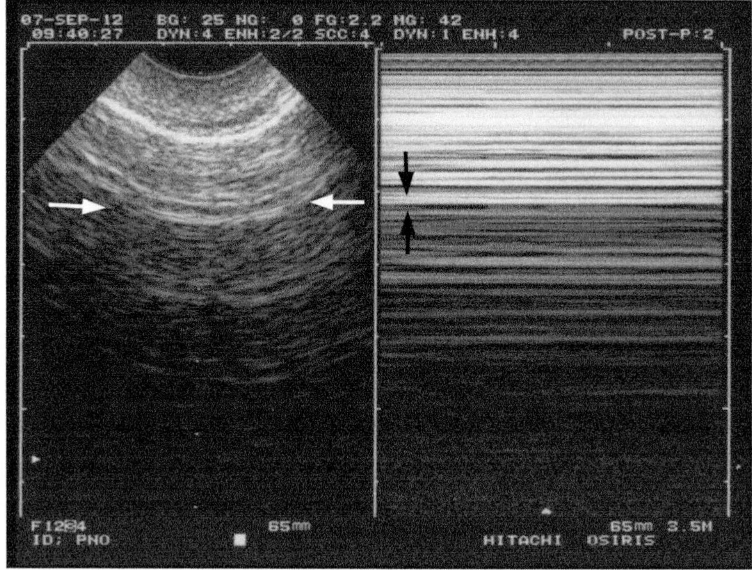

Figure 21.5 Pneumothorax and the A′-profile. Left (real time): below the pleural line (arrows), one can see an A-line (between the pleural line and the A-line is another horizontal line, called sub-A-line). Right (M-mode): even without video, one can perfectly see the abolition of lung sliding. Unlike Figure 21.2, the pattern below the pleural line (arrows) and above it is strictly the same: stratified pattern labelled the stratosphere sign. This combination of A-lines (left image) and abolished lung sliding (right image) at the anterior chest wall has been labelled the A′-profile. The A′-profile is highly suggestive of pneumothorax.

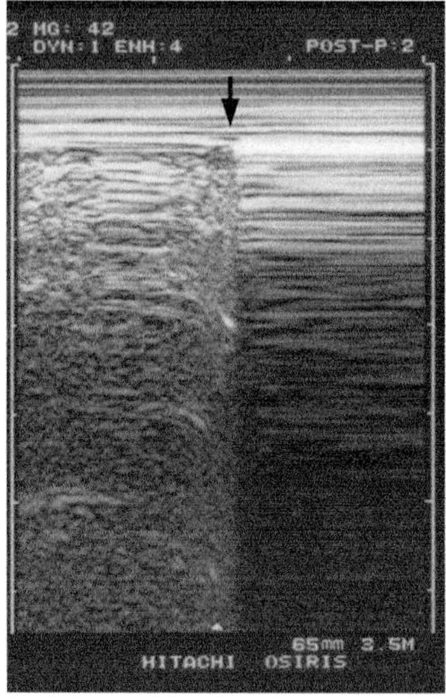

Figure 21.6 Pneumothorax and lung point. On this M-mode image, an ON/OFF pattern can be seen, in rhythm with breathing: the seashore sign of lung sliding is suddenly replaced by a stratospheric pattern. Or reversely an A′-profile is suddenly replaced by any other pattern. This pattern, seen at the very location where the lung, inflated by inspiration, slightly increases its contact with the chest wall, is specific to pneumothorax. Modern filters are not welcome for recording this subtle change. Found laterally in a patient with exacerbated COPD, this case indicated a moderate volume, here with the need for drainage.

THE USE OF LUCI IN THE VENTILATED PATIENT WITH ARDS: THE PINK-PROTOCOL

Acute respiratory distress syndrome (ARDS) patients are not dyspnoeic, they are not blue, but they have no more lung function. For them, the 'Pink-protocol' has been created. It is based on the fact that the profiles of the BLUE-protocol can be used in ventilated patients (with here the quiet variant of lung sliding). The Pink-protocol can be used at various steps.

On admission: the diagnosis. Roughly, the four profiles of pneumonia are found with no difference in ARDS (the B-profile is seen on occasion). Withdrawing pleural fluid for analysis before any antibiotherapy is an opportunity.

On the first few days: LUCI helps for bedside quantitative data of all disorders (read figure captions). This includes the volume of pleural effusion,[18,19] lung consolidations[20] and pneumothorax.[21–23] Relieving the patient from pleural effusions is a simple and safe procedure, provided basic criteria are followed.[13,24–28] Here, pneumothorax can be complex and septated, because of frequent adhesions. In these cases, the lung point cannot be seen: traditional imaging (radiography or CT) is sometimes useful. Some authors use PEEP (positive end-expiratory pressure) for assessing alveolar recruitment. For those who follow this policy, we advise the use of a simple ruler, showing the decrease of volume of lung consolidation in the case of successful recruitment.[29A]

During the first weeks: the patient can have many troubles, most pertaining to ultrasound: DVT (plus pulmonary embolism), maxillary sinusitis, gastrointestinal tract disorders, hypovolaemia or hypervolaemia. Ventilator-acquired pneumonia and atelectases are classical issues. Typically and apart from clinical and biological signs, pneumonia generates in 60% of cases a specific sign, the dynamic air bronchogram, not seen in obstructive atelectasis.[30] Infectious consolidations do not decrease the lung volume, as opposed to atelectases (with signs of attraction of cupola, heart, ribs, etc.).

When the patient has survived from ARDS, this is time for weaning. The diaphragm is a popular target today,[31,32] although one can use instead lung sliding, or even liver or spleen motion, to assess its function. A paradoxical phrenic movement is not a big deal to diagnose. We consider as important to check for all these radioccult troubles: pleural effusion, pneumothorax, interstitial syndrome from any cause (haemodynamic oedema, inflammatory oedema), pneumonia, atelectasis and possibly occult pulmonary embolism. All these causes can delay spontaneous breathing trials. Diagnosing weaning induced pulmonary oedema during weaning is one simple application among so many.[33]

BRIEFLY, OTHER POTENTIALS OF LUCI

FALLS-protocol

It uses the potential of LUCI to promptly detect a direct parameter of volaemic: the saturation of the interstitial compartment (interstitial oedema). It occurs at an infra-clinical, infra-radiological, infra-biological step, before the alveolar oedema. This potential allows a diagnosis in a specific sequence: FALLS-protocol begins by ruling out obstructive shock (pericardial tamponade, right ventricle enlargement, pneumothorax) and then left cardiogenic shock (B-profile). Then, fluid is administrated, a regular tendency since the remaining diagnoses are hypovolaemic and distributive (i.e. usually septic) shock. The FALLS-protocol analyses here the lung artefacts as an endpoint for fluid therapy: a hypovolaemic patient should recover once adequate fluid volume has been given, schematically, and an initial A-profile is not altered. In a distributive shock, the fluid therapy would not result in erasing the signs of shock, and fluid would eventually saturate the interstitial compartment, generating a transformation from A-lines to B-lines, *very schematically*.[15]

SESAME-protocol: Targeted whole-body ultrasound in cardiac arrest

This is a fast protocol used in cardiac arrest of unknown origin, for diagnosing reversible ones. It requires strict technical criteria, all present in the machine we have been using since 1992. Here are some of these criteria (see the first principle of LUCI): a really small lateral size, a 7-s start-up time, a universal probe and a simple knobology: *no button* is used during the first four of five steps. The setting is the natural image without filter, the best for the lung. The depth is settled by default at 85 mm in the adult, allowing the best compromise for the first four steps. The gain does not need to be touched. The machine is, by default, in 'SESAME-protocol' setting. Most protocols (BLUE, FALLS and all routine assessments) are done with this setting.[34]

The first step checks for pneumothorax. The second searches for a free DVT, at a specific location positive in half of the cases (on submission). The third step evaluates an abdominal fluid collection (can be extended to pleural and other spaces). The fourth step looks at, and only at, the pericardium. At the fifth step, the depth is increased to 140 mm, and the heart is now under analysis, windows permitting. The answers to many questions can be seen in Lichenstein (2016).[29B]

All these applications were already validated, so the SESAME-protocol does not require validation, it just asks the user to think different, to use machines optimising the speed, and work just fast – really fast. A single, universal probe is a mandatory requirement.

The LUCIFLR project (Lung Ultrasound in the Critically Ill Favouring Limitation [not *Eradication*] of Radiations)

The bedside radiograph is not very accurate. With a 60%–70% sensitivity, it appears as a suboptimal tool in critical care.[35,36] CT is better, but more dangerous (irradiation, transportation and delay are among the many drawbacks).[5–8] LUCI has quite similar accuracy in most cases.[13,14,23,37,38] LUCI is clearly superior for detecting the following: pleural septations,[29C] necrosis within a consolidation,[39] the dynamic of the lung using lung sliding,[38] the dynamic air bronchogram[30] and diaphragmatic function.[31,32] CT is unable to explore these items.

The LUCIFLR project aims at reducing 1/3 of urgent bedside radiographs and 2/3 of urgent CTs in the next three decades, a reasonable target.[29C] It is of major interest in children and pregnant women. Each time the clinical question is focused, for example, checking for the absence of a pneumothorax, and each time anterior lung sliding has been detected, pneumothorax is ruled out. From just this single example, one can imagine the number of spared x-rays and CTs.

All these applications are validated, so the LUCIFLR project does not require validation. Any physician using LUCI instead of irradiating imaging modalities (x-rays, CT) takes part in the LUCIFLR program.

FAT-protocol

LUCI can easily provide basic contribution at the anterior wall of these bariatric patients. The posterior wall is probably more difficult, but our equipment makes it easier (small microconvex probe), and the concept of PLAPS simplifies again: the detection of an image ill-defined but structural, that is, not an artefact, allows one to diagnose a PLAPS, with the same consequences as those described in the BLUE-protocol.[17]

ULTRASOUND IN THE VENTILATED PATIENT IS ALSO…

The title assigned to us was 'Ultrasound in the ventilated patient'. We assumed that it regarded the lung, yet the whole body benefits from this approach. We just evoke some of the countless potentials that our simple unit allows, from head to feet.

Heart. Echocardiography is usually a 'masterpiece' in the ICU, yet the rules of holistic ultrasound indicate that one can begin from a simple, basic approach, combined with LUCI, for answering precise clinical questions (see Question 5 below). Those who just want to know the 'cardiac function' per se should use traditional Doppler echocardiography.[40]

DVT. A DVT can be sought for at the legs (in any standstill patient) and at the sites of catheter insertions: the CLOT-protocol (catheter-linked occult thrombosis).[29D] We use a microconvex probe, more suitable for the whole venous network.

Venous cannulation can be done very simply using our microconvex probe: it allows all angulations and is really suitable for long-axis approaches, which is preferable but is not used because of the geometry of the so-called vascular probes. We cannulate the infra-clavicular subclavian vein.[41]

Maxillary sinusitis. Its detection is routine in the ventilated patient.[29E]

Abdomen. Ultrasound can show disorders that require urgent therapy (a huge field that cannot be developed in this volume).

VARIOUS CONSIDERATIONS AND LIMITATIONS

LUCI can affect the routine of many settings, briefly evoked here. It can be used in the critically ill neonate, where the signs are the same,[42,43] and in anesthesiology, emergency medicine, cardiology (lung data complement cardiac data) and others (simple pediatrics, nephrology, neurology, internal medicine, pulmonology, etc.). It can be used from sophisticated ICUs to out-of-hospital settings.[44] The SHUFLES (Simple Holistic Ultrasound for Low Economy Settings) program advocates simple equipments too. There is no required adaptation for these uses.

Note a peculiarity of LUCI: once the basics is mastered, this should be one of the less operator-dependent exercises of ultrasound. Today, the number of publications reproducing the signatures of LUCI is countless; we can cite very few of them.[45–59] For the lung (a superficial organ), the feasibility is >98%.[60] All this allows the proposal of a short and efficient training to lung ultrasound before other basic targets that need more time (e.g. heart).

We briefly define here holistic ultrasound. A discipline is holistic when it is necessary to understand each of its components for being able to understand the whole.[29F] LUCI makes critical ultrasound a holistic discipline. Adding the lung allows simplifying the heart (see Question 5 below), the equipment (Doppler and facilities become less necessary) and the probe (one probe for the whole body in our daily life).

The limitations are really limited. The subcutaneous emphysema is a hindrance in the most severe cases only. Large dressings can be limited by a smart policy. Let us always keep some place for humility: in exceptional cases, finding the standardised signs of LUCI may be challenging.

CONCLUSIONS

LUCI can be used in multiple disciplines and multiple conditions at any step of management of a critically ill patient. The case of the ventilated patient is a perfect application. We still advocate simple equipments for achieving the usual protocols of LUCI, as well as whole body critical ultrasound. We intentionally repeat that the simplicity of the used machine/probe is the best warrant for a short learning curve and the best efficiency. All in all, LUCI appears as a reasonable, bedside gold standard, using a visual approach to the critically ill patient.[61]

ACKNOWLEDGEMENTS

The author thanks François Jardin, who made everything possible.

COMMON CLINICAL QUESTIONS AND ANSWERS

When we lecture on LUCI, these questions are the most frequently asked:

1. *Is lung ultrasound easily learned?* Not that easy. Medicine is a profession for the elite. Within these elite, those who are willing to learn step by step will be able to understand and correctly apply lung ultrasound. Our work is to provide a standardized approach and standardized signs using a simple machine, in order not to add difficulties or confusion. Note that for defining the normal, only two signs are used, wherever the probe is applied, which makes lung ultrasound much more simple than echocardiography, abdominal ultrasound or foetal ultrasonography (the peak).
2. *Can I practice lung ultrasound with a standard laptop machine with a traditional probe?* Yes. These machines will generate an approach more difficult than ours.

This difficulty can be slight using certain equipments. When all issues are superadded, it can be substantial (large machine, long start-on time, filters, very large probe, etc.). We advise to bypass all filters, and we advise for those who do not have the universal probe the use of the abdominal probe, the less worst choice (then linear if needed).

3. *Is the comet-tail artefact the sign of haemodynamic pulmonary oedema?* Not at all. Only a certain kind of comet-tail artefact, the B-line, is the elementary sign. Then, B-lines must be multiple (more than two between two ribs), that is, lung rockets. Then, lung rockets must be associated with lung sliding. Then, this association must be diffuse at the anterior wall (supine, semi-recumbent patients). This defines the B-profile, 97% sensitive, 95% specific.
4. *In a patient with the B-profile, should I always treat a haemodynamic pulmonary oedema?* No. The BLUE-protocol is only a protocol and should not prevent the doctor to think. The doctor should pilot this protocol with clinical elements in mind in order to find the B-profile consistent with his or her own feeling. The B-profile comes (rarely) from an interstitial pneumonia (including ARDS); the physician should be alerted by clinical signs (as well as ultrasound signs, considered in the Extended BLUE-protocol[29G]). In exceptional instances, the physician will face a chronic interstitial disease in acutization (idiopathic pulmonary fibrosis [IPF], etc.). Given the history, the diagnosis can be very simple. In the first episode (of IPF), the E-BLUE-protocol will provide simple clues (including simple cardiac sonography).
5. *Why isn't the heart included in the decision tree of the BLUE-protocol?* A respiratory failure is a disease of the lung, coming from the lung, sometimes from the veins. This is why the BLUE-protocol considers the direct target. The heart is analysed once the BLUE-protocol is over. It is associated, not included, because the performances of the BLUE-protocol are usually high enough for not requiring urgent expert echocardiography. As simple examples, the B-profile is 95% specific to haemodynamic pulmonary oedema, and the A-profile plus DVT is 99% specific to pulmonary embolism. When cardiac windows are missing, when transesophageal echocardiography is contraindicated or not available, the BLUE-protocol provides precious pieces of information.

VIDEOS

Videos of profiles usually linked with diseases (the A-profile seen in pulmonary embolism among others); the B-profile (haemodynamic pulmonary oedema), the B′-profile of pneumonia, the C-profile of pneumonia, the A′-profile and the lung point of pneumothorax are freely accessible at www.CEURF.net, section BLUE-protocol, click on underlined words.

REFERENCES

1. Laënnec RTH. *Traité de l'auscultation médiate, ou traité du diagnostic des maladies des poumons et du cœur.* Paris: J.A. Brosson & J.S. Chaudé, 1819. New York: Hafner, 1962.
2. Roentgen WC. Ueber eine neue Art von Strahlen. Vorlaüfige Mittheilung, Sitzungsberichte der Wurzburger Physik-mediz Gesellschaft, December 28 1895:132–41.
3. Williams FH. A method for more fully determining the outline of the heart by means of the fluoroscope together with other uses of this instrument in medicine. *Boston Med Surg J.* 1896;135:335–7.
4. Hounsfield GN. Computerized transverse axial scanning. *Brit J Radiol.* 1973;46:1016–22.
5. Brenner DJ, Hall EJ. Computed tomography – An increasing source of radiation exposure. *New Engl J Med.* 2007;357(22):2277–84.
6. Berrington de Gonzales A, Darby S. Risk of cancer from diagnostic X-rays: Estimates for the UK and 14 other countries. *Lancet.* 2004;363(9406):345–51.
7. Lauer MS. Elements of danger – The case of medical imaging. *N Engl J Med.* 2009;361:841–3.
8. Scott MV, Fujii AM, Behrman RH, Dillon JE. Diagnostic ionizing radiation exposure in premature patients. *J Perinatol.* 2014;34:392–5.
9. Szem JW, Hydo LJ, Fischer E et al. High-risk intrahospital transport of critically ill patients: Safety and outcome of the necessary "road trip". *Crit Care Med.* 1995;23:1660–6.
10. Fuhlbrigge A, Choi A. Diagnostic procedures in respiratory disease. In *Harrison's Principles of Internal Medicine.* 18th Ed. New York: McGraw-Hill, 2012. p. 2098.
11. Lichtenstein D, Mezière G. The BLUE-points: Three standardized points used in the BLUE-protocol for ultrasound assessment of the lung in acute respiratory failure. *Crit Ultrasound J.* 2011;3:109–10.
12. Lichtenstein D, Mezière G, Biderman P, Gepner A. The comet-tail artifact, an ultrasound sign ruling out pneumothorax. *Intensive Care Med.* 1999;25:383–8.
13. Lichtenstein D, Hulot JS, Rabiller A et al. Feasibility and safety of ultrasound-aided thoracentesis in mechanically ventilated patients. *Intensive Care Med.* 1999;25:955–8.
14. Lichtenstein D, Lascols N, Mezière G, Gepner A. Ultrasound diagnosis of alveolar consolidation in the critically ill. *Intensive Care Med.* 2004;30:276–81.
15. Lichtenstein D. BLUE-protocol and FALLS-protocol, two applications of lung ultrasound in the critically ill (Recent advances in chest medicine). *Chest.* 2015;147:1659–70.
16. Lichtenstein D, Mezière G, Biderman P, Gepner A. The lung point: An ultrasound sign specific to pneumothorax. *Intensive Care Med.* 2000;26:1434–40.

17. Lichtenstein D, Mezière G. Relevance of lung ultrasound in the diagnosis of acute respiratory failure. The BLUE-protocol. *Chest.* 2008;134:117–25.
18. Vignon P, Chastagner C, Berkane V et al. Quantitative assessment of pleural effusion in critically ill patients by means of ultrasonography. *Crit Care Med.* 2005;33:1757–63.
19. Balik M, Plasil P, Waldauf P et al. Ultrasound estimation of volume of pleural fluid in mechanically ventilated patients. *Intensive Care Med.* 2006;32:318–21.
20. Bouhemad B, Brisson H, Le-Guen M et al. Bedside ultrasound assessment of positive end-expiratory pressure-induced lung recruitment. *Am J Respir Crit Care Med.* 2011;183:341–7.
21. Soldati G, Testa A, Silva FR et al. Chest ultrasonography in lung contusion. *Chest.* 2006;130(2):533–8.
22. Oveland NP, Lossius HM, Wemmelund K et al. Using thoracic ultrasonography to accurately assess pneumothorax progression during positive pressure ventilation. A comparison with CT scanning. *Chest.* 2013;43(2):415–22.
23. Lichtenstein D, Mezière G, Lascols N et al. Ultrasound diagnosis of occult pneumothorax. *Crit Care Med.* 2005;33:1231–8.
24. Talmor M, Hydo L, Gershenwald JG, Barie PS. Beneficial effects of chest tube drainage of pleural effusion in acute respiratory failure refractory to PEEP ventilation. *Surgery.* 1998;123:137–43.
25. Roch A, Bojan M, Michelet P et al. Usefulness of ultrasonography in predicting pleural effusion > 500 mL in patients receiving mechanical ventilation. *Chest.* 2005;127:224–32.
26. Depardieu F, Capellier G, Rontes O et al. Conséquence du drainage des épanchements liquidiens pleuraux chez les patients de réanimation ventilés. *Ann Fr Anesth Réanim.* 1997;16:785.
27. Ahmed SH, Ouzounian SP, Dirusso S et al. Hemodynamic and pulmonary changes after drainage of significant pleural effusions in critically ill, mechanically ventilated surgical patients. *J Trauma.* 2004;57:1184–8.
28. Nishida O, Arenallo R, Cheng DCH et al. Gas exchange and hemodynamics in experimental pleural effusion. *Crit Care Med.* 1999;27:583–7.
29. Lichtenstein D. *Lung Ultrasound in the Critically Ill.* Berlin: Springer, 2016. A, p. 206 (Pink-protocol). B, p. 261 (SESAME-protocol). C, p. 217 (LUCIFLR project). D, p. 209 (CLOT-protocol). E, p. 213 (Fever-protocol). F, p. 355 (Holistic ultrasound). G, p. 309 (Extended-BLUE-protocol).
30. Lichtenstein D, Mezière G, Seitz J. The dynamic air bronchogram. An ultrasound sign of alveolar consolidation ruling out atelectasis. *Chest.* 2009;135:1421–5.
31. Lerolle N, Guérot E, Dimassi S et al. Ultrasonographic diagnosis criterion for severe diaphragmatic dysfunction after cardiac surgery. *Chest.* 2009;135:401–7.
32. Matamis D, Soilemezi E, Tsagourias M et al. Sonographic evaluation of the diaphragm in critically ill patients. Technique and clinical applications. *Intensive Care Med.* 2013;39(5):801–10.
33. Ferré A, Guillot M, Teboul JL et al. Lung ultrasound enables the detection of weaning-induced pulmonary oedema. *Ann Intensive Care* 2016; 6(Suppl 1):50.
34. Lichtenstein D, Malbrain ML. Critical care ultrasound in cardiac arrest. Technological requirements for performing the SESAME-protocol – A holistic approach. *Anaesthesiol Intensive Ther.* 2015;47(5):471–81.
35. Hendrikse K, Gramata J, ten Hove W et al. Low value of routine chest radiographs in a mixed medical-surgical ICU. *Chest.* 2007;132:823–8.
36. Lichtenstein D, Goldstein I, Mourgeon E et al. Comparative diagnostic performances of auscultation, chest radiography and lung ultrasonography in ARDS. *Anesthesiology.* 2004;100:9–15.
37. Lichtenstein D, Mezière G, Biderman P et al. The comet-tail artifact, an ultrasound sign of alveolar-interstitial syndrome. *Am J Respir Crit Care Med.* 1997;156:1640–6.
38. Lichtenstein D, Menu Y. A bedside ultrasound sign ruling out pneumothorax in the critically ill: Lung sliding. *Chest.* 1995;108:1345–8.
39. Lichtenstein D, Peyrouset O. Lung ultrasound superior to CT? The example of a CT-occult necrotizing pneumonia. *Intensive Care Med.* 2006; 32:334–5.
40. Jardin F, Farcot JC, Boisante L et al. Influence of positive end-expiratory pressure on left ventricle performance. *New Engl J Med.* 1981;304(7):387–92.
41. Lichtenstein D, Saïfi R, Mezière G, Pipien I. Cathétérisme écho-guidé de la veine sous-clavière en réanimation. *Réan Urg.* 2000;9 Suppl 2:184s.
42. Lichtenstein D, Mauriat P. Lung ultrasound in the critically ill neonate. *Curr Pediatr Rev.* 2012;8(3):217–23.
43. Lichtenstein D. Ultrasound examination of the lungs in the intensive care unit. *Pediatr Crit Care Med.* 2009;10:693–8.
44. Lichtenstein D, Courret JP. Feasibility of ultrasound in the helicopter. *Intensive Care Med.* 1998;24:1119.
45. Reissig A, Kroegel C. Transthoracic sonography of diffuse parenchymal lung disease: The role of comet tail artifacts. *J Ultrasound Med.* 2003;22:173–80.
46. Kirkpatrick AW, Sirois M, Laupland KB et al. Hand-held thoracic sonography for detecting post-traumatic pneumothoraces: The Extended Focused Assessment with Sonography for Trauma (EFAST). *J Trauma.* 2004;57(2):288–95.

47. Mayo PH, Goltz HR, Tafreshi M, Doelken P. Safety of ultrasound-guided thoracentesis in patients receiving mechanical ventilation. *Chest.* 2004;125(3):1059–62.
48. Blaivas M, Lyon M, Duggal S. A prospective comparison of supine chest radiography and bedside ultrasound for the diagnosis of traumatic pneumothorax. *Acad Emerg Med.* 2005;12(9): 844–9.
49. Mathis G, Blank W, Reissig A et al. Thoracic ultrasound for diagnosing pulmonary embolism. A prospective multicenter study of 352 patients. *Chest.* 2005;128:1531–8.
50. Volpicelli G, Mussa A, Garofalo G et al. Bedside lung ultrasound in the assessment of alveolar-interstitial syndrome. *Am J Emerg Med.* 2006; 24:689–96.
51. Bouhemad B, Zhang M, Lu Q, Rouby JJ. Clinical review: Bedside lung ultrasound in critical care practice. *Crit Care.* 2007;11:205.
52. Fagenholz PJ, Gutman JA, Murray AF et al. Chest ultrasonography for the diagnosis and monitoring of high-altitude pulmonary edema. *Chest.* 2007;131:1013–8.
53. Soldati G, Testa A, Sher S et al. Occult traumatic pneumothorax: Diagnostic accuracy of lung ultrasonography in the emergency department. *Chest.* 2008;133:204–11.
54. Gargani L, Doveri M, d'Errico L et al. Ultrasound lung comets in systemic sclerosis: A chest sonography hallmark of pulmonary interstitial fibrosis. *Rheumatology.* 2009;48:1382–7.
55. Noble VE, Murray AF, Capp R et al. Ultrasound assessment for extravascular lung water in patients undergoing hemodialysis: Time course for resolution. *Chest.* 2009;135:1433–9.
56. Via G, Lichtenstein D, Mojoli F et al. Whole lung lavage: a unique model for ultrasound assessment of lung aeration changes. *Intensive Care Med.* 2010;36:999–1007.
57. Caiulo VA, Gargani L, Caiulo S et al. Lung ultrasound in bronchiolitis: Comparison with chest X-ray. *Eur J Pediatr.* 2011;170:1427–33.
58. Tsung JW, Kessler DP, Shah VP. Prospective application of clinician-performed lung ultrasonography during the 2009 H1N1 influenza A pandemic: Distinguishing viral from bacterial pneumonia. *Crit Ultrasound J.* 2012;4:16.
59. Xirouchaki N, Kondili E, Prinianakis G et al. Impact of lung ultrasound on clinical decision making in critically ill patients. *Intensive Care Med.* 2014;40:57–65.
60. Lichtenstein D, Biderman P, Chironi G et al. Faisabilité de l'échographie générale d'urgence en réanimation. *Réan Urg.* 1996;5(6):788 (SP 50).
61. van der Werf TS, Zijlstra JG. Ultrasound of the lung: Just imagine. *Intensive Care Med.* 2004;30:183–4.

22

Patient and caregiver education

OLE NORREGAARD

KEY MESSAGES

- Training of caregivers should be well structured, goal directed and competence based.
- Training should be sensitive to the individual ventilator user's and caregiver's specific and unique needs. The ventilator user's autonomy must be respected.
- It is recommended that the required knowledge and skills are presented as specific competencies, so it can be verified that the attendant has acquired the necessary qualifications, and if not where training should be reinforced.
- Attention should be paid also to the workload and working conditions of caregivers including also the mental and emotional stress the job can include.

Home mechanical ventilation (HMV) is an option for individuals with chronic respiratory insufficiency who cannot be weaned from respiratory assistance.[1] HMV has a long history dating back to the 1930s and was utilised in particular in the 1950s during the poliomyelitis epidemic. The major expansion, however, has taken place during the last two to three decades, especially in Western Europe and North America.[2–5]

The overall goal is to improve quality of life, to improve survival and to save money as the cost of HMV is considerably lower than that of an intensive care unit (ICU) stay. Data indicate that the cost of HMV is in the range of 20% to 50% of the cost of a stay at an ICU.[6] The cost associated with HMV is mainly related to the wages of caregivers, in some studies amounting to around two-thirds.[7]

The practice of HMV includes, among various issues, the balance between quality of life[8–10] and the level of risk.[11] Although data on adverse events are scarce and may be underreported, documented cases do exist.[12–15] To what extent the risks are due to poorly trained caregivers is not totally clear. However, a few studies[14,15] indicate that caregiver training may help reduce morbidity and mortality, and recent guidelines[16,17] emphasise the importance of caregiver education.

The attendants are obviously an integral part of HMV. Motivation and preparation of the ventilator user, family and caregivers are crucial for a successful transition to HMV.[18] Without attendants in some form, the practice of HMV would be generally impossible, at least for the most severely disabled patients, and the recent expansion in HMV would not have been possible.

Caregiving is managed in ways that vary a great deal from place to place. In some countries, the task is performed primarily by family members and relatives, while in others, it is handled by professional healthcare personnel or trained lay individuals.[19,20] Education of the ventilator-assisted individual (VAI) and their care team is crucial to the success of HMV.

LEGAL AND ETHICAL ISSUES

There is, to the author's knowledge, no legal framework to regulate HMV and caregivers' work, much less any common international regulation of the area.

In the absence/paucity of legal regulations, ethical standards may help guide the practice of HMV.

The Appleton Consensus[21] stated more than 20 years ago the four principles of ethics:

- Beneficence (do good)
- Non-maleficence (do not do bad)
- Autonomy (self-determination)
- Distributive justice

Patient autonomy has gained priority during the last few decades, to some extent at the cost of the other three principles.

This has, in some countries, resulted in the patient's right to choose or not to choose a specific treatment, and also to choose to terminate this treatment, even if this will result in the (immediate) death of the patient. Translated into the area of HMV, this means that a patient in some countries can ask for a termination of a life-sustaining ventilator treatment.

Little or no attention has been paid to the caregivers' rights. However, their rights and responsibilities should be an area of interest. In the absence of legal regulations, the caregiver may be left lost and unprotected, in some cases not even with a centre for HMV or a similar institution to rely on.

In some countries, the health authorities mandate the daily use of a logbook to assure the quality of treatment and to document (and safeguard) the activities of the caregivers, comparable to the compulsory use of hospital records when HMV users are hospitalised.

Funding varies tremendously, ranging from state-financed arrangements including attendants, equipment, modifications of the home and a vehicle as is the case in some of the Nordic countries, to scenarios where funding is very limited (in some parts of the world, nonexistent), and the financial burden is placed largely on the family, who may experience life as a struggle for economic support.

EDUCATION

Purpose

The overall purpose of HMV should be addressed, and it should be made clear to the VAI and to the attendants that an active self-directed life based on independence is a core issue in HMV. If that is not an option, for instance, because of an advanced malignant condition, amyotrophic lateral sclerosis (ALS)[22] or chronic obstructive pulmonary disease (COPD),[23] it should be made clear that palliation with HMV is the main goal of the treatment, so attendants do not develop a sense of guilt when the VAI deteriorates and ultimately dies.

It is important that acceptance of agreed upon goals is in place, as motivation is a critical element in the learning process, in addition to reinforcement and retention of knowledge and skills.[24] A structured learning process should be the aim, and it has been reported that formal training programmes for caregivers have led to an improvement in the caregivers' skills as well as in their satisfaction with the educational programme.[25] Evidence is in addition emerging that patient self-management is associated with improved patient satisfaction and outcome,[26] underlining the importance of involvement of the VAI. This involvement should preferably also include participation in training for HMV, to the extent that the VAI can participate.

Setting

Education of the VAI and attendants will usually take place in the hospital, preferably in a centre for HMV, or depending on how extensively the ventilator user is disabled, possibly in the patient's home or at some alternate outpatient setting.

A recent Dutch study[27] reported successful initiation of HMV in the home of a group of selected users. Initiation in the ventilator user's home was comparable to initiation in the hospital with respect to quality, but more than 3000 € cheaper per ventilator user.

Ideally, the educational process should start before admission to the hospital, by provision of detailed information, what can and cannot be expected of HMV through talks with hospital staff and, in the author's experience, also rewardingly with individuals already on HMV. This was confirmed in a group of patients suffering from ALS.[28] Education of ventilator users and their caregivers in advance of initiating HMV resulted in more accurate prediction of the ventilator users' later choice in real life, in decision assistance and in reduction of anxiety among patients compared to caregivers. This service should be facilitated by the hospital clinic. The experience is that the more realistic the expectations that the VAI has before starting HMV, the smoother the educational process and the discharge will be.

Education should initially, during a joint session with all involved parties present, clarify the responsibilities of each of these parties:

- The responsibility of the ventilator user can vary from being the employer who can direct, hire and fire their attendants, to an individual with very limited competencies and more or less total dependence on others.
- The responsibility of the caregiver would typically be to behave in a professional manner including respect for the ventilator user's autonomy, individual requirements and needs, and to practice the skills and attitudes acquired during the training programme – and in principle no further. It is advisable to make the limits of responsibility clear to the attendants as well as to the VAI.
- The responsibility of the hospital/HMV centre is to educate, to treat medical and technical problems, to achieve a safe discharge and subsequently to provide backup through, for instance, a 24-hour hotline and regular follow-up visits at the hospital and/or in the VAI's living site.

It is important that adequate time is allowed for the process to unfold. Depending on the local programme, usually 2–5 days is needed for the establishment of NIV, and 2–6 weeks for implementing complex invasive HMV. Ideally, a programme should be so organised that the process is continually moving forward to the benefit of the individual VAI and to optimise the use of all the available resources and of the facility, enabling it to maximise the number of VAIs it can accommodate.

Methodology

The learning atmosphere should not be stressful, but supportive and encouraging, and learning objectives should be clear to promote original learning and to facilitate subsequent retention of skills.[24] The learning process should preferably be **goal directed** and **competence based**.

The educational programme could be divided into a **theoretical** and a **practical** part.

The theoretical part will, depending on the specific equipment the individual VAI will be using, explain the rationale for long-term noninvasive and invasive ventilation (Box 22.1).

If the VAI raises other problems that need attention, this should be included in the programme. For the more disabled users, attention should possibly be paid to nutritional support typically via a percutaneous endoscopic gastrostomy (PEG) tube, to pressure sores and contractures and to communication equipment and techniques.

The practical part can be structured in three steps:

1. Instruction by the staff.
2. Assisted and supervised performance by the attendant (Figure 22.3).
3. Independent performance by the attendant and signed approval by the staff of each specified competency. This documents the HMV centre's approval of acquired skills.

When the required competencies are outlined in detail, it will be possible to a large extent to (1) document progress and thus stimulate motivation and self-assurance of the attendant (and of the VAI), to (2) verify that the knowledge and practical skills required are retained. Documentation and quality assurance are important aspects that are required increasingly by health authorities. This method easily provides that in a valid manner and offers in addition a structured framework that is accessible for stepwise adjustments as techniques and equipment change and develop over time.

The acquisition of practical skills should best be performed at the bedside. The details of a typical list of practical skills are given in Box 22.2.

This range of skills and competencies is not comprehensive and should be tailored to fit the individual VAI's requirements. Some of the issues that may require modification of the standard educational programme are listed in Box 22.3.

BOX 22.1: Rationale for HMV – issues to be covered with patient and carers

- Basic anatomy and physiology of the airways
- Explain the working principles of the ventilator(s) the individual ventilator user will use in his home
- Explain the importance of appropriate humidification
- Explain the rationale for choosing different types of masks. This includes knowledge of the importance of minimal leaks and transparency of mask material (Figures 22.1 and 22.2).

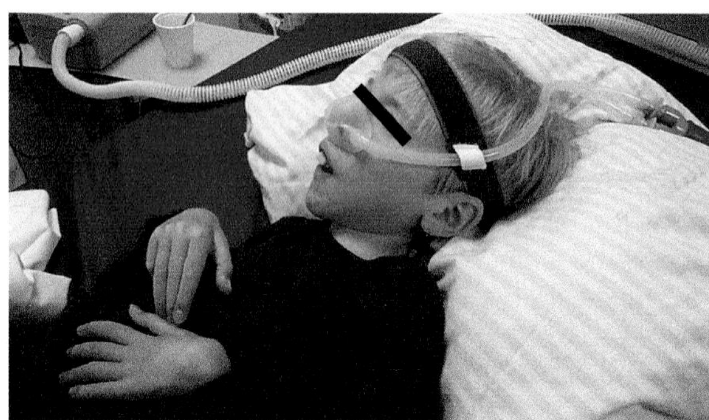

Figure 22.1 Boy with SMA II with transparent nasal mask.

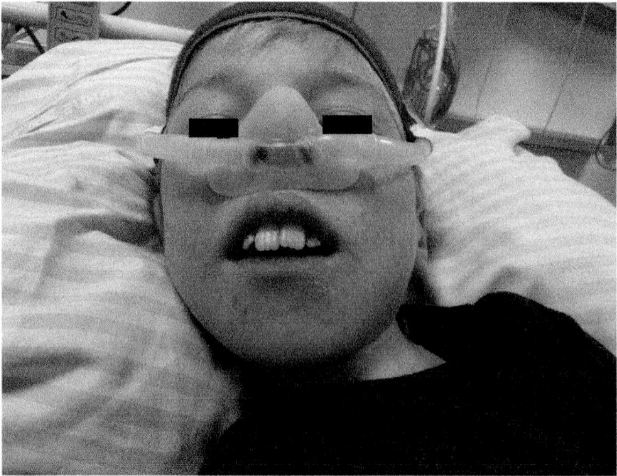

Figure 22.2 Boy with SMA II with transparent nasal mask.

- Explain the adverse effects of noninvasive ventilation, in particular leakage, irritation to mucous membranes and the eyes, gastrointestinal inflation, skin lesions and, very important, pressure-induced malformation of the facial bony structures in children
- Explain the rationale for choosing different types of tracheostomy tubes, in particular cuffed versus uncuffed and fenestrated versus non-fenestrated types and the significance of and risk from high cuff pressure
- Explain the adverse effects of invasive ventilation, in particular leakage around the tube via the stoma during uncuffed ventilation, pneumothorax during cuffed ventilation, mucous plugging, pneumonia, lesions to the tracheal mucous membrane, tracheal scarring, tracheal stenosis and tracheomalacia
- Explain the risk of accidental disconnection from the ventilator
- Explain the risk of accidental extubation and the reinsertion procedure, possibly using a smaller tube and/or using a suctioning catheter as a guide wire during intubation
- Explain the fundamental importance of preserving and optimising speech, whenever possible
- Explain possible detrimental effects of a tracheostomy tube on swallowing

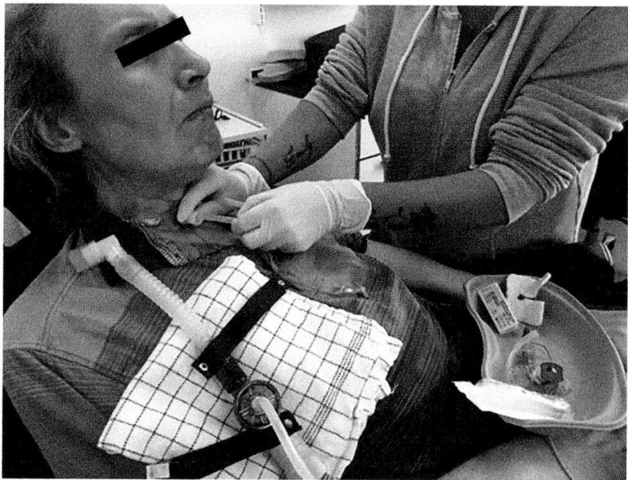

Figure 22.3 Lay attendant training change of tracheostomy inner cannula.

BOX 22.2: Practical skills needed depending on the nature of ventilator support

- Positioning of the mask and securing an unobstructed airway, selection of headgear and the balanced tightening that will, on one hand, prevent or minimise leaks and, on the other hand, exert minimal pressure on the face. The latter is very important in neonates and the very young where the bony structure of the skull is compliant and sensible to deformation from applied pressure.
- Forced expiration technique, breath-stacking using a one-way valve, cough assist via a mask.
- Suctioning procedures via a tracheostomy tube using a suctioning catheter or use of a cough-assist device, changing of inner cannula and, in some cases of the tracheostomy tube itself, tracheostomy tube cleaning and maintenance, assessment and cleaning of the stoma.
- Manual ventilation with a self-inflating ventilation bag, typically in relation to suctioning procedures in the invasively ventilated patient or in case of ventilator failure.
- Recognition of signs of infection of the airways and elsewhere.
- Hygienic precautions when dealing with the ventilator, masks, cannulae, circuits, humidifiers and disposables.
- Understanding ventilator settings and troubleshooting, understanding alarms and what action to take in response, in particular to understand the significance of low-pressure (or flow) alarms versus high-pressure (or flow) alarms.
- Assemble and disassemble relevant equipment such as masks, the ventilator circuit and the humidifier.
- Knowledge about who to call, and what to do, in an emergency.
- Patient care including helping with personal hygiene, dressing, handling special beds, handling use of hoists to ensure safe transfer from bed to wheelchair, driving the VAI's vehicle and more.
- In some cases, additional skills including handling a PEG tube, catheterisation of the urinary bladder, use of computer-assisted communication, physical exercises to mobilise limbs and so on.
- Handle specific needs in the technology-dependent neonate or child (and its parents), including familiarity with downscaled interfaces, downscaled equipment generally, low FRC leading to low oxygen reserves and short response time in hypoxemic conditions, delicate balance with respect to fluids and nutrition, possibly tension and anxiety of parents.
- Resuscitation skills are sometimes included. At the author's institution, we have chosen not to include that responsibility in the attendant's curriculum. However, if an attendant already possesses the skills to resuscitate, that attendant is allowed to resuscitate if needed.

When one further takes into account the physiologic differences between different conditions like ALS, cystic fibrosis, COPD, neuromuscular diseases (Duchenne, Limb-Girdle, SMA-II), quadriplegia, obesity hypoventilation syndrome and others, it is clear that the generic plan for caregiver training has to be modified – sometimes quite markedly – to the individual case.

The practical outline and format of a training programme will vary from place to place, depending also on economy, culture, geography and other factors.

BOX 22.3: Issues that may lead to modification of the training programme

- Cognitive impairment or a complex psychological profile
- VAI's inability to communicate
- VAI's degree of bulbar and general motor weakness
- Consequences of severe obesity
- Comorbidities (cardiac, nutritional problems, urinary and fecal incontinence, skin lesions, painful contractures of limbs and the jaw, spasms, etc.)
- Foreign language, religious beliefs and habits, family characteristics, strain or crisis caused by the disease or failed expectations
- 'Invisible' siblings while the technology-dependent child gets all attention, divorce, and so on

CAREGIVERS

The importance of caregiver education is widely accepted.[14,15] There is no agreed upon standard for minimal requirements for caregivers, and previous consensus statements barely comment on the topic.[29] Recently, this issue has been addressed in detail in different guidelines,[16,18,30] which, to some extent, document the size of the problem. Attendants express the desire and need for formal training,[31] as well as parents who care for their medically complex children in the home, although they express satisfaction but also report challenges, including the impact on their own health.[32,33] In addition, they may feel as if they are the 'lifeline' for the child.[34] In a group of well-educated North American mothers caring for ventilator-assisted children at home, 45% had a questionnaire score indicating depression.[35] Similar signs of caregiver burden is reported among those caring for chronically ill patients generally[36] and from a mixed population in Norway.[37] Recently, the ventilator users themselves[38,39] have expressed 'significant concerns about the risk of ventilator failure or mucous plugging', or fear that the ventilator hose will pop off the tracheostomy tube.[30,40]

The stress and strain associated with looking after an individual on HMV can lead to exhaustion, anxiety and depression and to a compromised quality of life.[41,42]

Ventilator users have hoped that properly trained attendants/PSWs (personal support workers) could at least partly ameliorate problems[40] and it has been reported that 'competence and continuity of healthcare personnel are factors for success'.[43]

It may not be a surprise that the main focus will be on the health of the ventilator user (sometimes with visible physical disabilities) and not on the health of the caregiver, but caregivers themselves often not only neglect their own health, but actually experience a decline in health over time.[44,45] This occurs across a series of different disabilities where caregivers report depression,[35,46,47] overload and burden.[36,37,41,42,48] The rate of some degree of depression among caregivers has at some time been reported to exceed 50%, and 6 months after discharge, 15% of caregivers were classified as having symptoms consistent with severe depression. This again may be explained on the basis of, or triggered by, social isolation[37,49] and a heavy workload of 12 to 14 hours a day.[50] Thirty per cent of caregivers working with patients suffering from advanced ALS have rated their quality of life as lower than that of their patient, and 60% of them left their job. If the caregiver at the same time is also a parent or a spouse to the ventilator user, it is conceivable that the strain may be even stronger.[33,49] It is a paradox that even today the interest in the health of caregivers is so limited[51] considering the crucial role they play in supporting the whole system of HMV. As mentioned before, caregivers themselves express a desire for training and the cost of HMV is favourable compared to that of a stay in a hospital ward.

Considering these premises, it is not difficult to propose that securing reasonable training and working conditions for caregivers may be the best and cheapest way to secure survival and quality of life in this vulnerable population of patients. This is to some extent already in place in some countries and has recently been suggested in a Canadian report on chronic ventilation, accompanied with proposals for improving the supporting community network of healthcare professionals and allied partners.[52]

A generic matrix for the global process including referral of a patient, education of caregivers and discharge to permanent living site is presented in Table 22.1.

Table 22.1 Example of a very summary generic matrix for orchestration of actors involved in training and discharge of HMV user and attendants

Time point	1	2	3	4	5	6
Patient	Symptoms	Hires attendants	Education begins	Education completed	Moves home	Checkup
Department of Neurology/Pulmonary Medicine/Paediatrics/ other	Refers patient to HMV					Checkup
Centre for HMV	Validates patient for HMV	Initiates 'global' plan	Education of attendants begins	Education completed	VAI is discharged	Checkup
Municipality/insurance	Asked for funding by HMV	Agrees funding				
Agent responsible for change of home		Contacted by HMV centre and begins change of home	Change of home continues		Home is ready	
Other relevant parties						

CONCLUSIONS

The purpose of HMV is to secure sufficient respiration and a self-directed life for individuals suffering from respiratory insufficiency or failure. The responsibilities of the ventilator user, the caregiver and the health professionals should be defined. Educational programmes should be well structured, goal directed and competency based and respect the ventilator user's autonomy. The caregiver's knowledge and practical skills should be measurable so that progress can be acknowledged and deficiencies be identified and improved. The educational programme should in addition be sensitive to the caregiver's needs and burdens.

REFERENCES

1. Bonnici DM, Sanctuary T, Warren A et al. Prospective observational cohort study of patients with weaning failure admitted to a specialist weaning, rehabilitation and home mechanical ventilation centre. *BMJ Open*. 2016;6:e010025 doi:10.1136/bmjopen-2015-010025.
2. Duiverman ML, Bladder G, Meinesz AF, Wijkstra PJ. Home mechanical ventilatory support in patients with restrictive ventilatory disorders: A 48 year experience. *Respir Med*. 2006;100:56–65.
3. Lloyd-Owen SJ, Donaldson GC, Ambrosino N et al. Patterns of home mechanical ventilation use in Europe: Results from the Eurovent survey. *Eur Respir J*. 2005;25:1025–31.
4. Jeppesen J, Green A, Steffensen BF, Rahbek J. The Duchenne muscular dystrophy population in Denmark, 1977-2001: Prevalence, incidence and survival in relation to the introduction of ventilator use. *Neuromusc Disord*. 2003;13:804–12.
5. Laub M, Berg S, Midgren B. Swedish Society of Chest Medicine. Home mechanical ventilation in Sweden—Inequalities within a homogenous health care system. *Respir Med*. 2004;98:38–42.
6. Final report of the Ontario Chronic Ventilation Strategy Task Force. 2006; June 30: 54–6.
7. Dranove D. What impact did the programs have on the costs of care for ventilator assisted childen? In: Aday LA, Aitken MJ, Wegener DH. *Pediatric Home Care: Results of a National Evaluation of Programs for Ventilator Assisted Children*. Chicago: Pluribus Press, University of Chicago, 1988:295–321.
8. Lumeng JC, Warschausky SA, Nelson VS, Augenstein K. The quality of life of ventilator-assisted children. *Pediatr Med*. 2001;4:21–7.
9. Moss AH, Oppenheimer EA, Casey P et al. Patients with amyotrophic lateral sclerosis receiving long-term mechanical ventilation. Advance care planning and outcome. *Chest*. 1996;110:249–55.
10. Bourke CB, Tomlinson M, Williams TL et al. Effects of non-invasive ventilation on survival and quality of life in patients with amyotrophic lateral sclerosis: A randomized controlled trial. *Lancet Neurol*. 2006;5:140–7.
11. Srinivasan S, Doly SM, White TR et al. Frequency, causes and outcomes of home ventilator failure. *Chest*. 1998;114:1363–7.
12. Lang A, Edwards N, Hoffman C et al. Broadening the patient safety to include home care issues. *Healthcare Q*. 2006;9 (Special Issue):124–6.
13. Edwards JD, Kun SS, Keens TG. Outcomes and causes of death in children on home mechanical ventilation via tracheostomy: An institutional and literature review. *J Pediatr*. 2010:157:955–9.e2.
14. Boroughs D, Dougherty JA. Decreasing accidental mortality of ventilator-dependent children at home: A call to action. *Home Health Nurse*. 2012;30:103–11; quiz 112–3.
15. Kun SS, Edwards JD, Ward SL, Keens TG. Hospital readmissions for newly discharged pediatric home mechanical ventilation patents. *Pediatr Pulmonol*. 2012;47:409–14.
16. Sterni LM, Collaco JM, Baker CD et al. An Official American Thoracic Society Clinical Practice Guideline: Pediatric Chronic Home Invasive Ventilation. *Am J Respir Crit Care Med*. 2016;193(8).e16–e35.
17. Mitchell BB, Hussey HM, Setzen G et al. Clinical consensus statement: Tracheostomy care. *Otolaryngol Head Neck Surg*. 2013;148:6–20.
18. McKim D, Road J, Avendano M et al. Home mechanical ventilation: A Canadian Thoracic Society clinical practice guideline. *Can Respir J*. 2011;18(4):201–2.
19. Brooks D, Gibson B, DeMatteo D. Perspectives of personal support workers and ventilator-users on training needs. *Patient Educ Counsel*. 2008;71:244–50.
20. Norregaard O. Home mechanical ventilation in Denmark. Paper presented at the 43rd Nordic Lung Congress, Uppsala, Sweden, May 2007.
21. Stanley JM. The Appleton Consensus: Suggested international guidelines for decisions to forego medical treatment. *J. Med Ethics*. 1989;15:129–36.
22. Laub M, Midgren B. Survival of patients on home mechanical ventilation: A nationwide prospective study. *Respir Med*. 2007;101:1074–8.
23. Escarrabill J. Discharge planning and home care for end-stage COPD patients. *Eur Respir J*. 2009; 34:507–12.
24. Lieb S. Principles of adult learning. Arizona Department of Health Services. South Mountain Community College. Vision. 1991.
25. Tearl DK, Hertzog JH. Home discharge of technology-dependent children: Evaluation of a respiratory-therapist driven family education program. *Respir Care*. 2007;52:171–6.
26. Holman H, Lorig K. Patient self-management: A key to effectiveness and efficiency in care of chronic disease. *Public Health Rep*. 2004;119:239–43.

27. Hazenberg A, KJerstjens HAM, Prins SCL, Vermeulen KM, Wijkstra PJ. Initiation of home mechanical ventilation at home: A randomized controlled trial of efficacy, feasibility and costs. *Respir Med.* 2014;108:1387–95.
28. McKim DA, King J, Walker K et al. Formal ventilation patient education for ALS predicts real-life choices. *Amyotroph Lateral Scler.* 2012;13:59–65.
29. Wallgren-Pettersson C, Bushby K, Mellies U, Simonds A. 117th ENMC Workshop: Ventilatory Support in Congenital Neuromuscular Disorders—Congenital Myopathies, Congenital Muscular Dystrophies, Congenital Myotonic Dystrophies and SMA (II). 4–6 April 2003 Naarden, The Netherlands. *Neuromusc Disord.* 2004;14:56–69.
30. Rose L, Douglas A, McKim MD et al. Home mechanical ventilation in Canada: A national survey. *Respir Care.* 2015:60(5):695–704.
31. Yamada K, Sugai K, Fukumizu M et al. The parents' assessment and needs for home mechanical ventilation in patients with pediatric neurologic disorders. *No To Hattatsu.* 2003;35:147–52.
32. Wang K-WK, Bernard A. Technology-dependent children and their families: A review. *J Adv Nurs.* 2004;45:36–46.
33. Carnevale FA, Alexander E, Davis M et al. Daily living with distress and enrichment: The moral experience of families with ventilator-assisted children at home. *Pediatrics.* 2006:117:e48–e60.
34. Mah JK, Tannhauser JE, McNeil DA, Dewey D. Being the lifeline: The parent experience of caring for a child with neuromuscular disease on home mechanical ventilation. *Neuromusc Disord.* 2008;18:983–8.
35. Kuster PA, Badr LK. Mental health of mothers caring for ventilator-assisted children at home. *Issues Mental Health Nurs.* 2006;7:817–35.
36. Douglas SL, Daly BJ, O'Toole E. Depression among white and nonwhite caregivers of the chronically ill. *J Crit Care.* 2010;25:364.e11–365.e19.
37. Dybwik K, Nilesen EW, Brinchmann BS. Home mechanical ventilation and specialized care in the community: Between a rock and a hard place. *BMC Health Services Res.* 2011;11:115.
38. Gibson BE, Upshur REG, Young NL, McKeever P. Disability, technology and place: Social and ethical implications on long-term dependency on medical devices. *Ethics Place Environ.* 2007:10:7–28.
39. Gibson BE, Upshur REG, Young NL, McKeever P. Men on the marg. Bourdiesian examination of living into adulthood with muscular dystrophy. *Soc Sci Med.* 2007;65:505–17.
40. Sarvey SI. Living a machine: The experience of the child who is ventilator dependent. *Mental Health Nurs.* 2008;29:179–86.
41. Van Pelt DC, Milbrandt EB, Qin L, Weissfeld LA, Rotondi AJ et al. Informal caregiver burden among survivors of prolonged mechanical ventilation. *Am J Respir Crit Care Med.* 2007;175:167–73.
42. Kim CH, Kim MS. Ventilator use, respiratory problems, and caregiver well-being in Korean patients with amyotrophic lateral sclerosis receiving home based care. *J Neurosci Nurs.* 2014;46(5):E25–32.
43. Ballangrud R, Bogsti WB, Johansson IS. Clients' experiences of living at home with a mechanical ventilator. *J Adv Nurs.* 2009;65:425–34.
44. Douglas SL, Daly BJ. Caregivers of long-term ventilator patients. Physical and psychological outcomes. *Chest.* 2003;123:1073–81.
45. Sexton DL, Munro BH. Impact of a husband's chronic illness (COPD) on the spouse's life. *Res Nurs Health.* 1985;8:83–90.
46. Miller B, Townsend A, Carpenter E et al. Social support and caregiver stress: A replication analysis. *J Gerontol B Psychol Sci Soc Sci.* 2001;56:S249–56.
47. Pilisuk M, Parks SH. Caregiving: Where families need help. *Soc Work.* 1988;33:436–40.
48. Pearlin LI, Mullan JT, Semple SJ et al. Caregiving and the stress process: An overview of concepts and their measures. *Gerontologist.* 1990;30:583–94.
49. Ibañez M, Aguilar JJ, Maderal MA et al. Sexuality in chronic respiratory failure: Coincidences and divergences between patient and primary caregiver. *Respir Med.* 2001;95:975–9.
50. Kaub-Wittemer D, Steinbüchel N, Wasner M, Laier-Groeneveld G, Borasio GD. Quality of life and psychosocial issues in ventilated patients with amyotrophic lateral sclerosis and their caregivers. *J Pain Symptom Manage.* 2003;26:890–6.
51. Talley RC, Crews JE. Framing in the public health of caregiving. *Am J Public Health.* 2007;97:224–8.
52. Final Report of the Ontario Chronic Ventilation Strategy Task Force. 2006; June 30:72.

23

Discharging the patient on home ventilation

JOAN ESCARRABILL AND OLE NORREGAARD

KEY MESSAGES

- Teamwork and coordination of multiple stakeholders are the core issue of transitional care.
- Discharge planning is a process that restarts every time circumstances change.
- The challenge is to be proactive and to identify in advance unmet needs of patients and caregivers.
- Zero risk doesn't exist, but with appropriate discharge planning, it can be minimised.
- One size does not fit all: an individualised package of care should be designed, with the agreement of the patient and caregivers, and this must be appropriate to their local situation.

TRANSITIONAL CARE

Transitional care (TC) is a set of organisational frameworks and actions designed to ensure the coordination and continuity of healthcare as patients transfer between different locations or different levels of care.[1] In home mechanical ventilation (HMV), TC refers, generically, to different situations:

- From intensive care unit (ICU) to general ward
- From hospital to home
- From hospital to a less complex health facility (from hospital to a community hospital or hospice, for example)
- From outpatient initiation of HMV to home[2,3]
- For patients on HMV admitted to the hospital for an acute exacerbation or to regulate the ventilatory settings

Discharge of a patient from the hospital to home or to a different healthcare facility is one of the most complex transitions of care. Discharge of a patient is a process that may take a few days (in most cases) or can be extended even to a few months (in the case of complex patients with long stays in the ICU). Generally, we speak of 'discharge plan' if it develops a strategy that allows the patient to adapt to a new treatment outside the hospital setting (in this case, a treatment involving ventilatory support). The purpose of the discharge plan is to achieve maximum independence for the patient using therapeutic resources and technology to suit their needs, taking into account the efficacy and safety of treatment.

In all these circumstances, discharge should be planned carefully. The discharge plan is not formulated just once at the time of establishment of HMV and is never 'final'. It must be revisited whenever circumstances lead to change in the ventilatory requirements: worsening of the disease, weight gain or loss or change of device.

DISCHARGE PLANNING IN HMV

In their classic article on the discharge of patients, Bertoye et al.[4] described how a patient with sequelae of polio began the process of transfer from hospital to the patient's home. Patients require a short period of adaptation, and in this case, a temporary transfer was made from the hospital to the patient's home, but the patient quickly decided to stay home with the ventilator. As illustrated in this classic experience, return home is possible if there is an agreement between the caregiver, patient and the care team. It is essential that the caregiver is competent and he or she accepts the workload of caring for a patient with HMV; finally, the home conditions should be adequate for this kind of therapy. Technical support should cover emergencies around the clock, with a short response time.

At the time of discharge, the recommendations concerning the use of the ventilator must be clearly written down, including the patient monitoring scheme.[5] Table 23.1 summarises the key elements in the patient-centred discharge plan.

In the discharge plan, there is a 'D-Day', which is agreed between the ventilator-assisted individual (VAI) and the caregiver and case manager. It is imperative to take time to decide the 'D-Day', especially in patients who have been in hospital for a long period of time. In such patients, it is not appropriate to plan the discharge at a weekend. The first hours at home are crucial for adaptation and it is preferable that the patient can communicate directly with the care team if there is any problem. Box 23.1 summarises specific points that should be clarified before discharge.

Moreover, the discharge plan is not a journey without return. The patient should be assured that the return to the previous situation is possible (though in most cases it will not be necessary or desired by the patient or caregiver).

It has been recognised for many years that without a discharge plan in place, the risk for failure is high.[7] Discharge planning should start as early as possible, and is best started at the beginning of the educational process. The plan should be comprehensible and ideally include all needs and actors in the often very complex scenario that the education of an HMV candidate with attendants constitutes. At the same time, it is advisable to try to make things as simple as possible.

Table 23.1 Key elements in patient-centered discharge planning

Key element	Basic content
Decision-making process	Appropriate information and time to allow patient (and caregiver) to be involved in the decision-making process. Patient's values (deliberative model)
Feasibility	Deciding the appropriate place for the patient. There is no place like home, but it is not always feasible to return home.
Education and training	Promoting self-care with three clear objectives: safety, excellence (achieve maximum effectiveness) and positive patient experience.
Needs	The care plan is a balance between the needs and the resources available at a local level: 'Appropriate package of care for individual patients at a local level'.[6]
Follow-up	Clarify the roles of all the stakeholders.
Risk management	Zero risk doesn't exist. The aim of the care plan is risk minimisation through training, availability of health data for all stakeholders and clear emergency plans (phone and transfer to hospital if it is needed).

BOX 23.1: Specific point that should be clarified before discharge

- VAI and caregivers are ready and motivated.
- Inpatients with rapidly progressive conditions end-of-life issues should preferably have been discussed, and clarified.
- VAI individual is stable, or as stable as possible.
- All caregivers and the VAI have completed the specific education and training programme.
  - Written and illustrated individualised material to take home, reinforcing what has been learned during the training period
- Supplementary material and adaptations (if needed):
  - Extra ventilator if needed
  - Secretion management devices if needed
  - Modification of the wheelchair
  - Modification of the home (access, transfers, toileting)
  - Mobility and modification of the vehicle
  - Communication support devices
- A plan for regular delivery of disposables is ready.
- Arrangements for school or other institution if relevant have been completed.
- Arrangements for risk management and emergencies:
  - Backup for supply of electricity in case of power cuts.
- Plans for follow-up.
- Detailed plan for transfer from hospital to home.

It is recommended to organise the planning in each case as a matrix including all involved parties and carried out in a well-defined temporal sequence with clearly defined actions, and to appoint a case manager for the job. This will increase the chances that all relevant questions are addressed, minimum time is wasted and the whole process will be seen as forward moving and experienced more satisfactorily by all parties including the ventilator user, his or her attendants and the staff. This might add to a better start and a more optimistic outlook to the future life of the HMV user.

The whole arrangement can include a multitude of players such as the funding agency, centre for HMV, agencies delivering the equipment (special bed, modified wheelchair, oxygen, lift, equipment for communication, disposals), the physiotherapist, the occupational therapist, the social worker, the nurse and the physician. Specific points that should be clarified and settled before discharge are presented in Box 23.1.

If the VAI will be taken care of by a professional agency whose employees are not trained at the centre for HMV, it is recommended to specify in detail the required qualifications of the hired staff and also to arrange a signed contract with the agency, and if possible also with the individual employee, to ensure that they possess the claimed knowledge, skills and experience.

No HMV programme is complete without a well-structured follow-up programme. In fact, this is the lifelong 'companion' that is supposed to ensure survival, safety and quality of life. Without this, the initiation of HMV carries the risk of being the beginning of the end.

ORGANISATION OF CARE IN HMV

Nobody questions the role of the ventilators, supplementary materials and technical services, but education, training and coaching are also crucial for successful HMV (see Chapter 22). Also, the availability of resources and local circumstances are relevant in the development of the package of care. There are four elements in the general framework of the organisation of care for effective HMV: the team, the care coordinator, the place where the patient will be cared for and the healthcare networks.

Team working and coordination of care

The care of patients with chronic diseases is an example of a complex system involving many actors. Decisions are made at different levels of the healthcare system and it is very difficult to control all the details. A decision taken at a point in the health system (e.g. in the emergency department) can have an enormous impact on the overall treatment plan. The global response to the needs of a patient requires teamwork and a very significant effort to coordinate care.

Wagner defines the characteristics of the care team very well: 'A patient care team is a group of diverse clinicians who communicate with each other regularly about the care of a defined group of patients and participate in that care'.[8] In patients with HMV, we can distinguish the 'core team' and other professionals also involved in patient care. The core team is usually made of a mix of individuals from the hospital expert team (doctors, nurses and physiotherapists) and the community care team (family physician and nurses). Physicians from many different specialties may be involved in HMV: chest physicians, paediatricians, anaesthetists or specialists in intensive care. But around this core team, we must consider the participation of many other professionals: hospital specialists (e.g. speech therapist, nutritionist, ENT, neurologists) and both the hospital and the community can develop relationships with the patient's social worker, occupational therapists, psychologists, technicians supply companies, and so on (see Figure 23.1).

The general characteristics that define a team are shown in Box 23.2[9] and the team skills to care for patients with HMV are shown in Box 23.3.[10]

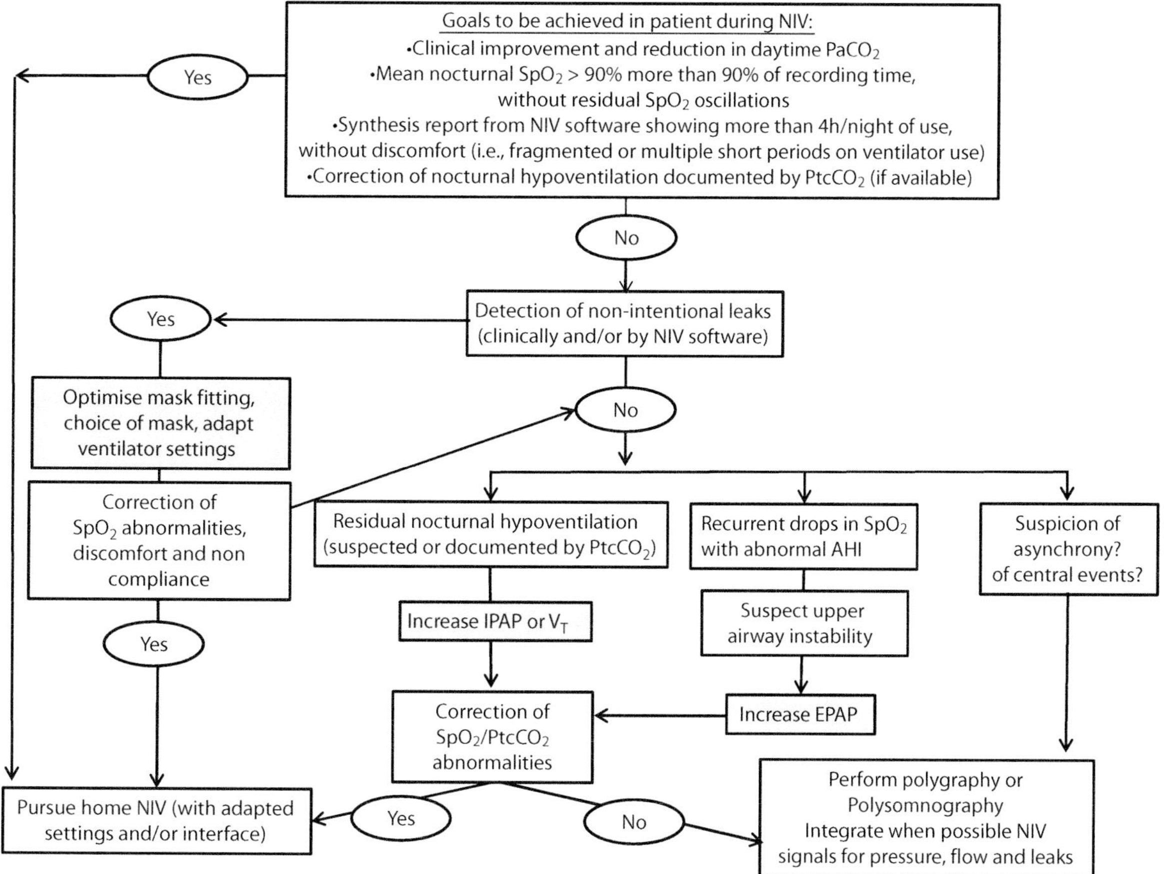

Figure 23.1 Core team.

BOX 23.2: Characteristics that define a team

- Heterogeneous group of individuals
- Shared leadership roles
- Individual and mutual accountability
- Specific purpose that the team delivers
- Team members working together to achieve an output—'Collective outputs'
- Encourages open-ended discussion and active problem-solving meetings (feel free to criticise)
- Supportive and informal atmosphere
- Measures performance directly by assessing collective outputs
- Discusses, decides and does real work together

Adapted from Katzenbach JR, Smith DK. The discipline of teams. *HBR*, July–August 2005.

BOX 23.3: Team skills to care for patients with HMV

- Clear ideas about the meaning of patient-centred care
- Empathic attitude and capacity for decision making through a deliberative process
- Skills related to HMV and home care
- Ability to assess the adequacy of caregivers
- Knowledge of community resources
- Capacity to integrate home, outpatient and hospital care
- Designing of guidelines-based care plans and integrating the technical needs and preferences of the patient
- Behavioural counselling and teaching of self-management
- Teamwork skills

Adapted from Escarrabill J, Goldberg A. Training the home health team. In: Ambrosino N, Goldstein R. *Ventilatory support for chronic respiratory failure*. Oxford: Informa Health Care, 2008.

Care coordinator

The organisation of complex care cannot be achieved simply by adding up the individual actions of each professional. Spontaneous coordination is impossible. Specialists, particularly physicians, have difficulty getting an overview of the problems of patients. The role of nurses is crucial because they are more holistic in outlook and they are more focused on care coordination by training.[12] Moreover, patients clearly value this nursing role and it is obvious that coordination has a direct impact on perceived quality of care.[13]

The role of 'care manager'[14] makes sense from several perspectives. From the perspective of the patient and caregiver, it builds confidence and provides competence assurance (it also identifies a single contact in case of problems); from the perspective of other team members, it helps to identify the targets; from the perspective of the physician who prescribes the HMV, it ensures that all patient needs are covered; and from the perspective of the financier, it ensures efficient use of resources. To achieve effective care coordination is essential, in that the professional in charge has the highest decision-making capacity in terms of care organisation, planning of visits and the establishment of priorities. The care manager should have the knowledge and skills to organise the care of patients with different diseases but with common problems (in this case, the common denominator would be the ventilation), and he or she focuses its critical role in coordinating the different health resources. The care manager must be very accessible to the patient.

Caregiver training and coaching are very important, and the appropriate skills should be assessed by the care coordinator. With HMV, as in most chronic conditions, the care plan cannot be finalised without the active participation of the patient (and caregiver) in their own treatment.[15] The role of the informal (or formal) caregiver is crucial because as Crimi et al. showed, more than 40% of patients on noninvasive ventilation (NIV) in Europe don't have any formal home support programme.[16] Becoming an expert carer is a process[17] that needs support from health professionals (predominantly nurses) but, in parallel, carers develop their own experience and use additional sources of information (Internet).

It is very important to note that the number of potential caregivers involved may be very high. In designing the training, the wide range of those involved in care should be taken into account.

Finally, evaluation of healthcare should specifically include an assessment of this coordination.[18]

Alternatives when home is not possible for the VAI

The alternatives to home in HMV sometimes are related to prolonged mechanical ventilation (PMV) or to patients with a high degree of dependence. PMV has been defined as 'ventilation for 21 or more consecutive days and medical stability'. In Canada, these patients occupied 11% of ventilator-capable beds.[19] Patients with tracheostomy, even without requiring round the clock ventilation, are the most problematic patients at home.

The first consequence of this situation is the increase in hospital stay[20] followed by the financial problems this causes institutions and patients.[21] Some countries have weaning centres where it is easier to make this transition. Weaning units, organised on a regional basis, play a role both in weaning and in long-term home care.[22] In long-term home care, weaning centres play a transitional role in the discharge plan for patients requiring HMV,[23] but in general, they should not be considered as the long-term solution for most patients.[24]

Some countries have centres that, while not specifically prepared to receive patients with HMV, can look after certain types of patients. The nomenclature may differ—hospices, nursing homes or long-stay facilities and so on—but they are all characterised by assurance of basic care in an environment with minimal medical supervision or nursing. The transfer of patients to such centres often requires monitoring by experts, since the caring professionals are not familiar with the use of ventilators. The transfer from hospital to these facilities is particularly difficult in patients with amyotrophic lateral sclerosis (ALS) and/or tracheostomy.

The success of the discharge plan depends largely on the availability of a skilled team that can support the patient and caregivers, both at home and in other healthcare facilities. A good example of this teamwork is in the French non-profit associations that have been working in this field for more than 50 years. The ALLP (*Association Lyonnaise de Logistique Posthospitalière,* formerly *Association Lyonnais de Lutte Contre la Poliomyélite*) was established more than 50 years ago to facilitate the return home of polio patients requiring long-term ventilatory support.[25] This kind of organisation allows support at home, support for ventilated patients who cannot return to their homes and must live in apartments supervised by nurses, as well as the education of both the formal and informal caregivers.

Networks: Strong and weak relationships

From a practical standpoint, the relationship between HMV prescribing centres and local hospitals or primary care teams is not always easy and clear-cut. In some countries, the physician who prescribes does not follow the patient and, therefore, once decisions are made, health professionals who are sometimes not familiar with this complex treatment must assume responsibility for the long-term follow-up. In other cases, the prescribing team establishes hierarchical relationships with health professionals in the community; this attitude is not the best strategy to promote collaboration. Neither of these two extreme positions is a guarantee of good patient care. There is no health organisation (from the high-tech centre to the primary care team) that can single-handedly deal with all the patient's needs in all the possible circumstances.

In addition, although greater centralisation improves knowledge, it possibly makes access harder for the patient. Several studies have shown that the best results are achieved by hospitals working as referral centres for the diagnosis and treatment of patients with serious diseases such as ALS. Farrero et al.[26] showed that early respiratory evaluation of patients with ALS, performed immediately after diagnosis, improves survival. The care provided by multidisciplinary teams is associated with a better quality of life and increased survival.[27] Traynor et al.[28] note that multidisciplinary intervention reduced mortality by 29.7% and, even in patients with bulbar involvement, survival improved by almost 10 months. However, this is not always the case. In one study, this lack of benefit has been attributed to a 'weak' intervention (although the percentage of patients with NIV or percutaneous endoscopic gastrostomy was very low in these studies with negative findings) rather than the team per se.[29]

This discussion about the benefits of a referral centre (with a lot of experience and a large number of patients) versus the benefits of a smaller centre (with greater accessibility to the patient but with more limited skills and knowledge) was discussed in the Eurovent survey.[30] This survey revealed a great diversity of strategies in Europe: some countries have fewer facilities with many patients in each (in Denmark, there are only two centres that coordinate HMV), whereas others have multiple centres with fewer patients. Moreover, the number of patients does not necessarily reflect the centre's experience in treating critically ill patients. Key skills in HMV are more related to the experience in the care of patients with neuromuscular diseases with or without tracheostomy. The technique of HMV, especially NIV, is not particularly difficult. More and more professionals are becoming familiar with the use of NIV in acute patients, and this experience can be transferred in part to the care of chronic patients. The difficulties in HMV are related to the decision-making process: choosing the best treatment (which, in many cases, is not necessarily related to the correction of gas exchange), solving problems and making complex decisions (such as performing tracheostomy in a patient with ALS). The balance between the efficiency of ventilation (measured from the perspective of physiology) and its acceptance by and the comfort of the patient is based more on a holistic view than rather just a focus on $PaCO_2$ or some other physiological variable.

A network is an alternative to a single centre doing everything. But networks should be cooperative rather than hierarchical, and replacing the referral centre by centralised networks is very limited in progress. In this sense, the so-called distributed networks are more stable[31] and help to identify the roles of each of the components.

In the last 15 years, the advent of telemonitoring has raised expectations as it could theoretically solve some of the problems of patients who require long-term ventilation or patients with a high burden of care at home (see Chapter 25), but these theoretical benefits are yet to be realised.

Lessons learned from big projects like 'Whole System Demonstrator' were as follows:[32]

- Local factors are important.
- An RCT does not allow iterative incorporation of lessons learned until the end of study.
- No expected organisational changes were generated (such as more integration of care or more penetration of eHealth).
- It wasn't possible to determine if any changes were due to the technology or how service was provided.
- No information on scalability was provided.

The systematic use of telemonitoring in HMV is very low. In Canada,[33] follow-up in the home was conducted via telemedicine by only 1 provider out of 142. Regarding telemonitoring, Chatwin et al.[34] suggested that 'More data can be helpful, but can also add to clinical uncertainty and therefore precipitate more activity' without adding any benefit to conventional care.

The conclusions of the ERS Telemonitoring of Ventilator-Dependent Patients Task Force[35] were as follows:

- Variable models of care exist.
- Research is needed before considering telemonitoring as real improvement in the management of these patients.
- The impact of telemonitoring is difficult to assess without considering the other services received by patients (homecare, access to hospital, social care).
- Telemonitoring should only be included as part of the full 'care package'.[36]

At the end of the day, patients on HMV need a comprehensive system of services (or care package)[37] at the local and regional level with a clear definition of responsibilities of each stakeholder.

PATIENT SAFETY

The negative health effects of medical interventions have been known since ancient times. The term 'iatrogenic' refers precisely to this effect: 'produced by the doctor'. Hippocrates (460–370 BC) dictated '*primum non nocere*'. However, the concern about clinical safety developed only recently, after the publication of the report *To Err Is Human* by the Institute of Medicine in the United States.[38]

Concern about clinical safety makes sense for several reasons. Errors can cause much inconvenience to the patient and are associated with inappropriate stays in hospital, injury, suffering and death. Whether or not they have an impact on the patient, they satisfy no one and are difficult to explain to an increasingly demanding society.

An important aspect related to clinical safety is that there has been a significant qualitative change in the interpretation: the avoidance of blaming individuals for past mistakes and focusing on the organisation as the source of the error. Errors do not occur because of 'bad people' but because of bad organisation that ignores the formation or the establishment of a protective barrier for the patient. Learnings from safety as developed in industrial activities should be applied to healthcare. A clear example is the safety in all matters relating to air travel.[39]

From a non-health organisational perspective, Spear[40] indicates that hospitals are usually organised by functions. This type of organisation tends to lead to fragmentation and, therefore, to the creation of ambiguities. Ensuring their proper functioning requires a high degree of coordination. Therefore, concerns about clinical safety require the redesign of health systems. The issues around clinical safety are especially relevant in the case of HMV. This is a complex treatment (use of equipment, adaptation of the ventilator, changes in settings in relation to the evolution of the disease, etc.) delivered by various professionals with different degrees of involvement. It is a treatment that takes place beyond the direct control of clinicians and most of the time is supervised by informal caregivers.

During patient care in hospital and when we prepare the discharge plan, we can identify hotspots that could compromise safety.[41] Box 23.4 identifies some of these points.

The transfer of information or changes to the care team are very important elements for patient safety. A patient with a chronic disease can see up to 16 different medical specialists in a year.[42] The method of transferring information is crucial when it involves many professionals. Visits to the emergency services are another source of risk. Some patient associations have made recommendations for ventilator users when in the emergency department,[43] and these are summarised in Box 23.5.

Fatalities have been reported in patients receiving HMV due to electricity supply problems.[45,46] It is also well documented that patients sometimes change the settings of the ventilator, with no apparent clinical consequences. Farré et al.[47] showed that the percentage of patients with a discrepancy between the prescribed and actual measured main ventilator variable (minute ventilation or inspiratory pressure) was higher than 20% in 13% of the cases and higher than 30% in 4%. Clearly, HMV carries a risk, but zero risk does not exist even in ICUs, but as Simonds said,[48] the risk can be minimised by sharing clinical information, properly training patients and families and ensuring technical support at home.

In this context, it is easy to overlook some critical points in patient safety. The discharge process is one of these points. Neale et al.[49] reported that 10.8% of patients admitted to two large hospitals in Greater London experienced one or more adverse events (most of them preventable) and 18% of adverse events were related to the care at the time of discharge. These figures suggest that the discharge should not just be regarded as a bureaucratic procedure. The pressure

BOX 23.4: Risk associated situations related to patients on HMV

- Unplanned admission.
  - Long stay in the emergency department
  - Contact with professionals unfamiliar with HMV
  - Admission to an inappropriate ward
- Transfer (even in emergency circumstances) is a high-risk period:
  - From another acute care hospital
  - From a monitored setting (e.g. ICU) to general ward
  - Any nocturnal transfer
- Discharge during the weekend carries an added risk.
- Long hospital stays involve risk of infections, additional medication, disconnection with the usual environment and overload for the caregiver.

BOX 23.5: Recommendations for patients on HMV while attending the emergency department

- Provide all available information (clinical reports, ventilator settings) and identify the care team.
- Oxygen can be dangerous for unventilated patients with neuromuscular diseases.
- Anaesthesia may have added risks for patients with neuromuscular diseases.
  - Intubation may be difficult.
  - Avoid respiratory depressants, cough medications and opiates.
- Insist on being placed in the best position for their stay in the emergency department (in some cases, patients are better off in the wheelchair than on a trolley). In case of paralysis of the diaphragm, the patient should be placed in a seated or semi-seated position.
- The patient should be autonomous with regard to the equipment (ventilator, assisted cough devices, masks, etc.) until he or she is assured that the health centre can look after their specific needs. It is advisable to avoid hospital admission whenever possible.
- Collect all the data related to the care in the emergency department (or be assured that this information will be sent to the care team).

From AFMTElethon. Urgences médicales et maladies neuromusculaires. Janvier 2014. http:// www.afm-telethon.fr/sites/default/files /flipbooks/urgences_medicales_et _maladies_neuromusculaires_01_14/index.htm#/8 (accessed 24 September 24 2016.

for short stays (reasonable from the viewpoint of preventing risks to the patient and also to avoid unnecessary costs) generates another source of risk. Sometimes, when discharging the patient, clinicians do not have all the information of the procedures performed in the hospital and some of these results can be crucial. Wise et al.[6] observed that in 41% of patients, results become available after discharge and that 9% of these results will require immediate action. This fact highlights the need for improved communication between hospital and community health services.[50] Learning from complaints, especially if they relate to the organisation of care, is a good way to improve clinical safety.[51]

Finally, it should be noted that, in many cases, deterioration of the patient with HMV can be very subtle. Kripalani et al.[50] analysed home visits due to a suspected malfunction of the ventilator. In 13%, no abnormality was detected, but in half the cases, the patients did not feel well and were admitted to hospital and two patients died in the course of a month. Perhaps this shows the difficulties faced by patients (and health professionals) in identifying early, subtle changes that suggest a deterioration in lung function or in the general condition. Changes in clinical condition were misinterpreted as equipment malfunction. In short, to improve clinical safety, organised care is required to operate unambiguously, as is the continued reinforcement of the training given to patients and caregivers and maintaining a high index of suspicion for potential problems.

DISCHARGE PLANNING IN PALLIATIVE CARE

In some circumstances, the discharge plan is designed without a long-term view. This can happen when prescribing HMV in patients in the advanced stage of their disease. In the patient on long-term HMV, it is sometimes difficult to identify the final stage of the disease, especially in patients with neuromuscular diseases that progress slowly or restrictive respiratory diseases. Despite these difficulties, recognition of the end-of-life stages has a major impact on patients and caregivers[52] from the emotional, workload and economic viewpoints. In ALS, the problems associated with the end-of-life stage are more severe and occur more rapidly than in other patients on HMV.[53] There are situations in which clinical management is especially difficult, for example, in ALS patients intubated before the diagnosis is known.

In some cases, HMV could also be the only strategy to allow the return home of critically ill patients who cannot be disconnected from the ventilator. In these cases, we talk more about 'rescue ventilation' than HMV itself. Rady and Johnson showed that 15% of patients admitted to the ICU were more than 85 years old[54] and 35% of survivors could not return to their homes, requiring admission to a care facility at discharge (the percentage of patients is twice that of the younger patient group).

It can be difficult to provide an individualised prognosis for a COPD patient. Discharge plans for more severe COPD patients require careful identification of suitable candidates, a precise definition of the care needed and a realistic plan to ensure provision of that care.[55] In COPD, there is no accepted definition of 'final stage of the disease', so it is difficult to compare different studies.[56] Moreover, the use of a cancer model to predict the need for palliative care of COPD patients is unhelpful.[57] In addition, there are no clear criteria for identifying patients with COPD who might benefit from long-term HMV. In some cases, it is clear that HMV is 'rescue ventilation' rather than a formal indication of HMV.

Admission to a hospice (or a centre for chronic patients) is also an alternative in the final stages of life. It is very important to identify the limits of treatment,[58] especially in regard to artificial nutrition, readmission to hospital and resuscitation. These decisions should be written into the medical record. Discharge planning of older patients or patients on palliative care and HMV poses challenges different from those in patients with classic indications. In these cases, the comfort and return to the home are as important as survival. Moreover, in many cases, the return home can be very difficult and the patient may require temporary or permanent stay in an institution such as a hospice.

CONCLUSION

Any transition in healthcare is potentially a period of uncertainty. Discharge from hospital to home is one of the most important transitions for ventilator users. The discharge process is a key element in the healthcare continuum for most seriously ill patients, and it going well is crucial to allow safe independent living for ventilator users.

Teamwork is essential and it is imperative to include all services in the hospital and in the community. Because this integration is so complex, the role of a care coordinator is mandatory.

During the life of ventilator users, a lot of circumstances will arise that require an adaptation of treatment or changes in the home environment. Caregiver changes, shift to another house or intercurrent surgical procedures are examples of the need to adapt the patient to new unmet needs.

REFERENCES

1. Wee S-L, Vrijhoef HJM. A conceptual framework for evaluating the conceptualization, implementation and performance of transitional care programmes. *J Eval Clin Pract.* 2015;21:221–8.
2. Luján M, Moreno A, Veigas C et al. Non-invasive home mechanical ventilation: Effectiveness and efficiency of an outpatient initiation protocol compared with the standard in-hospital model. *Respir Med.* 2007;101:1177–82.
3. Chatwin M, Nickol AH, Morrell MJ et al. Randomised trial of inpatient versus outpatient initiation of home mechanical ventilation in patients with nocturnal hypoventilation. *Respir Med.* 2008;102:1528–35.
4. Bertoye MMA, Garin JP, Vincent P et al. Le retour à domicile des insuffisants respiratoires chroniques appareillés. *Lyon Méd.* 1965;38:389–410.
5. Fiorenza D, Vitacca M, Clini E. Home hospital monitoring, setting and training for home non invasive ventilation. *Monaldi Arch Chest Dis.* 2003;59:119–22.
6. Wise M, Hart N, Craig D et al. Home mechanical ventilation. *BMJ.* 2011;342:d1687. http://doi.org/10.1136/bmj.d1687.
7. American Association for Respiratory Care. Clinical practice guideline: Discharge planning of the respiratory care patient. *Respir Care.* 1995;40:1308–12.
8. Wagner EH. The role of patient care teams in chronic disease management. *BMJ.* 2000;320:569–72.
9. Finlayson MP, Raymont A. Teamwork—General practitioners and practice nurses working together in New Zealand. *J Prim Health Care.* 2012;4:150–5.
10. Escarrabill J, Goldberg A. Training the home health team. In: Ambrosino N, Goldstein R. *Ventilatory Support for Chronic Respiratory Failure.* Oxford: Informa Health Care, 2008.
11. Katzenbach JR, Smith DK. The discipline of teams. *HBR*, July–August 2005.
12. Aiken LH. Achieving an interdisciplinary workforce in health care. *N Engl J Med.* 2003;348:164–6.
13. Kutney-Lee A, McHugh MD, Sloane DM et al. Nursing: A key to patient satisfaction. *Health Aff (Millwood).* 2009;28:w669–77.
14. Warren ML, Jarrett C, Senegal R et al. An interdisciplinary approach to transitioning ventilator-dependent patients to home. *J Nurs Care Qual.* 2004;19:67–73.
15. Ballangrud R, Bogsti WB, Johansson IS. Clients' experiences of living at home with a mechanical ventilator. *J Adv Nurs.* 2009;65:425–34.
16. Crimi C, Noto A, Princi P et al. Domiciliary non-invasive ventilation in COPD: An international survey of indications and practices. *COPD.* 2015;13:483–90.
17. McDonald J, McKinlay E, Keeling S, Levack W. Becoming an expert carer: The process of family carers learning to manage technical health procedures at home. *J Adv Nurs.* 2016;72:2173–84.
18. Tearl DK, Cox TJ, Hertzog JH. Hospital discharge of respiratory-technology-dependent children: Role of a dedicated respiratory care discharge coordinator. *Respir Care.* 2006;51:744–9.
19. Rose L, Fowler RA, Fan E et al. Prolonged mechanical ventilation in Canadian intensive care units: A national survey. *J Crit Care.* 2015;30:25–31.
20. MacIntyre NR, Epstein SK, Scheinhorn D et al. Management of patients requiring prolonged mechanical ventilation: Report of a NAMDRC consensus conference. *Chest.* 2005;128:3937–54.
21. White AC, O'Connor HH, Kirby K. Prolonged mechanical ventilation: Review of care settings and an update on professional reimbursement. *Chest.* 2008;133:539–45.
22. Lone NI, Walsh TS. Prolonged mechanical ventilation in critically ill patients: Epidemiology, outcomes and modelling the potential cost consequences of establishing a regional weaning unit. *Crit Care.* 2011;15:R102.
23. Carpenè N, Vagheggini G, Panait E, Gabbrielli L, Ambrosino N. A proposal of a new model for long-term weaning: Respiratory intensive care unit and weaning center. *Resp Med.* 2010;104:1505–11.
24. Unroe M, Kahn JM, Carson SS et al. One-year trajectories of care and resource utilization for recipients of prolonged mechanical ventilation: A cohort study. *Ann Internal Med.* 2010;153:167–75.
25. Association Lyonnaise de Logistique Posthospitalière. Available at: www.allp-sante.com/ (accessed 26 September 2016).
26. Farrero E, Prats E, Povedano M et al. Survival in amyotrophic lateral sclerosis with home mechanical ventilation: The impact of systematic respiratory assessment and bulbar involvement. *Chest.* 2007;127:2132–8.

27. Mitsumoto H, Rabkin JG. Palliative care for patients with amyotrophic lateral sclerosis: 'Prepare for the worst and hope for the best'. *JAMA*. 2007;298:207–16.
28. Traynor BJ, Alexander M, Corr B et al. Effect of a multidisciplinary amyotrophic lateral sclerosis (ALS) clinic on ALS survival: A population based study, 1996–2000. *J Neurol Neurosurg Psych*. 2003;74:1258–61.
29. Zoccolella S, Beghi E, Palagano G et al. ALS multidisciplinary clinic and survival. Results from a population-based study in Southern Italy. *J Neurol*. 2007;254:1107–12.
30. Lloyd-Owen SJ, Donaldson GC, Ambrosino N et al. Patterns of home mechanical ventilation use in Europe: Results from the Eurovent survey. *Eur Respir J*. 2005;25:1025–31.
31. Escarrabill J. Health care support for home mechanical ventilation: Networking versus centralization. *Arch Bronconeumol*. 2007;43:527–9.
32. Hendy J, Chrysanthaki T, Barlow J et al. An organisational analysis of the implementation of telecare and telehealth: The whole systems demonstrator. *BMC Health Services Res*. 2012;12:403.
33. Rose L, McKim DA, Katz SL et al. Home mechanical ventilation in Canada: A national survey. *Respir Care*. 2015;60(5):695–704.
34. Chatwin M, Hawkins G, Panicchia L et al. Randomised crossover trial of telemonitoring in chronic respiratory patients (TeleCRAFT trial). *Thorax*. 2016;71:305–11.
35. Ambrosino N, Vitacca M, Dreher M et al. Telemonitoring of ventilator-dependent patients: A European Respiratory Society Statement. *Eur Respir J*. 2016 Jul 7. pii: ERJ-01721-2015. doi: 10.1183/13993003.01721-2015.
36. Vitacca M. Telemonitoring in patients with chronic respiratory insufficiency: Expectations deluded? *Thorax*. 2016;71:299–301.
37. Leasa D. Elson S. Building a comprehensive system of services to support adults living with long-term mechanical ventilation. *Can Respir J*. 2016 (doi: 10.1155/2016/318538). http://doi.org/10.1155/2016/3185389
38. Institute of Medicine. *To Err Is Human. Building a Safer Health System*. Washington: National Academy Press, 2000.
39. Pronovost PJ, Goeschel CA, Olsen KL et al. Reducing health care hazards: Lessons from the commercial aviation safety team. *Health Aff (Millwood)*. 2009;28:w479–89.
40. Spear SJ. Fixing health care from the inside, today. *HBR*, September 2005.
41. Forster AJ, Asmis TR, Clark HD et al. Ottawa Hospital Patient Safety Study: Incidence and timing of adverse events in patients admitted to a Canadian teaching hospital. *CMAJ*. 2004;170:1235–40.
42. Pham HH, Schrag D, O'Malley AS et al. Care patterns in Medicare and their implications for pay for performance. *N Engl J Med*. 2007;356:1130–9.
43. International Ventilation Users Network. Home ventilator user's emergency preparation checklist. Available at: www.ventusers.org/vume/HomeVentuserChecklist.pdf (accessed 29 September 2009).
44. AFM-TElethon. Urgences médicales et maladies neuromusculaires. Janvier 2014. http://www.afm-telethon.fr/sites/default/files/flipbooks/urgences_medicales_et_maladies_neuromusculaires_01_14/index.htm#/8 (accessed 24 September 24 2016).
45. Lechtzin N, Weiner CM, Clawson L. A fatal complication of noninvasive ventilation. *N Engl J Med*. 2001;344:533.
46. Towlson S. Power cut kills man on home ventilator. *The Times*, 14 August 2000.
47. Farré R, Navajas D, Prats E et al. Performance of mechanical ventilators at the patient's home: A multicentre quality control study. *Thorax*. 2006;61:400–4.
48. Simonds AK. Risk management of the home ventilator dependent patient. *Thorax*. 2006; 61:369–71.
49. Neale G, Woloshynowych M, Vincent C. Exploring the causes of adverse events in NHS hospital practice. *J R Soc Med*. 2001;94:322–30.
50. Kripalani S, LeFevre F, Phillips CO et al. Deficits in communication and information transfer between hospital-based and primary care physicians: Implications for patient safety and continuity of care. *JAMA*. 2007;297:831–41.
51. Vincent C, Davy C, Esmail A et al. Learning from litigation. The role of claims analysis in patient safety. *J Eval Clin Pract*. 2006;12:665–74.
52. Vitacca M, Grassi M, Barbano L et al. Last 3 months of life in home-ventilated patients: The family perception. *Eur Respir J*. 2010;35:1064–71.
53. Laub M, Midgren B. Survival of patients on home mechanical ventilation: A nationwide prospective study. *Respir Med*. 2007;101:1074–8.
54. Rady MY, Johnson DJ. Hospital discharge to care facility: A patient-centered outcome for the evaluation of intensive care for octogenarians. *Chest*. 2004;126:1583–91.
55. Escarrabill J. Discharge planning and home care for end-stage COPD patients. *Eur Respir J*. 2009;34:507–12.
56. Habraken JM, Willems DL, de Kort SJ et al. Health care needs in end-stage COPD: A structured literature review. *Patient Educ Couns*. 2007;68:121–30.
57. Simonds AK. Living and dying with respiratory failure: Facilitating decision making. *Chron Respir Dis*. 2004;1:56–9.
58. Creechan T. Combining mechanical ventilation with hospice care in the home: Death with dignity. *Crit Care Nurs*. 2000;20:49–53.

24

Monitoring during sleep during chronic non-invasive ventilation

JEAN-PAUL JANSSENS,* JEAN-CHRISTIAN BOREL, DAN ADLER AND JEAN-LOUIS PÉPIN

INTRODUCTION

Long-term domiciliary non-invasive ventilation (NIV) in patients with chronic hypercapnic respiratory failure (CHRF) aims to normalise arterial blood gases (ABGs) and improve symptoms related to CHRF, health-related quality of life (HRQL) and survival.

NIV is most often used during sleep and thus must be monitored at night. Because patient–ventilator interactions and chronic respiratory failure are dynamic processes, regular monitoring of NIV is necessary not only when initiating NIV, but also during follow-up to ensure that NIV reaches predefined goals (ABG, nocturnal SpO_2, correction of nocturnal hypoventilation), that nocturnal respiratory events related to upper airway instability and/or variations in ventilatory command are controlled, that compliance is satisfactory, that leaks are minimal and that patient comfort is ensured.

Two recent developments may have an important influence on future management of patients under chronic NIV: (1) the rapidly increasing availability of telemonitoring, strongly promoted by ventilator manufacturers, derived from experience related to the management of continuous positive airway pressure (CPAP) in sleep-disordered breathing (SDB), and allowing not only a longitudinal assessment of relevant parameters but also the possibility of a remote adjustment of ventilator settings, and (2) recent data supporting the idea that daily use of ventilator and changes in patterns of parameters recorded by built-in software of ventilators may be associated with clinical exacerbations.[1,2]

The following chapter will detail tools available for monitoring patients using home bi-level pressure support or multimodal home ventilators and suggest a practical algorithm (Figure 24.1).

MONITORING NIV: THE BASICS

The minimal requirement for assessing the efficacy of NIV is measuring daytime ABG and nocturnal oxygen saturation (SpO_2). ABG can be measured either by puncture of the radial artery or by arterialised capillary blood analysis, which can be less painful and easier to perform in some patients, with a possible underestimation of PaO_2, but reliable values of $PaCO_2$.[3,4] Correction of nocturnal SpO_2 is mandatory to prevent progression of pulmonary hypertension and cor pulmonale. Patterns of desaturation may suggest different physiological mechanisms (central or obstructive events, hypoventilation), but are never specific.

DETECTING AND QUANTIFYING NOCTURNAL HYPOVENTILATION

Relying on daytime ABG and nocturnal pulse oximetry alone has been shown to underestimate the presence of nocturnal hypoventilation (defined as a mean nocturnal $PtcCO_2$ $\geq$ 50 mmHg).[5] Two non-invasive tools for assessing nocturnal arterial carbon dioxide (CO_2) tension have been studied in NIV: Peak expired CO_2 ($P_{ET}CO_2$) and transcutaneous measurement of CO_2. $P_{ET}CO_2$ measurements are considered unreliable for nocturnal monitoring of NIV patients with parenchymal or airway diseases. Indeed, the [$PaCO_2$ – $P_{ET}CO_2$] gradient varies according to the physiological dead space (VD and VD/V_T ratio), and to heterogeneity of alveolar ventilation. It is also technically difficult to measure because of the continuous flow through the mask related to bi-level pressure support and thus not recommended.[6]

Transcutaneous measurement of CO_2 ($PtcCO_2$) was developed in the early 1950s: the Severinghaus electrode on which $PtcCO_2$ measurements rely has three components: (1) the collar

* On behalf of the SomnoNIV group.

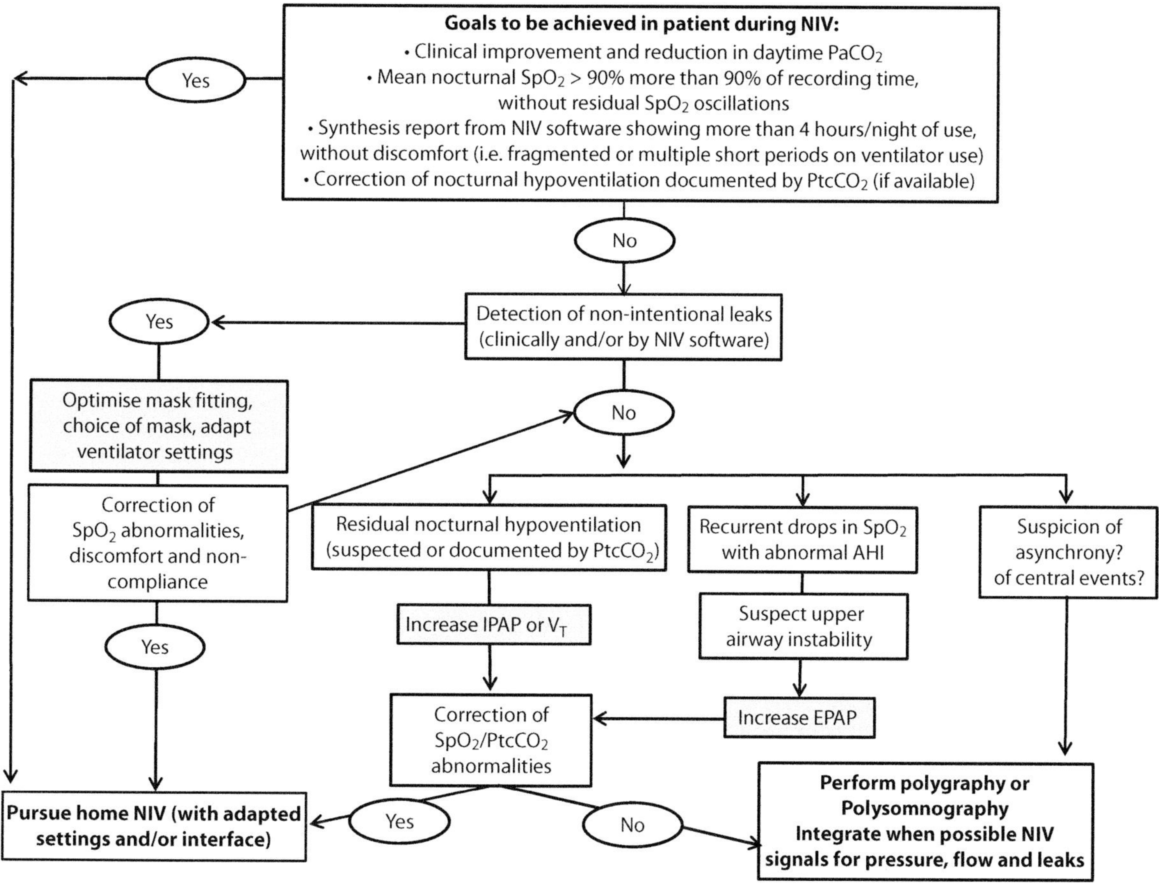

Figure 24.1 Proposed algorithm for monitoring of home NIV. See text for further details. $PtcCO_2$, transcutaneous carbon dioxide partial pressure; SpO_2, oxygen saturation by pulse oximetry.

of the sensor heats the skin to increase local perfusion, 'arterialise' capillary blood, and increase skin permeability to gas diffusion; (2) a pH-sensitive glass electrode, a buffer solution, and (3) a reference silver/silver chloride electrode. Basically, the sensor reacts to changes in pH of the buffer solution induced by CO_2 diffusing through the skin (CO_2 reacts with water to form H_2CO_3, which, in turn, dissociates into H^+ and HCO_3^-).[7] At a temperature of 42°C–43°C, $PtcCO_2$ measurements allow continuous overnight recordings with minimal drift and good agreement with $PaCO_2$ values.[8–11] Recent devices do not require recalibration during recordings and have improved software, as well as compatibility with certain polygraphy (PG) devices. The largest study performed on the reliability of $PtcCO_2$ overnight recordings in long-term NIV included 67 patients under NIV for CHRF related to restrictive lung disorders.[12] The authors found a low [$PaCO_2$/$PtcCO_2$] bias when comparing arterial and transcutaneous measurements (0.23 ± 0.28 kPa): none of the paired samples differed by more than 1 kPa. Mean overnight drift (assessed by comparing morning and evening readings of a calibration gas) was 0.14 ± 0.54 kPa, with three samples having a drift >1 kPa. Another clinical trial reported a similar bias but slightly wider limits of agreement, testing three different $PtcCO_2$ devices.[11]

However, $PtcCO_2$ devices have limitations. Several conditions may impair the reliability of $PtcCO_2$ readings: skin vasoconstriction, vasopressor treatment, haemodynamic instability, acidaemia, unstable clinical situations and low probe temperatures all increase [$PaCO_2$/$PtcCO_2$] bias and limits of agreement to a point where $PtcCO_2$ becomes unreliable.[12,13] In stable patients under NIV, higher $PaCO_2$ values tend to increase [$PaCO_2$/$PtcCO_2$] bias.[8] A lag time of 1–3 min limits detection of rapid changes in $PaCO_2$.[14] There are three other noteworthy limitations to use of $PtcCO_2$: (1) the occurrence of occasional unexplained errant values, which can be confusing for the clinician; (2) the importance of an experienced team when using $PtcCO_2$ and, conversely, the high rate of failures or poor-quality recordings when the device is used by inexperienced personnel; (3) the price and fragility of the devices. Visual inspection of the overnight graphic display is helpful for the detection of unreliable recordings.[6,12] Taking into account these important caveats, $PtcCO_2$ is a very useful technique for quantifying nocturnal $PaCO_2$ in stable patients under NIV; it is most often reliable in experienced hands, with a minimal drift.

DATA PROVIDED BY SOFTWARE OF HOME VENTILATORS

Most home ventilators provide longitudinal information regarding items such as compliance, ventilator performance (pressure, tidal volume [V_T], estimated minute ventilation [VE], percentage of respiratory cycles triggered and cycled by the ventilator), leaks and respiratory rate (RR). They may also estimate respiratory events related to upper airway or respiratory drive instability, providing indices of number of apnoeas and hypopnoeas per hour, and for some devices, further classifying these events as central or obstructive. Detailed (cycle by cycle) analysis of flow and pressure signals is also available with most software.

Compliance

Medical history is often unreliable to assess compliance, and thus recorded data from the ventilator are helpful to quantify precisely average daily use, variability of use over time and patterns of ventilator use (continuous vs. fragmented), which may suggest patient discomfort or impact of medication (i.e. diuretics).[15]

Estimated tidal volume and minute ventilation

Ventilator settings usually target a tidal volume of 8–10 mL/kg of ideal body weight in CHRF, and thus V_T is an important parameter for adjusting pressure support.[16] However, accuracy of estimated V_T has been shown to be highly variable from one device to another and to be influenced by leaks. Two bench studies have shown that V_T tends to be underestimated by ventilator software, with differences that can be substantial (range of bias between ventilator estimation and measured leaks: 66–236 mL, with only 2/7 devices having a bias <100 mL).[17,18] Clinicians must therefore consider this parameter as possibly unreliable. A high variability of V_T on graphic display may suggest leaks or, if the pattern is consistent, periodic breathing. Estimated VE is subject to the same limitations as VT.

Respiratory rate

Several home ventilator software provide mean and/or median RR (with 5th and 95th centiles) as well as percentage of 'controlled' respiratory cycles. Ventilator backup rate is often set approximately two cycles below the patient's spontaneous RR, although in certain indications (i.e. neuromuscular disorders), it is common practice to 'capture' the patient's RR and thus simulate a controlled mode. American Academy of Sleep Medicine (AASM) guidelines recommend the use of a spontaneous mode unless the patient presents central events with this setting.[19] However, the impact of backup RR on respiratory events in patients with obesity hypoventilation syndrome (OHS) has been studied by Contal et al.: the absence of backup rate increased central apnoeas or hypopnoeas, whereas a backup RR close to or slightly above the patients' RR stabilised both upper airway and respiratory drive.[20] Reliability of RR provided by the ventilator may be compromised by leaks or respiratory events that hinder detection of inspiratory efforts by the ventilator (i.e. upper airway closure): in this case, percentage of cycles triggered by the patient as reported by the device may be underestimated. Similarly, unrewarded efforts related to intrinsic positive end-expiratory pressure in COPD may be associated with a decrease in triggered cycles and a paradoxically low RR provided by the software.[21]

Ventilator software also often provides the percentage of respiratory cycles cycled by the device (or patient). Practical implications of this parameter is not yet fully clarified: for instance, a high percentage of cycling by the patient may be an index of patient–ventilator synchrony; conversely, a low percentage of cycling by the patient may be indicative of leaks, upper airway obstruction or patient–ventilator asynchrony. This information must be integrated with other available parameters.

Leaks

Leaks are a major problem in NIV and are always present to some extent. They can compromise efficacy of NIV, disrupt sleep and result in patient–ventilator asynchrony.[22] Reporting of estimated leaks varies from one device to another, which can be confusing for the clinician: data may indicate either total leaks or unintentional leaks (i.e. after subtracting intentional leaks associated with expiratory valve).[17] Furthermore, leaks may be averaged over the whole respiratory cycle or only during the expiratory phase. Finally, averaging of leaks may underreport short bursts of important leaks, causing patient discomfort, although not appearing in the 'synthesis report'. Rabec et al. showed, with one specific home ventilator, an excellent agreement between estimated leaks and bench test values.[23] Another bench test study showed that biases and limits of agreement for leaks varied substantially between devices for home NIV; also, bias for leaks increased with importance of leaks in some devices.[17] Many software report a threshold value of 24 L/min as a lower threshold for significant unintentional leaks: this value, first mentioned by Teschler et al. in a study on mouth leaks in NIV,[22] is arbitrary, has no demonstrated significance per se and has not been reevaluated for recent devices with high pressurisation capacities: leaks are a problem only if they cause patient discomfort, desaturations or patient–ventilator asynchrony.

Apnoea–hypopnoea indices

Undesired respiratory events may occur under NIV: among these are decreases or interruption of respiratory flow with upper airway obstruction and persistence of ventilatory command (i.e. obstructive apnoeas and hypopnoeas) or decreases or interruption of respiratory flow with simultaneous reduction or interruption of respiratory command (i.e. central apnoeas and hypopnoeas).[24] There are a certain number of uncertainties related to the definitions of these respiratory events used by manufacturers and thus as to the relevance of apnoea–hypopnoea index (AHI) values reported. Differentiating central from obstructive events relies on estimation of upper airway resistance either by the forced oscillation technique or by flow curve analysis. Bench tests in CPAP devices have shown to what extent events can be misclassified by either technique. For physicians following patients with CPAP for SDB, relying on AI, HI and AHI provided by home devices is common practice despite the few independent reports of the reliability of this information. In fact, an ATS consensus publication stated that, in obstructive sleep apnoea syndrome, CPAP devices estimated apnoeas and hypopnoeas using different algorithms according to the manufacturer, all definitions being different from AASM consensus definitions.[25] Available studies for CPAP showed good agreement between devices and PSG for AI, but lower agreement for HI.[26–31]

For NIV devices, there is very little information on the reliability of data provided by ventilator software. A pragmatic study compared AHI provided by ventilator software to AHI measured by polysomnography (PSG) in patients with OHS ($n = 10$, 27 paired tracings).[32] Correlation between ventilator and PSG was high ($r^2 = 0.89$, $p < 0.001$); furthermore, a threshold value of 10 for AHI correctly classified patients under NIV with a sensitivity of 90.9%, a specificity of 100%, and a negative predictive value of 71.4%.

Estimation of AHI may vary according to devices, and leaks, and requires further validation.

Flow and pressure tracings (coupled with SpO_2)

Ventilator software of most home ventilators allows a detailed graphic analysis of pressure and flow curves, which can be coupled with tidal volume, leaks and pulse oximetry (SpO_2). This analysis can be very helpful for analysing recurrent or prolonged drops in SpO_2, although determining a definite cause may be difficult without any indication of inspiratory effort (i.e. oesophageal pressure, pulse transit time [PTT] and—with limitations—thoracic and abdominal belts). Some software include a graphic code to distinguish controlled versus triggered breaths. Detailed analysis of these curves can clarify the temporal relationship between drops in SpO_2 and leaks for instance. Unrewarded inspiratory efforts, upper airway instability, double triggering and auto-triggering can also be detected through these graphs.

HEALTH-RELATED QUALITY OF LIFE (HRQL)

Improving HRQL is a major goal of NIV in CHRF. However, correlation between physiological parameters commonly used to monitor chronic respiratory failure and HRQL is poor. Therefore, the use of valid and reliable instruments to assess HRQL is of importance, although still not routine practice for respiratory physicians. Most generic (i.e. SF-36, Nottingham Health Profile) or condition-specific (Chronic Respiratory Questionnaire [CRQ]; St George Respiratory Questionnaire [SGRQ]; Severe Respiratory Insufficiency Questionnaire [SRI]; Maugeri Respiratory Failure Questionnaire [MRF-28/MRF-26]) are designed for study purposes, and not for longitudinal use in individuals.[33] Furthermore, generic questionnaires (i.e. SF-36) may not be appropriate to assess the impact of disease in patients treated with NIV, whereas condition-specific questionnaires such as MRF-28[34] and The Severe Respiratory Insufficiency (SRI)[35] questionnaire are specifically designed for measuring HRQL in patients with CRF (with or without NIV). Such questionnaires are sensitive to changes induced by treatment. Responsiveness of the SRI to changes induced by introduction of NIV is superior to that of the SF-36.[36] Broader use of such questionnaires may be limited by their length and the need to recode many items in order to compute a final score. There are ongoing efforts to develop shorter questionnaires and to provide reference norms in a population of NIV patients to facilitate the wider use of such tools by clinicians. Symptom scores or short technical questionnaires may be of help to identify specific problems and side effects related to NIV, which should be sought for in all follow-up visits.[37]

COMPLEX ASSESSMENTS SUCH AS NOCTURNAL VENTILATORY POLYGRAPHY (PG) OR POLYSOMNOGRAPHY (PSG) UNDER NIV

AASM guidelines recommend the use of PSG for titrating and following NIV, although, in most countries, this is not technically and/or financially feasible.[19] The SomnoNIV group proposed a more restrictive algorithm for monitoring NIV during sleep (Figure 24.1).[6] According to this approach, use of ventilatory PG or PSG should be limited to patients in whom empirical adjustments for leaks, upper airway instability or persistent nocturnal hypoventilation have failed. Whenever possible, PG or PSG should include tracings provided by the ventilator for leaks, pressure and flow, coupled to an external pneumo-tachograph, and ideally, $PtcCO_2$. Events occurring under NIV (either insufficiently corrected or resulting from NIV) have been extensively described.[24,38] Basically, these events fall into the following categories:

- Decrease or interruption of respiratory flow with simultaneous decrease or interruption of ventilatory command (i.e. central apnoea or hypopnoea)[39–41]
- Decrease or interruption of respiratory flow with persistence of ventilatory command (i.e. upper airway instability)
- Patient–ventilator asynchrony: includes events such as double triggering, auto-triggering, delayed triggering, unrewarded inspiratory efforts, total patient–ventilator uncoupling (dissociation), premature or delayed cycling[42]

PG, while providing very useful information as to the physiological process causing the undesired respiratory event, does not allow assessment of sleep structure. Surrogate markers of microarousals—autonomic activations detected by pulse wave amplitude (PWA) reductions ≥30%—have been compared to PSG as possible markers of sleep fragmentation under NIV: PWA had a sensitivity of 83% and a positive predictive value of 81% but a specificity of only 47% for detecting microarousals related to respiratory events.[43]

With both PG and PSG, distinction between central and obstructive events may be challenging. This is often the case in neuromuscular disorders, in which detection of inspiratory effort may be difficult. Markers of respiratory effort are sometimes mandatory to be sure to appropriately identify the underlying physiological process. Gold standard tools for the detection and quantification of inspiratory effort are oesophageal pressure (invasive and source of patient discomfort) and electroneuromyography (strongly dependent on expertise of investigators). PTT parallels changes in oesophageal pressure and reflects unloading of inspiratory effort by NIV as well as increases in inspiratory muscle effort induced by leaks. Analysis of PTT during PG or PSG under NIV is a promising tool for distinguishing between central and obstructive events in this setting: choice of software is however critical, and use of PTT requires validation in different groups of patients.[44] More recently, assessment of mandibular movements has been suggested as a reliable marker of respiratory effort during sleep.[45] Mandibular movements can be assessed using two magnetic sensors that measure the distance between two parallel coupled resonant circuits placed on the forehead and on the chin of the patient (one transmitter; one receiver). The transmitter generates a pulsed magnetic wave. The change in the magnetic field recorded by the receiver is inversely related to the cube of the distance between the chin and forehead probe. Analysis of mandibular movements has been developed for the scoring of apnoea or hypopnoea,[46] sleep/wake phases[47] and microarousals.[48] A recent version of a type 3 polygraph (SomnoHolter, Nomics, Liege, Belgium) has been specifically developed to easily monitor patients under NIV (or CPAP) and offers the possibility to simultaneously analyse mandibular behaviour and leaks.[49] This information might be of interest not only to detect leaks but also to choose the most appropriate mask.

Although these non-invasive markers of respiratory effort are helpful for interpreting PG, new automated ventilator modes (adaptive servo-ventilation [ASV], auto-titrating EPAP and pressure support) increase considerably the difficulty of interpretation of PG and PSG under NIV and require specific expertise in ventilator algorithms: adaptive changes in pressure support tend to confuse the analysis either because they mask the underlying event (such as in central hypopnoea and ASV) or because changes in ventilator settings are not the consequence but the cause of the undesired respiratory events.

CONCLUSION: A SYSTEMATIC APPROACH TO MONITORING OF CHRONIC NIV FOR CHRF

Assessment should systematically include a targeted medical history, a standardised questionnaire for ventilator-related symptoms and sleepiness (i.e. Epworth Sleepiness Scale), daytime ABGs without NIV, nocturnal pulse oximetry and the 'synthesis report' from ventilator software (Figure 24.1) with a focus on compliance, pattern of ventilator use, leaks and AHI.[6] Use of $PtcCO_2$ recordings should be standard procedure but depends on availability, which is highly variable, mainly because of high costs. Detailed inspection of cycle-by-cycle tracings provided by ventilator software may also be helpful to detect upper airway instability or central events. When leaks are detected or strongly suspected, their correction is a priority. Requirements for PG or PSG according to this approach are limited to situations in which initial assessment and empirical adjustments for leaks, upper airway instability or residual hypoventilation did not suffice. This pragmatic approach differs from that suggested by the AASM mainly because—albeit for a few expert centres—availability of systematic PSG for NIV titration or monitoring is much lower in most European countries than in the United States.

The increasing interest in telemonitoring for chronic NIV requires careful evaluation of cost–benefit ratio and management strategies, because of the considerable burden that data provided may represent for clinicians and healthcare providers.

REFERENCES

1. Borel JC, Pelletier J, Taleux N et al. Parameters recorded by software of non-invasive ventilators predict COPD exacerbation: A proof-of-concept study. *Thorax*. 2015 Mar;70(3):284–5.
2. Borel JC, Pepin JL, Pison C et al. Long-term adherence with non-invasive ventilation improves prognosis in obese COPD patients. *Respirology*. 2014 Aug;19(6):857–65.
3. Hollier CA, Maxwell LJ, Harmer AR et al. Validity of arterialised-venous PCO_2, pH and bicarbonate in obesity hypoventilation syndrome. *Respir Physiol Neurobiol*. 2013 Aug 15;188(2):165–71.
4. Sauty A, Uldry C, Debetaz LF et al. Differences in PO_2 and PCO_2 between arterial and arterialized earlobe samples. *Eur Respir J*. 1996 Feb;9(2):186–9.
5. Georges M, Nguyen-Baranoff D, Griffon L et al. Usefulness of transcutaneous PCO_2 to assess nocturnal hypoventilation in restrictive lung disorders. *Respirology*. 2016 May 17.
6. Janssens JP, Borel JC, Pepin JL. Nocturnal monitoring of home non-invasive ventilation: The contribution of simple tools such as pulse oximetry, capnography, built-in ventilator software and autonomic markers of sleep fragmentation. *Thorax*. 2011 May;66(5):438–45.
7. Severinghaus J. Transcutaneous blood gas analysis. *Respir Care*. 1982;27:152–9.
8. Cuvelier A, Grigoriu B, Molano LC, Muir JF. Limitations of transcutaneous carbon dioxide measurements for assessing long-term mechanical ventilation. *Chest*. 2005 May;127(5):1744–8.

9. Hazenberg A, Zijlstra JG, Kerstjens HA, Wijkstra PJ. Validation of a transcutaneous CO_2 monitor in adult patients with chronic respiratory failure. *Respiration.* 2011;81(3):242–6.
10. Janssens JP, Perrin E, Bennani I et al. Is continuous transcutaneous monitoring of PCO_2 ($TcPCO_2$) over 8 h reliable in adults? *Respir Med.* 2001 May;95(5):331–5.
11. Storre JH, Magnet FS, Dreher M, Windisch W. Transcutaneous monitoring as a replacement for arterial PCO_2 monitoring during nocturnal non-invasive ventilation. *Respir Med.* 2011 Jan;105(1):143–50.
12. Aarrestad S, Tollefsen E, Kleiven AL et al. Validity of transcutaneous PCO_2 in monitoring chronic hypoventilation treated with non-invasive ventilation. *Respir Med.* 2016 Mar;112:112–8.
13. Bendjelid K, Schutz N, Stotz M et al. Transcutaneous PCO_2 monitoring in critically ill adults: Clinical evaluation of a new sensor. *Crit Care Med.* 2005 Oct;33(10):2203–6.
14. Janssens JP, Howarth-Frey C, Chevrolet JC et al. Transcutaneous PCO_2 to monitor noninvasive mechanical ventilation in adults: Assessment of a new transcutaneous PCO_2 device. *Chest.* 1998 Mar;113(3):768–73.
15. Pasquina P, Adler D, Farr P et al. What does built-in software of home ventilators tell us? An observational study of 150 patients on home ventilation. *Respiration.* 2012;83(4):293–9.
16. Pepin JL, Timsit JF, Tamisier R et al. Prevention and care of respiratory failure in obese patients. *Lancet Respir Med.* 2016 May;4(5):407–18.
17. Contal O, Vignaux L, Combescure C et al. Monitoring of noninvasive ventilation by built-in software of home bilevel ventilators: A bench study. *Chest.* 2012 Feb;141(2):469–76.
18. Lujan M, Sogo A, Pomares X et al. Effect of leak and breathing pattern on the accuracy of tidal volume estimation by commercial home ventilators: A bench study. *Respir Care.* 2013 May;58(5):770–7.
19. Berry RB, Chediak A, Brown LK et al. Best clinical practices for the sleep center adjustment of noninvasive positive pressure ventilation (NPPV) in stable chronic alveolar hypoventilation syndromes. *J Clin Sleep Med.* 2010 Oct 15;6(5):491–509.
20. Contal O, Adler D, Borel JC et al. Impact of different backup respiratory rates on the efficacy of noninvasive positive pressure ventilation in obesity hypoventilation syndrome: A randomized trial. *Chest.* 2013 Jan;143(1):37–46.
21. Adler D, Perrig S, Takahashi H et al. Polysomnography in stable COPD under non-invasive ventilation to reduce patient–ventilator asynchrony and morning breathlessness. *Sleep Breath.* 2012 Dec;16(4):1081–90.
22. Teschler H, Stampa J, Ragette R et al. Effect of mouth leak on effectiveness of nasal bilevel ventilatory assistance and sleep architecture. *Eur Respir J.* 1999 Dec;14(6):1251–7.
23. Rabec C, Georges M, Kabeya NK et al. Evaluating noninvasive ventilation using a monitoring system coupled to a ventilator: A bench-to-bedside study. *Eur Respir J.* 2009 Oct;34(4):902–13.
24. Gonzalez-Bermejo J, Perrin C, Janssens JP et al. Proposal for a systematic analysis of polygraphy or polysomnography for identifying and +scoring abnormal events occurring during non-invasive ventilation. *Thorax.* 2012 Jun;67(6):546–52.
25. Schwab RJ, Badr SM, Epstein LJ et al. An official American Thoracic Society statement: Continuous positive airway pressure adherence tracking systems. The optimal monitoring strategies and outcome measures in adults. *Am J Respir Crit Care Med.* 2013 Sep 1;188(5):613–20.
26. Berry RB, Kushida CA, Kryger MH et al. Respiratory event detection by a positive airway pressure device. *Sleep.* 2012 Mar;35(3):361–7.
27. Cilli A, Uzun R, Bilge U. The accuracy of autotitrating CPAP-determined residual apnea-hypopnea index. *Sleep Breath.* 2013 Mar;17(1):189–93.
28. Desai H, Patel A, Patel P et al. Accuracy of autotitrating CPAP to estimate the residual Apnea-Hypopnea Index in patients with obstructive sleep apnea on treatment with autotitrating CPAP. *Sleep Breath.* 2009 Nov;13(4):383–90.
29. Ikeda Y, Kasai T, Kawana F et al. Comparison between the apnea-hypopnea indices determined by the REMstar Auto M series and those determined by standard in-laboratory polysomnography in patients with obstructive sleep apnea. *Intern Med.* 2012;51(20):2877–85.
30. Prasad B, Carley DW, Herdegen JJ. Continuous positive airway pressure device-based automated detection of obstructive sleep apnea compared to standard laboratory polysomnography. *Sleep Breath.* 2010 Jun;14(2):101–7.
31. Ueno K, Kasai T, Brewer G et al. Evaluation of the apnea-hypopnea index determined by the S8 auto-CPAP, a continuous positive airway pressure device, in patients with obstructive sleep apnea-hypopnea syndrome. *J Clin Sleep Med.* 2010 Apr 15;6(2):146–51.
32. Georges M, Adler D, Contal O et al. Reliability of apnea-hypopnea index measured by a home bi-level pressure support ventilator versus a polysomnographic assessment. *Respir Care.* 2015 Jul;60(7):1051–6.
33. Janssens JP. When and how to assess quality of life in chronic lung disease. *Swiss Med Wkly.* 2001 Nov 10;131(43–4):623–9.
34. Carone M, Bertolotti G, Anchisi F et al. Analysis of factors that characterize health impairment in patients with chronic respiratory failure. Quality of Life in Chronic Respiratory Failure Group. *Eur Respir J.* 1999 Jun;13(6):1293–300.

35. Windisch W, Freidel K, Schucher B et al. The Severe Respiratory Insufficiency (SRI) Questionnaire: A specific measure of health-related quality of life in patients receiving home mechanical ventilation. *J Clin Epidemiol.* 2003 Aug;56(8):752–9.
36. Windisch W. Impact of home mechanical ventilation on health-related quality of life. *Eur Respir J.* 2008 Nov;32(5):1328–36.
37. Janssens JP, Metzger M, Sforza E. Impact of volume targeting on efficacy of bi-level non-invasive ventilation and sleep in obesity-hypoventilation. *Respir Med.* 2009 Feb;103(2):165–72.
38. Rabec C, Rodenstein D, Leger P et al. Ventilator modes and settings during non-invasive ventilation: Effects on respiratory events and implications for their identification. *Thorax.* 2011 Feb;66(2):170–8.
39. Jounieaux V, Aubert G, Dury M et al. Effects of nasal positive-pressure hyperventilation on the glottis in normal sleeping subjects. *J Appl Physiol.* 1995 Jul;79(1):186–93.
40. Parreira VF, Delguste P, Jounieaux V et al. Glottic aperture and effective minute ventilation during nasal two-level positive pressure ventilation in spontaneous mode. *Am J Respir Crit Care Med.* 1996 Dec;154(6 Pt 1):1857–63.
41. Parreira VF, Jounieaux V, Aubert G et al. Nasal two-level positive-pressure ventilation in normal subjects. Effects of the glottis and ventilation. *Am J Respir Crit Care Med.* 1996 May;153(5):1616–23.
42. Vignaux L, Vargas F, Roeseler J et al. Patient–ventilator asynchrony during non-invasive ventilation for acute respiratory failure: A multicenter study. *Intensive Care Med.* 2009 May;35(5):840–6.
43. Adler D, Bridevaux PO, Contal O et al. Pulse wave amplitude reduction: A surrogate marker of micro-arousals associated with respiratory events occurring under non-invasive ventilation? *Respir Med.* 2013 Dec;107(12):2053–60.
44. Contal O, Carnevale C, Borel JC et al. Pulse transit time as a measure of respiratory effort under noninvasive ventilation. *Eur Respir J.* 2013 Feb;41(2):346–53.
45. Martinot JB, Senny F, Denison S et al. Mandibular movements identify respiratory effort in pediatric obstructive sleep apnea. *J Clin Sleep Med.* 2015 May;11(5):567–74.
46. Senny F, Destine J, Poirrier R. Midsagittal jaw movement analysis for the scoring of sleep apneas and hypopneas. *IEEE Trans Biomed Eng.* 2008 Jan;55(1):87–95.
47. Senny F, Destine J, Poirrier R. Midsagittal jaw movements as a sleep/wake marker. *IEEE Trans Biomed Eng.* 2009 Feb;56(2):303–9.
48. Maury G, Cambron L, Jamart J et al. Added value of a mandible movement automated analysis in the screening of obstructive sleep apnea. *J Sleep Res.* 2013 Feb;22(1):96–103.
49. Lebret M, Arnol N, Contal O et al. Nasal obstruction and male gender contribute to the persistence of mouth opening during sleep in CPAP-treated obstructive sleep apnoea. *Respirology.* 2015 Oct;20(7):1123–30.

25

Continuity of care and telemonitoring

MICHELE VITACCA

KEY MESSAGES

1. Chronic diseases increase dramatically the burden on healthcare systems, and hospitalisation of chronically ill patients is a 'failure' for healthcare systems.
2. Home care programmes and telemonitoring may provide an opportunity for health organisations to develop new strategies and clinical procedures.
3. Telemonitoring alone is not sufficient in itself to yield a better outcome—while considering the overall care 'package' received by the patient, telemonitoring may be included as one of the services offered within the package.
4. The key point is to identify correctly who the ideal candidates are, and at what time they should receive it and for how long.

INTRODUCTION

The demographics and consequently the health profile of the population are changing. The greatest challenge that we face over the next 20 years is the management of chronic diseases in an ageing population.[1–5] At present, about 80% of ill health, disability and premature deaths are due to chronic diseases. In highly developed countries, the per-capita healthcare costs are threefold higher in people aged ≥65 years than the rest of the population.[1–6] By the year 2020, the costs for chronic diseases are anticipated to increase the total health budget by 70%–80%.[1–6] Older adults in poor health are at risk of negative outcomes and are the major consumers of health resources both in hospital and in community settings.[3] This socioeconomic trend has resulted in markedly increased interest in delivering effective care to elderly and chronically ill patients in the home.[3,5,6] In particular, in chronic obstructive pulmonary disease (COPD) patients, the cost for hospitalisation is >40% of the overall cost of COPD care (in the most severe, it is >60%).[7] Mortality during hospitalisation is high and 63% of patients are readmitted in the year following an exacerbation.[7]

Challenges facing healthcare professionals in the care of elderly people with poor health include the organisation of the management programme and sustainability of the continuum of services, resource allocation and cultural competence in service delivery in partnerships with families.[3,5,6] All chronic patients have complex individual needs with a prognosis that is difficult to predict, have progressive functional decline, have frequent episodes of serious acute exacerbations and experience systemic effects and comorbidities that negatively affect outcome.[7] Finally, there is the vicious circle of inactivity with reduced effort tolerance[8] and the high risk of depression in these patients.[9]

In patients using home mechanical ventilation (HMV), the underlying diseases, the level of dependency, the hours spent using mechanical ventilation, presence of tracheostomy, distance from home to hospital and hospital access are all part of the care burden[10] for the family and the healthcare system. Caregivers need to spend a very large amount of time with the patient to provide assistance with activities of daily living;[11] furthermore, the time spent by caregivers transporting patients to hospitals is usually not included in the cost analysis.[11] The family burden for HMV patients has been reported to be particularly high with regard to finance, and is reported to be disproportionate in >17% of cases.[12] A significant number of HMV patients do not receive adequate supportive care at the end of life[12] and 50% of caregivers face problems in social relationships as well as in the level of care they can deliver.[13] Last, technical problems such as ventilator malfunction or blockage of ventilator circuit or tracheostomy tube can also occur in HMV patients.[14]

The aim of this chapter is to provide some insights into how telemonitoring might complement home care follow-up systems for patients on HMV.

TECHNICAL AND CLINICAL CONSIDERATIONS

Home care depends on the patient's needs, which result from an acute or chronic illness, permanent disability or terminal illness.[15] In particular, home care should have a patient-centred focus; fewer complications while in hospital, maintenance of an acceptable quality of life and assurance of a comfortable and dignified death have been advocated as major endpoints.[15]

There is no universal consensus regarding what type of a home care followup programme would be most effective in chronic patients. It covers a complex range of services in a setting in which patients and families are primary members of the healthcare team.[15] The lack of direct professional control and the possibility of acute exacerbations of chronic conditions contribute to the difficulty in organising home care assistance.[15] Box 25.1 summarises the main benefits of a well-organised follow-up programme in a home-based care system.

HMV has a high prevalence in European countries:[16] in patients receiving HMV, follow-up programmes should be well structured and well integrated with technology.[15,17–19] Traditional nurse-based home follow-up programmes have limitations relating to the number of patients who can be included, costs and logistical problems, such as the distances involved and the time needed to reach the patient at their home. Various follow-up models to prevent hospitalisations and exacerbations have been proposed, including self-management, home care and dedicated chronic care models, which may or may not be supported by information technologies.

BOX 25.1: Benefits of a well-organized follow-up system in a home-based care system

- Delivery of care tailored to the individual patient
- Improved access to effective healthcare by reducing barriers
- Empowerment of patients for self-care and healthcare decision-making
- Fewer responsibilities for the referral centre
- Provision of more information for the people involved
- Development of an educational model
- Accurate and timely transmission of data and opportunities for real-time consultation
- Complementary to classical models of care
- Increasing continuity of care
- Increasing effectiveness of care
- Prompt attention to emergencies
- Improved patient satisfaction

In the United States, Medicare-certified home health agencies provide this service; nurses or other home health personnel provide skilled care according to federal regulations. In Europe, new models of home care support programmes after discharge are being formulated and implemented: patients are discharged early from hospital or the emergency department with follow-up by a healthcare professional using frequent telephone contact, telemedicine (see below) or home visits when the patient's condition or reduced ability to manage the care makes it necessary. Studies have focused on the effectiveness of home care provided by specialised nurses, but there are scant data on visits by specialists and, in particular, on the feasibility and safety of medical intervention at home. Physicans and/or nurses may perform home visits, participating in the multidisciplinary team providing the home care.[15] Figure 25.1 summarises the organisational complexity required at home after discharge of a patient with HMV; a multidisciplinary team, including physicians, nurses, respiratory therapists, social services and psychologists, should be established to give support after discharge, for periodic assistance and for making home visits.[20] Careful selection of patients, a documented diagnosis and indications and an adequate setting, together with the patient's ability to pay close attention to and comply with the education and training, are essential; all these factors facilitate the development of better-quality and cost-saving home care.[20–23]

How often patients should be visited by the home care team, and what needs to be measured during the visits, varies greatly between the home care programmes in different environments and countries. Unfortunately, there are countries where a home care programme is not a reality: in some cases, patients are left totally alone or have to pay for all interventions. Monitoring and care over time require periodic clinical visits, prevention of clinical instability, evaluation and care of comorbidities, continuous education and self-management and psychological, economic and social support.[22–24]

Published data offer several different follow-up models of home care in COPD patients as a prototype for chronic patients. Reduction in hospitalisation[25,26] and use of other acute healthcare services,[26,27] reduction in mortality rate,[28] improvement in the sickness impact profile scores[28,29] and patient satisfaction[29] have all been reported with programmes providing chronic home care interventions and patient education. These programmes are based on strict adherence to interventions enhancing symptom self-monitoring by patients and their caregivers and increasing their understanding of drug therapy, symptom and treatment monitoring, as well as acting as a liaison between primary care providers and hospital services. This involves the delivery of time-intensive education by nurses and other personnel, such as respiratory therapists.[25,27–29]

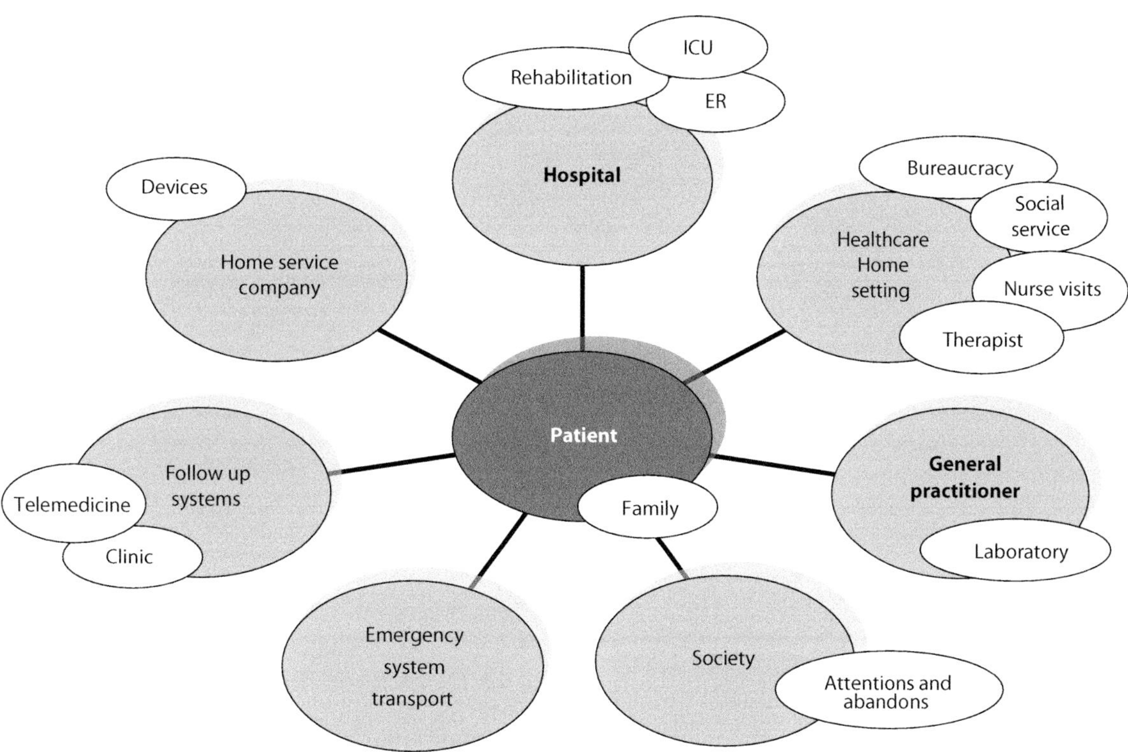

Figure 25.1 The complexity of a CRF patient when discharged at home.

In summary, home care[15] includes intermittent, often post-acute, healthcare, palliative and end-of-life care, medical equipment prescription, a protected discharge protocol or the more recent use of technology that allows reaching patients in their homes, termed e-health, with various kinds of tele-support or telemedicine. All these are components of the integrated home care 'puzzle' with different patients requiring different degrees of each component in the continuum of care (Figure 25.2). Figure 25.3 shows tools, techniques and outcomes for respiratory patients followed at home.

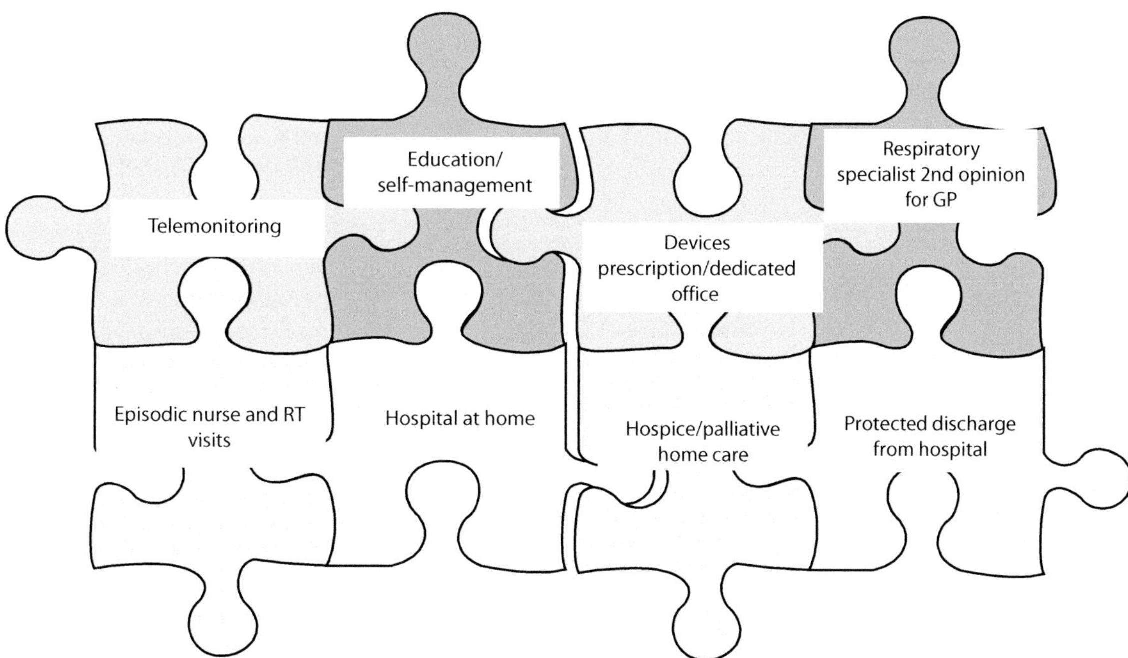

Figure 25.2 The puzzle of home integrated services for respiratory conditions.

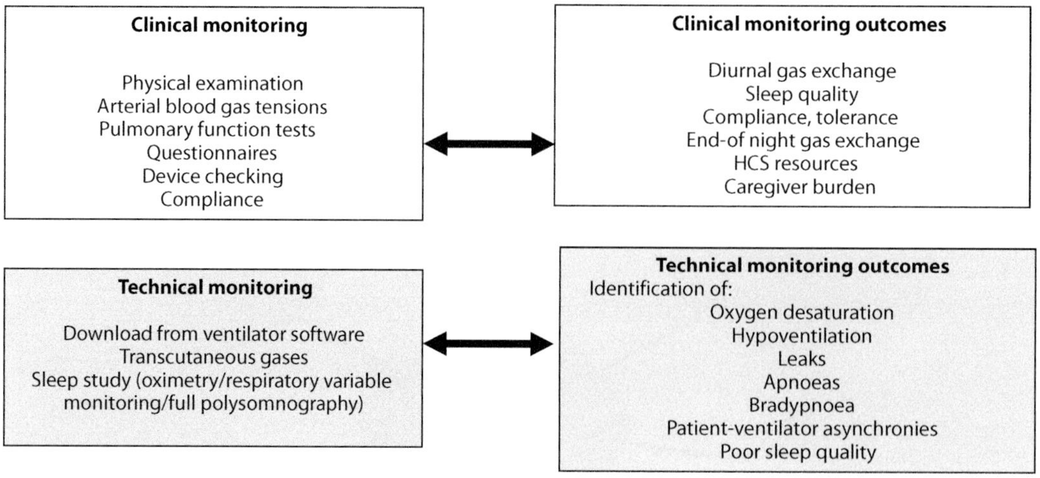

Clinical monitoring		Clinical monitoring outcomes
Physical examination Arterial blood gas tensions Pulmonary function tests Questionnaires Device checking Compliance	⟷	Diurnal gas exchange Sleep quality Compliance, tolerance End-of night gas exchange HCS resources Caregiver burden
Technical monitoring		**Technical monitoring outcomes**
Download from ventilator software Transcutaneous gases Sleep study (oximetry/respiratory variable monitoring/full polysomnography)	⟷	Identification of: Oxygen desaturation Hypoventilation Leaks Apnoeas Bradypnoea Patient-ventilator asynchronies Poor sleep quality

Figure 25.3 Tools, techniques and outcomes for respiratory patients.

TELEMONITORING

Modern information communication technologies offer new options to deliver specialised healthcare remotely, amongst which telemonitoring, a complex intervention that includes both the electronic transmission of patient information to the healthcare system and the follow-up response by a healthcare professional. The rationale for telemonitoring in patients with chronic respiratory insufficiency with or without HMV is related to (i) the increasing number of HMV patients across Europe;[16] (ii) difficulties associated with hospital discharge, with tremendous physical and psychological burden for caregivers of HMV patients;[12] and (iii) the opportunity that telemonitoring offers early remote detection of signs and symptoms of clinical decompensation,[30] and remote tailoring and monitoring of ventilator settings and education reinforcement for the patient and caregiver. Given the cost of telemonitoring in terms of human resources, equipment and patients' time, strong evidence of its cost-effectiveness is required, in particular as regards the impact of an earlier detection of relapses of chronic conditions. Unfortunately, decision-makers, for example, the healthcare authorities, are rushing to introduce telemonitoring in response to the pressure to reduce hospitalisations among patients with chronic diseases, without first carefully weighing up all the evidence.

In the last decade, several studies focusing on the effects of various telemanagement programmes for patients with chronic respiratory insufficiency (with COPD being the main diagnosis) have been published.[30–57] Table 25.1 shows a summary of the main published papers presenting studied population, time of telemonitoring use, outcomes and costs.

A few years ago, Wootton[58] concluded that the evidence base for telemedicine in managing chronic diseases is at present weak and contradictory. The conflicting results could be due to the fact that, to date, the literature on telemonitoring in patients with chronic respiratory insufficiency consists mainly of single-centre experiences carried out in small patient cohorts with different diseases and different levels of disease severity and followed up only in the short term. In addition, the studies have different settings, rationales, definition of the control group (i.e. usual care) and methodology. To date, the evidence as to whether telemonitoring is really effective in chronic respiratory insufficiency patients seems inconclusive. The 'one glove fits all' approach in offering telemonitoring for chronic respiratory insufficiency seems to be too simplistic for such a heterogeneous population. Factors that would be important for the successful implementation of telemonitoring are an individually tailored approach, flexibility and a service that is locally responsive. There are a number of possible explanations why the telemonitoring approach may not be superior to standard management carried out at home:

1. The patients who may benefit most from telemonitoring have not yet been identified. In fact, it is not clear which patients would benefit from other types of care delivery and, more importantly, what preferences patients have. Although many studies have included patients with severe disease, they vary in terms of the inclusion and exclusion criteria regarding baseline diagnosis, history of exacerbations, previous use of healthcare services such as home visits, hospitalisations or rehabilitation, as well as requirements for supplemental oxygen or HMV. Patients with severe symptoms, frequent exacerbations, multi-morbidity and limited community support might well benefit from telemonitoring. In the case of patients with multi-morbidity and very severe disease, telemonitoring needs to be able to deal flexibly with all the conditions that affect the patient's well-being. The crucial factor in preventing a hospital admission, or improving the patient's quality of life, may be relief of the distressing symptoms due to other comorbidities rather than monitoring of the chronic respiratory disease. Real-life studies of telemonitoring could help clarify this issue, first, by highlighting the subgroups of patients in whom telemonitoring is most used (and thus presumably of most benefit) and those for whom it is of little advantage,

Table 25.1 Summary of main published studies on telemonitoring

Study	Population	Time of TM use	Outcomes	Costs
Johnston[31]	102 TM vs. 102 controls; CHF, COPD, cerebral vascular accident, cancer, diabetes, anxiety	NA	QOL >	27% <
Farrero et al.[32]	COPD under LTOT; 46 TM vs. 48 controls	1 year	H and ER <	Total saving $46,823
Agha et al.[33]	Mixed; TM vs. controls vs. onsite care	NA	Costs	43% < in TM group
Hernandez et al.[34]	COPD exacerbations at ER; 121 TM vs. 101 controls	8 weeks	QOL >; H and ER <	NA
Bourbeau et al.[35]	COPD	2 months	QOL >; ER and GP calls <	NA
Paré et al.[36]	COPD; 19 TM vs. 10 controls	NA	H <	15% <
Casas et al.[37]	COPD at discharge; 65 TM vs. 90 controls	1 year	No effect on survival; H <	NA
Miyasaka et al.[38]	7 pediatric patients for home ventilatory care	NA	GP calls, visits, H <	NA
Pinto et al.[39]	ALS (N = 40, all ventilated)	3 years	Good adaptation to NIV; visits and ER <	NA
Vitacca et al.[40]	ALS (n = 73: 18 on NIV; 18 on invasive ventilation)	4 years	TM timing, TM feasibility, team time consuming, costs	TM costs 105€/ patient/month
Vitacca et al.[41]	ALS (n = 40: 19 on NIV; 12 on invasive ventilation)	1–12 months	TM use, patient requests for TM, TM staff activities, TM satisfaction	NA
Zamith et al.[42]	Asthma n = 21 + CRF n = 51, 41 on LTOT; 32 on NIV	9 months	TM use and acceptance; H < and QOL >	NA
Bertini et al.[43]	16 HMV (5 invasive MV, 11 NIV; 3 COPD, 4 RTD, 8 NMD, 1 Ondine syndrome)	2 years	TM use and acceptance; ER <; good satisfaction	NA
Vontetsianos et al.[44]	COPD (n = 18) + at least 4 H in previous 2 years	9 months	H and ER <	NA
Trappenburg et al.[45]	COPD (study n = 59; controls n = 56)	6 months	H and relapses <; QOL =	NA
Segrelles Calvo et al.[46]	30 home telehealth, 30 controls; FEV1 < 50%, age ≥ 50 years, LTOT, non-smokers, with at least one H for respiratory illness in the previous year	7 months	H, H days, need for NIV <; good satisfaction	NA
Jódar-Sánchez et al.[47]	TM (n = 24) control group (n = 21) on usual care. Under LTOT and with at least one hospitalisation for respiratory illness in the previous year	4 months	ER <; H >; QOL >; good satisfaction	NA
Maiolo et al.[48]	20 COPD patients on LTOT+3 RTD	1 year	QOL >; H and relapses <	17% <
Moreira et al.[49]	35 patients (OSA 40.0%, COPD 22.8%, NMD 11.4%, TB sequelae 2.9%, kyphoscoliosis 2.9%; 20.0% other CRF causes	3 months	In TM group hours use and % of usage days >	NA
Pinnock et al.[50]	128 patients randomised to TM; 128 to usual care	1 year	H, H days, QOL = to controls	NA

(Continued)

Table 25.1 (Continued) Summary of main published studies on telemonitoring

Study	Population	Time of TM use	Outcomes	Costs
Pedone et al.[51]	50 COPD patients in the TM group, 49 controls	9 months	Relapses and H <	NA
Vitacca et al.[52]	CRF patients needing LTOT or HMV+ at least one H for respiratory illness in the previous year. COPD: 56%, RTD: 15%, NMD: 10%, ALS: 9%, other 10%. 46% on NIV, 21.4% IMV, 63% LTOT	1 year	No effect on survival; QOL >; H, ER, GP visits, relapses <	33% <
Borel et al.[30]	COPD on home NIV	6 months	Relapses prediction with TM monitoring of breathing pattern; 21 exacerbations were correctly detected	NA
Lopes de Almeida et al.[53]	ALS patients; age 18–75 years; 40 patients: 20 TM; 20 controls	3 months	Intention-to-treat analysis considering three different type of costs; costs	TM of NIV in ALS is cost-effective. 700€ patient/year estimated long-term annual cost-saving
Cartwright et al.[54]	CHF, COPD or diabetes; 845 were randomised to TM and 728 to controls	1 year	Cost per quality adjusted life year gained	Quality adjusted life year gain was similar between TM and controls Costs associated with TM were higher
Chatwin et al.[55]	1211 adult and paediatric patients with neuromuscular disease, chronic obstructive pulmonary disease or chest wall disease receiving HMV	6 months	TM time consuming: 528 daytime calls/month Home visits from internal staff: <2/month	NA
Hazenberg et al.[56]	77 patients were included, of whom 38 patients started HMV at home (neuromuscular or thoracic cage disease)	1 month	Home initiation of HMV with TM improves ABG and QoL not inferior to controls TM is safe, feasible and cheaper	TM is safe, feasible; 3000 €/patient can be saved
Chatwin et al.[57]	68 CRF patients (38 COPD) with or without home mechanical ventilation	3 months	No differences for risk of H; H and home visits > in TM group; GP visits unchanged; self-efficacy fell during TM	NA

Note: TM, telemonitoring; CHF, chronic congestive failure; COPD, chronic obstructive pulmonary disease; NA, not available; QOL, quality of life; >, increased; <, decreased; LTOT, long-term oxygen therapy; H, hospitalisations; ER, emergency room; GP, general practitioner; ALS, amyotrophic lateral sclerosis; NIV, non-invasive ventilation; CRF, chronic respiratory failure; FEV1, forced expiratory volume at the first second; MV, mechanical ventilation; HMV, home mechanical ventilation; RTD, restrictive thoracic disease; NMD, neuromuscular diseases; OSA, obstructive sleep apnoea; TB, tuberculosis; IMV, invasive mechanical ventilation; ABG, arterial blood gases.

so that the health authorities can adjust their inclusion criteria accordingly. Second, through classifying patients according to the level of need so that different levels of telemonitoring (more or less technology and/or type of personnel) and duration (hours/day, months of follow-up) can be allocated to different categories of patients: that is, a more aggressive service for exacerbators and other major users of healthcare, while a less aggressive service for the others. Otherwise, whilst it is tempting to assume that in the more severe patients their clinical condition is such that some hospital admissions may be inevitable, people with less severe disease might be better targets for telemonitoring to reduce unnecessary hospitalisations. In any case, telemonitoring does not have the aim of avoiding hospitalisation per se but rather to control the progression of the disease, which sometimes in fact will mean increasing hospitalisation, through face-to-face hospital or home care visits to prevent catastrophic clinical worsening, and subsequent need for intensive care unit admission or mechanical ventilation.
2. The absence of standardised interventions in controlled trials with a minimum of 1 year of follow-up, which include a cost–benefit analysis, makes it impossible to be confident about the role of telemonitoring in the overall care of patients with chronic respiratory insufficiency.
3. The use of different generations of the telemonitoring and e-health devices and platforms may explain substantial differences in the findings between studies. Available telemonitoring devices[59] range from basic first-generation systems to the far more complete third-generation systems. First-generation systems allow non-reactive data collection with measurements transferred to the care provider asynchronously; second-generation systems, on the other hand, are equipped with a delayed analytical or decision-making structure with synchronous data transfer regulated by automated algorithms in which care providers can recognise important changes; however, delays can occur if the systems are only active during office hours. Third-generation systems are the most complete and provide constant analytical and decision-making support where monitoring centres are led by a physician, are staffed by specialist nurses and have full therapeutic authority 24 hours/day, 7 days/week. The role of the case manager/care manager during telemonitoring use may also vary among different countries depending on the current policy of each country's health system.
4. To evaluate the real cost-effectiveness of new methods such as telemonitoring in this population, it is important to understand what is meant by 'standard care' and 'usual care'. Standard care varies greatly not only between European countries, but also within each country.[60] Unfortunately, high level 'standard' care is not a common or mandatory care approach in all European Union (EU) countries. If an extensive home care package with strong community links exists, telemonitoring may add little additional benefit, whereas in the trials with less community support, telemonitoring seems to show more benefit in terms of team expertise, and the patient's (or carer's) self-efficacy. Now, the question to evaluate is if the superiority of telemonitoring to the gold standard is really the goal. Equivalence between telemonitoring and the gold standard may be a more appropriate goal; indeed, an intervention that cost-effectively improves a sub-optimal service bringing it on a par with the gold standard would be a success. Cost-effectiveness could be the 'gold standard' for each new service. It is not important for each health organisation to push for a 'unique modality' of continuity of care but to press for the 'most efficient' one, respecting shared and standardised clinical and scientific targets for chronic care.
5. Last but not least, negative or positive results clearly depend on the expected outcomes of the study (e.g. health resource use, patient-related outcomes, adherence, mechanical ventilation initiation and adaptation, need for palliative care) and corresponding methodological development, which differ from one study to the next.

Four factors influence the design and acceptance of telemonitoring processes: the patients, the healthcare systems, doctors (hospital and home domestic staff) and technology companies. Finally, telemonitoring programmes for a mechanical ventilation user should be well-designed, with clear aims and a well-structured service portfolio; be used with a clearly defined group of patients; have clear and well-organised protocols and procedures; be based on adequate technology for different conditions, well-established call centres and sustainable costs; and be safe and simple to use with a facility for continuous documentation.

The potential of and the availability of technology in this field is enormous (from basic to sophisticated tools: cards sent by post, telephone systems and modems, mobile and video phones, electromedical devices, computers, wireless and Internet technologies, in general). However, until now, stakeholders have offered solutions based on heterogeneous sensors and devices, and data security, protection and privacy have been lacking. Standards for telemonitoring need continuous review for accuracy, safety and ease of access for patients. Implementation of the system should run in parallel with its standardisation and harmonisation, which are the key issues for optimising e-health and telemonitoring.

FUTURE RESEARCH

More attention needs to be focused on how to accommodate the increasing number of chronic respiratory insufficiency patients in a post-discharge telemonitoring management programme with real integration between hospital and primary care professionals according to quality standards. The self-management support must also become more integrated, with standardised decision support and outcome measures plus electronic information so that critical information is shared among the various health professionals involved in the home programmes. In addition, more research is required on the organisational implications of introducing telemonitoring to avoid a new service duplicating a traditional system with more inefficiency and increased costs, on the security and confidentiality of patient data, on the responsibilities and potential obligations of health professionals and on EU jurisdictional problems regarding e-health systems. Finally, we need to provide a useful benchmarking picture of different telemonitoring practices around Europe as an aid to those who fund telemonitoring services in their decisions and investment in personnel, reduction of redundancy and duplication of care services, as well as prioritisation of services.

To establish evidence-based guidelines for the design and implementation of disease management applications employing telemonitoring, further research is needed on long-term effect, cost-effectiveness, effect on quality of life and the reduction in the public health burden. The 'model' to be implemented is the patient as a person, the product as a service and the service 'validated' by the person; a cooperative working model will lead to a 'service-oriented approach' rather than a 'product-oriented strategy'.

Nowadays, many applications of home care and telemonitoring are possible and operational. Designing tailored programmes for local situations and for specific diseases with different levels of severity will have a key role in reducing care costs. The future goals of such programmes should include patient and family satisfaction, maintenance of an acceptable quality of life and a dignified death at home.

CONCLUSIONS

Chronic diseases increase the burden on healthcare systems. Primary care needs to be sustained in the face of increasing demands: home care and telemonitoring may help primary care professionals and specialists to reduce the expected burden. Hospitalisation of chronically ill patients is a 'failure' for healthcare systems and chronic diseases, exemplifying the case for the large-scale deployment of follow-up programmes. For these reasons, home care programmes and telemonitoring may provide an opportunity for health organisations to develop new strategies and clinical procedures.

In conclusion, at the moment, the fundamental prerequisite for the efficacy of telemonitoring in the management of chronic respiratory insufficiency is to establish common standardised protocols rather than determine how to deliver the care.[61] The absence of conclusive evidence for the benefit of telemonitoring in chronic respiratory insufficiency should, however, not be taken as evidence of an absence of benefit. It is clear that telemonitoring alone is not sufficient in itself to yield a better outcome; telemonitoring could be a key element in management of chronic respiratory insufficiency patients, but it is difficult to evaluate its benefit without considering the other services received by patients (home care, access to hospital, social care).[61] Considering the overall care 'package' received by the patient, telemonitoring may be included as one of the services offered within the package. But other aspects—quality improvement, integration of programmes and services, increased collaboration and communication across the different care settings and the development of a shared vision, goals and priorities—are needed to improve the efficiency of the healthcare services provided for chronic patients. Successful implementation of telemonitoring can change how things are done and, in turn, the configuration of services.[61]

The key point in optimising the use of telemonitoring is to identify correctly who the ideal candidates are, and at what time they should receive it andnhjb for how long.[61] In other words, oscillating between expectations and disillusionment, the current dilemma is not 'telemonitoring—yes or no?', but how to use it in a mature and balanced manner in such a way as to enhance the health outcomes for our chronic patients.

REFERENCES

1. American College of Physicians. E-Health and its impact on medical practice. Philadelphia: American College of Physicians, 2008; Position Paper.
2. Meystre S. The current state of telemonitoring: A comment on the literature. *Telemed J E Health.* 2005;11:63–9.
3. Young HM. Challenges and solutions for care of frail older adults. *Online J Issues Nurs.* 2003;8:5.
4. World Health Organization Global Observatory for eHealth. Global eHealth Survey. Geneva, July 2005.
5. EHTEL. Sustainable telemedicine: Paradigms for future-proof healthcare. A briefing paper, 20 February 2008. Available at: www.ehtel.org (acscessed April 2008).
6. Ministers of EU Member States Ministerial Declaration. eHealth. Brussels, 22 May 2003.
7. Celli BR, MacNee W. Committee members. Standards for the diagnosis and treatment of patients with COPD: A summary of the ATS/ERS position paper. *Eur Respir J.* 2004;23:932–56.
8. Pitta F, Troosters T, Spruit MA et al. Characteristics of physical activities in daily life in chronic obstructive pulmonary disease. *Am J Respir Crit Care Med.* 2005;171:972–7.
9. de Voogd JN, Wempe JB, Koëter GH et al. Depressive symptoms as predictors of mortality in patients with COPD. *Chest.* 2009;135:619–25.
10. Vitacca M, Escarrabill J, Galavotti G et al. Home mechanical ventilation patients: A retrospective survey to identify level of burden in real life. *Monaldi Arch Chest Dis.* 2007;67:142–7.
11. Langa KM, Fendrick AM, Flaherty KR et al. Informal caregiving for chronic lung disease among older Americans. *Chest.* 2002;122:2197–203.
12. Vitacca M, Grassi M, Barbano L et al. Last three months of life in home ventilated patients: The family perception. *Eur Respir J.* 2010;35:1–8.

13. Tsara V, Serasli E, Voutsas V et al. Burden and coping strategies in families of patients under noninvasive home mechanical ventilation. *Respiration.* 2006;73:61–7.
14. Simonds AK. Risk management of the home ventilator dependent patient. *Thorax.* 2006;61:369–71.
15. ATS Documents. Statement on home care for patients with respiratory disorders. *Am J Respir Crit Care Med.* 2005;171:1443–64.
16. Lloyd-Owen SJ, Donaldson GC, Ambrosino N et al. Patterns of home mechanical ventilation use in Europe: Results from the Eurovent survey. *Eur Respir J.* 2005;25:1025–31.
17. Report of a Consensus Conference of the American College of Chest Physicians. Mechanical ventilation beyond the intensive care unit. *Chest.* 1998;113:289S–344S.
18. Farre R, Lloyd-Owen SJ, Ambrosino N et al. Quality control of equipment in home mechanical ventilation: A European survey. *Eur Respir J.* 2005;26:86–94.
19. ATS Consensus Statement. Care of the child with a chronic tracheostomy. *Am J Respir Crit Care Med.* 2000;161:297–308.
20. Haynes N, Raine SF, Rushing P. Discharging ICU ventilator-dependent patients to home healthcare. *Crit Care Nurse.* 1990;10:39–47.
21. Spence A. Home ventilation: How to plan for discharge. *Nurs Stand.* 1995;9:38–40.
22. Muir JF, Voisin C, Ludot A. Organization of home respiratory care: The experience in France with ANTADIR. *Monaldi Arch Chest Dis.* 1993;48: 462–7.
23. Douglas SL, Daly BJ. Caregivers of long-term ventilator patients: Physical and psychological outcomes. *Chest.* 2003;123:1073–81.
24. Dettenmeier PA. Planning for successful home mechanical ventilation. *AACN Clin Issues Crit Care Nurs.* 1990;1:267–79.
25. Tougaard L, Krone T, Sorknaes A et al. Economic benefits of teaching patients with chronic obstructive pulmonary disease about their illness. *Lancet.* 1992;339:1517–20.
26. Adams SG, Smith PK, Allan PF et al. Systematic review of the chronic care model in chronic obstructive pulmonary disease prevention and management. *Arch Intern Med.* 2007;167:551–61.
27. Haggerty MC, Stockdale-Woolley R, Nair S. Respicare: An innovative home care program for the patient with chronic obstructive pulmonary disease. *Chest.* 1991;100:607–12.
28. Littlejohns P, Baveystock CM, Parnell H et al. Randomized controlled trial of the effectiveness of a respiratory health worker in reducing impairment, disability, and handicap due to chronic airflow limitation. *Thorax.* 1991;46:559–64.
29. Cockcroft A, Bagnall P, Heslop A et al. Controlled trial of respiratory health worker visiting patients with chronic respiratory disability. *BMJ.* 1987;294:225–8.
30. Borel JC, Pelletier J, Taleux N et al. Parameters recorded by software of non-invasive ventilators predict COPD exacerbation: A proof-of-concept study. *Thorax.* 2015;70:284–5.
31. Johnston B, Wheeler L, Deuser J et al. Outcomes of the Kaiser Permanente tele-home health research project. *Arch Fam Med.* 2000;9:40–5.
32. Farrero E, Escarrabill J, Prats E et al. Impact of a hospital-based home-care program on the management of COPD patients receiving long-term oxygen therapy. *Chest.* 2001;119:364–9.
33. Agha Z, Schapira RM, Maker AH. Cost effectiveness of telemedicine for the delivery of outpatient pulmonary care to a rural population. *Telemed J E Health.* 2002;8:281–91.
34. Hernandez C, Casas A, Escarrabill J et al. Home hospitalisation of exacerbated chronic obstructive pulmonary disease patients. *Eur Respir J.* 2003;21:58–67.
35. Bourbeau J, Julien M, Maltais F et al. Reduction of hospital utilization in patients with chronic obstructive pulmonary disease: A disease-specific self-management intervention. *Arch Intern Med.* 2003;163:585–91.
36. Paré G, Sicotte C, St-Jules D et al. Cost-minimization analysis of a telehomecare program for patients with chronic obstructive pulmonary disease. *Telemed J E Health.* 2006;12:114–21.
37. Casas A, Troosters T, Garcia-Aymerich J et al. Integrated care prevents hospitalisations for exacerbations in COPD patients. *Eur Respir J.* 2006;28:123–30.
38. Miyasaka K, Suzuki Y, Sakai H, Kondo Y. Interactive communication in high-technology home care: Videophones for pediatric ventilatory care. *Pediatrics.* 1997;99:E1.
39. Pinto A, Almeida JP, Pinto S et al. Home telemonitoring of non-invasive ventilation decreases healthcare utilisation in a prospective controlled trial of patients with amyotrophic lateral sclerosis. *J Neurol Neurosurg Psychiatry.* 2010;81:1238–42.
40. Vitacca M, Comini L, Assoni G et al. Tele-assistance in patients with amyotrophic lateral sclerosis: Long term activity and costs. *Disabil Rehabil Assist Technol.* 2012;7:494–500.
41. Vitacca M, Comini L, Tentorio M et al. A pilot trial of telemedicine-assisted, integrated care for patients with advanced amyotrophic lateral sclerosis and their caregivers. *J Telemed Telecare.* 2010;16:83–88.
42. Zamith M, Cardoso T, Matias I, Marques Gomes MJ. Home telemonitoring of severe chronic respiratory insufficient and asthmatic patients. *Rev Port Pneumol.* 2009;15:385–417.

43. Bertini S, Picariello M, Gorini M et al. Telemonitoring in chronic ventilatory failure: A new model of survellaince, a pilot study. *Monaldi Arch Chest Dis.* 2012;77:57–66.
44. Vontetsianos TH, Giovas P, Katsaras TH et al. Telemedicine-assisted home support for patients with advanced chronic obstructive pulmonary disease: Preliminary results after nine-month follow-up. *J Telemed Telecare.* 2005;11 Suppl 1:S1,86–8.
45. Trappenburg JC, Niesink A, de Weert-van Oene GH et al. Effects of telemonitoring in patients with chronic obstructive pulmonary disease. *Telemed J E Health.* 2008;14:138–46.
46. Segrelles Calvo G, Gómez-Suárez C, Soriano JB et al. A home telehealth program for patients with severe COPD: The PROMETE study. *Respir Med.* 2014;108:453–62.
47. Jódar-Sánchez F, Ortega F, Parra C et al. Implementation of a telehealth programme for patients with severe chronic obstructive pulmonary disease treated with long-term oxygen therapy. *J Telemed Telecare.* 2013;19:11–7.
48. Maiolo C, Mohamed EI, Fiorani CM et al. Home tele-monitoring for patients with severe respiratory illnesses: The Italian experience. *J Telemed Telecare.* 2003;9:67–71.
49. Moreira J, Freitas C, Redondo M et al. Compliance with home non-invasive mechanical ventilation in patients with chronic respiratory failure: Telemonitoring versus usual care surveillance—A randomized pilot study. *Eur Respir J.* 2014;44 Suppl 58:447.
50. Pinnock H, Hanley J, McCloughan L et al. Effectiveness of telemonitoring integrated into existing clinical services on hospital admission for exacerbation of chronic obstructive pulmonary disease: Researcher blind, multicentre, randomised controlled trial. *BMJ.* 2013;347:f6070.
51. Pedone C, Chiurco D, Scarlata S, Incalzi RA. Efficacy of multiparametric telemonitoring on respiratory outcomes in elderly people with COPD: A randomized controlled trial. *BMC Health Serv Res.* 2013;13:82.
52. Vitacca M, Bianchi L, Guerra A et al. Tele-assistance in chronic respiratory failure patients: A randomised clinical trial. *Eur Respir J.* 2009;33:411–8.
53. Lopes de Almeida JP, Pinto A, Pinto S et al. Economic cost of home-telemonitoring care for BiPAP-assisted ALS individuals. *Amyotroph Lateral Scler.* 2012;13:533–7.
54. Cartwright M, Hirani SP Sr, Rixon L et al. Effect of telehealth on quality of life and psychological outcomes over 12 months (Whole Systems Demonstrator telehealth questionnaire study): Nested study of patient reported outcomes in a pragmatic cluster randomised controlled trial. *BMJ.* 2013;346:f653.
55. Chatwin M, Heather S, Hanak A et al. Analysis of home support and ventilator malfunction in 1,211 ventilator-dependent patients. *Eur Respir J.* 2010 Feb;35(2):310–6. doi: 10.1183/09031936.00073409. Epub 2009 Jul 30.
56. Hazenberg A, Kerstjens HA, Prins SC et al. Initiation of home mechanical ventilation at home: A randomised controlled trial of efficacy, feasibility and costs. *Respir Med.* 2014 Sep;108(9):1387–95. doi: 10.1016/j.rmed.2014.07.008. Epub 2014 Jul 22.
57. Chatwin M, Hawkins G, Panicchia L et al. Randomised crossover trial of telemonitoring in chronic respiratory patients (TeleCRAFT trial). *Thorax.* 2016 Mar 9. pii: thoraxjnl-2015-207045. doi: 10.1136/thoraxjnl-2015-207045.
58. Wootton R. Twenty years of telemedicine in chronic disease management—An evidence synthesis. *J Telemed Telecare.* 2012;18(4):211–20.
59. Scalvini S, Vitacca M, Paletta L et al. Telemedicine: A new frontier for effective healthcare services. *Monaldi Arch Chest Dis.* 2004;61:4,226–33.
60. European Commission. Commission staff working document on the applicability of the existing EU legal framework to telemedicine services. Brussels 6.12.2012
61. Vitacca M. Telemonitoring in patients with chronic respiratory insufficiency: Expectations deluded? *Thorax.* 2016 Mar 9. pii: thoraxjnl-2015-208211. doi: 10.1136/thoraxjnl-2015-208211.

PART 4

The diseases

26 Pathophysiology of respiratory failure 234
Paul P. Walker and Peter M. Calverley

26

Pathophysiology of respiratory failure

PAUL P. WALKER AND PETER M. CALVERLEY

KEY MESSAGES

1. Respiratory failure occurs where arterial blood gas homeostasis is inadequate to meet the body's metabolic needs. Knowledge of how and why respiratory failure develops is important to help determine the cause(s) and provide effective treatment quickly.
2. Type 1 or hypoxaemic respiratory failure is a failure of gas exchange caused by abnormalities of the lung parenchyma, pulmonary vasculature or both. The predominant physiological mechanism is ventilation perfusion mismatching.
3. Type 2 or hypercapnic respiratory failure is a failure of ventilation and occurs when the respiratory muscles are unable to provide sufficient ventilation to meet metabolic demands. The predominant physiological mechanism is alveolar ventilation.
4. There are multiple causes of type 2 respiratory failure and include central nervous system, neuromuscular, thoracic wall and lung abnormalities. They often co-exist and each should be considered when establishing the cause of type 2 respiratory failure and how to treat it.
5. Patients with COPD who develop type 2 respiratory failure usually have a normal or increased respiratory drive and normal intrinsic respiratory muscle function. Type 2 respiratory failure develops due to mechanical disadvantage from airflow obstruction, hyperinflation and intrinsic PEEP, all of which typically worsen during an acute exacerbation leading to respiratory muscle fatigue.

INTRODUCTION

The maintenance of stable arterial blood gas tensions and a normal arterial pH are prerequisites for a healthy life. Although respiration is ultimately an intracellular process, in a clinical context, most attention focuses on the uptake of oxygen and elimination of carbon dioxide, which, in turn, depend on a number of processes:

- Effective alveolar ventilation reflecting the bulk transfer of air in the airways
- Diffusion of gases from the lung to the circulation
- Passage of blood through the pulmonary circulation
- Transport of gases in blood, which reflects the oxygen and carbon dioxide content of the blood

By convention, the first three mechanisms are the focus of respiratory failure due to pulmonary diseases, although in practice, the systems are intimately linked and cannot be neatly separated. Respiratory failure exists when the body is unable to maintain arterial blood gas homeostasis adequate to meet the needs of metabolism. More specifically, failure to maintain gas exchange causes inadequate oxygenation of arterial blood and, consequently, the tissues. In some cases, the body additionally fails to eliminate carbon dioxide adequately from mixed venous blood.

In health, gas exchange can be maintained over a wide range of metabolic requirements from basal levels of oxygen consumption during stage III sleep to heavy exercise. Even under conditions when the inspired oxygen falls, as in ascent to high altitude, compensatory mechanisms still defend safe levels of arterial oxygenation (and hence tissue oxygen delivery) with hypoxic vasoconstriction within the lung and an increased total alveolar ventilation tending to mitigate the initial effects of hypoxaemia. In disease, the same range of physiological mechanisms come into play, but their effectiveness is often compromised.

Conventionally, gas exchange has been analysed using the three-compartment model developed almost 50 years ago by Riley and colleagues[1] and which is discussed in some detail below. This approach has the virtue of clarity and can be applied relatively easily to clinical situations. However, it is an oversimplification as the wide heterogeneity in pulmonary pathology within an individual can produce quite complex gas exchange abnormalities. Considerable insights into these complex problems have come from applying the multiple inert gas elimination (MIGET) method to analyse gas exchange in a wide range of settings. This is a mathematically complex and intellectually rigorous approach that involves the analysis of the uptake and excretion of six different gases of variable solubility. Although this has helped our understanding of gas exchange, and especially the complex causes of hypoxaemia, we will devote most of this chapter to illustrating the general principles of gas exchange using the older approach with some comments on one area in which the MIGET data have changed our understanding of disease.

DEFINITION OF RESPIRATORY FAILURE

Conventionally, respiratory failure is split into two types depending on whether hypercapnia is present.[2] This division is more than simply arbitrary, as it potentially provides important information about the pathophysiological mechanisms leading to respiratory failure. Combined with knowledge of the clinical situation, this may help the clinician determine the most appropriate treatment strategy.

Type 1 or hypoxaemic respiratory failure occurs where there is an abnormally low arterial oxygen tension (PaO_2) of <8 kPa (<60 mmHg) with a normal or low arterial carbon dioxide tension ($PaCO_2$) of <6 kPa (<45 mmHg)[3] (Table 26.1). This can be considered to be a failure of gas exchange sometimes described as 'lung failure' (Figure 26.1). Type 1 respiratory failure is most often caused by abnormalities of the lung parenchyma, the pulmonary vasculature or a combination of both, and several pathophysiological mechanisms might contribute, including the following:

- Ventilation–perfusion (V/Q) mismatch
- Intrapulmonary (right to left) shunt
- Impaired alveolar–capillary diffusion
- Hypoventilation

Table 26.1 Definition of respiratory failure based on level of PaO_2 and $PaCO_2$

	Type of respiratory failure	
	Type 1	**Type 2**
PaO_2 level	<8 kPa = <60 mmHg	<8 kPa = <60 mmHg
$PaCO_2$ level	<6 kPa = <45 mmHg	>6 kPa = >45 mmHg

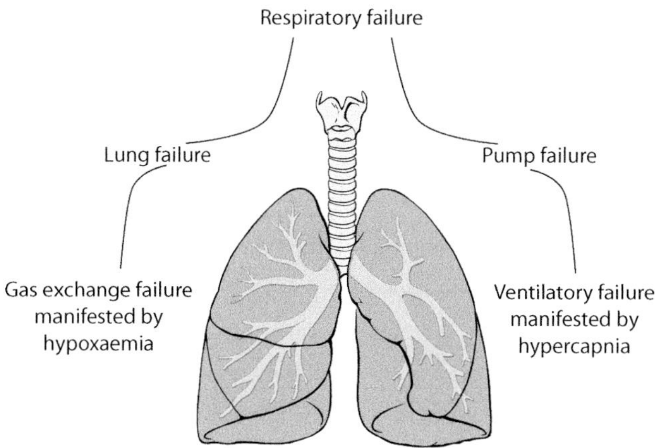

Figure 26.1 Types of respiratory failure described by Roussos and Koutsoukou. (From Roussos C, Koutsoukou A. Respiratory failure. *Eur Respir J Suppl.* 2003;47:3s–14s.)

A commonly used index of gas exchange is the alveolar-arterial oxygen gradient where the measured arterial PO_2 is subtracted from the ideal alveolar PO_2. In individuals without lung disease, hypoventilation leads to hypoxaemia with a normal alveolar-arterial gradient ($P_{A\text{-}a}O_2$), whereas in people with lung disease, for example, chronic obstructive pulmonary disease (COPD), any of the other mechanisms, in particular alveolar hypoventilation, may also be present, which normally results in widening of the $P_{A\text{-}a}O_2$ gradient and can accentuate the degree of hypoxaemia.

Type 2 or hypercapnic (hypercarbic) respiratory failure occurs where there is an abnormally low arterial oxygen tension (PaO_2) of <8 kPa (<60 mmHg) with an abnormally raised arterial carbon dioxide tension ($PaCO_2$) of >6 kPa (>45 mmHg) (Table 26.1). Hence, there is a failure of ventilation that has been described as 'pump failure' (see Figure 26.1).

The common causes of type 1 and type 2 respiratory failure are detailed in Table 26.2. In some cases, multiple pathologies may be present in the same individual, while in others, a single condition may lead to respiratory failure by a number of different mechanisms. For example, when an individual with COPD develops respiratory failure, often the respiratory muscles cannot maintain sufficient alveolar ventilation to prevent hypercapnia in the face of a significantly increased dead space-to-tidal volume ratio. However, on an intensive care unit, there can be respiratory muscle fatigue and use of opiates can contribute to hypoventilation. The presence of pulmonary hypertension or an acute insult such as pneumonia could additionally contribute to respiratory failure in the individual.

The degree to which arterial oxygen and carbon dioxide concentrations are regulated differs significantly, with regulation of PaO_2 significantly less tight. The normal PaO_2 for an individual is age dependent and expressed by the following equation:

$$PaO_2 = 13.3\ \text{kPa} - (0.04 \times \text{age}(\text{years}))$$

Table 26.2 The causes of type 1 and type 2 respiratory failure

Type 1 respiratory failure	Type 2 respiratory failure
Failure of the Pulmonary Vasculature • Pulmonary embolism • Pulmonary artery hypertension **Failure of Alveolar Gas Exchange** • Pulmonary oedema • Pneumonia • Pulmonary haemorrhage • Acute lung injury • Pulmonary fibrosis • Airway disease - acute asthma and COPD	**Central Nervous System** • Head injury • Reduced consciousness/coma • Sedative drugs, e.g. opiates **Neuromuscular** • Cervical spinal cord injury or disease - trauma, tumour, polio • Peripheral nerve injury - Guillain-Barre syndrome, critical illness polyneuropathy • Muscular - myasthenia gravis, muscular dystrophy **Thoracic Wall** • Kyphoscoliosis • Chest wall trauma (flail chest) • Ruptured diaphragm • Morbid obesity **Pulmonary** • Airway disease - COPD, acute severe asthma and bronchiectasis • Upper airway obstruction including obstructive sleep apnoea

Hence, a normal PaO_2 may range from 10 kPa (75 mmHg) to 13.5 kPa (95 mmHg), and for PaO_2 to stimulate ventilation, it would need to be below about 8 kPa (60 mmHg), the level used to define 'hypoxaemic' respiratory failure. In contrast, $PaCO_2$ is much more tightly coupled to ventilation with an acute rise in $PaCO_2$ to above 6 kPa (45 mmHg) quickly stimulating ventilation, hence the level used to define 'hypercapnic' respiratory failure.

TYPE 1 RESPIRATORY FAILURE

This is the most common type of respiratory failure. Hypoxia (low oxygen) is quantified by the partial pressure of oxygen, and it differs according to the compartment in which it is measured. The partial pressure of oxygen decreases from the atmosphere to tissue mitochondria, and this is illustrated by the oxygen cascade (Figure 26.2). In essence, the lungs, heart and circulation will act to maintain adequate oxygen delivery to tissue mitochondria, and measurement of the arterial partial pressure of oxygen (PaO_2) via arterial blood gas assessment is a surrogate of this. If the level of oxygenation falls acutely, the heart will increase cardiac output and peripheral vessels will vasodilate to maintain tissue oxygen delivery. In a more chronic situation, erythropoiesis will produce more oxygen-carrying red blood cells and tissues can extract more oxygen from blood, lowering the oxygen content of venous blood (P_VO_2) returning to the lungs.

Gas exchange in the 'ideal' lung (a lung where there was no V/Q mismatch) can be represented by the alveolar gas equation:

$$P_AO_2 = P_IO_2 - P_ACO_2/R + F$$

where P_IO_2 = F_IO_2 (P_b − $P_{water\ vapour}$), P_AO_2 = partial pressure of oxygen in the alveolus, P_IO_2 = partial pressure of inspired oxygen, P_ACO_2 = partial pressure of carbon dioxide in the alveolus, R = the respiratory quotient (moles of CO_2 produced per mole of O_2 consumed) and F is a small correction factor. F_IO_2 = the fraction of inspired oxygen, P_b = barometric pressure at sea level (101 kPa/760 mmHg) and $P_{water\ vapour}$ = the vapour pressure of water (6.3 kPa/47 mmHg) within the lungs. The respiratory quotient is also called the respiratory exchange ratio and is determined by tissue metabolism. It represents the ratio of carbon dioxide production to oxygen consumption and varies according to dietary consumption and metabolism. With fat metabolism, the ratio is 0.7; with carbohydrate metabolism, it is 1.0; and in most healthy people, it is around 0.8.

From this, it is clear that different factors can contribute to hypoxia. The following mechanisms contribute to this:

Low inspired oxygen fraction

As can be seen from the alveolar gas equation, if the inspired oxygen concentration (F_IO_2) falls, then the alveolar oxygen concentration (P_AO_2) will also fall. This can be seen if supplementary oxygen is disconnected, if hypoxic gas mixture is administered and if dead space is increased and re-breathing of exhaled gases is increased (see below).

Low barometric pressure

As can also be seen from the alveolar gas equation, the partial pressure of oxygen in inspired air (P_IO_2) is determined by the F_IO_2, which falls with a reduction in barometric pressure (P_b). This explains the fall in P_AO_2 with high altitude including during flight, albeit these effects are ameliorated by pressurisation of an aircraft cabin.

Ventilation–perfusion mismatch

This is the most important cause of hypoxaemia and can also contribute to hypercapnia. Ventilation–perfusion mismatching is both physiological and pathological. Physiological mismatch is fairly modest and occurs in the upright, normal lung with the ratio of ventilation to perfusion increasing from the base of the lungs to the apex. This is due to gravity/posture, cardiac output and pulmonary artery pressure. Perfusion and ventilation are highest at the bases as pulmonary artery pressure is highest there and there is a regional increase in ventilation due to the weight of the lung compressing the

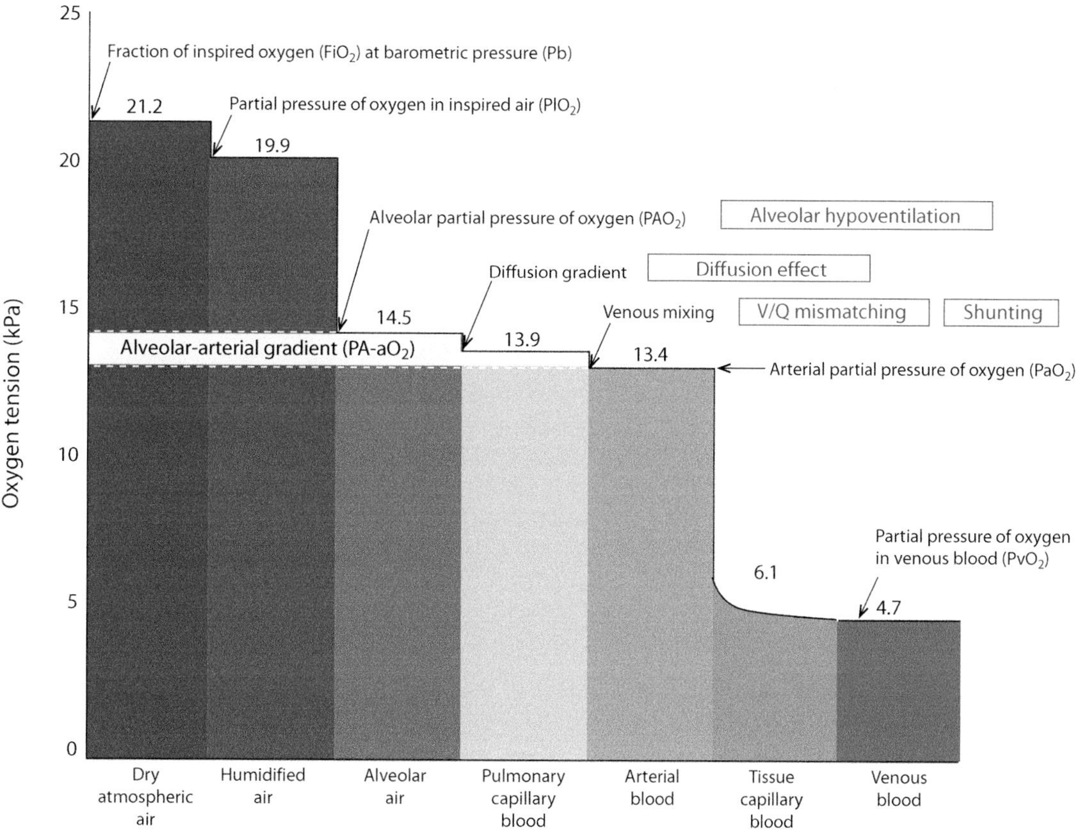

Figure 26.2 The oxygen cascade illustrating the alveolar–arterial gradient and the impact of physiological processes including alveolar hypoventilation, diffusion abnormality, ventilation–perfusion mismatching and shunting.

basal lung tissue both lowering negative intra-pleural pressure and reducing operating lung volumes. This is shown in Figure 26.3.

Ventilation–perfusion mismatch is most easily explained using the three-compartment model of dead space ventilation, ideal matching and shunting, but it should be remembered that mismatch is a continuum where each alveolus will have a different relationship. Hence, descriptions of V/Q mismatch in the overall lung are a summation of all individual units and the partial pressure of oxygen and carbon dioxide in arterial blood reflect this. Any pathological process that affects the airways, lung parenchyma or pulmonary vasculature will affect the V/Q relationship of the lungs, and different combinations of these exist in people with different lung diseases and all three can co-exist, for example, in individuals with COPD.

The three-compartment model is illustrated in Figure 26.4. In a normal lung, ventilation and perfusion are equally matched and the V/Q ratio is 1. In some disease states, there is normal ventilation, but reduced perfusion and the V/Q ratio is high (greater than 1), and at the extreme, it is infinity (where blood flow is absent), known as physiological dead space. In another situation, there is reduced ventilation but normal perfusion and the V/Q ratio is low (less than 1), and at the other extreme, it is zero (where ventilation is absent), called physiological shunting. It might be supposed that where ventilation–perfusion mismatch is patchy, then areas of normal lung and well-perfused lung would compensate for under-perfused areas. However, the oxygen–haemoglobin dissociation curve, which represents haemoglobin's affinity for oxygen, can be seen to be sigmoid shaped (Figure 26.5), and this means that well-perfused areas cannot increase blood oxygen saturation above 100%. Hence, PaO_2 will fall in the presence of V/Q mismatch. The oxygen–haemoglobin dissociation curve is influenced by a number of factors that shift or reshape the curve, and these include body temperature, pH (hydrogen ion concentration), carbon dioxide concentration and 2,3-diphosphglycerate. The effect is shown in Figure 26.5 with a shift of the curve to the left increasing haemoglobin's affinity for oxygen and a shift to the right decreasing haemoglobin's affinity for oxygen.

Using COPD as an example, predominantly emphysematous patients have been shown to ventilate large areas with a high V/Q ratio and hardly any areas with a very low V/Q ratio or shunt areas. This probably involves a reduction in blood flow to areas of the lung due to emphysematous destruction of alveoli in addition to inequality of ventilation. Where low V/Q patterns are seen, the likely causes are a reduction in ventilation due to mechanical bronchial obstruction due to airway oedema, mucus and airway narrowing, closure and/or collapse. However, perfusion to these areas is also likely to be reduced due to chronic hypoxic vasoconstriction in these areas.[4]

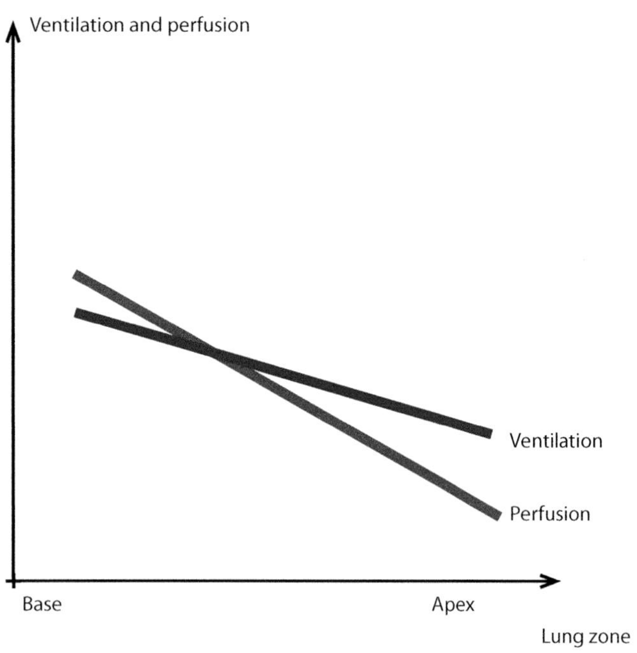

Figure 26.3 Illustration of the difference in ventilation and perfusion between the lung apex and lung base.

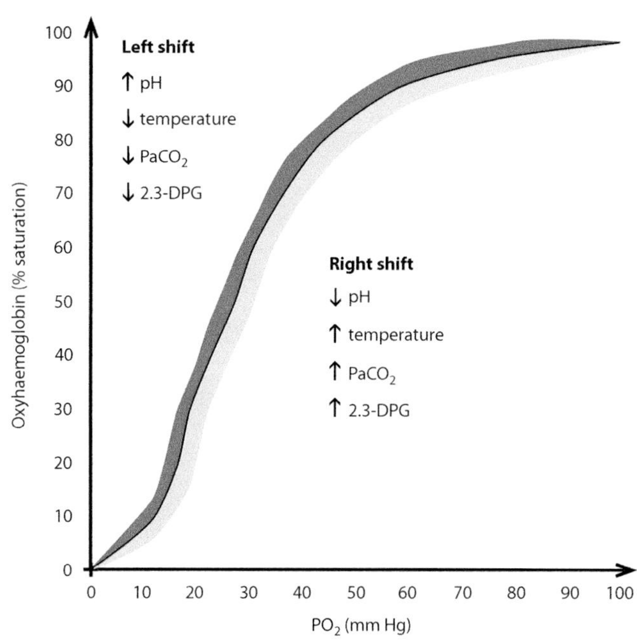

Figure 26.5 The oxygen–haemoglobin dissociation curve illustrating the effect of $PaCO_2$, pH, temperature and 2,3-DPG concentration.

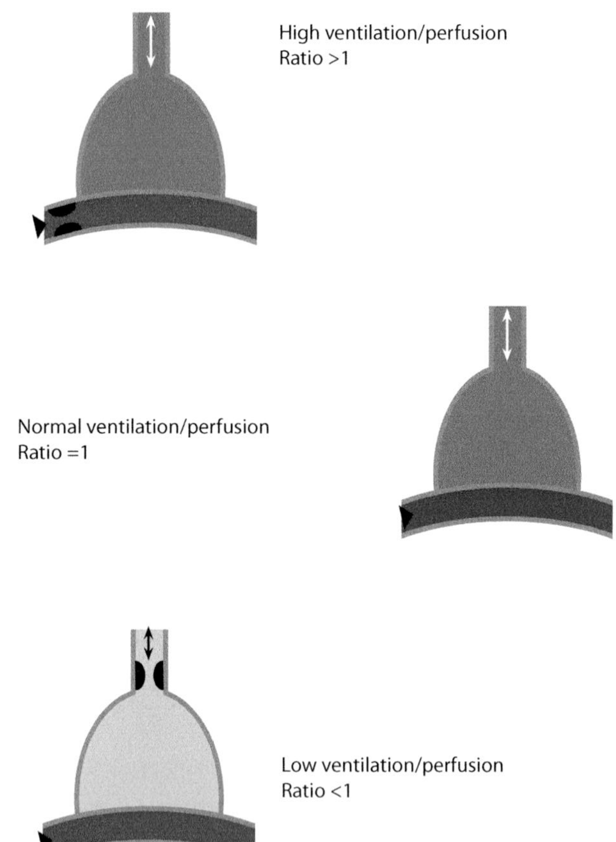

Figure 26.4 The three-compartment model of ventilation and perfusion illustrating ventilation–perfusion mismatch, physiological dead space and shunting. (Adapted from West JB. *Respiratory Physiology: The Essentials*, 8th edition. Lippincott Williams & Wilkins, 2008.)

The process is not unique to COPD, and any lung disease that causes significant architectural distortion will lead to impaired ventilation–perfusion matching, for example, interstitial lung disease. It is very difficult to directly measure ventilation–perfusion mismatching in the lung, and consequently, we tend to measure indices of gas exchange that are representative. The alveolar gas equation, described earlier, describes gas exchange in the 'ideal' lung (a lung where there was no V/Q mismatch). An increased alveolar-arterial oxygen difference is normally caused by abnormally low ventilation–perfusion ratios within the lung but can be caused by high ratios. It is possible to separate these two situations by calculating the physiological shunt (for low ratios) and the physiological dead space (for high ratios), though in many patients with COPD, both exist to a varying degree. In general, hypoxaemia associated with V/Q mismatch caused by deficits in ventilation can be improved by increasing inspired oxygen fraction.

Intrapulmonary shunting

Shunting is one end of the spectrum of ventilation–perfusion mismatch, a situation where deoxygenated blood passes through the pulmonary vascular bed without exposure to ventilation and therefore reduces the PaO_2 of arterial blood. A small shunt of about 2% of cardiac output exists in the normal lung due to blood from the bronchial arteries and the coronary circulation entering the arterial circulation without passing through the ventilated lung.

In patients with COPD, and other airway diseases such as asthma, the majority of pathological shunting relates to mechanical bronchial obstruction and closure and/or collapse of alveoli. This contrasts with airways filled with fluid or exudates as seen in conditions such as pulmonary oedema and pneumonia. Extrapulmonary conditions such as liver failure and intracardiac right-to-left shunts, for example, from an atrial septal defect, can also cause significant shunting.

An important feature of a shunt is that it cannot be completely abolished by administering 100% oxygen as shunted blood will never be exposed to oxygen—albeit the PaO_2 will rise because of the higher fraction of inspired oxygen (F_IO_2) delivered to functioning alveoli.

Impaired alveolar capillary diffusion

Effective and efficient gas exchange depends on the interface between the alveoli and the bloodstream, and diseases affecting this interface, such as pulmonary fibrosis, pulmonary oedema or acute respiratory distress syndrome, cause impairment in diffusion. Emphysema is also associated with alveolar destruction (see Figure 26.6), which can greatly reduce the surface area available for gas diffusion.

In the normal alveolar–capillary unit at rest, oxygen diffusion has equilibrated no more than a third of the way along the unit, and so even with significant diffusion impairment, there is rarely any impact on oxygenation at rest (see Figure 26.7). In theory, during exercise, cardiac output increases and the speed with which blood passes through the capillaries is increased. In these circumstances, diffusion impairment could reduce the rate of rise of partial pressure of oxygen in the capillary and contribute to hypoxaemia. However, detailed experiments have shown that ventilation–perfusion inequality and shunt account for all of the hypoxaemia at rest and during exercise, and there is no evidence for hypoxaemia caused by diffusion impairment.[4] The solubility of a gas is important and carbon dioxide is 20 times more soluble in water than oxygen, and therefore, a diffusion defect rarely affects carbon dioxide exchange.

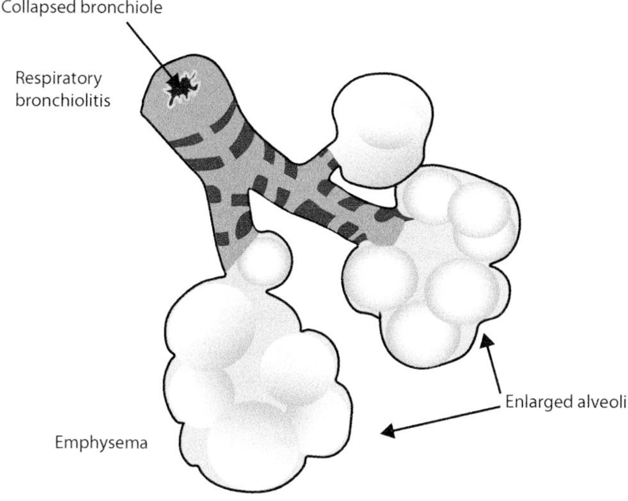

Figure 26.6 Emphysematous destruction of the alveoli and collapse/closure of the respiratory bronchioles seen in respiratory bronchiolitis.

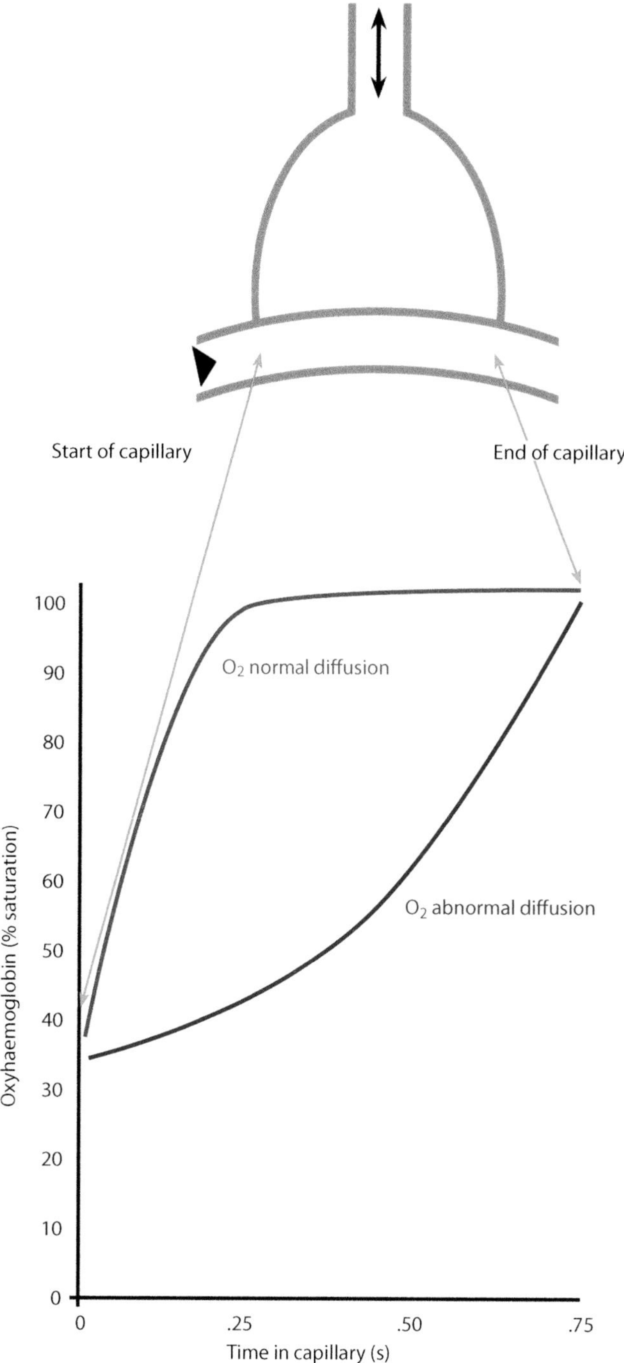

Figure 26.7 Oxygen time course in the pulmonary capillary in conditions where diffusion is normal and abnormal. (Adapted from West JB. *Respiratory Physiology: The Essentials*, 8th edition. Lippincott Williams & Wilkins, 2008.)

TYPE 2 RESPIRATORY FAILURE

Alveolar hypoventilation is the predominant mechanism leading to hypercapnia, but other mechanisms also contribute.

Alveolar hypoventilation

The amount of carbon dioxide eliminated per minute (VCO_2) is a function of the concentration of CO_2 in the alveoli multiplied by alveolar ventilation (V_A); hence,

$$\text{Alveolar } CO_2 \text{ concentration} = VCO_2/V_A$$

By converting the equation to pressures and using factor k (the constant of proportionality), the respiratory equation is obtained, which relates arterial $PaCO_2$ to alveolar ventilation:

$$PaCO_2 = k \times (VCO_2/V_A)$$

Since alveolar ventilation (V_A) is equivalent to minute ventilation (V_E) minus dead space ventilation (V_D), then:

$$PaCO_2 = k \times [VCO_2/(V_E - V_D)]$$

Physiological dead space includes anatomical dead space and a component due to dilution of resident gas in the airways. This can then be expressed as

$$PaCO_2 = k \times VCO_2/V_T \times f \times [1-(V_D - V_T)]$$

where V_T is tidal volume and f is breathing frequency.

Type 2 respiratory failure is reflected by hypercapnia, and it is clear from these equations that at a constant VCO_2, as alveolar ventilation (V_A) is reduced, the partial pressure of carbon dioxide in the arterial circulation ($PaCO_2$) increases. Hence, alveolar hypoventilation is a significant cause of type 2 respiratory failure. Reduced alveolar ventilation also results in a fall in PaO_2, but this can be overcome by increasing the concentration of oxygen inspired. The equation also illustrates that decrease in alveolar ventilation can result from a rise in $V_D - V_T$ (by an increase in V_D, a reduction in V_T or both), a decrease in V_E or a combination of these factors. This situation is seen in many patients with more severe COPD where hypercapnic respiratory failure is common.

An increase in carbon dioxide production will also result in a rise in $PaCO_2$. This is most commonly seen during exercise, in which VCO_2 can increase multifold, and can also occur during hyperthermia. In normal lungs, this would be compensated by a proportional rise in minute ventilation. However, in patients with COPD, this increase in minute ventilation may be significantly limited as V_E will represent a much higher proportion of maximum voluntary ventilation. In some patients with severe COPD, $PaCO_2$ increases during exercise and has been shown to relate to dynamic hyperinflation.[5] Individuals with marked abnormalities of the chest wall, for example, kyphoscoliosis, have impaired ventilatory mechanics, which results in alveolar hypoventilation.

The causes of type 2 respiratory failure are shown in Table 26.2. Factors that affect central respiratory drive, such as sedative drugs, head injury, raised intracranial pressure and central nervous system infection, will reduce respiratory drive and consequently minute ventilation. Damage to the spinal cord above the level of phrenic nerve innovation (C3–5) will impair or eliminate diaphragm function, causing hypoventilation, reduce tidal volume and lead to increased secretions due to a reduced ability to clear them. Similar effects are seen with motor neurone disease and poliomyelitis. Guillain–Barre syndrome leads to an ascending polyneuropathy, which can lead to respiratory muscle weakness and hypoventilation. Congenital myopathies, such as the muscular dystrophies, can lead to ventilatory failure due to progressive muscle weakness and hypoventilation, and a similar situation can occur with an acute crisis of myasthenia gravis.

Ventilation–perfusion mismatch

Ventilation–perfusion mismatch is a cause of hypercapnia, although this mechanism is less common than hypoventilation. Ventilation–perfusion mismatch delivers carbon dioxide-rich blood to the arterial circulation, but in the normal lung, it does not increase $PaCO_2$ as any increase in $PaCO_2$ is sensed by the chemoreceptors that increase ventilation until the $PaCO_2$ is again normal. This occurs because the transport of carbon dioxide from the blood to the alveoli is linear; hence, when minute ventilation is increased, areas where ventilation–perfusion ratio is normal can increase CO_2 removal and compensate for mismatching regions. Hence, V/Q mismatch is far more important as a cause of hypoxaemia than hypercapnia.

As is evident from the above equations, the situation where it does contribute to hypercapnia is in patients who have an increase in physiological dead space and consequently increased dead space ventilation. This is seen commonly in COPD patients, particularly those with predominant emphysema.

Acid–base balance

The concentration of hydrogen ions (H^+) is extremely important to cellular metabolism, and in particular, an increased level impairs normal cell function. The concentration of hydrogen ions is normally expressed as the pH that represents the negative logarithm of H^+. It should be remembered that with a logarithmic scale, relatively small changes in pH represent large changes in the concentration. In light of the importance to the body, pH is normally very tightly controlled.

Tissue metabolism is the main source of hydrogen ions as a molecule of carbon dioxide produced combined with water is equivalent to a hydrogen ion and bicarbonate. The body has an effective buffering system to maintain homeostasis. Haemoglobin, proteins and phosphate can all act as buffers, but the most important component of the

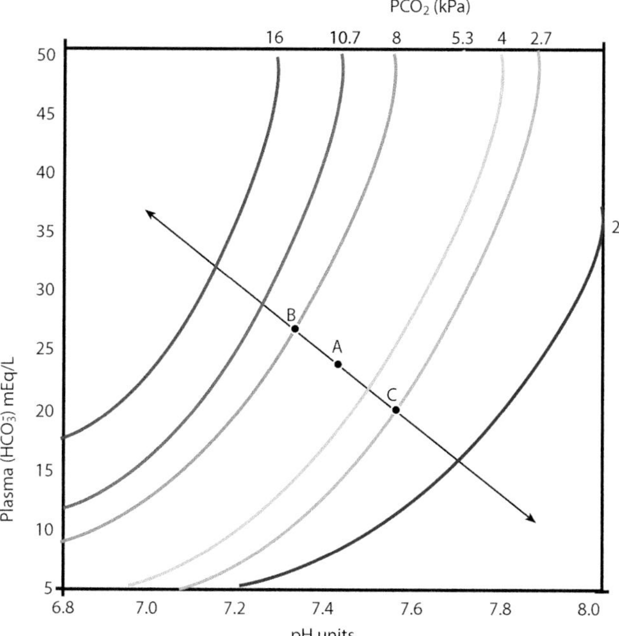

Figure 26.8 The relationship between pH, $PaCO_2$ and HCO_3 where A represents the buffer line, B represents respiratory acidosis and C represents respiratory alkalosis. (From West JB. *Respiratory Physiology: The Essentials*, 8th edition. Lippincott Williams & Wilkins, 2008.)

buffering system is the bicarbonate–carbonic acid system expressed as the Henderson–Hasselbalch equation:

$$CO_2 + H_2O \leftrightarrows H_2CO_3 \leftrightarrows H^+ + HCO_3^-$$

Balance is maintained by excretion of carbon dioxide through the lungs and excretion of fixed acid by the kidney. More than 100 times more carbon dioxide is excreted by the lungs each day compared with the amount of fixed acids excreted by the kidney; hence, mechanical ventilatory abnormalities significantly affect acid–base balance.

The relationship between pH, $PaCO_2$ and HCO_3^- can be seen in Figure 26.8.[6] If hypercapnia continues but acidosis does not progress, then renal buffering will normalise the pH by excreting hydrogen ions through the kidney (compensation), resulting in chronic type 2 respiratory failure.

In COPD, chest wall abnormalities and neuromuscular diseases, hypercapnia is the principal cause of any acidosis. In stable disease, this is compensated as described above, but it will usually worsen during exacerbations, where it is a marker of a worse prognosis (although not necessarily the most sensitive one).[7]

PATHOPHYSIOLOGY OF VENTILATORY FAILURE IN PATIENTS WITH COPD

As discussed earlier, ventilatory failure is primarily failure of the respiratory pump. Type 2 respiratory failure results when the respiratory muscles are unable to provide sufficient ventilation to meet metabolic demands. In stable COPD patients, this does not usually relate either to abnormalities of central respiratory muscle control/drive, to nerve signalling of the respiratory muscles or to intrinsic defects in respiratory muscle function. On the contrary, current evidence supports a marked increase in respiratory drive consistent with the structural and functional mechanical disadvantage seen in COPD patients that increases ventilatory requirements and relates to disease severity.[8] The combination of airflow obstruction and static and dynamic hyperinflation and presence of intrinsic positive end-expiratory pressure (PEEPi) increase the load on the respiratory muscles. Respiratory muscles operate at a mechanical disadvantage due to geometrical changes in the chest wall and diaphragm in addition to reduced compliance and elastic recoil of the respiratory system and are less able to produce the negative intrathoracic pressure necessary for respiration.[9] In addition, acute changes such as at the time of an exacerbation[10] and during exercise[11] accentuate these mechanical disadvantages by further worsening hyperinflation and airflow obstruction and increasing PEEPi.

Fatigue occurs when the respiratory muscles are unable to generate sufficient pressure to maintain ventilation. The respiratory muscles are relatively resistant to fatigue[12] at rest and at high-intensity exercise,[13,14] but changes seen at the time of an exacerbation may lead to fatigue and inadequate pleural pressure generation despite this increased drive. The mechanical changes that occur at the time of an exacerbation are accentuated by a decrease in cardiac output, a worsening of oxygenation and a reduction in nutritional intake at a time of increased energy requirement leading to an acute imbalance of energy supply and demand.

Fundamentally, there are a number of pathophysiological processes that contribute to ventilatory failure in COPD patients by increasing load on the respiratory system, and these will be examined in turn.

Increased inspiratory resistance

Inspiratory resistance consists of both airway resistance and the resistance of the lung tissue. In patients with COPD, the causes of increased inspiratory resistance have been elegantly described by Hogg et al.[15] The causes include airway wall thickening due to inflammation (inflammatory cell infiltration) and oedema, enlargement of mucous glands and airway wall smooth muscle (in the larger airways) and the existence of mucus within the airway (in particular the small, sub-2 mm airways). In addition, emphysema reduces the number of airway wall to parenchymal attachments, which are important in keeping small airways open. Combined with destruction and fibrosis of the respiratory bronchioles and hyperinflation, this predisposes to dynamic airway collapse and closure, further increasing resistance. Increases in inspiratory resistance of an extent seen in

COPD patients can markedly increase work of breathing, contributing to fatigue and ventilatory failure.

Increased static compliance and reduced elastic recoil

Lung elastance reflects the recoil of the lung and is defined by a change in pressure over a particular change in lung volume. It is the sum of the elastances of the lung and chest wall and the reciprocal of compliance. Emphysema leads to hyperinflation, destroys parenchymal tissue and reduces airway to parenchymal connections, consequently decreasing static lung elastance and increasing compliance. This results in reduced radial traction applied to the airways, airway collapse and closure and increased inspiratory resistance. In addition, it leads to a reduction in maximum expiratory flow, flow limitation and dynamic hyperinflation.

Increased expiratory resistance and expiratory flow limitation

Ventilatory limitation in COPD patients primarily relates to expiratory flow limitation. Conductance through an airway, at a set lung volume, is a function of alveolar pressure and flow, with increases in alveolar pressure (without forced expiration) increasing flow until maximum expiratory flow is reached. It occurs when, at a specific lung volume, an increase in pressure either does not increase or leads to a reduction in expiratory flow. Individuals with COPD, in particular emphysema, have static hyperinflation and reduced elastic recoil pressures from the lung. With unchanged chest wall recoil pressures acting outwards, the functional residual capacity (FRC) is increased and individuals breathe at a higher lung volume, which reduces airway distensibility and affects the driving force from the alveoli.[16] Compared with normal subjects, equal pressure points are now seen in the more peripheral airways,[17] reducing maximal expiratory flow. Such an individual is only able to increase expiratory flow by breathing at a lower lung volume resulting in dynamic hyperinflation, evidenced by an increase in FRC during exercise. Flow limitation can occur during resting tidal breathing in some patients, whereas in others, it only occurs during exercise[18] and exacerbations.[10] The impact of worsening hyperinflation on respiratory muscle function and consequently respiratory failure is discussed below.

Mechanical disadvantage due to chest wall and diaphragm position

Pulmonary hyperinflation has significant geometrical effects on the main muscles of respiration, the diaphragm and intercostal muscles. The diaphragm is shortened and flattened and the thoracic cage is expanded, and consequently, both diaphragm and intercostal muscles are shortened and operate at a mechanical disadvantage. Maximum force generation is achieved at lower lung volume, usually close to FRC, but shortened muscles[19] have a less favourable length–tension relationship and are able to produce less force for a specific degree of muscle activation.[20] In addition, the change in diaphragm shape reduces the number of muscle fibres that are arranged parallel to the chest wall as more are arranged perpendicularly or in series. A result of this is some muscles work isometrically; that is, they consume energy but do not contribute to force generation.

The change in the shape of the diaphragm reduces potential force generation (Figure 26.9). The zone of apposition, the area of the costal diaphragm that is in contact with the lateral chest wall, is reduced, which, in turn, reduces the impact of abdominal pressure generation on the thoracic cage, thereby limiting thoracic cage expansion.[21] At rest, the changes described have relatively little impact on the tidal volume generated, but they significantly reduce capacity to increase V_T, which is important at the time of an exacerbation or during exercise in particular because a majority of COPD patients dynamically inflate during exercise.[22]

Hyperinflation and intrinsic PEEP

When end-expiratory lung volume exceeds FRC, this leads to an elevation of recoil pressure and results in a positive recoil pressure being applied to the alveoli at end-expiration. This is seen in COPD patients with hyperinflation, particularly when exercising, and is called PEEPi. It is usually caused by airway compression and reduced expiratory time (discussed further below). When this is present, the inspiratory muscles have to overcome this applied pressure before inspiratory airflow can commence, which requires increased effort, increases the work of breathing and can contribute to respiratory muscle fatigue.

DEVELOPMENT OF HYPERCAPNIC RESPIRATORY FAILURE

The effect of the above different and interacting pathophysiological abnormalities seen in isolation, or usually in combination, contributes to the development of ventilatory (hypercapnic) respiratory failure. The mean tidal pressure (P_I), which needs to be developed for each breath by the inspiratory muscles, is increased and relates to the increased inspiratory load; however, the ability to generate pressure is compromised by impaired diaphragm and intercostal muscle position and function, and both static and dynamic hyperinflation. Furthermore, it also decreases as the duty cycle (T_i/T_{tot}) increases. In essence, expiratory time (T_e) is decreased, which has the effect of increasing end-expiratory lung volume and promoting dynamic hyperinflation. This situation is worsened by an increase in breathing frequency (f), which reduces T_{tot} and T_e, further promoting dynamic hyperinflation. The decrease in duty cycle also reduces maximum power generated by the respiratory muscles. The changes all lead to

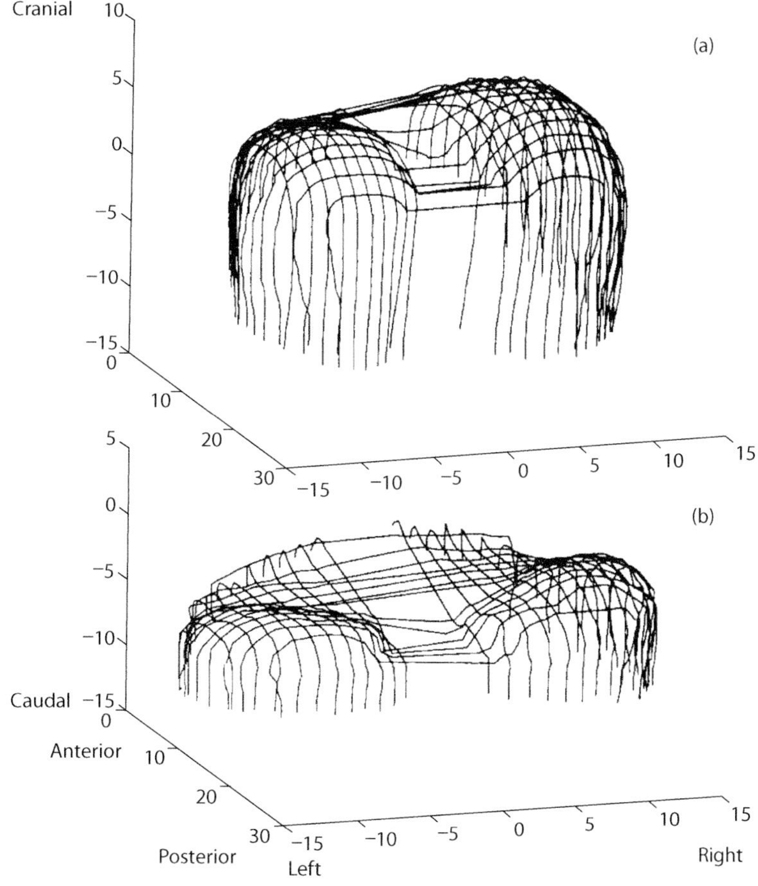

Figure 26.9 Changes in the diaphragm shape due to pulmonary hyperinflation comparing a normal subject **(a)** and a subject with COPD **(b)**. A marked reduction in muscle surface area is seen. (Taken from Cassart M, Pettiaux N, Gevenois PA et al. Effect of chronic hyperinflation on diaphragm length and surface area. *Am J Respir Crit Care Med.* 1997;156:504–8.)

muscle dysfunction and an inability to maintain V_T while weak muscles have greater energy requirements to perform a defined level of work and are more susceptible to fatigue.

DEVELOPMENT OF CHRONIC HYPERCAPNIC RESPIRATORY FAILURE

Development of chronic, compensated type 2 respiratory failure is a poor prognostic factor for COPD patients.[23] Why this occurs remains unclear. The earlier description of distinct patterns of V/Q abnormalities in hypercapnic disease with a bimodal distribution of low and high V/Q units[4] has not been consistently supported by subsequent papers using the same methodology. The most consistent abnormality has been the 'rapid shallow' breathing pattern described above, but why this should be adopted to different degrees in subjects with apparently similar degrees of mechanical impairment is unknown. It is tempting to speculate that these differences arise from inherent differences in the neural response to mechanical loading, but until more specific imaging methods like functional magnetic resonance imaging are applied to these problems, such explanations must remain a simple conjecture.

ACUTE OR ACUTE-ON-CHRONIC RESPIRATORY FAILURE

The development of acidosis due to either the development of hypercapnic respiratory failure or worsening of pre-existing compensated hypercapnic respiratory failure is a poor prognostic sign at the time of a COPD exacerbation and is associated with a worse mortality.[24] At the time of an exacerbation, inspiratory resistance is increased due to bronchospasm and airway inflammation leading to airway narrowing plus frequently a marked increase in airway mucus when a lower respiratory tract infection is present (which is commonly the case). Hyperinflation worsens, which increases expiratory flow resistance, promotes or increases PEEPi and disadvantages diaphragm, intercostal and even accessory muscle function. Increase in breathing frequency to maintain V_E reduces expiratory time and further promotes hyperinflation. Tidal breathing occurs at a steeper part of the pressure–volume curve, which is disadvantageous. In addition, the increased energy requirements needed to maintain ventilatory function often correspond with a time of relative anorexia and reduced cardiac output, which potentiates muscle fatigue and promotes acute hypercapnic respiratory failure. These extrapulmonary factors are important during exacerbations, with 50% of the abnormal gas exchange assessed using the MIGET methodology being explained by increases in metabolic demand, reductions in mixed venous oxygen tension secondary to reduced cardiac output and a fall in minute ventilation relative to these metabolic needs.[25]

CONCLUSIONS

A wide variety of cardiorespiratory conditions lead to respiratory failure, both acute and chronic. There is now greater clarity as to how to manage individuals with respiratory failure successfully, both with the use of oxygen in patients who are hypoxaemic and with non-invasive ventilation in patients who have hypercapnia. The acute use of non-invasive ventilation is among the most successful treatment options, in particular for COPD, and one of the few that reduce the risk of the individual dying. Knowledge of the pathophysiology and potentially modifiable effects of gas exchange abnormalities is important for any clinician involved in managing these situations.

CHAPTER SUMMARY

Respiratory failure is a common consequence of respiratory and cardiac disease and usually results in symptoms that are unpleasant and burdensome to the individual. Respiratory failure can be purely hypoxaemic or hypercapnic and the mechanisms through which this develops differ albeit with some overlap. Knowledge of how respiratory failure develops can help determine the cause(s), and this insight can help determine how it can be treated both acutely and chronically, particularly treatment with oxygen and use of ventilation. This chapter reviews the pathophysiology of both type 1 and type 2 respiratory failure and reflects on many important physiological principles. The latter part of the chapter addresses specific pathophysiology that contributes to the development of respiratory failure in people with chronic obstructive pulmonary disease.

REFERENCES

1. Riley RL, Cournard A. Ideal alveolar air and the analysis of ventilation–perfusion relationships in the lungs. *J Appl Physiol.* 1949;1:825–47.
2. Campbell EJ. Respiratory failure. *Br Med J.* 1965;i:1451–60.
3. Roussos C, Koutsoukou A. Respiratory failure. *Eur Respir J Suppl.* 2003;47:3s–14s.
4. Wagner PD, Dantzker DR, Dueck R et al. Ventilation–perfusion inequality in chronic obstructive pulmonary disease. *J Clin Invest.* 1977;59:203–16.
5. O'Donnell DE, D'Arsigny C, Fitzpatrick M et al. Exercise hypercapnia in advanced chronic obstructive pulmonary disease: The role of lung hyperinflation. *Am J Respir Crit Care Med.* 2002;166:663–8.
6. West JB. *Respiratory Physiology: The Essentials*, 8th edition. Lippincott Williams & Wilkins, 2008.
7. Chakrabarti B, Angus RM, Agarwal S et al. Hyperglycaemia as a predictor of outcome during non-invasive ventilation in decompensated COPD. *Thorax.* 2009;64:857–62.
8. Jolley CJ, Luo YM, Steier J et al. Neural respiratory drive in healthy subjects and in COPD. *Eur Respir J.* 2009;33:289–97.
9. Polkey MI, Kyroussis D, Hamnegard CH et al. Diaphragm strength in chronic obstructive pulmonary disease. *Am J Respir Crit Care Med.* 1996;154:1310–7.
10. Stevenson NJ, Walker PP, Costello RW et al. Lung mechanics and dyspnea during exacerbations of chronic obstructive pulmonary disease. *Am J Respir Crit Care Med.* 2005;172:1510–6.
11. Sinderby C, Spahija J, Beck J et al. Diaphragm activation during exercise in chronic obstructive pulmonary disease. *Am J Respir Crit Care Med.* 2001;163:1637–41.
12. McKenzie DK, Gandevia SC. Recovery from fatigue of human diaphragm and limb muscles. *Respir Physiol.* 1991;84:49–60.
13. Polkey MI, Kyroussis D, Keilty SEJ et al. Exhaustive treadmill exercise does not reduce twitch transdiaphragmatic pressure in patients with COPD. *Am J Respir Crit Care Med.* 1995;152:959–64.
14. Mador MJ, Kufel TJ, Pineda LA et al. Diaphragmatic fatigue and high-intensity exercise in patients with chronic obstructive pulmonary disease. *Am J Crit Care Med.* 2000;161:118–23.
15. Hogg JC, Chu F, Utokaparch S et al. The nature of small-airway obstruction in chronic obstructive pulmonary disease. *N Engl J Med.* 2004;350:2645–53.
16. Leaver DG, Tattersfield AE, Pride NB. Contributions of loss of lung recoil and of enhanced airways collapsibility to the airflow obstruction of chronic bronchitis and emphysema. *J Clin Invest.* 1973;52:2117–28.
17. Hogg JC, Macklem PT, Thurlbeck WM. Site and nature of airways obstruction in chronic obstructive lung disease. *N Engl J Med.* 1968;278:1355–60.
18. Koulouris NG, Dimopoulou I, Valta P et al. Detection of expiratory flow limitation during exercise in COPD patients. *J Appl Physiol.* 1997;82:723–31.
19. Gorman RB, McKenzie DK, Pride NB et al. Diaphragm length during tidal breathing in patients with chronic obstructive pulmonary disease. *Am J Respir Crit Care Med.* 2002;166:1461–9.
20. Roussos C, Macklem PT. The respiratory muscles. *N Engl J Med.* 1982;307:786–97.
21. Cassart M, Pettiaux N, Gevenois PA et al. Effect of chronic hyperinflation on diaphragm length and surface area. *Am J Respir Crit Care Med.* 1997;156:504–8.

22. O'Donnell DE, Revill SM, Webb KA. Dynamic hyperinflation and exercise intolerance in chronic obstructive pulmonary disease. *Am J Respir Crit Care Med.* 2001;164:770–7.
23. Burrows B, Earle RH. Course and prognosis of chronic obstructive lung disease: A prospective study of 200 patients. *N Engl J Med.* 1969;280: 397–404.
24. Seneff MG, Wagner DP, Wagner RP et al. Hospital and 1-year survival of patients admitted to intensive care units with acute exacerbation of chronic obstructive pulmonary disease. *JAMA*. 1995;274:1852–7.
25. Barberà JA, Roca J, Ferrer A et al. Mechanisms of worsening gas exchange during acute exacerbations of chronic obstructive pulmonary disease. *Eur Respir J.* 1997;10:1285–91.

PART 5

COPD

27 Non-invasive ventilation for exacerbation of COPD 247
Martin Dres, Alexandre Demoule and Laurent Brochard

28 NIV in chronic COPD 258
Enrico M. Clini, Nicolino Ambrosino, Ernesto Crisafulli and Guido Vagheggini

29 Non-invasive ventilation in COPD: The importance of comorbidities and phenotypes 266
Jean-Louis Pépin, Jean-Paul Janssens, Renaud Tamisier, Damien Viglino, Dan Adler and Jean-Christian Borel

30 High-intensity non-invasive positive pressure ventilation 272
Sarah Bettina Schwarz, Friederike Sophie Magnet and Wolfram Windisch

27

Non-invasive ventilation for exacerbation of COPD

MARTIN DRES, ALEXANDRE DEMOULE AND LAURENT BROCHARD

INTRODUCTION

In less than two decades, non-invasive ventilation (NIV) has become the cornerstone therapy of acute respiratory failure resulting from exacerbation of a chronic obstructive pulmonary disease (COPD). NIV is nowadays a routine clinical approach in these acutely ill patients.[1,2] The technique of NIV to support decompensated COPD patients began to be used in the early 1990s, when physiological knowledge and technical advances merged[3,4] and clinicians felt that there was a real need to prevent conventional invasive ventilation.

In this chapter, we will review the pathophysiology, the clinical applications and the technical aspects of NIV delivery. Finally, we will offer some comments regarding the future avenues of research in this field.

PHYSIOLOGIC EFFECTS OF NIV IN COPD

Patients with severe COPD generate much less maximal inspiratory pressure and transdiaphragmatic pressure compared to patients without COPD.[5] Weakness of the diaphragm can be explained by hyperinflation-induced diaphragm shortening, which places the diaphragm on a sub-optimal position on its force–length relationship.[5] Even at residual volume, the diaphragm remains flat and inspiratory force generation is not optimal. The presence of dynamic hyperinflation related to expiratory flow limitation implies that alveolar pressure remains positive throughout expiration. At the end of the expiration, this positive pressure is named intrinsic positive end-expiratory pressure (PEEPi) or auto-PEEP.[6] PEEPi further increases the workload, requiring that the inspiratory muscles reduce alveolar pressure to a subatmospheric level to initiate airflow for the next breath. In most severe patients, the capacity/load balance leads to chronic alveolar hypoventilation, leading to CO_2 retention with chronic bicarbonate reabsorption to maintain a normal pH.

During a COPD exacerbation, this precarious situation becomes more unstable, as these patients have no respiratory 'reserve', yet they can hardly increase inspiratory volumes in case of increased ventilatory demand. On the contrary, due to increased airway resistances (secretions, bronchospasm, expiratory flow limitation, etc.) or decreased lung compliance (pneumonia, atelectasis, etc.), inspiratory volumes are decreased and alveolar hypoventilation worsens despite increased needs. The respiratory drive is highly increased, leading to an increased respiratory rate and consequently to a decreased inspiratory time (and an increased mean inspiratory flow resulting in a higher burden on the inspiratory muscles).[7] This phenomenon generated reduced tidal volumes and increased respiratory rate ('rapid-shallow breathing pattern'). The patient's respiratory pattern of rapid shallow breathing is responsible for the two main issues during COPD exacerbation: (i) increased work of breathing (WOB) related to high respiratory rate and increased PEEPi, (ii) reduced alveolar ventilation related to low tidal volumes and increased dead space effect (Figure 27.1).

This vicious circle that is responsible for progressive respiratory muscle exhaustion, increased CO_2 with decreased level of consciousness and hypoxaemia may lead to death, unless therapeutic interventions interrupt the cycle. The first-line treatments frequently include bronchodilators, oxygen supplementation, diuretics, anticoagulant agents or antibiotics based on the suspected cause of COPD decompensation.[8] Every time, respiratory acidosis is present (pH $\geq$ 7.35 and high $PaCO_2$); the application of NIV is now part of the first-line recommended treatment with the objective to reverse this cycle:[8] to reduce the WOB and restore adequate alveolar ventilation by increasing tidal volume and reducing the respiratory rate.

Reduction of the WOB with NIV application

Many studies demonstrated the impact of positive pressure through NIV on WOB during COPD exacerbation with or

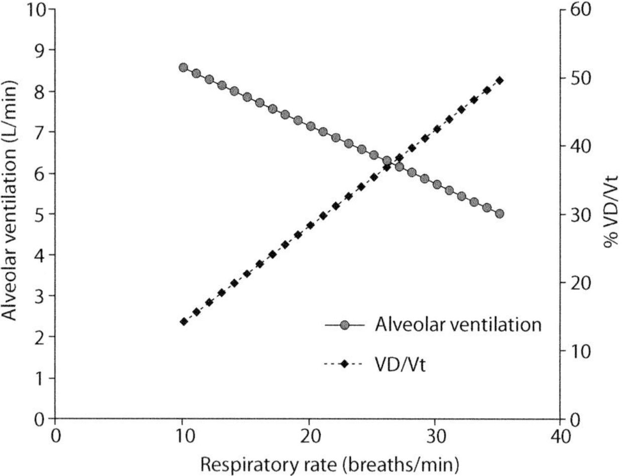

Figure 27.1 Estimated impact of the respiratory rate (from 10 to 35 breaths/min) on alveolar ventilation for a constant minute ventilation. In this example, minute ventilation is stable at 10 L/min in a male patient measuring 175 cm, and the estimated physiologic dead space is 142 mL. The alveolar ventilation decreases when the respiratory rate increases and the impact of dead space is proportional to the respiratory rate.

without positive end-expiratory pressure.[9–12] In most of the studies, baseline WOB before NIV application was very high, with negative deflections in esophageal pressure (ΔP_{es}) or transdiaphragmatic pressure (ΔP_{di}), frequently above 10 cmH_2O and with values up to 30 cmH_2O;[4,11,12] WOB was frequently above 1 J/L (expressed per liter of ventilation), or 10 J/min (expressed as power). Similarly, markers of effort to breathe, pressure–time product (PTP) of the inspiratory muscles (PTP_{es}), are frequently above 200 cmH_2O*s/min in this specific population (a normal value would be below 100 cmH_2O*s/min). Mean values for dynamic intrinsic PEEP (PEEPi) (the minimum alveolar pressure that must be overcome by the inspiratory muscles to initiate inspiratory gas flow) typically exceeded 3 cmH_2O and sometimes 5 cmH_2O in critically ill patients.[4,12] By comparison, in healthy subjects, ΔP_{es} is <5 cmH_2O, WOB <0.5 J/L, and PEEPi is absent at baseline.[13]

With NIV, all indexes of efforts are reduced in comparison with baseline. WOB is reduced by 30% to 70%, and ΔP_{es} and ΔP_{di} are reduced by 50% to 75%. In the first clinical study, WOB assessed by transdiaphragmatic pressure was reduced from 19.1 ± 5.4 cmH_2O before NIV to 10.1 ± 5.5 cmH_2O after 45 min of NIV.[4]

Modality of NIV during COPD exacerbation

The effect of the inspiratory support (pressure support level) and expiratory support (PEEP) must be differentiated. The inspiratory pressure support reduces the WOB by supplying a greater proportion of transpulmonary pressure during inspiration, leading to greater tidal volumes.[12] In their seminal paper, Brochard et al. used a range of pressure support from 12 to 20 cmH_2O and reported a significant decrease in diaphragm activity as assessed by the decrease in transdiaphragmatic pressure from 19 to 10 cmH_2O.[4] Vanpee et al. found that stepwise application of pressure support in 5-cmH_2O increments between 5 and 20 cmH_2O progressively reduced the indexes of effort.[14] Pressure support of 5 cmH_2O had minor impact in PTPdi and WOB reduction, while further incremental steps of 5 cmH_2O were associated with substantial reductions of approximately 15%–20% at each step.[14]

The application of PEEP reduces the WOB counterbalancing PEEPi, thereby reducing the threshold load to inspiration.[12] In COPD patients with exacerbation, continuous positive airway pressure (CPAP) of 5 cmH_2O alone can reduce the WOB in comparison with baseline before NIV application.[12] However, the addition of 10 cmH_2O of inspiratory pressure support is more efficient than CPAP alone or PSV alone[12] (Figure 27.2). Vanpee et al showed that when keeping peak inspiratory pressure constant, adding PEEP of 5 cmH_2O and 10 cmH_2O generally caused a greater decrease in PTPdi than did the same level of peak inspiratory pressure without PEEP.[14]

Altogether, these findings suggest applying both PEEP and pressure support. The level of pressure support should be considered as a positive pressure added to the negative pressure generated by the diaphragm to increase tidal volume. For this reason, the best target to titrate pressure

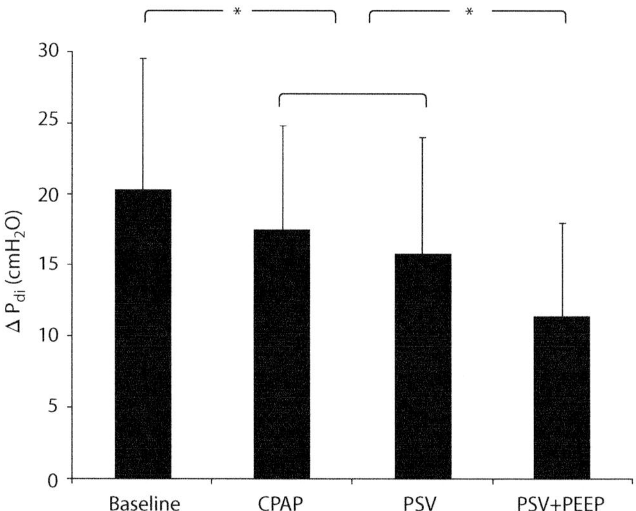

Figure 27.2 Reduction of the transdiaphragmatic pressure (ΔP_{di}) with different noninvasive ventilatory support in comparison with baseline. CPAP alone, PSV and PSV+PEEP all significantly reduced transdiaphragmatic pressure in comparison with baseline. PSV+PEEP was the most efficient ventilatory support and reduced the ΔP_{di} significantly more than PSV alone. (From Appendini L, Patessio A, Zanaboni S et al., *Am J Respir Crit Care Med.* 1994;149(5):1069–76.)

support should be expired tidal volume. Pressure support should increase until reaching an expired tidal volume around 6 to 8 mL/kg. If tolerance is good, pressure support level can be increased further but attention has to be paid to avoid hyperinflation and potential asynchrony.[15] The addition of external PEEP (3 to 5 cmH_2O) may be necessary to overcome intrinsic PEEP, which is, however, challenging to measure in practice.

Impact of NIV on cardiac performance

Located in the same closed area, the heart and lungs interact continuously. A given change in the performance of the respiratory system will affect the performance of the cardiovascular system as well as a left ventricular failure could induce an authenticable exacerbation of COPD. In some extent, the two diseases are sometimes difficult to distinguish.[16] Therefore, it is likely that during COPD exacerbation, beneficial effects of NIV can be explained by an improvement in left[17] and right[18] ventricle performance. The positive pressure generated by NIV will increase the pressure gradient of venous return, decrease right cardiac preload and decrease cardiac filling pressures. A decreased cardiac output with NIV has been described but it was not clear whether it was a deleterious effect of intrathoracic pressure or, more likely, an adaptation to a reduced demand in O_2 consumption.[19]

Obesity hypoventilation and overlap syndrome

Obesity hypoventilation syndrome (OHS) refers to the appearance of awake hypercapnia ($PaCO_2$ > 45 mm Hg) in obese patients (body mass index > 30 kg/m^2) after other causes such as lung or neuromuscular disease have been excluded.[20] Although obesity is frequent in patients with COPD, only a minority of obese subjects develop OHS and/or obstructive sleep apnoea–hypopnoea syndrome.[20] COPD and obstructive sleep apnoea–hypopnoea syndrome are both common diseases gathered into a so-called overlap syndrome whenever they are both present in the same patient.[20] Patients with OHS often present exacerbations of their respiratory symptoms that, like COPD, require hospitalisation because of acute hypercapnic respiratory failure that may require ventilatory support. There are only a few studies reporting the clinical effects of NIV in this population. Using a similar protocol to that used in patients with severe COPD exacerbation, a Spanish group reported that NIV was highly effective in patients with OHS.[21] Importantly, this group reported better outcomes for patients with OHS than for COPD.[21]

Impact of NIV on arterial blood gases

The short-term effects of NIV on arterial blood gases in patients with exacerbation of COPD are well documented.[4,9,12,22] In several studies, the reduction of $PaCO_2$ during NIV in comparison with baseline values was predictive of success of the technique, in opposition to patients in which $PaCO_2$ was stable or deteriorated while on NIV.[23,24]

The increase in alveolar ventilation with inspiratory pressure support is related to increased tidal volumes due to increased transpulmonary pressure and to the decrease of the dead space effect with respiratory rate reduction (Figure 27.1).

CLINICAL APPLICATIONS

In 1965, Sadoul et al. reported that administering positive pressure ventilation through a face mask instead of a tracheal prosthesis was a very efficient way to manage hypercapnic respiratory failure in patients suffering from chronic respiratory disorders and had little untoward effects.[25] This was rediscovered during the second half of the 1980s, and in less than 15 years, non-invasive mechanical ventilation (NIV) has become a major therapy of acute-on-chronic respiratory failure. The succeeding paragraph will focus on the evidence supporting the use of NIV in acute exacerbation of COPD, which includes the prevention of intubation, but also the facilitation of extubation and the prevention of reintubation. Future challenges will be highlighted.

NIV TO PREVENT INTUBATION IN ACUTE-ON-CHRONIC RESPIRATORY FAILURE

Strong evidence supports the benefit of NIV in COPD exacerbations

The positive results of the first randomised trials that evidenced the benefit of NIV on the risk of endotracheal intubation in the early 1990s[26,27] were further confirmed later (Table 27.1). NIV also bypasses the weaning phase, which contributes to increased duration of mechanical ventilation, and NIV decreases intensive care unit (ICU) and hospital length of stay in COPD exacerbation.[26,28] Finally, a matched controlled study showed that compared to endotracheal intubation, NIV is associated with a lower risk of nosocomial infections (pneumonia, urinary tract and bacteraemia).[29]

As a consequence of these multiple benefits, NIV significantly and consistently reduces the hospital mortality rate of patients admitted for COPD exacerbation (Table 27.1).

The results of these trials have been confirmed by three meta-analyses, which have clearly shown that, in acute exacerbation of COPD, NIV reduces intubation rate, hospital length of stay and hospital mortality.[30–32] However, these meta-analyses have pointed out that the benefit of NIV on intubation and mortality applies only to exacerbations associated with respiratory acidosis (pH < 7.35) and not to mild exacerbations without respiratory acidosis.[33]

Table 27.1 Benefit of non-invasive mechanical ventilation (NIV) in acute respiratory failure related to COPD exacerbation

	Intubation (%)			Hospital mortality (%)		
Studies	Standard therapy	NIV	p	Standard therapy	NIV	p
Bott et al.[27]	7	0	NS	30	10	NS
Brochard et al.[26]	74	26	0.001	29	9	<0.05
Barbe et al.[77]	0	0	NS	0	0	NS
Celikel et al.[78,a]	13	7	NA	7	0	NS
Plant et al.[39]	27	15	<0.05	20	10	0.05
Dikensoy et al.[28]	41	12	<0.05	12	6	NS
Conti et al.[40,b]	100	52	<0.01	19	26	NS
Thys et al.[22]	30	0	NA	20	10	NA

Note: NA, not applicable; NS, nonsignificant.

[a] In the study by Celikel et al., patients in the control group could cross over and receive NIV in case of failure of the standard medical therapy.

[b] In the study by Conti et al., intubation was the standard therapy.

The benefit of NIV is translated from randomised controlled trials to the clinical settings

The multiple benefits of NIV in COPD exacerbations observed in randomised controlled trials are translated to the daily practice. This actual translation is suggested by the results of various monocentric and multicentric studies. In recent years, several large retrospective database surveys, using strong methodology to compare NIV-treated and non-treated patients out of the context of trials, have confirmed the increased use of NIV and the related benefits on outcome.[34–36]

Physicians have adopted NIV

As a consequence of the multiple benefits of NIV, NIV use has increased over the years. Perceived NIV efficacy, which is obvious in many patients, might be a major reason for this large and progressive adoption by physicians across the last 25 years.[1,34–36] For instance, using a large retrospective cohort study, Lindenauer et al. reported that a total of 17,978 patients (70%) admitted for acute exacerbations of COPD were initially treated with NIV on hospital day 1 or 2.[36] Interestingly, a Francophone survey observed that between 2002 and 2011, NIV use did not increase any more in patients with acute-on-chronic respiratory failure who received ventilatory assistance,[1] suggesting a need for further efforts to promote NIV in this indication.

New challenges for NIV in exacerbation of COPD

The benefit of NIV in COPD exacerbation is now well established. Many questions remain, however, and the physicians have to solve various issues regarding NIV practice. They also need to face new challenges.

TO FURTHER IMPROVE THE PROPORTION OF PATIENTS WHO REALLY RECEIVE NIV

Since 1998, NIV use in the ICU has improved over the world.[2] However, in the specific context of exacerbation of COPD, NIV use rate is still lower than expected considering the high level of evidence.[1,34,35] Surveys have shown that lack of physician knowledge and inadequate equipment were the top two reasons resulting in low rate NIV.[41] These data underlie the necessity to develop and implement strategies aiming at increasing appropriate use of NIV in COPD exacerbations. Among these strategies are educational programmes and guidelines. In this direction, a consensus conference on NIV was organised in France in 2006 and gave a high recommendation to NIV in COPD exacerbation.[42] International guidelines recommend NIV in this indication.[8] The American Thoracic Society and the European Respiratory Society have recently revised their recommendations.[43]

TO IMPROVE NIV SUCCESS RATE

For the last 15 years, the NIV success rate seemed to increase,[1] although the success rate varies among centres (from 65% to 80%).[34,35,44] In addition, during the same period, the severity of patients receiving NIV has increased.[35]

Late failure, defined as persisting signs of respiratory distress after more than 48 or 72 hours of NIV, concerns a substantial number of patients probably because of the increasing severity of these patients. In a multicentre study, conducted in 137 patients who responded initially to NIV, 23% experienced a new episode of respiratory failure.[45] These patients were more likely to have a poor functional status as well as medical complication. Their prognosis was poor.[45] Here is clearly a major challenge for the forthcoming years. In a recent study, a strong association between sleep disturbances and late NIV failure was found.[46] Specifically, late NIV failure was associated with early sleep disturbances. Taking more attention to sleep quality of COPD patients treated by NIV may therefore be important for their outcome. The data do not tell, however, whether sleep disturbances pre-existed and represent a marker of severity or whether the patient's management in the ICU was responsible for part of these abnormalities.

TO USE NIV AS AN ALTERNATIVE TO INTUBATION

In the 1990s, trials that demonstrated the benefit of NIV actually compared NIV to conventional treatment and not to intubation. Two randomised controlled trials showed that NIV administered after failure of standard medical therapy to patients with intubation criteria could reduce the rate of intubation.[40,47] Moreover, a case–control matched study strongly suggested that these results can also apply to patients with moderate to severe encephalopathy (Kelly score of 3 or higher).[48] Altogether, these data suggest that NIV might still be beneficial as an alternative to intubation. Alteration of consciousness is not anymore a contraindication of NIV in acute exacerbation of COPD. In these patients, NIV should be attempted in the ICU and pursued in case of rapid improvement of the level of consciousness. A prospective non-controlled study designed to assess the outcome of NIV in patients with a Glasgow coma scale (GCS) score of <8 points due to acute respiratory failure showed that an improvement of the GCS or of hypercapnic acidosis within the first hour of NIV was highly predictive of NIV success.[49] Future studies are needed to better determine the criteria of selection of these patients.

TO CONTINUE NIV AFTER THE ACUTE PHASE IN SOME PATIENTS

Preventing relapse of exacerbation of COPD after ICU discharge is a major therapeutic goal. Obviously, prevention involves optimisation of the global treatment of COPD, including medical and physical therapy. Funk et al. randomised 26 consecutive COPD patients who remained hypercapnic after acute respiratory failure requiring mechanical ventilation.[50] Twelve months after randomisation, 10 patients (77%) in the withdrawal group, but only 2 patients (15%) in the ventilation group, experienced clinical worsening ($p < 0.01$). Another study prospectively allocated COPD patients after exacerbation requiring NIV in two groups: CPAP versus home NIV.[51] Authors reported a significant reduction in the recurrence of new exacerbation requiring NIV in patients treated with home NIV (38.5% vs. 60.2% at 1 year [$p = 0.039$]). These findings are very preliminary but suggest that pursuing ventilatory support after resolution of acute exacerbation of COPD may be beneficial.

TO DEFINE MORE PRECISELY THE ROLE OF NIV IN PALLIATIVE CARE SETTINGS

The role of NIV when patients and families have decided to forgo intubation remains controversial. In a 2004 European Respiratory Survey, NIV was the ceiling of ventilatory care in 31% of patients with an end-of-life decision.[52] COPD is a predictor of favourable outcome in this context. Survival in a patient with exacerbation of COPD who declined intubation but accepted NIV is about 50% to 60%.[53,54] However, 1-year survival is 30%, which is compared to more than 60% in COPD patients with no care limitation.[55] It is noticeable that providing NIV in do-not-intubate patients is not associated with a decrease in quality of life 3 months after ICU admission as assessed by the Short Form 36 and is comparable to patients with no limitation.[56] Although it is even more challenging, NIV may also be administered as a palliative measure when patients and families have chosen to forgo all life support, receiving comfort measures only.[57] A conceptual framework with three categories has been proposed to describe the possible uses of NIV for patients with acute respiratory failure.[58] For category 1, the main goal will be to avoid intubation, whereas for category 2, the main goal will be to improve gas exchanges and clinical variables. Finally, for category 3, NIV can be considered as a form of palliative care, to attempt to reduce dyspnoea and discomfort.

TO BETTER DEFINE THE ENVIRONMENT THAT IS REQUIRED TO SAFELY AND EFFICIENTLY ADMINISTER NIV OUT OF THE ICU

For safety reasons as well as to improve the chances of success, NIV requires an appropriate environment. Elliott et al. defined this environment as follows: location of staff with training and expertise in NIV, adequate staff available throughout a 24-hour period, facilities for monitoring, rapid access to endotracheal intubation and invasive ventilation.[59] Obviously, the ICU setting fulfils all these criteria. Unfortunately, there is often an imbalance between ICU beds and the number of patients that need NIV. According to forecasts, this imbalance should increase in the future. Indeed, the number of patients requiring mechanical ventilation will grow continuously, while workforce shortage currently forces ICU bed closure. The strong pressure on ICU beds combined with their high cost has made NIV outside the ICU an attractive option.

Two different locations for delivering NIV outside the ICU have been mostly studied: the emergency department and the respiratory ward. Many patients with acute respiratory failure enter the hospital through the emergency department where cares are initiated. It seemed therefore logical to evaluate the benefit of NIV in the emergency department. Such benefit stays controversial in general delivery of NIV.[60–62] Achieving a safe and successful NIV in wards is another challenge.[63] Of course, this is more feasible if the respiratory ward is close to a respiratory ICU. Carlucci et al. have thus shown that while the severity of patients treated in their respiratory ICU for acute exacerbations of COPD was increasing, more and more less severely ill patients were treated in the nearby ward.[44] For some authors, a pH cutoff could be used to safely provide NIV in the ward.[62,63] Without the vicinity of a respiratory ICU, it is suggested that with adequate staff training, NIV can be applied with benefit in the general respiratory ward with the usual ward staff.[39] Furthermore, recent Canadian surveys showed that although NIV was primarily used in monitored areas, initiation or continuation of NIV in general medical or surgical wards was not uncommon.[41] This observation raises the questions of staffing and training. Finally, preliminary reports show that NIV might be successfully and safely administered in the ward under the supervision of a medical emergency team,[61,64,65] but further studies are needed.

NIV TO FACILITATE EXTUBATION IN COPD PATIENTS

There is now strong evidence that NIV may be used to facilitate extubation and shorten the duration of intubation in COPD patients intubated for an episode of acute respiratory failure. For a better understanding, it is important to precisely determine what is exactly meant by *facilitate*. This indication for NIV means that the patient meets all the readiness criteria but fails the spontaneous breathing trial. The concept of a facilitation NIV strategy is to reduce the duration of invasive mechanical ventilation by providing non-invasive rather than invasive ventilation, which can have a similar physiological efficacy.[66] To make this strategy safe and effective, it is important to ensure (1) that patients are not exposed to an increased risk of reintubation and (2) that the strategy is associated with a reduction of intubation-related complications such as ventilator-associated pneumonia, ICU length of stay and ideally ICU mortality.

Three multicentric[67–69] randomised controlled trials support this strategy. These trials have included intubated COPD patients who have failed one to three spontaneous breathing trials. Their results have shown the benefit of NIV, which reduced the duration of intubation and mechanical ventilation, hospital length of stay and hospital mortality[67,69] without increasing the reintubation rate.[68] One study, however, did not observe any benefit in hard outcomes including the subgroup with COPD.[68]

Although there is enough scientific evidence to support this indication of NIV, there is no actual quantification of its use in ICUs.

NIV IN POST-EXTUBATION RESPIRATORY FAILURE

Respiratory failure after extubation occurs in about 15% of extubated patients with 30% or higher mortality.[70] Preventing and treating post-extubation respiratory failure is thus a major concern. NIV in post-extubation failure actually includes two completely different concepts: prophylactic NIV to prevent post-extubation respiratory failure/distress on one hand and therapeutic NIV to treat post-extubation respiratory failure on the other hand. Although the benefit of the former is clearly well demonstrated, the benefit of the latter is still debated.

Prophylactic NIV to prevent post-extubation respiratory failure

NIV seems beneficial if instituted immediately after intubation in a prophylactic way in patients 'at risk' of extubation failure. Three multicentre randomised trials have included patients considered at high risk of extubation failure.[71–73] Nava et al. enrolled patients deemed to be at 'high risk' of extubation failure and reported a significant decrease in the reintubation rate from 24% to 8%.[73] Later, Ferrer et al. designed a study where prophylactic NIV was applied in patients with a priori risk factors of extubation failure (age >65, APACHE II >12, intubation for cardiac failure).[71] In this study, there was a significant reduction in the occurrence of post-extubation respiratory failure (33% to 16%, $p = 0.029$) but without effect on the reintubation rate.[71] Nevertheless, hypercapnic patients had a significant improvement of the survival in the ICU, in the hospital and at 90 days in patients treated with NIV.[71] Logically, the same group conducted a randomised controlled trial that included only patients with hypercapnia.[74] This study confirmed the previous results by showing a reduction of the post-extubation respiratory failure and of the mortality at 90 days. Interestingly, there was no effect on the reintubation rate or the ICU mortality.[74] In these studies, sequential NIV (around 8 hours a day) was administered during the first 24[71] or 48 hours[73] after extubation. The NIV prophylactic strategy reduced the incidence of post-extubation respiratory failure,[71] the rate of reintubation,[73] and ICU mortality in a subgroup of patients with hypercapnia.[71] To evaluate to what extent the results of these randomised controlled trials translate to daily practice, Thille et al. investigated the effect of post-extubation prophylactic NIV in patients at high risk of reintubation.[75] They found that the reintubation rate significantly decreased from 28% (no NIV) to 15% (with NIV) ($p = 0.02$) in high-risk patients.[75]

Taken together, these results suggest that post-extubation prophylactic NIV may be beneficial in patients with hypercapnia or at risk of extubation failure.

Therapeutic NIV to treat post-extubation respiratory failure

Since the benefit of NIV on hypercapnic acute respiratory failure is well established, very few patients have been enrolled in studies investigating the effect of NIV to treat post-extubation respiratory failure in COPD patients. A case matched study in COPD patients gave encouraging results in the late 1990s.[76] However, two further randomised controlled studies did not confirm these results.[77,78] Moreover, one study reported a higher mortality in the NIV group, which was associated with a much longer delay in reintubation than in the control group.[77] However, these negative studies suffer from various limitations: inexperienced centres, low levels of assistance and higher NIV success rate in the patients of the control group who were crossed over to late NIV and eventually received NIV for acute respiratory failure. Moreover, these two studies included only 10% of COPD patients, who are among those who really get a benefit of NIV. Further studies in COPD are therefore needed on this topic.

PERSPECTIVES

Use of high flow oxygen cannula therapy

Heated, humidified, high flow nasal cannula (HFNC) oxygen is a technique that can deliver up to 100% heated and humidified oxygen at a maximum flow rate of 60 L/min of gas via nasal prongs or cannula.[79] These high flow rates generate low levels of positive pressure in the upper airways and the FiO_2 can be adjusted by changing the fraction of oxygen in the driving gas.[79] In acute hypercapnic respiratory failure, the use of HFNC could have important benefits by decreasing the WOB and performing a washout of anatomical dead space, thereby enhancing CO_2 clearance.[80] Nevertheless, no study has been conducted in the specific setting of acute exacerbation of COPD.[81]

Use of CO_2 removal

Extracorporeal circuits designed to remove CO_2 ($ECCO_2R$) have been used in patients with acute hypercapnic respiratory failure since $ECCO_2R$ should enhance the efficacy of NIV to remove CO_2 and avoid the worsening of respiratory acidosis. According to the findings of a recent meta-analysis,[82] initiation of $ECCO_2R$ seems to improve very quickly and significantly blood gas–related variables and breathing patterns. After initiation of $ECCO_2R$, pH increases by 0.07 at the first hour, by 0.11 after 6 hours and by 0.15 after 24 hours.[82] Accordingly, $PaCO_2$ decreases around 25 mmHg similarly between H1 and H6, and between H6 and 24 hours.[82] A case–control study published after the meta-analysis by Sklar et al. reported that half of patients refractory to NIV and treated with $ECCO_2R$ needed intubation.[82] Importantly, $ECCO_2R$ was associated with relevant adverse events, in particular related to bleeding complications.[83] Finally, this study reports discrepancy with the findings of Sklar et al. who found a very high proportion (93%) of patients avoiding intubation when treated with $ECCO_2R$.[82] In this context, predefined NIV failure and/or intubation criteria and NIV management are important issues to take into account that could explain heterogeneity observed in existing studies.

Altogether, these findings suggest that $ECCO_2R$ is an efficient technique to remove CO_2 but that the exact clinical indication and the overall benefits still remain undetermined (NIV failure prevention, intubation prevention, difficult weaning). Indeed, the technique seems to be associated with bleeding complications precluding its generalisation into routine use.

Improving NIV tolerance and patient–ventilator interaction

From a practical point of view, NIV intolerance could be defined as the need to discontinue NIV because the patient is no longer able to tolerate NIV. This definition was used in a recent prospective study that enrolled 961 patients receiving NIV as first-line treatment of acute respiratory failure, mostly related to an exacerbation of COPD or pneumonia.[84] The main finding of their study was the low level of NIV intolerance (5.2%). However, patients who experienced NIV intolerance had a higher risk of NIV failure and subsequent intubation. These findings highlight that the use of NIV with face mask should be done carefully and tightly monitored to avoid patient intolerance. Among the reasons of NIV intolerance, patient–ventilator asynchrony should be considered first. An observational study of 60 patients treated with NIV for acute respiratory failure, 55% of them being hypercapnic, showed that 43% of the patients had a high rate of patient–ventilator asynchronies.[85] In this study, ICU ventilators with non-NIV modes were used, which may explain the high rates of asynchrony. Recent studies suggest that the use of NIV modes in case of ICU ventilators reduces asynchronies.[85,86] Also, the use of specific NIV-dedicated turbine ventilators may be associated with significantly less asynchronies.[87] Moreover, modern ventilators are equipped with specific NIV algorithms aimed at compensating leaks occurring around the mask. Using NIV-dedicated ventilators, NIV algorithms improve slightly but significantly triggering and cycling off synchronisation.[88] Recent modes such as NAVA (Neurally Adjusted Ventilatory Assist, a ventilatory mode that synchronises the ventilator cycle to the diaphragm electrical activity) or PAV (Proportional Assist Ventilation, another adjustable ventilatory mode) have shown that a better synchrony is reachable in COPD patients by using proportional modes.[89,90] Whether the improvement in patient–ventilator synchrony is or is not associated with better outcomes deserves further studies. Another important aspect of the NIV technique is caregivers' personal beliefs and how their own perception of NIV may affect the patient's adhesion to care recommendations, communication, and empathy. A recent French multicentre questionnaire-based study reported that nurses generally reported more negative feelings and more frequent regrets about providing NIV compared to ICU physicians.[91] On the other hand, it is noteworthy that a significant proportion of patients and relatives perceived NIV as inefficient and reported regrets about having received NIV versus having received oxygen therapy or having been intubated.

CONCLUSION

NIV has become the gold standard for mild or severe forms of exacerbation of COPD, as a mean of improving alveolar ventilation, reducing patient's WOB and avoiding the need for endotracheal intubation and its related complications. Severe forms of exacerbations associated with hypercapnic coma can also be treated with this technique under careful monitoring. A possible risk of adverse outcome associated with delayed endotracheal intubation in patients who fail a trial of NIV has not been identified in COPD, by contrast to patients with *de novo* acute respiratory failure. Future avenues should consider improvements in patient–ventilator interfaces, reduction in asynchronies through more efficient algorithms for dealing with leaks and better understanding of late failures.

REFERENCES

1. Demoule A, Chevret S, Carlucci A et al. Changing use of noninvasive ventilation in critically ill patients: Trends over 15 years in francophone countries. *Intensive Care Med.* 2016;42:82–92.
2. Esteban A, Frutos-Vivar F, Muriel A et al. Evolution of mortality over time in patients receiving mechanical ventilation. *Am J Respir Crit Care Med.* 2013;188: 220–30.
3. Meduri GU, Conoscenti CC, Menashe P, Nair S. Noninvasive face mask ventilation in patients with acute respiratory failure. *Chest.* 1989;95:865–70.
4. Brochard L, Isabey D, Piquet J et al. Reversal of acute exacerbations of chronic obstructive lung disease by inspiratory assistance with a face mask. *N Engl J Med.* 1990;323:1523–30.
5. Similowski T, Yan S, Gauthier AP et al. Contractile properties of the human diaphragm during chronic hyperinflation. *N Engl J Med.* 1991;325:917–23.
6. Pepe PE, Marini JJ. Occult positive end-expiratory pressure in mechanically ventilated patients with airflow obstruction: The auto-PEEP effect. *Am Rev Respir Dis.* 1982;126:166–70.
7. Tobin MJ, Laghi F, Brochard L. Role of the respiratory muscles in acute respiratory failure of COPD: Lessons from weaning failure. *J Appl Physiol Bethesda Md. 1985.* 2009;107:962–70.
8. Vestbo J, Hurd SS, Agustí AG et al. Global strategy for the diagnosis, management, and prevention of chronic obstructive pulmonary disease: GOLD executive summary. *Am J Respir Crit Care Med.* 2013;187:347–65.
9. Ambrosino N, Nava S, Bertone P et al. Physiologic evaluation of pressure support ventilation by nasal mask in patients with stable COPD. *Chest.* 1992;101:385–91.
10. Nava S, Bruschi C, Rubini F et al. Respiratory response and inspiratory effort during pressure support ventilation in COPD patients. *Intensive Care Med.* 1995;21:871–9.
11. Vitacca M, Clini E, Pagani M et al. Physiologic effects of early administered mask proportional assist ventilation in patients with chronic obstructive pulmonary disease and acute respiratory failure. *Crit Care Med.* 2000;28:1791–7.
12. Appendini L, Patessio A, Zanaboni S et al. Physiologic effects of positive end-expiratory pressure and mask pressure support during exacerbations of chronic obstructive pulmonary disease. *Am J Respir Crit Care Med.* 1994;149(5):1069–76.
13. Chiumello D, Pelosi P, Taccone P et al. Effect of different inspiratory rise time and cycling off criteria during pressure support ventilation in patients recovering from acute lung injury. *Crit Care Med.* 2003;31(11):2604–10.
14. Vanpee D, El Khawand C, Rousseau L et al. Effects of nasal pressure support on ventilation and inspiratory work in normocapnic and hypercapnic patients with stable COPD. *Chest.* 2002;122(1):75–83.
15. Thille AW, Rodriguez P, Cabello B et al. Patient–ventilator asynchrony during assisted mechanical ventilation. *Intensive Care Med.* 2006;32(10):1515–22.
16. Abroug F, Ouanes-Besbes L, Nciri N et al. Association of left-heart dysfunction with severe exacerbation of chronic obstructive pulmonary disease: Diagnostic performance of cardiac biomarkers. *Am J Respir Crit Care Med.* 2006;174(9):990–6.
17. Lenique F, Habis M, Lofaso F et al. Ventilatory and hemodynamic effects of continuous positive airway pressure in left heart failure. *Am J Respir Crit Care Med.* 1997;155(2):500–5.
18. Thorens JB, Ritz M, Reynard C et al. Haemodynamic and endocrinological effects of noninvasive mechanical ventilation in respiratory failure. *Eur Respir J.* 1997;10(11):2553–9.
19. Diaz O, Iglesia R, Ferrer M et al. Effects of noninvasive ventilation on pulmonary gas exchange and hemodynamics during acute hypercapnic exacerbations of chronic obstructive pulmonary disease. *Am J Respir Crit Care Med.* 1997;156(6):1840–5. doi:10.1164/ajrccm.156.6.9701027.
20. Piper AJ, Grunstein RR. Obesity hypoventilation syndrome: Mechanisms and management. *Am J Respir Crit Care Med.* 2011;183(3):292–8.
21. Carrillo A, Ferrer M, Gonzalez-Diaz G et al. Noninvasive ventilation in acute hypercapnic respiratory failure caused by obesity hypoventilation syndrome and chronic obstructive pulmonary disease. *Am J Respir Crit Care Med.* 2012;186(12):1279–85. doi:10.1164/rccm.201206-1101OC.
22. Thys F, Roeseler J, Reynaert M et al. Noninvasive ventilation for acute respiratory failure: A prospective randomised placebo-controlled trial. *Eur Respir J.* 2002;20(3):545–55.
23. Ambrosino N, Foglio K, Rubini F et al. Non-invasive mechanical ventilation in acute respiratory failure due to chronic obstructive pulmonary disease: Correlates for success. *Thorax.* 1995; 50(7):755–57.
24. Putinati S, Ballerin L, Piattella M et al. Is it possible to predict the success of non-invasive positive pressure ventilation in acute respiratory failure due to COPD? *Respir Med.* 2000;94(10):997–1001.
25. Sadoul P, Aug M, Gay R. Traitement par ventilation instrumentale de 100 cas d'insuffisants respiratoires chroniques. *Bull Eur Physiopathol Respir Care.* 1965;1:549.
26. Brochard L, Mancebo J, Wysocki M et al. Noninvasive ventilation for acute exacerbations of chronic obstructive pulmonary disease. *N Engl J Med.* 1995;333(13):817–22.

27. Bott J, Carroll MP, Conway JH et al. Randomised controlled trial of nasal ventilation in acute ventilatory failure due to chronic obstructive airways disease. *Lancet.* 1993;341(8860):1555–7.
28. Dikensoy O, Ikidag B, Filiz A, Bayram N. Comparison of non-invasive ventilation and standard medical therapy in acute hypercapnic respiratory failure: A randomised controlled study at a tertiary health centre in SE Turkey. *Int J Clin Pr.* 2002;56(2):85–8.
29. Girou E, Schortgen F, Delclaux C et al. Association of noninvasive ventilation with nosocomial infections and survival in critically ill patients. *JAMA.* 2000;284(18):2361–7.
30. Keenan SP, Sinuff T, Cook DJ, Hill NS. Which patients with acute exacerbation of chronic obstructive pulmonary disease benefit from noninvasive positive-pressure ventilation? A systematic review of the literature. *Ann Intern Med.* 2003;138(11):861–70.
31. Lightowler JV, Wedzicha JA, Elliott MW, Ram FS. Non-invasive positive pressure ventilation to treat respiratory failure resulting from exacerbations of chronic obstructive pulmonary disease: Cochrane systematic review and meta-analysis. *BMJ.* 2003;326(7382):185.
32. Ram FS, Picot J, Lightowler J, Wedzicha JA. Non-invasive positive pressure ventilation for treatment of respiratory failure due to exacerbations of chronic obstructive pulmonary disease. *Cochrane Database Syst Rev.* 2004;(3):CD004104.
33. Keenan SP, Powers CE, McCormack DG. Noninvasive positive-pressure ventilation in patients with milder chronic obstructive pulmonary disease exacerbations: A randomized controlled trial. *Respir Care.* 2005;50(5):610–6.
34. Chandra D, Stamm JA, Taylor B et al. Outcomes of noninvasive ventilation for acute exacerbations of chronic obstructive pulmonary disease in the United States, 1998–2008. *Am J Respir Crit Care Med.* 2012;185(2):152–9.
35. Dres M, Tran T-C, Aegerter P et al. Influence of ICU case-volume on the management and hospital outcomes of acute exacerbations of chronic obstructive pulmonary disease. *Crit Care Med.* 2013;41(8):1884–92.
36. Lindenauer PK, Stefan MS, Shieh M-S et al. Outcomes associated with invasive and noninvasive ventilation among patients hospitalized with exacerbations of chronic obstructive pulmonary disease. *JAMA Intern Med.* 2014;174(12):1982–93. doi:10.1001/jamainternmed.2014.5430.
37. Barbe F, Togores B, Rubi M et al. Noninvasive ventilatory support does not facilitate recovery from acute respiratory failure in chronic obstructive pulmonary disease. *Eur Respir J.* 1996;9(6):1240–5.
38. Celikel T, Sungur M, Ceyhan B, Karakurt S. Comparison of noninvasive positive pressure ventilation with standard medical therapy in hypercapnic acute respiratory failure. *Chest.* 1998;114(6):1636–42.
39. Plant PK, Owen JL, Elliott MW. Early use of non-invasive ventilation for acute exacerbations of chronic obstructive pulmonary disease on general respiratory wards: A multicentre randomised controlled trial. *Lancet.* 2000;355(9219):1931–5.
40. Conti G, Antonelli M, Navalesi P et al. Noninvasive vs. conventional mechanical ventilation in patients with chronic obstructive pulmonary disease after failure of medical treatment in the ward: A randomized trial. *Intensive Care Med.* 2002;28(12):1701–7.
41. Maheshwari V, Paioli D, Rothaar R, Hill NS. Utilization of noninvasive ventilation in acute care hospitals: A regional survey. *Chest.* 2006;129(5):1226–33.
42. Robert R, Bengler C, Beuret P et al. Ventilation non invasive au cours de l'insuffisance respiratoire aigue (nouveau-né exclus). In: Conférence de Consensus Commune SFAR SPLR SRLF, 2006.
43. Rochwerg B, Brochard L, Elliott MW et al. Official ERS/ATS clinical practice guidelines: Noninvasive ventilation for acute respiratory failure. *Eur Respir J* 2017 Aug 31;50(2).
44. Carlucci A, Delmastro M, Rubini F et al. Changes in the practice of non-invasive ventilation in treating COPD patients over 8 years. *Intensive Care Med.* 2003;29(3):419–25.
45. Moretti M, Cilione C, Tampieri A et al. Incidence and causes of non-invasive mechanical ventilation failure after initial success. *Thorax.* 2000;55(10):819–25.
46. Roche Campo F, Drouot X, Thille AW et al. Poor sleep quality is associated with late noninvasive ventilation failure in patients with acute hypercapnic respiratory failure. *Crit Care Med.* 2010;38(2):477–85.
47. Honrubia T, García López FJ, Franco N et al. Noninvasive vs conventional mechanical ventilation in acute respiratory failure: A multicenter, randomized controlled trial. *Chest.* 2005;128(6):3916–24.
48. Scala R, Nava S, Conti G et al. Noninvasive versus conventional ventilation to treat hypercapnic encephalopathy in chronic obstructive pulmonary disease. *Intensive Care Med.* 2007;33(12):2101–8.
49. Diaz GG, Alcaraz AC, Talavera JC et al. Noninvasive positive-pressure ventilation to treat hypercapnic coma secondary to respiratory failure. *Chest.* 2005;127(3):952–60.
50. Funk G-C, Breyer M-K, Burghuber OC et al. Long-term non-invasive ventilation in COPD after acute-on-chronic respiratory failure. *Respir Med.* 2011;105(3):427–34.

51. Cheung APS, Chan VL, Liong JT et al. A pilot trial of non-invasive home ventilation after acidotic respiratory failure in chronic obstructive pulmonary disease. *Int J Tuberc Lung Dis Off J Int Union Tuberc Lung Dis*. 2010;14(5):642–9.
52. Nava S, Sturani C, Hartl S et al. End-of-life decision-making in respiratory intermediate care units: A European survey. *Eur Respir J*. 2007;30(1):156–64.
53. Schettino G, Altobelli N, Kacmarek RM. Noninvasive positive pressure ventilation reverses acute respiratory failure in select "do-not-intubate" patients. *Crit Care Med*. 2005;33(9):1976–82.
54. Levy M, Tanios MA, Nelson D et al. Outcomes of patients with do-not-intubate orders treated with noninvasive ventilation. *Crit Care Med*. 2004;32(10):2002–7.
55. Chu CM, Chan VL, Wong IW et al. Noninvasive ventilation in patients with acute hypercapnic exacerbation of chronic obstructive pulmonary disease who refused endotracheal intubation. *Crit Care Med*. 2004;32(2):372–7.
56. Azoulay E, Kouatchet A, Jaber S et al. Noninvasive mechanical ventilation in patients having declined tracheal intubation. *Intensive Care Med*. 2013;39(2):292–301. doi:10.1007/s00134-012-2746-2.
57. Nava S, Ferrer M, Esquinas A et al. Palliative use of non-invasive ventilation in end-of-life patients with solid tumours: A randomised feasibility trial. *Lancet Oncol*. 2013;14(3):219–27. doi:10.1016/S1470-2045(13)70009-3.
58. Curtis JR, Cook DJ, Sinuff T et al. Noninvasive positive pressure ventilation in critical and palliative care settings: Understanding the goals of therapy. *Crit Care Med*. 2007;35(3):932–9.
59. Elliott MW, Confalonieri M, Nava S. Where to perform noninvasive ventilation? *Eur Respir J*. 2002;19(6):1159–66.
60. van Gemert JP, Brijker F, Witten MA, Leenen LPH. Intubation after noninvasive ventilation failure in chronic obstructive pulmonary disease: Associated factors at emergency department presentation. *Eur J Emerg Med Off J Eur Soc Emerg Med*. 2015;22(1):49–54.
61. Khalid I, Sherbini N, Qushmaq I et al. Outcomes of patients treated with noninvasive ventilation by a medical emergency team on the wards. *Respir Care*. 2014;59(2):186–92. doi:10.4187/respcare.02515.
62. Pastaka C, Kostikas K, Karetsi E et al. Non-invasive ventilation in chronic hypercapnic COPD patients with exacerbation and a pH of 7.35 or higher. *Eur J Intern Med*. 2007;18(7):524–30. doi:10.1016/j.ejim.2006.12.012.
63. Fiorino S, Bacchi-Reggiani L, Detotto E et al. Efficacy of non-invasive mechanical ventilation in the general ward in patients with chronic obstructive pulmonary disease admitted for hypercapnic acute respiratory failure and pH < 7.35: A feasibility pilot study. *Intern Med J*. 2015;45(5):527–37.
64. Cabrini L, Idone C, Colombo S et al. Medical emergency team and non-invasive ventilation outside ICU for acute respiratory failure. *Intensive Care Med*. 2009;35(2):339–43.
65. Masa JF, Utrabo I, Gomez de Terreros J et al. Noninvasive ventilation for severely acidotic patients in respiratory intermediate care units: Precision medicine in intermediate care units. *BMC Pulm Med*. 2016;16(1):97.
66. Vitacca M, Ambrosino N, Clini E et al. Physiological response to pressure support ventilation delivered before and after extubation in patients not capable of totally spontaneous autonomous breathing. *Am J Respir Crit Care Med*. 2001;164(4):638–41.
67. Ferrer M, Esquinas A, Arancibia F et al. Noninvasive ventilation during persistent weaning failure: A randomized controlled trial. *Am J Respir Crit Care Med*. 2003;168(1):70–6.
68. Girault C, Bubenheim M, Abroug F et al. Noninvasive ventilation and weaning in patients with chronic hypercapnic respiratory failure: A randomized multicenter trial. *Am J Respir Crit Care Med*. 2011;184(6):672–9.
69. Nava S, Ambrosino N, Clini E et al. Noninvasive mechanical ventilation in the weaning of patients with respiratory failure due to chronic obstructive pulmonary disease. A randomized, controlled trial. *Ann Intern Med*. 1998;128(9):721–8.
70. Epstein SK, Ciubotaru RL, Wong JB. Effect of failed extubation on the outcome of mechanical ventilation. *Chest*. 1997;112(1):186–92.
71. Ferrer M, Valencia M, Nicolas JM et al. Early noninvasive ventilation averts extubation failure in patients at risk: A randomized trial. *Am J Respir Crit Care Med*. 2006;173(2):164–70.
72. Ferrer M, Sellarés J, Valencia M et al. Non-invasive ventilation after extubation in hypercapnic patients with chronic respiratory disorders: Randomised controlled trial. *Lancet Lond Engl*. 2009;374(9695):1082–8.
73. Nava S, Gregoretti C, Fanfulla F et al. Noninvasive ventilation to prevent respiratory failure after extubation in high-risk patients. *Crit Care Med*. 2005;33(11):2465–70.
74. Ferrer M, Sellarés J, Valencia M et al. Non-invasive ventilation after extubation in hypercapnic patients with chronic respiratory disorders: Randomised controlled trial. *Lancet Lond Engl*. 2009;374(9695):1082–8.
75. Thille AW, Boissier F, Ben-Ghezala H et al. Easily identified at-risk patients for extubation failure may benefit from noninvasive ventilation: A prospective before-after study. *Crit Care Lond Engl*. 2016;20:48.

76. Hilbert G, Gruson D, Portel L et al. Noninvasive pressure support ventilation in COPD patients with postextubation hypercapnic respiratory insufficiency. *Eur Respir J.* 1998;11(6):1349–53.
77. Esteban A, Frutos-Vivar F, Ferguson ND et al. Noninvasive positive-pressure ventilation for respiratory failure after extubation. *N Engl J Med.* 2004;350(24):2452–60.
78. Keenan SP, Powers C, McCormack DG, Block G. Noninvasive positive-pressure ventilation for post-extubation respiratory distress: A randomized controlled trial. *JAMA.* 2002;287(24):3238–44.
79. Papazian L, Corley A, Hess D et al. Use of high-flow nasal cannula oxygenation in ICU adults: A narrative review. *Intensive Care Med.* 2016.
80. Möller W, Feng S, Domanski U et al. Nasal high flow reduces dead space. *J Appl Physiol* (1985) 2017;122(1):191–7.
81. Fraser J, Spooner AJ, Dunster KR et al. Nasal high flow oxygen therapy in patients with COPD reduces respiratory rate and tissue carbon dioxide while increasing tidal and end-expiratory lung volumes: A randomised crossover trial. *Thorax.* 2016 Aug;71(8)759–61.
82. Sklar MC, Beloncle F, Katsios CM et al. Extracorporeal carbon dioxide removal in patients with chronic obstructive pulmonary disease: A systematic review. *Intensive Care Med.* 2015;41(10):1752–62.
83. Braune S, Sieweke A, Brettner F et al. The feasibility and safety of extracorporeal carbon dioxide removal to avoid intubation in patients with COPD unresponsive to noninvasive ventilation for acute hypercapnic respiratory failure (ECLAIR study): Multicentre case-control study. *Intensive Care Med.* 2016.
84. Liu J, Duan J, Bai L, Zhou L. Noninvasive ventilation intolerance: Characteristics, predictors, and outcomes. *Respir Care.* 2016;61(3):277–84.
85. Vignaux L, Vargas F, Roeseler J et al. Patient–ventilator asynchrony during non-invasive ventilation for acute respiratory failure: A multicenter study. *Intensive Care Med.* 2009;35(5):840–6.
86. Schmidt M, Dres M, Raux M et al. Neurally adjusted ventilatory assist improves patient–ventilator interaction during postextubation prophylactic noninvasive ventilation. *Crit Care Med.* 2012;40(6):1738–44.
87. Lyazidi A, Thille AW, Carteaux G et al. Bench test evaluation of volume delivered by modern ICU ventilators during volume-controlled ventilation. *Intensive Care Med.* 2010;36(12):2074–80.
88. Carteaux G, Lyazidi A, Cordoba-Izquierdo A et al. Patient–ventilator asynchrony during noninvasive ventilation: A bench and clinical study. *Chest.* 2012;142(2):367–76.
89. Doorduin J, Sinderby CA, Beck J et al. Automated patient–ventilator interaction analysis during neurally adjusted non-invasive ventilation and pressure support ventilation in chronic obstructive pulmonary disease. *Crit Care Lond Engl.* 2014;18(5):550.
90. Wysocki M, Richard J-C, Meshaka P. Noninvasive proportional assist ventilation compared with noninvasive pressure support ventilation in hypercapnic acute respiratory failure. *Crit Care Med.* 2002;30(2):323–9.
91. Schmidt M, Demoule A, Deslandes-Boutmy E et al. Intensive care unit admission in chronic obstructive pulmonary disease: Patient information and the physician's decision-making process. *Crit Care.* 2014;18(3):R115.

28

NIV in chronic COPD

ENRICO M. CLINI, NICOLINO AMBROSINO, ERNESTO CRISAFULLI AND GUIDO VAGHEGGINI

KEY MESSAGES

- The indiscriminate use of domiciliary non-invasive ventilation (NIV) in patients with chronic obstructive pulmonary disease (COPD) cannot be justified by the available evidence.
- Domiciliary NIV should be *considered* in patients with COPD and hypercapnia ($PaCO_2$ > 7 kPa or 55 mmHg) when clinically stable and after optimisation of medical therapy including long-term oxygen therapy if indicated.
- It should not usually be initiated during an admission for an acute exacerbation of COPD; patients should be evaluated 2 to 6 weeks after discharge.
- The effectiveness of ventilation delivered should be confirmed by appropriate monitoring.

INTRODUCTION

Chronic obstructive pulmonary disease (COPD) is a preventable and treatable disease, characterised by persistent and progressive airflow limitation, caused by a mixture of small airways disease (obstructive bronchiolitis) and parenchymal destruction (emphysema), following an enhanced chronic inflammatory response to inhaled noxious particles or gases.[1] Chronic respiratory failure (CFR) develops very frequently in the late stage of the disease. When CRF ensues, one or both of the respiratory system functions fail, namely, gas exchange, leading to hypoxaemia, and/or pump function, leading to hypercapnia. Even when in a stable state, COPD patients often have daytime and/or nocturnal hypoxaemia and/or hypercapnia, as a result of impaired alveolar ventilation, sleep disorders and increased work of breathing, which in turn cause symptoms.[2]

At present, no medication has been shown to change the natural history of COPD. Long-term oxygen therapy (LTOT), when used ≥18 hours/day, is the only available therapy that has been shown to significantly improve survival of hypoxaemic COPD patients.[3] Non-invasive mask mechanical ventilation performed by means of intermittent positive pressure ventilation (NIV) has been proposed in patients with hypercapnic CRF and progressive worsening of their general and respiratory status. To date, there is strong evidence for the use of NIV to treat acute exacerbations of COPD,[4] and home NIV is widely accepted for the treatment of chronic hypercapnia due to restrictive thoracic or neuromuscular diseases.[5] The usefulness of long-term NIV in stable hypercapnic COPD patients is still debated, although it is widely prescribed across Europe.[6] This chapter describes the pathophysiological basis and presents the available clinical evidence to support the indication for domiciliary NIV in the stable COPD population.

PATHOPHYSIOLOGY AND EFFECT OF NIV

The pathophysiological features in COPD contribute to disadvantage of lung mechanics and respiratory muscle dysfunction. The latter is likely to contribute to acute and/or chronic respiratory muscle fatigue (diaphragm in particular), which, in turn, may lead to reduced alveolar ventilation, progressive hypercapnia and eventually respiratory acidosis. Hypercapnia is, therefore, the hallmark of chronic respiratory pump failure. The flattened diaphragm (with shortened muscle length and reduced maximal force) and the recruitment of additional inspiratory muscles (parasternal and accessory muscles, in particular) were thought to induce an energy supply to demand imbalance, thus producing a vicious cycle in maintaining and worsening CRF. The load on the respiratory muscles is also increased by the presence of intrinsic positive end-expiratory pressure (PEEPi) as the result of dynamic hyperinflation.[7]

There are four potential mechanisms explaining the effectiveness of NIV in these patients: (1) unloading of respiratory muscles, (2) improvement in sleep quality and correction of hypoventilation, (3) 'resetting' of respiratory centres and (4) cardiovascular effects.

1. *Respiratory muscle unloading.* NIV unloads the inspiratory muscles and the application of positive end-expiratory pressure (PEEP) counteracts the PEEPi associated with lung hyperinflation in these patients.[8]
2. *Sleep quality and correction of hypoventilation.* Physiological studies have shown that in stable hypercapnic COPD patients, NIV is able to improve alveolar ventilation by increasing the tidal volume and reducing the respiratory rate.[9] The sleep hypoventilation and the consequent night-to-morning change in CO_2, which may also partly be due to a reduced CO_2 responsiveness, could be an additional factor in the development of pulmonary hypertension.[10] Moreover, chronic hypercapnia may further impair diaphragmatic function[11] and also have a deleterious effect on the central respiratory drive.
3. *Resetting of the respiratory centres.* Compared with LTOT alone, addition of night NIV resulted in significant improvements in daytime arterial oxygen (PaO_2) and carbon dioxide ($PaCO_2$) tensions, total sleep time, sleep efficiency and overnight $PaCO_2$. The degree of improvement in daytime $PaCO_2$ was significantly correlated with the improvement in mean overnight $PaCO_2$.[12]
4. *Cardiovascular effects.* Nocturnal NIV applied over 3 months may improve heart rate variability, reduce circulating natriuretic peptide levels and enhance the functional performance of patients with advanced COPD, suggesting that NIV may reduce the impact of cardiac comorbidities in this population.[13] A recent study[14] has shown that long-term NIV with adequate pressure to improve gas exchange did not have an overall adverse effect on cardiac performance. Nevertheless, confirming an earlier study[15] in patients with pre-existing heart failure, the application of very high inspiratory pressures might reduce cardiac output.

CLINICAL EVIDENCE

Systematic reviews and meta-analysis have assessed the potential benefits ($PaCO_2$ level stabilisation, reduction in hospitalisation rate, etc.) of NIV in chronic stable COPD.[16–20] So far, randomised controlled trials (RCTs) with similar designs have provided different results. In a 3-month crossover study, Meecham-Jones et al.[12] compared the effect of NIV added to LTOT versus LTOT alone in 18 severely stable patients. In the NIV group, as compared with the LTOT group, the authors demonstrated a significant improvement in diurnal and nocturnal arterial blood gases, sleep architecture (total time and efficiency) and health-related quality of life (HRQL). In addition, good compliance with NIV was reported in up to 70% of patients completing the trial.[12] On the other hand, a similar study[21] in severe COPD patients did not find any advantage using NIV as compared to control therapy. Moreover, the authors reported a significantly high dropout rate with NIV (only 30% of patients completed the trial). One explanation for these different results might be differences in the baseline characteristics of COPD patients. Indeed, despite similar degrees of severity in airway obstruction, the $PaCO_2$ level at baseline in one trial[21] (47 mmHg) was much lower than that recorded in the other (57 mmHg).[12] Notably, patients in these two trials also had differences in sleep-related disturbances (hypopnoea and oxygen desaturation events). This suggests that only subgroups of patients with specific pathophysiological features (i.e. hypercapnia) might benefit from nocturnal home NIV.

Díaz et al.[22] reported increases in FEV1 (forced expiratory volume at 1 s) after NIV in a group of hypercapnic COPD patients. This raises the possibility that NIV may have an effect on the airways; possible mechanisms include a reduction in airway oedema or even stretching of chronically fibrosed airways. If correct, it is likely that this will require a level of inspiratory positive airway pressure (IPAP) to be delivered to the airways for a period of time. If this is an important mechanism, logic would suggest that the higher the IPAP and the longer it is applied to the airways, the better. Furthermore, it has been suggested that in hypercapnic COPD patients treated with long-term NIV over 6 months, a mass flow redistribution occurs, providing a better ventilation-perfusion match and hence better blood gases and lung function.[23]

Casanova et al.[24] studied severe COPD patients on LTOT in a 1-year RCT receiving nocturnal NIV plus standard care or standard care alone. Survival as well as the number of acute exacerbations did not differ between groups. The number of admissions to hospital fell significantly at 3 months in the NIV group but remained unchanged thereafter. The only marginal benefits observed at 6 months in the NIV group were reduction in dyspnoea and improvement in neuropsychological tests (psychomotor coordination).[24]

The Italian multicentre RCT[25] with 2-year follow-up and including a large sample of severe stable hypercapnic COPD patients compared the use of nocturnal NIV (in pressure support mode) plus LTOT versus LTOT alone. This trial aimed at assessing the long-term effect of NIV treatment on hypercapnia, use of healthcare resources and HRQL, measured by both the specific Maugeri Foundation Respiratory Failure Questionnaire (MRF-28) and the St George's Respiratory Questionnaire (SGRQ). There was no advantage with NIV on the mortality rate (18% and 17% in NIV and control groups, respectively). However, a marked trend towards a reduction in hospital admissions (when comparing the follow-up with the follow-back periods) was seen in favour of NIV, and the MRF-28 questionnaire (but not SGRQ) significantly improved in the NIV group alone.[25] The positive effect on

HRQL scores (both SGRQ and Nottingham Health Profile) with domiciliary NIV was also reported in a study by Perrin et al.[26] in patients followed up to 6 months; physical mobility, emotional reactions and energy component scores were those areas showing the best improvement over time. McEvoy et al. prospectively studied stable COPD patients.[27] They reported an effect on survival (mean follow-up, 2.21 years) with a 27% adjusted mortality risk reduction when using NIV in comparison with LTOT alone. Unfortunately, this effect appeared to be at the cost of worsening HRQL, suggesting that patients receiving NIV had poorer general and mental health status. A recent small retrospective study[28] confirms the usefulness of long-term NIV in reducing new episodes of acute on CRF in severe COPD patients.

Recently, the 'negative' results in survival of some of these studies have been challenged by a German RCT[29] and ascribed to the IPAP setting, which was considered 'low' and as such unable to improve hypercapnia in those studies. They performed a 12-month RCT with NIV added to standard medical treatment alone in severe and hypercapnic (daytime $PaCO_2$: 51.9 mmHg or higher) stable COPD patients; NIV was targeted to reduce baseline $PaCO_2$ level by at least 20% or to achieve $PaCO_2$ values lower than 48.1 mmHg. One-year mortality rate was 12% in the intervention group versus 33% in controls. Thus, authors concluded that the addition of long-term NIV to standard treatment improves survival of stable COPD patients with hypercapnia when IPAP is targeted to significantly reduce hypercapnia.[29]

The results of this study differ from those by Struik et al.[30] who investigated whether night home NIV, after discharging patients admitted to hospital for acute respiratory failure, prolongs the time to readmission for respiratory causes or death in the following year. Despite daytime $PaCO_2$ significantly improving following the use of NIV, the rate of readmission, survival rate and time to first event were similar. Moreover, number of exacerbations, lung function, mood state, daily activity and symptoms were not significantly different. Notably however, a similar improvement in $PaCO_2$ was seen in the control arm, reflecting the natural history of recovery from an acute exacerbation of COPD. Many patients hospitalised with hypercapnia due to an acute exacerbation of COPD revert to normocapnia during recovery and data support reversible hypercapnia as a distinct manifestation of respiratory failure in COPD, with a similar prognosis to that of normocapnic CRF.[31]

More recently, Murphy et al.[32] recruited from 13 UK centers and randomised patients with persistent hypercapnia ($PaCO_2$ > 53 mmHg) 2–4 weeks after resolution of respiratory acidemia, to home oxygen alone or to home oxygen plus home NIV. The median home ventilator settings were an IPAP of 24 cm H_2O, an EPAP of 4 cm H_2O and a backup rate of 14 breaths/minute. The median time to readmission or death was 4.3 months in the home oxygen plus home NIV group vs. 1.4 months in the home oxygen alone group. The 12-month risk of readmission or death was 63.4% in the home oxygen plus home NIV group vs. 80.4% in the home oxygen alone group.

Taken together, these studies using NIV in hypercapnic COPD patients[25,29,30,32] show some physiological benefits over 6–24 months. When considering the clinical results of NIV as related to change in $PaCO_2$, it must be considered whether improving hypercapnia is necessarily desirable. Hypercapnia is regarded as a poor prognostic indicator in COPD, but a large study from Japan, including patients with COPD, suggested that in patients receiving LTOT, hypercapnic patients had a better prognosis.[33] The advantage in survival as reported in trials might not be necessarily due only to the reduction in $PaCO_2$ levels. There is growing evidence that mortality in COPD patients is related to many factors other than hypercapnia, such as exercise capacity, comorbidities and systemic inflammation.[34–36] An improvement in $PaCO_2$ should not necessarily be taken as a surrogate for an improvement in prognosis, though it does seem to relate to changes in HRQL.

ECONOMIC CONSIDERATIONS

Even if the clinical role of long-term NIV is not clearly established yet, the presence of repeated hospital admissions due to hypercapnic acute respiratory failure seems to be a possible hallmark of a patient's disease progression and instability, and may be a useful indication for domiciliary NIV. This aspect also brings the possibility of a health–economic advantage from domiciliary NIV. Indeed, Tuggey et al.,[37] in a retrospective economic analysis in a selected population of COPD patients with recurrent acidotic exacerbations and admission to hospital, showed that following the adoption of long-term NIV, costs were dramatically reduced, primarily due to a reduction in hospitalisations and ICU admissions, which more than offset the costs of providing NIV. This finding has been further confirmed in a post hoc analysis[38] from the Italian RCT study.[25] In that study,[38] it was shown that, given similar charges for drug therapy and oxygen in the follow-up, the cost of acute care in the hospital was significantly lower in patients receiving also domiciliary NIV when compared to LTOT alone (8.25 ± 10.29 vs. 12.50 ± 20.28 €/patient/day).[38] A recent review suggests that reductions in the rate of hospital admissions per patient per year by 24% and 15% in the stable and post-hospital populations, respectively, are required for long-term NIV to be cost-effective.[20]

CLINICAL APPLICATION AND SELECTION OF CANDIDATES

Guidelines on the use of NIV in stable COPD were published in 1999, as the result of a Consensus Conference,[39] recommending that chronic ventilatory support **should not** be **systematically** prescribed in all COPD patients with CRF, which still remains true today. Those guidelines[39] considered that NIV may produce some benefits in selected symptomatic COPD patients with particular functional characteristics. Although this document considered chronic hypercapnia ($PaCO_2$ ≥ 55 mmHg) a necessary condition for indication (current opinion is that patients with $PaCO_2 \leq 55$ mmHg or no CO_2 retention with oxygen appear to gain little or no benefit from NIV), the presence of hypercapnia by itself, especially when stable and well tolerated by patients, was not considered a mandatory indication for NIV. Indeed, symptoms linked to nocturnal hypoventilation (very often under-estimated) are more likely to appear in patients' CRF, and these will not be helped by nocturnal oxygen therapy. Therefore, a recommendation was made that sleep monitoring should be performed during O_2 supplementation and that the failure to reverse nocturnal desaturation (at a level ≥90%) was a key point in deciding whether to apply nasal intermittent positive pressure ventilation during the night.[39] Since patients on supplemental oxygen, although adequately oxygenated, may develop symptomatic hypercapnia, addition of NIV should be considered, especially if adequate oxygenation cannot be maintained with a lower level of supplemental oxygen.

In 2010, the German Society of Pneumology[40] recommended that the presence of symptoms linked to CRF, poor HRQL, and at least one of the following criteria could indicate the need for long-term ventilatory support in COPD patients:

- Chronic daytime hypercapnia with $PaCO_2 \geq 50$ mmHg
- Nocturnal hypercapnia with $PaCO_2 \geq 55$ mmHg
- Stable daytime hypercapnia with $PaCO_2$ 46–50 mmHg and a rise in transcutaneous CO_2 ($TcCO_2$) ≥ 10 mmHg during sleep[41]
- Stable daytime hypercapnia with $PaCO_2$ 46–50 mmHg and at least two acute acidotic exacerbations with hospital admission in the last 12 months
- Need of prolonged ventilatory support following an acute exacerbation[42]

Poor compliance with medication intake and/or LTOT are relative contraindications. Complete cessation of nicotine abuse should be strongly advised.[40] These recommendations need to be revisited in the light of the results of the RCTs discussed above.

Table 28.1 compares the clinical and physiological parameters for NIV in COPD patients, as indicated by available international documents.

Despite the fact that all the clinical guidelines do not recommend the routine use of NIV in COPD patients with CRF, it is common practice in some countries.[6] Moreover, a recent international web survey among specialists dealing with NIV domiciliary programmes examined patterns of use in these patients.[43] Reduction in hospital admissions, improvement in HRQL and relief of dyspnoea were considered the main expected benefits. Nocturnal oxygen saturation recording was the most frequent procedure performed before prescription, whereas recurrent exacerbations requiring mechanical ventilation (>3) or weaning failure from in-hospital NIV were the most important reasons for starting home ventilation. Pressure support, with both 'low intensity' (44% of cases) or 'high intensity' (27%) settings, was the most popular ventilation mode adopted.[43]

Table 28.1 Clinical and functional indications for domiciliary NIV in severe COPD patients suggested on documents available

Criteria	ACCP	GSP
Presence of symptoms	Dyspnea	na
	Fatigue	na
	Morning headache	na
Physiology (at least one)	$PaCO_2 \geq 55$ mmHg	Daytime $PaCO_2 \geq 50$ mmHg
	$PaCO_2$ 50 > 54 mmHg and nocturnal $SatO_2$ ≤88% for 5 continuous minutes while receiving O_2 therapy with 2 ≥ L·min^{-1}	Nocturnal $PaCO_2 \geq 55$ mmHg
		Daytime $PaCO_2$ 46 > 50 mmHg and a rise in $TcCO_2 \geq 10$ mmHg during sleep
Clinical history	Hospitalisation related to recurrent episodes of hypercapnic respiratory failure (≥2 over 12 months)	At least 2 acidotic exacerbations with admission over 12 months
		Need of prolonged ventilatory support following an acute exacerbation

Sources: Adapted from ACCP Consensus report. *Chest.* 1999;116:521–34; Windisch W, Walterspacher S, Siemon K et al. German Society for pneumology. *Pneumologie.* 2010;64:640–52.

Abbreviations: ACCP, American College of Chest Physicians; GSP, German Society of Pneumology; $PaCO_2$, arterial carbon dioxide tension; $SatO_2$, oxygen saturation by pulsoxymetry; $TcCO_2$, transcutaneous carbon dioxide tension.

TECHNICAL CONSIDERATIONS

Although a pressure preset modality of ventilation allows the patient to retain considerable control of breathing pattern and tidal volume, both volume and pressure-limited modalities are considered as clinically equivalent and effective in CRF.[44] The usual advice in COPD patients with increased $PaCO_2$ is to utilise pressure-limited ventilators as the first-line mode of treatment, especially in the pressure-assisted mode such as pressure support that delivers a pre-set IPAP to help every spontaneous breathing effort. With this modality, the patient's capacity to vary inspiratory time breath by breath is then warranted, and this allows a close matching with the patient's breathing pattern.

When setting the ventilator, the level of IPAP is progressively raised according to patient tolerance, with a minimum level of EPAP around 4 cmH_2O in order to improve CO_2 removal by preventing rebreathing[45] and counterbalance the PEEPi (considered to be around 4–5 cmH_2O, in stable patients).[46] Once NIV has been optimised, oxygen supplementation is then adjusted to correct nocturnal hypoxaemia and to maintain arterial blood saturation ≥90%. During delivery of assisted/controlled NIV, a patient-initiated and adjustable trigger signal is able to synchronise the inspiratory phase, while a threshold reduction of inspiratory flow is, most commonly, the cause for the ventilator to cycle into expiration. It is possible, moreover, to select many other ventilator parameters such as 'rise time' (time required to reach peak pressure), inspiratory time, inspiratory to expiratory (I:E) ratio and backup respiratory rate in order to best match the patient's breathing pattern and characteristics. All these features may enhance the so-called *patient–ventilator synchrony* and the overall comfort of NIV.

Although the use of higher IPAP levels and higher backup respiratory rate has been associated with benefits,[29,32,47,48] a small physiological study showed that there was no additional benefits in terms of night-time adherence or in lung function, or gas exchange by the addition of high backup respiratory rate to high IPAP.[49]

Given that NIV is usually applied during sleep, overnight monitoring is mandatory. Ventilators without a timed backup are significantly cheaper and, in the absence of any data confirming that a timed backup is needed, these should be the machine of choice for domiciliary NIV in COPD. More recently, so-called *volume-assured modes*, pressure support ventilators that deliver a guaranteed tidal volume, have become available and these have theoretical advantages over existing devices.[50] Volume-assured NIV may improve compliance and ventilation during sleep by automatically titrating ventilatory pressures.[51] A prospective single-centre RCT comparing this modality and pressure preset NIV in COPD patients with CRF naïve to home NIV has shown that both modalities have similar effects on physiological outcomes and both are well tolerated.[52] In a randomised crossover trial, volume-assured servoventilation with automation of ventilation settings was as effective as pressure support ventilation initiated by a skilled healthcare professional in controlling nocturnal hypoventilation and produced better overnight adherence in patients naive to NIV.[53]

FUTURE RESEARCH

There is still discussion in which COPD patients' home NIV may have an adjunctive role on survival, when compared with the usual LTOT. This particular aspect clearly suggests the need to design future studies in order to finally answer the open questions. Future trials should include clear therapeutic endpoints and should consider technical aspects, such as the choice of ventilator mode, settings, duration of NIV[54] according to presence of comorbidities and the phenotype of the COPD patient.[55]

Clear benefits from home NIV in patients who remain hypercapnic after a COPD exacerbation are still discussed.[29,30,32,56] Further studies are needed to select the patients, the right moment to initiate home NIV, the optimal ventilatory settings and follow-up programme.

A lack of knowledge about the optimal ventilatory settings in the post-exacerbation period is still present. Furthermore, the contribution of the higher IPAP level and backup respiratory rate to both the positive (respiratory muscle unloading, improvement in gas exchange) and negative (increased hyperinflation, increased asynchrony, barotrauma) effects is still unknown.[57]

The cost-effectiveness of home NIV remains uncertain and the findings in this report are sensitive to emergent data. Further evidence is required to identify patients most likely to benefit from home NIV and to establish optimum time points for starting NIV and equipment settings.[20,37,38]

The best tool to evaluate the effects of long-term NIV on HRQL of these patients needs further studies.[58]

Finally, there is promising evidence on the usefulness of adding tele-assistance and monitoring to long-term care programmes in hypercapnic COPD patients on LTOT with or without night-time NIV, but the benefits remain to be proven.[59–61]

PRACTICAL RECOMMENDATIONS AND CONCLUSIONS

Several practical recommendations on home mechanical ventilation have been proposed and can be summarised as follows:

1. The physiological target of NIV (to correct hypoventilation and reduce or normalise daytime $PaCO_2$ during NIV and spontaneous breathing) must be defined and checked.
2. In COPD patients with chronic hypercapnia, NIV is effective in improving arterial blood gases and in unloading inspiratory muscles independent on whether it is set on the basis of patient comfort or physiologically

targeted. However, physiological setting of PEEP may improve the patient–ventilator synchrony.[46,62]

3. As a key component in the long-term management of underweight COPD under NIV, nutritional status and dietary intake-related problems should be addressed in these patients.[63]

To conclude, NIV may reduce re-admissions and mortality in COPD patients with acute hypercapnic respiratory failure. Once stable and prolonged hypercapnia is proven, NIV may improve survival and HRQL. Recent studies add something new in the comprehension of the role of domiciliary NIV; in the light of these, the authors of this chapter feel that although there is not enough evidence for a widespread **generalised** use of this therapeutic approach in all stable hypercapnic COPD patients, long-term NIV should be tailored to patients after appropriate evaluation of each individual case. Higher inspiratory airway pressure levels, better compliance and higher baseline $PaCO_2$ seem to improve $PaCO_2$.

REFERENCES

1. Vogelmeier CF, Criner GJ, Martinez FJ et al. Global strategy for the diagnosis, management and prevention of chronic obstructive lung disease 2017 report. GOLD Executive Summary. *Am J Respir Crit Care Med* 2017;195:557–82.
2. Ambrosino N, Guarracino F. Respiratory failure. In: *ERS Handbook of Respiratory Medicine* 2nd edition, 2013, ERS editions. pp. 162–5.
3. Nocturnal Oxygen Therapy Trial Group. Continuous or nocturnal oxygen therapy in hypoxemic chronic obstructive lung disease: A clinical trial. *Ann Intern Med.* 1980;93:391–8.
4. Rochwerg B, Brochard L, Elliott MW et al. Official ERS/ATS clinical practice guidelines: Noninvasive ventilation for acute respiratory failure. *Eur Respir J.* 2017;50: pii:1602426.
5. Ambrosino N, Carpenè N, Gherardi M. Chronic respiratory care in neuromuscular diseases for adults. *Eur Respir J.* 2009;34:444–51.
6. Lloyd-Owen SJ, Donaldson GC, Ambrosino N et al. Patterns of home mechanical ventilation use in Europe: Results from the Eurovent survey. *Eur Respir J.* 2005;25:1025–31.
7. Ambrosino N. Rationale of noninvasive ventilation. In: Esquinas AM (ed). *Noninvasive Mechanical Ventilation.* Switzerland: Springer International Publ, 2015. pp 3–6.
8. Ambrosino N, Nava S, Bertone P et al. Physiologic evaluation of pressure support ventilation by nasal mask in patients with stable COPD. *Chest.* 1992;101:385–91.
9. Nava S, Ambrosino N, Rubini F et al. Effect of nasal pressure support ventilation and external PEEP on diaphragmatic activity in patients with severe stable COPD. *Chest.* 1993;103:143–50.
10. Juan G, Calverley P, Talamo C et al. Effect of carbon dioxide on diaphragmatic function in human beings. *N Engl J Med.* 1984;310:874–9.
11. Elliott MW, Mulvey DA, Moxham J et al. Domiciliary nocturnal nasal intermittent positive pressure ventilation in COPD: Mechanisms and underlying changes in arterial blood gas tensions. *Eur Respir J.* 1991;4:1044–52.
12. Meecham-Jones DJ, Paul EA, Jones PW et al. Nasal pressure support ventilation plus oxygen compared to oxygen therapy alone in hypercapnic COPD. *Am J Respir Crit Care Med.* 1995;152:538–44.
13. Sin DD, Wong E, Mayers I et al. Effects of nocturnal noninvasive mechanical ventilation on heart rate variability of patients with advanced COPD. *Chest.* 2007;131:156–63.
14. Duiverman ML, Maagh P, Magnet FS et al. Impact of High-Intensity-NIV on the heart in stable COPD: A randomised cross-over pilot study. *Respir Res.* 2017;18:76.
15. Ambrosino N, Nava S, Torbicki A et al. Haemodynamic effects of pressure support and PEEP ventilation by nasal route in patients with stable chronic obstructive pulmonary disease. *Thorax.* 1993;48:523–8.
16. Wijkstra PJ, Lacasse Y, Guyatt GH et al. A meta-analysis of nocturnal noninvasive positive pressure ventilation in patients with stable COPD. *Chest.* 2003;124:337–43.
17. Kolodziej MA, Jensen L, Rowe B et al. Systematic review of non invasive positive pressure ventilation in severe stable COPD. *Eur Respir J.* 2007;30:293–306.
18. Struik FM, Lacasse Y, Goldstein R et al. Nocturnal non-invasive positive pressure ventilation for stable chronic obstructive pulmonary disease. *Cochrane Database Syst Rev.* 2013;6:CD002878.
19. Struik FM, Lacasse Y, Goldstein RS et al. Nocturnal noninvasive positive pressure ventilation in stable COPD: A systematic review and individual patient data meta-analysis. *Respir Med.* 2014;108: 329–37.
20. Dretzke J, Blissett D, Dave C et al. The cost-effectiveness of domiciliary non-invasive ventilation in patients with end-stage chronic obstructive pulmonary disease: A systematic review and economic evaluation. *Health Technol Assess.* 2015;19:1–246.
21. Strumpf DA, Millman RP, Carlisle CC et al. Nocturnal positive-pressure ventilation via nasal mask in patients with severe chronic obstructive pulmonary disease. *Am Rev Respir Dis.* 1991;144:1234–9.
22. Díaz O, Bégin P, Torrealba B et al. Effects of non invasive ventilation on lung hyperinflation in stable hypercapnic COPD. *Eur Respir J.* 2002;20:1490–8.
23. De Backer L, Vos W, Dieriks B et al. The effects of long-term noninvasive ventilation in hypercapnic COPD patients: A randomized controlled pilot study. *Int J COPD.* 2011;6:615–24.

24. Casanova C, Celli BR, Tost L et al. Long-term controlled trial of nocturnal nasal positive pressure ventilation in patients with severe COPD. *Chest.* 2000;118:1582–90.
25. Clini E, Sturani C, Rossi A et al. Rehabilitation and Chronic Care Study Group, Italian Association of Hospital Pulmonologists (AIPO). The Italian multicentre study on non invasive ventilation in chronic obstructive pulmonary disease patients. *Eur Respir J.* 2002;20:529–38.
26. Perrin C, El Far Y, Vandenbos F et al. Domiciliary nasal intermittent positive pressure ventilation in severe COPD: Effects on lung function and quality of life. *Eur Respir J.* 1997;10:2835–9.
27. McEvoy RD, Pierce RJ, Hillman D et al. on behalf of the Australian Trial of Non-invasive Ventilation in Chronic Airflow Limitation (AVCAL) Study Group. Nocturnal non-invasive nasal ventilation in stable hypercapnic COPD: A randomised controlled trial *Thorax.* 2009;64;561–6.
28. Ankjærgaard KL, Maibom SL, Wilcke JT. Long-term non-invasive ventilation reduces readmissions in COPD patients with two or more episodes of acute hypercapnic respiratory failure. *Eur Clin Respir J.* 2016;3:28303.
29. Kohnlein T, Windisch W, Kohler D et al. Non-invasive positive pressure ventilation for the treatment of severe stable chronic obstructive pulmonary disease: A prospective, multicentre, randomised, controlled clinical trial. *Lancet Respir Med.* 2014;2:698–705.
30. Struik FM, Sprooten RT, Kerstjens HA et al. Nocturnal non-invasive ventilation in COPD patients with prolonged hypercapnia after ventilatory support for acute respiratory failure: A randomised, controlled, parallel-group study. *Thorax.* 2014;69:826–34.
31. Costello R, Deegan P, Fitzpatrick M, McNicholas WT. Reversible hypercapnia in chronic obstructive pulmonary disease: A distinct pattern of respiratory failure with a favourable prognosis. *Am J Med.* 1997;102:239–44.
32. Murphy PB, Rehal S, Arbane G et al. Effect of home noninvasive ventilation with oxygen therapy vs oxygen therapy alone on hospital readmission or death after an acute COPD exacerbation. A randomized clinical trial. *JAMA.* 2017;317:2177–86.
33. Aida A, Miyamoto K, Nishimura M et al. Prognostic value of hypercapnia in patients with chronic respiratory failure during long-term oxygen therapy. *Am J Respir Crit Care Med.* 1998;158:188–93.
34. Stolz D, Meyer A, Rakic J et al. Mortality risk prediction in COPD by a prognostic biomarker panel. *Eur Respir J.* 2014;44:1557–70.
35. Yang H, Xiang P, Erming Zhang E et al. Is hypercapnia associated with poor prognosis in chronic obstructive pulmonary disease? A long-term follow-up cohort study. *BMJ Open.* 2015;5:e008909.
36. Paone G, Conti V, Biondi-Zoccai G et al. Long-term home noninvasive mechanical ventilation increases systemic inflammatory response in chronic obstructive pulmonary disease: A prospective observational study. *Mediators Inflamm.* 2014;2014:503145.
37. Tuggey JM, Plant PK, Elliott MW. Domiciliary non-invasive ventilation for recurrent acidotic exacerbations of COPD: An economic analysis. *Thorax.* 2003;58:867–71.
38. Clini EM, Magni G, Crisafulli E et al. Home non-invasive mechanical ventilation and long-term oxygen therapy in stable hypercapnic chronic obstructive pulmonary disease patients: Comparison of costs. *Respiration.* 2009;77:44–50.
39. ACCP Consensus report. Clinical indications for non invasive positive pressure ventilation in chronic respiratory failure due to restrictive lung disease, COPD, and nocturnal hypoventilation. *Chest.* 1999;116:521–34.
40. Windisch W, Walterspacher S, Siemon K et al. German Society for pneumology. Guidelines for non-invasive and invasive mechanical ventilation for treatment of chronic respiratory failure. *Pneumologie.* 2010;64:640–52.
41. Berry RB, Budhiraja R, Gottlieb DJ et al. Rules for scoring respiratory events in sleep: Update of the 2007 AASM Manual for the Scoring of Sleep and Associated Events. Deliberations of the Sleep Apnea Definitions Task Force of the American Academy of Sleep Medicine. *J Clin Sleep Med.* 2012;8:597–619.
42. Sancho J, Servera E, Jara-Palomares L et al. Noninvasive ventilation during the weaning process in chronically critically ill patients. *ERJ Open Res.* 2016;2:00061–2016.
43. Crimi C, Noto A, Princi P et al. Domiciliary non-invasive ventilation in COPD: An international survey of indications and practices. *COPD.* 2016;13:483–90.
44. Storre JH, Matrosovich E, Ekkernkamp E et al. Home mechanical ventilation for COPD: High-intensity versus target volume noninvasive ventilation. *Respir Care.* 2014;59:1389–97.
45. Ferguson GT, Gilmartin M. CO_2 rebreathing during BiPAP ventilatory assistance. *Am J Respir Crit Care Med.* 1995;151:1126–35.
46. Vitacca M, Nava S, Confalonieri M et al. The appropriate setting of non invasive pressure support ventilation in stable COPD patients. *Chest.* 2000;118:1286–93.
47. Dreher M, Ekkernkamp E, Walterspacher S et al. Non-invasive ventilation in COPD: Impact of inspiratory pressure levels on sleep quality. *Chest.* 2011;140:939–45.
48. Lukácsovits J, Carlucci A, Hill N et al. Physiological changes during low- and high-intensity noninvasive ventilation. *Eur Respir J.* 2012;39:869–75.

49. Murphy PB, Brignall K, Moxham J et al. High pressure versus high intensity noninvasive ventilation in stable hypercapnic chronic obstructive pulmonary disease: A randomized crossover trial. *Int J Chron Obstruct Pulmon Dis.* 2012;7:811–8.
50. Arellano-Maric MP, Gregoretti C, Duivermann M et al. Long-term volume-targeted pressure-controlled ventilation: Sense or nonsense? *Eur Respir J.* 2017;49: 1602193.
51. Crisafulli E, Manni G, Kidonias M et al. Subjective sleep quality during Average Volume Assured Pressure Support (AVAPS) ventilation in patients with hypercapnic COPD. A Physiological Pilot Study. *Lung.* 2009;187:299–305.
52. Oscroft NS, Chadwick R, Davies MG et al. Volume assured versus pressure preset non-invasive ventilation for compensated ventilatory failure in COPD. *Respir Med.* 2014;108:1508–15.
53. Kelly JL, Jaye J, Pickersgill RE et al. Randomized trial of 'intelligent' autotitrating ventilation versus standard pressure support non-invasive ventilation: Impact on adherence and physiological outcomes. *Respirology.* 2014;19:596–603.
54. Borel J-C, Pepin J-L, Pison C et al. Long-term adherence with non-invasive ventilation improves prognosis in obese COPD patients. *Respirology.* 2014;19:857–65.
55. Vanfleteren LE, Spruit MA, Groenen M et al. Clusters of comorbidities based on validated objective measurements and systemic inflammation in patients with chronic obstructive pulmonary disease. *Am J Respir Crit Care Med.* 2013;187:728–35.
56. Galli JA, Krahnke JS, James Mamary A et al. Home non-invasive ventilation use following acute hypercapnic respiratory failure in COPD. *Respir Med.* 2014;108:722–8.
57. Duiverman ML, Windisch W, Storre JH et al. The role of NIV in chronic hypercapnic COPD following an acute exacerbation: The importance of patient selection? *Ther Adv Respir Dis.* 2016;10:149–57.
58. Oga T, Taniguchi H, Hideo Kita H et al. Comparison of different disease-specific health-related quality of life measurements in patients with long-term noninvasive Ventilation. *Can Respir J.* 2017;2017:8295079.
59. Vitacca M, Paneroni M, Grossetti F, Ambrosino N. Is there any additional effect of tele-assistance on long-term care programs in hypercapnic COPD patients? A retrospective study. *COPD.* 2016;13:576–82.
60. Ambrosino N, Vitacca M, Dreher M et al. on behalf of the ERS "Tele-monitoring of ventilator-dependent patients" Task Force. Tele-monitoring of ventilator-dependent patients: A European Respiratory Society Statement. *Eur Respir J.* 2016;48:648–63.
61. Chatwin M, Hawkins G, Panicchia L et al. Randomised crossover trial of telemonitoring in chronic respiratory patients (TeleCRAFT trial). *Thorax.* 2016;71:305–11.
62. Vitacca M, Barbano L, D'Anna S et al. Comparison of five bilevel pressure ventilators in patients with chronic ventilatory failure: A physiologic study. *Chest.* 2002;122:2105–14.
63. Ambrosino N, Clini E. Long-term mechanical ventilation and nutrition. *Respir Med.* 2004;98:413–20.

29

Non-invasive ventilation in COPD: The importance of comorbidities and phenotypes

JEAN-LOUIS PÉPIN, JEAN-PAUL JANSSENS, RENAUD TAMISIER, DAMIEN VIGLINO, DAN ADLER AND JEAN-CHRISTIAN BOREL

TAKE-HOME MESSAGES

- Chronic obstructive pulmonary disease (COPD) comorbidities such as obesity, cardiovascular and metabolic diseases substantially contribute to recurrence of hospitalisations for exacerbations and significantly affect prognosis.
- Distinct pathophysiological mechanisms associated with COPD phenotypes underlie differences in non-invasive ventilation (NIV) settings and NIV tolerance and are associated with different categories of residual events when wearing the device.
- The settings for NIV in COPD are not unique and should be tailored to an individual patient's comorbidities and phenotype.
- NIV use is higher for obese COPD patients compared to non-obese COPD patients with a possible association with hospital readmission and mortality.
- In severe COPD with static hyperinflation, excessive pressure support might lead to dynamic hyperinflation and increased intrinsic positive end-expiratory pressure, which are major determinants of unrewarded efforts.

INTRODUCTION

Chronic obstructive pulmonary disease (COPD) is a growing global health concern, causing considerable health-related costs and increased mortality.[1,2] Although diagnosis is mainly based on the presence of chronic airflow limitation, as assessed by post-bronchodilator spirometry, COPD is nowadays considered a complex, heterogeneous and systemic condition. It is increasingly recognised that the presence of comorbidities, such as obesity and cardiovascular and metabolic diseases, substantially contributes to recurrence of hospitalisations for exacerbations and significantly affect prognosis.[3,4]

Heterogeneity in COPD clinical manifestations and disease progression has many implications for patient's health risk assessment, severity stratification and integrated management.[4–7] In the late stage of the disease, non-invasive ventilation (NIV) is widely prescribed either to treat acute hypercapnic respiratory failure during an exacerbation of COPD (AECOPD) or for the long term[8] even if definitive evidence for domiciliary NIV is lacking and this is demonstrated by large heterogeneity of practices in Europe.[8] The study of Kohnlein et al.[9] showed a substantial improvement in survival and quality of life when NIV was used in stable hypercapnic chronic respiratory failure. However, the study was not blinded and benefits might be attributed to higher standards of care in the arm receiving NIV.[10] Moreover, the authors took 6 years to recruit 200 patients from 36 centres. This strongly suggests selection biases and more studies are needed to target a population of best responders to NIV. Patients with specific COPD 'treatable characteristics' should be identified to indicate effective personalised treatments, including long-term NIV.[11]

In this chapter, we will discuss the importance and impact of obesity, comorbidities and COPD subtypes regarding NIV indications, tolerance and compliance. We will also discuss the NIV titration and setting adjustments in the different COPD subgroups of interest.

COPD SUBTYPES AND THEIR RELEVANCE FOR NIV MANAGEMENT (FIGURE 29.1)

The existing literature has identified three main different COPD subtypes that have been prospectively validated in terms of prognosis. The wording for designating clinical COPD subtypes varies between studies. However, 'frequent exacerbator', 'severe respiratory COPD' (with few comorbidities) and 'systemic COPD' (with moderate respiratory disease but associated with obesity and high rates of cardio-metabolic comorbidities) are the most reproducible phenotypes across studies.[4–6,12] The latter two COPD clinical subtypes differ primarily in terms of severity of alterations in respiratory function (e.g. emphysema and hyperinflation), body mass index, obstructive sleep apnoea (OSA) prevalence and muscle wasting (Figure 29.1). In systemic COPD, obesity will have an impact on respiratory mechanics, respiratory drive and upper airway patency.[13] The high prevalence of OSA and rapid eye movement (REM) sleep hypoventilation in this subgroup of COPD patients will require specific settings for both inspiratory and expiratory pressures during NIV. Also, in these patients with frequent pre-existing cardiac disease and especially cardiac failure, NIV may induce central apnoeas and reductions in cardiac output (CO). On the other hand (Figure 29.1), severe and cachectic 'respiratory COPD' are less prone to OSA but exhibit more hyperinflation that is going to increase intrinsic positive end-expiratory pressure (PEEPi). In these patients, inappropriate ventilator settings may lead to dynamic hyperinflation and increased PEEPi resulting in unrewarded inspiratory efforts and morning discomfort when NIV is discontinued.[14,15] These distinct pathophysiological mechanisms certainly underlie differences in NIV settings and NIV tolerance and are associated with different categories of residual events when wearing the device.

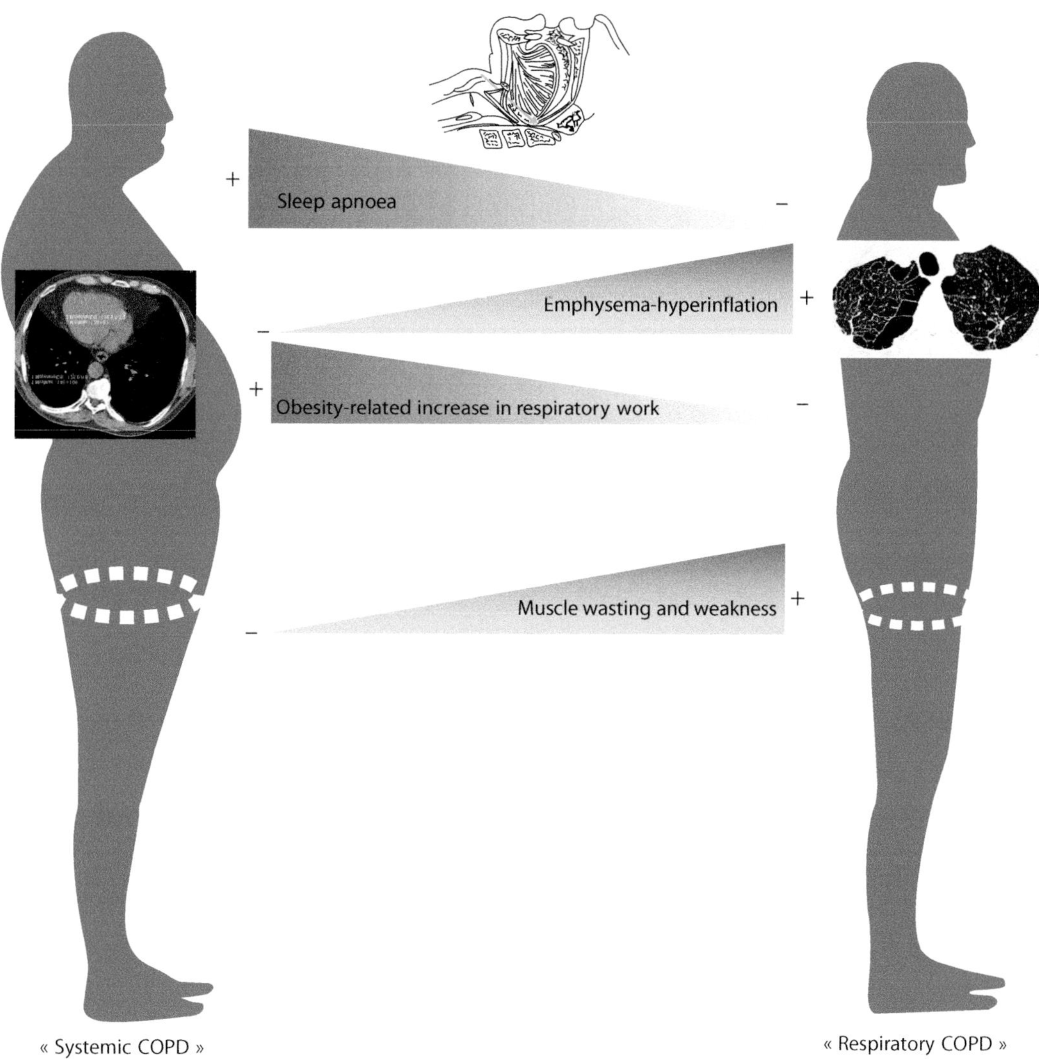

Figure 29.1 COPD subtypes and their relevance for non-invasive ventilation management.

COPD SUBTYPES AND COMORBIDITIES: IMPACT ON MORTALITY AND HOSPITALISATION OUTCOMES DURING LONG-TERM NIV (FIGURE 29.2)

Clinical cohort studies in COPD suggest that mortality and readmission rates are specific to different COPD subgroups. Severe respiratory COPD patients have more frequent hospitalisations due to respiratory exacerbations and higher all-cause mortality whereas systemic COPD patients have more admissions due to cardiovascular disease.[5,6] In existing studies, the effect of NIV on outcome has been poorly addressed across different COPD phenotypes. Studies[16,17] have shown that more than one-third of consecutive COPD patients admitted to the intensive care unit for acute respiratory failure requiring NIV were obese. The rate of late NIV failure was lower in obese COPD compared to non-obese patients. Moreover, obesity was associated with less hospital readmission at 1 year in COPD patients. This was potentially explained by a more frequent use of domiciliary nocturnal NIV in obese COPD patients. Studies in the field of long-term NIV in COPD have usually included patients with a body mass index in the normal or at the upper end of the normal weight range (see the table in the work of Elliott[10]; also see the study by O'Donoghue and Howard[18]). Patients with obesity or important comorbidities are frequently excluded from clinical trials. This is unfortunate since knowledge derived from a highly selected population cannot be generalised to the whole real-life clinical spectrum of COPD. Interestingly, in the study showing the lowest rate of mortality at 1 year in long-term domiciliary NIV for patients with COPD, 38% of the patients were obese,

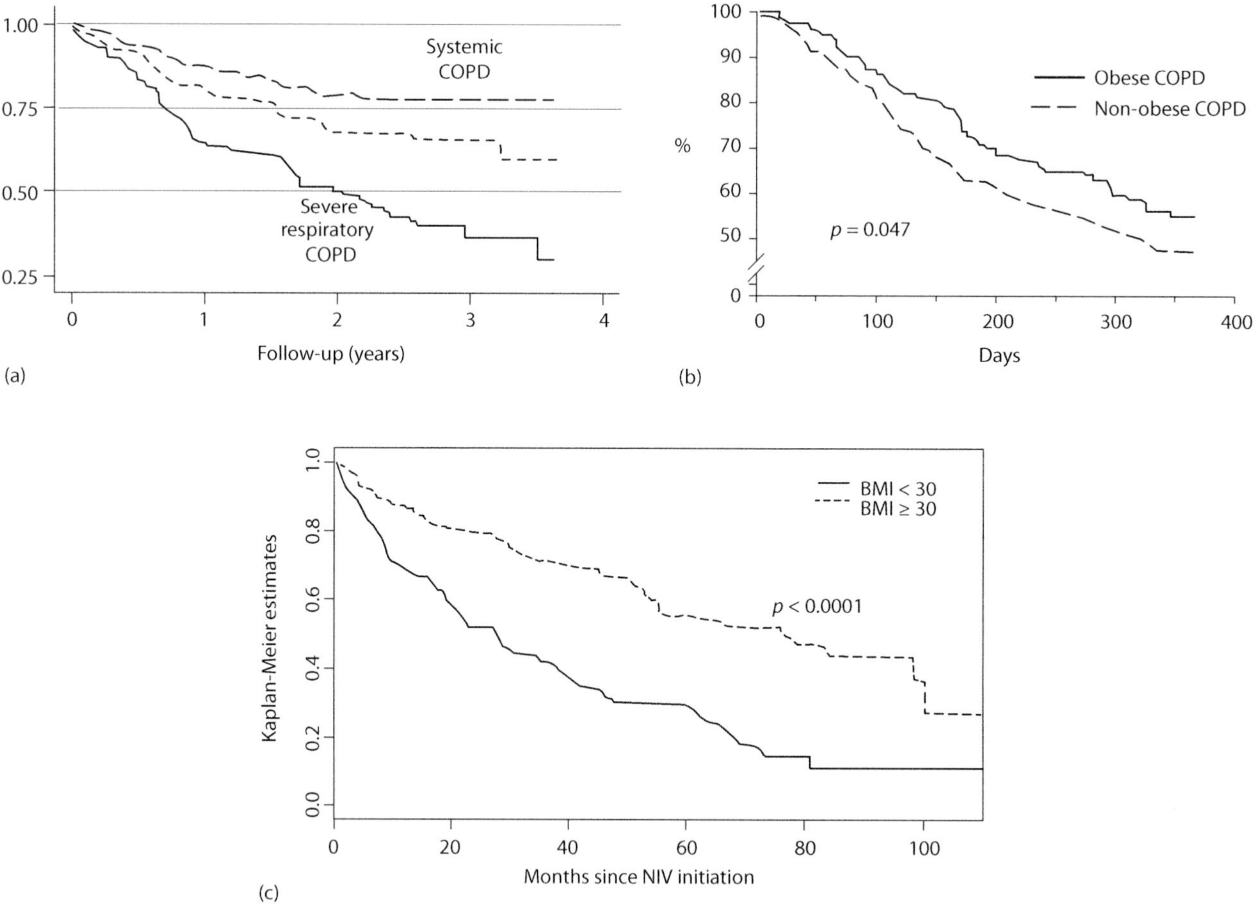

Figure 29.2 Impact of obesity and comorbidities on mortality and hospitalisation outcomes during long-term non-invasive ventilation. **(a)** COPD hospital free admissions in systemic and severe respiratory COPD subgroups. **(b)** Probability of remaining free from hospital readmission during the follow-up period of 1 year after ICU admission for hypercapnic acute respiratory failure in patients with COPD with and without obesity. **(c)** Kaplan–Meier estimates of survival without hospital readmission for acute exacerbation according to the two subtypes of chronic obstructive pulmonary disease (obese and non-obese). ([a] Modified from Garcia-Aymerich J, Gomez FP, Benet M, Farrero E, Basagana X, Gayete A et al., *Thorax.* 2011;66(5):430–7; [b] Modified from Carrillo A, Ferrer M, Gonzalez-Diaz G, Lopez-Martinez A, Llamas N, Alcazar M et al., *Am J Respir Crit Care Med.* 2012;186(12):1279–85; [c] Modified from Borel JC, Pepin JL, Pison C, Vesin A, Gonzalez-Bermejo J, Court-Fortune I et al., *Respirology.* 2014;19(6):857–65.)

with a mean body mass index for the whole population of 28.3 ± 7.3 kg/m^2 (range, 17.3 to 49.3).[19] In this study, there was a good tolerance of high-intensity ventilation that might also be explained by the requirement for higher pressure support in COPD individuals with associated obesity. Our own observations in a prospective multicentre cohort study including 213 COPD are in line with those results, that is, a significant positive association between obesity and survival in COPD patients treated with home NIV.[20] Obesity is an established risk factor for OSA. Overlap syndrome (e.g. COPD plus OSA) patients are potentially among the better responders to CPAP/NIV.[21–25] Unfortunately, most of the NIV studies in COPD[26–28] have excluded overlap syndrome patients, and this might partly explain negative results of some of these trials.

Acute exacerbations (AECOPD) are relevant events in the natural history of COPD with therapeutic and prognostic implications.[29] AECOPD are heterogeneous and related to different underlying mechanisms. Sudden and gradual onset are two distinct patterns in the natural history and time course of the onset of a COPD exacerbation.[30] Sudden exacerbations are associated with an abrupt increase in respiratory symptoms but shorter recovery times back to baseline health. Early detection to implement therapeutic interventions rapidly is a major goal in the management of frequent exacerbations in COPD patients. There are also economical concerns particularly in the United States with the Hospital Readmission Reduction Program penalising hospitals for 'excessive' readmission rates for COPD. In this context, we assessed whether day-to-day variation in parameters recorded by the ventilators can predict an imminent exacerbation in patients with COPD treated at home with NIV.[31] We showed that daily variations in respiratory rate and percentage of respiratory cycles triggered by the patient were convincing predictors of an exacerbation.[31] However, this highly specific strategy using NIV data was partly flawed by a low sensitivity owing to the difficulty to anticipate sudden exacerbations. These sudden exacerbations are mainly related to viral or acute cardiac dysfunction difficult to recognise in these patients. Severe respiratory COPD patients showing a gradual increase in respiratory symptoms might be better candidates than systemic COPD patients, who are more prone to admissions due to cardiovascular events, for this home remote monitoring allowing detection of exacerbation. This has to be confirmed in further studies (e.g. ongoing randomised controlled trial [RCT] comparing a telemedicine system driven by NIV daily remote monitoring versus standard care; clinical trials identifier: NCT02756533).

COPD SUBTYPES AND COMORBIDITIES: IMPACT ON NIV COMPLIANCE, TOLERANCE AND SETTINGS

Respiratory COPD patients have a worse prognosis, and in addition, they also have a lower mean daily NIV usage than obese systemic COPD patients.[20] A significant improvement in prognosis when NIV was used for more than 5 hours per day was found solely in the systemic COPD phenotype.[20] Such a dose–response relationship between NIV compliance and mortality was not found in the respiratory COPD subgroup. This underscores a potential interaction between COPD phenotypes and daily NIV use. Importantly, a meta-analysis has shown that $PaCO_2$ progressively deteriorates over time for COPD patients with NIV compliance of less than 5 hours, while it improves in the subgroup of patients using NIV for more than 5 hours per night.[32] In our study, average daily NIV use during follow-up was higher for obese COPD patients (6.9 hours) compared to non-obese COPD patients (5.3 hours) with a possible association with hospital readmission and mortality. In non-obese COPD patients with severely impaired respiratory function and hyperinflation, ventilator settings may be more difficult to adjust. In this case, the clinician will always have to balance the efficacy of treatment with high pressures on arterial blood gazes and subjective discomfort related to treatment. This is acknowledged in routine practice in Europe as only 25% of COPD patients are treated with high-intensity ventilation settings.[8,10,15]

There is still a debate regarding the most appropriate settings for NIV in COPD. Higher inspiratory pressures combined with high respiratory rates (high-intensity NIV) have been shown to improve blood gases and quality of life more than the traditional lower-pressure approach (low-intensity NIV),[33] although high backup rate does not improve blood gas further when added to high inspiratory pressures in a randomised trial. It has also been suggested that high-intensity NIV might induce a reduction in CO by decreasing venous return and then right atrial preload. This could limit its application in COPD patients with pre-existing cardiac disease.[3,34,35]

From a physiological point of view, obese COPD patients with moderate airway obstruction (e.g. systemic COPD patients) are more likely to hypoventilate, especially during sleep, owing to obesity-related abnormalities in respiratory mechanics. NIV can recruit peripheral airways and increase alveolar ventilation, reduce respiratory muscle work and suppress REM sleep hypoventilation. In the study of Carrillo et al.,[16,17] a similar titration protocol with high levels of expiratory pressures was used for NIV in acute conditions in COPD and in patients with obesity hypoventilation syndrome (OHS); among patients with COPD, 34% were obese, and 28% had associated OSA ('overlap syndrome'), which probably explains why the same titration protocol was in fact effective. This subgroup might also require, and tolerate, relatively high levels of inspiratory pressures.[20] In a recent study evaluating safety and efficacy of auto-titrating noninvasive ventilation in overlap syndrome, Murphy and colleagues[36] demonstrated that high levels of expiratory pressure (11 ± 2 cmH_2O) and elevated pressure support are actually required. In contrast, NIV could be less effective for addressing V/Q mismatching in non-obese COPD patients with more generalised emphysema. In selected subjects with severe COPD and static hyperinflation, excessive pressure support might lead to dynamic hyperinflation and increased PEEPi, which are major determinants of unrewarded efforts.[15] In such a clinical situation, a slight decrease in pressure support may change ventilation patterns to a more physiological mode for severe COPD, i.e. increase spontaneous respiratory rate with a slight decrease in tidal volume, without any deterioration of $PaCO_2$.[15] These data suggest that settings for NIV in COPD are not unique and should be tailored to the patient's comorbidities and phenotypes.

CONCLUSIONS

As recently stated in a cost-effectiveness analysis of home NIV,[37,38] a better description of patient characteristics or equipment settings that are predictive of a benefit of NIV remains to be established. We suggest that subsequent RCTs in the field be conducted on specific COPD subgroups that have higher likelihood of responding to NIV (i.e. obese patients with comorbidities and moderate to severe airflow obstruction). This might represent a new, more personalised approach in the challenging area of long-term NIV in stable COPD patients.

CONFLICTS OF INTEREST

None of the authors declare a conflict of interest in relation to this publication.

ROLE OF THE FUNDING SOURCE

Endowment fund 'AGIR pour les maladies chroniques' and 'Mutualia' provided unrestricted funding for the management of the Grenoble ECO-COPD cohort.

REFERENCES

1. Vanfleteren LE, Spruit MA, Wouters EF, Franssen FM. Management of chronic obstructive pulmonary disease beyond the lungs. *Lancet Respir Med.* 2016;4(11):911–24.
2. Sjoding MW, Cooke CR. Readmission penalties for chronic obstructive pulmonary disease will further stress hospitals caring for vulnerable patient populations. *Am J Respir Crit Care Med.* 2014;190(9):1072–4.
3. MacDonald MI, Shafuddin E, King PT et al. Cardiac dysfunction during exacerbations of chronic obstructive pulmonary disease. *Lancet Respir Med.* 2016;4(2):138–48.
4. Rennard SI, Locantore N, Delafont B et al. Identification of five chronic obstructive pulmonary disease subgroups with different prognoses in the ECLIPSE cohort using cluster analysis. *Ann Am Thorac Soc.* 2015;12(3):303–12.
5. Garcia-Aymerich J, Gomez FP, Benet M et al. Identification and prospective validation of clinically relevant chronic obstructive pulmonary disease (COPD) subtypes. *Thorax.* 2011;66(5):430–7.
6. Burgel PR, Roche N, Paillasseur JL et al. Clinical COPD phenotypes identified by cluster analysis: Validation with mortality. *Eur Respir J.* 2012;40(2):495–6.
7. Roca J, Vargas C, Cano I et al. Chronic obstructive pulmonary disease heterogeneity: Challenges for health risk assessment, stratification and management. *J Transl Med.* 2014;12 Suppl 2:S3.
8. Crimi C, Noto A, Princi P et al. Domiciliary non-invasive ventilation in COPD: An international survey of indications and practices. *COPD.* 2016;13(4):483–90.
9. Kohnlein T, Windisch W, Kohler D et al. Non-invasive positive pressure ventilation for the treatment of severe stable chronic obstructive pulmonary disease: A prospective, multicentre, randomised, controlled clinical trial. *Lancet Respir Med.* 2014;2(9):698–705.
10. Elliott M. Domiciliary NIV for COPD: Where are we now? *Lancet Respir Med.* 2014;2(9):672–3.
11. Agusti A. The path to personalised medicine in COPD. *Thorax.* 2014;69(9):857–64.
12. Burgel PR, Sethi S, Kim V. Chronic obstructive pulmonary disease phenotypes. Past, present, and future. *Ann Am Thorac Soc.* 2015;12(3):289–90.
13. Pepin JL, Timsit JF, Tamisier R et al. Prevention and care of respiratory failure in obese patients. *Lancet Respir Med.* 2016;4(5):407–18.
14. Vitacca M, Nava S, Confalonieri M et al. The appropriate setting of noninvasive pressure support ventilation in stable COPD patients. *Chest.* 2000;118(5):1286–93.
15. Adler D, Perrig S, Takahashi H et al. Polysomnography in stable COPD under non-invasive ventilation to reduce patient-ventilator asynchrony and morning breathlessness. *Sleep & breathing = Schlaf & Atmung.* 2012;16(4):1081–90. Epub 2011/11/05.
16. Carrillo A, Ferrer M, Gonzalez-Diaz G et al. Noninvasive ventilation in acute hypercapnic respiratory failure caused by obesity hypoventilation syndrome and chronic obstructive pulmonary disease. *Am J Respir Crit Care Med.* 2012;186(12):1279–85.
17. Pepin JL, Borel JC, Janssens JP. Obesity hypoventilation syndrome: An underdiagnosed and undertreated condition. *Am J Respir Crit Care Med.* 2012;186(12):1205–7.
18. O'Donoghue FJ, Howard ME. Obesity, COPD, NIV and reverse epidemiology. *Respirology.* 2014;19(6):777–9.
19. Windisch W, Kostic S, Dreher M et al. Outcome of patients with stable COPD receiving controlled noninvasive positive pressure ventilation aimed at a maximal reduction of Pa(CO2). *Chest.* 2005;128(2):657–62. Epub 2005/08/16.

20. Borel JC, Pepin JL, Pison C et al. Long-term adherence with non-invasive ventilation improves prognosis in obese COPD patients. *Respirology.* 2014;19(6):857–65.
21. Machado MC, Vollmer WM, Togeiro SM et al. CPAP and survival in moderate-to-severe obstructive sleep apnoea syndrome and hypoxaemic COPD. *Eur Respir J.* 2010;35(1):132–7.
22. Marin JM, Soriano JB, Carrizo SJ et al. Outcomes in patients with chronic obstructive pulmonary disease and obstructive sleep apnea: The overlap syndrome. *Am J Respir Crit Care Med.* 2010;182(3):325–31.
23. McNicholas WT, Verbraecken J, Marin JM. Sleep disorders in COPD: The forgotten dimension. *Eur Respir Rev.* 2013;22(129):365–75.
24. Jaoude P, Kufel T, El-Solh AA. Survival benefit of CPAP favors hypercapnic patients with the overlap syndrome. *Lung.* 2014;192(2):251–8.
25. Steveling EH, Clarenbach CF, Miedinger D et al. Predictors of the overlap syndrome and its association with comorbidities in patients with chronic obstructive pulmonary disease. *Respiration.* 2014;88(6):451–7.
26. Casanova C, Celli BR, Tost L et al. Long-term controlled trial of nocturnal nasal positive pressure ventilation in patients with severe COPD. *Chest.* 2000;118(6):1582–90.
27. Clini E, Sturani C, Rossi A et al. The Italian multicentre study on noninvasive ventilation in chronic obstructive pulmonary disease patients. *Eur Respir J.* 2002;20(3):529–38.
28. McEvoy RD, Pierce RJ, Hillman D et al. Nocturnal non-invasive nasal ventilation in stable hypercapnic COPD: A randomised controlled trial. *Thorax.* 2009;64(7):561–6.
29. Lopez-Campos JL, Agusti A. Heterogeneity of chronic obstructive pulmonary disease exacerbations: A two-axes classification proposal. *Lancet Respir Med.* 2015;3(9):729–34.
30. Aaron SD, Donaldson GC, Whitmore GA et al. Time course and pattern of COPD exacerbation onset. *Thorax.* 2012;67(3):238–43.
31. Borel JC, Pelletier J, Taleux N et al. Parameters recorded by software of non-invasive ventilators predict COPD exacerbation: A proof-of-concept study. *Thorax.* 2015;70(3):284–5.
32. Struik FM, Lacasse Y, Goldstein RS et al. Nocturnal noninvasive positive pressure ventilation in stable COPD: A systematic review and individual patient data meta-analysis. *Respir Med.* 2014;108(2):329–37.
33. Windisch W, Storre JH, Kohnlein T. Nocturnal non-invasive positive pressure ventilation for COPD. *Expert Rev Respir Med.* 2015;9(3):295–308.
34. Lukacsovits J, Carlucci A, Hill N et al. Physiological changes during low- and high-intensity noninvasive ventilation. *Eur Respir J.* 2012;39(4):869–75. Epub 2011/09/03.
35. Lahousse L, Verhamme KM, Stricker BH, Brusselle GG. Cardiac effects of current treatments of chronic obstructive pulmonary disease. *Lancet Respir Med.* 2016;4(2):149–64.
36. Murphy PB, Arbane G, Ramsay M et al. Safety and efficacy of auto-titrating noninvasive ventilation in COPD and obstructive sleep apnoea overlap syndrome. *Eur Respir J.* 2015;46(2):548–51.
37. Dretzke J, Blissett D, Dave C et al. The cost-effectiveness of domiciliary non-invasive ventilation in patients with end-stage chronic obstructive pulmonary disease: A systematic review and economic evaluation. *Health Technol Assess.* 2015;19(81):1–246.
38. Dretzke J, Moore D, Dave C et al. The effect of domiciliary noninvasive ventilation on clinical outcomes in stable and recently hospitalized patients with COPD: A systematic review and meta-analysis. *Int J Chron Obstruct Pulmon Dis.* 2016;11:2269–86.

30

High-intensity non-invasive positive pressure ventilation

SARAH BETTINA SCHWARZ, FRIEDERIKE SOPHIE MAGNET AND WOLFRAM WINDISCH

KEY MESSAGES

- High-intensity non-invasive positive pressure ventilation (NPPV) is defined as long-term NPPV aimed at achieving either normocapnia or the lowest $PaCO_2$ values possible if normocapnia cannot be achieved.
- For the purpose of high-intensity NPPV, ventilator settings are increased in a stepwise manner until normocapnia is achieved, or at least until the maximum tolerated by the individual patient is reached; here, NPPV is used in the assist/control mode typically with high backup rates allowing for controlled ventilation and levels of inspiratory positive airway pressure ranging between 20 and 30 cmH_2O.
- High-intensity NPPV is superior over the classical approach of low-intensity NPPV, which uses lower inspiratory positive airway pressures of typically <18 cmH_2O in the assisted mode. This refers to the capability of improving blood gases, breathing pattern, lung function, respiratory muscle resting, adherence to therapy and health-related quality of life.
- High-intensity NPPV but not low-intensity NPPV is capable of improving outcome in chronic hypercapnic chronic obstructive pulmonary disease (COPD) patients: (1) high-intensity NPPV improves long-term survival in patients with chronic hypercapnic COPD; (2) high-intensity NPPV improves admission-free survival in COPD patients with status post-acute exacerbation who required acute NPPV in hospital, and had persistent hypercapnia for at least 2 weeks after the cessation of acute NPPV in hospital.
- Future research should target the following: (1) outpatient commencement and control of NPPV aimed at reducing costs and overcoming hospital-bed shortages, (2) how to best select patients for high-intensity NPPV and (3) alternative/additional treatment strategies to treat chronic hypercapnic respiratory failure in COPD patients.

INTRODUCTION

Long-term non-invasive positive pressure ventilation (NPPV) delivered by a nasal or a full-face mask is increasingly being used in patients with chronic hypercapnic respiratory failure due to different conditions. While the rationale for long-term NPPV in thoracic restrictive and neuromuscular patients and also in those with obesity hypoventilation syndrome is undisputed, there is an ongoing debate about whether this treatment strategy is useful for patients with chronic hypercapnic chronic obstructive pulmonary disease (COPD).[1–3] A recent meta-analysis that covered seven trials (245 patients) concluded that there is still insufficient evidence to support the routine application of NPPV in patients with stable COPD, since no clear survival benefits could have been established. However, the authors of this report also pointed out that higher levels of inspiratory positive airway pressure (IPAP), better compliance and higher baseline $PaCO_2$ values were associated with improved alveolar ventilation. Thereby, it has been clearly acknowledged that both the settings and the techniques used for long-term NPPV application substantially influence clinical outcome.[3]

Importantly, two more recent randomised controlled trials (RCTs) using relatively different approaches to those in previous studies also produced positive outcomes, which were attributed to the ability of long-term NPPV to improve $PaCO_2$.[1,2] Thus, the time has now come to change the direction of questioning: the question for COPD patients is no longer whether long-term NPPV is beneficial. It is rather: What are the best settings and techniques for long-term NPPV?

These more aggressive forms of NPPV aimed at maximally improving elevated $PaCO_2$ values have been described as high-intensity NPPV.[4] This contrasts to the traditional approach to NPPV, which is referred to as low-intensity NPPV, since it comprises less aggressive ventilator settings. Today, high-intensity NPPV as used for COPD has been used in several trials. The current article provides an overview over this technique and summarises the current evidence when compared to low-intensity NPPV.

HIGH-INTENSITY NPPV: DEFINITION AND DESCRIPTION

Originally, high-intensity NPPV was described in 2009,[4] even though earlier studies had already reported the use of this technique in COPD patients.[5–8] The definition and description of high-intensity NPPV are summarised in Table 30.1.

High-intensity NPPV refers to a specific ventilatory approach in which NPPV settings are aimed at maximally improving reduced alveolar ventilation.[9] Thus, high-intensity NPPV is aimed at achieving either normocapnia or the lowest $PaCO_2$ values possible if normocapnia cannot be achieved. For the purpose of high-intensity NPPV, ventilator settings are increased in a stepwise manner until normocapnia is achieved, or at least until the maximum tolerated by the individual patient is reached.[10]

Although IPAP levels used for high-intensity NPPV are regularly higher than those used for low-intensity NPPV, it is emphasised that high-intensity NPPV is not defined by specific IPAP cutoff values; rather, it is driven by the physiologic aim of maximally improving alveolar ventilation, as described above.[10] Furthermore, despite IPAP levels being generally high, it should not be increased any further if it is not individually tolerated. In addition, subjective conditions such as symptoms, side effects, tolerance and adherence to treatment affect IPAP level selection.[4] This and given that IPAP levels also depend on the patient's baseline physiology explain why IPAP levels turn out to be severely heterogeneous across individuals. IPAP levels that typically range between 20 and 30 cmH_2O are chosen for the purpose of high-intensity NPPV.[9] This is first established in the hospital setting and subsequently used in the home environment as home mechanical ventilation.

It should also be noted that the term *high-intensity NPPV* does not refer to a specific ventilatory mode, even though the assist/control mode is most often chosen for high-intensity NPPV with the aim of achieving controlled ventilation.[4,9] In contrast to high-intensity NPPV, low-intensity NPPV typically uses lower IPAP settings of <18 cmH_2O during assisted ventilation. Here, ventilator settings are not increased for the purpose of reducing $PaCO_2$. Low-intensity NPPV has served as the primary approach to all of the outcome studies published before 2014.[11–13] Therefore, the low-intensity version is deemed to be the classic approach to NPPV in patients with COPD.[9] In contrast, more recent outcome studies used approaches related to the techniques of high-intensity NPPV.[1,2]

A synopsis of physiological and clinical considerations regarding high- and low-intensity NPPV is provided in Table 30.2.[9]

Table 30.1 Definition and description of high-intensity NPPV used in COPD patients

Definition	Long-term NPPV aimed at achieving either normocapnia or the lowest $PaCO_2$ values possible if normocapnia cannot be achieved.
Description	Ventilator settings are increased in a stepwise manner until normocapnia is achieved, or at least until the maximum tolerated by the individual patient is reached. For this purpose, NPPV is used in the assist/control mode typically with high backup rates allowing for controlled ventilation and IPAP levels ranging between 20 and 30 cmH_2O (sometimes even higher).

Note: IPAP, inspiratory positive airway pressure; NPPV, non-invasive positive pressure ventilation.

HIGH-INTENSITY NPPV: PHYSIOLOGICAL CONSIDERATIONS

As pointed out above, many studies have shown that low-intensity NPPV using IPAP levels of less than 18 cm H_2O is not capable of improving elevated $PaCO_2$ levels.[9,14] In contrast, high-intensity NPPV has been shown to be capable of improving $PaCO_2$ by numerous trials. Here, $PaCO_2$ reduction occurs not only during NPPV application but also during periods of subsequent spontaneous breathing.[4–6,8] In addition, in a randomised crossover study that directly compared long-term high- and low-intensity NPPV, mean IPAP for high- versus low-intensity NPPV was 29 versus 15 cmH_2O, respectively.[15] Low-intensity NPPV was applied using assisted ventilation, while the assist-control mode with mean respiratory rate settings of 18 per minute was chosen for high-intensity NPPV. As a main result, the mean treatment effect was 9.2 mmHg (95%CI, −13.7/−4.6 mmHg; $p < 0.001$) in favour of high-intensity NPPV for the reduction in $PaCO_2$ (primary outcome). Of note, high-intensity NPPV in this trial was associated with better adherence to therapy, health-related quality of life (HRQL), lung function and exercise-related dyspnoea.[15] Interestingly, one study was able to show that supplementing high IPAP levels with

Table 30.2 Synopsis of differences between low- and high-intensity long-term NPPV, as used for chronic hypercapnic COPD patients: physiological and clinical considerations

	Low-intensity NPPV	High-intensity NPPV
Adherence to therapy	–	+
Effects on lung function	–	+[a]
Hypercapnia		++
Inspiratory effort	+	++
Inspiratory muscle strength	–	–
Sleep quality	(+)	(+)
Cardiac function	–	–[b]
HRQL	+[c]	++
Initiation of NPPV during stable disease (outcome)	–	++
Initiation of NPPV following exacerbation with acute NPPV (outcome)	–	++[d]

[a] Improved FEV_1.
[b] High-intensity NPPV is more likely to reduce cardiac output compared to low-intensity NPPV. There are no contraindications in heart failure patients for either mode. Long-term reduction in proBNP has been reported only for high-intensity NPPV.
[c] Besides some positive effects on specific aspects of HRQL, general aspects of HRQL are not improved and can even decline.
[d] Patients with $PaCO_2$ >7 kPa at least 2 weeks after acute NPPV presented improved admission-free survival.
+, Advantage; –, disadvantage. HRQL, health-related quality of life; IPAP, inspiratory positive airway pressure; NPPV, non-invasive positive pressure ventilation; $PaCO_2$, arterial partial pressure of carbon dioxide; proBNP, pro-brain natriuretic peptide.

high backup rates did not result in further physiological improvements.[16] Based on this finding, it was suggested that it is the high-pressure component of high-intensity NPPV that plays a key therapeutic role. This is also supported by the most recent outcome studies reporting positive results in which NPPV was shown to improve $PaCO_2$ using higher IPAP levels compared to previous RCTs, but using lower mean respiratory rates compared to those in the original description of high-intensity NPPV.[1,2]

The improvement in $PaCO_2$ during daytime spontaneous breathing following nocturnal high-intensity NPPV has been attributed to an improved breathing pattern with increased tidal volume at an unchanged respiratory rate.[8] Another interesting theory for improved spontaneous breathing stems from recent studies showing that FEV_1 is reportedly improved in COPD patients following high-intensity NPPV.[4,6,15] This raises the possibility that high-intensity NPPV has an effect on the airways themselves. Whether this is due to an anti-inflammatory effect of NPPV, or is the result of chronically fibrosed airways being stretched open, remains speculative.[17]

Moreover, oedema in hypercapnic COPD patients can result from CO_2-associated vasodilatation and is therefore a common finding in these patients.[14,18] Therefore, a possible alternative mechanism to explain improved FEV_1 following high-intensity NPPV is a reduction in airway oedema. Since oedema is also likely to be present in the airways, reducing elevated $PaCO_2$ values after high-intensity NPPV would then reverse dilation of the precapillary sphincters, thereby positively affecting the oedema in the airways.[17] This, in turn, would eventually improve respiratory mechanics as well as FEV_1. This, however, remains to be investigated.

In another elegant physiological randomised crossover study, high-intensity NPPV established a greater reduction in the pressure–time product of the diaphragm, as assessed by oesophageal and gastric balloon catheters, and completely abolished spontaneous breathing activity in 9 out of 15 patients. From these data, it was concluded that high-intensity NPPV is more effective than low-intensity NPPV, both in improving gas exchange and in reducing inspiratory effort.[19] If so, resting the diaphragm could be another mechanism by which high- rather than low-intensity NPPV improves respiratory function.

Importantly, however, the aforementioned physiological study also showed that high-intensity NPPV was more likely to significantly reduce non-invasively measured cardiac output than low-intensity NPPV.[19] The authors accordingly emphasised that this effect needs to be taken into account when high-intensity NPPV is used in patients with pre-existing cardiac disease. Nevertheless, clinical data have revealed a reduction in proBNP values following either high- or low-intensity NPPV.[20,21] In addition, a very recent randomised crossover clinical RCT comparing long-term high- and low-intensity NPPV did not show an overall adverse effect of high-intensity NPPV on cardiac performance, although it could reduce cardiac output in patients with pre-existing heart failure.[22,23] Therefore, there is currently no reason to withhold high-intensity NPPV from COPD patients due to fear of adverse cardiac outcomes. However, heart function should be checked regularly in those patients with pre-existing cardiac disease.

HIGH-INTENSITY NPPV: CLINICAL CONSIDERATIONS

In one randomised crossover trial, considerably higher leak volumes were observed during high-intensity NPPV compared to the low-intensity approach.[15] This raised the question of whether high-intensity NPPV could disturb sleep quality, and whether the improvement in hypercapnia is achieved at the cost of reduced sleep quality. A subsequent randomised crossover RCT revealed that sleep quality is well preserved to a similar degree during both forms of NPPV.[24] Another randomised crossover trial confirmed that the sleep quality is acceptable during high-intensity NPPV. In addition, in this trial switching to target volume, NPPV did not provide any further benefits, in terms of both physiology and sleep quality.[25] Therefore, there are currently no data to suggest that high-intensity NPPV using more aggressive ventilator settings compared to the classical approach of low-intensity NPPV negatively affects sleep quality.

Of course, experience is inevitably needed to help patients get used to high-intensity NPPV. Furthermore, more time in hospital is necessary to establish high-intensity NPPV compared to low-intensity NPPV.[9,15] This, however, was deemed to be justified, given the physiological and clinical advantages.

In one large observational study, substantial improvements in HRQL were detected by both the Severe Respiratory Insufficiency Questionnaire (SRI) and the Short Form 36 (SF-36) following high-intensity NPPV in COPD patients, and these improvements were comparable to patients with restrictive thoracic diseases and those with neuromuscular disorders.[26] Here, the SRI is currently the most frequently used specific instrument for HRQL assessment in patients receiving NPPV.[27] The SRI has even been specifically validated for COPD patients under NPPV therapy[28] and has been shown to be capable of scoring the best in comparison to other established questionnaires in the specific subgroup of COPD patients receiving long-term NPPV.[29] Information about the current status of the international adaptation of the SRI can be found on the homepage of the German Society of Pneumology and Mechanical Ventilation.[30] Following, there are many studies in which the SRI reveals HRQL improvements in COPD patients following high-intensity NPPV commencement.[14]

In contrast, generic aspects of HRQL using the SF-36 were reduced in the NPPV group compared to controls, while the COPD-specific St Georges Respiratory Questionnaire revealed a lack of difference between the two groups in terms of specific aspects of HRQL. In this trial, NPPV did provide a small survival benefit. However, this was reportedly at the expense of HRQL.[13] Importantly, HRQL was not assessed with tools specific to chronic respiratory failure as the SRI. In addition, low-intensity NPPV, which is not capable of improving $PaCO_2$, was used in this trial. Therefore, it is suggested that NPPV techniques that do not have the capacity to improve alveolar ventilation are also incapable of improving HRQL. Furthermore, the generic aspects of HRQL can even deteriorate in association with low-intensity NPPV use. This may be attributed to the side effects of NPPV, or at least to the burden caused by the need to wear a mask every night without any subjective benefit. Accordingly, mean adherence to NPPV was low in this study (4.5 ± 3.2 hours per night). Finally, more recent RCTs showed that NPPV aimed at improving elevated $PaCO_2$ values is indeed capable of improving specific aspects of HRQL when compared to controls,[1,2] but also when compared to low-intensity NPPV.[15]

Regarding long-term survival, older outcome studies using low-intensity NPPV published between 2000 and 2009 have yielded conflicting results. The first two studies published in 2000[11] and 2002[12], respectively, showed no survival benefit, while the third one (2009)[13] showed a slight survival benefit for patients undergoing long-term NPPV.

In contrast, in 2014, Köhnlein et al. demonstrated both a substantial survival and HRQL benefit following NPPV commencement.[1] The key difference between the Köhnlein et al. study[1] and the three others mentioned above[11–13] is that the Köhnlein protocol required a 20% reduction in $PaCO_2$ during subsequent spontaneous breathing periods. In this large RCT, patients were randomly assigned to either the NPPV group (n = 102) or the control group (n = 93). The 1-year mortality rate was 12% (12 of 102 patients) in the intervention group and 33% (31 of 93 patients) in the control group (hazard ratio, 0.24; 95% CI, 0.11–0.49; $p = 0.0004$).[1]

In the most recent British trial,[2] long-term high-intensity NPPV was used in addition to long-term oxygen therapy (LTOT) compared to LTOT alone following exacerbation that required acute NPPV in hospital. Notably, patients were randomised in this trial if hypercapnia ($PaCO_2$ >7 kPa) persisted for at least 2 weeks. The primary outcome in the British study was admission-free survival. Of note, the number of patients needed to be treated with NPPV was 6 for this outcome parameter.[2] This is in contrast to the Dutch study where NPPV was also used after exacerbation that required acute NPPV in hospital, since long-term NPPV was already started if hypercapnia had persisted for only 2 days after acute NPPV could have been stopped.[30] Here, both the control group and the treatment group in the Dutch trial experienced a significant reduction in $PaCO_2$, but there was reportedly no outcome benefit for the NPPV-group. This suggests that NPPV was started too early and that not all patients require long-term NPPV following acute NPPV in hospital.[31]

Overall, based on the current findings, there is now increasing evidence that long-term high-intensity NPPV is capable of improving: (i) survival in stable hypercapnic COPD patients[1] and (ii) admission-free survival in COPD patients with status post-acute exacerbation who required acute NPPV in hospital, and had persistent hypercapnia for at least 2 weeks after the cessation of acute NPPV in hospital.[31]

HIGH-INTENSITY NPPV: FUTURE CONSIDERATIONS

Following the enduring discussion on the usefulness of long-term NPPV for chronic hypercapnic COPD patients, there is now increasing evidence to suggest that high-intensity NPPV is superior to low-intensity NPPV and confers both physiological and clinical benefits.[9] However, there are still some important issues that need to be addressed.

First, outpatient commencement and control of NPPV aimed at reducing costs and overcoming hospital-bed shortages should be investigated in the future. This is important considering the increasing numbers of patients with COPD and chronic hypercapnic respiratory failure. The process of acclimatising patients to NPPV in a hospital setting is expensive and dependent on the availability of a hospital bed, and this is particularly true for high-intensity NPPV.

Second, it remains unclear how to best select patients for high-intensity NPPV. It is particularly unknown how to treat older patients with difficulties in tolerating NPPV. Furthermore, even though there is growing evidence to suggest that patients with more severe hypercapnia benefit the most, it is not known how many of these patients are offered long-term NPPV, or how many of them end up not receiving it. This is crucial, since high-intensity NPPV in particular has been shown to be advantageous in clinical trials performed by experienced research groups. However, its feasibility in real life still remains to be elucidated.

Third, scientific research should also target alternative treatment strategies to treat chronic hypercapnic respiratory failure in COPD patients. This is particularly important as the establishment of high-intensity NPPV is complex and cost-intensive. Interestingly, two very recent short studies also demonstrated a potential role for high flow oxygen therapy as an alternative to NPPV in chronic hypercapnic COPD patients, since this approach improved $PaCO_2$, breathing pattern and inspiratory effort.[32,33] Even though these two studies were small, this calls for more research in this direction to verify the findings.

CONFLICT OF INTEREST

The authors SBS, FSM and WW have accepted speaking fees and/or travel funding from companies involved in mechanical ventilation. WW also received funds for research from the following companies: Weinmann, Germany; Vivisol, Germany; VitalAire, Germany and Heinen und Löwenstein, Germany.

REFERENCES

1. Köhnlein T, Windisch W, Köhler D et al. for the COPD study group. Non-invasive positive pressure ventilation for the treatment of severe stable chronic obstructive pulmonary disease. A prospective, multicentre, randomised, controlled clinical trial. *Lancet Respir Med.* 2014;2:698–705.
2. Murphy P, Arbane G, Bourke S et al. Improving admission free survival with home mechanical ventilation (HMV) and home oxygen therapy (HOT) following life threatening COPD exacerbations: HoT-HMV UK Trial. *Eur Respir J.* 2016;48(suppl 60).
3. Struik FM, Lacasse Y, Goldstein R et al. Nocturnal noninvasive positive pressure ventilation in stable COPD. A systematic review and individual patient data metaanalysis. *Respir Med.* 2014;108:329–37.
4. Windisch W, Haenel M, Storre JH, Dreher M. High-intensity non-invasive positive pressure ventilation for stable hypercapnic COPD. *Int J Med Sci.* 2009;6:72–6.
5. Windisch W, Vogel M, Sorichter S et al. Normocapnia during nIPPV in chronic hypercapnic COPD reduces subsequent spontaneous $PaCO_2$. *Respir Med.* 2002; 96:572–9.
6. Windisch W, Kostic S, Dreher M et al. Outcome of patients with stable COPD receiving controlled noninvasive positive pressure ventilation aimed at a maximal reduction of $PaCO_2$. *Chest.* 2005;128:657–62.
7. Windisch W, Storre JH, Sorichter S, Virchow JC Jr. Comparison of volume- and pressure-limited NPPV at night: A prospective randomized cross-over trial. *Respir Med.* 2005;99:52–9.
8. Windisch W, Dreher M, Storre JH, Sorichter S. Nocturnal non-invasive positive pressure ventilation: Physiological effects on spontaneous breathing. *Respir Physiol Neurobiol.* 2006;150:251–60.
9. Schwarz SB, Magnet FS, Windisch W. Why high-intensity NPPV is favourable to low-intensity NPPV: Clinical and physiological reasons. *COPD.* 2017;14:389–395.
10. Windisch W. Noninvasive positive pressure ventilation in COPD. *Breathe.* 2011;8:114–23.
11. Casanova C, Celli BR, Tost L et al. Long-term controlled trial of nocturnal nasal positive pressure ventilation in patients with severe COPD. *Chest.* 2000;118:1582–90.
12. Clini E, Sturani C, Rossi A et al. The Italian multicentre study on noninvasive ventilation in chronic obstructive pulmonary disease patients. *Eur Respir J.* 2002;20:529–38.
13. McEvoy RD, Pierce RJ, Hillman D et al. Nocturnal non-invasive nasal ventilation in stable hypercapnic COPD: A randomised controlled trial. *Thorax.* 2009;64:561–6.
14. Windisch W, Storre JH, Köhnlein T. Nocturnal non-invasive positive pressure ventilation for COPD. *Expert Rev Respir Med.* 2015;9:295–308.
15. Dreher M, Storre H, Schmoor C, Windisch W. High-intensity versus low-intensity noninvasive ventilation in stable hypercapnic COPD patients: A randomized cross-over trial. *Thorax.* 2010:65:303–8.
16. Murphy PB, Brignall K, Moxham J et al. High pressure versus high intensity noninvasive ventilation in stable hypercapnic chronic obstructive pulmonary disease: A randomized crossover trial. *Int J Chron Obstruct Pulmon Dis.* 2012;7:811–8.
17. Elliott MW. Domiciliary non-invasive ventilation in stable COPD? *Thorax.* 2009;64:553–6.
18. De Leeuw PW, Dees A. Fluid homeostasis in chronic obstructive lung disease. *Eur Respir J.* 2003; Suppl. 46,33–40.
19. Lukácsovits J, Carlucci A, Hill N et al. Physiological changes during low- and high-intensity noninvasive ventilation. *Eur Respir J.* 2012;39:869–75.
20. Sin DD, Wong E, Mayers I et al. Effects of nocturnal noninvasive mechanical ventilation on heart rate variability of patients with advanced COPD. *Chest.* 2007;131:156–63.

21. Dreher M, Schulte L, Müller T et al. Influence of effective noninvasive positive pressure ventilation on inflammatory and cardiovascular biomarkers in stable hypercapnic COPD patients. *Respir Med.* 2015;109:1300–4.
22. Duiverman ML, Arellano-Maric MP, Windisch W. Long-term noninvasive ventilation in patients with chronic hypercapnic respiratory failure: Assisting the diaphragm, but threatening the heart? *Curr Opin Pulm Med.* 2016;22:130–7.
23. Duiverman ML, Maagh P, Magnet FS et al. Impact of high-intensity NIV on the heart in stable COPD: A randomised cross-over pilot study. *Respir Res.* 2017;18:76.
24. Dreher M, Ekkernkamp E, Walterspacher S et al. Non-invasive ventilation in COPD: Impact of inspiratory pressure levels on sleep quality. *Chest.* 2011;140:939–45.
25. Storre JH, Matrosovich E, Ekkernkamp E et al. Home mechanical ventilation for COPD: High-intensity versus target volume noninvasive ventilation. *Respir Care.* 2014 Sep;59(9):1389–97.
26. Windisch W. Impact of home mechanical ventilation on health-related quality of life. *Eur Respir J.* 2008;32:1328–36.
27. Windisch W, Freidel K, Schucher B et al. The Severe Respiratory Insufficiency (SRI) Questionnaire: A specific measure of health-related quality of life in patients receiving home mechanical ventilation. *J Clin Epidemiol.* 2003;56:752–9.
28. Windisch W, Budweiser S, Heinemann F et al. The Severe Respiratory Insufficiency (SRI) Questionnaire was valid for patients with COPD. *J Clin Epidemiol.* 2008;61:848–53.
29. Struik FM, Kerstjens HA, Bladder G et al. The Severe Respiratory Insufficiency Questionnaire scored best in the assessment of health-related quality of life in chronic obstructive pulmonary disease. *J Clin Epidemiol.* 2013;66:1166–74.
30. Windisch W. The Severe Respiratory Insufficiency Questionnaire (SRI). [cited 5 April 2017]. Available from: https://www.pneumologie.de/service/patienteninformation/patienten-fragebogen-zur-befindlichkeit-bei-schwerer-respiratorischer-insuffizienz/
31. Struik FM, Sprooten RT, Kerstjens HA et al. Nocturnal non-invasive ventilation in COPD patients with prolonged hypercapnia after ventilatory support for acute respiratory failure: A randomised, controlled, parallel-group study. *Thorax.* 2014;69:826–34.
32. Fraser JF, Spooner AJ, Dunster KR et al. Nasal high flow oxygen therapy in patients with COPD reduces respiratory rate and tissue carbon dioxide while increasing tidal and end-expiratory lung volumes: A randomised crossover trial. *Thorax.* 2016;71:759–61.
33. Pisani L, Fasano L, Corcione N et al. Change in pulmonary mechanics and the effect on breathing pattern of high flow oxygen therapy in stable hypercapnic COPD. *Thorax.* 2017;72:373–5.

PART 6

Hypoxaemic respiratory failure

31	Home oxygen therapy in chronic respiratory failure *Jadwiga A. Wedzicha and Mark W. Elliott*	279
32	Acute oxygen therapy *Mark W. Elliott*	287
33	High-flow oxygen therapy: Physiological effects and clinical evidence *Nuttapol Rittayamai, Arnaud W. Thille and Laurent Brochard*	295
34	Equipment for oxygen therapy *Jane Slough*	307
35	Non-invasive ventilation for hypoxaemic respiratory failure *Massimo Antonelli and Giuseppe Bello*	315

31

Home oxygen therapy in chronic respiratory failure

JADWIGA A. WEDZICHA AND MARK W. ELLIOTT

KEY MESSAGES

- Long-term oxygen therapy (LTOT) corrects chronic hypoxaemia and is associated with reduction in mortality and a number of important physiological benefits if used for at least 15 hours daily.
- There is no evidence to support the use of LTOT in patients who are not hypoxic breathing spontaneously at rest by day.
- Ambulatory oxygen therapy may prolong the usage of home oxygen though the evidence for longer-term benefit on other outcomes is not strong.
- Short-burst oxygen therapy should not be prescribed for the relief of dyspnoea; other therapies are more appropriate.
- Effective LTOT requires comprehensive assessment of the underlying condition causing respiratory failure, and the therapy provided, together with determining oxygen flow rates, appropriate oxygen equipment to match the patient's lifestyle and long-term follow-up.

INTRODUCTION

Long-term oxygen therapy (LTOT) is an important therapy in patients with chronic respiratory failure as, to date, it is one of the few interventions that can improve survival in patients with chronic obstructive pulmonary disease (COPD) complicated by chronic respiratory failure. In the early 1980s, two important clinical trials of LTOT were reported,[1,2] which considerably advanced our understanding, prescription and provision of home oxygen therapy. The purpose of home oxygen therapy is to correct hypoxaemia and not primarily as a therapy for breathlessness for which other pharmacological and non-pharmacological interventions will be more appropriate.

There are three main types of oxygen therapy that can be prescribed for home use, and these will be discussed in this chapter.[3,4] Home oxygen therapy may also be used in infants and children but paediatric prescription is relatively small and has been covered in detail elsewhere.[5] This chapter will concentrate on home oxygen therapy for chronic respiratory failure in adults.

Long-term oxygen therapy

LTOT is prescribed for patients for continuous use at home usually through an oxygen concentrator with chronic hypoxaemia (PaO_2 at or below 7.3 kPa, or 55 mm Hg). In some circumstances, LTOT may also be indicated in patients with a PaO_2 between 7.3 and 8 kPa (55–60 mm Hg), if they have evidence of pulmonary hypertension, secondary hypoxaemia, oedema or significant nocturnal arterial oxygen desaturation. There is no benefit in the use of LTOT in COPD patients with a PaO_2 above 8 kPa.[6] Once started, this therapy is likely to be lifelong. LTOT is usually given for at least 15 hours daily, to include the overnight period, as arterial hypoxaemia worsens during sleep.

Ambulatory oxygen therapy

Ambulatory oxygen therapy refers to the provision of oxygen therapy with a portable device during exercise and daily activities. It is usually prescribed in conjunction with LTOT, although a small group of normoxaemic patients may benefit from ambulatory oxygen if they have significant arterial oxygen desaturation on exercise.

Short-burst oxygen therapy

Short-burst oxygen therapy (SBOT) refers to the intermittent use of supplemental oxygen at home usually provided by static cylinders and normally for periods of about 10–20 min at a time to relieve dyspnoea. Although a considerable amount of SBOT is used, the evidence for benefit of SBOT is weak[7,8] and other treatments for dyspnoea should be used. However, some patients on rare occasions may develop 'intermittent hypoxaemia', for example, during a COPD exacerbation, and then use of short-term or intermittent oxygen may be appropriate.

INDICATIONS FOR LTOT

There are three main indications for the prescription of LTOT: chronic hypoxaemia, nocturnal hypoventilation and palliative use (Box 31.1).

Chronic hypoxaemia

Identification of patients with chronic hypoxaemia is important, as LTOT is one of the few treatments that can improve prognosis in patients with COPD. Chronic hypoxaemia, with or without carbon dioxide retention, can occur in several respiratory and cardiac disorders, including COPD, chronic severe asthma, interstitial lung disease such as fibrosing alveolitis and asbestosis, cystic fibrosis and pulmonary hypertension. Approximately 60% of prescriptions for home oxygen therapy are for chronic respiratory failure due to COPD. Chronic hypoxaemia leads to an increase in pulmonary arterial pressure, secondary polycythaemia and neuropsychological changes, and these complications can be improved with LTOT.

Although two randomised controlled trials showed survival benefit of LTOT in patients with COPD, when used for at least 15 hours daily,[1,2] the precise mechanism of the improvement in survival with oxygen therapy is unknown (Figure 31.1). Epidemiological data have suggested that lack of home oxygen prescription in hypoxaemic patients may predispose to hospital admissions.[9] The two large home oxygen trials did not evaluate systematically the effects of LTOT on exacerbations, though it is possible that the mortality reduction with LTOT may be due to correction of increasing hypoxaemia at exacerbation.

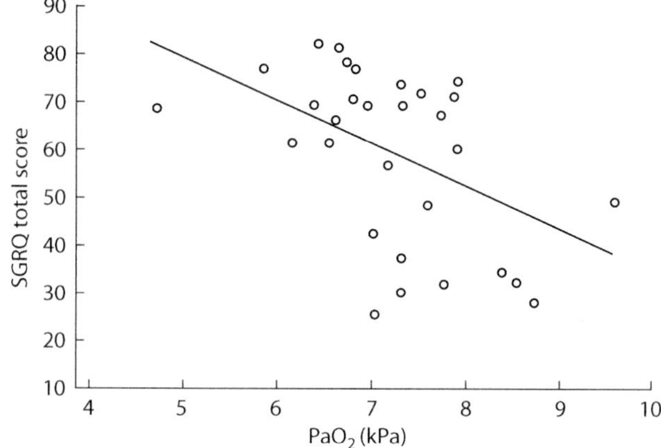

Figure 31.1 Relation between quality of life and arterial hypoxaemia in chronic obstructive pulmonary disease (COPD). (Reproduced from Okubadejo AA, Paul EA, Jones PW et al. *Thorax*. 1996;51:44–7.)

Previous studies have shown that effects of LTOT on pulmonary artery pressure (PAP) have been small, though PAP may be more useful prognostically and reflect disease severity. Both randomised controlled trials evaluated changes in PAP with LTOT. In the Nocturnal Oxygen Therapy Trial (NOTT), survival was related to the decrease in mean PAP during the first 6 months of treatment.[10] In the UK Medical Research Council (MRC) trial, LTOT prevented a rise of PAP of 3 mm Hg, seen in the control group, though a fall in PAP was not found.[2] Patients who have daytime hypoxaemia may develop further arterial oxygen desaturation at night during nocturnal hypoventilation, and this will contribute to the observed rise in PAP.[3] Thus, LTOT is always prescribed to include the night time as it will reduce the nocturnal hypoxia episodes and thus reduce the peaks of pulmonary hypertension.

The MRC trial showed that only patients who were hypercapnic and who had had a previous documented episode of oedema (cor pulmonale) had benefits after LTOT.[2] On the contrary, the NOTT showed that the benefits of LTOT were present in relatively normocapnic patients.[1] It is thus a reasonable assumption that improvements in survival are likely in the presence of chronic hypoxaemia, irrespective of chronic hypercapnia or previous episodes of oedema. This assumption is reflected in the advice of all current international guidelines on the prescription of LTOT. Patients should be prescribed LTOT for at least 15 hours daily, although survival improves further when

BOX 31.1: Indications for long-term oxygen therapy

- Chronic COPD
- Severe chronic asthma
- Interstitial lung disease
- Cystic fibrosis
- Bronchiectasis
- Pulmonary vascular disease
- Primary pulmonary hypertension
- Pulmonary malignancy
- Chronic heart failure

LTOT is used for more than 20 hours daily.[2] Thus, the hours of LTOT use should not be restricted, especially in severe COPD.

Secondary polycythaemia is another complication of chronic hypoxaemia, though elevation in haematocrit is not consistent in patients in that some develop polycythaemia and others do not. This variability in haematocrit levels may be reflected by the variable erythropoietin levels found in these patients.[11] LTOT as shown in the MRC trial reduces polycythaemia with reductions in haematocrit and red cell mass.[2] Cigarette smoking predisposes to secondary polycythaemia and the variable haematocrit levels may be due to an interaction with smoking. The effect of LTOT on reducing haematocrit may be offset by raised carboxyhaemoglobin levels from cigarette smoking.[12] Patients on home oxygen should stop smoking as the use of oxygen, which supports combustion, in the presence of smoking can cause burns and is a fire hazard. Any patient who persists in smoking despite using any form of home oxygen must be warned of the potential risks. It is important to note that oxygen may be retained in clothing and petroleum-based ointments; for a period of time after discontinuing oxygen, there is still an increase in the risk of burns. A risk assessment must be performed for any smoker prescribed oxygen, and this will sometimes involve other agencies such as the fire service, housing officials and so on; others may be put at risk by an individual smoking while using oxygen. However, there is no objective evidence available that patients who continue smoking have worse outcomes on LTOT.

Important relationships have been found between chronic hypoxaemia and health-related quality of life. In moderate and severe hypoxaemia, the quality of life score is related to the degree of hypoxaemia, when measured using the St George's Respiratory Questionnaire, a disease-specific questionnaire[13] (Figure 31.1). Anxiety and depression are also related to hypoxaemia, and this accounts for psychological comorbidity seen in these patients. Improvements have been found in both anxiety and health status after LTOT. COPD patients have impaired sleep quality with frequent arousals.[14] LTOT corrects nocturnal SaO_2, decreases sleep latency and improves sleep quality.[15,16]

Patients with chest wall or neuromuscular diseases who develop hypercapnic respiratory failure usually require ventilatory support with non-invasive ventilation rather than LTOT alone. Use of LTOT in these patients may lead to a potentially dangerous rise in carbon dioxide overnight with morning headaches. However, if chronic hypoxaemia persists while the patient is on ventilatory support, then LTOT should be prescribed initially at a low oxygen flow rate, for example, 1 L/min, and titrated to maintain SpO_2 >90% and with monitoring of transcutaneous CO_2. If overnight monitoring is not available, measuring early morning arterial blood gases for the presence of hypercapnia may be useful.

Benefits of LTOT are listed in Box 31.2.

BOX 31.2: Benefits of long-term oxygen therapy

- Increased survival and quality of life
- Prevention of deterioration of pulmonary haemodynamics
- Reduction of secondary polycythaemia
- Neuropsychological benefit with reduction in symptoms of anxiety and depression
- Improved sleep quality
- Reduction in cardiac arrhythmias
- Increase in renal blood flow

Sleep or exercise induced oxygen desaturation, but with daytime PaO_2 above threshold for LTOT

There is a question as to what should be done for the patient who is above the PaO_2 criterion for LTOT but desaturates during sleep or exercise. Chaouat et al.[17] studied COPD patients with a daytime PaO_2 of 56–69 mmHg. Sleep-related oxygen desaturation was defined as spending more than 29% of the nocturnal recording time with SpO_2 <90%. Of the 64 patients, 35 were desaturators and 29 were non-desaturators. At baseline, patients with sleep-related desaturation had a significantly higher daytime (mean ± SD) $PaCO_2$ (44.9 ± 4.9 mmHg vs. 41.0 ± 4.1 mmHg, p = 0.001); mean PAP (mPAP) was similar in the two groups. After 2 years, none of the non-desaturator patients became desaturators. The mean changes in mPAP at 2 years were similar between the two groups, as were the rates of death or requirement for LTOT during follow-up of up to 6 years. They concluded that sleep-related oxygen desaturation is not a transitional state before the worsening of daytime arterial blood gases but is a characteristic of some COPD patients who have a higher daytime arterial carbon dioxide partial pressure. Such isolated nocturnal hypoxaemia or sleep-related worsening of moderate daytime hypoxaemia does not appear to favour the development of pulmonary hypertension or to lead to worsening of daytime blood gases. In another study,[18] looking at the endpoints of pulmonary haemodynamics, survival and requirement for LTOT after 2 years of follow-up 76 patients were randomised, to nocturnal oxygen, prescribed to maintain SpO_2 >90% or control. Nocturnal oxygen therapy did not modify the evolution of pulmonary haemodynamics and did not prevent progression to LTOT. No effect on survival was observed, but the small number of deaths precludes any firm conclusion. An RCT powered for survival is planned.[19] These results suggest that the prescription of nocturnal oxygen therapy in isolation is probably not justified in COPD patients who do not meet the criteria for LTOT.

Recently, a randomised controlled trial[20] of LTOT for patients with an oxygen saturation between 89% and 93% or who developed oxygen saturation during a 6-min walking test showed that patients were randomised to long-term supplemental oxygen either given for 24 hours a day (n = 224) or during sleep and exercise (n = 148) or to no supplemental oxygen (n = 370). In total, 738 patients from 42 centres were followed for 1 to 6 years. Self-reported compliance was 15.1 ± 6.2 hours/day in those on the 24-hour prescription and 11.3 ± 5 hours/day on the sleep/exercise prescription. The no prescribed supplemental oxygen group received a mean of 1.8 ± 3.9 hours/day of supplemental oxygen. The authors found no significant difference between the two groups in the time to death or first hospitalisation, hospitalisation rate COPD exacerbation rate and COPD related hospitalisations. There were no consistent differences in measures of quality of life lung function or 6-min walking distance. A total of 51 adverse events were attributed to the use of supplemental oxygen; there were 23 reports of tripping over equipment, with two patients requiring hospitalisation, and five patients reported fires or burns, with one patient requiring hospitalisation. These data do not suggest that existing guidelines for the prescription of LTOT in patients with COPD should be changed to include those with milder or intermittent hypoxia; furthermore, there is a risk with the use of oxygen at home.

Palliative use

Oxygen may also be prescribed for palliation of severe dyspnoea in patients with lung cancer[21,22] and other causes of disabling dyspnoea such as in patients with severe COPD or interstitial lung disease. However, evidence shows that oxygen is only beneficial in a palliative setting when there is also evidence of chronic hypoxaemia. A systematic review concluded that oxygen is not beneficial to non-hypoxaemic patients with cancer.[22]

ASSESSMENT FOR LTOT

It essential that all patients as candidates for LTOT undergo a full assessment in a specialist centre with experience in assessing patients for home oxygen therapy. The purpose of assessment is to confirm the presence of hypoxaemia and to ensure that the correct oxygen flow rate is provided to correct the hypoxaemia adequately. Assessment for LTOT requires measurement of arterial blood gases. Either blood gases from a radial or femoral artery or arterialised ear lobe capillary blood gases can be used for assessments. The advantage of ear lobe gases is that samples can be obtained by various healthcare professionals.[23] Before LTOT assessment and prescription, it is essential that there has been optimum medical management of the underlying condition causing hypoxia and patients should be clinically stable. Patients should not be assessed for LTOT during an acute exacerbation of their disease. As exacerbation recovery may be prolonged,[24] hypoxaemia can persist after exacerbation and thus assessment should occur no sooner than at around 5–6 weeks after the patient has recovered from an exacerbation. As a general rule, patients should not be assessed for LTOT during a period of hospitalisation, though it should be appreciated that some patients do not stay out of hospital long enough to meet the above criterion. It is usual to start with a supplemental oxygen flow rate of 2 L/min via nasal cannulae, or from a 24% controlled oxygen face mask, and to aim for a PaO_2 value of at least 8 kPa.[4]

Blood gases must be measured, rather than SpO_2, with a pulse oximeter, as assessment of hypercapnia and its response to oxygen therapy is required for safe prescription of LTOT. Pulse oximetry has also poor specificity in the crucial PaO_2 range for LTOT prescription and thus is unsuitable when used alone for assessment.[25] However, oximetry may prove valuable in screening or case finding of patients with chronic respiratory disease and selecting those patients who require further blood gas analysis.

Patients on LTOT require follow-up after prescription to ensure that there is adequate correction of hypoxaemia and that they are adherent to their oxygen treatment.[26]

INDICATIONS FOR AMBULATORY OXYGEN THERAPY

Patients with COPD who have chronic hypoxaemia frequently develop worsening arterial oxygen desaturation on exercise, considered significant when the SpO_2 falls at least 4% to be below 90% with exercise. A small group of patients without resting hypoxaemia can also develop significant desaturation during exercise and may benefit from ambulatory oxygen. Patients with interstitial fibrosis may develop more severe exercise desaturation for a given level of PaO_2. Administration of supplemental oxygen therapy on exercise to patients with hypoxaemia reduces ventilatory demand, may improve operational lung volumes and alleviates dyspnoea. Although ambulatory oxygen can correct exercise hypoxaemia, reduce breathlessness and increase exercise capacity, short-term responses to ambulatory oxygen are variable among patients.[27] However, most of the studies of the effects of ambulatory oxygen are relatively short-term studies and there is less evidence that ambulatory oxygen improves quality of life over the longer term.[28] Indeed, short-term responses to ambulatory oxygen with respect to dyspnoea and exercise capacity do not relate to longer-term benefits.[29] More recently, a Cochrane systematic review[30] of patients with COPD who did not qualify for home oxygen therapy included 44 studies with 1195 participants; 33 were included in the meta-analysis. Most included small numbers of patients and were short term. The primary aim was to reduce dyspnoea and the requirement for exercise-induced oxygen desaturation was variable. Breathlessness during exercise was reduced by oxygen compared to air. There was no effect of short-burst oxygen given before exercise. Oxygen reduced breathlessness measured during exercise tests, whereas an effect on breathlessness measured in daily life was limited. There was no clear effect on quality of life. The authors concluded that oxygen can relieve breathlessness when given during exercise to mildly and non-hypoxic patients with COPD who would not otherwise qualify for home oxygen therapy. Most of the benefits were seen during exercise. There is another Cochrane systematic review[31] of longer-term studies (with a maximum of only 12 weeks) of ambulatory oxygen for patients with COPD but no resting hypoxia. In only two of the studies was confirmation of oxygen desaturation during exercise required. Two studies showed a statistically significant benefit in favour of oxygen for dyspnoea after exercise. There was a statistically significant benefit for subcategories of dyspnoea and fatigue in the quality-of-life domains. No evidence of any effect was reported for survival, and there were limited benefits for exercise capacity. One problem with both of these meta-analyses was the failure to distinguish between oxygen desaturators and non-desaturators. As for LTOT, the purpose of ambulatory oxygen is to correct exercise hypoxaemia and not as a therapy with the sole aim of reduction in dyspnoea.

The addition of oxygen to pulmonary rehabilitation is theoretically attractive. If patients desaturate during exercise, the training effect of rehabilitation may be reduced. Correcting the oxygen desaturation will allow patients to exercise more, thereby gaining greater benefit from the programme. In a randomised controlled trial of 45 patients who desaturated by more than 4%, and to less than 90%, during a walking test, the addition of oxygen made no difference to outcomes at the end of a 20-week supervised training programme followed by 13 weeks unsupervised exercise at home. Endpoints were the endurance shuttle walk test, St George's Respiratory Questionnaire and number of hospitalisations or dropout.[32]

Ambulatory oxygen therapy is indicated in a number of respiratory conditions, with COPD being the most common. Ambulatory oxygen is not indicated in patients with no evidence of arterial hypoxaemia and is not indicated in patients with chronic heart failure.[33] This has been confirmed in a recent RCT[34] of patients with chronic heart failure randomised to conventional therapy or LTOT for at least 15 hours/day. Mean usage was poor at 5.4 hours/day, and there was no impact on quality of life. However, patients were included on the basis of severity of heart failure and hypoxia was not required; indeed, the median saturation before a 6-min walk was 97% and very few patients desaturated to <90% with exercise. It is difficult to see why oxygen should help. Given that the usage was so poor, it is still possible that oxygen could have had an effect if used as prescribed; however, in reality, if patients are only going to use it for that amount of time, then on an intention-to-treat basis, no survival benefit will accrue.

The other indications are listed in Box 31.3.

Ambulatory oxygen can be prescribed in three broad groups of patients:[4]

Grade 1 – Some patients on LTOT are already housebound and unable to leave the home unaided. In this group, ambulatory oxygen will be used for short periods only and intermittently. These patients will generally use ambulatory oxygen at the same flow rate as with their LTOT.

Grade 2 – Some patients on LTOT are mobile and need to or can leave the home on a regular basis. In this patient group, assessment will need to include a review of activity and oxygen flow rate required to correct hypoxaemia.

Grade 3 – These are patients without chronic hypoxaemia (PaO_2 > 7.3 kPa), who are not on LTOT, but who show evidence of arterial oxygen desaturation on exercise, with a fall of SpO_2 of at least 4% to below 90%. Ambulatory oxygen should only be prescribed if there is evidence of exercise desaturation that is corrected by the proposed ambulatory device.

BOX 31.3: Indications for ambulatory oxygen

- Chronic COPD
- Severe chronic asthma
- Interstitial lung disease
- Cystic fibrosis
- Pulmonary vascular disease
- Primary pulmonary hypertension
- Chest wall disease, for example, kyphoscoliosis

A major issue with ambulatory oxygen is usage of the oxygen outside the home. There is little information on compliance with ambulatory oxygen therapy, though when assessed, compliance has been found to be generally poor, with most patients only using it occasionally to go out of the house or into their gardens and much less than instructed by their healthcare professionals.[35] In an early crossover study of oxygen cylinders and liquid systems, Lock et al. showed that patients preferred the liquid systems and use them more but did not increase the time outside the home.[36] A number of other studies have reported poor adherence to therapy with ambulatory oxygen therapy.[28,37] Sandland and colleagues have recently shown that in the short term, ambulatory oxygen therapy is not associated with improvements in physical activity, or time spent away from home.[38] However, the use of cylinder oxygen increased over the 8 weeks compared to cylinder air. The authors conclude that patients need time to learn how to use the ambulatory oxygen and thus may then enhance activity.

ASSESSMENT FOR AMBULATORY OXYGEN

The type of ambulatory oxygen assessment will depend on the patient's grade and thus on the patient's activity and ability to leave the home (Box 31.4). Traditionally, assessments for ambulatory oxygen therapy use short-term response to supplemental oxygen therapy during an exercise test (e.g. 6-min walking test). However, it is now recognised that short-term responses do not predict benefit over a longer period of time and thus the short-term response cannot be used to select patients for ambulatory oxygen. In some cases, the weight of the ambulatory device has been shown to

BOX 31.4: Ambulatory oxygen therapy: Patient assessment based on the British Thoracic Society (BTS) working group on home oxygen services

- Grade 1 oxygen requirements – same flow rate as for static source
- Grade 2 oxygen requirements – evaluate oxygen flow rate to correct exercise SaO_2 above 90% using exercise test, for example, 6-min walk
- Grade I oxygen requirements – exercise test required, performed on air and oxygen; require evidence of exercise desaturation and improvement with oxygen

Source: British Thoracic Society (BTS) Working Group on Home Oxygen Services. *Clinical Component for the Home Oxygen Service in England and Wales.* London: BTS, 2006.

negate the benefit of the therapy on the short-term response. Thus, the ambulatory oxygen assessment should be used as an opportunity to assess the patient's activity, to set the optimal oxygen flow rate and introduce the patient to the ambulatory device. The assessment should ideally be performed after a course of exercise training as part of a pulmonary rehabilitation programme. The initial assessment should be followed by a review after approximately 2 months of oxygen usage and ambulatory oxygen withdrawn if unhelpful.

Before prescription of ambulatory oxygen, it is important to determine the level of outside activity that the patient is likely to perform, so that the most effective and economic device is provided. Most ambulatory oxygen is provided with lightweight portable cylinders, though small cylinders provide oxygen for a short duration and oxygen-conserving devices may be useful in prolonging oxygen availability. However, patient responses to these conserving devices vary owing to varying inspiratory flow rates, and patients should be assessed on the same equipment that they will eventually use when at home. Liquid oxygen systems can provide a longer period of ambulatory oxygen usage but are generally more expensive to provide and not so widely available.

SHORT-BURST OXYGEN THERAPY

Despite extensive prescription of short-burst therapy, there is no evidence available for the benefit of this oxygen modality and other interventions should be used for control of dyspnoea.[7,8] SBOT has traditionally been used for pre-oxygenation before exercise, recovery from exercise and control of breathlessness at rest.[39,40] It has also been used after a COPD exacerbation when a patient has not yet recovered from hypoxaemia, though in that case, temporary LTOT would be more appropriate.

FUTURE RESEARCH

Despite widespread use of home oxygen therapy, there are a number of issues that require further study. More information is required on the mechanisms of long-term benefit with LTOT, especially if LTOT reduces the severity of exacerbations. However, further randomised controlled studies of LTOT in hypoxaemic patients are not appropriate, in view of the beneficial effects seen on mortality. Studies must be in well-defined populations with accurate classification of oxygen desaturation during exercise, sleep and so on. If oxygen is to be given to patients without evidence of hypoxia, and it is hard to see a rationale for this, they must not be lumped together with patients who become hypoxic, for instance, during sleep or exercise. Beneficial effects in the whole group may just be because of benefits in the desaturators.

Attention is needed to the problem of poor adherence to ambulatory oxygen therapy and how much support and education is required in order that patients use the therapy on a daily basis. Withdrawal of home oxygen in patients with inappropriate short-burst prescriptions also requires evaluation. The goal of a comprehensive home oxygen service for patients with chronic respiratory failure is to ensure that the right person is treated with home oxygen for the correct indications and thus optimal benefits will be obtained with this important but costly therapy.

REFERENCES

1. Nocturnal Oxygen Therapy Trial Group. Continuous or nocturnal oxygen therapy in hypoxaemic chronic obstructive lung disease. *Ann Intern Med.* 1980; 93:391–8.
2. Medical Research Council Working Party. Long term domiciliary oxygen therapy in chronic hypoxic cor pulmonale complicating chronic bronchitis and emphysema. *Lancet.* 1981;i:681–6.
3. Royal College of Physicians. Domiciliary Oxygen Therapy Services. *Clinical Guidelines and Advice for Prescribers.* London: Royal College of Physicians, 1999.
4. British Thoracic Society (BTS) Working Group on Home Oxygen Services. *Clinical Component for the Home Oxygen Service in England and Wales.* London: BTS, 2006.
5. Balfour-Lynn M, Field DJ, Gringras P et al. On behalf of the paediatric section of the Home Oxygen Guideline Development Group of the BTS Standards of Care Committee. BTS Guidelines for home oxygen in children. *Thorax.* 2009;64 Suppl 2:ii1–ii26.
6. Gorecka D, Gorzelak K, Sliwinski P et al. Effect of long term oxygen therapy on survival in chronic obstructive pulmonary disease with moderate hypoxaemia. *Thorax.* 1997;52:674–9.

7. Stevenson NJ, Calverley PMA. Effect of oxygen on recovery from maximal exercise in patients with chronic obstructive pulmonary disease. *Thorax.* 2004;59:668–72.
8. Eaton W, Fergusson J, Kolbe CA et al. Short-burst oxygen therapy for COPD patients: A 6-month randomised, controlled study. *Eur Respir J* 2006;27:697–704.
9. Garcia-Aymerich E, Farrero MA, Félez J et al. Risk factors of readmission to hospital for a COPD exacerbation: A prospective study. *Thorax.* 2003;58:100–5.
10. Timms RM, Khaja FU, Williams GW et al. Hemodynamic response to oxygen therapy in chronic obstructive pulmonary disease. *Ann Intern Med.* 1985;102:29–36.
11. Wedzicha JA, Cotes PM, Empey DW et al. Serum immunoreactive erythropoietin in hypoxic lung disease with and without polycythaemia. *Clin Sci.* 1985;69:413–22.
12. Calverley PMA, Leggett RJ, McElderry L et al. Cigarette smoking and secondary polycythaemia in hypoxic cor pulmonale. *Am Rev Respir Dis.* 1982; 125:507–10.
13. Okubadejo AA, Paul EA, Jones PW et al. Quality of life in patients with chronic obstructive pulmonary disease and severe hypoxaemia. *Thorax.* 1996;51:44–7.
14. Brezinova V, Catterall JR, Douglas NJ et al. Night sleep of patients with chronic ventilatory failure and age matched controls: Number and duration of the EEG episodes of intervening wakefulness and drowsiness. *Sleep* 1982;5:123–30.
15. Calverley PMA, Brezinova V, Douglas NJ et al. The effect of oxygenation on sleep quality in chronic bronchitis and emphysema. *Am Rev Respir Dis.* 1982;126:206–10.
16. Goldstein RS, Ramcharan V, Bowes G et al. Effect of supplemental nocturnal oxygen on gas exchange in patients with severe obstructive lung disease. *N Engl J Med.* 1984;310:425–9.
17. Chaouat A, Weitzenblum E, Kessler R et al. Outcome of COPD patients with mild daytime hypoxaemia with or without sleep-related oxygen desaturation. *Eur Respir J.* 2001;17(5):848–55. Epub 2001/08/08.
18. Chaouat A, Weitzenblum E, Kessler R et al. A randomized trial of nocturnal oxygen therapy in chronic obstructive pulmonary disease patients. *Eur Respir J.* 1999;14(5):1002–8.
19. Lacasse Y, Bernard S, Series F et al. Multi-center, randomized, placebo-controlled trial of nocturnal oxygen therapy in chronic obstructive pulmonary disease: A study protocol for the INOX trial. *BMC Pulmon Med.* 2017;17(1):8. Epub 2017/01/11.
20. Albert RK, Au DH, Blackford AL et al. A randomized trial of long-term oxygen for COPD with moderate desaturation. *N Engl J Med.* 2016;375(17):1617–27. Epub 2016/10/27.
21. Bruera E, de Stoutz N, Valsco-Leiva A et al. Effects of oxygen on dyspnoea in hypoxaemic terminal-cancer patients. *Lancet.* 1993;342:13–14.
22. Uronis HE, Currow DC, McCrory DC et al. Oxygen for the relief of dyspnoea in mildly or non hypoxaemic patients with cancer: A systematic review and meta-analysis. *Br J Cancer.* 2008;98:294–9.
23. Pitkin AD, Roberts CM, Wedzicha JA. Arterialised ear lobe blood gas analysis: An underused technique. *Thorax.* 1994;49:364–6.
24. Seemungal TAR, Donaldson GC, Bhowmik A et al. Time course and recovery of exacerbations in patients with chronic obstructive pulmonary disease. *Am J Respir Crit Care Med.* 2000;161: 1608–13.
25. Roberts CM, Bugler JR, Melchor R et al. Value of pulse oximetry in screening for long-term oxygen requirement. *Eur Respir J.* 1993;6:559–62.
26. Restrick LJ, Paul EA, Braid GM et al. Assessment and follow-up of patients prescribed long term oxygen treatment. *Thorax.* 1993;48:708–13.
27. Bradley JM, Lasserson T, Elborn S et al. A systematic review of randomized controlled trials examining the short-term benefit of ambulatory oxygen in COPD. *Chest.* 2007;131:278–85.
28. Eaton T, Garrett JE, Young P et al. Ambulatory oxygen improves quality of life of COPD patients: A randomised controlled study. *Eur Respir J.* 2002;20:306–12.
29. Garrod R, Paul EA, Wedzicha JA. Supplemental oxygen during pulmonary rehabilitation in patients with COPD with exercise hypoxaemia. *Thorax.* 2000;55:539–44.
30. Ekstrom M, Ahmadi Z, Bornefalk-Hermansson A et al. Oxygen for breathlessness in patients with chronic obstructive pulmonary disease who do not qualify for home oxygen therapy. *Cochrane Database Syst Rev.* 2016;11:CD006429. Epub 2016/11/26.
31. Ameer F, Carson KV, Usmani ZA, Smith BJ. Ambulatory oxygen for people with chronic obstructive pulmonary disease who are not hypoxaemic at rest. *Cochrane Database Syst Rev.* 2014(6):CD000238. Epub 2014/06/25.
32. Ringbaek T, Martinez G, Lange P. The long-term effect of ambulatory oxygen in normoxaemic COPD patients: A randomised study. *Chron Respir Dis.* 2013;10(2):77–84. Epub 2013/02/23.
33. Restrick LJ, Davies SW, Noone L et al. Ambulatory oxygen in chronic heart failure. *Lancet.* 1992;340:1192–3.

34. Clark AL, Johnson M, Fairhurst C et al. Does home oxygen therapy (HOT) in addition to standard care reduce disease severity and improve symptoms in people with chronic heart failure? A randomised trial of home oxygen therapy for patients with chronic heart failure. *Health Technol Assess*. 2015;19(75): 1–120. Epub 2015/09/24.
35. Lock AH, Paul EA, Rudd RM et al. Portable oxygen therapy: Assessment and usage. *Respir Med*. 1991;85:407–12.
36. Lock SH, Blower G, Prynne M et al. Comparison of liquid and gaseous oxygen for domiciliary portable use. *Thorax*. 1992;47:98–100.
37. Lacasse Y, Lecours R, Pelletier C et al. Randomised trial of ambulatory oxygen in oxygen-dependent COPD. *Eur Respir J*. 2005;25:1032–8.
38. Sandland CJ, Morgan MDL, Singh SJ. Patterns of domestic activity and ambulatory oxygen usage in COPD. *Chest*. 2008;134:753–60.
39. Woodcock AA, Gross ER, Geddes DM. Oxygen relieves breathlessness in 'pink puffers'. *Lancet*. 1981;i:907–9.
40. Evans TW, Waterhouse JC, Carter A et al. Short burst oxygen treatment for breathlessness in chronic obstructive airways disease. *Thorax*. 1986;41:611–5.

32

Acute oxygen therapy

MARK W. ELLIOTT

KEY MESSAGES

- Oxygen therapy may be harmful.
- The clinician must make assessments of both oxygenation and ventilation – if ventilation is reduced, there will be no signs of respiratory distress and cyanosis may be overlooked.
- Pulse oximeters have limitations; clinicians should be aware of what they are.
- Oxygen should be *prescribed* to both a lower and an upper target oxygen saturation.
- In patients with lung disease, end tidal CO_2 monitors do not provide useful information about absolute CO_2 levels or trends. *They should never be used, except to confirm correct placement of an endotracheal tube.*

INTRODUCTION

Oxygen is one of the commonest drugs used in medical emergencies. Most breathless patients and a large number of patients with other acute conditions are given supplementary oxygen. Dogma is that a high FIO_2 is protective and gives a margin of safety and therefore practitioners should err on the side of generous oxygen supplementation. However, this is not without risk (Table 32.1) and there are occasional deaths due to under- or overuse of oxygen.[1] Audits of oxygen use have consistently shown poor performance.[2–5]

Tissue hypoxia and cell death can occur, especially in the brain, after just a few minutes of profound hypoxaemia, such as occurs during cardiac arrest. The degree of hypoxia that will cause cellular damage is not well established and subjects can acclimatise to even very severe hypoxaemia.[6] Patients with chronic lung diseases may tolerate low levels of blood oxygen when in a clinically stable condition, but these levels may not be adequate during acute illness, when the tissue oxygen demand may increase. Unfortunately, there are few randomised controlled trials (RCTs) to guide practice, which is largely guided by precedent; when RCTs have been performed, they show harm.[7–9]

CLINICAL ASSESSMENT OF THE POTENTIALLY HYPOXIC PATIENT

Clinical assessment of hypoxaemia involves inspection of the tongue for central cyanosis. This is difficult, especially in poor lighting conditions, and is made even more unreliable by the presence of anaemia or polycythaemia. Peripheral cyanosis, without central cyanosis, is due to poor peripheral circulation and does not indicate arterial hypoxaemia. Hypoxaemia may occur with increased or decreased ventilation, but the majority of patients have increased ventilation in an attempt to increase the blood oxygen level. However, some patients with marked hypoxaemia may present with non-specific findings, such as restlessness and confusion. If ventilation is reduced, for example, because of opiate overdose, there will be no signs of respiratory distress and cyanosis may be overlooked.[10–11] The clinician must make assessments of both oxygenation and ventilation.

In patients with lung disease, hypercapnia is usually accompanied by visible respiratory distress, because minute ventilation is increased; carbon dioxide levels rise because alveolar ventilation is reduced. This is a consequence of the adoption of a rapid shallow pattern of breathing to protect overloaded respiratory muscles from developing fatigue.

Table 32.1 Risks associated with supplemental oxygen therapy

- Masking of a decline in the gas exchanging function of the lung, giving a false sense of security
- Worsening hypercapnia in patients with COPD
- Hyperoxaemia may cause direct damage
  - It can cause vasoconstriction, which may cause paradoxical myocardial hypoxia in a patient with already narrowed coronary arteries.[7]
  - Reactive oxygen species are generated in the presence of high tissue PO_2, causing oxidative stress and free radical damage.
  - Hazardous to patients with paraquat poisoning[12]
  - Potentiates
    - Bleomycin lung injury[13]
    - Injury from aspiration of acids[14–15]

Patients may have a flushed face, a full and bounding pulse and muscle twitching together with a flap of the outstretched hands. In severe cases, consciousness may be depressed and convulsions may occur. Coma will usually occur when the $PaCO_2$ is in the range of 12 to 16 kPa (90 to 120 mmHg).[16]

INVESTIGATIONS (TABLE 32.2)

Oximetry is the cornerstone in the assessment of a possibly hypoxic patient, but it is important to recognise its limitations. Haemoglobin oxygen saturation is measured by determining the absorption of light at two wavelengths, corresponding to the absorption peaks of oxygenated and de-oxygenated haemoglobin. Anything that will affect transmission of light should be removed, in particular nail varnish and false nails. Accuracy is also reduced in patients with poor peripheral perfusion. Most oximeters give an indication of the pulse signal strength, and if it is low, the probe may need to be moved. A finger generally gives the best signal, but toes or earlobes are alternatives. If the quality of the signal remains poor, the results should be interpreted with caution. Although oximeters are less accurate at low saturations, modern devices are accurate at oxygen saturations (SpO_2) above about 88%. Inaccuracies at lower levels should not affect management in most clinical situations as values greater than this will usually be targeted. A SpO_2 of 92% or above has a sensitivity of 100% and a specificity of 86% for detecting an arterial oxygen tension below 60 mmHg (8 kPa) in fair-skinned individuals,[17]

Table 32.2 Evaluation of the potentially hypoxic patient

	Indication	Limitations
History and clinical examination	**Mandatory** in all patients to ascertain cause	Cyanosis an unreliable clinical sign Absence of respiratory distress may deflect clinician from considering possibility of hypoxia and respiratory compromise
Pulse oximetry	**Mandatory** in all cases of possible hypoxia or critical illness when available (may not be in an out-of-hospital emergency)	Less reliable if pigmented skin Less reliable if poor perfusion Less accurate at low levels (but usually will not affect clinical management) Caution if CO poisoning, severe anaemia, methaemoglobinaemia
Arterial blood gas analysis Alternatives Arteriolised capillary sampling Venous sampling	Should be performed • In most patients with oxygen saturation <92% • In **all** patients with features of life-threatening respiratory illness regardless of the SpO_2 • In **all** patients at risk for hypercapnia • **Whenever there is clinical doubt**	May be technically difficult to obtain May be painful – reduced by use of local anaesthetic or thin needles Small risk of arterial trauma Technically more difficult and time consuming Not validated in shock patients No information about oxygenation
Non-invasive CO_2 monitors		
End tidal	**NO** role in acute situation except to confirm correct position of endotracheal tube in intubated patient	
Transcutaneous	May have a role in monitoring trends following initial blood sample	

but for those with pigmented skin, a saturation of 94% is recommended.[18] Oximetry will give no information concerning CO_2 or pH levels; normal pulse oximetry may provide false reassurance in patients, who may have unexpected hypercapnia or acidosis. Oximetry gives a normal reading for SpO_2 in patients with anaemia because the oxygen saturation of the available haemoglobin is normal, though the total oxygen content of the blood may be markedly reduced. The accuracy of oximetry is unreliable in the presence of carbon monoxide or methaemoglobin because these substances have similar light absorption characteristics to oxyhaemoglobin. Carboxyhaemoglobin levels above 2% may cause falsely elevated SpO_2 measurements.[19] Many smokers will have carboxyhaemoglobin levels above this level shortly after smoking a cigarette and the carboxyhaemoglobin level may be elevated to 15% chronically in some smokers.

Blood gas tensions should be measured as soon as possible in most emergency situations in which patients are potentially hypoxaemic and should be checked (and the clinical situation reviewed) if the SpO_2 falls by a few percentage points, even if it remains within the target range; because of the shape of the oxygen dissociation curve at higher oxygen saturations, small falls in SpO_2 indicate large falls in PaO_2.[20] Blood gas measurements are not mandatory for patients with no risk factors for hypercapnic respiratory failure and a SpO_2 above 92% breathing air, provided there are no clinical pointers to life-threatening illness.[21] Blood gas sampling may be required for other reasons, for example, acid–base analysis. An arterial sample is considered to be the gold standard, but there are alternatives. Pain can be reduced by the use of local anaesthetic,[22] but this is seldom used by ward doctors.[23] Arterialised capillary gases from the earlobe (but not from the finger) can provide an assessment of pH and $PaCO_2$ that is almost identical to that obtained from an arterial sample.[24,25] In both acute and stable situations, the earlobe specimen gives a PO_2 measurement that is 0.5 to 1 kPa (4–7.5 mmHg) lower than the simultaneous arterial measurement, with most of the divergence occurring at oxygen tensions above 8–10 kPa.[24,26] However, obtaining a capillary sample is not straightforward and staff must be fully trained if inaccuracies are to be minimised.[27] A venous PCO_2 level can be used to screen for hypercapnia in patients with acute respiratory disease.[28,29] In one study[28] for pH, there was very good agreement with venous samples being an average of 0.034 pH units lower than arterial samples. With respect to PCO_2, there was only fair agreement, with the PCO_2 on average 5.8 mmHg higher in venous samples and 95% limits of agreement −8.8 to +20.5 mmHg. The receiver operating characteristic curve analysis showed that a venous PCO_2 level of 45 mmHg was a potential screening cutoff (sensitivity for the detection of hypercarbia of 100%, specificity of 57%). In another study, McKeever et al.[29] found good agreement between arterial and venous measures of pH and HCO_3^- (mean difference, 0.03 and −0.04; limits of agreement, −0.05 to 0.11 and −2.90 to 2.82, respectively) and between SaO_2 and SpO_2 (in patients with an SpO_2 of >80%) in 234 subjects having paired arterial and venous blood gas analysis. Arterial sampling required more attempts and was more painful than venous sampling.

End-tidal CO_2 measurements correlate poorly with arterial CO_2 levels in patients,[30] particularly with airways disease and should not be used in clinical practice, other than to confirm correct placement of an endotracheal tube. Transcutaneous monitors of both oxygen and carbon dioxide are available and have been shown to be reliable in the acute situation.[31–35] They are particularly useful for monitoring trends. Drift correction of $PtcCO_2$ measurements improves the accuracy compared to $PaCO_2$. There is a lag time of approximately 2 min between $PtcCO_2$ and $PaCO_2$.[31]

In a pilot study, van Oppen et al.[34] demonstrated that $PtcCO_2$ monitoring also allows pH prediction (derived from the $PtcCO_2$ and a single measurement of serum bicarbonate).

OXYGEN THERAPY

The mitochondrion is the final destination of oxygen, where it is required for aerobic ATP synthesis. The PO_2 in the mitochondrion is dependent on variables other than PaO_2 and it is not possible to monitor mitochondrial PO_2 clinically. Lactate concentration in venous blood is the only clinically available surrogate of mitochondrial hypoxia, but it is a late marker and insensitive. Oxygen therapy is therefore usually directed at the PaO_2 and arterial oxygen saturation, but oxygen therapy is only one of several strategies that may be used to increase oxygen concentration in the mitochondrion. Supplementary oxygen increases alveolar PO_2 (PAO_2) and is therefore only effective when there is some functional alveolar ventilation. In poorly ventilated units, PAO_2 will remain low but increasing FIO_2 will still increase PAO_2 and therefore PaO_2. When there is diffusion limitation, due to increased alveolar–capillary membrane thickness, such as in fibrotic lung disease, increasing PAO_2 will augment the rate of diffusion across the alveolar–capillary membrane by increasing the concentration gradient. It is ineffective if there is a pure shunt (such as pulmonary arterio-venous malformations), where mixed venous blood bypasses the alveolar–capillary units.

The partial pressure of O_2 in air at sea level is 21.2 kPa (160 mmHg), but at the mitochondrion, PO_2 is in the range of 0.5–3.0 kPa (4–22 mmHg), depending on tissue type and local metabolic activity. The gradient from atmosphere to mitochondrion is known as the oxygen cascade (Table 32.3). Under pathological conditions, any change in one step in this cascade may result in mitochondrial hypoxia. Although not necessarily addressing the underlying cause of tissue hypoxia, increasing FIO_2 is the simplest and quickest way of avoiding hypoxic tissue damage. In critically ill patients, other steps are usually necessary to improve the delivery of oxygen (DO_2) to the tissue (Table 32.3).

An adequate concentration of haemoglobin is necessary to maximise the oxygen content (CaO_2) of blood as the majority of oxygen is carried bound to haemoglobin. Previously, most physicians maintained the haemoglobin close to 10 g/dL in critically ill patients. However, an RCT in

Table 32.3 Intervention points in the oxygen cascade

The oxygen cascade	Physiological aim	Clinical intervention
Oxygen in inspired gas	Increase	Supplementary oxygen
Airway	Ensure patent	Remove obstruction
Lungs	Ensure adequate alveolar ventilation	Assisted ventilation
	Optimise V/Q matching	Treat reversible pathology Positioning (good side down)
Circulation	Adequate blood flow	Maintain cardiac output • Volume expansion • Inotropes
	Adequate oxygen carriage	Transfuse
Mitochondrion	Reduce oxygen demand	Hypothermia Treat sepsis etc.

critically ill patients showed that a restrictive strategy (Hb target 7 g/dL) was associated with a better outcome than a liberal strategy (Hb target 10 g/dL).[36] However, non-leukocyte depleted blood was used and it is possible that some of the infective complications in the group who were given more transfusions might have been avoided by the use of leukocyte-depleted blood. The optimal Hb target for the generality of critically ill patients remains uncertain, but at least in patients with coronary artery disease, haemoglobin levels of 10 g/dL are recommended. DO_2 to the tissues depends on adequate blood flow, which is dependent on an adequate cardiac output, which should be optimised.

Oxygen has traditionally been given at a fixed FIO_2 or flow rate, but oxygen requirements may vary over time so that the prescribed oxygen dose may be too high or too low even a short time after the prescription was written. It is now recommended that oxygen should be prescribed to a target saturation range.[37] The prescriber should indicate a starting dose, device and flow rate and a system for adjusting the oxygen dose according to a patient's needs. Targeting an upper and lower limit avoids the possibility of tissue hypoxia in most patients and the potential deleterious effects of hyperoxia, and oxygen should usually be prescribed to a saturation (or PaO_2) rather than in terms of FIO_2.[37] The normal arterial oxygen levels decline with age and SpO_2 94%–98% reflects the range of normal across most situations. This has therefore been recommended as the target saturation range for patients not at risk of hypercapnia. The lower limit of 94% allows a margin of error in the oximeter measurement, thus minimising the risk of any patient being allowed to desaturate below 90% due to inaccurate oximetry.

The majority of patients with modest hypoxaemia can be treated with nasal cannulae or a simple face mask. Venturi masks are an alternative for low-dose oxygen therapy; they deliver a more reliable oxygen concentration than nasal cannulae or variable flow masks. However, patients tend to wear masks for less of a 24-hour period than cannulae.[38] The theoretical advantages of a Venturi mask are lost when oxygen is titrated against an upper as well as a lower limit and nasal cannulae are preferred for most patients. The mask and/or flow rate should be changed if the target saturation is not achieved. A non-rebreathe, reservoir mask with an oxygen flow rate of 10–15 L/min should usually be used for severely hypoxaemic patients without risk factors for hypercapnic respiratory failure and in cardiac arrest. High flow oxygen therapy is discussed in Chapter 33. The delivery system and FIO_2 may be adjusted subsequently to a lower dose of oxygen as a patient improves or towards assisted ventilation if they deteriorate.

WHO SHOULD RECEIVE SUPPLEMENTARY OXYGEN?

Supplementary oxygen is required for all acutely hypoxaemic patients. There are some other clinical situations in which a patient may benefit from oxygen as a therapy in its own right, for example, carbon monoxide (CO) poisoning, though usually hyperbaric oxygen is prescribed.[39,40] Hyperoxaemia may also be used to accelerate the resolution of a pneumothorax in patients who do not require a chest drain.[41]

Oxygen is traditionally given to all patients with myocardial infarction, angina or stroke, in an attempt to increase oxygen delivery to the heart or brain. A systematic[42] and a historical[43] review of oxygen therapy in acute myocardial ischaemia have both concluded that there is no evidence to support this practice in non-hypoxaemic patients and there is some evidence of harm; this is confirmed in a more recent RCT.[7] The administration of supplemental oxygen to normoxaemic patients has very little effect on blood oxygen content and may reduce myocardial blood flow, by causing vasoconstriction and reduced myocardial oxygen supply with worsened systolic myocardial performance.[44] There is also a theoretical possibility that high oxygen levels might exacerbate reperfusion injury to the heart. One study showed that hypoxia did not affect the availability of oxygen for myocardial metabolism until the oxygen saturation fell to about 50% in normal subjects, but evidence of myocardial ischaemia was seen at saturations of 70%–85% in subjects with coronary artery disease.[45] Generally, oxygen should only be given to patients with myocardial infarction or suspected angina if hypoxaemia is present, usually due to complications such as heart failure or co-existent lung disease and targeted to maintain a saturation of 94%–98%. Future RCTs will help clarify management in patients with myocardial infarction.[46,47] A randomised trial of oxygen therapy in stroke[9] found no difference in 1-year survival for the entire cohort of stroke patients, but for patients with minor or moderate strokes, the outcome was worse in patients who received oxygen: 1-year mortality of 18% in the group given oxygen versus 9% in the group given air (p = 0.023). Again, oxygen should be targeted to the saturations suggested for other conditons.[37]

Oxygen can also be given to patients with dyspnoea, though there is no evidence that it reduces dyspnoea more than air (placebo effect or due to flow across face) unless the patient is hypoxic.[48]

Patients who may be vulnerable to oxygen

It is well recognized that patients with chronic obstructive pulmonary disease (COPD) can develop hypercapnic (Type II) respiratory failure with injudicious oxygen therapy, especially if the PaO_2 is elevated above 10 kPa or 75 mmHg.[49] This has been shown to lead to an increased mortality. Austin et al.[8] performed an RCT of oxygen given to patients with a presumptive diagnosis of an acute exacerbation of COPD during ambulance transfer to hospital in Tasmania, Australia. The risk of death was significantly lower in the group in which oxygen was titrated to an SpO_2 of 88% to 92%, 4% (7 deaths), compared with the high flow oxygen group, 9% (21 deaths). Titrated oxygen treatment reduced mortality compared with high flow oxygen by 58% for all patients (relative risk, 0.42; 95% CI, 0.20 to 0.89; $p = 0.02$) and by 78% for the patients with confirmed COPD (0.22, 0.05 to 0.91; $p = 0.04$). Patients with COPD who received titrated oxygen according to the protocol were significantly less likely to have respiratory acidosis or hypercapnia (mean difference in arterial carbon dioxide pressure −33.6 (16.3) mmHg; $p = 0.02$; $n = 29$) than were patients who received high flow oxygen.

There are a number of other conditions (Box 32.1) that may predispose patients to hypercapnic respiratory failure. The emphasis for all such patients is to avoid clinically harmful levels of hypoxia or hypercapnia by giving carefully titrated oxygen therapy or, if necessary, by supporting ventilation non-invasively or invasively.

The recommended usual initial target of 88%–92%[37] can be modified subsequently, based on blood gas results. A lower starting saturation range, for example, 85%–90%, may be chosen based on previous experience for an individual patient; alert cards or wrist bands (Figure 32.1), may be helpful in such patients. If a patient with COPD remains acidotic (pH < 7.35) despite appropriate oxygen therapy, non-invasive ventilation (NIV) should be considered.[51] Although there are no RCTs, NIV should be started for hospitalised hypercapnic patients with chest wall deformity or neuromuscular disease, even if they are not acidotic. Patients with obesity hypoventilation should probably be managed using the same criteria as COPD patients.

BOX 32.1: Patients at risk of hypercapnic respiratory failure

- COPD
- Severe chest wall deformity
  - Early-onset kyphoscoliosis
  - Thoracoplasty
- Morbid obesity
- Neuromuscular disease (NMD) – consider possibility in *any* patient with generalised NMD – respiratory muscle weakness may be a feature in most/all patients (e.g. amyotrophic lateral scoliosis, Duchenne muscular dystrophy) or occasional patients (fascioscapular humeral muscular dystrophy, Charcot–Marie–Tooth, etc).[50]
- Overdose of opiates, benzodiazepines or other respiratory depressant drugs
- Reduced central respiratory drive
  - Brainstem pathology

Oxygen is known to be hazardous to patients with paraquat poisoning[10] and potentiates lung injury from bleomycin[11] and following aspiration of acids.[12,13] Bleomycin lung injury can be potentiated by high-dose oxygen therapy, even if given many years after the initial lung injury. Because of these risks, oxygen should be given to patients with these conditions only if the oxygen saturation falls below 90%. Some authors have suggested the use of hypoxic ventilation with 14% oxygen as a specific treatment for paraquat poisoning.[52]

Prescription, administration and monitoring (Box 32.2)

Medical oxygen is a drug and should always be prescribed. The quality of oxygen prescription can be improved with the use of an oxygen prescription chart.[3] The clinicians who administer oxygen (usually nurses) should be trained to adjust the oxygen dose upwards and downwards as necessary to maintain the patient in the target range based on continuous monitoring of the oxygen saturation by pulse oximetry. Falls in oxygen saturation below the lower limit of the target range should prompt an increase in the oxygen dose and also consideration of medical review. In most instances, failure to achieve the desired oxygen saturation is due to the severity of the patient's illness, but the oxygen delivery device and flow rate should be checked. Blood gas analysis should be repeated if clinical progress is not satisfactory and in all cases of hypercapnia

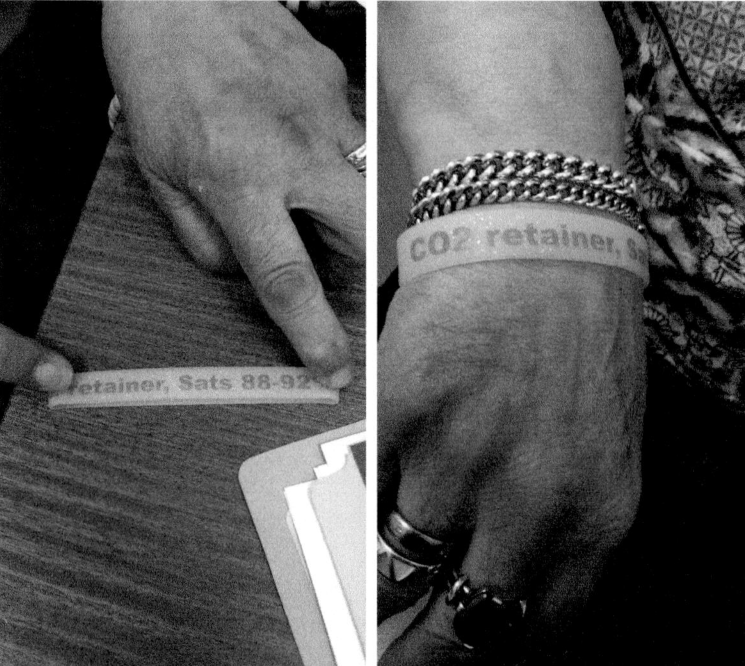

Figure 32.1 An example of a wrist band worn by a patient to alert healthcare professionals to potential problems with oxygen therapy.

and acidosis. Most conditions that require supplemental oxygen therapy will improve with treatment and it will be possible to reduce the oxygen dose; if the saturation is above the upper limit of the target range, the dose should be reduced. Even if not above the upper limit, the dose should be reduced if the patient is stable and the oxygen saturation has been in the upper zone of the target range for some time (usually 4–8 hours). Saturations should be observed for 5 min following a change of oxygen therapy and readjusted if they change. Some patients with chronic lung diseases will already be established on long-term oxygen therapy (LTOT) and should be tapered slowly to their usual maintenance dose of oxygen. Others can be weaned off continuous oxygen, but may still require short-burst oxygen, for instance during mobilisation. A small proportion of patients may require LTOT to permit safe discharge from hospital. However, many patients with a low PaO_2 on discharge from hospital have a PaO_2 above the threshold for LTOT at a subsequent clinic visit so usually decisions about long-term oxygen should not be made on the basis of blood gas measurements made during acute exacerbations of chronic lung disease.[53]

BOX 32.2: Prescribing oxygen

Select target oxygen saturation
- Usually 94% to 98%
- 88% to 92% if at risk for hypercapnic respiratory failure
- No more than 90% for paraquat/bleomycin-induced lung injury
- Individualised
  - Based on clinical situation
  - Previous experience (alert card)

Prescribe oxygen – device, initial flow rate and document target range

If falls below target range or falls by a few points within target range
- Increase oxygen until back in range
- **CLINICAL REVIEW** ± blood gas sampling (why has oxygenation deteriorated?)

If remains within range but increase in respiratory rate, pulse rate or respiratory distress
- **CLINICAL REVIEW** ± blood gas sampling

If remains in range for a few hours and clinical improvement or above upper target level
- Reduce oxygen dose or discontinue
- Continue to monitor oxygen saturation

FUTURE RESEARCH

Much of the guidance about oxygen therapy is based on theoretical analysis rather than controlled trial data. Further research is required about the use of supplementary oxygen. The suggested target ranges are reasonable given current understanding, but should be underpinned by more evidence. For instance, as with haemoglobin concentration, the correct target may prove to be lower than theory would suggest. Further research is needed about the effects of hyperoxia and whether it is harmful or could still be beneficial. The effectiveness of strategies to prevent oxygen-induced hypercapnia, such as the use of personalised alert cards, need to be evaluated.

CONCLUSION

Oxygen is a drug and should be prescribed with the same rigour and monitoring of effect as pharmaceutical preparations and should usually be prescribed to a target. All clinicians should be trained to recognise and treat hypoxia; this must include understanding of the role and limitations of pulse oximetry and interpretation of blood gas samples.

REFERENCES

1. Downs JB. Has oxygen administration delayed appropriate respiratory care? Fallacies regarding oxygen therapy. Respir Care. 2003;48(6):611–20.
2. Cook DJ, Reeve BK, Griffith LE et al. Multidisciplinary education for oxygen prescription. A continuous quality improvement study. Arch Int Med. 1996;156(16):1797–801.
3. Dodd ME, Kellet F, Davis A et al. Audit of oxygen prescribing before and after the introduction of a prescription chart. *BMJ*. 2000;321(7265):864–5.
4. Kbar FA, Campbell IA. Oxygen therapy in hospitalized patients: The impact of local guidelines. *J Eval Clin Pract*. 2006;12(1):31–6.
5. Boyle M, Wong J. Prescribing oxygen therapy. An audit of oxygen prescribing practices on medical wards at North Shore Hospital, Auckland, New Zealand. *New Zealand Med J*. 2006;119(1238):U2080.
6. Grocott MP, Martin DS, Levett DZ et al. Arterial blood gases and oxygen content in climbers on Mount Everest. *N Engl J Med*. 2009;360(2):140–9. Epub 2009/01/09.
7. Stub D, Smith K, Bernard S et al. Air versus oxygen in St-segment-elevation myocardial infarction. *Circulation*. 2015;131(24):2143–50.
8. Austin MA, Wills KE, Blizzard L et al. Effect of high flow oxygen on mortality in chronic obstructive pulmonary disease patients in prehospital setting: Randomised controlled trial. *BMJ*. 2010;341:c5462.
9. Ronning OM, Guldvog B. Should stroke victims routinely receive supplemental oxygen? A quasi-randomized controlled trial. *Stroke*. 1999;30(10):2033–7.
10. Bota GW, Rowe BH. Continuous monitoring of oxygen saturation in prehospital patients with severe illness: The problem of unrecognized hypoxemia. *J Emerg Med*. 1995;13(3):305–11.
11. Brown LH, Manring EA, Kornegay HB, Prasad NH. Can prehospital personnel detect hypoxemia without the aid of pulse oximeters? *Am J Emerg Med*. 1996;14(1):43–4.
12. Smith LL. Mechanism of paraquat toxicity in lung and its relevance to treatment. *Human Toxicol*. 1987;6(1):31–6.
13. Cersosimo RJ, Matthews SJ, Hong WK. Bleomycin pneumonitis potentiated by oxygen administration. *Drug Intell Clin Pharm*. 1985;19(12):921–3.
14. Nader-Djalal N, Knight PR, III, Thusu K et al. Reactive oxygen species contribute to oxygen-related lung injury after acid aspiration. *Anest Analg*. 1998;87(1):127–33.
15. Knight PR, Kurek C, Davidson BA et al. Acid aspiration increases sensitivity to increased ambient oxygen concentrations. *Am J Physiol Lung Cell Mol Physiol*. 2000;278(6):L1240–L7.
16. Sieker HO, Hickam JB. Carbon dioxide intoxication: The clinical syndrome, its etiology and management with particular reference to the use of mechanical respirators. *Medicine*. 1956;35(4):389–423.
17. Kelly AM, McAlpine R, Kyle E. How accurate are pulse oximeters in patients with acute exacerbations of chronic obstructive airways disease? *Respir Med*. 2001;95(5):336–40.
18. Jubran A, Tobin MJ. Reliability of pulse oximetry in titrating supplemental oxygen therapy in ventilator-dependent patients. *Chest*. 1990;97(6):1420–5. Epub 1990/06/01.
19. Lee WW, Mayberry K, Crapo R, Jensen RL. The accuracy of pulse oximetry in the emergency department. *Am J Emerg Med*. 2000;18(4):427–31.
20. Collins JA, Rudenski A, Gibson J et al. Relating oxygen partial pressure, saturation and content: The haemoglobin-oxygen dissociation curve. *Breathe*. 2015;11(3):194–201.
21. British Thoracic S. British guideline on the management of asthma. *Thorax*. 2008;63 Suppl 4:iv1–121.
22. Lightowler JVJ, Elliott MW. Local anaesthetic infiltration prior to arterial puncture: A survey of current practice and a randomised double blind placebo controlled trial. *J R Coll Phys London*. 1997;31(6):645–6.
23. Sado DM, Deakin CD. Local anaesthesia for venous cannulation and arterial blood gas sampling: Are doctors using it? *J R Soc Med*. 2005;98(4):158–60.
24. Murphy R, Thethy S, Raby S et al. Capillary blood gases in acute exacerbations of COPD. *Respir Med*. 2006;100(4):682–6.

25. Zavorsky GS, Cao J, Mayo NE et al. Arterial versus capillary blood gases: A meta-analysis. *Respir Physiol Neurobiol.* 2007;155(3):268–79.
26. Pitkin AD, Roberts CM, Wedzicha JA. Arterialised earlobe blood gas analysis: An underused technique. *Thorax.* 1994;49:364–6.
27. Wimpress S, Vara DD, Brightling CE. Improving the sampling technique of arterialized capillary samples to obtain more accurate PaO_2 measurements. *Chron Respir Dis.* 2005;2(1):47–50.
28. Kelly AM, Kyle E, McAlpine R. Venous pCO(2) and pH can be used to screen for significant hypercarbia in emergency patients with acute respiratory disease. *J Emerg Med.* 2002;22(1):15–9.
29. McKeever TM, Hearson G, Housley G et al. Using venous blood gas analysis in the assessment of COPD exacerbations: A prospective cohort study. *Thorax.* 2016;71(3):210–5.
30. Lermuzeaux M, Meric H, Sauneuf B et al. Superiority of transcutaneous CO_2 over end-tidal CO_2 measurement for monitoring respiratory failure in nonintubated patients: A pilot study. *J Crit Care.* 2016;31(1):150–6.
31. Storre JH, Steurer B, Kabitz HJ et al. Transcutaneous PCO_2 monitoring during initiation of noninvasive ventilation. *Chest.* 2007;132(6):1810–6.
32. Nicolini A, Ferrari MB. Evaluation of a transcutaneous carbon dioxide monitor in patients with acute respiratory failure. *Ann Thoracic Med.* 2011;6(4):217–20.
33. Kelly AM, Klim S. Agreement between arterial and transcutaneous PCO_2 in patients undergoing noninvasive ventilation. *Respir Med.* 2011;105(2):226–9.
34. van Oppen JD, Daniel PS, Sovani MP. What is the potential role of transcutaneous carbon dioxide in guiding acute noninvasive ventilation? *Respir Care.* 2015;60(4):484–91.
35. McVicar J, Eager R. Validation study of a transcutaneous carbon dioxide monitor in patients in the emergency department. *Emerg Med J.* 2009;26(5):344–6.
36. Hebert PC, Wells G, Blajchman MA et al. A multicenter, randomized, controlled clinical trial of transfusion requirements in critical care. Transfusion Requirements in Critical Care Investigators, Canadian Critical Care Trials Group. *New Engl J Med.* 1999;340(6):409–17.
37. O'Driscoll BR, Howard LS, Davison AG. BTS guideline for emergency oxygen use in adult patients. *Thorax.* 2008;63 Suppl 6:vi1–68.
38. Agusti AG, Carrera M, Barbe F et al. Oxygen therapy during exacerbations of chronic obstructive pulmonary disease. *Eur Respir J.* 1999;14(4):934–9.
39. Norkool DM, Kirkpatrick JN. Treatment of acute carbon monoxide poisoning with hyperbaric oxygen: A review of 115 cases. *Ann Emerg Med.* 1985;14(12):1168–71.
40. Thom SR, Keim LW. Carbon monoxide poisoning: A review epidemiology, pathophysiology, clinical findings, and treatment options including hyperbaric oxygen therapy. *J Toxicol Clin Toxicol.* 1989;27(3):141–56.
41. Northfield TC. Oxygen therapy for spontaneous pneumothorax. *BMJ.* 1971;4(5779):86–8.
42. Nicholson C. A systematic review of the effectiveness of oxygen in reducing acute myocardial ischaemia. *J Clin Nurs.* 2004;13(8):996–1007.
43. Beasley R, Aldington S, Weatherall M et al. Oxygen therapy in myocardial infarction: An historical perspective. *J R Soc Med.* 2007;100(3):130–3.
44. McNulty PH, King N, Scott S et al. Effects of supplemental oxygen administration on coronary blood flow in patients undergoing cardiac catheterization. *Am J Physiol Heart Circul Physiol.* 2005;288(3):H1057–H62.
45. Neill WA. Effects of arterial hypoxemia and hyperoxia on oxygen availability for myocardial metabolism. Patients with and without coronary heart disease. *Am J Cardiol.* 1969;24(2):166–71.
46. Hofmann R, James SK, Svensson L et al. DETermination of the role of OXygen in suspected Acute Myocardial Infarction trial. *Am Heart J.* 2014;167(3): 322–8.
47. Khoshnood A, Carlsson M, Akbarzadeh M et al. The effects of oxygen therapy on myocardial salvage in ST elevation myocardial infarction treated with acute percutaneous coronary intervention: The Supplemental Oxygen in Catheterized Coronary Emergency Reperfusion (SOCCER) Study. *Cardiology.* 2015;132(1):16–21.
48. Gallagher R, Roberts D. A systematic review of oxygen and airflow effect on relief of dyspnea at rest in patients with advanced disease of any cause. *J Pain Palliative Care Pharmacother.* 2004;18(4):3–15.
49. Joosten SA, Koh MS, Bu X et al. The effects of oxygen therapy in patients presenting to an emergency department with exacerbation of chronic obstructive pulmonary disease. *Med J Austral.* 2007;186(5):235–8.
50. Shahrizaila T, Kinnear W. Recommendations for respiratory care of adults with muscle disorders. *Neuromusc Disord.* 2007;17(1):13–5.
51. Davidson AC, Banham S, Elliott M et al. BTS/ICS guideline for the ventilatory management of acute hypercapnic respiratory failure in adults. *Thorax.* 2016;71 Suppl 2:ii1–35.
52. Demeere JL. Paraquat toxicity. The use of hypoxic ventilation. *Acta Anaesthesiol Belgica.* 1984;35(3):219–30.
53. Hardinge M, Suntharalingam J, Wilkinson T. Guideline update: The British Thoracic Society Guidelines on home oxygen use in adults. *Thorax.* 2015;70(6):589–91.

33

High-flow oxygen therapy: Physiological effects and clinical evidence

NUTTAPOL RITTAYAMAI, ARNAUD W. THILLE AND LAURENT BROCHARD

INTRODUCTION

The use of standard oxygen delivering a gas flow rate between 10 and 15 L/min through a reservoir mask has long been the first-line therapy in patients with acute hypoxaemic respiratory failure. However, this oxygenation strategy does not enable a reduction in work of breathing and/or improvement in alveolar ventilation, and the FiO_2 delivered to the patient does not exceed 70% on average. Moreover, oxygen provided by an outlet hospital or a tank is a particularly dry gas that may be irritating for airways and troublesome for patient comfort. All these disadvantages may lead to failure of the technique and subsequent need for intubation.

The use of non-invasive ventilation (NIV) is the main alternative to standard oxygen in patients with acute respiratory failure before endotracheal intubation. The gas delivered to the patient can be heated and humidified, via a heat and moisture exchanger or a heated humidifier, with a FiO_2 up to 100% in the absence of leaks, and provides positive pressure, which improves gas exchange and reduces patient inspiratory effort. However, tolerance to NIV is sometimes poor due to a tight-fitting mask and to frequent leaks around the mask leading to patient–ventilator asynchronies. Moreover, deleterious effects of NIV may happen, such as delayed intubation by masking signs of respiratory distress or potential lung injury promoted by high tidal volumes that may occur with pressure-support ventilation in case of high respiratory drive.

High-flow oxygen therapy through nasal cannula (HFOT) is a more recent technique of oxygenation that could have many beneficial effects. The gas delivered to the patient is humidified and heated, while FiO_2 can easily reach more than 80%. Although there is no pressure support *per se*, the high flow enables the generation of low levels of positive end-expiratory pressure (PEEP) and provision of continuous washout of dead space in the airways. These two mechanisms may contribute to improve gas exchange and to reduce patient effort without increased risk of barotrauma. Finally, oxygen is delivered through nasal cannula, which may facilitate patient comfort and tolerance.

The use of HFOT is growing and we focus our review first on physiological aspects to understand its potential benefits and second on clinical evidence regarding its use in clinical practice.

CHARACTERISTICS AND PHYSIOLOGICAL EFFECTS OF HIGH-FLOW OXYGEN THERAPY

The high flow rate of gas delivered with HFOT enables an increase in the FiO_2, providing continuous positive pressure and washing out the dead space in the upper airways. This oxygenation strategy seems particularly comfortable for the patient thanks to nasal cannula delivering a warmed and humidified gas similar to physiological conditions and allowing the patient to continue to talk, drink and eat.

Warming and humidification of delivered gas

In physiological conditions and regardless of the external environment, the inspired gas needs to be heated and humidified in the upper airways to reach the lower airways and alveoli with a temperature of 37°C and containing 44 mg of H_2O/L of gas, that is, completely saturated in water (relative humidity of 100%). At high altitude, it is more difficult to breathe for a normal subject, not only due to low O_2 partial pressure but also because ambient air is dry and cold, which irritates the airways and requires a more efficient humidification. Similarly, oxygen delivered from a hospital outlet or from a tank is a particularly dry gas with humidity less than 5 mg H_2O/L.[1] Consequently, it is recommended that a heat and moisture exchanger or a heated humidifier be used during mechanical ventilation, to maintain minimal absolute humidity between 25 and 30 mg H_2O/L and to avoid endotracheal tube obstruction or atelectasis. However, even during spontaneous breathing, standard oxygen may dry airways, and it has been shown that it could increase airway resistance.[2] By contrast, high-flow oxygen is delivered via a heated humidifier, allowing one to approach physiological conditions and possibly to contribute to promote comfort to breathe and to decrease the sensation of dryness and of dyspnoea observed when switching from standard to HFOT oxygen therapy.[3,4]

Mismatch between patient's inspiratory flow rate and oxygen flow rate: Impact of high flow on FiO_2

Whereas the inspired fraction of oxygen (FiO_2) delivered to the patient can reach up to 100% of oxygen using NIV and in the absence of leaks, the maximal FiO_2 does not usually exceed 70% with standard oxygen despite a reservoir mask and a flow rate of 15 L/min.[4,5] Indeed, the inspiratory peak flow generated by a patient suffering from acute respiratory failure reaches at least 30–40 L/min in mean and can even exceed 60 L/min in more severe patients,[6] which is markedly higher than the flow rate delivered with standard oxygen. Oxygen is consequently mixed with room air, dropping the delivered FiO_2 to the patient. Using HFOT, the high flow of oxygen delivered allows minimising its dilution with room air and reaching a maximal FiO_2 of more than 80%.[5] In a physiological study, Sim et al. measured FiO_2 in healthy subjects ventilated using a standard mask, a non-rebreathing mask with reservoir and high-flow oxygen through nasal cannula.[5] Using a standard mask, FiO_2 was less than 60% despite a flow of 12 L/min and dropped below 50% by simulating acute respiratory failure by thoracic contention. Although the non-rebreathing mask enabled the avoidance of FiO_2 drop during acute respiratory failure, the FiO_2 was less than 70% even with a flow rate of 15 L/min. By comparison, FiO_2 reached 85% using HFOT set with a flow rate of 40 L/min.[5] It is obvious that this effect directly contributes to oxygenation improvement observed when switching from standard to HFOT.

Positive pressure generated by high gas flow rate

The use of HFOT could generate a PEEP directly proportional to the delivered gas flow: the higher is the flow, the higher is the pressure. The high flow continuously delivered creates a certain degree of resistance during expiration. This PEEP effect is due to an increase in expiratory resistance generated by the high gas flow continuously delivered during the expiration phase but also because HFOT is delivered by large nasal prongs that promote a certain degree of nasal obstruction. Consequently, the PEEP effect is markedly reduced when the patient opens the mouth. Parke et al. measured nasopharyngeal pressure in patients at different levels of flow using HFOT.[7] The PEEP level exceeded 3–5 cmH_2O with a gas flow rate of 50 L/min and with a closed mouth whereas it dropped at less than 2 cmH_2O with an open mouth.[7] Although the PEEP level seems only moderate, this PEEP effect could help improve gas exchange and decrease work of breathing in patients with intrinsic PEEP. In a physiological study that measured pulmonary volumes after cardiac surgery using inductance plethysmography, the authors found an increase in end-expiratory lung volume using HFOT compared to standard oxygen, due to its PEEP effect.[8]

Washout of dead space in the airways induced by high gas flow rate

The high flow rate of gas continuously delivered in the airways may generate a washout of dead space from the oropharyngeal cavity, flushing the carbon dioxide (CO_2) out of the upper airways.[9] This phenomenon may contribute to reduce ventilator requirement, improve alveolar ventilation[10] and reduce the work of breathing.[11] In a recent study comparing the short-term physiological response to oxygen, the respiratory rate and transcutaneous CO_2 were rapidly reduced with HFOT as compared to standard oxygen in stable chronic obstructive pulmonary disease (COPD) patients.[10] In hypoxaemic patients, standard oxygen is usually delivered with a reservoir mask, which includes a supplemental dead space and may promote rebreathing of CO_2. The supplemental dead space could be even larger during NIV according to the type of mask used and the humidification device.[12–14] By contrast, high-flow oxygen is delivered through nasal prongs reducing the dead space potentially induced by a usual mask, with less risk of rebreathing.

CLINICAL EFFECTS OF HIGH-FLOW OXYGEN THERAPY

All physiological effects abovementioned together enable oxygenation improvement and probably explain the significant reduction in respiratory rate and patient's effort and a better comfort with less sensation of dryness of the mouth and of dyspnoea (Figure 33.1).

Improvement of oxygenation

In patients with acute respiratory failure, it has been observed that PaO_2 significantly increased by switching from standard oxygen to HFOT.[3,15–17] This oxygenation improvement could be due to a higher amount of oxygen delivered to the patient (the higher is the flow, the higher is the FiO_2) or due to the PEEP effect and of possible recruitment. The impact of PEEP effect on oxygenation is probably often negligible and oxygenation increase seems mainly driven by higher delivered FiO_2. In a pilot study assessing successively standard oxygen, HFOT and then NIV in patients with acute respiratory failure, PaO_2 increased from standard oxygen to HFOT without changes in the PaO_2/set FiO_2, suggesting that oxygenation improvement was directly due to an increase in

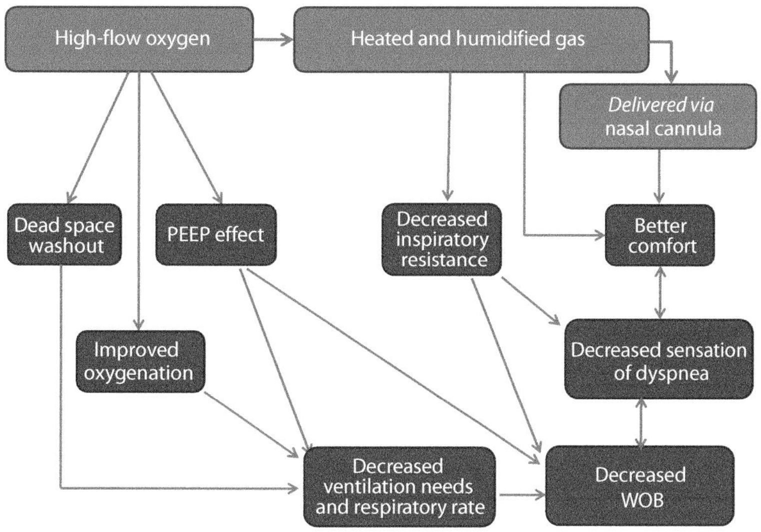

Figure 33.1 Physiological effects of high-flow oxygen therapy via nasal cannula. Abbreviations: PEEP = positive end-expiratory pressure; WOB = work of breathing.

delivered FiO_2.[17] By contrast, PaO_2 further increased with NIV with a significant increase in PaO_2/set FiO_2 ratio, suggesting alveolar recruitment induced by PEEP. Standard oxygen, HFOT and NIV were also compared in a large multicentre study.[4] At baseline, all patients received standard oxygen and FiO_2 was measured using an oxygen analyser. Again, FiO_2 and PaO_2 were increased from standard oxygen to HFOT without changes in PaO_2/delivered FiO_2 ratio, whereas it was markedly higher with NIV than with the two other strategies of oxygenation.

Decrease in respiratory rate and work of breathing

In patients with acute respiratory failure, it has been found that the work of breathing was lower with HFOT than with standard oxygen.[11] In this physiological study, the work of breathing was measured with a non-rebreathing mask, HFOT or continuous positive airway pressure (CPAP) at 5 cm H_2O.[11] The decrease in work of breathing observed with HFOT was of the same extent as that observed with a CPAP at 5 cm H_2O.[11] However, the mechanism by which the work of breathing is decreased is not fully elucidated. The overall work of breathing includes a resistive and an elastic portion, and mostly expressed per minute. Consequently, the decrease in work of breathing could be due to a decrease in airway resistance, to an improvement of pulmonary compliance or only to a decrease in respiratory rate and in ventilator requirement. Most studies observed a rapid decrease in respiratory rate when switching from standard oxygen to HFOT in healthy subjects,[18] as well as in patients with acute respiratory failure and tachypnea.[3,4,15–17] The respiratory rate in patients treated with HFOT was also lower than that of patients treated with NIV.[4] A recent study evaluating HFOT in postextubation found a reduced incidence of upper airway obstruction as compared to standard oxygen.[19] Although this finding may suggest a decrease in inspiratory resistance of the upper airways, until now, no physiological study supports this finding. The use of HFOT may also increase the tidal volume and therefore could decrease elastic work of breathing.[18] However, the tidal volumes should theoretically remain lower than those observed with NIV. Recently, it has been suggested that the large tidal volumes generated by the pressure support may generate high transpulmonary pressures and worsen lung injury in patients with acute respiratory failure and high respiratory drive.[20,21]

Improvement of patient comfort and breathlessness

Most studies that assessed HFOT in acute respiratory failure found that the patients felt better comfort, less sensation of dyspnoea and less dryness of mouth as compared to standard oxygen through a non-reservoir mask.[3,15,22,23] As compared to NIV, patients treated with HFOT had also less discomfort and less breathlessness.[4,17] This improvement in comfort probably has a major impact on clinical benefits of HFOT that we will list in the following section.

CLINICAL EVIDENCE FOR THE USE OF HFOT IN CLINICAL PRACTICE

As already mentioned, HFOT improves breathing pattern, gas exchange and dyspnoea symptoms and also reduces patient's work of breathing via several mechanisms including (1) a modest PEEP effect, (2) dead space washout, (3) reduced inspiratory resistance, (4) providing a high flow rate of gas that matches patient's demand and (5) the effect of heat and humidity to protect airway mucosa and reduce dryness symptom. Using HFOT in clinical practice might improve the patient's outcome in some specific population and particularly in critically ill patients.

Acute hypoxaemic respiratory failure

Oxygen therapy is routinely used in patients with acute hypoxaemic respiratory failure via a low-flow oxygen delivery system such as a simple nasal cannula or a non-rebreathing face mask. However, these devices can provide maximum flow rate up to 15 L/min that might not be compatible with the patient's flow demand. In addition, FiO_2 varies depending on how much room air is entrained. HFOT is therefore an attractive method for delivering oxygen in patients with acute hypoxaemic respiratory failure by providing a high flow rate of gas and constant FiO_2 and creating some positive airway pressure.

Several clinical studies of HFOT in critically ill patients admitted in intensive care units (ICUs) with acute hypoxaemic respiratory failure demonstrated that HFOT improved oxygenation and dyspnoea and decreased respiratory rate.[3,15,16] However, the impact of most of these studies is limited due to the methodology and there has been no report on major clinical outcomes such as mortality or intubation rate until recently. A first pilot, randomised comparative study in 60 mild-to moderate hypoxaemic patients showed that patients receiving HFOT had less use of NIV than the conventional oxygen therapy group (10% vs. 30%; $p = 0.009$).[24]

A multicentre randomised controlled study by Frat et al.[4] compared HFOT with conventional oxygen therapy and NIV in 310 patients with acute hypoxaemic respiratory failure (FLORALI study). Approximately 75% of patients in this study had pneumonia and moderate-to-severe hypoxaemia with an average PaO_2/FiO_2 ratio <150 mmHg. They found that HFOT did not reduce the overall intubation rate in comparison to the two other groups (38% vs. 47% vs. 50% with HFOT, standard oxygen therapy and NIV, respectively; $p = 0.18$ for all comparisons), but in the subgroup of patients with PaO_2/FiO_2 ratio ≤200 mmHg, the intubation rate was significantly lower with HFOT. In addition, the 90-day mortality rate was significantly lower with HFOT (hazard ratio = 2.01 for standard oxygen vs. HFOT, $p = 0.046$, and hazard ratio = 2.50 for NIV vs. HFOT, $p = 0.006$). Interestingly, patients in the NIV group tended to have the highest mortality, higher than HFOT but not different from conventional oxygen therapy. The presence of higher tidal volumes (9.0 ± 3.0 mL/kg predicted body weight) may have explained a greater risk of ventilator-induced lung injury.

HFOT has also been tested in immunocompromised patients with acute hypoxaemic respiratory failure whether it is used as an alternative treatment to avoid endotracheal intubation. Lee et al.[12] investigated the feasibility of HFOT in 45 patients with haematologic malignancies and they found that 33% of patients successfully recovered without intubation, whereas bacterial pneumonia was a risk factor for HFOT failure. Another retrospective study comparing HFOT with conventional oxygen therapy in 37 lung transplant patients admitted to the ICU for acute respiratory failure demonstrated that absolute risk reduction for mechanical ventilation with HFOT was 29.8% and the number needed to treat to prevent one intubation with HFOT was 3.[25] However, a multicentre randomised controlled study by Lemiale and colleagues in 100 immunocompromised patients with acute respiratory failure who were randomly assigned to receive HFOT or Venturi masks for 2 hours showed no difference in the need for mechanical ventilation, either invasive or non-invasive, dyspnoea, respiratory rate and heart rate.[26] It was surprising in this study to see that HFOT could be used for only 2 hours. In contrast, an observational study comparing HFOT and NIV as a first-line treatment in 115 immunocompromised patients found that intubation and 28-day mortality rates were significantly lower in patients treated with HFOT than NIV (35% vs. 55%; $p = 0.04$ and 20% vs. 40%; $p = 0.02$, respectively).[27] Lemiale et al. also recently performed a post hoc analysis of a randomised controlled trial of NIV in critically ill immunocompromised patients with hypoxaemic acute respiratory failure.[28] They did not find that HFOT, compared with standard oxygen, reduced intubation or survival rates. However, their results could be due to low statistical power or unknown confounders associated with the subgroup analysis. By contrast, the post hoc analysis of the FLORALI trial in the subgroup of patients with immunosuppression found a strong benefit of HFOT and a worsening with NIV.[29]

Another controversial issue is whether HFOT can be used for treating patients with acute respiratory distress syndrome (ARDS). Although the study by Frat et al.[4] enrolled patients who had a PaO_2/FiO_2 ratio below 300 mmHg and nearly 80% of patients had bilateral pulmonary infiltrates, the degree of hypoxaemia was evaluated without PEEP and thus these patients could not strictly be considered as having ARDS according to the Berlin definition.[30] A retrospective study in 45 patients (with an average PaO_2/FiO_2 ratio of 137 mmHg) who met the Berlin definition of ARDS receiving HFOT showed that 40% of them required endotracheal intubation, and the main reason for intubation was worsening hypoxaemia.[31] A prospective observation study in 28 patients including 23 (82%) with ARDS treated with HFOT and NIV found that oxygenation significantly improved after switching from standard oxygen therapy to HFOT and NIV and respiratory rate significantly decreased. Intubation rate in patients with ARDS in this study was 35%.[17] A previous multicentre survey on the use of NIV as first-line therapy for ARDS had shown that NIV was followed by intubation in 46% of patients.[32]

Regarding the evidence, HFOT is feasible and should be considered to be an effective and safe first-line therapy for patients with acute hypoxaemic respiratory failure (Table 33.1) as it is a life-saving therapy.[33] The role of HFOT in some specific entities such as immunocompromised patients or patients with ARDS, however, needs to be explored in larger clinical trials. Appropriate monitoring during HFOT use is crucial, and prompt intubation should not be delayed in patients without improvement in oxygenation and clinical parameters. Late intubation in such patients was associated with worse outcomes in a retrospective study.[34] The predictors of HFOT failure in acute hypoxaemic respiratory

Table 33.1 Main clinical studies of high-flow nasal oxygen cannula in adults with acute hypoxaemic respiratory failure

References	Population	Patients	Study design	Main outcomes
Intensive care unit				
Roca et al.[3]	ARF patients	20	Prospective comparative: HFOT 30 L/min vs. COT 15 L/min for 30 min	HFOT improved oxygenation, decreased respiratory rate and dyspnoea Better comfort with HFOT
Sztrymf et al.[15]	ARF patients	38	Prospective cohort: HFOT 50 L/min vs. HFFM 15 L/min for 48 hours	HFOT improved oxygenation and thoraco-abdominal synchrony, decreased respiratory rate, heart rate and dyspnoea Indicators of HFOT failure: absence of a decrease in respiratory rate, lower oxygenation and persistence of thoraco-abdominal asynchrony
Parke et al.[24]	Mild to moderate ARF patients	60	Randomised RCT: HFOT vs. COT	Fewer desaturations with HFOT Trend toward decrease in the rate of NIV use with HFOT compared to COT (10% vs. 30%; $p = 0.10$)
Rello et al.[35]	ARF patients due to influenza A/H1N1	20	Post hoc analysis of prospective cohort	9/20 of patients (45%) succeeded HFOT (no intubation). All 8 patients on vasopressor required intubation within 24 hours. Non-responders had lower PaO_2/FiO_2 ratio and required higher delivered flows
Sztrymf et al.[16]	ARF patients	20	Prospective observational study: HFOT 40 L/min vs. COT 15 L/min	HFOT improved oxygenation (SpO_2, PaO_2) and reduced lower respiratory rate
Frat et al.[4]	ARF patients	310	Multicentre RCT: HFOT vs. COT vs. NIV	Intubation rate was 38% in the HFOT group, 47% in the COT group and 50% in the NIV group ($p = 0.18$) Higher ventilator free day in the HFOT group ($p = 0.02$) Hazard ratio for death at 90 days was 2.01 (95% CI, 1.01 to 3.99; $p = 0.046$) with COT vs. HFOT and 2.50 (95% CI, 1.31 to 4.78; $p = 0.006$) with NIV vs. HFOT
Messika et al.[31]	ARDS patients according to Berlin definition	45	Retrospective study	Intubation rate was 40% with HFOT. Higher SAPII score was associated with HFOT failure from multivariate analysis
Frat et al.[17]	ARDS patients according to Berlin definition	23	Prospective observational study	Improved oxygenation and lower respiratory rate with HFOT Intubation rate was 35% and respiratory rate ≥ 30 was an early factor associated with intubation

(*Continued*)

Table 33.1 (Continued) Main clinical studies of high-flow nasal oxygen cannula in adults with acute hypoxaemic respiratory failure

References	Population	Patients	Study design	Main outcomes
Kang et al.[34]	ARF patients	175	Retrospective study of patients who failed HFOT and required intubation	Early intubation was associated with better ICU mortality (39.2% vs. 66.7%; *p* = 0.001), ventilator free days (8.6 ± 10.1 vs. 3.6 ± 7.5 days; *p* = 0.011) and extubation success (37.7% vs. 15.6%; *p* = 0.006)
Lee et al.[12]	ARF patients with haematologic malignancies	45	Retrospective study	33.3% of patients receiving HFOT successfully recovered without intubation Bacterial pneumonia was significantly higher in patients with HFOT treatment failure
Roca et al.[25]	ARF patients after lung transplantation	37	Retrospective study	Relative risk of mechanical ventilation in patients with COT was 1.50 (95% CI, 1.02 to 2.21) Absolute risk reduction for mechanical ventilation with HFOT was 29.8% and the number needed to treat to prevent one intubation with HFOT was 3
Lemiale et al.[28]	Immunocompromised patients with ARF	100	Multicentre RCT, HFOT vs. Venturi mask for 2 hours	No differences in escalation of ventilator treatment, dyspnoea, respiratory rate and heart rate were found
Coudroy et al.[27]	Immunocompromised patients with ARF	115	Observational study: HFOT vs. NIV as a first-line therapy	Lower intubation rate and 28-day mortality rate with HFOT in comparison to NIV (35% vs. 55%, *p* = 0.04 and 20% vs. 40%, *p* = 0.02, respectively)
Emergency department				
Lenglet et al.[48]	ARF patients	17	Prospective observational study	HFOT improved SpO_2 and dyspnoea and reduced respiratory rate
Rittayamai et al.[49]	ARF patients	40	RCT: HFOT vs. COT for 1 hour	HFOT improved dyspnoea and comfort Rate of hospitalisation: 50% in the HFOT group vs. 65% in COT group (*p* = 0.34)
Bell et al.[50]	ARF patients	100	RCT: HFOT vs. COT for 2 hours	Significant reduction in respiratory rate, less escalation of ventilation therapy and dyspnoea and better comfort with HFOT
Jones et al.[51]	ARF patients	303	RCT: HFOT vs. COT	No differences in requiring mechanical ventilation, length of stay and mortality rate between groups HFOT improved dryness symptom

Note: ARF, acute respiratory failure; COT, conventional oxygen therapy; HFOT, high-flow oxygen therapy via nasal cannula; HHFM, high-flow face mask; L/min, liters per minute; NIV, non-invasive ventilation; RCT, randomised controlled trial.

failure patients were presence of shock, high severity score and absence of improvement including respiratory rate, lower oxygenation and persistent thoraco-abdominal asynchrony,[15,35] which should be considered and closely monitored during HFOT use.

Prevention of postextubation respiratory failure

Conventional oxygen therapy is commonly used especially during the first few hours after extubation to correct residual hypoxaemia and to reduce increased work of breathing. Reintubation occurs in some patients because of pulmonary congestion, laryngeal oedema or secretion obstruction, and it is associated with increased morbidity and mortality.[36] Whether NIV prevents postextubation respiratory failure has been tested, but the results have been inconclusive with positive effects observed only in the case of high-risk patients.[37–40]

HFOT has the potential to improve oxygenation and secretion clearance and to alleviate increased work of breathing after extubation (Table 33.2). However, some studies in extubated patients comparing HFOT with non-rebreathing face masks had conflicting results.[41,42] A randomised comparative single-centre study in 105 patients who had a PaO_2/FiO_2 ratio of <300 before extubation observed that HFOT resulted in better oxygenation and lower intubation rate in comparison to the Venturi mask.[23] More recently, a multicentre randomised study comparing HFOT and conventional oxygen therapy in 527 patients at low risk for reintubation (e.g. age <65 years, APACHE II <12, body mass index [BMI] <30 kg/m^2, and absence of major comorbidities) found that HFOT reduced intubation rate (absolute risk reduction, 7.2%; 95% CI, 2.5% to 12.2%; $p = 0.004$) and postextubation respiratory failure (absolute risk reduction, 6.1%; 95% CI, 0.7% to 11.6%; $p = 0.03$).[19] The same group also compared HFOT in 604 patients considered at high risk with NIV for 24 hours after extubation and found a similar efficacy to prevent reintubation with a lower rate of side effects.[43]

Although HFOT has been shown to prevent postextubation respiratory failure in critically ill patients in the ICU, the effectiveness of HFOT following extubation after cardiothoracic surgery remains controversial. A pragmatic randomised controlled study comparing HFOT and usual care in 340 patients did not find any difference in SpO_2/FiO_2 ratio between groups, but patients in the HFOT group had less requirement for escalation of respiratory support than the usual care group (28.7% vs. 45%; odds ratio, 0.47; 95% CI, 0.29 to 0.7; $p = 0.001$).[44] Another randomised controlled study by Corley and colleagues included 150 patients with BMI $\geq$ 30 kg/m^2 who were randomly assigned to HFOT or standard oxygen therapy after extubation following cardiac surgery. The study showed that HFOT did not improve respiratory rate, oxygenation, atelectasis and dyspnoea.[45] In contrast, a recent large multicentre randomised study in 830 hypoxaemic patients after cardiothoracic surgery comparing HFOT and NIV found that HFOT was not inferior to NIV in terms of treatment failure (risk difference, 0.9%; 95% CI, −4.9% to 6.6%; $p = 0.003$) and ICU mortality (6.8% in HFOT group vs. 5.5% in NIV group; $p = 0.66$). HFOT was better tolerated whereas more skin breakdown and nursing workload were found in the NIV group.[46] Last, a randomised study involved 59 patients who underwent elective lung resection and were assigned to immediately receive either HFOT or standard oxygen therapy after extubation. The study showed that prophylactic HFOT therapy did not improve postoperative 6-min walk test distance but was associated with reduced hospital length of stay and improved patient satisfaction.[47]

In sum, HFOT does not seem to be inferior to NIV in situations where some evidence existed in favour of NIV (at risk patients after extubation, post cardiothoracic surgery). The good tolerance of the technique makes it a very attractive alternative.

Using HFOT in the Emergency Department

HFOT is generally implemented in the ICU; however, using HFOT outside the ICU in particular in an emergency department (ED) has increasingly grown (Table 33.1). Acute hypoxaemic respiratory failure is a common cause of ED admission, and oxygen therapy is an essential supportive treatment. NIV has also been used in many conditions (e.g. cardiogenic pulmonary oedema and acute exacerbation of COPD), but there are some limitations (e.g. patient unable to speak or eat and patient discomfort). A small cohort study showed that HFOT alleviated dyspnoea and improved oxygenation in patients who were admitted in the ED due to hypoxaemic respiratory failure.[48] Later, two prospective randomised studies comparing HFOT and conventional oxygen therapy demonstrated that HFOT significantly improved dyspnoea and patient's comfort[49,50] and decreased the need for escalation in ventilation treatment.[50]

In contrast, a recent randomised controlled study performed in 303 hypoxaemic patients admitted in the ED did not find any difference in mortality rate, hospital length of stay and need for mechanical ventilation between HFOT and standard oxygen therapy.[51] However, this study had important limitations: the enrolment rate was lower than the estimated sample size and severe hypoxaemic patients were excluded at the beginning of the study, which led to the very low rate of ventilator support requirement. The reasons why HFOT has conflicting results in the ED may be explained by different patient population and confounding by some co-treatments such as diuretics and bronchodilators.

HFOT is feasible and efficient to improve oxygenation in patients who were admitted in the ED due to acute hypoxaemic respiratory failure, but the impact on clinical outcome needs to be better evaluated in the future and explored in the specific patient population.

Table 33.2 Main clinical studies of high-flow nasal oxygen cannula following extubation

References	Population	Patients	Study design	Main outcomes
Intensive care unit				
Tiruvoipati et al.[41]	Postextubation	50	Randomised crossover study: HFOT vs. HFFM for 30 min	No difference in gas exchange, respiratory rate, or haemodynamics were found Better tolerance with HFOT
Rittayamai et al.[42]	Postextubation	17	Randomised crossover study: HFOT vs. COT for 30 min	Less dyspnoea and lower respiratory rate and heart rate with HFOT Better comfort with HFOT
Maggiore et al.[23]	Patients with $PaO_2/FiO_2 \leq 300$ before extubation	105	RCT: HFOT vs. Venturi mask for 48 hours	Higher PaO_2/FiO_2 (287 ± 74 vs. 247 ± 81, $p = 0.03$) and better comfort with HFOT Lower intubation rate (4% vs. 21%, $p = 0.01$) and less requiring ventilator support (7% vs. 35%, $p < 0.001$) with HFOT
Hernández et al.[19]	Patients with low risk of reintubation	527	Multicentre RCT: HFOT vs. COT for 24 hours	Lower reintubation rate within 72 hours (4.9% vs. 32%, $p = 0.004$) and postextubation respiratory failure (8.3% vs. 14.4%, $p = 0.03$) with HFOT
Hernández et al.[43]	Patients with high risk of reintubation	604	Multicentre RCT: HFOT vs. NIV for 24 hours	Similar reintubation rate within 72 hours and time to reintubation
After cardiothoracic surgery				
Parke et al.[44]	Cardiac surgery	340	RCT: HFOT vs. usual care for 48 hours	No difference in SpO_2/FiO_2 ratio between group but $PaCO_2$ was significantly lower with HFOT Lower rate of escalation in respiratory support with HFOT (27.8% vs. 45%, $p = 0.001$)
Corley et al.[45]	Cardiac surgery patients with BMI ≥30 kg/m^2	155	RCT: HFOT vs. standard oxygen therapy	No differences in atelectasis scores, PaO_2/FiO_2 ratio and respiratory rate between groups Lower dyspnoea levels with HFOT
Stéphan et al.[46]	Cardiothoracic surgery	830	Multicentre RCT: HFOT vs. BiPAP	HFOT was not inferior to BIPAP regarding treatment failure (absolute difference 0.9%, 95% CI −4.9% to 6.6%; $p = 0.003$) and ICU mortality (absolute difference 1.2%, 95% CI −2.3% to 4.8%; $p = 0.66$) Skin breakdown was more common with BIPAP
Ansari et al.[47]	Lung resection surgery	59	RCT: HFOT vs. standard oxygen therapy	No difference in 6-min walk test distance between groups Lower hospital length of stay with HFOT (2.5 vs. 4.0 days, $p = 0.03$)

Note: BiPAP, bilevel positive airway pressure; BMI, body mass index; COT, conventional oxygen therapy; HFOT, high-flow oxygen therapy via nasal cannula; HFFM, high-flow face mask; ICU, intensive care unit; RCT, randomised clinical trial.

Preoxygenation before endotracheal intubation

Endotracheal intubation is a life-saving procedure that can be associated with morbidity and mortality.[52,53] Preoxygenation via an oxygen mask with a bag is routinely used to prevent desaturation during intubation, but hypoxaemia may still occur. NIV has been shown to be more effective to reduce the incidence of desaturation;[54] however, this technique may be interrupted during the procedure. HFOT continuously provides a high flow rate of gas without any interruption and constant FiO_2, which may also be beneficial before endotracheal intubation (Table 33.3).

A quasi-experimental before–after study in 101 patients with mild-to-moderate hypoxaemia requiring endotracheal intubation observed that HFOT significantly improved oxygenation and reduced prevalence of severe hypoxaemia during intubation from 14% with a standard oxygen face mask to 2% with HFOT.[55] In contrast, a randomised study in more severe hypoxaemic patients did not find any significant differences between HFOT and oxygen face mask in preventing hypoxaemia and reducing mortality rate during endotracheal intubation.[56] Thus, the current evidence does not support using HFOT to preoxygenate before endotracheal intubation and further study is needed.

HFOT during fiberoptic bronchoscopy

Fiberoptic bronchoscopy is widely used as a diagnostic or therapeutic tool in pulmonary and critical care medicine. Oxygen supplement with a total oxygen flow of 6–15 L/min via a conventional oxygen device is routinely used to prevent hypoxaemia during bronchoscopy, but some patients, particularly critically ill patients, still develop severe hypoxaemia and need escalation of ventilatory support.[57] Few randomised studies used NIV or CPAP in patients with acute hypoxaemic respiratory failure undergoing fiberoptic bronchoscopy, and the results showed that NIV or CPAP was superior to conventional oxygen therapy in terms of preventing hypoxaemia during the procedure.[58,59] HFOT may be an alternative method for delivering oxygen in patients at risk for bronchoscopy-induced respiratory deterioration because it provides high flow of gas, constant FiO_2 and some PEEP (Table 33.3). Lucangelo et al.[60] compared HFOT at a flow rate of 40 and 60 L/min with a Venturi mask in 45 patients without hypoxaemia undergoing fiberoptic bronchoscopy. The results at the end of bronchoscopy showed that HFOT at 60 L/min had higher PaO_2, PaO_2/FiO_2 ratio and SpO_2 than the two other groups. In contrast, Simon and colleagues[61] compared HFOT and NIV in 40 patients with hypoxaemic respiratory failure during bronchoscopy. They found that oxygenation was significantly better in patients receiving NIV, but no

Table 33.3 Main clinical studies of high-flow nasal oxygen cannula during invasive procedures

References	Population	Patients	Study design	Main outcomes
Preoxygenation before endotracheal intubation				
Miguel-Montanes et al.[55]	Mild to moderate hypoxaemic patients	101	Prospective quasi-experimental before (HFFM) and after (HFOT) study	Higher SpO_2 at the end of preoxygenation with HFOT HFOT reduced prevalence of severe hypoxaemia during intubation (2% vs. 14%, $p = 0.03$)
Vourc'h et al.[56]	Patients with acute hypoxaemic respiratory failure	124	Multicentre RCT: HFOT vs. HFFM	No difference in the lowest saturation, difficult intubation, ventilation-free days, intubation-related adverse events between groups
During fibreoptic bronchoscopy				
Lucangelo et al.[60]	Elective bronchoscopy	45	Randomised crossover study: HFOT at 40 and 60 L/min and Venturi mask	HFOT at 60 L/min presented higher PaO_2, PaO_2/FiO_2 and SpO_2 than the two other groups
Simon et al.[61]	Acute hypoxaemic respiratory failure patients in ICU	40	RCT: HFOT vs. NIV	NIV had better oxygen levels No significant differences regarding heart rate, mean arterial pressure, respiratory rate, and intubation rate between groups

Note: HFOT, high-flow oxygen therapy via nasal cannula; HFFM, high-flow face mask; ICU, intensive care unit; L/min, liters per minute; NIV, non-invasive ventilation; RCT, randomised controlled trial.

difference in intubation rate was found. Thus, we cannot recommend the use of HFOT during fibreoptic bronchoscopy particularly in hypoxaemic patients because limited data and more research are required to assess the role of HFOT during such procedure.

Hypercapnic respiratory failure

A common cause of hypercapnic respiratory failure is COPD. NIV has been proven to reduce intubation and mortality rates in patients with acute exacerbation of COPD requiring ventilator support.[62,63] The mechanism of action of HFOT to wash out dead space that may reduce CO_2 rebreathing should have benefit, but the evidence of HFOT in patients with hypercapnic respiratory failure is scant. A retrospective study of 46 patients with acute hypercapnic respiratory failure (65.2% of patients had acute exacerbation of COPD) who visited the emergency room found that $PaCO_2$ significantly reduced from 73 ± 20 mmHg with standard oxygen therapy to 67 ± 23 mmHg with HFOT ($p = 0.02$), and pH also increased from 7.28 ± 0.08 to 7.31 ± 0.08 ($p < 0.01$).[64] A recent randomised crossover study by Fraser et al.[10] investigated the short-term effects of HFOT in comparison to low-flow oxygen supplement (2–4 L/min) in 30 patients with stable COPD using long-term oxygen therapy. The study showed that HFOT significantly improved gas exchange by reducing transcutaneous CO_2 and respiratory rate and increasing transcutaneous oxygen and tidal volume but also worsened hyperinflation. We clearly need larger clinical studies to assess the efficacy of HFOT in patients with hypercapnic respiratory failure.

REFERENCES

1. Lellouche F, Maggiore SM, Lyazidi A et al. Water content of delivered gases during non-invasive ventilation in healthy subjects. *Intensive Care Med.* 2009;35:987–95.
2. Fontanari P, Burnet H, Zattara-Hartmann MC, Jammes Y. Changes in airway resistance induced by nasal inhalation of cold dry, dry, or moist air in normal individuals. *J Appl Physiol.* 1996;81:1739–43.
3. Roca O, Riera J, Torres F, Masclans JR. High-flow oxygen therapy in acute respiratory failure. *Respir Care.* 2010;55:408–13.
4. Frat JP, Thille AW, Mercat A et al. High-flow oxygen through nasal cannula in acute hypoxemic respiratory failure. *N Engl J Med.* 2015;372:2185–96.
5. Sim MA, Dean P, Kinsella J et al. Performance of oxygen delivery devices when the breathing pattern of respiratory failure is simulated. *Anaesthesia.* 2008;63:938–40.
6. Katz JA, Marks JD. Inspiratory work with and without continuous positive airway pressure in patients with acute respiratory failure. *Anesthesiology.* 1985;63:598–607.
7. Parke RL, Eccleston ML, McGuinness SP. The effects of flow on airway pressure during nasal high-flow oxygen therapy. *Respir Care.* 2011;56:1151–55.
8. Corley A, Caruana LR, Barnett AG et al. Oxygen delivery through high-flow nasal cannulae increase end-expiratory lung volume and reduce respiratory rate in post-cardiac surgical patients. *Br J Anaesth.* 2011;107:998–1004.
9. Moller W, Celik G, Feng S et al. Nasal high flow clears anatomical dead space in upper airway models. *J Appl Physiol.* 2015;118:1525–32.
10. Fraser JF, Spooner AJ, Dunster KR et al. Nasal high flow oxygen therapy in patients with COPD reduces respiratory rate and tissue carbon dioxide while increasing tidal and end-expiratory lung volumes: A randomised crossover trial. *Thorax.* 2016.
11. Vargas F, Saint-Leger M, Boyer A et al. Physiologic effects of high-flow nasal cannula oxygen in critical care subjects. *Respir Care.* 2015;60:1369–76.
12. Lee HY, Rhee CK, Lee JW. Feasibility of high-flow nasal cannula oxygen therapy for acute respiratory failure in patients with hematologic malignancies: A retrospective single-center study. *J Crit Care.* 2015;30:773–7.
13. Lellouche F, Maggiore SM, Deye N et al. Effect of the humidification device on the work of breathing during noninvasive ventilation. *Intensive Care Med.* 2002;28:1582–9.
14. Boyer A, Vargas F, Hilbert G et al. Small dead space heat and moisture exchangers do not impede gas exchange during noninvasive ventilation: A comparison with a heated humidifier. *Intensive Care Med.* 2010;36:1348–54.
15. Sztrymf B, Messika J, Bertrand F et al. Beneficial effects of humidified high flow nasal oxygen in critical care patients: A prospective pilot study. *Intensive Care Med.* 2011;37:1780–6.
16. Sztrymf B, Messika J, Mayot T et al. Impact of high-flow nasal cannula oxygen therapy on intensive care unit patients with acute respiratory failure: A prospective observational study. *J Crit Care.* 2012;27:324 e329–313.
17. Frat JP, Brugiere B, Ragot S et al. Sequential application of oxygen therapy via high-flow nasal cannula and noninvasive ventilation in acute respiratory failure: An observational pilot study. *Respir Care.* 2015;60:170–8.
18. Mundel T, Feng S, Tatkov S, Schneider H. Mechanisms of nasal high flow on ventilation during wakefulness and sleep. *J Appl Physiol.* 2013;114:1058–65.
19. Hernandez G, Vaquero C, Gonzalez P et al. Effect of postextubation high-flow nasal cannula vs conventional oxygen therapy on reintubation in low-risk patients: A randomized clinical trial. *JAMA.* 2016;315:1354–61.
20. Slutsky AS, Ranieri VM. Ventilator-induced lung injury. *N Engl J Med.* 2014;370:980.

21. Carteaux G, Millan-Guilarte T, De Prost N et al. Failure of noninvasive ventilation for de novo acute hypoxemic respiratory failure: Role of tidal volume. *Crit Care Med.* 2016;44:282–90.
22. Cuquemelle E, Pham T, Papon JF et al. Heated and humidified high-flow oxygen therapy reduces discomfort during hypoxemic respiratory failure. *Respir Care.* 2012;57:1571–7.
23. Maggiore SM, Idone FA, Vaschetto R et al. Nasal high-flow versus Venturi mask oxygen therapy after extubation. Effects on oxygenation, comfort, and clinical outcome. *Am J Respir Crit Care Med.* 2014;190:282–8.
24. Parke RL, McGuinness SP, Eccleston ML. A preliminary randomized controlled trial to assess effectiveness of nasal high-flow oxygen in intensive care patients. *Respir Care.* 2011;56:265–70.
25. Roca O, de Acilu MG, Caralt B et al. Humidified high flow nasal cannula supportive therapy improves outcomes in lung transplant recipients readmitted to the intensive care unit because of acute respiratory failure. *Transplantation.* 2015;99:1092–8.
26. Lemiale V, Mokart D, Mayaux J et al. The effects of a 2-h trial of high-flow oxygen by nasal cannula versus Venturi mask in immunocompromised patients with hypoxemic acute respiratory failure: A multicenter randomized trial. *Crit Care.* 2015;19:380.
27. Coudroy R, Jamet A, Petua P et al. High-flow nasal cannula oxygen therapy versus noninvasive ventilation in immunocompromised patients with acute respiratory failure: An observational cohort study. *Ann Intensive Care.* 2016;6:45.
28. Lemiale V, Resche-Rigon M, Mokart D et al. High-flow nasal cannula oxygenation in immunocompromised patients with acute hypoxemic respiratory failure: A Groupe de Recherche Respiratoire en Reanimation Onco-Hematologique Study. *Crit Care Med.* 2017 Mar;45(3):e274–80.
29. Frat JP, Ragot S, Girault C et al. Effect of non-invasive oxygenation strategies in immunocompromised patients with severe acute respiratory failure: A post-hoc analysis of a randomised trial. *Lancet Respir Med.* 2016;4:646–52.
30. Force ADT, Ranieri VM, Rubenfeld GD et al. Acute respiratory distress syndrome: The Berlin Definition. *JAMA.* 2012;307:2526–33.
31. Messika J, Ben Ahmed K, Gaudry S et al. Use of high-flow nasal cannula oxygen therapy in subjects with ARDS: A 1-year observational study. *Respir Care.* 2015;60:162–9.
32. Antonelli M, Conti G, Esquinas A et al. A multiple-center survey on the use in clinical practice of noninvasive ventilation as a first-line intervention for acute respiratory distress syndrome. *Crit Care Med.* 2007;35:18–25.
33. Matthay MA. Saving lives with high-flow nasal oxygen. *N Engl J Med.* 2015;372:2225–6.
34. Kang BJ, Koh Y, Lim CM et al. Failure of high-flow nasal cannula therapy may delay intubation and increase mortality. *Intensive Care Med.* 2015;41:623–32.
35. Rello J, Perez M, Roca O et al. High-flow nasal therapy in adults with severe acute respiratory infection: A cohort study in patients with 2009 influenza A/H1N1v. *J Crit Care.* 2012;27:434–9.
36. Thille AW, Richard J-CM, Brochard L. The decision to extubate in the intensive care unit. *Am J Respir Crit Care Med.* 2013;187:1294–1302.
37. Thille AW, Boissier F, Ben-Ghezala H et al. Easily identified at-risk patients for extubation failure may benefit from noninvasive ventilation: A prospective before–after study. *Crit Care.* 2016;20:48.
38. Ferrer M, Sellares J, Valencia M et al. Non-invasive ventilation after extubation in hypercapnic patients with chronic respiratory disorders: Randomised controlled trial. *Lancet.* 2009;374:1082–8.
39. Ferrer M, Valencia M, Nicolas JM et al. Early non-invasive ventilation averts extubation failure in patients at risk: A randomized trial. *Am J Respir Crit Care Med.* 2006;173:164–70.
40. Nava S, Gregoretti C, Fanfulla F et al. Noninvasive ventilation to prevent respiratory failure after extubation in high-risk patients. *Crit Care Med.* 2005;33:2465–70.
41. Tiruvoipati R, Lewis D, Haji K, Botha J. High-flow nasal oxygen vs high-flow face mask: A randomized crossover trial in extubated patients. *J Crit Care.* 2010;25:463–8.
42. Rittayamai N, Tscheikuna J, Rujiwit P. High-flow nasal cannula versus conventional oxygen therapy after endotracheal extubation: A randomized crossover physiologic study. *Respir Care.* 2014;59:485–90.
43. Hernandez G, Vaquero C, Colinas L et al. Effect of postextubation high-flow nasal cannula vs noninvasive ventilation on reintubation and postextubation respiratory failure in high-risk patients: A randomized clinical trial. *JAMA.* 2016;316:1565–74.
44. Parke R, McGuinness S, Dixon R, Jull A. Open-label, phase II study of routine high-flow nasal oxygen therapy in cardiac surgical patients. *Br J Anaesth.* 2013;111:925–31.
45. Corley A, Bull T, Spooner AJ et al. Direct extubation onto high-flow nasal cannulae post-cardiac surgery versus standard treatment in patients with a BMI ≥30: A randomised controlled trial. *Intensive Care Med.* 2015;41:887–94.
46. Stephan F, Barrucand B, Petit P et al. High-flow nasal oxygen vs noninvasive positive airway pressure in hypoxemic patients after cardiothoracic surgery: A randomized clinical trial. *JAMA.* 2015;313:2331–9.

47. Ansari BM, Hogan MP, Collier TJ et al. A randomized controlled trial of high-flow nasal oxygen (Optiflow) as part of an enhanced recovery program after lung resection surgery. *Ann Thorac Surg.* 2016;101:459–64.
48. Lenglet H, Sztrymf B, Leroy C et al. Humidified high flow nasal oxygen during respiratory failure in the emergency department: Feasibility and efficacy. *Respir Care.* 2012;57:1873–8.
49. Rittayamai N, Tscheikuna J, Praphruetkit N, Kijpinyochai S. Use of high-flow nasal cannula for acute dyspnea and hypoxemia in the emergency department. *Respir Care.* 2015;60:1377–82.
50. Bell N, Hutchinson CL, Green TC et al. Randomised control trial of humidified high flow nasal cannulae versus standard oxygen in the emergency department. *Emerg Med Australas.* 2015;27:537–41.
51. Jones PG, Kamona S, Doran O et al. Randomized controlled trial of humidified high-flow nasal oxygen for acute respiratory distress in the emergency department: The HOT-ER Study. *Respir Care.* 2016;61:291–9.
52. Schwartz DE, Matthay MA, Cohen NH. Death and other complications of emergency airway management in critically ill adults. A prospective investigation of 297 tracheal intubations. *Anesthesiology.* 1995;82:367–76.
53. Jaber S, Amraoui J, Lefrant JY et al. Clinical practice and risk factors for immediate complications of endotracheal intubation in the intensive care unit: A prospective, multiple-center study. *Crit Care Med.* 2006;34:2355–61.
54. Baillard C, Fosse JP, Sebbane M et al. Noninvasive ventilation improves preoxygenation before intubation of hypoxic patients. *Am J Respir Crit Care Med.* 2006;174:171–7.
55. Miguel-Montanes R, Hajage D, Messika J et al. Use of high-flow nasal cannula oxygen therapy to prevent desaturation during tracheal intubation of intensive care patients with mild-to-moderate hypoxemia. *Crit Care Med.* 2015;43:574–83.
56. Vourc'h M, Asfar P, Volteau C et al. High-flow nasal cannula oxygen during endotracheal intubation in hypoxemic patients: A randomized controlled clinical trial. *Intensive Care Med.* 2015;41:1538–48.
57. Cracco C, Fartoukh M, Prodanovic H et al. Safety of performing fiberoptic bronchoscopy in critically ill hypoxemic patients with acute respiratory failure. *Intensive Care Med.* 2013;39:45–52.
58. Maitre B, Jaber S, Maggiore SM et al. Continuous positive airway pressure during fiberoptic bronchoscopy in hypoxemic patients. A randomized double-blind study using a new device. *Am J Respir Crit Care Med.* 2000;162:1063–7.
59. Antonelli M, Conti G, Rocco M et al. Noninvasive positive-pressure ventilation vs. conventional oxygen supplementation in hypoxemic patients undergoing diagnostic bronchoscopy. *Chest.* 2002;121:1149–54.
60. Lucangelo U, Vassallo FG, Marras E et al. High-flow nasal interface improves oxygenation in patients undergoing bronchoscopy. *Crit Care Res Pract.* 2012;2012:506382.
61. Simon M, Braune S, Frings D et al. High-flow nasal cannula oxygen versus non-invasive ventilation in patients with acute hypoxaemic respiratory failure undergoing flexible bronchoscopy—A prospective randomised trial. *Crit Care.* 2014;18:712.
62. Brochard L, Mancebo J, Wysocki M et al. Noninvasive ventilation for acute exacerbations of chronic obstructive pulmonary disease. *N Engl J Med.* 1995;333:817–22.
63. Keenan SP, Sinuff T, Cook DJ, Hill NS. Which patients with acute exacerbation of chronic obstructive pulmonary disease benefit from noninvasive positive-pressure ventilation? A systematic review of the literature. *Ann Intern Med.* 2003;138:861–70.
64. Jeong JH, Kim DH, Kim SC et al. Changes in arterial blood gases after use of high-flow nasal cannula therapy in the ED. *Am J Emerg Med.* 2015;33:1344–9.

34

Equipment for oxygen therapy

JANE SLOUGH

INTRODUCTION

An oxygen delivery system is used to normalise or increase arterial oxygen pressure by regulating the oxygen supply to a patient. The oxygen supply depends on a combination of delivery equipment, oxygen flow, breathing pattern, tidal volume and respiratory rate. It has to be correlated with the patient's oxygenation and arterial blood gas value.

Oxygen is given not only to relieve dyspnoea and to maintain oxygenation, but also to improve normal daily activity, to increase endurance exercise capacity and to decrease exacerbations and thus hospitalisations. A fine balance between device comfort, ability to continue normal daily activity and therapeutic effect will determine the choice of a specific oxygen delivery device. If one of these conditions is not fulfilled, lack of compliance will be the consequence.

The choice of a device also depends on many individual factors, including quality of life, age, comorbidity, next of kin and social history. Good education of the patient, family and/or carers is essential for good compliance. In this chapter, an overview of the different available systems is provided, to enable the reader to make appropriate choices with regard to correct equipment for oxygen delivery, to achieve therapeutic success.

OXYGEN-PROVIDING SYSTEMS

There are several oxygen delivery systems: cylinders, concentrators and liquid oxygen. The choice of the system depends on the following factors:[1]

- Expected duration of the therapy
- Type of pathology
- Breathing pattern of the patient
- Need for humidification of the delivered oxygen
- Patient preference
- The needs, restrictions and mobility of the patient[2,3]

Supply of oxygen in the hospital

In most hospitals, a centralised storing system is used to supply piped oxygen to wall-mounted flow meters by the patient bedside. The oxygen has a concentration of at least 99.5% and can be used at all times. Flow meters allow the oxygen flow rate to be adjusted to a specific rate depending on the patient requirements. Most wall-mounted flow meters have a floating ball to indicate the flow rate; the centre of the ball should be aligned with the correct flow rate marking.[2] When a patient has to be transported in the hospital, a small cylinder of oxygen is usually used.[2]

The correct flow meters and connections must be used and the equipment of the different systems should not be mixed.[2] The oxygen tubing should not exceed 12 m in length; preferably not more than 5 m. A long tube or a large internal diameter cause a decrease in oxygen flow and thus in oxygen concentration.[2,4]

Supply of oxygen at home

CYLINDERS

Cylinders contain compressed gaseous oxygen, stored at 200 bar. Oxygen cylinders can be identified by the label and the colour coding on the shoulder or the curved part at the top of the cylinder. On oxygen cylinders, this is usually colour coded white.[2,5,6] All oxygen cylinders are provided with a pressure and flow regulator, to decompress the compressed oxygen to atmospheric pressure at a specific flow rate before being administered to a patient.[2] Oxygen cylinders have a pressure gauge that usually forms part of the regulator, it indicates the pressure within the cylinder. This allows the operator to know how much oxygen is left in the cylinder. When the cylinder is almost empty, the needle on the gauge will be in the red zone. Each connection has to be airtight and free of lubricant or dust.

Oxygen cylinders come in a range of sizes and capacity. Larger cylinders tend to be used in hospitals when piped oxygen is not available or in the home as a backup in case of a power cut when using an electrical concentrator as they are always ready to use. If a patient requires more than 2 L/min for more than 8 hours a day, other oxygen systems such as an oxygen concentrator are more suitable and more economical.[2,7,8] Large cylinders are unwieldy and should be secured to a wall or on a trolley with a chain. Small portable cylinders are available for ambulatory use and patient transportation. Patients requiring ambulatory oxygen should be assessed and provided with the lightest cylinder that can operate for the longest period of time to meet the patient's need.[9] There is a balance to be struck between the weight of the cylinder and the length of time the cylinder will last. Smaller oxygen cylinders that are considered portable cylinders can be used with a suitable backpack or a trolley.[6] Unfortunately, without the addition of an oxygen-conserving device, many of the portable cylinders only last 2 to 3 hours at a continuous flow rate of 2 L/min.

STATIC OXYGEN CONCENTRATORS

A static oxygen concentrator is an electric apparatus that filters ambient air through a molecular sieve, thus absorbing nitrogen and carbon dioxide and delivering high oxygen concentrations[2,7,9] (Figure 34.1). It generates an average oxygen concentration of between 85% and 95%.[10–12] Oxygen concentrators are compact, reliable and cheap, and are used mainly in the home. One of the main advantages of a concentrator is that as long as there is an electrical source, they deliver a continuous supply of oxygen and eliminate the need for repeat delivery as in the case of oxygen cylinders and liquid oxygen systems.[13] Oxygen concentrators can deliver a range of flow rates. Standard concentrators deliver between 0.5 and 5 L/min. Low flow meters can be added to standard concentrators to deliver lower flows where needed. High flow concentrators can deliver up to 8 L/min. If even higher flow rates are required, concentrators can be connected in series with each concentrator set at the same flow rate: for example, in order to deliver oxygen at a 14 L/min flow rate, two concentrators can be set to deliver 7 L/min each.[6]

Some concentrators have an added reservoir system on the top and have the ability to refill small ambulatory cylinders; they are known as 'homefill oxygen delivery systems'.[10,14] This obviously is beneficial to the healthcare provider by reducing cost as a result of eradicating the need for cylinder deliveries and to the patient by promoting independence.[14]

The oxygen concentrator should be placed in a well-ventilated area away from open fires and cooking areas. In order to increase patient freedom around the home and reduce the trip hazard from long lengths of tubing, a 'piped' or fixed oxygen system may be used. This involves connecting the clear oxygen tubing from an oxygen concentrator to multiple outlet points within the home.[8,11] Fire breaks should be inserted into the tubing to reduce the risk of catastrophic fire.[6] Concentrators do have some drawbacks, in particular their inability to work without an electrical power source, which requires the patient to swap to a backup system, usually a cylinder, in the event of electrical power failure. Some patients find that the noise from the concentrator is annoying and can be a reason for decreased compliance overnight when trying to sleep.[13] Concentrators can also generate heat when in operation and in turn increase the ambient temperature within a room.[13]

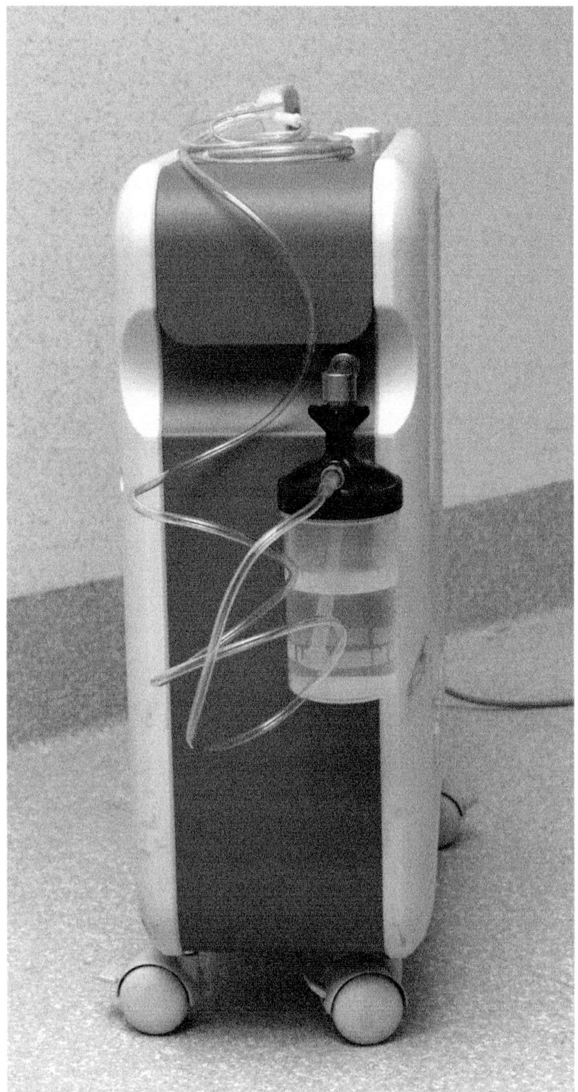

Figure 34.1 Oxygen concentrator.

TRANSPORTABLE AND PORTABLE CONCENTRATORS

Transportable oxygen concentrators are similar to static concentrators but are smaller in size and can operate from batteries as well as mains electric. They provide both continuous oxygen flow and pulsed, demand or intermittent oxygen delivery. Pulsed, demand or intermittent oxygen flow is referred to as the delivery of oxygen during the inspiration phase of breathing only. The term *pulsed flow* will be used within this text. This type of concentrator can be used as a static concentrator as well as an ambulatory device. The battery life depends on the flow rate and delivery mode, continuous or pulsed, and varies from device to device. This can be a limiting factor for their use outside the home.[9,10,15]

Portable oxygen concentrators are a developing technology and are generally much smaller than transportable concentrators. They are much lighter in weight but their features vary from model and/or manufacture. Many portable devices tend only to deliver pulsed oxygen and are therefore not suitable for use while sleeping.[6] As with all oxygen equipment, its suitability to meet a patient's requirements needs to be assessed on an individual basis.[9,10,15]

LIQUID OXYGEN

Liquid oxygen systems provide the most flexible oxygen delivery equipment at home. It allows the storage of large amounts of gas compared to gaseous oxygen. One litre of liquid oxygen provides 860–900 L of gaseous oxygen when evaporated.[4,7,12] The system consists of two different units: a large dewar, which is a big metal tank containing a large amount of liquid oxygen, and a smaller, portable and refillable flask used for ambulatory oxygen[4,7] (Figure 34.2). The liquid oxygen is stored at −183°C, The dewar can only be installed in a suitable ground floor area. The stationary home dewars can vary in size, and portable flasks can be filled as needed in the patient home. Liquid oxygen is ideal for patients requiring larger amounts of portable ambulatory oxygen or a higher flow rate. Some liquid oxygen systems can provide 15 L/min of continuous oxygen and are capable of delivering pulsed oxygen. Users require training in decanting oxygen from the dewar into the flasks, which some patients with poor dexterity may find difficult to do. Liquid oxygen can cause accidental burns when the equipment is wrongly manipulated. One drawback of liquid oxygen systems is the steady evaporation of the liquid oxygen that occurs whether the system is used or not.[13]

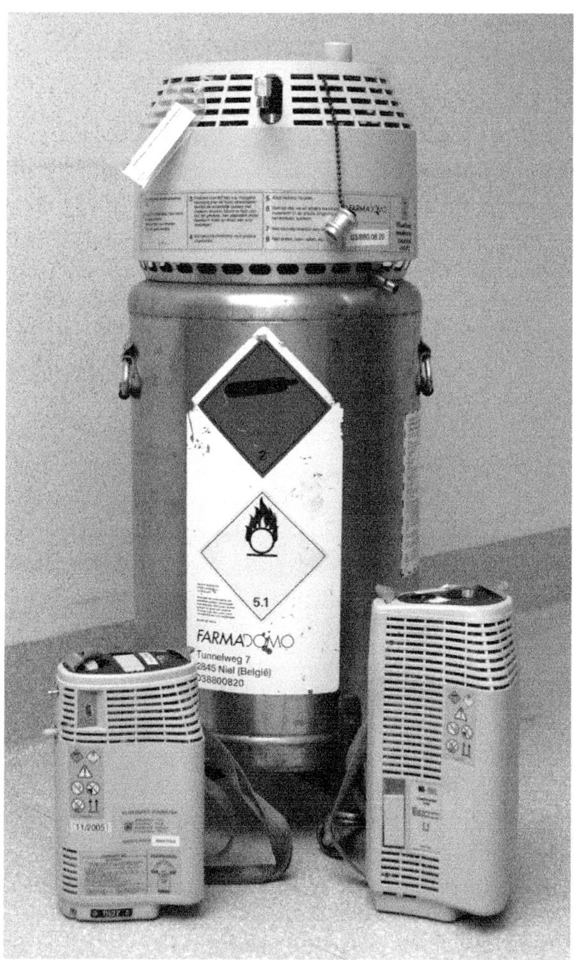

Figure 34.2 Liquid oxygen.

OXYGEN-CONSERVING DEVICE

An oxygen-conserving device can either be stand-alone or be an integral part of an oxygen cylinder. They were developed to enhance the duration that a cylinder would last, allowing a smaller and lighter cylinder to be used and in turn reducing the overall oxygen consumption and cost.[9] They have been reported to reduce oxygen usage by as much as 50%.[6] They work by only delivering oxygen on the inhalation phase of breathing, thus avoiding the waste of oxygen during the expiration phase. This may alter the desired oxygen concentration compared to continuous flow.[10] Some patients find the sudden on and off delivery of oxygen and the noise within the cannulae uncomfortable.[10] The specification and characteristics of the different oxygen-conserving devices are very varied, and their rationale and efficacy need to be considered on an individual basis.[3,9,10]

Nasal cannulae with a reservoir are also considered an oxygen-conserving device and are discussed later.

OXYGEN DELIVERY SYSTEMS

There are three different delivery systems used to supply oxygen to a patient, depending on the needed oxygen concentration, the patient and the pathology.[2] These are nasal cannulae or a nasal catheter, a face mask and a transtracheal catheter.[1,2,7,11,16]

The terms *low-flow system* and *high-flow system* are not well defined. Sometimes, low flow is defined as a flow of less than 5 L/min of oxygen, whereas others define it as a flow lower than the tidal breathing flow of the patient. The same ambiguity exists for the definition of the high-flow systems.[17–19]

If an oxygen flow administered is lower than tidal breathing flow, ambient air will be inhaled as well during inhalation, leading to variable oxygen concentrations. The oxygen concentration depends on the dilution with ambient air, respiratory rate and velocity. Using an oxygen flow higher than tidal breathing flow results in a more stable inhaled oxygen concentration.[17,18]

Nasal systems

NASAL CATHETER

The nasal catheter is a small tube, inserted via the nose until the tip of the tube is visible behind the uvula in the oropharynx. The distance between the tip of the nose and the ear correlates well with the length needed to insert the catheter.[2,16,18,20,21] Correct positioning of the catheter is essential for successful oxygenation, since wrong positioning of the catheter can lead to oxygen delivery into the oesophagus. Symptoms of incorrect positioning are nausea, bloating, vomiting and burping.[2,18,22]

NASAL CANNULAE

Nasal cannulae consist of a tube that divides at one end with two pronged extensions, which are placed into the nostrils.[2,16,18,23] To fix the prongs under the nose, the tubing has to be fitted tightly underneath the chin after positioning it behind the ears. If the tube is fixed too tight, it is not well tolerated, and after a while, it can lead to pressure sores. Nasal cannulae cannot be used with patients with nasal obstruction.[2,18,25]

Although some patients do report an unpleasant and uncomfortable feeling when oxygen is delivered by nasal cannulae, it is the preferred method for long-term use and is generally well tolerated and preferred by patients in preference to oxygen masks.[2,16,18,23,24,25]

NASAL SYSTEM WITH A RESERVOIR

Nasal reservoir cannulae were the first oxygen-conserving device to be developed.[6,13] There are two nasal systems with an oxygen reservoir. The first system is the so-called 'moustache', consisting of nasal prongs with an enlargement of the diameter of the tubing between the two prongs, thus creating a small reservoir for approximately 20 mL of oxygen (Figure 34.3a).[7,26] The second system is the 'pendant', which is an enlargement of the tubing a few centimetres below the nasal prongs and which hangs near the chest of the patient as a reservoir for approximately 30 mL of oxygen (Figure 34.3b).[26] Both systems are filled during exhalation and provide an extra boost of oxygen at the beginning of the following inhalation. This can reduce oxygen consumption by 25%–75%, depending on the used flow when compared to a nasal system without reservoir. They are suitable for the supply of oxygen with a flow of 2–4 L/min, providing an oxygen concentration of 24%–50%, respectively.[7,26]

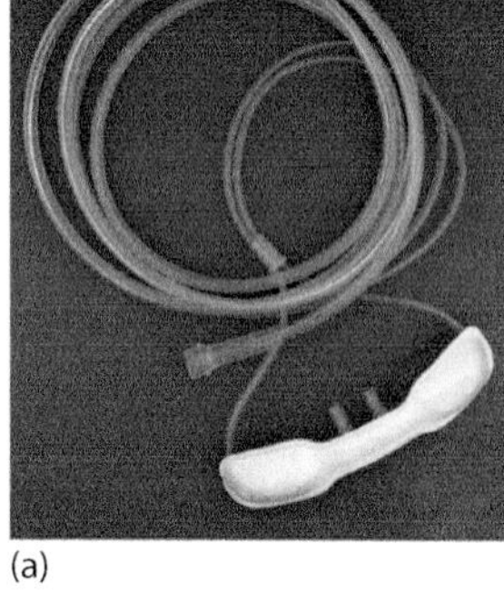
(a)

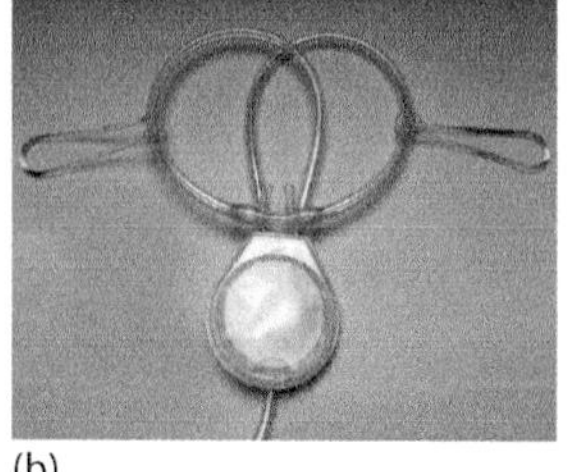
(b)

Figure 34.3 **(a)** Moustache. **(b)** Chest reservoir.

THE USE OF NASAL SYSTEMS

For the majority of patients, adequate oxygenation is achieved with 2–3 L/min of oxygen delivered by nasal systems. The inhaled oxygen concentration increases with approximately 4% for each litre per minute of delivered oxygen, starting at 24% for a flow of 1 L/min. Oxygen flows above 4 L/min often give an uncomfortable feeling with headache and dryness of the nose, especially if the oxygen therapy exceeds 24 hours.[2,11,18]

Although patients with dyspnoea tend to breathe more by mouth, the inhaled oxygen concentration does not vary much between nasal and mouth breathing. However, the oxygen concentration strongly depends on the breathing frequency and the flow rate.[2,11,20,27]

The big advantages of the nasal systems are that patients are able to continue normal daily activities and do not interfere with their ability to eat, drink and speak.[2,7,11,20] Furthermore, because patients feel less claustrophobic than with mask systems, nasal systems are well tolerated.[2,11,16–18,20] Occasionally, a patient needs to switch to a face mask, if the nose is too irritated.

Mask systems

SIMPLE FACE MASK

Simple face masks deliver an oxygen concentration of between 40% and 60%. The concentration of oxygen delivered to the patient will be variable depending on the oxygen flow rate and the patient's depth and rate of breathing. The oxygen flow rate is adjusted up or down depending on the required concentration. The characteristics of simple face masks vary between manufacturers so differing oxygen concentrations are achieved at differing flow rates. This type of mask requires oxygen flow rates greater than 5 L/min to avoid the possibility of rebreathing the exhaled carbon dioxide remaining in the mask.[2,24] This type of mask should be avoided for patients at risk of type 2 respiratory failure.

FACE MASKS WITH A RESERVOIR BAG

There are two types of reservoir mask, a partial rebreather and non-rebreather, both with a reservoir bag at the inhalation port of the mask that fills with oxygen and must be kept inflated. The patient breathes directly out of the reservoir; therefore, the volume of the reservoir bag needs to be larger than the tidal volume of the patient.[2,7,16,18,20,28]

The non-rebreathing mask has a one-way valve at the entrance of the bag and two on the side of the mask. The coordination of these valves avoids mixing inhaled and exhaled air and delivers an oxygen concentration up to 90%.[2,16,28,29] The partial rebreathing mask enables the patient to exhale into the bag so that the following inhalation will be a mixture of the exhaled air diluted with pure oxygen.[2,16,30,31]

As these masks can deliver high concentrations of oxygen, they tend to be used for short term in patients who are critically ill. Unfortunately, the oxygen cannot be humidified when using this type of mask.

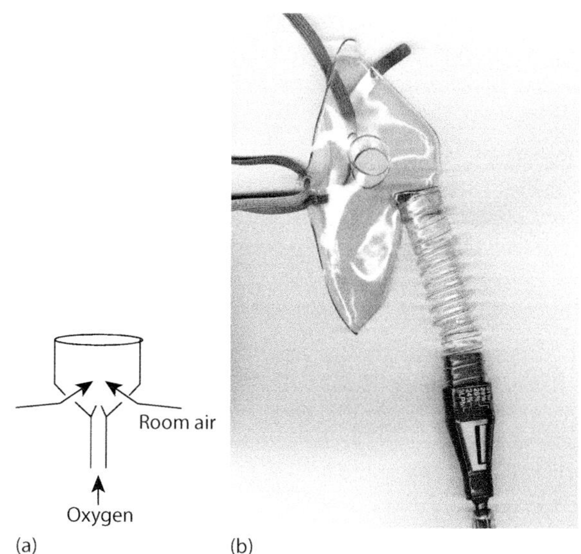

Figure 34.4 **(a)** Mechanism of action of the Venturi system. **(b)** Venturi mask.

VENTURI MASKS

This mask has a so-called 'Venturi system' at the inhalation port. The Venturi system gives an accurate oxygen concentration regardless of the respiratory flow rate.[2,32] Oxygen is delivered at high velocity as a jet flow through a narrow orifice, thus creating a negative pressure. The negative pressure sucks in ambient air via the Venturi adaptor into the system, thus diluting the gas flow (Figure 34.4a). The degree of dilution depends on the flow of the delivered oxygen and the diameter of the Venturi system and therefore provides a fixed oxygen concentration for each Venturi mask.[2,32] The main advantage of this mask, when compared to traditional masks, is a higher oxygen concentration for the same oxygen flow rate.[2,32]

Venturi masks are available for different oxygen concentrations (e.g. 24%, 28%, 35% and 40%) (Figure 34.4b). Another advantage of the Venturi mask, besides the fixed oxygen concentration, is that the flow delivered by the system is usually higher than the inhalation flow of the patient. If the respiratory rate exceeds 30 breaths per minute, the oxygen flow rate may need to be adjusted above the minimum flow rate indicated on the mask for patient comfort and according to blood gas values.

There are two major disadvantages of the Venturi mask. First, inhaled oxygen concentration decreases quickly if the mask is not well adjusted to nose and mouth. Second, the constant blowing of air into the face is considered as very unpleasant by patients. These disadvantages may lead to failure in compliance by some patients.[2,18,32]

TRACHEOSTOMY MASK

This is a small mask especially designed to place over a tracheostomy and fixed with a rubber ribbon around the neck. Because natural humidification via the nose is bypassed, the oxygen supply has to be humidified.[2]

THE USE OF MASK SYSTEMS

The mask is placed over the mouth and nose and fixed with a rubber ribbon behind the patient's head. The mask is often provided with a metal strip on top of the nose. Use of the mask may lead to irritation and open wounds on the nose and/or behind the ears.[2,18,28,33] The face mask is considered as less user friendly, because of poor fitting to the face and the inability to eat, drink and speak while in use. Furthermore, it impedes vision during reading, smells, is noisy and irritates the eyes.[16,18,31]

This system is not suited for disoriented, confused or agitated patients. Compliance of the patient regarding a mask system is influenced by understanding its necessity and by its comfort, since uncomfortable devices are usually abandoned after a while.[2,33]

Tracheal systems

TRANSTRACHEAL CATHETER

The transtracheal catheter is a small plastic tube placed between the first and second tracheal ring. It is inserted through a narrow incision, thus bypassing the dead space of the upper airway (Figure 34.5).[7,13,34,35] It creates an oxygen reservoir in the mouth, larynx and trachea, which leads to a savings of 50% of oxygen at rest and 30% during exercise. A supply of 0.5 L/min of oxygen by the catheter is equivalent to 4 L/min of oxygen given by nasal cannulae.[7,34] There is no irritation or discomfort at the nose, mouth and throat, and it is less visible than nasal systems and may lead to better therapy compliance.[13,34]

The procedure to place this catheter takes several weeks. First, a stent is placed into the trachea. After 1 week, it is replaced by the catheter. At 6–8 weeks later, when the fistula is mature and the wound is fully healed, the patient is able to remove the catheter and to clean the fistula. For safety reasons, it is better to hospitalise the patient for at least 24 hours to ensure the correct position of the catheter. This procedure is well tolerated by most patients.[34,35]

However, this catheter is only an option in long-term oxygen therapy since it is accompanied by a higher incidence of complications. Possible complications are cough, subcutaneous oedema, closure of the fistula, loss of a broken

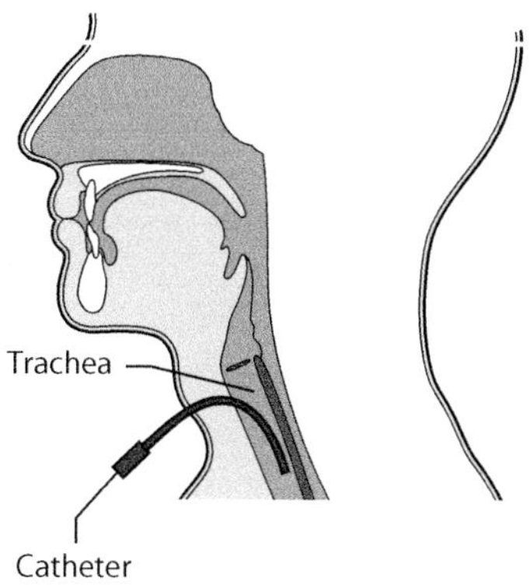

Figure 34.5 A transtracheal system.

catheter and clotting of mucus around the catheter.[13,34,35] Frequent manipulation of the catheter may cause granulation tissue formation. Other complications mostly involve catheter position and problems reinserting the catheter. Nevertheless, most of these complications are temporary and can be solved relatively easy.[7,34,35] The patient's ability to receive training and education remains the restricting factor in the use of this system.[11,18,34,35]

Enclosures

OXYGEN TENT

This is a large tent that is placed over the bed of a patient. It is seldom used nowadays due to high cost and substantial loss of oxygen.[1,36–38]

OXYGEN HAT OR HOOD

This is a system that covers the head of a patient to create an enriched oxygen environment.[36,38] It is often used in neonatal and/or paediatric wards because there is no immediate body contact with the infant.[37]

The OxyArm

The OxyArm is a minimal-contact oxygen delivery device, consisting of a headset and a semi-rigid, in-position adjustable boom, with an oxygen diffuser placed approximately 2 cm in front of both the nose and the mouth (Figure 34.6).[39–41] It generates a so-called 'oxygen cloud' with an oxygen concentration of 28%–35%, depending on the flow. In comparison with other systems such as face masks or nasal systems, it is more comfortable for the patient; that is, there is no claustrophobic feeling and especially there is almost no direct contact between device and face.[39–41] This avoids pressure lesions and is therefore better tolerated than other systems.[39,41]

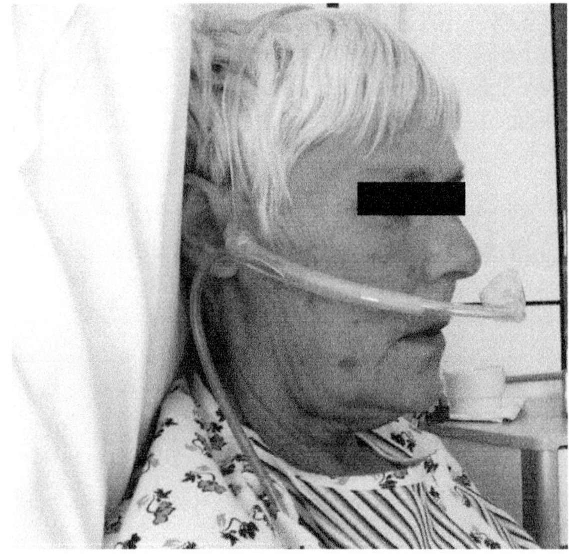

Figure 34.6 OxyArm.

HIGH-FLOW HUMIDIFIED NASAL CANNULAE OXYGEN THERAPY SYSTEMS

High-flow humidified nasal cannulae oxygen therapy systems consist of an air/oxygen blender, an active humidifier, a single heated circuit and nasal cannulae.[42,43] The air/oxygen blender can be set to deliver a concentration of 21% to 100% oxygen in a humidified flow of up to 60 L/min.[42] It is thought to have a number of physiological effects, including the reduction of the anatomical dead space, some positive end-expiratory pressure, a relatively constant inspiratory fraction of oxygen as well as warmed humidified flow, which promotes mucociliary clearance.[42] It is generally well tolerated and reported to be more comfortable than a face mask and has been associated with better oxygenation and lower respiratory rates.[44]

OXYGEN DELIVERY AND NON-INVASIVE VENTILATION SYSTEMS

In patients in respiratory distress, non-invasive ventilation (NIV) is recommended to be used, as long as possible for postponing intubation, in order to avoid all complications of invasive mechanical ventilation, weaning problems and infection.[45–47]

The success rate of NIV depends not only on the knowledge of healthcare professionals regarding the use of different ventilation modes but also on each patient's compliance and acceptance. These key factors are strongly influenced by training and experience of the clinical team.[45–49] The oxygen supply during NIV is not well validated and has to be clarified more in detail.[49]

Several NIV ventilators do not have a blender to deliver a precise inspired oxygen fraction, but it is always possible to add oxygen supply in the circuit or directly at the mask.[50] There are various factors that can cause oxygen concentration fluctuations during NIV.[49,50] The position of the oxygen injection in the respiration circuit can affect the oxygen concentration. The best place to connect the oxygen is directly before the exhalation valve and not near the ventilator or close to the mask.[49] The mixing of the exhaled air with the inhaled air during respiration in the semi-closed system is the cause of decrease in the fraction of inspired oxygen (FiO_2).[49] Oxygen concentrations below 21% are to be expected when no oxygen supply is connected, due to rebreathing into the dead space tubing circuit of the ventilator.[49] Furthermore, the oxygen concentration changes by using different respiration modes and, more specifically, by changing the level of the inspiratory positive airway pressure.[49] Finally, different oxygen flow rates can influence the oxygen concentration without changing other ventilation parameters or settings.[49]

OXYGEN SAFETY

Oxygen is considered relatively safe when handled with care. It is important, however, to recognise that oxygen supports combustion. It is therefore imperative that patients are advised not to smoke and to avoid naked flames, when wearing oxygen therapy. Other sources of ignition also need to be avoided such as electronic cigarettes, hair dryers, electric razors, cookers, heaters and so on. Oxygen users should be cautioned against using petroleum/oil and alcohol-based products such as petroleum gel, face creams and sun lotions on the skin, as they are flammable and there is the potential for a spark to ignite.[6,13]

Equipment should be stored in a well-ventilated area. Concentrators and oxygen cylinder valves should be switched off when not in use. As discussed earlier, consideration should be given to the position of the equipment and the length of tubing to reduce the trip hazard. Oxygen cylinders can be unwieldy and should be secured to ensure they don't fall over.[6,13]

REFERENCES

1. Pruitt W, Jacobs M. Breathing lessons: Basics of oxygen therapy. *Nursing.* 2003;33:43–5.
2. O'Driscoll B, Howard L, Davison A. On behalf of the British Thoracic Society. BTS guideline for emergency oxygen use in adult patients. *Thorax.* 2008;63 Suppl VI:vi1–vi68.
3. O'Neill, Dodd M E. Oxygen on the move: Practical considerations for physiotherapists. *Phys Ther Rev.* 2006;11:28–36.
4. Kampelmacher M, Cornelisse P, Alsbach G et al. Accuracy of oxygen delivery by liquid oxygen canisters. *Eur Respir J.* 1998;12:204–7.
5. British Compressed Gases Association: Cylinder Identification. Colour and labelling Requirements. 2012 Technical Information Sheet 6 Revision 2: 2012.
6. Hardinge M, Annandale J, Bourne S et al. British Thoracic Society Home Oxygen Guideline Group. BTS Guideline for home oxygen use in Adults. *Thorax.* 2015;70 Suppl 1:i1–i43.
7. Rees P, Dudely F. Provision of oxygen at home. *BMJ.* 1998;317:935–8.
8. Pfister S. Home oxygen therapy: Indications, administration, recertification and patient education. *Nurse Pract.* 1995;20:44–7.
9. Murphie P. Oxygen delivery devices: Exploring the options. *Pract Nurs.* 2014;25(3):124–8.
10. McCoy E. Options for home oxygen therapy equipment: Storage and metering of oxygen within the home. *Respir Care.* 2013;58(1):65–81.
11. Stretton T. Provision of long term oxygen therapy. *Thorax.* 1985;40:801–5.
12. Nasilowski J, Przybylowski T, Zielinski J et al. Comparing supplementary oxygen benefits from a portable oxygen concentrator and a liquid oxygen portable device during a walk test in COPD patients on long term oxygen therapy. *J Respir Med.* 2008;102:1021–5.
13. McInturff SL, Dunne PJ. In: Dunne PJ, McInturff SL, eds. *Respiratory Home Care, The Essentials.* 1st edition. Philadelphia: FA Davis Company, 1998. pp. 43–83.
14. Murphie P, Hex N, Setters J et al. Self-fill oxygen technology: Benefits for healthcare providers and the environment. *Breathe.* 2016;12:113–9.
15. Christopher KL, Porte P. Long term oxygen therapy. *Chest.* 2011;139(2):430–4.
16. Goldmann, K. Oxygenation and airway management. *Nursecom Educ Technol.* 2004;3:54–76.
17. Naresh A, Dewan MD, William C. Effect of low flow and high flow oxygen delivery on exercise tolerance and sensation of dyspnoea. A study comparing the transtracheal catheter and nasal prong. *Chest.* 1994;105:1061–5.
18. Eastwood G, O'Connell B, Gardner A et al. Patients' and nurses' perspectives on oxygen therapy: A qualitative study. *J Adv Nurs.* 2009;65:634–41.
19. Agarwal R, Singhal A, Gupta D. What are high-flow and low-flow oxygen delivery systems? *Stroke.* 2005;36:2066–7.
20. Singh C, Singh N, Singh J et al. Emergency medicine: Oxygen therapy. *J Indian Acad Clin Med.* 2001;3:181–3.
21. Eastwood GM, Reeves JH, Cowie BS. Nasopharyngeal oxygen in adult intensive care—Lower flows and increased comfort. *Anaesth Intensive Care.* 2004:32(5):670–1.
22. Cigada M, Gavazzi A, Assi E et al. Gastric rupture after nasopharyngeal oxygen administration. *Intensive Care Med.* 2001;27:939.
23. Eastwood G, Gardner A, O'Connell B. Low flow oxygen therapy: Selecting the right device. *Austral Nurs J.* 2007;15(4):27–30.
24. Olive S. Practical procedures: Oxygen therapy. *Nurs Times.* 2016;112(1/2):12–14.
25. Costello R, Liston R, McNicholas W. Compliance at night with low flow oxygen therapy: A comparison of nasal cannulae and venture masks. *Thorax.* 1995;50(4):405–6.
26. Hagarty E, Skorodin M, Stiers W et al. Performance of a reservoir nasal cannulae (Oxymizer®) during sleep in hypoxemic patients with COPD. *Chest.* 1993;103:1129–34.
27. McConnell EA. Administrating oxygen by nasal cannulae. *Nursing.* 1996;26:14–5.
28. Higgings D. Oxygen therapy. *Nurs Times.* 2005; 101:30–1.
29. Sim M, Dean P, Kinsella J et al. Performance of oxygen delivery devices when the breathing pattern of respiratory failure is simulated. *Anaesthesia.* 2008;63:938–40.
30. Jevon P. Respiratory procedures: Use of a non-rebreathing oxygen mask. *Nurs Times.* 2007; 103(32):26.

31. McConnell E. Administering oxygen by masks. *Nursing*. 1997;27:26.
32. Adock CJ, Dawson JS. The Venturi® mask: More than moulded plastic. *Br J Hosp Med (Lond)*. 2007;68:28–9.
33. Nerlich S. Oxygen therapy. *Austral Nurs J*. 1997;5:23–4.
34. Kampelmacher M, Deenstra M, van Kesteren R et al. Transtracheal oxygen therapy: An effective and safe alternative to nasal oxygen administration. *Eur Respir J*. 1997;10:828–33.
35. Walsh D, Govan J. Long term continuous domiciliary oxygen therapy by transtracheal catheter. *Thorax*. 1990;45:478–81.
36. Amirav I, Balanov I, Gorenberg M et al. Nebulizer hood compared to mask in wheezy infants: Aerosol therapy without tears. *Arch Dis Child*. 2003;88:719–23.
37. Sherwood B, Indyk L, Indyk LN. Danger of plexiglass oxygen hood: Query and clarification. *Pediatrics*. 1971;48:333–5.
38. Ambalavanan N, St John E, Carlo W et al. Feasibility of nitric oxide administration by oxygen hood in neonatal pulmonary hypertension. *J Perinatol*. 2002;22:50–6.
39. Ling E, McDonald L, Dinesen T et al. The OxyArm®: A new minimal contact oxygen delivery system for mouth or nose breathing. *Can J Anesth*. 2002; 49:297–301.
40. Futrell J, Moore J. The OxyArm®: A supplemental oxygen delivery system. *Anesth Analg*. 2006;102:491–4.
41. Dinesen T, McDonnald L, McDonnald S et al. A comparison of the OxyArm® oxygen delivery device and standard nasal cannulae in chronic obstructive pulmonary disease patients. *Respir Care*. 2003;48:120–3.
42. Nishimura M. High-flow nasal cannula oxygen therapy in adults. *J Intensive Care*. 2015;3(1):15. Available from doi:10.1186/s40560-015-0084-5
43. Turnbull B. High-flow humidified oxygen therapy used to alleviate respiratory distress. *Br J Nurs*. 2008;17(19):1226–30.
44. Roca O, Riera J et al. High-flow oxygen therapy in acute respiratory failure. *Resp Care*. 2010; 55(4):408–13.
45. Nava S, Navalesi P, Conti G. Time of noninvasive ventilation. *Intensive Care Med*. 2006;32:361–70.
46. Nava S, Ceriana P. Cause of failure of noninvasive mechanical ventilation. *Respir Care*. 2004;49:295–303.
47. Plant P, Eliott M. Chronic obstructive pulmonary disease: Management of ventilatory failure in COPD. *Thorax*. 2003;58:537–42.
48. Ambrosino N, Vagheggini G. Noninvasive ventilation in exacerbations of COPD. *Int J COPD*. 2007;2:471–6.
49. Thys F, Liistro G, Dozin O et al. Determinants of FiO_2 with oxygen supplementation during noninvasive two-level positive pressure ventilation. *Eur Respir J*. 2002;19:653–7.
50. Eliott MW, Ambrosino N, Schönhofer B et al. Equipment needs for noninvasive mechanical ventilation. *Eur Respir J*. 2002;20:1029–36.

35

Non-invasive ventilation for hypoxaemic respiratory failure

MASSIMO ANTONELLI AND GIUSEPPE BELLO

INTRODUCTION

Patients with hypoxaemic acute respiratory failure (ARF) are defined as those with a ratio of the partial pressure of arterial oxygen (PaO_2) to the fraction of inspired oxygen (FiO_2) of 300 mmHg or less, acute dyspnoea (with a respiratory rate >25 breaths/min and/or active contraction of accessory respiratory muscles) and a partial pressure of carbon dioxide ($PaCO_2$) below or equal to 45 mmHg. In contrast to chronic obstructive pulmonary disease (COPD), the efficacy of non-invasive ventilation (NIV) in patients with hypoxaemic ARF is less clear.

The following sections describe the use of NIV in the heterogeneous group of hypoxaemic ARF patients.

CONTINUOUS POSITIVE AIRWAY PRESSURE AND NIV

The terms CPAP (continuous positive airway pressure) and NIV should not be used interchangeably. CPAP delivers a constant pressure throughout spontaneous inspiration and exhalation without assisting inspiration. Because spontaneous breathing is not assisted during CPAP, this technique requires an intact respiratory drive and adequate alveolar ventilation. Unlike CPAP, NIV provides a pressure during the inspiratory phase greater than the pressure given during exhalation, thus providing ventilatory support and unloading respiratory muscles. NIV is generally delivered by using a combination of pressure support ventilation (PSV) plus positive end-expiratory pressure (PEEP).

RATIONALE

The pathophysiologic mechanisms that underlie hypoxaemic ARF include shunt, ventilation/perfusion abnormalities, and impairment of alveolar–capillary diffusion. The application of positive airway pressure opens underventilated alveoli and increases functional residual capacity, thus decreasing right-to-left intrapulmonary shunt and improving lung mechanics.[1] Furthermore, by lowering left ventricular transmural pressure in patients with left congestive heart failure, positive airway pressure may reduce left ventricular afterload without compromising cardiac index.[2,3]

In hypoxaemic patients, NIV is able to improve dyspnoea and gas exchange, lowering neuromuscular drive and inspiratory muscle effort.[4] On the other hand, CPAP used alone can improve oxygenation, but is less effective in unloading the respiratory muscles.[4]

EVIDENCE BASE

Great caution must be exercised when applying NIV in patients with hypoxaemic ARF, as trials on NIV in these patients have yielded conflicting results. The first application of positive airway pressure (via face mask CPAP) in hypoxaemic patients was reported by Barach et al.[5] in 1938. In 1982, Covelli et al.[6] applied face mask CPAP in 35 patients with hypoxaemia of various aetiologies, with all patients improving their oxygenation within the first hour of therapy. Only five patients were ultimately intubated, due to mask discomfort and lack of cooperation. In 1989, Meduri et al.[7] described one of the first clinical applications of NIV in patients with hypoxaemic ARF. Subsequently, in 1994, Pennock et al.[8] reported a 50% success rate in a large group of patients with ARF of different aetiologies, and similar good results were achieved by Lapinsky et al.[9] using nasal mask.

Surveys

In a multiple centre survey, Antonelli et al.[10] investigated the application of NIV as first-line intervention in 147 patients admitted to the intensive care unit (ICU) with early acute respiratory distress syndrome (ARDS).[11] NIV improved gas exchange and avoided endotracheal intubation (ETI) in 54% of the treated patients. NIV success was associated with less pneumonia (2% vs. 20%, $p < 0.001$) and a lower ICU mortality rate (6% vs. 53%, $p < 0.001$) compared with failures.

A large observational multicentre Italian survey conducted by Gristina et al.[12] on the clinical impact of NIV in 1302 haematological patients admitted to the ICU with ARF confirmed the role of NIV treatment *ab initio* as an independent predictor of survival.

A prospective survey on the use of NIV in 70 French ICUs showed that NIV success was independently associated with survival either in patients with de novo hypoxaemic ARF or in those with cardiogenic pulmonary oedema (CPO) or COPD exacerbation.[13] Interestingly, in that study, NIV failure was associated with ICU mortality only in those patients with de novo hypoxaemic ARF.

A more recent study of NIV in 54 French and Belgian ICUs over a 15-year period found an increase in the overall use of NIV over time and a decline in NIV use in patients with de novo ARF.[14] The study showed an increase in NIV success rate and an overall decrease in mortality. It is worth noting that, in patients with de novo ARF, NIV failure remained more common than in other causes of ARF but was no longer associated with mortality as in previous years, thus suggesting a better selection of patients for NIV therapy and greater expertise of caregivers in the application of NIV during the last few years.

Another large survey performed in the United States from 2000 to 2009 and comparing NIV utilisation trends and failure rates in more than 11 million cases of ARF with or without a diagnosis of COPD showed that the rate of increase in the use of NIV was significantly greater in patients without COPD.[15] Also, in this study, non-COPD patients were more likely to experience NIV failure requiring ETI. Furthermore, patients who required ETI after NIV failure had higher hospital mortality than patients who received invasive mechanical ventilation without a preceding trial of NIV.

Similarly, in their retrospective study on 235 patients, Mosier et al.[16] showed an increased risk of a composite complication (desaturation, hypotension or aspiration) associated with the intubation of critically ill patients who failed NIV compared to patients intubated primarily without a trial of NIV.

A prospective, observational, Italian study aimed to assess the 1-year survival rate of 220 patients treated with NIV outside the ICU because of ARF of heterogeneous causes and to identify the predictors of long-term mortality.[17] Mortality rates at 30 days, 90 days and 1-year follow-up were 20%, 26% and 34%, respectively. These rates, registered in ordinary wards, were similar to those reported for ICU settings. The multivariate analyses identified solid cancer, pneumonia in haematologic patients, and do-not-resuscitate order as independent predictors of mortality, and postoperative ARF associated with improved survival.

Randomised controlled trials

In randomised controlled trials (RCTs), NIV has been compared with either usual medical treatment or conventional mechanical ventilation through an endotracheal tube (Table 35.1).[18–30] The first RCT on NIV in hypoxaemic ARF was reported by Wysocki et al.[18] who randomised 41 non-COPD patients with ARF to NIV delivered by face mask versus conventional medical therapy. NIV reduced the need of ETI, the duration of ICU stay, and mortality rate only in those patients with hypercapnia ($PaCO_2$ > 45 mmHg).

Antonelli et al.[19] compared NIV use to invasive mechanical ventilation in 64 patients with hypoxaemic ARF and showed that patients randomised to invasive ventilation more frequently developed septic complications including pneumonia or sinusitis ($p = 0.003$). Also, in that study, NIV patients had a lower duration of mechanical ventilation ($p = 0.006$) and a shorter ICU stay ($p = 0.002$).

Substantially negative results were reported from an RCT of 27 patients admitted to the emergency department with hypoxaemic respiratory failure who received NIV or conventional medical therapy.[20] The 16 patients in the NIV group had an ETI rate and duration of ICU stay similar to the 11 patients who received medical treatment alone, with a trend toward a greater rate of hospital mortality.

Delclaux et al.[24] randomly assigned 123 patients with hypoxaemic ARF ($n = 102$ with ARDS and $n = 21$ with cardiac disease) to receive standard medical therapy or CPAP. CPAP provided rapid but transient improvements in oxygenation and dyspnoea but failed to reduce ETI rate, hospital mortality or ICU stay compared with standard therapy.

A subset analysis of 29 patients with non-COPD–related ARF showed that patients treated by non-invasive bilevel positive airway pressure (BiPAP) ventilation had a lower ETI rate per 100 ICU days compared to the usual care group (8.5 vs. 30.3; $p = 0.01$), even though no difference in ICU mortality rates was observed between groups.[23]

Ferrer et al.[26] prospectively randomised 105 patients with severe hypoxaemic ARF to receive NIV or high-concentration oxygen. Compared with oxygen therapy, NIV decreased the need for ETI (25% vs. 52%), the incidence of septic shock (12% vs. 31%) and the ICU mortality (18% vs. 39%), and increased the cumulative 90-day survival ($p < 0.05$ for all the variables).

In ARDS, transient loss of positive pressure during mechanical ventilation may seriously compromise lung recruitment and gas exchange. For this reason, most NIV studies have excluded patients with ARDS, and limited data are currently available on this topic. A subset analysis of two RCTs showed that in patients with ARDS ($n = 31$), NIV avoided ETI in 60% of the cases.[19,22] A multicentre RCT on 40 patients with hypoxaemia (200 mmHg < $PaO_2/FIO_2 \leq$ 300 mmHg) in 10 Chinese ICUs reported that NIV was associated with a lower incidence of ETI or organ failure compared with high-concentration oxygen therapy through a Venturi mask.[27]

Complications associated with ETI in immunosuppressed patients have been widely described.[31–33] In these patients, the use of NIV has provided positive results.

Table 35.1 Randomised controlled studies using NIV in hypoxaemic respiratory failure

First author	Year	Population	Intervention		Sample size (NIV/control)	Need for ETI (NIV/control, %)	ICU LOS (NIV/control, days)	ICU mortality (NIV/control, %)	Hospital mortality (NIV/control, %)
			NIV	Control					
Wysocki[18]	1995	Varied	PSV	UMC	21/20	62/70	17 ± 19/25 ± 23	33/50	
Antonelli[19]	1998	Varied	PSV	Invasive MV	32/32	31.3/NA	9 ± 7/16 ± 17[a]	28/47	
Wood[20]	1998	Varied, emergency dep.	BiPAP	UMC	16/11	45.5/43.8	5.8 ± 5.5/4.9 ± 3.2		25/0
Confalonieri[21,b]	1999	CAP	PSV	UMC	16/17	37.5/47.1	2.9 ± 1.8/4.8 ± 1.7		37.5/23.5[a]
Antonelli[22]	2000	IC	PSV	UMC	20/20	20/70[a]	5.5 ± 3/9 ± 4[a]	20/50[a]	35/55
Martin[23,b]	2000	Varied	BiPAP	UMC	16/13	37.5/77[a]		25/54	
Delclaux[24]	2000	Mild[c] ARDS/ cardiac disease	CPAP	UMC	62/61	34/39	6.5 (1–57)/6 (1–36)	21/25	31/30
Hilbert[25]	2001	IC	PSV	UMC	26/26	46/77[a]	7 ± 3/9 ± 4	38/69[a]	50/81[a]
Ferrer[26]	2003	Varied	BiPAP	UCM	51/54	25/52[a]	9.6 ± 12.6/11.3 ± 12.6	9.2/21.4[a]	
Zhan[27]	2012	Mild[c] ARDS	BiPAP	UCM	21/19	4.8/36.8[a]	5.9 (4–10)/7.8 (6–13)	4.8/26.3	4.8/26.3
Brambilla[28]	2014	Pneumonia	CPAP	UCM	40/41	15/63[a]			5/17.1
Lemiale[29]	2015	IC	PSV	UCM	191/183	44.8/38.2	7 (3–16)/6 (3–16)		
Jaber[30]	2016	Postoperative	PSV	UCM	148/145	33.1/45.5[a]	7 (5–14)/8 (5–15)		

Abbreviations: ARDS, acute respiratory distress syndrome; BiPAP, bilevel positive airway pressure; CAP, community-acquired pneumonia; ETI, endotracheal intubation; IC, immunocompromised; ICU, intensive care unit; LOS, length of stay; MV, mechanical ventilation; NA, not applicable; NIV, non-invasive ventilation; PSV, pressure support ventilation; UMC, usual medical care.

[a] Significant difference.

[b] Subset analysis.

[c] 200 mmHg < PaO_2:FiO_2 ≤ 300 mmHg.

Antonelli et al.[22] randomised 40 recipients of solid organ transplantation with ARF to receive NIV versus conventional therapy, showing that patients treated with NIV more often achieved a better oxygenation (60% vs. 25%, $p = 0.03$), with lower ETI (20% vs. 70%, $p = 0.002$) and ICU mortality rates (20% vs. 50%, $p = 0.05$). In another RCT of 52 ARF patients with pneumonia and immunosuppression of various origin, Hilbert et al.[25] showed reductions of ETIs (46% vs. 77%, $p = 0.03$) and lower mortality rate (50% vs. 81%, $p = 0.02$) when NIV patients were compared to controls. Also, CPAP has been used in oncologic patients with ARF in order to prevent their admission to the ICU. Squadrone et al.[34] randomised 40 patients with haematological malignancy recruited in the haematological ward during the early phases of ARF, with PaO_2/FiO_2 levels between 200 and 300 mmHg and without a secure diagnosis of infection, to receive helmet CPAP or standard supplemental oxygen. In that study, patients treated with helmet CPAP were less frequently admitted to the ICU and their ETI rate was lower than that in the control group. In view of this, it would be reasonable to consider NIV as a useful tool to avoid intubation and associated infectious complications in selected patients with immunocompromised states. However, contrasting results were reported by Lemiale et al.[29] in a more recent study on 374 immunocompromised subjects in whom early NIV, compared with standard oxygen therapy, was not associated with any clinical advantage in terms of mortality, ICU-acquired infections, duration of mechanical ventilation and length of ICU stay.

The application of NIV to treat pneumonia has yielded no definitive conclusions. In a multicentre RCT comparing face mask NIV with standard medical treatment by supplemental oxygen in 56 patients with ARF caused by severe community-acquired pneumonia (CAP), Confalonieri et al.[21] found that NIV was associated with a significant reduction in the rate of ETI and duration of ICU stay. Interestingly, in that study, a post hoc analysis showed that among COPD patients with similar severity of illness, those randomised to NIV had a significant reduction in 2-month mortality. Another RCT conducted in four Italian centres showed a reduction of the risk of meeting predefined criteria for intubation and a faster and greater improvement in oxygenation with helmet CPAP in comparison to oxygen therapy in 81 patients with severe hypoxaemic ARF due to pneumonia.[28]

Among studies on the effectiveness of NIV interfaces, a single-centre, randomised clinical trial showed that NIV delivered by helmet significantly reduced the intubation rate among 83 patients with ARDS compared with the patients receiving NIV by face mask.[35] NIV via helmet also was associated with improved ventilator-free days and significantly reduced ICU length of stay as well as 90-day mortality.

Finally, among 293 patients with hypoxaemic respiratory failure following abdominal surgery, use of NIV compared with standard oxygen therapy reduced the risk of ETI within 7 days.[30]

NIV IN SPECIAL CONDITIONS

Cardiogenic pulmonary oedema

Non-invasive use of positive airway pressure should be strongly considered as a first-line treatment in patients with CPO. Both NIV and CPAP have been proven to efficiently improve respiratory distress and metabolic alterations during CPO.[36–38] BiPAP delivered non-invasively has the potential advantage over CPAP of assisting the respiratory muscles during inspiration, which would result in faster alleviation of dyspnoea and exhaustion. However, according to all available data, there is no evidence to suggest superiority of CPAP compared to BiPAP in terms of intubation or mortality, even in patients with CPO and hypercapnia.[39–42] In the management of suspected acute CPO in the pre-hospital setting, helmet CPAP has been used as first-line treatment, allowing prompt improvement in respiratory and haemodynamic parameters.[43] However, favorable results on the use of NIV or CPAP for CPO before hospitalisation are not consistent among studies, thus preventing a firm recommendation regarding the use of positive pressure techniques in this setting.

Immunocompromission

NIV plays a central role in the management of immunocompromised patients, as respiratory failure is the main indication for ICU admission in these patients. Currently available literature is, for the most part, supportive of the use of NIV as the first-line approach for treating mild/moderate ARF in selected patients with immunosuppression of various origins. However, while several studies have proven the clinical benefits of NIV or CPAP in immunocompromised patients,[12,22,34,44] in a more recent multicentre RCT, some investigators could not confirm the benefits of NIV over standard oxygen therapy in these patients.[29]

Post-operative

CPAP or NIV application may be considered a suitable option for the management of patients after thoracic and upper abdominal surgery who frequently develop prolonged postoperative gas exchange deterioration and reduction in functional residual capacity. A systematic review summarised the results of 29 articles where the use of preventive and therapeutic NIV was investigated in post-surgical patients after thoraco-abdominal/bariatric surgical interventions and solid organ transplants.[45] Arterial blood gas improvement and intubation rate reduction were the main benefits associated with the use of NIV. A more recent multicentre RCT on post-operative patients after abdominal surgery confirmed the benefits of NIV in this setting.[30] Thus, accumulating evidence supports the use of NIV/CPAP in reducing respiratory post-operative complications in selected patients.

Trauma

Post-traumatic ARF usually results from reduced pulmonary compliance and functional residual capacity, and subsequent restrictive defects. In a meta-analysis of 10 studies addressing the use of NIV in patients with chest trauma associated with mild to severe respiratory failure, there was no difference between CPAP and PS NIV in terms of mortality, but the latter could significantly increase arterial oxygenation, leading to a reduction in intubation rate and infectious complications incidence.[46] Despite the favorable results obtained, however, large randomised studies are still needed before definitive recommendations on the use of NIV in post-traumatic ARF can be made.

Weaning

NIV use has been proposed as prophylaxis to prevent re-intubation (preventive NIV) or as rescue intervention in case of established post-extubation respiratory failure (rescue NIV). Importantly, in patients with specific risk factors for ARF after extubation, early application of NIV, immediately after extubation, was efficiently used as a tool to prevent post-extubation ARF.[47,48] However, no benefits were found in avoiding reintubation in patients who had developed ARF after extubation, as they showed higher mortality rates as compared with patients treated according to standard treatment.[49,50] Hence, even though NIV approach can be helpful in preventing post-extubation ARF, more data are needed to better define which patient categories may most benefit from its use in such field.

Bronchoscopy

In non-intubated patients, severe hypoxaemia is an accepted contraindication to fiberoptic bronchoscopy. As oxygenation routinely decreases even after uncomplicated bronchoscopy, hypoxaemic patients are at high risk for developing ARF or serious cardiac arrhythmias. Bronchoscopy during NIV has been performed either in patients who were already receiving NIV and were scheduled to perform bronchoscopy or in at-risk patients who were initially breathing spontaneously and who started NIV to assist bronchoscopy.[51,52] Both the facial mask and the helmet may be adopted during fiberoptic bronchoscopy. The bronchoscope is passed through a T adapter applied to the mask and then advanced transnasally; otherwise, the specific seal connector placed in the plastic ring of the helmet may be used as external access for the device.[53]

End of life

NIV may have a role in the management of terminal patients with respiratory failure. In these patients, caregivers should remember that not assuring a quality death to the patient is a serious and irreparable error. Use of NIV in patients with do-not-resuscitate order remains a matter of concern, with some warning of the potential ethical and economic cost of delaying the inevitable in patients with terminal respiratory failure.[54,55] In end-of-life patients with ARF, NIV may be of benefit as it may alleviate dyspnoea and prolong life for a period of time sufficient to possibly carry out personal tasks or realise end-of-life desires. Before initiation of NIV in terminally ill patients, family members and clinicians should have a clear understanding of the possible outcomes of NIV. Controversy remains about which is the most appropriate setting to deliver palliative NIV in end-of-life care.

HOW TO APPLY NIV IN THE HYPOXAEMIC PATIENT

NIV should be considered early when patients first develop signs of incipient respiratory failure needing ventilatory assistance. Clinical criteria for selecting appropriate candidates to receive NIV of the acute care setting include dyspnoea, tachypnoea, accessory muscle use, paradoxical abdominal breathing and gas exchange deterioration. NIV should be avoided in some clinical conditions (Table 35.2), and criteria for ETI and NIV discontinuation must be thoroughly considered to prevent dangerous delays of invasive ventilation (Table 35.3).

Once it has been decided to start NIV, the initial approach should consist in illustrating the various pieces of equipment to the patient and fitting the NIV interface. Patients should be motivated and reassured by the clinician, instructed to coordinate their breathing with the ventilator and encouraged to communicate any discomfort or fears. Although sedation is infrequently required during NIV, caution is advised if benzodiazepines or opiates are administered to prevent hypoventilation or loss of airway protection. During the last few years, dexmedetomidine use has been widely implemented in the clinical practice as a sedative agent, although few data are available in patients undergoing NIV.[56] After an initial period of continuous administration, NIV can be intermittently applied, with variable periods of discontinuation, depending on the patient's respiratory conditions. Collaboration among caregivers including physicians, respiratory therapists and nurses is critical to the success of NIV.

Table 35.2 Criteria for NIV discontinuation and endotracheal intubation

- Technique intolerance (pain, discomfort or claustrophobia)
- Inability to improve gas exchanges and/or respiratory mechanics
- Haemodynamic instability or evidence of cardiac ischaemia or severe arrhythmia
- Severe neurological deterioration or inability to improve mental status in agitated/confused patients

Table 35.3 Contraindications to NIV

- Coma, seizures or severe central neurological disturbances
- Inability to cooperate with fitting and wearing the interface
- Apnoea
- Inability to protect the airway or clear respiratory secretions
- Unstable haemodynamic conditions (blood pressure or rhythm instability)
- Severe upper gastrointestinal bleeding
- Recent facial surgery or significant facial trauma, burns or deformity (unless a helmet is used)
- Recent gastro-oesophageal surgery
- Undrained pneumothorax
- Vomiting

Predictors of success or failure

Identification of predictors of success or failure may help in recognising patients who are likely to benefit from NIV and exclude those for whom NIV would be unsafe or ineffective.

Predictors of NIV failure observed in hypoxaemic patients with ARF are the following:

1. Higher severity score (Simplified Acute Physiology Score [SAPS] II ≥ 35[57]/SAPS II > 34[10]/higher SAPS II[12])
2. Older age (> 40 years)[57]
3. Presence of ARDS or CAP[12,44,57]
4. Failure to improve oxygenation after 1 hour of treatment (PaO_2:FiO_2 ≤ 146 mmHg[57]/PaO_2:FiO_2 ≤ 175 mmHg[10])
5. Higher respiratory rate under NIV[44]
6. Need for vasopressors[37]
7. Need for renal replacement therapy[37]
8. Expired tidal volume above 9.5 mL/kg predicted body weight (PBW) in patients with PaO_2:FiO_2 ≤ 200 mmHg[58]

Lung stretching during NIV

Some concepts should be taken into account when NIV is used. Preserved spontaneous breathing during mechanical ventilation may have either beneficial or detrimental effects on the lung. When a patient is undergoing NIV, measurement of respiratory mechanics cannot be reliably achieved using conventional manoeuvres. Thus, much of the knowledge about respiratory mechanics during NIV comes from experimental or clinical studies conducted in spontaneously breathing subjects under invasive mechanical ventilation.

Compared with fully controlled mechanical ventilation, spontaneous breathing during ventilatory assistance has several beneficial effects, including decreased diaphragmatic atrophy,[59] reduced ventilator-induced lung injury,[60] improved cardiac function,[61] better ventilation–perfusion distribution (with improved tidal ventilation of dependent lung regions)[62,63] and less cyclic collapse in the lung zones close to the diaphragm.[63] However, spontaneous breathing during mechanical ventilation can also be responsible for detrimental effects on lung tissue and clinical outcomes.

Tidal volume is of relevant importance during assisted spontaneous breathing. In a multicentre study on 62 patients with hypoxaemic ARF, Carteaux et al.[58] sought to assess the association between expired tidal volume and NIV outcome. In their study, NIV was started with a pressure support level of 8 cmH_2O and then adjusted in an attempt to target a predefined tidal volume of 6–8 PBW. They found that a higher expired tidal volume was independently associated with NIV failure. In particular, an expired tidal volume above 9.5 mL/kg PBW could accurately predict NIV failure when patients had a PaO_2:FiO_2 ratio ≤ 200 mmHg. Interestingly, in this study, targeting a 6–8 PBW range of expired tidal volume could not be achieved in the majority of the patient population. In fact, the pressure support level used to deliver NIV was often the lowest value (7 cmH_2O) allowed by the study protocol, suggesting that the persistently high tidal volume was mainly driven by continued strong patient's inspiratory efforts, more than the respiratory muscle pressure generated by the patient. In this context, possible strategies to decrease spontaneous breathing efforts might be the early intubation or the administration of sedative drugs, but that is not currently supported by clear evidence.

Limiting transpulmonary pressure during mechanical ventilation is an accepted approach to avoid lung overdistention. By convention, transpulmonary pressure is the difference between the pressure at the airway opening and the pleural or esophageal pressure.[64] The total transpulmonary pressure comprises the pressure needed to generate the airflow across the airway, yielding an inspiratory flow, and the pressure needed to expand the terminal airways, that is, the transalveolar pressure (product of lung elastance and volume), which is the only part of transpulmonary pressure that is dissipated across the alveoli and is considered to contribute to functional and histologic lung damage.[65]

When a patient is breathing spontaneously under mechanical ventilation, addition of spontaneous effort to a mechanical breath results in a further effect to the transpulmonary pressure because positive ventilator pressure in the alveoli is increased with the negative pleural pressure caused by diaphragmatic excursion, resulting in higher pressure across the whole lung. Measuring transpulmonary pressure has been commonly used to assess lung stretching during mechanical ventilation in experimental and clinical research.

Animal studies have pointed out the risks associated with spontaneous breathing during ventilatory assistance. In an ARDS animal model, Yoshida et al.[66] demonstrated that, even when plateau pressure is limited to <30 cmH_2O, transpulmonary pressure generated by strenuous breathing efforts may exceed plateau pressure and, combined with increased respiratory rate and tidal volume, exacerbate lung damage. In another animal study, these investigators showed that in the injured lung, local negative pleural pressure generated by diaphragmatic contraction is not uniformly transmitted, but is concentrated in dependent lung regions.[67] This causes a 'pendelluft' phenomenon, with shift of gas from nondependent to dependent lung regions, without gain in tidal volume and with a transient overstretching of dependent lung and a concurrent deflation of nondependent lung.[67] In a more recent study on a severe ARDS animal model, the same authors showed that spontaneous effort at low PEEP improved oxygenation but promoted the pendelluft phenomenon, whereas higher PEEP levels could reduce the intensity of inspiratory effort, thus reducing pendelluft and its potential consequences.[68]

Bellani et al.[69] compared the amplitude of the change in transpulmonary pressure during spontaneous assisted breathing and fully controlled ventilation, trying to match similar conditions of airflow and volume, in 10 patients undergoing different levels of PSV followed by a phase of controlled mechanical ventilation. They showed that under similar conditions of flow and volume, transpulmonary pressure change was similar between controlled mechanical ventilation and PSV. Predictably, transpulmonary pressure was positive during controlled mechanical ventilation, whereas decreasing levels of pressure support assistance led to progressively more negative changes in transpulmonary pressure, causing remarkably negative swings also in alveolar pressure, a mechanism by which spontaneous breathing might potentially induce lung damage. From a haemodynamic standpoint, these negative pressure swings during assisted spontaneous breathing can lead to increased vascular pressure in the pulmonary circulation, which is associated with extravascular lung water accumulation and constitutes one of the known factors contributing to lung injury.[70]

In view of the above, when spontaneous breathing is preserved during mechanical ventilation as in the case of NIV, caregivers should be aware that the presence of strong inspiratory effort can result in a non-protective ventilation, with excessive levels of transpulmonary pressure and a hidden lung overstretch even if airway pressures are not high.

NIV VERSUS HIGH-FLOW NASAL CANNULA OXYGENATION

High-flow nasal cannula oxygenation (HFNCO) is increasingly being utilised in critically ill patients. Use of nasal prongs to deliver high heated and humidified flow (maximum 60 L/min) at a prescribed FiO_2 is an attractive alternative to conventional oxygen therapy. The main potential mechanisms through which HFNCO may alleviate symptoms of respiratory distress and enhance gas exchange include deadspace washout with subsequent facilitation of CO_2 removal, provision of a moderate flow-dependent positive airway pressure that may result in alveolar recruitment, reduction in inspiratory nasopharyngeal resistance and a better tolerance and comfort with the technique.[71] Levels of airway pressure (generally <4 cmH_2O) measured in the nasopharynx or the trachea increase as flow increases and are higher during breathing with mouth closed compared with mouth open.[72,73] Over the last years, HFNCO use has been compared with NIV in the critical care setting. HFNCO and NIV are two technically different methods (Table 35.4) and use different mechanisms to achieve clinical outcomes.

In an RCT, 310 patients with hypoxaemic ARF were randomised to receive nasal high-flow oxygen therapy, standard oxygen through a face mask or NIV. Interestingly, among the three interventions, no significant differences were observed in terms of intubation rate, but the treatment with high-flow oxygen was associated with a significant lower number of ventilator-free days at day 28 and 90-day mortality rate.[74] Similarly, in a larger cohort of cardiothoracic surgical patients, deemed at risk for respiratory failure after extubation, high-flow nasal oxygen therapy was not inferior to NIV delivered as bilevel positive airway pressure in terms of reintubation and ICU mortality.[75] On the other hand, delayed intubation after HFNCO therapy failure has been found to be associated with adverse outcomes, including increased overall ICU mortality, poorer extubation success and ventilator weaning and fewer ventilator-free days.[76]

Table 35.4 Technical differences between high-flow nasal cannula oxygenation and NIV

	HFNCO	NIV
Ability to apply a predefined level of PEEP	No	Yes
Ability to apply positive pressure during inspiratory phase	No	Yes
Additional dead space	No	Yes (depending on the interface or the use of HME)
Risk for skin breakdown	No	Yes (depending on the interface)
Compromised ability to speak or eat	No	Yes (depending on the interface)
Problems of asynchrony	No	Yes (depending on the interface or ventilation mode)
Need of ventilator	No	Yes
Availability of respiratory monitoring (e.g. TV and MV)	No	Yes
Availability of respiratory alarms (e.g. TV and MV)	No	Yes

Abbreviations: HFNCO, high-flow nasal cannula oxygenation; HME, heat and moisture exchanger; MV, minute ventilation; NIV, non-invasive ventilation; PEEP, positive end-expiratory pressure; TV, tidal volume.

Hence, despite the above recent encouraging results, strong data are still lacking before suggesting HFNCO instead of NIV or CPAP as first-line treatment for critically ill patients in whom supplemental oxygen is not sufficient.

CONCLUSIONS

NIV can be used to treat hypoxaemic patients without hypercapnia. However, an extremely prudent approach is needed, limiting the application of NIV to haemodynamically stable patients who can be closely monitored in the ICU, where ETI is promptly available. Patients at high risk of failure should be closely managed only by experienced personnel and with a low threshold for ETI.

Further studies may be useful in clarifying the actual role of HFNCO, compared with NIV, in the management of patients with hypoxaemic ARF.

REFERENCES

1. Katz JA, Marks JD. Inspiratory work with and without continuous positive airway pressure in patients with acute respiratory failure. *Anesthesiology*. 1985; 63:598–607.
2. Räsänen J, Heikkilä J, Downs J et al. Continuous positive airway pressure by face mask in acute cardiogenic pulmonary edema. *Am J Cardiol*. 1985;55:296–300.
3. Naughton MT, Rahman MA, Hara K et al. Effect of continuous positive airway pressure on intrathoracic and left ventricular transmural pressures in patients with congestive heart failure. *Circulation*. 1995;91:1725–31.
4. L'Her E, Deye N, Lellouche F et al. Physiologic effects of noninvasive ventilation during acute lung injury. *Am J Respir Crit Care Med*. 2005;172:1112–8.
5. Barach AL, Martin J, Eckman M. Positive-pressure respiration and its application to the treatment of acute pulmonary edema. *Ann Intern Med*. 1938;12:754–95.
6. Covelli HD, Weled BJ, Beekman JF. Efficacy of continuous positive airway pressure administered by face mask. *Chest*. 1982;81:147–50.
7. Meduri GU, Conoscenti CC, Menashe P et al. Noninvasive face mask ventilation in patients with acute respiratory failure. *Chest*. 1989;95:865–70.
8. Pennock BE, Crawshaw L, Kaplan PD. Noninvasive nasal mask ventilation for acute respiratory failure. Institution of a new therapeutic technology for routine use. *Chest*. 1994;105:441–4.
9. Lapinsky SE, Mount DB, Mackey D, Grossman RF. Management of acute respiratory failure due to pulmonary edema with nasal positive pressure support. *Chest*. 1994;105:229–31.
10. Antonelli M, Conti G, Esquinas A et al. A multiple-center survey on the use in clinical practice of noninvasive ventilation as a first-line intervention for acute respiratory distress syndrome. *Crit Care Med*. 2007;35:18–25.
11. ARDS Definition Task Force, Ranieri VM, Rubenfeld GD, Thompson BT et al. Acute respiratory distress syndrome: The Berlin Definition. *JAMA*. 2012; 307:2526–33.
12. Gristina GR, Antonelli M, Conti G et al. Noninvasive versus invasive ventilation for acute respiratory failure in patients with hematologic malignancies: A 5-year multicenter observational survey. *Crit Care Med*. 2011;39:2232–9.
13. Demoule A, Girou E, Richard JC, Taille S, Brochard L. Benefits and risks of success or failure of non-invasive ventilation. *Intensive Care Med*. 2006;32: 1756–65.
14. Demoule A, Chevret S, Carlucci A et al; oVNI Study Group; REVA Network (Research Network in Mechanical Ventilation). Changing use of noninvasive ventilation in critically ill patients: Trends over 15 years in francophone countries. *Intensive Care Med*. 2016;42:82–92.
15. Walkey AJ, Wiener RS. Use of noninvasive ventilation in patients with acute respiratory failure, 2000–2009: A population-based study. *Ann Am Thorac Soc*. 2013; 10:10–7.
16. Mosier JM, Sakles JC, Whitmore SP et al. Failed non-invasive positive-pressure ventilation is associated with an increased risk of intubation-related complications. *Ann Intensive Care*. 2015;5:4.
17. Cabrini L, Landoni G, Bocchino S et al. Long-term survival rate in patients with acute respiratory failure treated with noninvasive ventilation in ordinary wards. *Crit Care Med*. 2016. DOI: 10.1097 /CCM.0000000000001866.
18. Wysocki M, Tric L, Wolff MA et al. Noninvasive pressure support ventilation in patients with acute respiratory failure: A randomized comparison with conventional therapy. *Chest*. 1995;107:761–8.
19. Antonelli M, Conti G, Rocco M et al. A comparison of noninvasive positive-pressure ventilation and conventional mechanical ventilation in patients with acute respiratory failure. *N Engl J Med*. 1998;339:429–35.
20. Wood KA, Lewis L, Von Harz B, Kollef MH. The use of noninvasive positive pressure ventilation in the emergency department. *Chest*. 1998;113:1339–46.
21. Confalonieri M, Potena A, Carbone G et al. Acute respiratory failure in patients with severe community-acquired pneumonia. A prospective randomized evaluation of noninvasive ventilation. *Am J Respir Crit Care Med*. 1999;160:1585–91.
22. Antonelli M, Conti C, Bufi M et al. Noninvasive ventilation for treatment of acute respiratory failure in patients undergoing solid organ transplantation. *JAMA*. 2000;283:235–41.
23. Martin TJ, Hovis JD, Costantino JP et al. A randomized prospective evaluation of noninvasive ventilation for acute respiratory failure. *Am J Respir Crit Care Med*. 2000;161:807–13.

24. Delclaux C, L'Her E, Alberti C et al. Treatment of acute hypoxemic nonhypercapnic respiratory insufficiency with continuous positive airway pressure delivered by a face mask: A randomized controlled trial. *JAMA*. 2000;284:2352–60.
25. Hilbert G, Gruson D, Vargas F et al. Noninvasive ventilation in immunosuppressed patients with pulmonary infiltrates, fever, and acute respiratory failure. *N Engl J Med*. 2001;344:481–7.
26. Ferrer M, Esquinas A, Leon M et al. Noninvasive ventilation in severe hypoxemic respiratory failure: A randomized clinical trial. *Am J Respir Crit Care Med*. 2003;168:1438–44.
27. Zhan Q, Sun B, Liang L et al. Early use of noninvasive positive pressure ventilation for acute lung injury: A multicenter randomized controlled trial. *Crit Care Med*. 2012;40:455–60.
28. Brambilla AM, Aliberti S, Prina E et al. Helmet CPAP vs. oxygen therapy in severe hypoxemic respiratory failure due to pneumonia. *Intensive Care Med*. 2014;40:942–9.
29. Lemiale V, Mokart D, Resche-Rigon M et al.; Groupe de recherche en réanimation respiratoire du patient d'onco-hématologie (GRRR-OH). Effect of noninvasive ventilation vs oxygen therapy on mortality among immunocompromised patients with acute respiratory failure: A randomized clinical trial. *JAMA*. 2015;314:1711–9.
30. Jaber S, Lescot T, Futier E et al. Effect of noninvasive ventilation on tracheal reintubation among patients with hypoxemic respiratory failure following abdominal surgery: A randomized clinical trial. *JAMA*. 2016;315:1345–53.
31. Estopa R, Torres Marti A, Kastanos N et al. Acute respiratory failure in severe hematologic disorders. *Crit Care Med*. 1984;12:26–8.
32. Blot F, Guignet M, Nitenberg G et al. Prognostic factors for neutropenic patients in an intensive care unit: Respective roles of underlying malignancies and acute organ failures. *Eur J Cancer*. 1997;33:1031–7.
33. Ewig S, Torres A, Riquelme R et al. Pulmonary complications in patients with haematological malignancies treated at a respiratory ICU. *Eur Respir J*. 1998;12:116–22.
34. Squadrone V, Massaia M, Bruno B et al. Early CPAP prevents evolution of acute lung injury in patients with hematologic malignancy. *Intensive Care Med*. 2010;36:1666–74.
35. Patel BK, Wolfe KS, Pohlman AS et al. Effect of noninvasive ventilation delivered by helmet vs face mask on the rate of endotracheal intubation in patients with acute respiratory distress syndrome: A randomized clinical trial. *JAMA*. 2016;315:2435–41.
36. Crane SD, Elliott MW, Gilligan P et al. Randomised controlled comparison of continuous positive airways pressure, bilevel non-invasive ventilation, and standard treatment in emergency department in patients with acute cardiogenic pulmonary oedema. *Emerg Med J*. 2004;21:155–61.
37. Bellone A, Vettorello M, Monari A et al. Noninvasive pressure support ventilation vs. continuous positive airway pressure in acute hypercapnic pulmonary edema. *Intensive Care Med*. 2005;31:807–11.
38. Gray A, Goodacre S, Newby DE et al.; 3CPO Trialists. Noninvasive ventilation in acute cardiogenic pulmonary edema. *N Engl J Med*. 2008;359:142–51.
39. Wysocki M. Noninvasive ventilation in acute cardiogenic pulmonary edema: Better than continuous positive airway pressure? *Intensive Care Med*. 1999;25:1–2.
40. Masip J, Roque M, Sanchez B et al. Noninvasive ventilation in acute cardiogenic pulmonary edema: Systematic review and meta-analysis. *JAMA*. 2005;294:3124–30.
41. Collins SP, Mielniczuk LM, Whittingham HA et al. The use of noninvasive ventilation in emergency department patients with acute cardiogenic pulmonary edema: A systematic review. *Ann Emerg Med*. 2006;48:260–9.
42. Ho KM, Wong K. A comparison of continuous and bi-level positive airway pressure non-invasive ventilation in patients with acute cardiogenic pulmonary oedema: A meta-analysis. *Crit Care*. 2006;10:R49.
43. Foti G, Sangalli F, Berra L et al. Is helmet CPAP first line pre-hospital treatment of presumed severe acute pulmonary edema? *Intensive Care Med*. 2009;35:656–62.
44. Adda M, Coquet I, Darmon M et al. Predictors of noninvasive ventilation failure in patients with hematologic malignancy and acute respiratory failure. *Crit Care Med*. 2008;36:2766–72.
45. Chiumello D, Chevallard G, Gregoretti C. Noninvasive ventilation in postoperative patients: A systematic review. *Intensive Care Med*. 2011;37:918–29.
46. Chiumello D, Coppola S, Froio S et al. Noninvasive ventilation in chest trauma: Systematic review and meta-analysis. *Intensive Care Med*. 2013;39:1171–80.
47. Nava S, Gregoretti C, Fanfulla F et al. Noninvasive ventilation to prevent respiratory failure after extubation in high-risk patients. *Crit Care Med*. 2005;33:2465–70.
48. Ferrer M, Valencia M, Nicolas JM et al. Early noninvasive ventilation averts extubation failure in patients at risk: A randomized trial. *Am J Respir Crit Care Med*. 2006;173:164–70.
49. Keenan SP, Powers C, McCormack DG, Block G. Noninvasive positive-pressure ventilation for postextubation respiratory distress: A randomized controlled trial. *JAMA*. 2002;287:3238–44.
50. Esteban A, Frutos-Vivar F, Ferguson ND et al. Noninvasive positive-pressure ventilation for respiratory failure after extubation. *N Engl J Med*. 2004;350:2452–60.

51. Antonelli M, Conti G, Riccioni L et al. Noninvasive positive-pressure ventilation via face mask during bronchoscopy with BAL in high-risk hypoxemic patients. *Chest.* 1996;110:724–8.
52. Antonelli M, Conti G, Rocco M et al. Noninvasive positive-pressure ventilation vs. conventional oxygen supplementation in hypoxemic patients undergoing diagnostic bronchoscopy. *Chest.* 2002;121:1149–54.
53. Antonelli M, Pennisi MA, Conti G et al. Fiberoptic bronchoscopy during noninvasive positive pressure ventilation delivered by helmet. *Intensive Care Med.* 2003;29:126–9.
54. Clarke DE, Vaughan L, Raffin TA. Noninvasive positive pressure ventilation for patients with terminal respiratory failure: The ethical and economic costs of delaying the inevitable are too great. *Am J Crit Care.* 1994;3:4–5.
55. Azoulay E, Kouatchet A, Jaber S et al. Noninvasive mechanical ventilation in patients having declined tracheal intubation. *Intensive Care Med.* 2013;39: 292–301.
56. Huang Z, Chen YS, Yang ZL, Liu JY. Dexmedetomidine versus midazolam for the sedation of patients with non-invasive ventilation failure. *Intern Med.* 2012; 51:2299–305.
57. Antonelli M, Conti G, Moro ML et al. Predictors of failure of noninvasive positive pressure ventilation in patients with acute hypoxemic respiratory failure: A multi-center study. *Intensive Care Med.* 2001;27:1718–28.
58. Carteaux G, Millán-Guilarte T, De Prost N et al. Failure of noninvasive ventilation for de novo acute hypoxemic respiratory failure: Role of tidal volume. *Crit Care Med.* 2016;44:282–90.
59. Futier E, Constantin JM, Combaret L et al. Pressure support ventilation attenuates ventilator-induced protein modifications in the diaphragm. *Crit Care.* 2008;12:R116.
60. Xia J, Zhang H, Sun B et al. Spontaneous breathing with biphasic positive airway pressure attenuates lung injury in hydrochloric acid–induced acute respiratory distress syndrome. *Anesthesiology.* 2014;120:1441–9.
61. Putensen C, Zech S, Wrigge H et al. Long-term effects of spontaneous breathing during ventilatory support in patients with acute lung injury. *Am J Respir Crit Care Med.* 2001;164:43–9.
62. Putensen C, Mutz NJ, Putensen-Himmer G, Zinserling J. Spontaneous breathing during ventilatory support improves ventilation-perfusion distributions in patients with acute respiratory distress syndrome. *Am J Respir Crit Care Med.* 1999;159:1241–8.
63. Wrigge H, Zinserling J, Neumann P et al. Spontaneous breathing with airway pressure release ventilation favors ventilation in dependent lung regions and counters cyclic alveolar collapse in oleic-acid-induced lung injury: A randomized controlled computed tomography trial. *Crit Care.* 2005;9:R780–9.
64. Akoumianaki E, Maggiore SM, Valenza F et al. The application of esophageal pressure measurement in patients with respiratory failure. *Am J Respir Crit Care Med.* 2014;189:520–31.
65. Slutsky AS, Ranieri VM. Ventilator-induced lung injury. *N Engl J Med.* 2013;369:2126–36. Erratum in: *N Engl J Med.* 2014;370:1668–9.
66. Yoshida T, Uchiyama A, Matsuura N et al. Spontaneous breathing during lung-protective ventilation in an experimental acute lung injury model: High transpulmonary pressure associated with strong spontaneous breathing effort may worsen lung injury. *Crit Care Med.* 2012;40:1578–85.
67. Yoshida T, Torsani V, Gomes S et al. Spontaneous effort causes occult pendelluft during mechanical ventilation. *Am J Respir Crit Care Med.* 2013; 188:1420–7.
68. Yoshida T, Roldan R, Beraldo MA et al. Spontaneous effort during mechanical ventilation: Maximal injury with less positive end-expiratory pressure. *Crit Care Med.* 2016;44:e678–88.
69. Bellani G, Grasselli G, Teggia-Droghi M et al. Do spontaneous and mechanical breathing have similar effects on average transpulmonary and alveolar pressure? A clinical crossover study. *Crit Care.* 2016;20:142.
70. Dreyfuss D, Saumon G. Ventilator-induced lung injury: Lessons from experimental studies. *Am J Respir Crit Care Med.* 1998;157:294–323.
71. Papazian L, Corley A, Hess D et al. Use of high-flow nasal cannula oxygenation in ICU adults: A narrative review. *Intensive Care Med.* 2016;42:1336–49.
72. Parke RL, McGuinness SP. Pressures delivered by nasal high flow oxygen during all phases of the respiratory cycle. *Respir Care.* 2013;58:1621–4.
73. Chanques G, Riboulet F, Molinari N et al. Comparison of three high flow oxygen therapy delivery devices: A clinical physiological cross-over study. *Minerva Anestesiol.* 2013;79:1344–55.
74. Frat JP, Thille AW, Mercat A et al.; FLORALI Study Group; REVA Network. High-flow oxygen through nasal cannula in acute hypoxemic respiratory failure. *N Engl J Med.* 2015;372:2185–96.
75. Stéphan F, Barrucand B, Petit P et al.; BiPOP Study Group. High-flow nasal oxygen vs noninvasive positive airway pressure in hypoxemic patients after cardiothoracic surgery: A randomized clinical trial. *JAMA.* 2015;313:2331–9.
76. Kang BJ, Koh Y, Lim CM et al. Failure of high-flow nasal cannula therapy may delay intubation and increase mortality. *Intensive Care Med.* 2015; 41:623–32.

PART 7

Cardiac failure

36 Acute heart failure syndrome 326
Ross S. Archibald and Alasdair J. Gray
37 Ventilation in chronic congestive cardiac failure 341
Matthew T. Naughton

36

Acute heart failure syndrome

ROSS S. ARCHIBALD AND ALASDAIR J. GRAY

KEY POINTS

1. In patients with acute heart failure syndrome (AHFS) and significant respiratory compromise, non-invasive ventilation (NIV) is now widely used either as a primary intervention or as an adjunctive treatment if there has been failure to respond to standard medical therapy.
2. NIV has a number of potentially beneficial physiological effects in AHFS, including the following:
   - Splinting alveoli open at the end of expiration, thereby improving lung compliance, ventilation/perfusion (V/Q) ratio and gas exchange
   - Improvement of cardiac output, via a reduction in both preload and afterload
   - Pushing fluid out of the alveoli and preventing further transfer of fluid inward in pulmonary oedema
3. NIV provides significant early improvement in patient symptoms and physiological parameters in AHFS.
4. The mortality benefit of NIV in AHFS remains unclear.
5. Despite theoretical advantages, there is no evidence demonstrating additional benefit of bilevel positive airway pressure over continuous positive airway pressure in AHFS.

DEFINITION AND CLASSIFICATION

Acute heart failure syndrome[1] (AHFS) is a clinical condition characterised by the rapid onset or deterioration in the signs and/or symptoms of heart failure.[2] It is a potentially life-threatening medical condition requiring urgent assessment and management, and typically requires hospital admission.[2]

AHFS may be the first manifestation, or more frequently, a consequence of acute decompensation of known chronic heart failure. It may be precipitated by acute cardiac dysfunction secondary to ischaemia, arrhythmias, inflammation or toxins, or extrinsic factors such as infection, uncontrolled hypertension, non-adherence with medications or diet.[2,3] Patients typically present with signs and symptoms that relate to isolated pulmonary congestion or generalised systemic congestion, occurring as a result of elevated ventricular filling pressures, accompanied by dyspnoea.[4] Twenty-five to fifty per cent of patients will present with acute pulmonary oedema as part of the clinical syndrome, and this may occur with or without systemic congestion and fluid overload.[5–8]

Historically, the classification of heart failure has been based on measurement of left ventricular ejection fraction (LVEF).[2] Patients with heart failure may have normal LVEF (typically considered as ≥50%), mid-range LVEF (40%–49%) or reduced LVEF (<40%). Differentiation of heart failure based on LVEF is important due to differing associated aetiologies, demographics, comorbidities and potential response to therapies.[2]

A number of overlapping classifications and criteria for AHFS have been proposed.[2] In practice, it is most useful to classify AHFS by the signs and symptoms at initial presentation, allowing therapy to be directed appropriately.[2] One approach is defined by the presence or absence of the clinical symptoms and signs of congestion and hypoperfusion, allowing four clinical groups to be established[2] (Figure 36.1): *warm and wet* (well perfused and congested, the most common); *cold and wet* (hypoperfused and congested); *cold and dry* (hypoperfused without congestion); and *warm and dry* (compensated, well perfused without congestion).

More recently, a number of authorities, most notably Collins and colleagues,[9] advocate that clinical classification and initial treatment of AHFS is based on blood pressure.

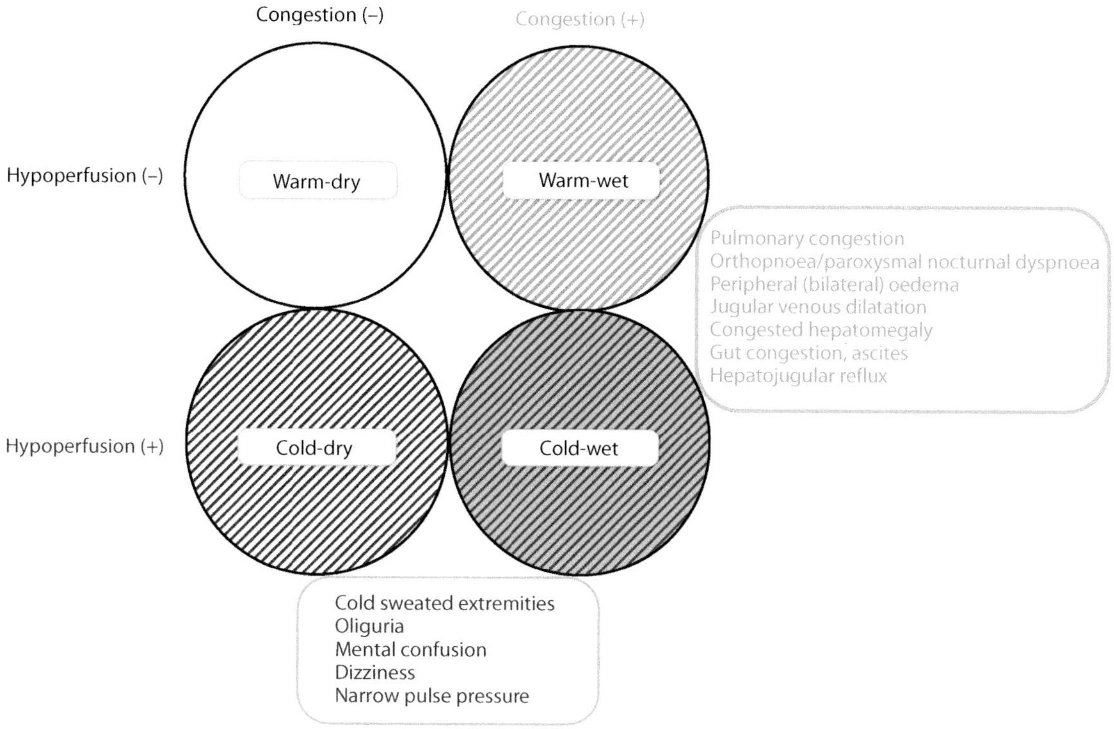

Congestion (–) Congestion (+)

Hypoperfusion (–) Warm-dry Warm-wet

Pulmonary congestion
Orthopnoea/paroxysmal nocturnal dyspnoea
Peripheral (bilateral) oedema
Jugular venous dilatation
Congested hepatomegaly
Gut congestion, ascites
Hepatojugular reflux

Hypoperfusion (+) Cold-dry Cold-wet

Cold sweated extremities
Oliguria
Mental confusion
Dizziness
Narrow pulse pressure

Figure 36.1 Clinical grouping of patients with acute heart failure based on the presence/absence of congestion and/or hypoperfusion. (Adapted from Ponikowski et al. 2016 European Society of Cardiology Guidelines for the diagnosis and treatment of acute and chronic heart failure.)

Hypertensive acute heart failure (H-AHF) is defined as the rapid onset of pulmonary congestion in the setting of a systolic blood pressure over 140 mmHg and comprises a significant proportion of patients with AHFS, with large registries showing that 50% of patients with AHFS have elevated blood pressure upon presentation.[9] H-AHF is characterised by distinct underlying pathophysiological mechanisms resulting in elevated left ventricular filling pressures, rather than solely volume overload. It is proposed that treatment in this clinical subgroup should be reflective of this, with a focus on preload and afterload reduction with vasodilators rather than volume removal with diuretics.[9]

ASSESSMENT, DIAGNOSIS AND PROGNOSTICATION

The diagnosis of AHFS is primarily based on clinical evaluation, including a clear history and examination, supported by appropriate initial investigations including a 12-lead electrocardiogram (ECG) and plain radiograph of the chest.[8,10] Symptoms typically include breathlessness at rest, orthopnoea, paroxysmal nocturnal dyspnoea or increased dyspnoea on exercise, in conjunction with clinical findings of a third heart sound, pulmonary crackles, raised jugular venous pressure and leg oedema. These, together with a history of heart failure or ischaemic heart disease, all increase the likelihood of a diagnosis of acute heart failure.[11]

However, in reality, the diagnosis of AHFS remains challenging. A recent systematic review and meta-analysis of 57 studies by Martindale and colleagues[12] assessed the ability of standard clinical information and diagnostic tests to predict AHFS as a cause of undifferentiated dyspnoea in adult patients in the emergency department. It was found that, on their own, commonly sought elements of clinical history, physical examination and investigations, including chest radiography and electrocardiography, lack discriminatory value in the confirmation or exclusion of a diagnosis of acute heart failure.[12] For example, S3 gallop was the examination finding with the highest specificity for AHFS, at 0.97 (0.97–0.98 95% CI), but with a sensitivity of only 0.13 (0.11–0.14 95% CI), while pulmonary crackles and peripheral oedema had even poorer test characteristics.[12] Echocardiography and bedside lung ultrasound were found to have the best test characteristics for confirming the presence of AHFS, with the presence or absence of diffuse B-lines on ultrasound the most useful finding (sensitivity, 0.85 [0.82–0.87 95% CI]; specificity, 0.92 [0.90–0.94 95% CI]). The review did not evaluate the diagnostic utility of these elements in combination.

Serum natriuretic peptides (NPs), including brain natriuretic peptide (BNP), N-terminal pro-B-type natriuretic peptide (NT-proBNP) and mid-regional pro-atrial natriuretic peptide (MR-proANP), are increasingly used to support the diagnosis of AHFS in emergency patients.[13] National and international guidance[2,14] currently recommends that in people presenting with suspected acute heart failure, a single measurement of one of these NPs may be used to rule out the diagnosis of heart failure, with the following thresholds: BNP < 100 ng/L, NT-proBNP < 300 ng/L and MR-proANP <120 pg/mL. A recent large systematic review and meta-analysis by Roberts and colleagues[13] including 42 studies with a total of 15,263 test results found that at these recommended thresholds, BNP, NT-proBNP and MR-proANP have excellent ability to exclude a diagnosis of acute heart failure. At the above recommended thresholds, sensitivities ranged from 0.95 for BNP (0.93–0.96 95% CI), 0.99 for NT-proBNP (0.97 to 1.0 95% CI) and 0.95 for MR-proANP (0.90–0.98 95% CI). The specificity of NPs is variable, so further investigations, such as echocardiogram, chest radiograph and lung ultrasound, are required to confirm a diagnosis of heart failure.[13] Introduction of NP measurement in the investigation of patients with suspected AHFS therefore has the potential to allow rapid and accurate exclusion of the diagnosis.[13] This is likely to be particularly helpful in the intermediate clinical risk group of patients, where a very low result effectively rules out a diagnosis of AHFS. However, it is important to note that elevated levels of NPs do not automatically confirm a diagnosis of AHF, as they may also be associated with a wide variety of other cardiac and non-cardiac conditions, including chronic obstructive pulmonary disease (COPD) and pulmonary embolism.[2]

Please see the e-book for details of biomarkers, which have been suggested to be of prognostic importance in AHFS.

CLINICAL MANAGEMENT

In patients with acute pulmonary oedema and respiratory failure, non-invasive ventilation (NIV) is now widely used in emergency and critical care settings either as the primary intervention or as an adjunctive treatment if pharmacological therapies in conjunction with oxygen are failing to deliver clinical improvement.[15–17] The evidence base supporting the use of NIV will be discussed in detail later in the chapter. Although continuous positive airway pressure support (CPAP) is not technically a mode of ventilation, it will be included with bilevel positive airway pressure (BiPAP) support as NIV for ease of discussion in this chapter.

The principal pharmacological agents used in the treatment of AHFS have changed little in recent years and comprise loop diuretics, intravenous vasodilators (usually nitrate) and cautiously titrated intravenous opiates. The international Acute Heart Failure Global Survey of Standard Treatment (ALARM-HF)[18] collected data from 4953 patients with acute heart failure from 666 hospitals across nine countries (France, UK, Germany, Turkey, Italy, Spain, Greece, Australia and Mexico). The median age of patients was between 66 and 70 years, and 62.4% were male.[18] Clinical presentations included the following: decompensated congestive heart failure (38.6%), pulmonary oedema (36.7%) and cardiogenic shock (11.7%).[18] It compared patients with de novo acute heart failure (36.2%) to those with a pre-existing episode of AHFS (63.8%), and distinguished subgroups hospitalised in intensive care units (ICU), cardiac care units and ward environments. Overall, intravenous diuretics were given in 89.7%, vasodilators in 41.1%, and inotropic agents (dobutamine, dopamine, adrenaline, noradrenaline and levosimendan) in 39% of cases. Another large database, the Acute Decompensated Heart Failure National Registry (ADHERE),[19] characterised more than 100,000 patients from 274 hospitals across the United States. The mean age of patients was 72 years, and 48% were male.[19] A lower proportion of patients (23.4%) than ALARM-HF received intravenous vasoactive treatment, consisting of nesiritide (10.0%), milrinone (3.1%) or dobutamine (6.4%).[19] Recently, many of these established pharmacological agents have been questioned.[15,20,21] There remains a paucity of evidence to support their effectiveness and there are observational data suggestive of an association with worse outcomes.[22–25] A detailed review of the mechanism of action, evidence base and role in management of the main pharmacological agents used to treat AHFS can be found in the e-book.

A number of novel pharmacological agents have been evaluated for the management of AHFS. In general, they are of unclear benefit, are only used in specialist settings, vary in their use depending on country or continent or are experimental. A brief overview of these agents can also be found in the e-book.

The immediate treatment goals in AHFS are improvement of symptoms and haemodynamic status.[8] Traditional primary therapeutic goals of reducing pulmonary capillary wedge pressure (PCWP) and/or increasing cardiac output have been de-emphasised.[5] More recently, a number of other treatment targets have been highlighted, including management of the underlying precipitant, improvement in physiological derangement, blood pressure control, respiratory support and prevention of secondary harm to the heart and kidneys.[5,8]

Non-invasive ventilation

Although many patients with AHFS respond adequately to pharmacological therapy, some require ventilatory support in the form of non-invasive or invasive ventilation. The potential clinical benefit of NIV was first described in the 1930s by Barach and Poulton.[26,27] Following the publication of experimental studies and small randomised controlled trials in the 1980s, NIV has become increasingly employed in the treatment of AHFS in the pre-hospital, emergency department and critical care settings.[28–32] The discussion of invasive ventilation in AHFS is beyond the scope of this chapter.

MECHANISM OF ACTION

NIV includes types of mechanical ventilation that do not require the use of an endotracheal tube. There are two principal forms of NIV used in AHFS: CPAP and BiPAP. CPAP provides a constant additional positive airway pressure to a spontaneously breathing patient throughout their respiratory cycle. BiPAP delivers a similar constant airway pressure to CPAP, as well as additional positive pressure during the inspiration phase.

NIV has a number of potentially beneficial physiological effects. The increased airway pressure delivered by NIV (both CPAP and BiPAP) 'splints' open collapsed or under-ventilated alveoli at the end of expiration, thereby improving lung compliance and the ventilation/perfusion (V/Q) ratio. This reduces work of breathing, helping to alleviate respiratory muscle fatigue. Keeping alveoli open also results in improvement of gas exchange, increasing blood levels of oxygen and decreasing levels of carbon dioxide. Positive airway pressure also serves to counteract the increased interstitial and capillary hydrostatic pressure occurring in pulmonary oedema, pushing fluid out of the alveoli and preventing further transfer inward.[33–37]

Cardiac output is also improved in the failing heart, via a reduction in both preload and afterload. Normally, changes in preload (venous filling pressures) have a dominant effect on cardiac output, as described by Starling's law. In pulmonary oedema due to heart failure, right heart pressure is already high, so changes in afterload become significant in determining cardiac output. With NIV, intrathoracic pressure is increased, reducing venous return and decreasing ventricular preload, serving to offload the overloaded ventricle. Increased intrathoracic pressure also serves to reduce afterload by facilitating left ventricle ejection, increasing cardiac output. If intrathoracic pressure is too high, however, preload to the right side of the heart will be reduced, in turn reducing cardiac output and blood pressure.[38–43]

EVIDENCE BASE

Initial studies assessing CPAP against standard oxygen therapy demonstrated significant improvements in oxygenation, and decreases in heart rate, respiratory rate and blood pressure.[44] A number of these studies also reported significant improvements in cardiopulmonary indices such as PCWP, stroke volume, cardiac output or cardiac index.[44]

A number of randomised trials have investigated the effectiveness of NIV in the management of acute cardiogenic pulmonary oedema.[45–64] Most of these trials have been small and none have in isolation, demonstrated mortality benefit. Their comparison is made difficult by variability in inclusion criteria, medical management and NIV administration.[44] These studies also used a variety of endpoints, such as physiological parameters, intubation or pre-defined treatment failure. They investigated the comparative effectiveness of CPAP and standard oxygen therapy,[51–55,62,63] BiPAP and standard oxygen therapy,[56,57] BiPAP and CPAP[47–49,58,59,64] or either intervention compared with standard oxygen therapy alone.[45,46,50,60,61] The majority of these trials showed improvement in physiological indices or a reduction in endotracheal intubation rate or other markers of treatment failure in the NIV arm. Despite theoretical physiological benefits of BiPAP over CPAP, no difference has been found to date in head-to-head comparisons.[45–50] Two of the more significant in-hospital trials,[45,46,49] as well as two more recent trials investigating pre-hospital NIV in AHFS,[62,63] are discussed in more detail below, in addition to the evidence from pooled data studies.

IN-HOSPITAL TRIALS

The 3CPO trial[45,46] remains the largest trial of NIV in AHFS to date. In this multicentre, prospective randomised controlled trial, 1069 patients with cardiogenic pulmonary oedema were recruited from 26 UK emergency departments. Patients were randomised to one of three arms: standard oxygen therapy delivered by variable delivery oxygen mask with a reservoir bag, CPAP (5–15 cmH_2O) or BiPAP (inspiratory pressure 8–20 cmH_2O, expiratory pressure 4–10 cmH_2O). NIV (both CPAP and BiPAP) was delivered through a mid-range portable ventilator. The primary endpoint for the comparison between NIV (CPAP or BiPAP) and standard oxygen was 7-day mortality. The primary endpoint for the comparison between CPAP and BiPAP was 7-day mortality or intubation. Patients with a clinical and radiological diagnosis of cardiogenic pulmonary oedema were included if they were tachypnoeic (respiratory rate >20 breaths/min) and acidotic (pH <7.35) at presentation. Additional management was at the discretion of the treating clinician. As this was a pragmatic trial, there was no pre-defined treatment failure and patients could, if necessary, cross over between treatment arms. A total of 1069 patients (mean age [±SD] 78 ± 10 years; 43% male) were recruited to standard oxygen therapy (n = 367), CPAP (n = 346; 10 ± 4 cmH_2O) or BiPAP (n = 356; 14 ± 5/7 ± 2 cmH_2O). The mean ± SD duration of CPAP therapy was 2.2 ± 1.5 hours and that of NIV was 2.0 ± 1.3 hours. There was no difference between 7-day mortality for standard oxygen therapy (9.8%) and NIV (9.5%; p = 0.87). The combined endpoint of 7-day death or intubation rate was similar irrespective of NIV modality (11.7% vs. 11.1%, CPAP vs. NIV, respectively; p = 0.81). In comparison with standard oxygen therapy, NIV was associated with greater reductions in breathlessness, heart rate, acidosis and hypercapnia at 1 hour. There were no differences between NIV and standard oxygen therapy in other secondary outcomes such as myocardial infarction rate, intubation, length of hospital stay or critical care admission rate. It has been suggested that the ability to cross over between treatment arms may have been an influence in the lack of mortality difference between either NIV modality or standard oxygen therapy.

Moritz and colleagues[49] recruited 120 patients from three French emergency departments to either CPAP or BiPAP. There was no standard oxygen therapy arm. Patients had either a clinical or a radiological diagnosis of pulmonary oedema and two out of three of the following criteria: respiratory rate >30 breaths per minute, oxygen saturations of <90% with standard oxygen delivered at least 5 L/min by a variable delivery mask with reservoir or, last, use of accessory musculature. CPAP was increased to 10 cmH_2O and BiPAP to obtain a tidal volume of 8–10 mL/kg and expiratory pressure support was set at 5 cmH_2O. A combined primary endpoint of death, myocardial infarction or intubation in the first 24 hours of hospital admission was used. Secondary outcomes included physiology, arterial blood gas analysis, length of hospital stay, in-hospital mortality and work of breathing. During the intervention, mean CPAP levels were 7.7 and 12/4.9 cmH_2O for BiPAP. Respiratory distress and physiology improved in both arms and there was no difference found between interventions for any outcome. Only 3% of patients required intubation and only one person died within the first 24 hours. It is notable that 68 potentially eligible but non-recruited patients had NIV applied pre-hospital and another 11 were intubated.

PRE-HOSPITAL NIV

Plaisance and colleagues[63] recruited 124 patients to a randomised single-centre pre-hospital study in France, aiming to assess the benefit of CPAP as a first-line treatment of acute cardiogenic pulmonary oedema in the pre-hospital environment. Primary endpoints were effect of early CPAP on a dyspnoea clinical score and on arterial blood gases. Secondary endpoints were incidence of tracheal intubation, inotropic support and in-hospital mortality. It concluded that when compared to usual medical care and delayed application of CPAP (15–30 min) for acute cardiogenic pulmonary oedema, immediate application of CPAP (0–15 min) alone pre-hospital is significantly better in improving physiological variables and symptoms. Additionally, tracheal intubation incidence, requirement for inotropic support and in-hospital mortality were found to be higher in the delayed CPAP group. Overall, 22 patients required tracheal intubation during or after the study period; 6 in the immediate CPAP group versus 16 in the delayed group; $p = 0.01$, OR = 0.30, 0.09–0.89 95% CI. Two patients died during their hospital stay in the immediate group versus 8 in the delayed group; $p = 0.05$, OR = 0.22, 0.04–1.0 95% CI. It is uncertain whether the results constituted a clear benefit with early administration of CPAP, given the limitations of the study, which included relatively low patient numbers and unblinded design, meaning that bias stemming from investigators delaying intubation in the early CPAP group could not be ruled out. There is limited further evidence relating to the influence the specific timing of NIV initiation has on outcomes in AHFS.

ASSOCIATION WITH MYOCARDIAL INFARCTION

Historically, there has been concern regarding an increase in myocardial infarction rates in patients administered BiPAP,[47] but this was subsequently shown to be unfounded.[45,46,64] One of the first trials comparing CPAP with BiPAP in cardiogenic pulmonary oedema was prematurely terminated because of an increase in myocardial infarction rate in the BiPAP arm.[47] Subsequent reanalysis of data suggested that this finding was due to confounding factors rather than a direct effect of the intervention. A subsequent study[64] demonstrated no effect of BiPAP on myocardial infarction rate when patients with ischaemic ECGs or raised cardiac biomarkers were excluded before randomisation. A systematic review by Peter and colleagues[31] reported a weak relationship between the delivery of BiPAP and an increase in myocardial infarction rate. This finding was largely the result of the weighting of the study by Mehta and colleagues.[47] The 3CPO trial has subsequently demonstrated that there is no relationship between myocardial infarction rate and the application of either CPAP or BiPAP.[45]

HEALTH ECONOMICS

Little data exist regarding the cost-effectiveness of NIV in AHFS. The cost-utility analysis conducted alongside the 3CPO trial[45] suggested that NIV is likely to be cost-effective compared to standard oxygen therapy for treating patients with severe acute cardiogenic pulmonary oedema. The same analysis showed that BiPAP was not cost-effective in the same respect. Recent national guidance[14] has expressed caution over these results as they are driven by small differences in health-related quality of life, and they have concluded that the cost-effectiveness of NIV is most certain in patients with cardiogenic pulmonary oedema with severe dyspnoea and acidaemia.

POOLED DATA

A number of systematic reviews and meta-analyses have been completed in order to establish whether NIV improves outcomes including mortality in AHFS.[30–32,65–71] The aggregate evidence is predominately drawn from small-scale trials and generally suggests a mortality benefit for patients with AHFS treated with NIV, although this was contradicted by the 3CPO trial, a large multicentre trial in the UK in 2008.[45,46] The following section reviews some of the more significant and up-to-date meta-analyses and reviews.[30,31,69–71]

Masip and co-investigators[30] conducted a systematic review of 15 randomised controlled trials from 10 countries comparing NIV (CPAP or BiPAP) to standard oxygen or CPAP with BiPAP. The primary outcomes for the systematic review were in-hospital mortality and treatment failure (this was inconsistently categorised and defined arbitrarily as the 'need to intubate'). Data on myocardial infarction rate during hospital admission were collected and analysed. All other parameters such as physiology, length of stay, co-treatments and critical care admission were variably reported across the trials. The majority of trials were small and single centre (sample size, 26–130) and based in either the ICU or the emergency department. The majority used full face masks and CPAP or BiPAP. The complexity of the ventilator used varied considerably. Pooled data included 727 patients for the comparison of NIV (CPAP or BiPAP) to standard oxygen. Patients receiving NIV had a significant reduction in in-hospital mortality and endotracheal intubation. Results remained significant if CPAP was analysed independently for both in-hospital mortality and 'need for intubation'. Results for BiPAP remained significant for intubation and showed reduction in mortality, but not to a statistically significant level, possibly reflecting the number of patients included in these particular trials ($n = 315$). There was no difference in outcomes between CPAP and BiPAP, but these comparisons only included a total of 219 patients. There was no difference in myocardial infarction rates between arms. The review concluded that NIV should be considered as a first-line treatment for patients presenting with acute cardiogenic pulmonary oedema.

Peter and co-investigators[31] identified 23 eligible randomised controlled studies from 14 countries over an 18-year period, in order to compare: CPAP with standard therapy (oxygen by face mask, diuretics, nitrates and other supportive care), BiPAP with standard therapy and BiPAP with CPAP. The primary outcomes were in-hospital mortality and the need for intubation and mechanical ventilation. Secondary outcomes included treatment failure, length of hospital stay, length of time on NIV and myocardial infarction rate. When compared with standard care, there was a significant mortality reduction for those patients treated with CPAP and there was also a non-significant mortality reduction with BiPAP. Both CPAP and BiPAP showed a reduction in need for endotracheal intubation when compared with standard therapy. There was no difference in any outcome when CPAP was compared with BiPAP. As discussed above, there was a trend toward increased myocardial infarction rate with BiPAP but this related to the weighting of a single study.[47]

A more recent meta-analysis by Weng[69] included 31 randomised controlled trials involving 2887 patient randomised trials comparing CPAP and BiPAP (bilevel ventilation) with standard therapy or each other. They found that compared with standard therapy, CPAP reduced mortality and need for intubation but not incidence of new myocardial infarction. These effects were noted despite the inclusion of the 3CPO trial[45] in the aggregate data and were more prominent in trials where myocardial ischaemia or infarction caused acute cardiogenic pulmonary oedema in higher proportions of patients. BiPAP reduced the need for intubation but did not reduce mortality or new myocardial infarction. No differences were detected between CPAP or BiPAP in any clinical outcomes. The authors noted that the quality of the evidence base was limited and studies varied in terms of definitions, cause and severity of acute cardiogenic pulmonary oedema, as well as in patient characteristics and clinical settings.

In their systematic review, Vital and colleagues[70,71] identified 32 randomised trials, consisting of 2916 adult patients with acute cardiogenic pulmonary oedema, where NIV (CPAP or BiPAP) plus standard medical care was compared with standard medical care alone. It found that compared with standard medical care, NIV significantly reduced hospital mortality and endotracheal intubation rate, and modestly reduced ICU stay, but there was no difference in overall length of hospital stay. They did not observe any significant increase in the incidence of myocardial infarction. The authors again found a persistent mortality benefit with NIV despite the inclusion of the 3CPO trial data[45] in their analysis. They concluded that NIV in addition to standard medical care is an effective and safe treatment for adults with acute cardiogenic pulmonary oedema. After comparison of CPAP and BiPAP, it was suggested that CPAP be the first option in selection of NIV modality due to better evidence for efficacy and safety, as well as lower costs compared to BiPAP.

The recent systematic review by Pandor and colleagues[72] aimed to determine the clinical effectiveness and cost-effectiveness of pre-hospital NIV compared with standard care for adults with acute respiratory failure, with 10 studies (with sample sizes ranging from 23 to 207 participants) meeting its inclusion criteria. It concluded that pre-hospital CPAP may reduce mortality and intubation rates compared with standard care, but the effectiveness of pre-hospital BiPAP remains uncertain. It was noted that while CPAP was more expensive than standard care, its cost-effectiveness remains uncertain.

DISCREPANCIES IN EVIDENCE

There are a number of potential reasons why the discrepancies between the 3CPO trial and other trials and systematic reviews may have arisen. Most of the individual trials assessing NIV in AHFS have consisted of small patient group sizes (<100 patients), limiting the generalisability of their findings. This is in addition to the more general issue of meta-analyses compounding the effect of any bias in reporting, publication and recruitment present in its constituent studies.

It has been suggested that there may have been significant differences in patient population in the 3PO trial in terms of patient age, severity of illness and comorbidities, when compared to the smaller trials. However, like previous studies, strict patient selection criteria were applied, enabling recruitment of patients most likely to benefit from NIV (i.e. those with respiratory distress and acidosis). Baseline characteristics and event rates in the NIV arms were similar to previous studies and demonstrate that recruited patients had severe disease. Also, given the identical 7-day mortality in non-recruited patients, there was no evidence of selection bias. It has been suggested that the 3CPO mortality rate indicated that the recruited patient population was less sick than previous studies.[73,74] However, the 3CPO trial used 7-day and 30-day mortality, whereas most other comparable studies have used the less well-defined criteria of in-hospital mortality or composite endpoints with endotracheal intubation or mortality.[14] Additionally, patient age, male-to-female ratio and comorbidities were also similar to previous primary trials. As around 15% of patients in the 3CPO trial crossed over between treatment arms, it is possible that this was an influencing factor in the absence of significant mortality difference between either NIV modality or standard oxygen therapy.

Previous trials indicated that NIV is associated with a reduction in intubation rates,[30,31,62] in contradiction to the findings of the 3CPO trial. Reasons for this are unclear but may reflect differing patient populations, concomitant therapies and thresholds for intubation and mechanical ventilation across different countries, clinical environments and time periods. Intubation rates vary widely across studies, despite comparable illness severity, in-hospital mortality and length of hospital stay. Notably, the trial by Moritz and colleagues[49] reported an intubation rate almost identical to that in the 3CPO trial (3%). Given that trials have been by necessity 'open', there is concern of treatment bias with the threshold for intervention varying according to treatment allocation (e.g. patients on standard oxygen may be more likely to undergo intubation than those already gaining the apparent benefit of NIV, and conversely, clinicians may persevere with patients slow to improve with NIV if they believe in its efficacy).

Given that around 90% of the patients in the 3CPO trial received a standard set of co-treatments, which included nitrates, it is possible that the cardiovascular benefits of NIV were masked by the effect of another treatment. Co-treatments are incompletely characterised and documented in smaller trials, so their consistency and influence on trial results is unclear.

SUMMARY OF EVIDENCE

NIV is widely used in clinical practice and advocated by specialty organisations,[2,6,14] with unequivocal data to support early symptomatic and physiological benefit in patients with cardiogenic pulmonary oedema. This is evident in both large primary trials[45] and pooled data.[28–32,65–68,72] Previous and more recent meta-analyses and systematic reviews[28–32,65–68,72] have also concluded that NIV (CPAP or BiPAP) delivers mortality benefit and reduces endotracheal intubation when compared to standard oxygen therapy. One such study reported a 47% reduction in mortality.[31] This is at odds with the results of the 3CPO trial,[45] a large multicentre trial that recruited more patients than those previously assimilated in published systematic reviews. This trial reported no difference in 7-day or 30-day mortality between standard oxygen therapy and NIV in emergency department patients with severe acute cardiogenic pulmonary oedema and acidosis. This was despite early improvements in symptoms and patient physiological parameters. To date, no data support the additional benefit of BiPAP over CPAP, despite the likely mechanistic advantages,[31,49] although there are potential reasons why a true benefit may not have been detected.[51] Last, despite continuing concerns[31,47] regarding the potential for an increase in myocardial infarction rates in patients treated with NIV, subsequent trials have confirmed the safety of the intervention.[45,64]

PRACTICAL CONSIDERATIONS

There are a number of considerations required for the implementation of NIV into clinical practice. Various systems factors may inform the specifics of how NIV is utilised and where in the pre-hospital or hospital setting NIV is initiated for AHFS. These include hospital setup, availability of equipment and trained staff, location of specialties and both local and national guidelines and practice. Specific equipment choices will be influenced by many of the above factors as well as the equipment already in use in the hospital and local procurement policies.

Most patients with cardiogenic pulmonary oedema requiring NIV do not need a complex ventilator. The principal features should be a suitable patient interface, the ability to deliver up to 100% oxygen and simple functionality. NIV can be delivered through devices designed for invasive mechanical ventilation, as used in critical care units, and portable ventilators. The former tend to be less tolerant of circuit leaks but are generally preferred due to superior monitoring and control functionality and the availability of oxygen blenders.[67] Numerous comparative studies, however, demonstrate that portable devices perform as well as more complex critical care ventilators.[75]

NIV is most commonly delivered to the patient using a tight-fitting face (oronasal) mask, but nasal attachments, full face masks and hoods are also used. Nasal masks are theoretically more comfortable and less claustrophobic, allowing eating and speech more easily, as well as less buildup of secretions. However, face masks tend to be better tolerated due to improved control of mouth leak and have been shown to deliver better quality ventilation, in terms of improved minute ventilation and blood gas pressures.[76,77] There is insufficient evidence to demonstrate that either interface is superior with respect to outcome measures such as intubation rate or mortality. When fitting an interface for NIV, it is important that it is the correct size and fits comfortably, with care taken not to over-tighten straps, in order to avoid pressure sores.

A patient on NIV will require a more intensive level of nursing care and monitoring than a conventionally managed patient, ideally, in an environment with continuous monitoring (a minimum of oxygen saturations, heart rate, ECG, respiratory rate, blood pressure), resuscitation facilities, access to a blood gas analyser and adequate levels of appropriately trained nursing staff. All services that use NIV should audit practice, have clear clinical guidelines and have established training programmes.

PLACE IN CLINICAL MANAGEMENT

National and international guidelines[2,14] recommend consideration of NIV as part of first-line therapy in patients who have AHFS with severe dyspnoea and acidaemia. NIV should also be considered as an adjunct if there has been failure to respond to standard medical therapy. Management should be aimed at reducing respiratory distress and improving physiological parameters. It should be noted that NIV can reduce blood pressure and should be used with caution in hypotensive patients, with blood pressure regularly monitored during use.[2] An algorithm for the early management of acute heart failure based largely on the initial blood pressure, can be seen in the 2012 European Society for Cardiology Guidelines for the diagnosis and management of acute and chronic heart failure.[78]

CONCLUSIONS

NIV is widely used for patients who have AHFS with significant respiratory compromise. There are clear mechanistic reasons why these interventions work in acute pulmonary oedema. Indeed, multiple trials have shown that physiological parameters improve quickly with the use of NIV, and this reduces the need for endotracheal intubation and potentially in-hospital mortality. Despite theoretical advantages for BiPAP over CPAP, no trial data support additional benefits of this modality. The 3CPO trial unequivocally demonstrated the safety of both BiPAP and CPAP and clearly shows that there is no increased risk of myocardial infarction with BiPAP. Recent data support the use and benefit of NIV use in sophisticated pre-hospital systems.

In the majority of patients, medical therapy, in particular, loop diuretics and nitrates, should be instigated as the primary treatment of AHFS. NIV should be reserved for those patients who have significant respiratory distress and failure, or those not improving with standard medical therapy. Further research is required to investigate whether certain subgroups of patients will gain particular benefit from NIV. These may include patients with normal or low blood pressure, valvular heart disease or patients with co-existing chronic respiratory disease such as COPD.

NIV (CPAP or BiPAP) provides significant early improvement in patient symptoms and markers of disease severity but this does not clearly translate into a reduction in subsequent mortality.

APPENDIX

Prognostic variables in AHFS

A number of factors have been identified as having prognostic implications for AHFS patients. These include age, blood pressure, BNP rise, troponin rise, hyponatraemia, renal dysfunction, previous ischaemic heart disease, ejection fraction and function at discharge.[3,79–82] Some of these have been evaluated together in clinical prediction rules.[83] Table 36.1, adapted from a review by Collins and Storrow,[84] provides a summary of these risk variables. The majority of these factors have been identified using registry data encompassing the complete spectrum of AHFS.[3,80] Moreover, most relate to longer-term outcomes and have not been used to identify those patients at immediate risk of death or need for intervention on presentation. In a large primary multicentre study, the 3CPO investigators found that age, systolic blood pressure and the patient's ability to obey commands were factors clearly associated with 7-day mortality in patients with severe cardiogenic pulmonary oedema.[85]

Table 36.1 Risk variables in acute heart failure from selected emergency department-based risk stratification studies

Clinical variables	Laboratory variables	Other variables
BP, Oxygen saturation, pulse, ECG findings	WBC, Glucose, Sodium, pH, Creatinine, Troponin, CRP, NT-proBNP, BNP, MR-proANP, ST2, MR-proADM and Blood urea nitrogen	History of TIA/CVA, History of cancer, Home metolazone, EMS transport.

Numerous novel biomarkers, including those reflecting inflammation, oxidative stress, neuro-hormonal dysfunction and myocardial re-modelling, have been investigated for their diagnostic and prognostic value in AHFS, although none of these have yet become established in routine clinical practice. A recent review by Rosenbaum and Miller[86] examines the various biomarkers studied to date and their respective clinical practicalities.

Pharmacological treatment of AHFS

DIURETICS

Mechanism of action

Diuretics increase renal excretion of salt and water and have a moderate vasodilatory action. They remain the mainstay of therapeutic management in AHFS. Although not all patients with AHFS are volume overloaded,[9] the majority of patients presenting with acute heart failure have some degree of either pulmonary or peripheral oedema.[18] In AHFS, diuretics are thought to achieve an improvement in patient symptoms through a reduction in intravascular volume, inducing a shift in alveolar transudate back into the intravascular space. Although contentious, small studies have suggested that diuretics also produce symptomatic relief via a direct effect on vascular smooth muscle, resulting in a vasodilatory effect and a reduction in preload.[87–89]

Evidence base

There is a lack of a rigorous evidence base supporting the clinical benefit of loop diuretics in AHFS. However, almost 90% of patients in the large international ADHERE[90] and ALARM-HF[18] registries, as well as the 3CPO trial,[45] received loop diuretics. There are no randomised clinical trials evaluating the clinical benefit of intravenous furosemide alone, the most commonly used first-line diuretic in AHFS.[44]

The use of loop diuretics causes sympathetic nervous system and renin–angiotensin–aldosterone system (RAAS) activation,[91] which may be associated with adverse effects such as hypotension, reduced renal function and electrolyte imbalance.[8] This is important, given the link between reduced renal function and increased mortality in AHFS. Observational data from the ADHERE registry[25] show no clear benefit in patients receiving early low-dose loop diuretic, although the majority received the agent. Additionally, data suggest that increased adverse outcomes (length of hospital stay and mortality) are associated with loop diuretic therapy in patients admitted with AHFS, even after controlling for potential confounding factors.[25] In a randomised study by Cotter and colleagues[92] of patients presenting with severe pulmonary oedema and oxygen saturations below 90%, those treated with high-dose furosemide and low-dose nitrate had a higher rate of intubation and myocardial infarction, and a slower improvement in pulse rate, respiratory rate and oxygen saturation than patients treated with high-dose nitrate and low-dose furosemide. The Digoxin Intervention Group study[93] showed that chronic heart failure patients receiving diuretics had increased all-cause and cardiovascular mortality, and heart failure-related hospitalisation, independent of illness severity. This effect is likely to be related to volume depletion activating the RAAS in conjunction with electrolyte imbalance.[94]

Data relating to optimal dosing, timing and mode of delivery are inconclusive.[2,14] In the prospective, randomised, double-blind, controlled Diuretic Optimization Strategies Evaluation trial,[95] various diuretic strategies were investigated in 308 patients with acute decompensated heart failure enrolled across 26 hospital sites in the United States and Canada. Patients were assigned to receive intravenous furosemide by means of either a bolus every 12 hours or continuous infusion and at either a low dose (equivalent to the patient's previous oral dose) or a high dose (2.5 times the previous oral dose).[95] Administration of furosemide at 2.5 times the pre-existing oral dose resulted in greater improvement in dyspnoea, larger weight change and fluid loss at the cost of transient worsening in renal function.[95] A recent meta-analysis by Wu and colleagues[96] of the existing limited studies comparing continuous infusion versus bolus injection of intravenous loop diuretics in acute decompensated heart failure showed no significant differences in terms of safety or efficacy.

Role in management

Loop diuretics are widely used and recommended by guidelines for the management of patients with AHFS, using either a bolus or infusion strategy.[2,14] In the absence of unequivocal randomised controlled trial evidence relating to the safety and efficacy of diuretics in AHFS, guidance proposes that diuretics should be carefully titrated to promote effective diuresis and symptom improvement, while avoiding significantly deteriorating renal function.[2,14,44]

VASODILATORS: NITRATES AND SODIUM NITROPRUSSIDE

Mechanism of action

Nitrates are principally venodilators, although at higher dose, they cause both coronary and systemic arterial vasodilatation.[97] Nitroprusside is an alternative, potent, combined venous and arterial dilator, which is not widely used in clinical practice due to its side effect profile. In acute heart failure, nitrates have a dual benefit through decreasing venous tone (reducing preload) and arterial tone (reducing afterload),[98] which consequently may result in an increase in cardiac output. These effects are thought to contribute to relief of pulmonary oedema and make vasodilators particularly useful in patients with hypertensive acute heart failure,[9] whereas they should be avoided in those with symptomatic hypotension.

Evidence base

Nitrates are the second most commonly used agents in AHFS, but again there is no robust evidence defining their beneficial effects or impact on clinical outcomes.[2,14] In the 3CPO trial,[45] 90% of patients received nitrate therapy during initial management in the emergency department. A retrospective analysis from the ADHERE database[19] showed a lower rate of mortality in patients receiving intravenous glyceryl trinitrate (GTN) than in patients receiving either milrinone or dobutamine. There was no difference in outcomes when GTN was compared with nesiritide.[19] There are no placebo-controlled trials of nitrates alone in acute heart failure, but a literature review[99] reveals a few small randomised controlled trials of nitrates versus furosemide, all of which showed better or comparable haemodynamic responses with nitrates. Recent systematic reviews suggest that intravenous nitrates, including GTN, improve short-term symptoms in acute heart failure,[100] but do not appear to affect mortality.[100,101] There is evidence that a single pre-hospital sublingual dose may be associated with improved clinical outcomes.[102] Further primary trials are needed to evaluate the safety and efficacy of nitrates in acute heart failure.

Role in management

Recent international guidelines[2] advocate nitrate use for symptomatic relief in AHFS in the absence of hypotension, while UK guidance advises that nitrates should not routinely be offered in AHFS.[14] In patients who are oxygenated with high-flow oxygen and hypertensive, early nitrate use may prevent the need for NIV. Nitrates may be administered sublingually, transdermally or by intravenous bolus or infusion. Most commonly, GTN is used as a bolus or continuous infusion, allowing titration against symptomatic response and blood pressure. Both are generally well tolerated in the context of normal (systolic BP above 110 mmHg) or high initial blood pressure (140/90 mmHg or above).[9,103] Nitrate dosing should be carefully controlled to avoid hypotension, its principal side effect, which is related to poor outcomes.[2,9,103] Other side effects include headache and rarely, methaemoglobinaemia.

VASODILATORS: NESIRITIDE

Mechanism of action

Nesiritide, a recombinant form of BNP, is a potent arterial and venous dilator, reducing preload and afterload, and has a natriuretic effect.[104] It was approved in North America for use in patients with AHFS after early studies demonstrated dose-related reductions in PCWP, increased stroke volume and cardiac index, as well as improvement in symptoms.[105,106]

Evidence base

Approximately 8% of patients in the ADHERE registry received nesiritide.[19] Several prospective, randomised, placebo-controlled trials have evaluated nesiritide in AHFS. The Vasodilatation in the Management of Acute CHF investigators[107] compared GTN with nesiritide and placebo in 489 patients with AHFS and dyspnoea at rest. The trial demonstrated small reductions in PCWP and greater improvement in 'global clinical status' in patients receiving nesiritide, although no mortality difference was demonstrated.[107] However, a number of limitations in this study have been noted. Patients received standard management (usually including morphine and furosemide) before randomisation, concomitant therapies were not controlled for and 'global clinical status' was poorly described and unvalidated. Subsequent pooled analyses[108,109] of data from small randomised trials have raised concerns regarding the safety of nesiritide, demonstrating both increased 30-day mortality and renal dysfunction with nesiritide compared to controls, although these estimates were associated with wide confidence intervals. The more recent multicentre Acute Study of Clinical Effectiveness of Nesiritide and Decompensated Heart Failure trial[110] randomised 7141 patients hospitalized with acute decompensated heart failure to receive nesiritide or placebo, in addition to standard care. Results showed that nesiritide was associated with an increase in the rate of hypotension and had minimal effects on dyspnoea, renal function and rates of death and re-hospitalisation.[110]

Role in management

Owing to the lack of evidence demonstrating superiority of nesiritide over nitrates and the uncertainty regarding its safety in AHFS, nesiritide is not supported by clinical guidelines.[2,14,44]

OPIATES

Mechanism of action

Patients presenting with acute heart failure are often considerably distressed by their symptoms, so opiates are frequently employed to provide anxiolysis. There are some data to demonstrate that opiates also have a venodilatory effect, as a result of venous pooling, which is postulated to occur due to either histamine release or an alternative action on opioid receptors in vascular smooth muscle.[111,112] No central effect on PCWP has been elicited, but there is some evidence to suggest an increase in heart filling pressures and a reduction in cardiac index due to a direct myocardial depressant effect.[113,114] Additionally, opiates may have an indirect beneficial effect on symptoms and physiology via a reduction in anxiety and pain, therefore ameliorating the adverse effects of excess catecholamine drive. The benefits of opiates need to be carefully balanced with their depressant effect on the central respiratory and central nervous systems, particularly in those patients with co-existent respiratory disease such as COPD.

Evidence base

It is unclear whether opiates improve clinical outcomes in acute heart failure.[14] Indeed, a number of observational studies have reported poorer outcomes associated with opiate use.[17,45,115–117] Sacchetti and colleagues[115] found a significant increase in endotracheal intubation and ICU admission in patients with pulmonary oedema receiving morphine. This may have been related to underlying disease severity rather than a direct drug effect. In a retrospective analysis of ADHERE data, Tallman and colleagues[17] found that in patients with acute heart failure given morphine, there was an increase in breathlessness and respiratory rate, as well as an increased requirement for mechanical ventilation, longer median hospitalisation, more ICU admissions and greater mortality. Data from the 3CPO trial[45,116] suggest that opioid administration is associated with increased 7-day mortality. Similarly, in a recent study, Iakobishvili and colleagues[117] found that intravenous morphine administration was independently associated with increased in-hospital mortality. Whether morphine has a causative or merely associative relationship with these effects is unclear, as AHFS patients who are administered morphine may be more unwell as a starting point, predisposing them to a poorer outcome. There is no evidence relating to the association of opiate use in AHFS with major cardiovascular events, length of hospital stay or quality of life.[14]

Role in management

Opioids are commonly used in the initial management of patients with AHFS. However, current UK,[14] European[2] and US[6] guidelines do not promote their routine use. It has been suggested that given the potential detrimental effects of these agents, it may be preferable to use alternative agents such as benzodiazepines if anxiolysis is desired.[21]

OTHER AGENTS

Recombinant human relaxin-2 (Serelaxin), a vasoactive peptide hormone, has been investigated by Teerlink and colleagues in the international randomised placebo-controlled RELAX-AHF trial.[118] A total of 1161 patients with acute heart failure were randomly assigned to standard care plus 48-hour intravenous infusions of placebo (n = 580) or Serelaxin (n = 581) within 16 hours of presentation.[118] The primary endpoint was dyspnoea improvement, evaluated with a change from baseline in the visual analogue scale area under the curve (VAS AUC) up to day 5, and Likert scale measurement of the proportion of patients with moderate or marked dyspnoea improvement during the first 24 hours. Serelaxin improved the VAS AUC primary dyspnoea endpoint compared with placebo, but had no significant effect on the other primary endpoint, or the secondary endpoints of cardiovascular death or readmission to hospital for heart failure or renal failure.[118] Serelaxin was, however, associated with significantly reduced 180-day mortality, with fewer signs of organ damage and more rapid relief of congestion in the short term.[118,119] Results are awaited for the multi-centre, randomised, double-blind, placebo-controlled phase III RELAX-2 study, which aims to evaluate the efficacy, safety and tolerability of Serelaxin when added to standard therapy in acute heart failure patients.

Tolvaptan, a V_2 receptor antagonist, blocks the action of arginine vasopressin at the V_2 receptor in renal tubules, increasing water loss. In the multicentre, randomised, placebo-controlled Efficacy of Vasopressin Antagonism in Heart Failure Outcome Study With Tolvaptan study,[120] it was found that Tolvaptan significantly improved secondary endpoints of day 1 dyspnoea, day 1 body weight, and day 7 oedema in patients with AHFS.[69] There was no difference in cardiovascular mortality, cardiovascular death or hospitalisation, worsening heart failure or long-term mortality.[120]

Levosimendan is a calcium sensitizer, with both positive inotropic and vasodilatory effects. In a meta-analysis of 19 randomised controlled trials enrolling 3650 patients,[121] levosimendan improved haemodynamics but not survival in comparison to placebo, as well as haemodynamics and survival in comparison to dobutamine.[121] Use of inotropes in AHFS is generally reserved for hypotensive acute heart failure associated with severely reduced cardiac output resulting in compromised vital organ perfusion and is not recommended in international guidance for cases of hypotensive AHF where the underlying cause is hypovolaemia or other reversible factors.[2]

Further agents studied for use in AHFS include phosphodiesterase inhibitors (milrinone), inotropes (dobutamine), endothelin antagonists (tezosentan), A_1-adenosine receptor antagonists (rolofylline) and ACE inhibitors (captopril).[14,122–125] A comprehensive review of these agents is beyond the scope of this chapter.

REFERENCES

1. Adams KF Jr, Fonarow GC, Emerman CL et al. Characteristics and outcomes of patients hospitalized for heart failure in the United States: Rationale, design, and preliminary observations from the first 100,000 cases in the Acute Decompensated Heart Failure National Registry (ADHERE). *Am Heart J.* 2005;149:209–16.
2. Ponikowski P, Voors AA, Anker SD et al. 2016 European Society of Cardiology Guidelines for the diagnosis and treatment of acute and chronic heart failure. First published online: 20 May 2016.
3. Gheorghiade M, Pang PS. Acute heart failure syndromes. *J Am Coll Cardiol.* 2009;53:557–73.
4. De Luca L, Fonarow GC, Adams KF Jr et al. Acute heart failure syndromes: Clinical scenarios and pathophysiologic targets for therapy. *Heart Fail Rev.* 2007;12:97–104.
5. Gheorghiade M, Zannad F, Sopko G et al. Acute heart failure syndromes: Current state and framework for future research. *Circulation.* 2005;112:3958–68.
6. 2013 ACCF/AHA Guideline for the Management of Heart Failure. A Report of the American College of Cardiology Foundation/American Heart Association Task Force on Practice Guidelines. *Circulation.* 2013;128:e240–e327.
7. Collins S, Storrow AB, Kirk JD et al. Beyond pulmonary edema: Diagnostic, risk stratification, and treatment challenges of acute heart failure management in the emergency department. *Ann Emerg Med.* 2008;51:45–57.
8. Nieminen MS, Bohm M, Cowie MR et al. Executive summary of the guidelines on the diagnosis and treatment of acute heart failure: The Task Force on Acute Heart Failure of the European Society of Cardiology. *Eur Heart J.* 2005;26:384–416.
9. Collins SP, Levy PD, Martindale JL et al. Clinical and research considerations for patients with hypertensive acute heart failure: A consensus statement from the Society for Academic Emergency Medicine and the Heart Failure Society of America Acute Heart Failure Working Group. *J Card Fail.* 2016;22:618–27.
10. Wang CS, Fitzgerald JM, Schulzer M et al. Does this dyspnoeic patient in the Emergency Department have congestive heart failure. *JAMA.* 2005;294:1944–56.
11. American College of Emergency Physicians Clinical Policies Subcommittee (Writing Committee) on acute heart failure syndromes, Silvers SM, Howell JM et al. Clinical policy: Critical issues in the evaluation and management of adult patients presenting to the emergency department with acute heart failure syndromes. *Ann Emerg Med.* 2007;49:627–69.
12. Martindale JL, Wakai A, Collins SP et al. Diagnosing acute heart failure in the emergency department: A systematic review and meta-analysis. *Acad Emerg Med.* 2016;23:223–42.
13. Roberts E, Ludman AJ, Dworzynski K et al. The diagnostic accuracy of the natriuretic peptides in heart failure: Systematic review and diagnostic meta-analysis in the acute care setting. *BMJ.* 2015;350.
14. National Institute for Health and Care Excellence. Acute heart failure: Diagnosis and management. (NICE CG187). Published October 2014.
15. Graham CA. Pharmacological therapy of acute cardiogenic pulmonary oedema in the emergency department. *Emerg Med Australas.* 2004;16:47–54.
16. Browning J, Atwood B, Gray A. CPO trial group. Use of non-invasive ventilation in UK emergency departments. *Emerg Med J.* 2006;23:920–1.
17. Tallman TA, Peacock WF, Emerman CL et al. Noninvasive ventilation outcomes in 2430 acute decompensated heart failure patients: An ADHERE Registry analysis. *Acad Emerg Med.* 2008;15:355–62.

18. Follath F, Yilmaz MB, Delgado JF et al. Clinical presentation, management and outcomes in the Acute Heart Failure Global Survey of Standard Treatment (ALARM-HF). *Intensive Care Med.* 2011;37:619–26.
19. Abraham WT, Adams KF, Fonarow GC et al. In-hospital mortality in patients with decompensated heart failure requiring vasoactive medications: An analysis of the Acute Decompensated Heart Failure National Registry (ADHERE). *J Am Coll Cardiol.* 2005;46(1):57–64.
20. Mattu A, Martinez JP, Kelly BS. Modern management of cardiogenic pulmonary oedema. *Emerg Med Clin North Am.* 2005;23:1105–25.
21. Northridge D. Frusemide or nitrates for acute heart failure. *Lancet.* 1996;247:667–8.
22. Hoffman JR, Reynolds S. Comparison of nitroglycerin, morphine and furosemide in the treatment of presumed pre-hospital pulmonary edema. *Chest.* 1987;92:923–7.
23. Sacchetti A, Ramoska E, Moakes ME et al. Effect of ED management on ICU use in acute pulmonary edema. *Am J Emerg Med.* 1999;17:571–4.
24. Peacock WF, Hollander JE, Diercks DB et al. Morphine and outcomes in acute decompensated heat failure: An ADHERE analysis. *Emerg Med J.* 2008;25:205–9.
25. Peacock WF, Costanzo MR, De Marco T et al. for the ADHERE Scientific Advisory Committee and Investigators. Impact of intravenous loop diuretics on outcomes of patients hospitalized with acute decompensated heart failure: Insights from the ADHERE registry. *Cardiology.* 2009;13:12–9.
26. Barach AL, Martin J, Eckman M. Positive pressure respiration and its application to the treatment of acute pulmonary edema. *Ann Intern Med.* 1938;12:754–95.
27. Poulton EP, Oxon DM. Left-sided heart failure with pulmonary oedema its treatment with the 'pulmonary plus pressure machine'. *Lancet.* 1936;228:981–3.
28. Pang D, Keenan SP, Cook DJ et al. The effect of positive pressure airway support on mortality and the need for intubation in cardiogenic pulmonary edema: A systematic review. *Chest.* 1998;114:1185–92.
29. Kelly C, Newby DE, Boon NA et al. Support ventilation versus conventional oxygen. *Lancet.* 2001;357:1126.
30. Masip J, Roque M, Sanchez B et al. Noninvasive ventilation in acute cardiogenic pulmonary edema: Systematic review and meta-analysis. *JAMA.* 2005;294:3124–30.
31. Peter JV, Moran JL, Phillips-Hughes J et al. Effect of non-invasive positive pressure ventilation (BIPAP) on mortality in patients with acute cardiogenic pulmonary oedema: A meta-analysis. *Lancet.* 2006;367:1155–63.
32. Collins SP, Mielniczuk LM, Whittingham HA et al. The use of noninvasive ventilation in emergency department patients with acute cardiogenic pulmonary edema: A systematic review. *Ann Emerg Med.* 2006;48:260–9.
33. Naughton MT, Rahman MA, Hara K et al. Effect of continuous positive airway pressure on intrathoracic and left ventricular transmural pressures in patients with congestive heart failure. *Circulation.* 1995;91:1725–31.
34. Lenique F, Habis M, Lofaso F et al. Ventilatory and hemodynamic effects of continuous positive airway pressure in left heart failure. *Am J Respir Crit Care Med.* 1997;155:500–5.
35. Katz JA. PEEP and CPAP in perioperative respiratory care. *Respir Care.* 1984;29:614–29.
36. Katz JA, Marks JD. Inspiratory work with and without continuous positive airway pressure in patients with acute respiratory failure. *Anesthesiology.* 1985;63:598–607.
37. Branson RD, Hurst JM, DeHaven CB Jr. Mask CPAP: state of the art. *Respir Care.* 1985;30:846–57.
38. Pinsky MR, Summer WR, Wise RA et al. Augmentation of cardiac function by elevation of intrathoracic pressure. *J Appl Physiol.* 1983; 54:950–5.
39. Pinsky MR, Summer WR. Cardiac augmentation by phasic high intrathoracic pressure support in man. *Chest.* 1983;84:370–5.
40. Pinsky MR, Marquez J, Martin D et al. Ventricular assist by cardiac cycle-specific increases in intrathoracic pressure. *Chest.* 1987;91:709–15.
41. Grace MP, Greenbaum DM. Cardiac performance in response to PEEP in patients with cardiac dysfunction. *Crit Care Med.* 1982;10:358–60.
42. De Hoyos A, Liu PP, Benard DC et al. Haemodynamic effects of continuous positive airway pressure in humans with normal and impaired left ventricular function. *Clin Sci.* 1995;88:173–8.
43. Acosta B, DiBenedetto R, Rahimi A et al. Hemodynamic effects of noninvasive bilevel positive airway pressure on patients with chronic congestive heart failure with systolic dysfunction. *Chest.* 2000;118:1004–9.
44. Silvers SM, Howell JM, Kosowsky JM et al. from the American College of Emergency Physicians clinical policies subcommittee. Clinical policy: Critical issues in the evaluation and management of adult patients presenting to the emergency department with acute heart failure syndromes. *Ann Emerg Med.* 2007;49:627–69.
45. Gray A, Goodacre S, Newby DE et al. Noninvasive ventilation in acute cardiogenic pulmonary edema. *New Engl J Med.* 2008;359(2):142–51.
46. Gray A, Goodacre S, Newby D et al. on behalf of the 3CPO trialists. Noninvasive ventilation in acute cardiogenic pulmonary edema. *Health Technol Assess.* 2009;13.

47. Mehta S, Jay GD, Woolard RH et al. Randomized, prospective trial of bilevel versus continuous positive airway pressure in acute pulmonary oedema. *Crit Care Med.* 1997;25:620–8.
48. Nava S, Carbone G, DiBattista N et al. Noninvasive ventilation in cardiogenic pulmonary edema: A multi-center randomized trial. *Am J Respir Crit Care Med.* 2003;168:1432–7.
49. Moritz F, Brousse B, Gellee B et al. Continuous positive airway pressure versus bilevel noninvasive ventilation in acute cardiogenic pulmonary edema: A randomized multicenter trial. *Ann Emerg Med.* 2007;50:666–75.
50. Crane SD, Elliott MW, Gilligan P et al. Randomised controlled comparison of continuous positive airways pressure, bilevel non-invasive ventilation, and standard treatment in emergency department patients with acute cardiogenic pulmonary oedema. *Emerg Med J.* 2004;21:155–61.
51. Bersten AD, Holt AW, Vedig AE et al. Treatment of severe cardiogenic pulmonary edema with continuous positive airway pressure delivered by face mask. *N Engl J Med.* 1991;325:1825–30.
52. Rasanen J, Heikkila J, Downs J et al. Continuous positive airway pressure by face mask in acute cardiogenic pulmonary edema. *Am J Cardiol.* 1985;55:296–300.
53. Lin M, Yang YF, Chiang HT et al. Reappraisal of continuous positive airway pressure therapy in acute cardiogenic pulmonary edema. Short-term results and long-term follow-up. *Chest.* 1995;107:1379–86.
54. Takeda S, Nejima J, Takano T et al. Effect of nasal continuous positive airway pressure on pulmonary edema complicating acute myocardial infarction. *Jap Circ J.* 1998;62:553–8.
55. Kelly CA, Newby DE, McDonagh TA et al. Randomised controlled trial of continuous positive airway pressure and standard oxygen therapy in acute pulmonary oedema; effects on plasma brain natriuretic peptide concentrations. *Eur Heart J.* 2002;23:1379–86.
56. L'Her E, Duquesne F, Girou E et al. Noninvasive continuous positive airway pressure in elderly cardiogenic pulmonary edema patients. *Intensive Care Med.* 2004;30:882–8.
57. Masip J, Betbese AJ, Paez J et al. Non-invasive pressure support ventilation versus conventional oxygen therapy in acute cardiogenic pulmonary oedema: A randomised trial. *Lancet.* 2000;356:2126–32.
58. Bellone A, Vettorello M, Monari A et al. Noninvasive pressure support ventilation vs. continuous positive airway pressure in acute hypercapnic pulmonary edema. *Intensive Care Med.* 2005;31:807–11.
59. Levitt MA. A prospective, randomized trial of BiPAP in severe acute congestive heart failure. *J Emerg Med.* 2001;21:363–9.
60. Park M, Lorenzi-Filho G, Feltrim MI et al. Oxygen therapy, continuous positive airway pressure, or non-invasive bilevel positive pressure ventilation in the treatment of acute cardiogenic pulmonary edema. *Arq Bras Cardiol.* 2001;76:221–30.
61. Park M, Sangean MC, Volpe MS et al. Randomized, prospective trial of oxygen, continuous positive airway pressure, and bilevel positive airway pressure by face mask in acute cardiogenic pulmonary edema. *Crit Care Med.* 2004;32:2407–15.
62. Ducros L, Logeart D, Vicaut E et al. CPAP for acute cardiogenic pulmonary oedema from out-of-hospital to cardiac intensive care unit: A randomised multicentre study. *Intensive Care Med.* 2011;37(9):1501–9.
63. Plaisance P, Pirracchio R, Berton C et al. A randomized study of out-of-hospital continuous positive airway pressure for acute cardiogenic pulmonary oedema: Physiological and clinical effects. *Eur Heart J.* 2007;28(23):2895–2901.
64. Bellone A, Monari A, Cortellaro F et al. Myocardial infarction rate in acute pulmonary edema: Noninvasive pressure support ventilation versus continuous positive airway pressure. *Crit Care Med.* 2004;32:1860–5.
65. Ho KM, Wong K. A comparison of continuous and bi-level positive airway pressure non-invasive ventilation in patients with acute cardiogenic pulmonary oedema: A meta-analysis. *Crit Care.* 2006;10:R49.
66. Winck JC, Azevedo LF, Costa-Pereira A et al. Efficacy and safety of non-invasive ventilation in the treatment of acute cardiogenic pulmonary edema—A systematic review and meta-analysis. *Crit Care.* 2006;10:R69.
67. Agarwal R, Aggarwal AN, Gupta D et al. Non-invasive ventilation in acute cardiogenic pulmonary oedema. *Postgrad Med J.* 2005;81:637–43.
68. Nadar S, Prasad N, Taylor RS et al. Positive pressure ventilation in the management of acute and chronic cardiac failure: A systematic review and meta-analysis. *Int J Cardiol.* 2005;99:171–85.
69. Weng CL, Zhao YT, Liu QH et al. Meta-analysis: Noninvasive ventilation in acute cardiogenic pulmonary edema. *Ann. Internal Med.* 2010; 152(9):590–600.
70. Vital FM, Ladeira MT, Atallah AN. Non-invasive positive pressure ventilation (CPAP or bilevel NPPV) for cardiogenic pulmonary oedema. *Cochrane Database Syst Rev.* 2013;(3).
71. Vital FM, Saconato H, Ladeira MT et al. Non-invasive positive pressure ventilation (CPAP or bilevel NPPV) for cardiogenic pulmonary edema. *Cochrane Database Syst Rev.* 2008;(Issue 3):CD005351.
72. Pandor A, Thokala P, Goodacre S et al. Pre-hospital non-invasive ventilation for acute respiratory failure: A systematic review and cost-effectiveness evaluation. *Health Technol Assess.* 2015 Jun;19(42):v–vi, 1–102.

73. McDermid RC, Bagshaw S. Noninvasive ventilation in cardiogenic pulmonary edema. *N Engl J Med.* 2008;359:2068–9.
74. Masip J, Mebazaa A, Filippatos G. Noninvasive ventilation in cardiogenic pulmonary edema. *N Engl J Med.* 2008;359:2068–9.
75. Hess DR. The evidence for noninvasive positive-pressure ventilation in the care of patients in acute respiratory failure: A systematic review of the literature. *Respir Care.* 2004 Jul;49(7):810–29.
76. Navalesi P, Fanfulla F, Frigerio P et al. Physiologic evaluation of noninvasive mechanical ventilation delivered with three types of masks in patients with chronic hypercapnic respiratory failure. *Crit Care Med.* 2000;28:1785–90.
77. Kwok H, McCormack J, Cece R et al. Controlled trial of oronasal versus nasal mask ventilation in the treatment of acute respiratory failure. *Crit Care Med.* 2003;31:468–73.
78. McMurray JJ, Adamopoulos S, Anker D et al. ESC Guidelines for the diagnosis and treatment of acute and chronic heart failure 2012: The Task Force for the Diagnosis and Treatment of Acute and Chronic Heart Failure 2012 of the European Society of Cardiology. Developed in collaboration with the Heart Failure Association (HFA) of the ESC. *Eur Heart J.* 2012;33(14):1787–1847.
79. Gheorghiade M, Abraham WT, Albert NM et al. For the OPTIMIZE-HF investigators. Systolic blood pressure at admission, clinical characteristics, and outcomes in patients hospitalized with acute heart failure. *JAMA.* 2006;296:2217–26.
80. Mueller C, Scholer A, Laule-Kilian K et al. Use of B-type natriuretic peptide in the evaluation and management of acute dyspnea. *N Engl J Med.* 2004;350:647–54.
81. Fonarow GC, Abraham TW, Nancy MA et al. for the OPTIMIZE-HF investigators. Factors Identified as precipitating hospital admissions for heart failure and clinical outcomes. *Arch Int Med.* 2008;168:847–54.
82. Fonarow GC, Adams KF, Abraham TW et al. for the ADHERE scientific advisory committee, study group and investigators. Risk stratification for in-hospital mortality in acutely decompensated heart failure. Classification and regression tree analysis. *JAMA.* 2005;293:572–80.
83. Auble TE, Hsleh M, McCausland JB et al. Comparison of four clinical prediction rules for estimating risk in heart failure. *Ann Emerg Med.* 2007;50:127–35.
84. Collins SP, Storrow AB. Moving toward comprehensive acute heart failure risk assessment in the emergency department. *JACC Heart Fail.* 2013;1(4):273–80.
85. Gray A, Goodacre S, Masson M et al. A simple risk score to predict early outcome in acute cardiogenic pulmonary oedema. Circulation: *Heart Failure*; published online ahead of print 30 October 2009.
86. Rosenbaum AN, Miller WL. Biomarkers in acute decompensated heart failure. *Clin Med Insights: Therapeutics.* 2015;7:33–42.
87. Dormans TPJ, Pickkers P, Russel FGM et al. Vascular effects of loop diuretics. *Cardiovasc Res.* 1996;32:988–97.
88. Pickkers P, Dormans TPJ, Smits P. Direct vasoactivity of frusemide. *Lancet.* 1996;347:1338–9.
89. Sinoway L, Minotti J, Musch T et al. Enhanced metabolic vasodilation secondary to diuretic therapy in decompensated congestive heart failure secondary to coronary artery disease. *Am J Cardiol.* 1987;60:107–11.
90. Fonarow GC, Heywood JT, Heidenreich PA et al. Temporal trends in clinical characteristics, treatments, and outcomes for heart failure hospitalizations, 2002 to 2004: Findings from Acute Decompensated Heart Failure National Registry (ADHERE). *Am Heart J.* 2007;153:1021–8.
91. Kubo SH, Clark M, Laragh JH et al. Identification of normal neurohormonal activity in mild congestive heart failure and stimulating effect of upright posture and diuretics. *Am J Cardiol.* 1987;60:1322–8.
92. Cotter G, Metzkor E, Kaluski E et al. Randomised trial of high-dose isosorbide dinitrate plus low-dose furosemide versus high-dose furosemide plus low-dose isosorbide dinitrate in severe pulmonary oedema. *Lancet.* 1998;355:389–93.
93. Domanski M, Tian X, Haigney M et al. Diuretic use, progressive heart failure, and death in patients in the DIG study. *J Card Fail.* 2006;12:327–32.
94. Krum H, Cameron P. Diuretics in the treatment of heart failure: Mainstay of therapy or potential hazard. *J Card Fail* 2006;12:333–5.
95. Felker GM, Lee KL, Bull DA et al. Diuretic strategies in patients with acute decompensated heart failure. *N Engl J Med.* 2011;364:797–805.
96. Wu MY, Chang NC, Su CL et al. Loop diuretic strategies in patients with acute decompensated heart failure: A meta-analysis of randomized controlled trials. *J Crit Care* 2014;29(1):2–9.
97. Imhof PR, Ott B, Frankhauser P et al. Differences in nitroglycerin dose response in the venous and arterial beds. *Eur J Clin Pharamacol.* 1980;18:455–60.
98. Haber HL, Siek CL, Bergin JD et al. Bolus intravenous nitroglycerin predominantly reduces afterload in patients with severe congestive heart failure. *J Am Coll Cardiol.* 1993;22:251–7.
99. Johnson A, Mackway-Jones K. Frusemide or nitrates in acute left ventricular failure. *Emerg Med J.* 2001;18:59–60.

100. Alexander P, Alkhawam L, Curry J et al. Lack of evidence for intravenous vasodilators in ED patients with acute heart failure: A systematic review. *Am J Emerg Med.* 2015;33(2):133–41.
101. Farag M. Nitrates for the management of acute heart failure syndromes, a systematic review. Published online before print May 25, 2016; *Cardiovasc Pharmacol Ther.* 2016.
102. Crane SD, Elliott MW, Gilligan P et al. Randomised controlled comparison of continuous positive airways pressure, bilevel non-invasive ventilation, and standard treatment in emergency department patients with acute cardiogenic pulmonary oedema. *Emerg Med J.* 2004;21:155–61.
103. Piper S, McDonagh T. The role of intravenous vasodilators in acute heart failure management. *Eur J Heart Fail.* 2014;16:827–34.
104. Hollenberg SM. Vasodilators in acute heart failure. *Heart Fail Rev.* 2007;12:143–7.
105. Colucci WS, Elkayam U, Horton DP et al. Intravenous nesiritide, a natiuretic peptide, in the treatment of decompensated congestive heart failure. *N Engl J Med.* 2000;343:246–53.
106. Moazemi K, Chana J, Willard AM et al. Intravenous vasodilator therapy in congestive heart failure. *Drugs Aging.* 2003;20:485–508.
107. Publication committee for the VMAC investigators. Intravenous nesiritide vs nitrogylcerin for treatment of decompensated congestive heart failure: A randomized controlled trial. *JAMA.* 2002;287:1531–40.
108. Sackner-Bernstein JD, Skopicki HA, Aaronson KD. Risk of worsening renal function with nesiritide in patients with acutely decompensated heart failure. *Circulation.* 2005;111:1487–91.
109. Sackner-Bernstein JD, Kowalski M, Fox M, Aaronson K. Short-term risk of death after treatment with nesiritide for decompensated heart failure: A pooled analysis of randomized controlled trials. *JAMA.* 2005;293:1900–5.
110. O'Connor CM, Starling RC, Hernandez AF et al. Effect of nesiritide in patients with acute decompensated heart failure. *N Engl J Med.* 2011;365:32–43.
111. Vismara LA, Leaman DM, Zelis R. The effects of morphine on venous tone in patients with acute pulmonary edema. *Circulation.* 1976;18:455–60.
112. Zelis R, Mansour EJ, Capone RJ, Mason DT. The cardiovascular effects of morphine. The peripheral capacitance and resistance vessels in human subjects. *J Clin Invest.* 1974;18:455–60.
113. Timmis AD, Rothman MT, Henderson MA et al. Haemodynamic effect of intravenous morphine on patients with acute myocardial infarction complicated by severe left ventricular failure. *BMJ.* 1980;280:980–2.
114. Amsterdam EA, Zelis R, Kohfeld DB et al. Effect of morphine on myocardial contractility negative inotropic action during hypoxia and reversal by isoproterenol. *Circulation.* 1971;135 Suppl II:43–4.
115. Sacchetti A, Ramoska E, Moakes ME et al. Effect of ED management on ICU use in acute pulmonary edema. *Am J Emerg Med.* 1999;17:571–4.
116. Gray A, Goodacre S, Seah M, Tilley S. Diuretic, opiate and nitrate use in severe acidotic acute cardiogenic pulmonary oedema: Analysis from the 3CPO trial. *QJM.* 2010;103(8):573–81.
117. Iakobishvili Z et al. Use of intravenous morphine for acute decompensated heart failure in patients with and without acute coronary syndromes. *Acute Card Care.* 2011;13:76–80.
118. Teerlink JR, Cotter G, Davidson BA et al. Serelaxin, recombinant human relaxin-2, for treatment of acute heart failure (RELAX-AHF): A randomised, placebo-controlled trial. *Lancet.* 2013;381(9860):29–39.
119. Metra M, Cotter G, Davison BA et al. Effect of Serelaxin on Cardiac, Renal, and Hepatic Biomarkers in the Relaxin in Acute Heart Failure (RELAX-AHF) Development Program. *J Am Coll Cardiol.* 2013;61(2):196–206.
120. Konstam MA, Gheorghiade M, Burnett JC Jr et al. Effects of Oral Tolvaptan in Patients Hospitalized for Worsening Heart Failure: The EVEREST Outcome Trial. *JAMA.* 2007;297(12):1319–31.
121. Delaney A, Bradford C, McCaffrey J et al. Levosimendan for the treatment of acute severe heart failure: A meta-analysis of randomised controlled trials. *Int J Cardiol.* 2010;138(3):281–9.
122. Cuffe MS, Califf RM, Adams KF Jr et al. Short-term intravenous milrinone for acute exacerbation of chronic heart failure. *JAMA.* 2002;287:1541–7.
123. McMurray JJ, Teerlink JR, Cotter G et al. Effects of tezosentan on symptoms and clinical outcomes in patients with acute heart failure: The VERITAS randomised controlled trials. *JAMA.* 2007;298:2009–19.
124. Massie BM, O'Connor CM, Metra M et al. Rolofylline, an adenosine A1-receptor antagonist, in acute heart failure. *N Engl J Med.* 2010;363:1419–28.
125. Hamilton RJ, Carter WA, Gallagher EJ. Rapid improvement of acute pulmonary edema with sublingual captopril. *Acad Emerg Med.* 1996;3:205–12.

37

Ventilation in chronic congestive cardiac failure

MATTHEW T. NAUGHTON

KEY MESSAGES

1. Sleep-disordered breathing occurs commonly in heart failure (HF) with an increasing prevalence with age, male gender, atrial fibrillation and worsening cardiac contractility.
2. Understanding the severity and aetiology of HF is as important as understanding the type and severity of sleep-disordered breathing.
3. Obstructive sleep apnoea is an important cause of HF.
4. Central sleep apnoea is a consequence of HF and is usually associated with hyperventilation and hypocapnia. Central sleep apnoea (CSA) may also be a compensatory mechanism to severe HF.
5. Positive airway pressure has a role to play in various HF types (i.e. acute pulmonary oedema, OSA and CSA), through upper airway, pulmonary and cardiac effects. However, its effects must be carefully monitored particularly if other therapies (e.g. medications) are also in use.

INTRODUCTION

Chronic congestive heart failure (HF) is a common and costly condition.[1] Acute cardiogenic pulmonary oedema (APO) is responsible for the majority of acute hospital admissions in people aged above 65 years, of whom ~50% are readmitted for the same reason within a year. Anaemia, renal failure, depression, skeletal myopathy and abnormal lung function tests are common, in addition to an array of associated medical problems (e.g. arthritis, infection, frailty). Both incidence and prevalence of chronic HF are increasing, due to an ageing population and improved management of most medical conditions (including ischaemic heart disease), such that >10% of people now aged 80 years have HF. The 5-year mortality, from the time of HF diagnosis, is 50%, which rivals many malignancies. Thus, new and imaginative HF management strategies are required.

One such strategy, namely, non-invasive positive airway pressure "assisted" ventilation (NIV), has been gaining momentum over the past 80 years.[2] In this review, the term *NIV* will encompass positive airway pressure (PAP) delivered by an electrically driven air pump (flow generator) via a mask to a spontaneously breathing patient. This will include "pressure" set devices in either continuous (i.e. fixed) (CPAP), bilevel (BPAP), auto-titrating (APAP) or adaptive servo-controlled ventilation (ASV) modes. Specifically, the review will not refer to other NIV techniques, such as "volume" set NIV, or to the outdated (but historically very interesting) mode of negative pressure (i.e. cuirasse) ventilation.

PATHOPHYSIOLOGY

Heart failure

Circulatory failure occurs when the heart is unable to pump sufficient blood to meet the metabolic needs of the body, caused by cardiac (i.e. HF) and non-cardiac causes (Table 37.1). The causes and classifications of HF are important to appreciate when one considers the role of NIV, as some types of HF will be more responsive to NIV than others. For example, cardiac pump dysfunction is more likely to be

Table 37.1 Causes of circulatory failure

A. Heart failure
Myocardial (systolic and diastolic)
Coronary artery disease (large and small vessel)
Hypertension
Infiltrative (e.g. sarcoid)
Inflammatory
Congenital
Associated with neuromuscular (e.g. Duchenne Myopathy)
Toxic (e.g. alcohol)
Post-partum (i.e. pregnancy associated)
Pericardial
Valvular
Rhythm and conduction
Fibrillation
Extreme tachycardia or bradycardia
Asynchrony
B. Non-cardiac
Thyroid (hypo or hyperthyroid)
Anaemia
Blood volume loss (e.g. haemorrhage)
Inadequate oxyhemoglobin (e.g. high altitude)
Increased capacity of vascular bed (e.g. infection, sepsis, anaphylaxis)
Increased venous return (e.g. excessive intravenous fluids)
Decreased peripheral resistance (e.g. arteriovenous fistula, cirrhosis)

responsive to PAP than would HF secondary to disorders of cardiac rhythm or rate.

Systolic HF is defined by impaired left ventricular contractility and measured by a left ventricular ejection fraction (LVEF) estimated by nuclear angiography or echocardiography of <55% or left ventricular fractional shortening measured by echocardiography of <28%.

Diastolic HF or heart failure with normal systolic function is defined by symptoms of HF[3] with elevated left ventricular filling pressures in the setting of impaired left ventricular relaxation, and normal systolic contraction is commonly due to "stiff" ventricular walls, which can result from hypoxia, tachycardia,[4] amyloid and hypertension. Objectively, diastolic HF is defined by an elevated left ventricular filling pressure measured during a right heart catheter study (i.e. pulmonary capillary wedge pressure [PCWP] of >12 mmHg) in the setting of normal systolic function (i.e. LVEF >55%).

Unfortunately, HF symptoms do not parallel well with the main objective marker of systolic and diastolic HF, namely, PCWP.[5] Moreover, the distinction between systolic and diastolic HF may not be clear in many patients (e.g. the frail patient with systolic HF plus atrial fibrillation, oral steroids and non-steroidal drugs for arthritis plus pneumonia).

Sleep-disordered breathing

About 1 in 3 patients with HF will have obstructive sleep apnoea (OSA) and another 1 in 3 will have central sleep apnoea (CSA). Both groups usually snore. Thus, the understanding of both sleep physiology and sleep apnoea pathophysiology is crucial if one wishes to manage HF optimally.

HEALTHY NORMALS

In contrast to exercise, in which *more* cardiac output (CO) is required, sleep is a time in which *less* CO is usually required. Sleep is an important time of recuperation and repair. In addition to a lower CO, sleep is characterised by a change in body posture (horizontal vs. upright; i.e. a change in lung volume) and neurochemical state of mind (sleep vs. wake; i.e. a change in autonomic drive). During sleep, heart rate, systemic blood pressure, minute ventilation, airway calibre and lung volumes are reduced by ~20%. In non-rapid eye movement (REM) sleep, the autonomic nervous system changes: sympathetic activity is usually withdrawn and parasympathetic activity is increased. In REM sleep, both sympathetic and parasympathetic activities become active, although regional blood flow differs from wakefulness (e.g. blood is directed away from skeletal muscles, which are actively inhibited during REM sleep). In normal circumstances, the above changes have no adverse effects as metabolic rate is also diminished.

OBSTRUCTIVE SLEEP APNOEA

In OSA, sleep-related loss of upper airway muscle tone and upper airway collapse contributes to hypopnoeas and apnoeas (partial and complete obstruction for >10 s, respectively) in concert with strong diaphragmatic contractions, large negative intrathoracic pressure (ITP) swings accompanied by hypoxaemia and hypercapnia, terminated by an arousal from sleep, an acute rise in systemic and pulmonary blood pressure and sympathetic activity.[6] Usually, OSA is associated with the greatest hypoxaemia in REM sleep when respiratory muscle activity is at a minimum. In slow wave sleep, which is characterised by a reduction in arousability, loud continuous uninterrupted snoring occurs with levels of ITP ~3 times greater than during wakefulness. The combined negative ITP and elevated systemic blood pressure result in elevated transmural pressure to which the cardiac chambers are exposed.[7] Recurring hypoxia and hypercapnia result in endothelial cell damage and oxygen radical formation, which may lead to premature or accelerated atherosclerosis. Left untreated, OSA may contribute to the development of HF through systemic hypertension, premature atherosclerosis and coronary artery disease and increased left ventricular transmural pressure.

CENTRAL SLEEP APNOEA

For patients with established systolic HF, elevated pulmonary capillary wedge pressure[8] and catecholamines[9] may occur with resultant hyperventilation and hypocapnia.[10] In HF, compared with normal ventilation during sleep,

CSA is associated with a greater minute volume of ventilation (~22%) and a lower $PaCO_2$ (38 to 33 mmHg).[10] This is an extremely important concept to grasp, as HF is causing the hyperventilation and then the CSA: therapies will result in a reduction in minute ventilation. In addition, the route of breathing often changes from nasal to oral when tidal volume increases: the clinical impact of this relates to choice of mask (oronasal vs. nasal). Moreover, if nasal pressure (rather than oronasal thermistor) is being measured, a swap from nasal to oral, with ongoing respiratory effort, can be confused with OSA. When hyperventilation is combined with lung to brain circulatory delay, advanced HF results in a waxing and waning pattern of ventilation known as Cheyne-Stokes respiration or CSA (Figure 37.1). Typically, CSA occurs in stages 1 and 2 non-REM sleep, with arousals occurring classically at the peak of ventilation associated with mild hypoxaemia. Patients may complain of fatigue, insomnia, orthopnoea and/or paroxysmal nocturnal dyspnoea. Some patients with HF have an overlap of CSA and OSA.[11] In one study of single night analyses of HF patients, the frequency of OSA dropped from 69% to 23% and CSA increased from 32% to 78%, associated with a ~2 mmHg fall in mean transcutaneous PCO_2 from the first to the last quarter of the night in 12 patients with HF.[12] It is important to note that CSA is very sensitive to changes in position. CSA severity is alleviated by more than 50% when in the lateral[13] and similarly by the elevated head position[14] compared with the horizontal supine position. Patients with CSA and HF do appear to have increased association with greater mortality, as indicated by 1374 patients followed over 3.5 years in three large trials[15–17] but not all studies.[18]

PULMONARY EFFECTS OF HF

The mechanisms of dyspnoea in HF cannot be explained purely by the severity of cardiac impairment. In addition to skeletal muscle changes, pulmonary changes are also very common.[19,20]

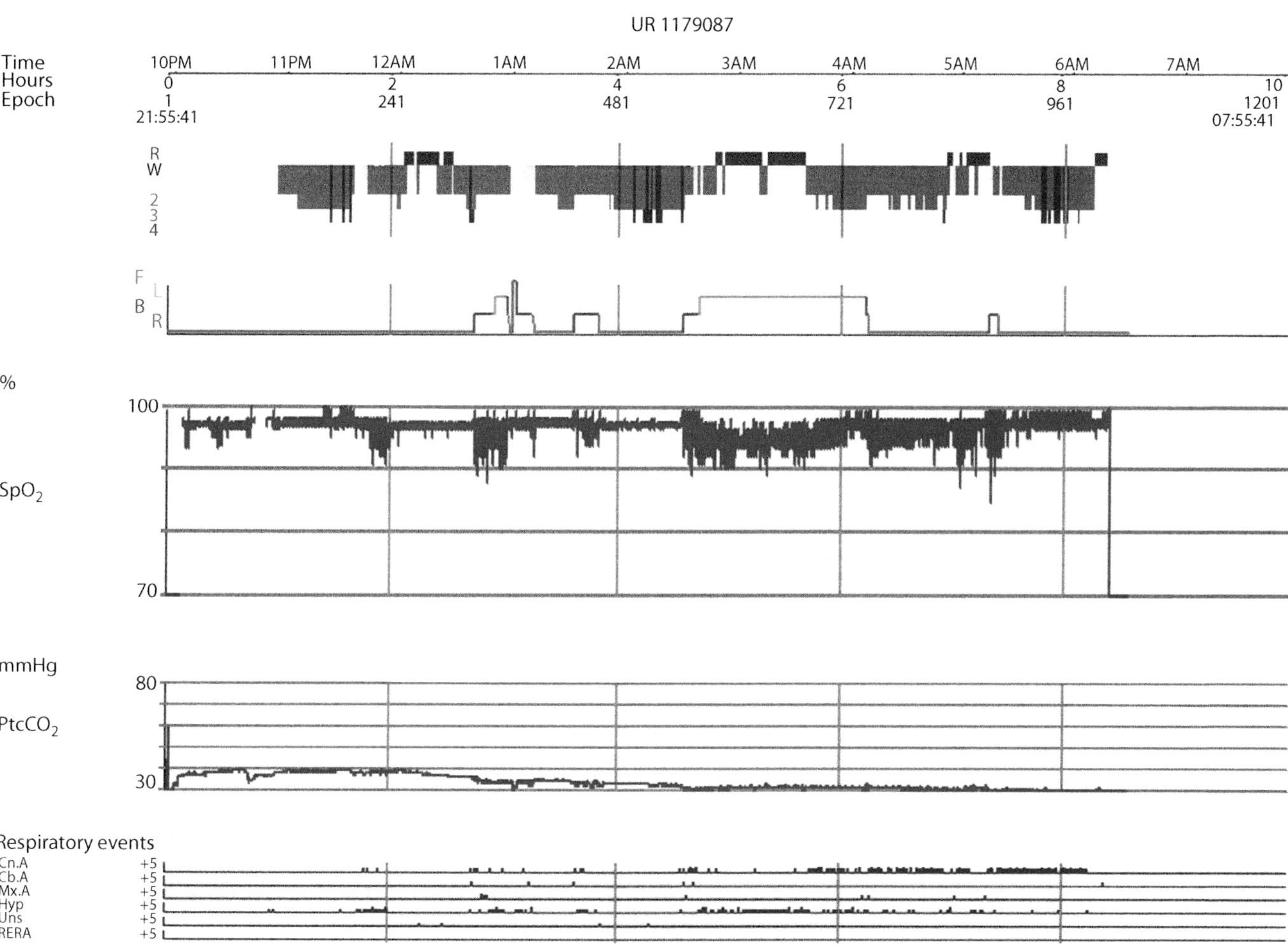

Figure 37.1 Typical polysomnogram illustrating hyperventilation during sleep in an HF patient with CSA. Note from top: time, colour-coded sleep stages (non-REM sleep: yellow, green and blue; REM sleep: red), colour-coded body position (front, left, back, right), SpO_2, transcutaneous PCO_2 and respiratory events (central and obstructive apnoeas and hypopnoeas). Note the episodic fall in SpO2 to values generally about 90%, peak values to 100%, and corresponding gradual reduction in $PtcCO_2$ to 30 mmHg. This indicates the presence of hyperventilation associated with CSA.

With HF, pulmonary capillary wedge pressure increases and fluid extravasates into the interstitium, then along the interlobular septa, toward the peribronchovascular space and thereafter toward the hila. In addition, fluid accumulates in the pleural spaces, where ~25% of the total body fluid accumulated in HF is deposited. In HF, the lymphatic drainage is estimated to increase 10-fold, allowing drainage of fluid from the pleural space and interlobar septa.

Pulmonary complications related to HF (Table 37.2) include a reduced total lung capacity (TLC) and functional residual capacity (FRC) and bronchial wall oedema with associated airflow obstruction. Pulmonary restriction correlates inversely with cardiac size. Respiratory muscle weakness occurs with HF, which in APO may lead to hypercapnia (~20%–45% of APO). Usually, <1% of CO is needed by respiratory muscles; however, this increases disproportionately with increased work of breathing (WOB) at a time of reduced CO.[21] In APO, the carbon monoxide diffusing capacity is usually elevated, related to increased pulmonary blood volume, but falls with medical management of APO.

Table 37.2 Pulmonary complications of heart failure

- Restrictive ventilatory defect
- Obstructive ventilatory defect
- Diffusing capacity increased (acute HF) and reduced (chronic HF)
- Respiratory muscle weakness
- Hyperventilation

Chronic HF with long-standing interstitial oedema and interstitial haemosiderosis may lead to ossific nodules.[22]

The pulmonary effects of HF described above are likely to be dependent on age at HF onset and duration. For example, HF effects related to mitral stenosis of rheumatic origin in youth may differ from hypertensive HF in the elderly. This may be due to the rate of deterioration and compensatory processes. Therefore, knowing the severity and temporal change in symptoms (hours vs. decades), the cause of HF, the age at symptom onset (youth vs. elderly), the response to treatment and the presence or absence of co-existing pulmonary conditions are important. Also, given the commonality of cigarette smoking in heart and lung disease plus the pulmonary side effects of cardiac treatment (e.g. amiodarone, beta blockers [BBs], pacemakers, thoracotomy), interpretation of lung function testing (including cardiopulmonary testing [Figure 37.2] and sleep studies) and the understanding of mechanisms of dyspnoea in HF can be challenging.

In normal subjects, acute volume loading results in reductions in TLC and forced vital capacity (FVC).[23] In stable HF, acute volume loading causes small airway obstruction.[24] Recovery from pulmonary oedema in non-smokers with HF is associated with a rise in TLC, FVC, forced expiratory volume in 1 s (FEV1) and FEV1/FVC ratio.[24]

With acute HF, capillary filtration of water leads to alveolar oedema. Over months to years, compensatory mechanisms may occur and reduce capillary filtration by as much as 50%. Therefore, a reduced pulmonary diffusing capacity in HF may indicate a compensatory thickening of the alveolar capillary membrane, which may prevent

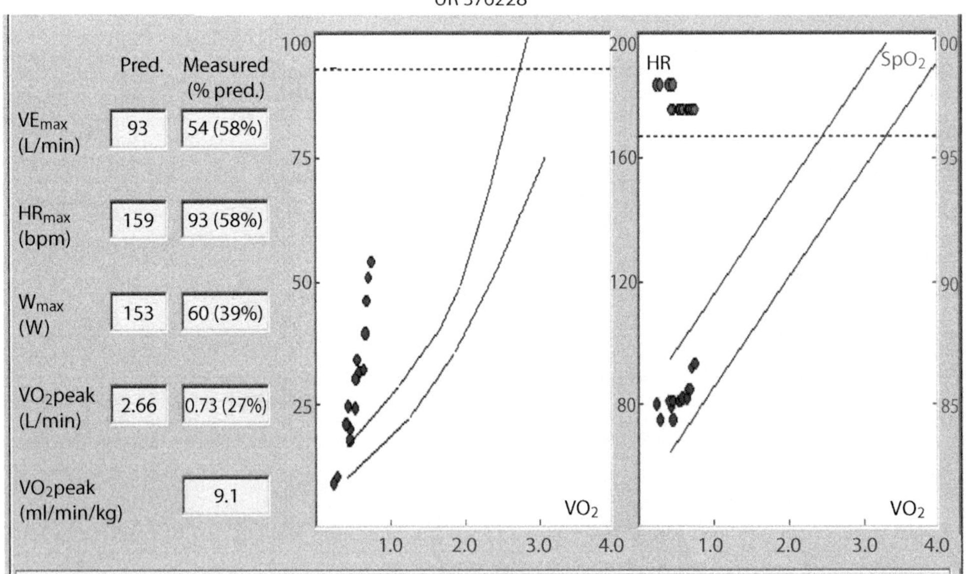

Figure 37.2 Typical cardiopulmonary exercise test illustrating hyperventilation during exercise in an HF patient. Note the left-hand graph of minute ventilation (VE) versus oxygen consumption (VO_2), the near-vertical display of blue dots (representing 30-s data points) to the left of the expected normal (parallel black lines). Patient's VE reaches only 58% predicted maximum (maximum displayed as dotted horizontal line). The right-hand graph displays heart rate (blue) versus VO_2 and SpO_2 (red) versus VO_2. Note little change in heart rate due to negative inotropic drugs with a maximum heart rate achieved of 58% predicted. Note also the absence of hypoxaemia (minimum SpO_2 97%).

alveolar oedema.[25] In support of this theory, reduced diffusing capacity with increased pulmonary dry weight suggesting an interstitial process made up of insoluble protein, lipid and cellular infiltrate, greater numbers of alveolar type 2 cells (source of surfactant) and an increase in surfactant was observed in a rodent model of HF.[26] The increase in alveolar surfactant would reduce surface tension and thereby reduce the WOB. In humans, it is also likely that recurring episodes of APO lead to interstitial thickening, responsible for a reduced diffusing capacity, perhaps as a defence against pulmonary oedema.[19] A downstream effect is that ventilation perfusion mismatch can be altered, leading to increased dead space and unnecessary hyperventilation (without hypoxaemia), which progresses during exercise.[27]

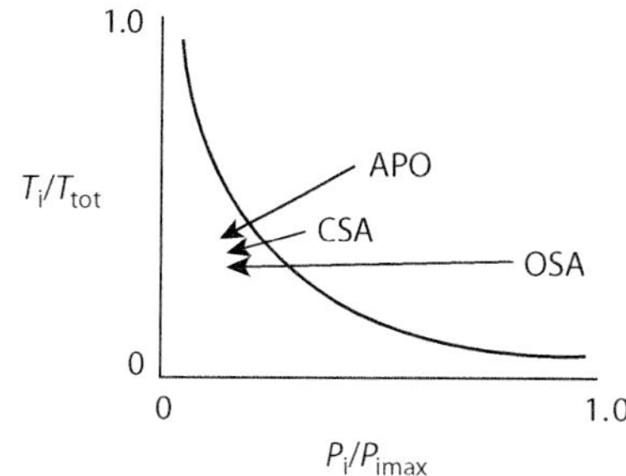

Figure 37.3 Schematic representation of respiratory muscle fatigue.[32] On the vertical axis is the ratio of inspiratory time/total inspiratory and expiratory time (i.e. T_i/T_{tot}). The horizontal axis is the inspiratory pressure/maximum inspiratory pressure (P_i/P_{imax}). The area to the right of the line represents a condition of high predisposition to fatigue, whereas the area to the left of the line denotes low chance of fatigue. Estimates of the positions of patients with HF and OSA, CSA and APO are marked. Arrows indicate the expected direction when CPAP is applied.

Mechanisms of NIV in HF

The proposed mechanisms of NIV in HF are listed in Table 37.3.

UPPER AIRWAY STABILISATION

The provision of NIV via a mask allows pneumatic splinting of the upper airway while breathing spontaneously. This action is most important during sleep in patients with OSA or when the sleep-deprived APO patient becomes drowsy and their neck flexes forward.

INCREASE IN LUNG VOLUME

HF, supine position and sleep are associated with a restrictive ventilatory defect. The lungs contain 50% of the body's oxygen stores; thus, a fall in total lung capacity will increase the propensity to tissue hypoxaemia. Ten cmH_2O CPAP increases lung volume (~0.5–1.0 L) and tidal volume[28,29] associated with a fall in rate of hypoxaemia (i.e. $dSpO_2/dt$ from 0.42 to 0.20%/s).[30]

Table 37.3 Effects of NIV in HF

1. Upper airway splinting
2. Pulmonary effects
   a. ↑ Lung volume
   b. Bronchodilatation
   c. ↑ V/Q
   d. Assist inspiratory respiratory muscles
   e. ↑ Dead space
3. Cardiac effects
   a. ↓ Afterload
      i. ↓ Transmural pressure
      ii. ↓ Cardiac chamber size
      iii. ↓ Systemic blood pressure
   b. ↓ Preload
4. Autonomic effects
   a. Attenuate sympathetic activity
   b. Accentuate parasympathetic activity

BRONCHODILATATION

PAP has a bronchodilating effect, particularly if the cause of bronchoconstriction is due to mechanical (obesity) or oedema (HF). Bronchogram studies indicate that CPAP is associated with a 30% increase in airway diameter.[31] Lenique et al.[30] estimated lung resistance to fall with CPAP in adults with subacute HF by 40%.

RESPIRATORY MUSCLE STRENGTH

Respiratory muscle weakness of HF may be overcome with CPAP by assisting inspiratory muscles and reducing increasing pulmonary compliance. Using the tension time index (Figure 37.3),[32] it is estimated that CPAP reduces P_i/P_{imax} and T_i/T_{tot} and thereby WOB and avoiding fatigue. In 3-month studies of CPAP in HF and CSA, respiratory muscle strength improves.[6]

LUNG MECHANICS

In patients with subacute APO, CPAP was associated with a 45% increase in lung compliance,[30] which is a similar effect to that seen with surfactant in the rodent model of HF.[25] WOB falls by 40% in stable HF patients with CPAP associated with a 35% reduction in pleural pressure amplitude and 7% reduction in respiratory rate.[33] Others have shown similar reductions in WOB following APO with CPAP compared with T piece breathing.[28] We have recently shown that the WOB (i.e. pressure × volume product) in a group of patients with HF is similarly elevated in periods of OSA and CSA, compared with normal ventilation; however, CSA is associated with a greater efficiency (pressure × time product) of ventilation compared with OSA and normal ventilation.[34]

VENTILATORY DRIVE

HF is associated with an increased respiratory drive during sleep and exercise[6,11,35] and CPAP during sleep causes a reduction in ventilation and a CO_2 rise.[36] The fall in ventilation and rise in CO_2 with CPAP are due to improved oxygenation (increased lung volume), improved CO and a reduction in sympathetic activity. CPAP may increase dead space (due to dilated conducting airways and mask volume) and thereby contribute to hypercapnia.

CARDIAC AFTERLOAD

In HF, CO is critically dependent on left ventricular afterload, defined by the Law of Laplace, namely

$$\text{Afterload} = \frac{(\text{Systolic blood pressure} - \text{Intrathoracic pressure}) \times \text{LV radius}}{\text{LV wall thickness}}$$

Thus, left ventricular afterload is increased when (a) systemic blood pressure is raised, (b) the ITPs are more negative, (c) the radius of the ventricle is increased and (d) the wall of the left ventricle is decreased. These variables will change to differing degrees during APO, OSA and CSA, as illustrated in Figure 37.4a through e.

In HF, the stroke volume is sensitive to changes in afterload: any factors that reduce afterload should increase stroke volume (unless there are conduction defects).[37]

CPAP at pressures of 5–10 cmH_2O has been shown to reduce systemic blood pressure acutely and chronically,[38] elevate ITPs and reduce LV chamber radius.[39] Due to reductions in left ventricular transmural pressure and heart rate, significant reductions in cardiac work have also been reported.[33,40,41] CPAP in stable HF patients has been associated with reductions in myocardial oxygen uptake[40] and cardiac sympathetic activity.[41]

The effects of CPAP directly on CO are variable. Increased stroke volume in stable HF patients with elevated filling pressures (PCWP > 18 mmHg) has been shown acutely,[42] whereas others could not confirm this if in atrial fibrillation.[43] Other studies have shown an increase in LVEF over 1–3 months in OSA[44,45] and CSA patients[46,47] with LV remodelling plus reductions in mitral regurgitation and cardiac chamber dimensions.[48]

PRELOAD

The elevation of ITP will impede venous return by up to 40% in canine models given 10 mmHg CPAP.[49] In normal

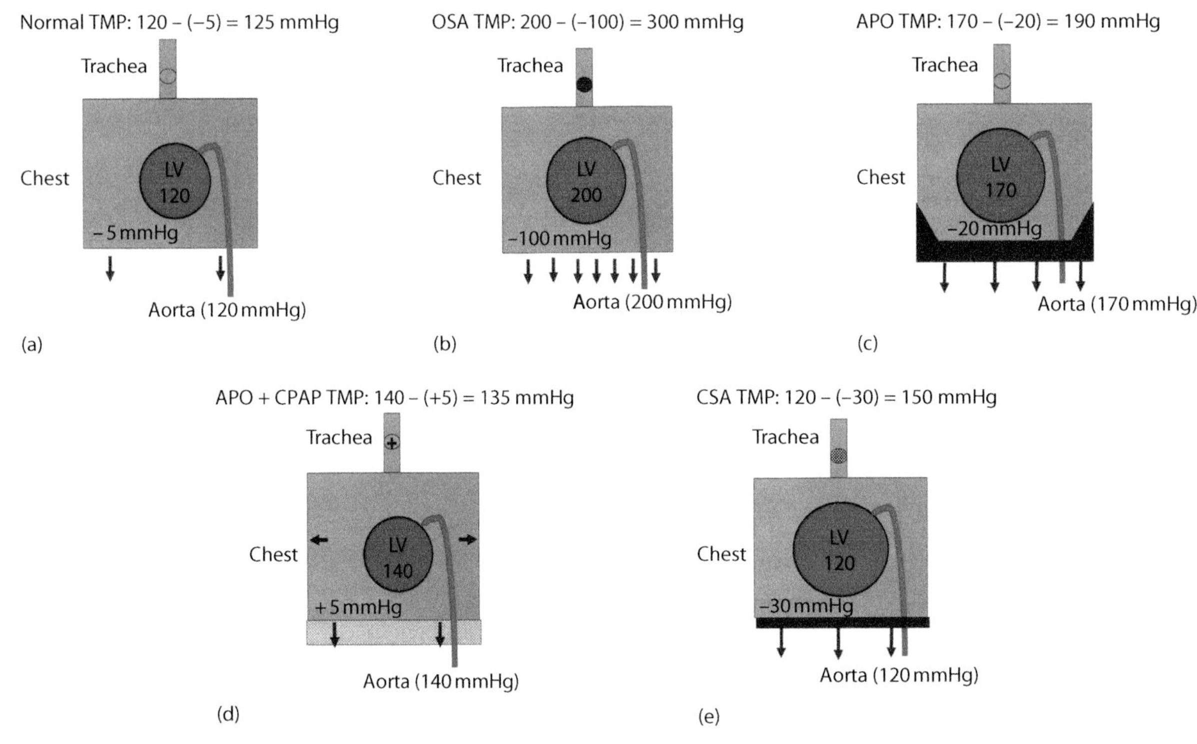

Figure 37.4 (**a** through **e**) These five figures illustrate the effects of intrathoracic and systemic blood pressure on left ventricular transmural pressure during systole (TMP). **(a)** A normal situation during inspiration and systole with systolic BP of 120 mmHg and normal inspiratory pressures of −5 mmHg, accounting for a TMP of 125 mmHg. **(b)** A patient with obstructive sleep apnoea (OSA) and HF: note very elevated systolic BP and very large negative ITPs with a corresponding TMP of 300 mmHg. **(c)** A patient with acute pulmonary oedema (APO): note elevated systolic BP and large negative ITPs with a corresponding TMP of 190 mmHg. Also note development of effusions and further loss of total lung capacity. **(d)** The patient with APO on 10 mmHg (~12 cmH_2O) CPAP: note fall in systolic blood pressure, positive change in ITPs and abolition of pleural effusions and reduction in left ventricular chamber size with overall reduction in TMP to 135 mmHg. **(e)** A patient with CSA and HF: note elevated systolic BP and large negative ITPs, greater cardiomegaly and elevated TMP of 150 mmHg. Also note loss of total lung capacity and left ventricular chamber dilatation.

subjects, this may result in elevation of heart rate to maintain CO. In HF, a small amount of CPAP (5–10 cmH_2O) may independently augment stroke volume. High levels of CPAP may impair venous return and reduce CO (e.g. HF with dehydration, sepsis), and in such circumstances, BPAP may be more beneficial.

AUTONOMIC EFFECTS

Based on heart rate variability analysis (both temporal and power spectral analysis), the acute effects of CPAP in HF have been shown to increase vagal and attenuate sympathetic activity.[41,50] Reductions in urinary and blood norepinephrine have been observed to be associated with improvement in cardiac function with CPAP in patients with HF and OSA[44,45] and CSA.[46,47] Baroreceptor function and heart rate variability have been shown to improve over 4 weeks with CPAP in HF and OSA patients.[51]

Evidence base for NIV in chronic HF

NIV has been used in various areas of HF. In acute HF (i.e. APO), NIV (mainly CPAP) has been shown to be effective in terms of improvement in physiology, reduced intubation risk and survival (CPAP only) in carefully selected patients.[52] In HF patients without sleep apnoea, CPAP was found to have no impact on cardiac function or survival over 5 years.[53] Thus, the balance of this section will be confined to chronic HF with OSA and CSA (Table 37.4).

OBSTRUCTIVE SLEEP APNOEA

OSA occurs in ~33% of HF patients,[11] and CPAP over 1–3 months has been shown to improve LVEF, autonomic control and quality of life[44,45] while improvements in long-term mortality are suggested in uncontrolled studies.[54,55]

In the first randomised controlled parallel designed trial of CPAP in stable HF with OSA,[44] 24 patients (~55 years) with HF (mean LVEF 27%, ~50% on BB therapy) and OSA (AHI 41 events per hour [eph], min SpO_2 80%) were randomised to CPAP or no CPAP for 1 month. Optimal medical therapy continued in both groups. Compared with the untreated control group, the CPAP-treated group (9 cmH_2O × 6 hours/night) experienced a significant improvement in LVEF (25% to 34%) associated with falls in heart rate, systolic blood pressure plus left ventricular end systolic and diastolic volumes. Similar changes were noted in the BB- and non-BB-treated groups. Sympathetic nerve activity, measured by muscle sympathetic nerve activity (MSNA) recordings, was taken during wakefulness from the common perineal nerve at baseline and 1 month follow-up in 17 patients;[56] the MSNA fell by ~15% with the CPAP-treated group. In 18 of the 24 patients, the frequency of premature ventricular beats also fell (170 to 70 per hour) with CPAP over 1 month whereas there was no significant change in the control group.[57] In a further retrospective study from the same investigators, the control group (i.e. stable HF with untreated OSA) had a significantly worse 3-year survival than the HF group without OSA.[53] Although there was no significant difference in survival between the OSA-treated and untreated groups, a trend for improved survival with CPAP emerged.

The second randomised controlled parallel designed trial of CPAP treatment for OSA in stable HF by Mansfield et al.[45] involved 55 patients (~57 years, LVEF 35%, BB use 78%, AHI 28 eph and min SpO_2 78%), of whom 40 completed the 3-month trial. They were randomised to CPAP (8 cmH_2O × 6 hours/night) or control. The change in mean LVEF was significant (38% to 43%), as was the 42% fall in overnight urinary noradrenaline and improved quality of life (SF-36 and chronic HF) with 3 months of nocturnal CPAP compared with the untreated control group. However, there was no significant change in maximum oxygen uptake during incremental cycle ergometry exercise. Although survival was not a primary endpoint, two deaths occurred in the CPAP group: one spontaneous and the other a complication of a pacemaker insertion, whereas there were no deaths in the control arm. Thus, the call for longer trials with death as an endpoint is warranted.

Table 37.4 Various actions of positive airway pressure (CPAP, BPAP, ASV) in different situations of HF (ITP, intrathoracic)

	OSA	CSA	APO
Upper airway stability	+++	+	–
Increase lung volume	+	++	+++
Increase alveolar pressure	+	++	+++
Decrease LV transmural pressure			
by alleviating negative ITP	+++		
by elevating ITP	–	++	+
Assist inspiratory muscles	–	++	+++
Bronchodilating	–	+	+++
Prevent expiratory muscle recruitment (e.g. BPAP)	–	–	+
Prevent fluctuation in tidal volume (e.g. ASV)	–	+	–

CENTRAL SLEEP APNOEA

CSA occurs in ~33% of HF patients.[11] Before considering PAP, one must consider that the HF is maximally managed (and the patient is compliant): this may include not only dietary (fluid, salt) and medical therapy toward the cardiac pump (BBs, digoxin, diuretics, ACE inhibition, etc) and arrhythmias (digoxin, amiodarone) but also consideration of various devices (cardiac resynchronisation therapy, left ventricular assist devices) and surgery (valve repair and transplantation). Given the variability of CSA, it may be prudent to repeat the sleep test (and assessment of fluid retention, e.g. body weight) after a period of therapy to ensure that the CSA persists. Note that long-term oxygen therapy has not been shown to be beneficial in routine HF and the evidence in support of its use in CSA is very limited and of dubious scientific merit.[58] Similarly, treatments that reduce arousability (sedative and narcotics) or stimulate ventilation (CO_2, dead space, theophylline) should be used with great caution and be considered experimental at this stage.

Based on the basic principles that PAP has upon cardiac, pulmonary and upper airway dynamics in HF, a single-centre randomised trial of CPAP in stable HF with CSA was undertaken.[46] This study enrolled 24 subjects with HF and CSA (before the routine use of BB) (~59 years, LVEF 20%, AHI 38 eph). Those randomised to CPAP (10 cmH_2O × 6 hours/night) experienced a significant improvement in LVEF (21% to 29%), quality of life and markers of neurohormonal activity[9] compared with a control group. Unlike CPAP for OSA (which responds immediately), CPAP for CSA was slowly titrated with careful inpatient observation for 2–3 nights, from 5 to 13 cmH_2O with the knowledge that CSA may take days to weeks to resolve. Importantly, in this group of patients, there was a fall in minute ventilation and a rise in transcutaneous CO_2 levels.[36] Taken together, these data suggested an improvement in cardiac function, a fall in sympathetic activity, a reduction in hyperventilation (with rise in $PaCO_2$) and resultant stabilisation of ventilation during sleep with CPAP over weeks to months.

This led to the larger CANPAP trial[47] with transplant-free survival as the primary outcome. This trial was conducted in 11 centres with 258 patients recruited (~63 years, LVEF 24%, BB use 77%, AHI 40 eph, min SpO_2 82%). Patients continued medical therapy and were randomised to CPAP or no CPAP. The mean follow-up period was 2.2 years and 85% completed the trial (CPAP 9 cmH_2O × 4 hours/night). There was no significant improvement in the primary outcome, namely, transplant-free survival, or in two secondary outcomes (hospitalisations and quality of life). However, there were significant improvements in other secondary outcomes (plasma norepinephrine, LVEF, nocturnal oxygenation, AHI, and 6-min walk distance).

A post hoc analysis[56] of transplant-free survival based on the "suppressability" of the AHI during a repeat sleep study at 3 months in 210 of the original 258 CANPAP patients indicated that AHI fell to <15 eph in 57% of patients randomised to CPAP. This CSA suppression with CPAP at 3 months was associated with a significant improvement in LVEF (25.6% to 29.2%). Most importantly, the transplant-free survival at 60 months follow-up was greater in the CSA suppressed group compared with the untreated control and non-suppressed CSA groups (~95% vs. ~50%, respectively).

ASV was developed for use in CSA.[59] This device detects and maintains a patient's ventilation at ~90% of their prior 3-min moving average by providing a small amount of CPAP (~5 cmH_2O) plus a small amount of inspiratory pressure support (~3 cmH_2O). During central apnoeas, it provides greater inspiratory support (5–8 cmH_2O) at 15 breaths per minute sufficient to maintain ventilation.

In a series of single-night studies, Teschler et al.[59] compared the effects of a single night of supplemental oxygen (2 L/min), CPAP (mean 9.3 cmH_2O), BPAP (IPAP 13.5 and EPAP 5.2 cmH_2O) and ASV (mean 7–9 cmH_2O) on consecutive nights, in random order in 14 HF patients with CSA. The AHI declined significantly from 45 (control) to 28 (oxygen) to 27 (CPAP) and 15 (BPAP) and 6 (ASV) eph. Improvements in sleep quality (combined SWS and REM sleep) occurred only in the BPAP and ASV treatment groups. The effects on cardiovascular function were not assessed. The group mean $PtcCO_2$ and arterialised $PaCO_2$ increased overnight with ASV and CPAP (2.0 and 3.6 mmHg with ASV and 2.5 and 4.2 mmHg with CPAP) compared with baseline control night. The rise in PCO_2 with ASV was attributed to a fall in minute volume of ventilation (although not measured) related to greater slow wave and REM sleep and less arousals. Alternatively, it may have been due to dead space provided by ASV.

A meta-analysis comparing the effects of ASV with CPAP in ~470 patients with HF and CSA indicated a similar effectiveness in terms of improvement in LVEF and reduction in AHI.[60]

Two meta-analyses comparing the effects of ASV with best care in HF were undertaken providing positive results for ASV in HF. The first, based on 14 trials, concluded ASV reduced AHI and improved LVEF and 6 MWD, but not QOL.[61] The second (5 RCTS, 395 subjects) concluded that ASV reduced mortality in HF with preserved or reduced LVEF and CSA.[62]

Two large long-term trials of ASV in HF with sleep apnoea were launched circa 2008: The Adaptive **Ser**vo **V**entilation in Patients with **H**eart **F**ailure (SERVE-HF, NCT00733343) and the Effect of **Ad**aptive Servo **Vent**ilation on Survival and Hospital Admissions in **H**eart **F**ailure (ADVENT-HF, NCT01128816) trials.[63,64]

The SERVE-HF trial (launched 2008) randomised 1325 patients from 91 centres with maximally treated HF (LVEF < 45%) with predominant CSA (>50% events central and AHI > 15) to either ASV or usual care.[63] The initial SERVE-HF trial publication in 2015 reported that ASV had no effect on the primary outcome (composite of death from any cause, lifesaving cardiovascular intervention or unplanned hospitalisation for HF) based on an intention-to-treat analysis.

Secondary outcomes were increased with ASV, namely, all-cause and cardiovascular mortality. Compared with the CANPAP trial, the SERVE-HF population was older (63 vs. 70 years), was less male dominated (97% vs. 90%), had similar body mass index (29 vs. 29 kg/m^2) and had a higher LVEF (24% vs. 33%) with less severe CSA (AHI 40 vs. 32 eph). Of note, the 5-year survival on treatment in the CANPAP trial appeared significantly better (50% vs. 90%) compared with the SERVE-HF trial (40% vs. 45%).

The SERVE-HF trial findings of increased mortality with ASV were most unexpected and contrary to meta-analyses and the understanding of PAP actions in HF. From a trial point of view, the analysis was undertaken as *intention to treat*, yet of patients randomised to ASV, 25% discontinued the therapy, the balance used ASV for only 3.7 hours/night. Also, 15% of the patients randomised to the control group crossed over to ASV. This highlights the vagaries of clinical trials of devices using drug trial designs! Follow-up correspondence from the authors suggests that similar findings were observed with *per-protocol analysis*.[63]

Why allocation to ASV was associated with increased mortality is not clear. Minute ventilation (or CO_2) was unfortunately not measured, nor pH. It is possible that ventilation increased on ASV, resulting in a respiratory alkalosis, hypokalemia, secondary arrhythmias and sudden death. Alternatively, patients with HF may have had dynamic CSA, such that those allocated to ASV may have had clearing of lung water, minimising CSA. This group may have become increasingly "preload" sensitive, creating a sympathetically driven state and subsequent arrhythmias. Unfortunately, heart rate during sleep was not reported. Frequency of contact with patients was 2 weeks, 3 months and 12 months in person (and 6 months by telephone), which may not have been of sufficient frequency: note that medical therapies designed to manage HF (and their response) frequently change. Finally, the ASV may have been operating in ASV or CPAP modes: this information would be valuable to know as suppression of (or disguised) CSA is difficult to determine on polysomnography; the output of the ASV device would assist in this regard. Persistent CSA needing ongoing ASV would differ from suppressed CSA needing a low level of CPAP (or no CPAP).

Finally, it was also noted that the presence of residual CSA on polysomnography was associated with an improved survival. This later observation is suggestive that CSA may be compensatory for severe HF as suggested over the past 16 years by this author.[65,66] From a physiological standpoint, CSA should assist HF by various mechanisms. First, in the setting of congested lungs, CSA provides ~30 s tachypnoea followed by ~30 s rest.[67] Second, during tachypnoea, the end expiratory lung volume increases[68] plus forward stroke volume is assisted.[69,70] Large tidal breaths attenuates sympathetic activity.[71] During central apnoea, there is in reality a prolonged expiration (not really an apnoea!) until the upper airway closes,[72] resulting in ~5 cmH_2O intrinsic positive end-expiratory pressure. The mild respiratory alkalosis has a twofold effect: it is a tolerant environment for hypoxia compared with acidosis[73] and there is a pH buffer in the event of an acute deterioration (e.g. APO) that protects the HF patients from developing hypercapnic acidotic respiratory failure.

The ADVENT-HF trial is underway[64] and expected to be completed by 2016. This study differs from the SERVE-HF trial above. First, there is a different proprietary device with differing algorithms and lower pressures. Second, they are including both CSA and (non sleepy) OSA.

LIMITATIONS OF STUDIES

The major concern with much of the published data relates to study design and absence of appropriate endpoints. When dealing with HF patients, it is important to include a control group and robust markers of cardiac function (e.g. mortality, admissions, LVEF, BNP) in addition to general and disease-specific quality of life (i.e. HF and sleep apnoea)—composite endpoints may be used. The level, duration and mode of NIV need to be adequate and include reporting of leak mask type and efficacy (i.e. follow-up AHI). It is noteworthy that the duration of NIV therapy is important: in the "positive" APO studies, NIV was used ~8 hours total,[52] whereas it was 2 hours total in the negative study.[74] In the positive OSA trials, CPAP was used ~6 hours/night.[44,45] In the CSA trials, the positive trial had CPAP in use ~6 hours/night,[46] whereas it was <4 hours in the negative[47,63] trials. NIV must be used for a modest period of time to obtain the benefit! Accurate descriptions of HF are also required and include cardiac rhythm, rate and any associated features of HF (e.g. anaemia, renal failure, etc). Duration of HF should also be included, as the features of mitral stenosis in youth may differ from ischemic cardiomyopathy in the elderly.

Technical aspects

SUPPLEMENTAL OXYGEN

The role of oxygen therapy in HF with SDB has been influenced by a number of studies that have shown marginal effects upon markers of CSA and no significant changes in cardiac function.[6,74] The alleviation of AHI may relate to attenuation of peripheral and central chemosensitivity, although this remains to be proven. Although avoidance of hypoxia is thought to be important, so too is the avoidance of hyperoxia: as it can impair pulmonary and cardiac function and cause coronary vasoconstriction.[6]

CPAP TITRATION IN CSA

Unlike CPAP for OSA (which usually responds immediately), CPAP for CSA should be slowly titrated with careful observation for 2–3 nights, from 5 to 13 cmH_2O with the knowledge that CSA may take days to weeks to resolve. Mask type is crucial as oral breathing will be common during the periods of hyperventilation.

SUMMARY

Patients with HF have dyspnoea and fatigue as their main symptoms. Understanding the relationship between lung function and polysomnography and the effects of PAP provides insight into the pathogenesis of HF.

It is likely that the severity and presence of either type of SDB is dependent on several factors including body weight, fluid accumulation, drugs, posture and head elevation.

Whether NIV remodels the failing heart, acutely or chronically, and for how long is unknown as is whether the trajectory of the underling HF prognosis and severity can be altered.

The effects of HF therapies (from medications, pacemakers to transplantation) on SDB need further investigation, as it is possible that HF treatment will attenuate SDB.

The optimal mode and duration of the various NIV settings and devices to treat sleep apnoea in HF remain unknown. Whether APAP and ASV devices are beneficial over commonplace and less expensive CPAP remains speculative. The additional risk of mortality with ASV in HF[63] appears to be related to sudden death (i.e. arrhythmias). Accordingly, HF patients on ASV need to be warned of the risk. Factors that might predispose to arrhythmias such as electrolyte change due to respiratory alkalosis (i.e. excessive ventilation) or medications now redundant (e.g. excessive diuretics) need to be carefully observed and considered. Anti-arrhythmic pacemakers also need to be considered. Finally, determining whether the CSA is disguised (i.e. ASV is working actively) or the CSA is suppressed (i.e. ASV is working similar to a CPAP device) would be worth considering. Suppressed CSA at 3 months appears to be associated with a survival benefit.[56]

Defining the best metric of improvement in patients with HF and SDB remains to be determined. The AHI may not be best suited for the CSA group as shorter cycle length (indicating better cardiac function) and less hypoxaemia (indicating increased oxygen stores) may be dismissed by a higher AHI. Cycle length, markers of oxygenation and CO_2, sleep quality, patient comfort and quality of life plus markers of autonomic control (e.g. heart rate, heart rate variability, overnight urinary noradrenaline) and BNP may be best.

The use of ASV may negate central apnoeas and hypopnoeas measured in the usual way, that is, by chest and abdominal plethysmography and oronasal airflow, and thus drop the AHI. However, the underlying pathophysiologic periodic breathing may persist and only be detected by measurement of the fluctuating swings in peak inspiratory pressures. Whether persistent underlying periodic breathing is of clinical importance remains to be determined.

A more intricate knowledge of cardiopulmonary interaction in HF is required particularly related to rest, exercise, posture and sleep with and without PAP and its effect on respiratory control, fatigue and changes in lung volume.

REFERENCES

1. Jessup M, Abraham WT, Casey DE et al. 2009 Focused Update: ACCF/AHA Guidelines for the Diagnosis and Management of Heart Failure in Adults: A Report of the American College of Cardiology Foundation/American Heart Association Task. *Circulation*. 2009;119:1977–2016.
2. Poulton EP. Left sided heart failure with pulmonary plus pressure machine. *Lancet*. 1936;2:981–3.
3. Maeder MT, Kaye DM. Heart failure with normal left ventricular ejection fraction. *J Am Coll Cardiol*. 2009;53:905–18.
4. Serizawa T, Vogel WM, Apstein CS, Grossman W. Comparison of acute alterations in left ventricular relaxation and diastolic chamber stiffness induced by hypoxia and ischemia. Role of myocardial oxygen supply–demand imbalance. *J Clin Invest*. 1981;68: 91–102.
5. Stevenson LW, Perloff JK. The limited reliability of physical signs for estimating hemodynamics in chronic heart failure. *JAMA*. 1989;261:884–8.
6. Naughton MT, Lorenzi Filho G. Sleep in heart failure: Cardiovascular implications of sleep disorders. *Prog Cardiovasc Dis*. 2009;51:339–49.
7. Usui K, Parker JD, Newton GE et al. Left ventricular structural adaptations to obstructive sleep apnea in dilated cardiomyopathy. *Am J Respir Crit Care Med*. 2006;173:1170–75.
8. Solin P, Bergin P, Richardson M et al. Influence of pulmonary capillary wedge pressure on central apnea in heart failure. *Circulation*. 1999;99:1574–9.
9. Naughton MT, Benard DC, Liu PP et al. Effects of nasal CPAP on sympathetic activity in patients with heart failure and central sleep apnea. *Am J Respir Crit Care Med*. 1995;152:473–9.
10. Naughton MT, Benard D, Tam A et al. Role of hyperventilation in the pathogenesis of central sleep apneas in patients with congestive heart failure. *Am Rev Respir Dis*. 1993;148:330–8.
11. Sin DD, Fitzgerald F, Parker JD et al. Risk factors for central and obstructive sleep apnea in 450 men and women with congestive heart failure. *Am J Respir Crit Care Med*. 1999;160:1101–6.
12. Tkacova R, Niroumand M, Lorenzi-Filho G, Bradley TD. Overnight shift from obstructive to central apneas in patients with heart failure role of PCO_2 and circulatory delay. *Circulation*. 2001;103: 238–42.
13. Szollosi I, Roebuck T, Thompson B, Naughton MT. Lateral sleeping position reduces severity of central sleep apnea/Cheyne Stokes respiration. *Sleep* 2006;29:1045–51.
14. Soll BAG, Yeo KK, Davis JW et al. The effect of posture on Cheyne Stokes respirations and hemodynamics in patients with heart failure. *Sleep*. 2009;32:1499–1506.

15. Corrà, U, Pistono M, Mezzani A et al. Sleep and exertional periodic breathing in chronic heart failure: Prognostic importance and interdependence. *Circulation*. 2006;113:44–50.
16. Luo Q, Zhang HL, Tao XC et al. Impact of untreated sleep apnea on prognosis of patients with congestive heart failure. *Int J Cardiol*. 2010;144(3):420–2.
17. Khayat R, Jarjoura D, Porter K et al. Sleep disordered breathing and post-discharge mortality in patients with acute heart failure. *Eur Heart J*. 2015 Jun 14; 36(23):1463–9.
18. Grimm W, Sosnovskaya A, Timmesfeld N et al. Prognostic impact of central sleep apnea in patients with heart failure. *J Cardiac Fail*. 2015 Feb 28;21(2):126–33.
19. Gehlbach BK, Geppert E. The pulmonary manifestations of left heart failure. *Chest*. 2004;125(2):669–82.
20. Kee K, Naughton MT. Heart failure and the lung. *Circ J*. 2010 Nov;74(12):2507–16.
21. Roberston CH, Foster GH, Johnson RL. The relationship of respiratory failure to the oxygen consumption of lactate production by and distribution of blood flow among respiratory muscles during increasing inspiratory resistance. *J Clin Investig*. 1977;59:31–42.
22. Galloway RW, Epstein EJ, Coulshed N. Pulmonary ossific nodules in mitral valve disease. *Br Heart J*. 1961;23:297–307.
23. Muir AL, Flenley DC, Kirby BJ et al. Cardiorespiratory effects of rapid saline infusion in normal man. *J Appl Physiol*. 1975;28:786–93.
24. Puri S, Dutka DP, Baker BL et al. Acute saline infusion reduces alveolar–capillary membrane conductance and increases airflow obstruction in patients with left ventricular dysfunction. *Circulation*. 1999;99:1190–6.
25. Noble WH, Kay JC, Obdrzalek J. Lung mechanics in hypervolemic pulmonary edema. *J Appl Physiol*. 1975;38:681–7.
26. Dixon DL, De Pasquale CG, De Smet HR et al. Reduced surface tension normalizes static lung mechanics in a rodent chronic heart failure model. *Am J Respir Crit Care Med*. 2009;180:181–7.
27. Kee K, Stuart-Andrews C, Ellis MJ et al. Increased dead space ventilation mediates reduced exercise capacity in systolic heart failure. *Am J Respir Crit Care Med*. First published online 06 Jan 2016 as DOI: 10.1164/rccm.201508-1555OC
28. Katz JA, Marks JD. Inspiratory work with and without continuous positive airway pressure in patients with acute respiratory failure. *Anaesthesiology*. 1985;63:598–607.
29. Krachman SL, Crocetti J, Berger TJ et al. Effects of nasal continuous positive airway pressure on oxygen body stores in patients with Cheyne Stokes respiration and congestive heart failure. *Chest*. 2003;123:59–66.
30. Lenique F, Habis M, Lofaso F et al. Ventilatory and hemodynamic effects of continuous positive airway pressure in left heart failure *Am J Respir Crit Care Med*. 1997;155:500–5.
31. Barach AL, Swenson P. Effect of breathing gases under positive pressure on lumens of small and medium-sized bronchi. *Arch Intern Med*. 1939;63:946–8.
32. Bellemare F, Grassino A. Effect of pressure and timing of contraction on human diaphragm fatigue. *J Appl Physiol*. 1982;53:1190–5.
33. Naughton MT, Rahman MA, Hara K et al. Effect of continuous positive airway pressure on intrathoracic and left ventricular transmural pressures in patients with congestive heart failure. *Circulation*. 1995;91:1725–31.
34. Kee K, Sands S, Stuart-Andrews C et al. The effect of sleep apnoea and inspired carbon dioxide on respiratory effort in patients with heart failure. *Respirology*. 2015;20:50.
35. Solin P, Roebuck T, Johns DP et al. Peripheral and central ventilatory responses in central sleep apnea with and without heart failure. *Am J Respir Crit Care Med*. 2000;162:2194–200.
36. Naughton MT, Benard DC, Rutherford R, Bradley TD. Effect of continuous positive airway pressure on central sleep apnea and nocturnal PCO_2 in heart failure. *Am J Respir Crit Care Med*. 1994;150:1598–604.
37. Pinsky MR, Matuschak GM, Klain M. Determinants of cardiac augmentation by elevations in intrathoracic pressure. *J Appl Physiol*. 1985;58:1189–98.
38. Haentjens P, Van Meerhaeghe A, Moscariello A et al. The impact of continuous positive airway pressure on blood pressure in patients with obstructive sleep apnea syndrome: Evidence from a meta-analysis of placebo-controlled randomized trials. *Arch Intern Med*. 2007;167(8):757–64.
39. Leithner C, Podolsry A, Globits S et al. Magnetic resonance imaging of the heart during positive pressure ventilation in normal subjects. *Crit Care Med*. 1994;22:426–32.
40. Kaye DM, Mansfield D, Naughton MT. Continuous positive airway pressure reduces myocardial oxygen consumption in congestive heart failure. *Clin Sci (Lond)*. 2004;106:599–603.
41. Kaye DM, Mansfield D, Aggarwal A et al. Acute effects of continuous positive airway pressure on cardiac sympathetic tone in congestive heart failure. *Circulation*. 2001;103:2336–8.
42. Bradley TD, Holloway RM, McLaughlin PR et al. Cardiac output response to continuous positive airway pressure in congestive heart failure. *Am Rev Resp Dis*. 1992;145:377–82.
43. Kiely JL, Deegan P, Buckley A et al. Efficacy of nasal continuous positive airway pressure therapy in chronic heart failure: Importance of underlying heart rhythm. *Thorax*. 1998;53:957–62.
44. Kaneko Y, Floras JS, Usui K et al. Cardiovascular effects of continuous positive airway pressure in patients with heart failure and obstructive sleep apnea. *N Engl J Med*. 2003;348(13):1233–41.

45. Mansfield DR, Gollogly NC, Kaye DM et al. Controlled trial of continuous positive airway pressure in obstructive sleep apnea and heart failure. *Am J Respir Crit Care Med.* 2004;169(3):361–6.
46. Naughton MT, Liu PP, Benard DC et al. Treatment of congestive heart failure and Cheyne-Stokes respiration during sleep by continuous positive airway pressure. *Am J Respir Crit Care Med.* 1995;151:92–7.
47. Bradley TD, Logan AG, Kimoff RJ et al. Continuous positive airway pressure for central sleep apnea and heart failure. *N Engl J Med.* 2005;135:2025–33.
48. Tkacova R, Liu PP, Naughton MT, Bradley TD. Effect of continuous positive airway pressure on mitral regurgitation and atrial natriuretic peptide in patients with heart failure and central sleep apnea. *J Am Coll Cardiol.* 1997;30:739–45.
49. Fessler HE, Brower RG, Wise RA, Permutt S. Effects of positive end-expiratory pressure on the canine venous return curve. *Am Rev Respir Dis.* 1992;146:4–10.
50. Butler GC, Naughton MT, Rahman MA et al. Continuous positive airway pressure increases heart rate variability in congestive heart failure. *J Am Coll Cardiol.* 1995;25:672–9.
51. Gilman MP, Floras JS, Usui K et al. Continuous positive airway pressure increases heart rate variability in heart failure patients with obstructive sleep apnoea. *Clin Sci (Lond).* 2008 Feb;114(3):243–9.
52. Peter JV, Moran JL, Phillips-Hughes J et al. Effect of non-invasive positive pressure ventilation (NIPPV) on mortality in patients with acute cardiogenic pulmonary oedema: A meta-analysis. *Lancet.* 2006;367(9517):1155–63.
53. Sin DD, Logan AG, Fitzgerald FS et al. Effects of continuous positive airway pressure on cardiovascular outcomes in heart failure patients with and without Cheyne-Stokes respiration. *Circulation.* 2000;102:61–6.
54. Wang H, Parker JD, Newton GE et al. Influence of obstructive sleep apnea on mortality in patients with heart failure. *J Am Coll Cardiol.* 2007;49(15):1625–31.
55. Kasai T, Narui K, Dohi T et al. Prognosis of patients with heart failure and obstructive sleep apnea treated with continuous positive airway pressure. *Chest.* 2008;133:690.
56. Arzt M, Floras JS, Logan AG et al. Suppression of central sleep apnea by continuous positive airway pressure and transplant-free survival in heart failure: A post hoc analysis of the Canadian Continuous Positive Airway Pressure for Patients with Central Sleep Apnea and Heart Failure Trial (CANPAP). *Circulation.* 2007;115(25):3173–80.
57. Ryan CM, Usui K, Floras JS, Bradley TD. Effect of continuous positive airway pressure on ventricular ectopy in heart failure patients with obstructive sleep apnea. *Thorax.* 2005;60:781–5.
58. Clark AL, Johnson MJ, Squire I. Practice uncertainties page. Does home oxygen benefit people with chronic heart failure? *BMJ.* 2011;342:d234.
59. Teschler H, Dohring J, Wang YM, Berthon-Jones M. Adaptive pressure support servo-ventilation: A novel treatment for Cheyne-Stokes respiration in heart failure. *Am J Respir Crit Care Med.* 2001;164:614–9.
60. Aurora RN, Chowdhuri S, Ramar K et al. The treatment of central sleep apnea syndromes in adults: Practice parameters with an evidence-based literature review and meta-analyses. *Sleep.* 2012;35:17–40.
61. Sharma BK, Bakker JP, McSharry DG et al. Adaptive servo-ventilation for treatment of sleep-disordered breathing in heart failure: A systematic review and meta-analysis. *Chest.* 2012;142:1211–21.
62. Nakamura S, Asai K, Kubota Y et al. Impact of sleep-disordered breathing and efficacy of positive airway pressure on mortality in patients with chronic heart failure and sleep-disordered breathing: A meta-analysis. *Clin Res Cardiol.* 2015 Mar;104(3):208–16.
63. Cowie MR, Woehrle H, Wegscheider K et al. Adaptive servo-ventilation for central sleep apnea in systolic heart failure. *N Engl J Med.* 2015;373: 1095–105. Plus correspondence: *N Engl J Med.* 2016;374:687–91.
64. Effect of Adaptive Servo Ventilation (ASV) on Survival and Hospital Admissions in Heart Failure (ADVENT-HF). https://clinicaltrials.gov/ct2/show/NCT01128816 (accessed 27 July 2018).
65. Naughton MT. Is Cheyne Stokes detrimental in heart failure? *Sleep Breathing.* 2000;4(3):127–8.
66. Naughton MT. Cheyne-Stokes respiration: Friend or foe? *Thorax.* 2012;67:357–60.
67. Levine M, Cleave JP, Dodds C. Can periodic breathing have advantages for oxygenation? *J Theor Biol.* 1995;172:355–68.
68. Brack T, Jubran A, Laghi F, Tobin MJ. Fluctuations in end-expiratory lung volume during Cheyne-Stokes respiration. *Am J Respir Crit Care Med.* 2005 Jun 15;171(12):1408–13.
69. Maze SS, Kotler MN, Parry WR. Doppler evaluation of changing cardiac dynamics during Cheyne–Stokes respiration. *Chest.* 1989;95:525–9.
70. Yumino D, Kasai T, Kimmerly D et al. Differing effects of obstructive and central sleep apneas on stroke volume in patients with heart failure. *Am J Respir Crit Care Med.* 2013 Feb 15;187(4):433–8.
71. Naughton MT, Floras JS, Rahman MA et al. Respiratory correlates of muscle sympathetic nerve activity in heart failure. *Clin Sci.* 1998 Sep 1;95(3):277–85.
72. Badr MS, Toiber FR, Skatrud JB, Dempsey JE. Pharyngeal narrowing/occlusion during central sleep apnea. *J Appl Physiol.* 1995 May 1; 78(5):1806–15.
73. Bing OH, Brooks WW, Messer JV. Heart muscle viability following hypoxia: Protective effect of acidosis. *Science.* 1973;180:1297–8.
74. Gray A, Goodacre S, Newby DE et al. Noninvasive ventilation in acute cardiogenic pulmonary edema. *Engl J Med.* 2008 Jul 10;359(2):142–51.

PART 8

Neuromuscular disease

38 Muscle disorders and ventilatory failure 354
David Hilton-Jones
39 Pathophysiology of respiratory failure in neuromuscular diseases 364
Franco Laghi, Hameeda Shaikh and Dejan Radovanovic
40 Slowly progressive neuromuscular diseases 375
Vikram A. Padmanabhan and Joshua O. Benditt
41 Amyotrophic lateral sclerosis 388
Stephen C. Bourke and John Steer
42 Duchenne muscular dystrophy 399
Anita K. Simonds
43 Central sleep apnoea 408
Shahrokh Javaheri and Mark W. Elliott
44 Mouthpiece ventilation for daytime ventilatory support 419
Miguel R. Gonçalves and Tiago Pinto

38

Muscle disorders and ventilatory failure

DAVID HILTON-JONES

INTRODUCTION

Ventilation is ultimately achieved through the contraction and relaxation of the muscles of the chest wall and diaphragm. They are voluntary muscles of the same general composition as the skeletal musculature. It is therefore not surprising that primary muscle disorders may be complicated by the development of ventilatory insufficiency. Given that many such myopathies are progressive in nature and have no specific treatment, it is unarguable that one of the greatest successes of management in the past 20 years has been the introduction of non-invasive ventilatory techniques that have given enormous benefit with respect to quality of life, together with, in some disorders, a very substantial increase in life expectancy.[1]

Much of the rest of this volume is devoted to the basics of clinical and laboratory assessment of ventilatory insufficiency and its subsequent management. Such details will not be repeated here except in so much that there may be specific issues concerning individual disorders. A major aim of this chapter is to educate respiratory specialists about the often individually very rare muscle disorders that they will come across while providing non-invasive ventilation. Their knowledge need not be encyclopaedic, but greater insight must help overall patient management.

Many individual myopathies are extremely rare but as the ventilatory consequences, and their management, are essentially independent of the pathological process causing the myopathy, there is no need for the respiratory specialist to have detailed knowledge of all forms of myopathy. This chapter will concentrate on the more common muscle diseases associated with ventilatory insufficiency and the need for ventilatory support, noting the rarer entities in passing.

At the clinical level, a fundamentally important distinction is between those conditions in which ventilatory insufficiency is invariably a late feature of the disease (by which time the patient has long been wheelchair dependent) and those conditions in which significant ventilatory insufficiency, requiring intervention, may develop while the patient is still ambulant. Arguably, these latter patients are at greatest risk because neither the patient nor the managing clinician, if not specialising in the area, may be aware of the risks or be attuned to the premonitory symptoms until problems ensue. In rare instances, ventilatory failure may be the first manifestation of a myopathy.

This chapter is concerned primarily with late-childhood and adult muscle disorders. It deals with conditions in which the pathological process involves some part of muscle fibre, including the neuromuscular junction. Most of the conditions covered will require long-term ventilatory support once insufficiency has developed, although in some instances, temporary non-invasive ventilation may be required to cover complications such as pneumonia or the post-operative period.

The other major part of the motor unit is the anterior horn cell and motor neurone. Brief comment will be made about spinal muscular atrophy, as in the clinic it is commonly seen alongside primary muscle disorders and shares similarities of management with muscular dystrophy. Acquired disorders such as poliomyelitis and neuropathies, such as Guillain–Barré syndrome, will not be covered here. Similarly, amyotrophic lateral sclerosis (motor neurone disease) will not be discussed, but is covered in Chapter 41. There are a number of neuromuscular disorders that present in the neonatal period and require invasive ventilation, and often have a poor prognosis (e.g. type 1 spinal muscular atrophy, Pompe's disease) and they will also not be discussed here.

CLASSIFICATION OF MUSCLE DISORDERS

There is no uniquely applicable or useful system of classification, but nevertheless, it is valuable to have a framework, particularly for those less familiar with the field of neuromuscular disorders. A fundamental distinction is between acquired and inherited disorders. At the time of writing, a fair generalisation is that there are no specific treatments for inherited disorders, and that most acquired disorders can either be treated successfully or will remit if the cause is withdrawn. Exceptions include enzyme replacement therapy for acid maltase deficiency (Pompe's disease), as a treatable inherited disorder,[2] and inclusion body myositis as an untreatable acquired disorder. Not surprisingly, therefore, the main burden with respect to the provision of non-invasive ventilation is for patients with inherited muscle disorders.

The main categories of acquired and inherited muscle disorders, and the more common conditions within each category, are shown in Boxes 38.1 and 38.2, respectively. Those conditions commonly associated with significant ventilatory problems are shown in italics. In other words, those conditions highlighted represent the bulk of the clinical workload.

BOX 38.1: Acquired muscle disorders

(Conditions commonly associated with ventilatory problems are in italics)

Endocrinopathies
- Hypothyroidism
- Hyperthyroidism
- Cushing's syndrome

Drug-induced: numerous but including the following:
- Any drug causing hypokalaemia (e.g. diuretic, liquorice)
- Penicillamine (causing myasthenic syndrome)
- Statins
- Anti-retroviral drugs (mitochondrial myopathy)
- Steroid/neuromuscular blocker acute quadriplegic myopathy

Idiopathic inflammatory myopathies
- Polymyositis (often with connective tissue disease)
- Dermatomyositis
- Inclusion body myositis

Metabolic myopathies
- Glycogenoses
- Disorders of lipid metabolism (e.g. carnitine palmitoyltransferase deficiency)

Infection
- Viruses (e.g. myalgia associated with flu)
- Bacteria (abscess formation)
- Numerous helminths and protozoa

BOX 38.2: Inherited muscle disorders

(Conditions commonly associated with ventilatory problems are in italics)

Muscular dystrophies
- X-linked recessive:
  - *Duchenne*
  - Becker
  - Emery–Dreifuss syndrome (Emerin deficiency)
- Autosomal dominant:
  - Facioscapulohumeral
  - Limb-girdle: Type 1B (allelic with autosomal dominant Emery–Dreifuss syndrome), Type 1C
  - Emery–Dreifuss syndrome (lamin A/C deficiency)
  - Oculopharyngeal
- Autosomal recessive: limb-girdle: numerous types numbered 2A–2O, *Type 2I (FKRP deficiency)*

Congenital muscular dystrophy
- Numerous subtypes

Myotonic dystrophy
- Type 1 (Steinert's disease, DMPK gene CTG repeat)
- Type 2 (Proximal myotonic myopathy, *ZNF9* gene CCTG repeat)

Myofibrillar myopathies
- Desminopathy

Congenital myopathies
- Collagen VI disorders (Bethlem and Ullrich myopathies)
- Central core disease
- Nemaline myopathy
- Rigid spine disorders (SEPN1 and RyR1 mutations)

Metabolic myopathies
- Glycogenoses:
  - *Acid maltase deficiency (Pompe's disease)*
  - McArdle's disease (myophosphorylase deficiency)
- Lipidoses: carnitine palmitoyltransferase deficiency)
- Mitochondrial cytopathies: numerous phenotypes

Muscle channelopathies
- Sodium
  - Hyperkalaemic periodic paralysis
  - Normokalaemic periodic paralysis
- Calcium
  - Hypokalaemic periodic paralysis

- Potassium
  - Andersen's syndrome
- Chloride
  - Autosomal dominant and recessive myotonia congenita

MUSCLE DISORDERS ASSOCIATED WITH LATE VENTILATORY INSUFFICIENCY

In the conditions discussed below, ventilatory insufficiency is inevitable in later stages of the disease. Early manifestations include increased susceptibility to chest infections (compounded by aspiration in those with pharyngeal muscle involvement) and delayed recovery following general anaesthesia. Either may precipitate ventilatory failure, which may be transient or permanent. In myotonic dystrophy, sleep-disordered breathing may contribute to excessive daytime sleepiness (EDS) (although central mechanisms are more important). All boys with Duchenne will eventually develop ventilatory failure, whereas only a small proportion of men with the allelic disorder Becker dystrophy will do so. Similarly, only a small proportion of patients with myotonic dystrophy require, or as will be mentioned will tolerate, long-term assisted ventilation.

Duchenne muscular dystrophy

That this was the first clearly defined dystrophy simply reflects the fact that it is the most common inherited myopathy presenting in childhood and has a stereotypic clinical presentation. It is an X-linked recessive disorder and thus typically affects males but is transmitted by carrier females. The incidence is 1 in 3500 live male births. Up to 10% of carrier females manifest muscle features, but they are generally mild and asymptomatic. Features in carriers include elevated serum creatine kinase levels, calf muscle hypertrophy, and proximal limb weakness; such weakness is very rarely severe.

MOLECULAR ASPECTS

Duchenne muscular dystrophy (DMD) is caused by mutations in the gene coding for the very large structural protein dystrophin,[3] whose main function is supporting the muscle fibre membrane. It is allelic with Becker muscular dystrophy (BMD), discussed below, and these and related conditions are sometimes referred to as the dystrophinopathies. The main consequence of the defect is increased membrane fragility, which leads to abnormal calcium homoeostasis, activation of proteases and muscle fibre necrosis. The commonest mutations are large deletions (about 70%), which are readily detected by relatively simple molecular tests. The remaining mutations include small deletions, duplications and point mutations, which, within an extremely large gene, had proved difficult to identify with conventional technology. Previously, the approach to diagnosis included testing for larger deletions, and if they were absent to demonstrate the absence of dystrophin by immunohistochemistry on a muscle biopsy specimen, more detailed (and expensive) mutational analysis could be undertaken when appropriate. Recent advances have meant that rapid, cost-effective laboratory testing is increasingly becoming available, with the imminent arrival of 'DNA-chip' diagnosis.

In DMD, the mutation is 'out of frame', resulting in disruption of the reading frame and failure of protein production.[4] Thus, muscle biopsy immunohistochemistry shows complete lack of dystrophin. In BMD, there is a mutation in the same gene, but it is 'in frame', allowing production of a truncated version of dystrophin that is partly functional. Muscle immunohistochemistry typically shows patchiness of dystrophin staining, and Western blotting shows reduced quantities of dystrophin of reduced molecular weight.

CLINICAL FEATURES

No clinical features are evident at birth, but if the serum creatine kinase is measured, it is invariably massively elevated – this has formed the basis of neonatal screening programmes.[5] Typically, motor milestones are slightly delayed, but often not by enough to cause any immediate concern. It gradually becomes apparent that the boy is not gaining motor skills. He appears clumsy in his movements, can walk but not run and cannot hop or jump. Speech delay is common. In some boys, learning difficulties are apparent, thought to relate to the fact that dystrophin is expressed in the brain.[6] Behavioural difficulties are common, which may again reflect abnormal dystrophin expression in the brain, but also may be a reaction to the physical consequences of the disorder. Despite the stereotypical nature of the presentation and the relative ease of diagnosis (a massively elevated serum creatine kinase together with such clinical features is essentially diagnostic), delayed diagnosis is common.[7]

The weakness invariably affects the proximal lower limb muscles first. Often there is hypertrophy of the calf muscles – this may initially be due to compensatory muscle fibre hypertrophy, but the end-stage process is replacement of muscle by fat and fibrous tissue, hence the commonly used term *pseudohypertrophy*. Such hypertrophy is particularly common in DMD and BMD, but can be seen in other dystrophies and spinal muscular atrophy.[8] Tongue hypertrophy is often striking. The proximal weakness is reflected in Gower's manoeuvre, in which the boy trying to rise from the floor has to use his hands against his legs in ladder fashion to push himself up. The boys pass through a period of maintaining mobility by the use of aids (in the 8- to 10-year age range) but become increasingly restricted and all are wheelchair dependent by the age of 12 years.

The weakness spreads to involve the proximal upper limb muscles, the paraspinal muscles and the respiratory muscles. Hand function is preserved late into the course of the disorder and computer keyboard and joystick control abilities remain vital assets. Paraspinal muscle weakness leads to lumbar lordosis, which, combined with the proximal lower limb weakness, gives a characteristic waddling gait. A major consequence of the dorsal kyphoscoliosis is further ventilatory compromise, in addition due to that caused by respiratory muscle weakness, due to mechanical restriction of movement.

The age of onset of significant ventilatory impairment is variable. In the early teens, forced vital capacity is substantially reduced. There is increased risk of chest infection. It is at this age that spinal surgery (insertion of rods to straighten the spine) is often considered – the potential benefits include improvement in ventilation due to correction of kyphoscoliosis and improvement of posture (and thus reduction of discomfort) in the wheelchair.[9] But the reduced vital capacity and nature of the surgery carry with them the risk of substantial peri- and post-operative complications requiring detailed pre-operative assessment. A further complicating issue for surgery is the presence, almost inevitably, of cardiomyopathy (see below). The symptomatology and management of hypoventilation are discussed in detail elsewhere in this volume.

Cardiac dystrophin expression is impaired and cardiomyopathy is inevitable. Initial features include electrocardiographic (ECG) changes followed by the development of a dilated cardiomyopathy. Despite the severity of the echocardiographic changes, symptomatic heart involvement is relatively uncommon probably because of the patient's profound immobility and lack of 'stress' on the heart. Given that the introduction of non-invasive ventilation has substantially lengthened life expectancy, cardiac involvement is likely to become a more important issue. Regular cardiac surveillance should start early in the second decade, and despite lack of evidence from specific trials, it is accepted practice to treat pre-symptomatic cardiomyopathy, for example, with angiotensin-converting enzyme inhibitors and β-blockers.[10] Some have advocated even more intensive prophylaxis.[11]

Becker muscular dystrophy

As discussed above, this disorder is allelic to DMD. Becker defined the disorder on the basis of a characteristic presentation with onset in childhood/adolescence, relatively slow progression and a distribution of weakness paralleling that seen in DMD. The pattern of inheritance was X-linked and there was debate for many years as to whether it was an allelic disorder to DMD or related to involvement of a different gene, the former eventually being proven when the dystrophin gene was identified. In one extensive study of BMD, about 10% of patients required a wheelchair by the age of 40 years, reflecting the much milder prognosis compared with DMD.[12]

The phenotypic variability of the dystrophinopathies (Box 38.3) relates to the nature of the underlying mutation. First, the position of the mutation within the gene is a major determinant of whether the phenotype is restricted to cardiomyopathy or also involves skeletal muscle or involves skeletal muscle alone. Second, the position of the mutation and the extent that the mutation leads to truncation of the protein product have a major effect on the severity of muscle involvement. This raises issues with respect to nosology. The disorder that Becker recognised is outlined above and discussed in more detail below. But some patients present with the same pattern of muscle involvement at a much earlier age, are wheelchair dependent by early teens and thus overlap with those patients with milder forms of DMD. Others are so mildly affected that they remain asymptomatic until they present with quadriceps weakness in late-middle age. Others never develop weakness but have a cramp/myalgia syndrome, and a very small number are asymptomatic but have an elevated creatine kinase. To use the eponym Becker for all of these variants, and some even include those with only cardiomyopathy, seems inappropriate and confusing, for doctors and patients. The more general term *dystrophinopathy* therefore has its merits.

BOX 38.3: Phenotypic expression of the dystrophinopathies

- Duchenne muscular dystrophy
- Becker muscular dystrophy
- Manifesting female carriers
- Cramp/myalgia syndrome
- Asymptomatic hypercapnia
- Late-onset quadriceps myopathy
- Isolated cardiomyopathy

The description below is the condition that Becker would have recognised and is indeed the most prevalent form of dystrophinopathy in adult life.

MOLECULAR ASPECTS

These were discussed above. From a practical point of view, a patient suspected of having BMD should have DNA analysis as the first approach to diagnosis (noting that as in DMD the serum creatine kinase is invariably elevated). The same issues with respect to deletions and smaller mutations apply. It has recently been recognised that autosomal recessive limb-girdle muscular dystrophy type 2I (due to mutations in the *FKRP* gene) can look exactly like BMD, including raised serum creatine kinase and cardiac involvement, and exclusion of that by DNA testing should be performed before considering muscle biopsy.

CLINICAL ASPECTS

Although the incidence of BMD is lower than DMD, the much longer survival means that its prevalence is higher than DMD. The diagnosis is typically made in adolescence with the history of symptoms dating back to very early teens. A history of calf cramps, often attributed to 'growing pains', and toe-walking is common. Calf hypertrophy may have been noted. The onset of weakness is invariably in the proximal lower limb/pelvic area and examination shows weakness of hip flexion and knee extension (quadriceps). The greater involvement of quadriceps than the hamstrings (knee flexors) is characteristic and distinguishes Becker from many forms of limb-girdle muscular dystrophy. As in DMD, a rather characteristic waddling gait develops. An oft repeated history is that the boy was poor at games, coming last in races and being clumsy during sporting activities. Subsequently, difficulties climbing stairs are noted, and then difficulty getting up from low chairs.

At a later stage, peri-scapular muscle involvement becomes evident with some winging of the shoulder blades. Rather strikingly, in some patients, weakness of grip can become troublesome. As the proximal lower limb weakness advances, rising from a chair becomes extremely difficult and stairs impossible without handrails. Falls, due mainly to quadriceps weakness and thus lack of knee support, are inevitable. There is an increasing need for walking aids and then occasional use of a wheelchair. However, the majority of patients retain a degree of independent ambulation into late middle age.

Significant ventilatory insufficiency is very much less common than in DMD, and few patients require long-term non-invasive ventilation – and then only in patients who have been wheelchair dependent for a long period (Figure 38.1). Chest infections and post-operative respiratory depression may require short-term ventilatory support. Many patients retain a normal, or only minimally reduced, forced vital capacity throughout their lives. Life expectancy is reduced in those with more severe muscle involvement, leading to wheelchair dependence, and in those with cardiomyopathy, but in many, it is normal.

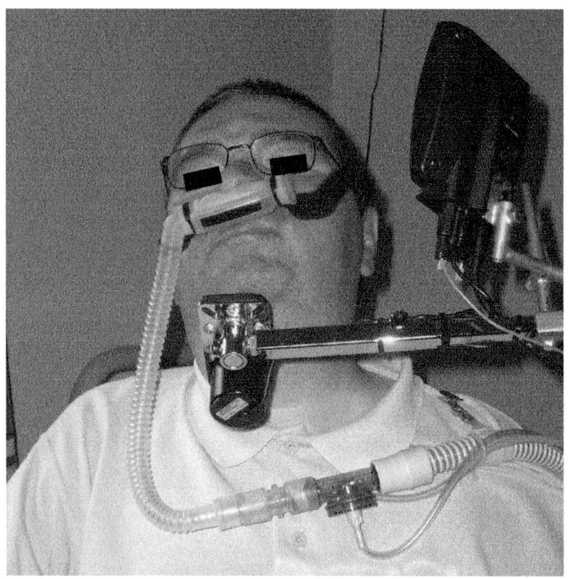

Figure 38.1 This patient with Becker muscular dystrophy developed ventilatory insufficiency after having been wheelchair dependent for many years. Initially, he required nocturnal ventilation only, but subsequently became dependent on daytime ventilation. His degree of immobility is profound and he uses an environmental control system operated by the chin apparatus.

The development of cardiomyopathy is highly variable and, unlike in DMD, is not inevitable.[13] But some patients may develop severe cardiomyopathy even in the presence of only mild limb muscle involvement, so cardiac surveillance is essential from diagnosis. There have been many reports of patients requiring cardiac transplantation while still fully ambulant.[14]

Myotonic dystrophies

Myotonic dystrophy type 1 (DM1) is the commonest inherited disorder seen in adult muscle clinics and has a prevalence of ~12/100,000 population.[15] It is clinically highly variable and has important systemic manifestations other than skeletal and cardiac muscle involvement.[16] For reasons that will be discussed, despite the almost inevitable involvement of the respiratory muscles, the use of long-term non-invasive ventilation is relatively uncommon.

Myotonic dystrophy type 2 (DM2) is, in most parts of the world, considerably less common than DM1. Although sharing some common features, the many differences mean that clinical confusion between the disorders is unlikely.[17] There are clear molecular similarities, with DM2 being associated with an unstable quadruplet expansion (in the *CNBP* gene, previously known as *ZNF9*). Onset is usually in middle age. The muscle weakness is proximal rather than distal. Myotonia is often subclinical. Premature cataracts and cardiac conduction defects can be seen as in DM1. A congenital form has not been described. EDS is common. Ventilatory insufficiency appears to be much less common than in DM1, but there are reports of significant sleep-related problems including apnoeas.[18,19]

MOLECULAR ASPECTS

DM1 occurs due to an unstable trinucleotide repeat expansion in a gene (*DMPK*) coding for a protein kinase. It is believed that most of the manifestations of this disorder, and those of DM2, are a consequence of disturbed RNA metabolism rather than dysfunction of the gene in which the mutation is located.[20] Thus, altered splicing of the chloride channel gene causes the characteristic myotonia, of the insulin receptor gene insulin resistance, and of cardiac and CNS genes the common conduction abnormalities and cognitive features.

The mutation is unstable and an increase in size in mitosis explains some of the progression of the disorder during life. More importantly, an increase in size, sometimes dramatic, in meiosis means that the offspring have a tendency to develop the condition at an earlier age (anticipation); earlier-onset cases are inclined to show a rather different pattern of clinical involvement with cognitive and behavioural problems initially predominating over muscle involvement. Although there is significant overlap it is convenient in clinical practice to recognise four major phenotypes:

- Asymptomatic/oligosymptomatic
- Adult-onset (classical Steinert's disease)
- Childhood onset
- Congenital onset

The size of the expansion increases down the group. Thus, most normal individuals have ~12 repeats. Up to ~100 repeats may be asymptomatic, typical adult-onset disease is seen with ~100–500 repeats, childhood-onset with somewhat larger repeats, and the most severe congenital form with more than 1000 repeats. The figures given are only a rough approximation such that a DNA result alone is of little use for prognostication. A major reason for this is that repeat size is determined from a blood sample (lymphocytes), and as a consequence of instability of the mutation during mitosis, different tissues from the same individual may show widely differing numbers of repeats.

CLINICAL ASPECTS

Those with very small expansions may be asymptomatic, but cataracts, often presenting at a relatively young age, are common. Significant skeletal muscle involvement is not seen, cardiac complications are rare and assisted ventilation is not an issue. Congenital myotonic dystrophy presents as a floppy infant with feeding and respiratory difficulties. Although both may need support, in most they settle down within a few days; more severe cases remain ventilator dependent and do not survive. The child then makes progress but milestones are somewhat delayed and learning difficulties are inevitable. Relatively mild skeletal involvement is evident, but the learning difficulties and behavioural problems present the major challenge. The facial appearance is characteristic due to facial muscle weakness and underlying skeletal dysmorphism, which in itself relates to the long-standing weakness. In early adulthood, the muscular manifestations progress, as in the adult-onset form, and there is a high morbidity and mortality in the third and fourth decades from cardiorespiratory problems.[21] The childhood-onset form presents in the first decade with cognitive and behavioural problems with little or no evidence of skeletal muscle involvement, such that the diagnosis is often missed for some considerable time.

The remainder of this section will deal with the multisystemic features seen in adult-onset myotonic dystrophy – by far and away the most common form encountered in clinical practice. Onset of symptoms is typically in adolescence and early adult life. Most commonly, it is limb skeletal muscle features that lead to presentation, more rarely EDS or cardiorespiratory problems. In women, the diagnosis may come to light following the birth of a congenitally affected child.

Skeletal muscle

Myotonia is a hallmark of the disease and describes the phenomenon of delayed muscle relaxation after contraction. The patient complains of stiffness of their hands and difficulty relaxing the hand after gripping something tightly. Myotonia may also affect the muscles in the throat region, causing difficulties swallowing and a feeling of clumsiness of the tongue when speaking.

The pattern of muscle weakness is essentially invariable involving the facial, neck flexor and distal limb muscles (and respiratory muscles as discussed below). Proximal limb weakness is a late feature and thus strikingly different to most myopathies. Before the patient is aware of symptoms, it is possible to show weakness of the facial muscles (incomplete burying of the eyelids), neck flexion and grip. Although the facial weakness may become quite severe, few patients complain of it – however, it may contribute to some of the difficulties in establishing non-invasive ventilation (Figure 38.2). The facial weakness, combined with ptosis and receding hairline, gives rise to the characteristic facies.

The respiratory muscles are involved early, and in our experience, many patients have a significantly reduced forced vital capacity (less than 50% predicted) even at first presentation when other features of skeletal muscle involvement may be minimal. The forced vital capacity falls with time and many adults have values below 2 L. This, combined with swallowing impairment due to pharyngeal muscle weakness, contributes to the high incidence of chest

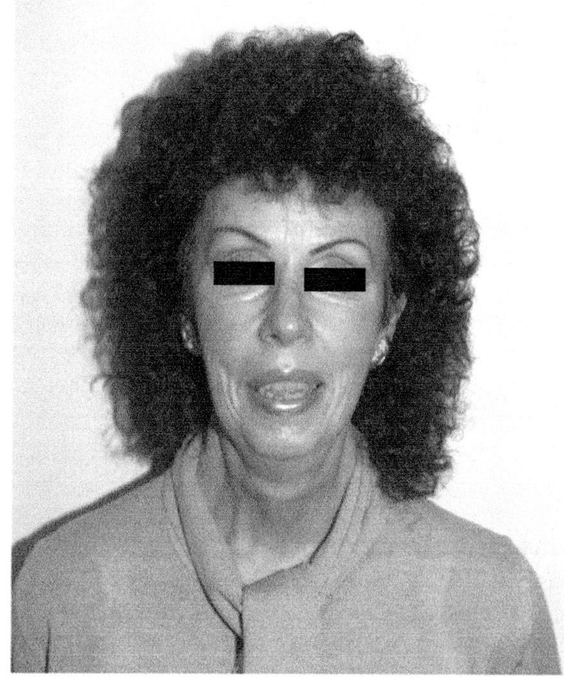

Figure 38.2 Myotonic dystrophy. Characteristic facial weakness due to atrophy of the facial and masticatory muscles, and ptosis. The facial muscle weakness, and in some patients dysmorphic features, may hinder use of masks for non-invasive ventilation.

infections, which are a major source of morbidity and mortality.[22] Many studies have shown nocturnal compromise of ventilation with associated sleep fragmentation.[23,24] While this might be thought to be a contributing factor to EDS, it is striking that treatment with non-invasive nocturnal ventilation may not help[25] and that EDS can be a major symptom in those with no evidence of respiratory compromise – all supporting the view that EDS largely relates to central nervous system dysfunction.

Delayed recovery of ventilation following anaesthesia is extremely common and undiagnosed patients may be first identified in this setting. At diagnosis, all patients should be advised of the risks of surgery and anaesthesia. The highest morbidity has been associated with gallbladder surgery, presumably because of additional direct effects of the surgery on the adjacent diaphragm.

Heart

Cardiac conduction abnormalities are extremely common,[26] whereas symptomatic cardiomyopathy is rare. Typical ECG changes include progressive lengthening of the PR interval, broadening of the QRS complex and the development of various forms of block including partial and complete bundle branch block and complete heart block. Bradyarrhythmias may be treated by pacemaker insertion, but there is increasing evidence that many patients die from tachyarrhythmias, which may appropriately be treated by insertion of an implantable defibrillator. Despite numerous publications, the best approach to cardiac surveillance and management remains unclear.[27] Annual ECG is a minimum requirement. Changes on the ECG and the development of cardiac symptoms indicate the need for further assessment, which will include 24-hour recording and possibly intracardiac electrophysiology.

Brain

As a group, these patients have a slightly lower IQ than average. More striking is a characteristic psychological profile that largely reflects frontal lobe dysfunction and practically is associated with apathy and impaired organisational skills.[28] Apathy and related behavioural issues have a profound effect for some individuals with respect to employment, social interactions and clinical management.[29] It partly explains why patients with myotonic dystrophy have a reputation for being poor attendees in clinic, although it can be argued that some clinics offer little benefit to the patients who therefore see no reason to attend. These factors are also relevant with respect to non-compliance with non-invasive ventilation.

EDS is extremely common but under-recognised.[30] It can be debilitating for the patient, and seriously compromise employability, and can be particularly irksome for family and friends, who may perceive it as the patient showing boredom and lack of interest. The fact that many patients show sleep-disordered breathing might suggest that it would respond to non-invasive ventilation, but it is striking that it rarely does so. On the other hand, stimulant drugs such as modafinil can be highly effective.[31]

Additional features

Cataracts develop at a younger age than normal. Fertility can be impaired, particularly in males, who may develop azoospermia. Premature, male pattern balding is more striking in males than in females. Insulin resistance is common, but frank diabetes is rare. It is more common in the older obese patient and essentially behaves like, and is managed in the same way as, maturity-onset diabetes. Irritable bowel symptoms are very common. Bladder involvement is probably underestimated.

Other dystrophies

Ventilatory failure may occur in the limb-girdle dystrophies, but as in BMD, this is rare other than in patients who have substantial limb weakness and have long been wheelchair dependent. The same is true for facioscapulohumeral dystrophy, one of the commonest dystrophies in adults, and overall, the need for non-invasive ventilation is very rare.

MUSCLE DISORDERS ASSOCIATED WITH EARLY VENTILATORY INSUFFICIENCY

In these disorders, ventilatory failure may occur while the patient is still ambulant. Non-invasive ventilation is life-saving, improves quality of life and allows long-term survival. Each is rare, and only the major clinical and management features will be described.

Acid maltase deficiency

This is an autosomal recessive disorder that may present in two major fashions, depending on the level of residual enzyme activity. The most severe form is classical Pompe's disease presenting early in the first decade and associated with ventilatory failure, widespread weakness and organomegaly. Death was inevitable until the recent introduction of enzyme replacement therapy.[32]

A later onset form is associated with proximal muscle weakness and respiratory muscle weakness selectively affecting the diaphragm.[33] Onset is typically in adolescence but can be much later, in early middle age. The pattern of proximal limb weakness is non-specific, and an incorrect initial diagnosis of limb-girdle dystrophy or myositis is often made. A proportion of patients first present in respiratory failure, but on closer assessment, nearly all have signs, and usually also previously unrecognised symptoms, of proximal limb weakness. In those presenting with limb weakness, evidence of diaphragmatic weakness (a significant fall in forced vital capacity when the patient is lying compared with standing) may be found and point toward the diagnosis. In those who develop ventilatory failure, non-invasive ventilation is highly effective. Most will require, at least initially, nocturnal ventilation only, but as the condition advances, daytime ventilation may become necessary. Those who are still ambulant are unlikely to require daytime ventilation.

The diagnosis is often not considered unless there is the additional clue of early respiratory muscle involvement. Once thought of, the diagnosis is established or refuted by enzymological studies that can be performed on a blood sample.[34,35] In some patients, the diagnosis is suggested by the appearance on muscle biopsy (accumulation of glycogen and increased acid phosphatase activity), but the biopsy can be normal.

Congenital myopathies

This title is misleading because many of these conditions (Box 38.2) are not truly congenital (evidence of disease at birth) but have their onset in the first few years of life. Although genetically and pathologically very heterogeneous, they share many clinical similarities. Perhaps the most striking attribute is that despite early onset, they are relatively non-progressive, unlike the dystrophies. Much of the apparent progression in childhood and adolescence is due to enlargement of the skeleton without the musculature keeping pace. Once the individual is fully grown, and throughout adult life, there is very little progression of weakness. What they also share in common is rather diffuse proximal and distal muscle involvement, without the marked proximal predilection seen in most myopathies. The weakness is typically modest, with the individual retaining independent ambulation. In many of these conditions, ventilatory failure, requiring the introduction of non-invasive ventilation, develops in childhood or adolescence.

Emery–Dreifuss syndrome

This rare syndrome was first described as an X-linked disorder and was subsequently shown to be due to mutations in a gene (*STA*) producing the nuclear envelope protein emerin. It was subsequently realised that most patients with this phenotype have an autosomal dominant disorder due to mutations in the *LMNA* gene coding for another nuclear envelope protein lamin A/C[36] and that it is allelic to autosomal dominant limb-girdle muscular dystrophy type 1B.

The phenotype is defined by the triad of early muscle contractures, a humero-pelvic distribution of muscle weakness and cardiac involvement (which carries high mortality). Contractures develop in the advanced stages of most myopathies, when the patient is very immobile, but in Emery–Dreifuss syndrome, they are an early feature, when the patient is fully ambulant, and characteristically affect the neck, elbows and ankles. Most patients retain ambulation but it becomes increasingly difficult because of the contractures and abnormal posture. Cardiac arrhythmias carry a high mortality, and current evidence supports the implantation of a defibrillator.[37,38] The development of ventilatory failure is relatively common.

LGMD 2I

As noted, this autosomal recessive limb-girdle dystrophy can mimic BMD, including cardiac involvement.[39] Unlike BMD, ventilatory insufficiency can develop while the patient is still ambulant and requires regular monitoring.

COMMENTS ON OTHER MYOPATHIES AND RELATED CONDITIONS

For the intensivist, the most common neuromuscular disorders that they will see on an intensive care unit (ICU) are Guillain–Barré syndrome and myasthenia gravis. They share in common the need for invasive ventilation during the acute stage (e.g. myasthenic crisis), but both are self-limiting. It is very rare for patients with myasthenia to need long-term non-invasive ventilation, although that need is slightly more common in patients with anti-MuSK antibodies as opposed to anti-acetylcholine receptor antibodies. Ventilatory failure is much less common in Lambert–Eaton myasthenic syndrome than in myasthenia gravis.

Another condition that is seen on ICU is acute quadriplegic myopathy due to the combined use of high-dose steroids and a neuromuscular blocking drug – typically in a patient with acute asthma.[40,41] Invasive ventilation is required, and sometimes non-invasive ventilation during the recovery period, but not long-term. Desmin mutations are one cause of so-called myofibrillar myopathies.[42] Slowly progressive proximal weakness develops from early middle age. Diaphragmatic involvement is common and ventilatory failure may develop in an ambulant patient. Although not a myopathy, spinal muscular atrophy is a common condition whose management is typically in the same clinic as those patients with muscular dystrophies. The commonest form, autosomal recessive proximal spinal muscular atrophy, is due to mutations affecting the *SMN* gene and four major categories are recognised:

- Type 1 – diagnosed by 6 months of age; ventilator dependence and early death
- Type 2 – diagnosed by 2 years of age; can sit but never walk
- Type 3 – diagnosed between 18 months and adolescence; can walk
- Type 4 – onset in adult life

As with DMD, patients with type 2 spinal muscular atrophy, and to a lesser extent type 3, have problems with kyphoscoliosis, which may, together with respiratory muscle weakness, contribute to ventilatory insufficiency requiring long-term non-invasive ventilation. Despite the early onset in some patients, and substantial early disability, progression throughout life is extremely slow and many with type 3 will have a normal life expectancy. The major cause of morbidity is chest infection.

RESPIRATORY CARE OF ADULTS WITH MUSCLE DISORDERS

The rest of this book is devoted to this! But it has been recognised that deficiencies exist in current services with the clinicians looking after patients with muscle diseases not being expert respiratory physicians and respiratory physicians managing non-invasive ventilation not having experience of other aspects of the patient's condition. With this in mind, Muscular Dystrophy UK (a UK charity devoted to patients with neuromuscular disorders) convened a workshop to develop 'best practice' guidelines, and some of the same authors reviewed the features of respiratory involvement in inherited myopathies.[43,44] These are useful documents to provide a framework for effective management of such patients.

From all of the above, it is apparent that there is an urgent need for cooperation between specialist chest physicians, neurologists and paediatricians to optimise the care of this particular population of patients.

REFERENCES

1. Strehle EM, Straub V. Recent advances in the management of Duchenne muscular dystrophy. *Arch Dis Child.* 2015;100(12):1173–7. Epub 2015/07/15.
2. Güngör D, Kruijshaar ME, Plug I et al. Impact of enzyme replacement therapy on survival in adults with Pompe disease: Results from a prospective international observational study. *Orphanet J Rare Dis.* 2013;8(1).
3. Muntoni F, Torelli S, Ferlini A. Dystrophin and mutations: One gene, several proteins, multiple phenotypes. *Lancet Neurol.* 2003;2:731–40.
4. Tuffery-Giraud S, Beroud C, Leturcq F et al. Genotype–phenotype analysis in 2,405 patients with a dystrophinopathy using the UMD–DMD database: A model of nationwide knowledge base. *Hum Mutat.* 2009;30:934–45.
5. Gatheridge MA, Kwon JM, Mendell JM et al. Identifying non-duchennemuscular dystrophy-positive and false negative results in prior Duchenne muscular dystrophy newborn screening programs: A review. *JAMA Neurol.* 2016;73(1):111–6.
6. Donders J, Taneja C. Neurobehavioral characteristics of children with Duchenne muscular dystrophy. *Child Neuropsychol.* 2009;15:295–304.
7. Ciafaloni E, Fox DJ, Pandya S et al. Delayed diagnosis in Duchenne muscular dystrophy: Data from the muscular dystrophy surveillance, tracking, and research network (MD STARnet). *J Pediatr.* 2009;155:380–5.
8. Reimers CD, Schlotter B, Eicke BM et al. Calf enlargement in neuromuscular diseases: A quantitative ultrasound study in 350 patients and review of the literature. *J Neurol Sci.* 1996;143:46–56.
9. Eagle M, Bourke J, Bullock R et al. Managing Duchenne muscular dystrophy—The additive effect of spinal surgery and home nocturnal ventilation in improving survival. *Neuromuscul Disord.* 2007;17:470–5.
10. Kaspar RW, Allen HD, Montanaro F. Current understanding and management of dilated cardiomyopathy in Duchenne and Becker muscular dystrophy. *J Am Acad Nurse Pract.* 2009;21:241–9.
11. Nigro G, Politano L, Passamano L et al. Cardiac treatment in neuro-muscular diseases. *Acta Myol.* 2006;25:119–23.
12. Bushby KM, Gardner-Medwin D. The clinical, genetic and dystrophin characteristics of Becker muscular dystrophy. I. Natural history. *J Neurol.* 1993;240:98–104.
13. Finsterer J, Stollberger C. Cardiac involvement in Becker muscular dystrophy. *Can J Cardiol.* 2008;24:786–92.
14. Finsterer J, Bittner RE, Grimm M. Cardiac involvement in Becker's muscular dystrophy, necessitating heart transplantation, 6 years before apparent skeletal muscle involvement. *Neuromuscul Disord.* 1999;9:598–600.
15. Harper PS. *Myotonic Dystrophy, 3rd edition. Major Problems in Neurology.* London: WB Saunders, 2001. 436 pp.
16. Harper PS, Van Engelen B, Eymard B et al. *Myotonic Dystrophy: Present Management, Future Therapy.* Oxford: Oxford University Press, 2004. 251 pp.
17. Ulane CM, Teed S, Sampson J. Recent advances in myotonic dystrophy type 2. *Curr Neurol Neurosci Rep.* 2014;14(2):429.
18. Romigi A, Albanese M, Placidi F et al. Sleep disorders in myotonic dystrophy type 2: A controlled polysomnographic study and self-reported questionnaires. *Eur J Neurol.* 2014;21(6):929–34.
19. Leonardis L, Blagus R, Dolenc Groselj L. Sleep and breathing disorders in myotonic dystrophy type 2. *Acta Neurol Scand.* 2015;132(1):42–8.
20. Machuca-Tzili L, Brook D, Hilton-Jones D. Clinical and molecular aspects of the myotonic dystrophies: A review. *Muscle Nerve.* 2005;32:1–18.
21. Reardon W, Newcombe R, Fenton I et al. The natural history of congenital myotonic dystrophy: Mortality and long term clinical aspects. *Arch Dis Child.* 1993;68:177–81.
22. de Die-Smulders CE, Howeler CJ, Thijs C et al. Age and causes of death in adult-onset myotonic dystrophy. *Brain.* 1998;121:1557–63.
23. Sansone VA, Gagnon C, Atalaia A et al. 207th ENMC Workshop on chronic respiratory insufficiency in myotonic dystrophies: Management and implications for research, 27–29 June 2014, Naarden, The Netherlands. *Neuromuscul Disord.* 2015;25(5):432–42.
24. Laberge L, Begin P, Dauvilliers Y et al. A polysomnographic study of daytime sleepiness in myotonic dystrophy type 1. *J Neurol Neurosurg Psychiatry.* 2009;80:642–6.
25. Guilleminault C, Philip P, Robinson A. Sleep and neuromuscular disease: Bilevel positive airway

pressure by nasal mask as a treatment for sleep disordered breathing in patients with neuromuscular disease. *J Neurol Neurosurg Psychiatry.* 1998;65:225–32.

26. Cudia P, Bernasconi P, Chiodelli R et al. Risk of arrhythmia in type I myotonic dystrophy: The role of clinical and genetic variables. *J Neurol Neurosurg Psychiatry.* 2009;80:790–3.
27. Dello Russo A, Mangiola F, Della Bella P et al. Risk of arrhythmias in myotonic dystrophy: Trial design of the RAMYD study. *J Cardiovasc Med (Hagerstown).* 2009;10:51–8.
28. Modoni A, Silvestri G, Vita MG et al. Cognitive impairment in myotonic dystrophy type 1 (DM1): A longitudinal follow-up study. *J Neurol.* 2008; 255:1737–42.
29. Rubinsztein JS, Rubinsztein DC, Goodburn S et al. Apathy and hypersomnia are common features of myotonic dystrophy. *J Neurol Neurosurg Psychiatry.* 1998;64:510–5.
30. Hilton-Jones D. Myotonic dystrophy—Forgotten aspects of an often neglected condition. *Curr Opin Neurol.* 1997;10:399–401.
31. Talbot K, Stradling J, Crosby J et al. Reduction in excess daytime sleepiness by modafinil in patients with myotonic dystrophy. *Neuromuscul Disord.* 2003;13(5):357–64.
32. Broomfield A, Fletcher J, Davison J et al. Response of 33 UK patients with infantile-onset Pompe disease to enzyme replacement therapy. *J Inherit Metab Dis.* 2016;39(2):261–71.
33. Muller-Felber W, Horvath R, Gempel K et al. Late onset Pompe disease: Clinical and neurophysiological spectrum of 38 patients including long-term follow-up in 18 patients. *Neuromuscul Disord.* 2007;17:698–706.
34. Goldstein JL, Young SP, Changela M et al. Screening for Pompe disease using a rapid dried blood spot method: Experience of a clinical diagnostic laboratory. *Muscle Nerve.* 2009;40:32–6.
35. Winchester B, Bali D, Bodamer OA et al. Methods for a prompt and reliable laboratory diagnosis of Pompe disease: Report from an international consensus meeting. *Mol Genet Metab.* 2008;93:275–81.
36. Bonne G, Di Barletta MR, Varnous S et al. Mutations in the gene encoding lamin A/C cause autosomal dominant Emery-Dreifuss muscular dystrophy. *Nat Genet.* 1999;21:285–8.
37. Sanna T, Dello Russo A, Toniolo D et al. Cardiac features of Emery-Dreifuss muscular dystrophy caused by lamin A/C gene mutations. *Eur Heart J.* 2003;24:2227–36.
38. Golzio PG, Chiribiri A, Gaita F. 'Unexpected' sudden death avoided by implantable cardioverter defibrillator in Emery Dreifuss patient. *Europace.* 2007;9:1158–60.
39. Poppe M, Cree L, Bourke J et al. The phenotype of limb-girdle muscular dystrophy type 2I. *Neurology.* 2003;60:1246–51.
40. Larsson L. Acute quadriplegic myopathy: An acquired 'myosinopathy'. *Adv Exp Med Biol.* 2008;642:92–8.
41. Argov Z. Drug-induced myopathies. *Curr Opin Neurol.* 2000;13:541–5.
42. Schroder R, Schoser B. Myofibrillar myopathies: A clinical and myopathological guide. *Brain Pathol.* 2009;19:483–92.
43. Shahrizaila T, Kinnear W. Recommendations for respiratory care of adults with muscle disorders. *Neuromuscul Disord.* 2007;17:13–15.
44. Shahrizaila N, Kinnear WJ, Wills AJ. Respiratory involvement in inherited primary muscle conditions. *J Neurol Neurosurg Psychiatry.* 2006;77:1108–15.

39

Pathophysiology of respiratory failure in neuromuscular diseases

FRANCO LAGHI, HAMEEDA SHAIKH AND DEJAN RADOVANOVIC

INTRODUCTION

According to the level of anatomical involvement, neuromuscular diseases (NMDs) can be grouped into those involving upper motor neurons, lower motor neurons, peripheral nerves, neuromuscular junction and peripheral muscles (Table 39.1). In patients affected by NMDs, respiratory failure is one of the most important causes of morbidity and mortality.[1] Ventilatory support is the only intervention known to extend survival in patients who develop respiratory failure as a result of NMDs.[1,2]

PATHOPHYSIOLOGY OF RESPIRATORY FAILURE IN NMD

Alveolar hypoventilation – defined as alveolar ventilation inappropriately low for the patient's level of carbon dioxide production – is the primary mechanism responsible for respiratory failure in NMDs. The rise in the partial pressure of carbon dioxide in the alveoli that accompanies hypoventilation causes a concurrent decrease in the partial pressure of oxygen. This means that hypoventilation can cause hypoxaemia even when the lung parenchyma is normal – that is, hypercapnia with normal alveolar-to-arterial oxygen gradient (A-aDO_2).* When NMDs cause pulmonary complications that impair gas exchange and increase A-aDO_2, hypoxaemia can be out of proportion to the degree of alveolar hypoventilation. In patients with increased A-aDO_2, the magnitude of neuromuscular derangement causing hypercapnia can be minor compared to patients with NMDs and normal gas exchange. When gas exchange is impaired – or when

* The A-aDO_2 is calculated as $PAO_2 - PaO_2$, where PAO_2 (alveolar O_2 tension) can be estimated according to the simplified alveolar gas equation. $PAO_2 = FIO_2 \bullet (PB - PH_2O) - PaCO_2/R$, where FIO_2 = fractional concentration of inspired O_2 (about 0.21 when breathing room air), PB = barometric pressure (about 760 mm Hg at sea level), PH_2O = water vapor pressure (usually taken as 47 mm Hg at 37°C) and R = respiratory exchange ratio of the whole lung. R is calculated as the ratio of CO_2 production over O_2 consumption (VCO_2/VO_2). R is normally ~0.8. In steady state, R is determined by the relative proportions of free fatty acids, protein, and carbohydrate consumed by the tissues. In this equation, it is assumed that the values of $PACO_2$ and $PaCO_2$ are the same (usually they nearly are). In healthy young subjects (≤30 years old) breathing air at sea level, A-aDO_2 is <10 mmHg and increases by ~ 3 mmHg per decade after 30.

Table 39.1 Examples of NMDs that can be associated with respiratory failure grouped according to the level of anatomical involvement

1. Upper motor neuron
   a. Amyotrophic lateral sclerosis
   b. Multiple sclerosis
   c. Stroke
   d. Trauma
   e. Post-polio syndrome
2. Lower motor neuron
   a. Spinal cord injury
   b. Post-polio syndrome
   c. Amyotrophic lateral sclerosis
   d. Spinal muscle atrophies
3. Peripheral nerves
   a. Guillain–Barré syndrome
   b. Critical illness polyneuropathy
   c. Acute porphyria
4. Neuromuscular junction
   a. Botulism
   b. Myasthenia gravis
   c. Tick paralysis
   d. Shellfish poisoning
   e. Drugs (neuromuscular blocking agents)
5. Muscle fibres
   a. Inflammatory/autoimmune myopathies (dermatomyositis, polymyositis)
   b. Myotonic dystrophies
   c. Duchenne's muscular dystrophy
   d. Metabolic myopathies (glycogen storage disease, abnormal lipid metabolism)
   e. Endocrine myopathies (hyperthyroidism)

the pattern of breathing is rapid and shallow – alveolar hypoventilation can occur despite normal or increased total minute ventilation.[3]

In the sections that follow, we will discuss mechanisms for alveolar hypoventilation and impaired gas exchange in NMDs. In addition, we will conclude with an overview on selected diagnostic tools that can be used to identify patients with NMDs who are at risk for the development of respiratory failure.

Alveolar hypoventilation

In patients with NMDs, alveolar hypoventilation can result from a combination of altered respiratory drive, increased mechanical load, diminished respiratory muscle performance and impaired cardiovascular performance.

ALVEOLAR HYPOVENTILATION: ALTERED RESPIRATORY DRIVE

Structural lesions of the central nervous system can contribute to, or cause, alveolar hypoventilation and hypercapnic respiratory failure (Table 39.1). In myotonic dystrophy, dysregulation of the control of breathing contributes to alveolar hypoventilation independent of the severity of respiratory muscle weakness.[4]

When it develops for whatever reason, severe hypercapnia depresses the central nervous system and decreases respiratory motor output. A vicious cycle can arise, whereby hypercapnia causes depressed drive leading to more hypercapnia.[1] Hypercapnia can decrease diaphragmatic contractility, although not consistently.[1] Acidosis may be more important than hypercapnia in causing respiratory muscle impairment as mortality is more closely related to acidosis than to hypercapnia.[5] In animal models, the decrease in diaphragmatic contractility is proportional to the degree of hypercapnia, but only in the case of respiratory acidosis.[6,7] Even this last possibility is uncertain because diaphragmatic contractility was not affected by acidosis in one study.[8]

ALVEOLAR HYPOVENTILATION: INCREASED MECHANICAL LOAD

In patients with NMDs, upper airway obstruction and reduced chest wall and lung compliance can limit the ability of the respiratory muscles to generate and sustain adequate alveolar ventilation.

Upper airway obstruction: Parkinson's disease, multiple system atrophy (a Parkinson-like syndrome that causes progressive degenerative disease of the central nervous system), amyotrophic lateral sclerosis (ALS) and botulism are some of the NMDs that can cause vocal cord dysfunction and frank vocal cord paralysis.[1] Presence of vocal cord dysfunction or paralysis can predispose to upper airway obstruction and contribute to ventilatory failure and death.[1] In some NMDs, macroglossia can contribute to upper airway obstruction and difficult intubation.[9,10]

Impaired chest wall and lung mechanics: Severe weakness of the inspiratory muscles produces a restrictive pattern with decreases in vital capacity (VC), total lung capacity and functional residual capacity.[1] When respiratory muscle strength is less than 50% of predicted, the loss in VC is greater than expected.[1] The decrease is secondary to decreases in compliance of the chest wall and lungs. Several factors can decrease chest wall compliance. Thoracic scoliosis can be particularly severe in those patients in whom respiratory and vertebral muscle weakness is present before spinal growth is complete. Obesity is a common occurrence in patients with spinal cord injury. In patients with NMDs, there is often stiffening of tendons and ligaments of the rib cage, and ankylosis of the costosternal and thoracovertebral joints.[1]

Decrease in lung compliance can result from inflammatory and fibrotic changes of the lung parenchyma. The last two processes can be triggered by recurrent aspiration of gastric contents and impaired cough. (Other factors that can decrease lung compliance include diffuse microatelectasis and, in patients with cardiac impairment, pulmonary congestion.[1])

ALVEOLAR HYPOVENTILATION: DECREASED RESPIRATORY MUSCLE PERFORMANCE DURING WAKEFULNESS

Respiratory muscle weakness may be present at birth (Type 1 spinal muscular dystrophy), arise later in the course of the disease (myotonic dystrophy, Duchenne muscular dystrophy) or be acquired (spinal cord injury, poliomyelitis, post-polio syndrome, Guillain–Barré Disease, ALS).[1,2] Respiratory muscle weakness frequently goes undetected in patients with NMDs until ventilatory failure is precipitated by aspiration pneumonia or cor pulmonale.[1,2] Diagnosis is delayed because limb muscle weakness prevents patients from exceeding their limited ventilatory capacity.[1] In specific cases such as multiple sclerosis or ALS, the apparent lack of dyspnoea may in fact reflect difficulty in communicating this symptom due to impaired phonation or compromised cognition.[1] Among patients with neuromuscular respiratory failure, those without known diagnosis of NMDs before admission to the intensive care unit (ICU) have the poorest outcomes.[11]

Severe respiratory muscle weakness and even complete diaphragmatic paralysis can occur despite little or no peripheral muscle weakness.[2,12] Lone diaphragmatic weakness or paralysis can occur with disease processes that damage the phrenic nerve such as trauma, mediastinal malignancies, alcoholism and diabetes.[12] In a substantial number of patients, the etiology of diaphragmatic paralysis remains elusive. Many of them are affected by neuralgic amyotrophy,[13] an idiopathic or, less often, an autosomal dominant neuropathy, probably autoimmune in nature, that is usually limited to the brachial plexus. In a few patients, neuralgic amyotrophy causes unilateral (about 5%) or bilateral (about 1%) diaphragmatic paralysis.[1] Dyspnoca usually occurs after a prodromal flu-like episode, followed by acute severe neck and shoulder pain with or without arm weakness.[1] The first episode of dyspnoea may also be precipitated by surgery. More than 90% of patients recover upper limb function within 3 years after the onset of symptoms. Recovery of diaphragmatic function, however, is slower and less complete.[1] Ten of 14 patients recovered some diaphragmatic strength over 2 to 11 years, but function was less than 50% of predicted in 7 of the 10 patients.[1] Recovery took 3 years or more in most patients.[3] Similar to limb muscles, diaphragmatic paralysis can recur after complete recovery. No specific therapy is available for patients with neuralgic amyotrophy. Plication of both hemidiaphragms improved ventilation and gas exchange and resolved orthopnoea in three patients with persistent bilateral paralysis who developed cor pulmonale.[3]

Patients with respiratory muscle weakness take rapid shallow breaths, possibly as a result of afferent signals arising from the weakened respiratory muscles, intrapulmonary receptors or both.[1] $PaCO_2$ may be reduced early in the disease, but hypercapnia is likely when respiratory muscle strength falls to 25% of predicted.[1] Reduction in strength, however, does not consistently predict alveolar hypoventilation, because factors such as elastic load and breathing pattern also contribute to it.[5] Abnormalities in respiratory muscle performance and alveolar ventilation may initially be evident only during exercise or sleep.[1] When inspiratory strength and VC are 50% of predicted, hypoventilation can occur even with minor upper respiratory tract infections.[1]

Orthopnoea that develops within seconds of lying down is often reported in bilateral and, less often, unilateral diaphragmatic paralysis.[12] This contrasts with the more gradual onset of orthopnoea in patients with congestive heart failure. In general, orthopnoea occurs when maximal transdiaphragmatic pressure is less than 30 cmH_2O[1] and when there is a supine drop in forced VC of more than 30%.[2]

When immersed in water, patients with severe diaphragmatic weakness or with diaphragmatic paralysis often complain of dyspnoea[1] and experience greater reductions in lung volumes and greater increases in reparatory drive than healthy subjects.[14] The increased hydrostatic pressure surrounding an individual immersed in water decreases chest wall compliance.[5] In addition, the movement of blood into the thorax decreases lung compliance.[5]

Patients with bilateral diaphragm paralysis often complain of dyspnoea when bending or lifting—activities that require expiratory muscle recruitment.[1] These symptoms may arise because the paralysed diaphragm cannot prevent the rise in intrathoracic pressure and thus cannot prevent the cessation of an ongoing inhalation caused by expiratory muscle recruitment.

In contrast to patients with diaphragmatic paralysis, patients with quadriplegia can experience platypnoea (dyspnoea when sitting and relieved in the supine position).[5] In this position, the area of apposition of the diaphragm with respect to the abdominal wall and its resting length are increased, and these two factors combined enhance the force generation capacity of the muscle.[15]

ALVEOLAR HYPOVENTILATION: DECREASED RESPIRATORY MUSCLE PERFORMANCE DURING SLEEP

Irrespective of the primary pathology, patients with NMDs commonly develop abnormalities during sleep including frequent arousals, increased Stage 1 sleep, decreased rapid eye movement (REM) sleep, hypoventilation[16,17] and hypoxaemia.[1] The earliest warning of respiratory muscle involvement causing hypoventilation is represented by a sawtooth pattern of the saturation tracing occurring during REM sleep.[18]

Patients with impaired diaphragmatic function, such as those affected by ALS, are at particular risk of developing hypoventilation during REM sleep (when rib cage muscle contribution to tidal breathing decreases due to GABAnergic and glycinergic-mediated inhibition of motor neurons).[19] To limit REM-related hypoventilation, the central nervous system can adopt two strategies: phasic recruitment of extradiaphragmatic inspiratory muscles during REM sleep or suppression of REM sleep.[18] Failure to develop these adaptive strategies in some patients may explain the divergent reports on desaturation during sleep in patients with isolated diaphragmatic paralysis.[1]

Sleep-disordered breathing usually precedes, and probably contributes to, daytime ventilatory failure.[1] Patients commonly report daytime symptoms such as excessive sleepiness, morning headaches, fatigue, poor concentration and memory problems. Often they also report nighttime symptoms such as sleep fragmentation, nocturia, leg cramps and restless legs, orthopnoea, snoring/choking and nightmares.[1,18] Sleep-disordered breathing usually develops when VC in the supine position is less than 60% of the predicted value or maximal inspiratory pressure is less negative than −34 cmH_2O.[20] Severity of sleep-disordered breathing tends to parallel the extent of respiratory weakness.[20]

Hypopnoeas and apnoeas in NMDs can be central, pseudo-central, or obstructive.[1] Central events can result from either Cheyne-Stokes breathing in association with cardiomyopathy, such as in patients with muscle dystrophies, or to an instability in control of breathing due to diaphragm weakness, as proposed for patients with spinal cord injury, postpolio syndrome or in myotonic dystrophy.[18] Obstructive events typically result from weakness of the upper airway musculature, more rarely macroglossia.[1] Pseudo-central events occur when the inspiratory efforts are too weak to be identified during polysomnography.[18] Hypoventilation and daytime hypercapnia may be aggravated by resetting of the chemoreceptors during sleep, which is reversible with chronic nocturnal mechanical ventilation.[1]

ALVEOLAR HYPOVENTILATION: DECREASED RESPIRATORY MUSCLE PERFORMANCE IN THE ICU

Although less than 2% of critically ill patients in the ICU receive mechanical ventilation because of NMDs,[21] most mechanically ventilated patients develop profound diaphragmatic and extra-diaphragmatic muscle weakness.[22,23] In recent years, studies have demonstrated a correlation between duration of mechanical ventilation and diaphragmatic atrophy or swelling, sarcomere injury, decreased diaphragmatic fibre specific force and upregulation of atrophic genes (Atrogin1 and MuRF1).[24,25] Diaphragmatic weakness has been associated with longer ventilator duration and higher mortality.[26] Whether sepsis contributes to diaphragmatic weakness remains controversial.[27,28] Similarly, the purported mechanistic link between respiratory weakness and weaning failure remains controversial.[26–29]

ALVEOLAR HYPOVENTILATION: IMPAIRED CARDIOVASCULAR PERFORMANCE

NMDs caused by genetic abnormalities such as myotonic dystrophy, Duchenne muscular dystrophy and mitochondrial syndromes can cause myocardial dysfunction.[30] Myocardial dysfunction, in turn, exacerbates respiratory muscle weakness by causing atrophy and structural damage of all types of rib cage and diaphragm muscle fibres and by decreasing the number of Type IIb fibres. (Type IIb fibres produce more force than Type I fibres.[1]) Potential mechanisms for muscle atrophy and structural damage include decreased regional blood flow and activation of the ubiquitin–proteasome proteolytic pathway by tumour necrosis factor. Finally, myocardial dysfunction can decrease the voluntary drive to the diaphragm during maximal inspiratory efforts.[1]

As with respiratory muscle strength, endurance is also reduced in heart failure.[1] Two factors may contribute to the decreased endurance: decreased circulatory supply of energy substrates and increased work of breathing caused by decreased static lung compliance (when pulmonary congestion or pleural effusions are present).[1]

Impaired gas exchange

Ventilation/perfusion inequalities and, less often, increased intrapulmonary shunt, can complicate the clinical course of NMDs. The mechanisms for such impairments in gas exchange include development of diffuse microatelectasis, ineffective cough with retention of secretions/bronchopneumonia and heart failure.

IMPAIRED GAS EXCHANGE: DIFFUSE MICROATELECTASIS

In the past, investigators considered the presence of diffuse microatelectasis a common occurrence in patients with NMDs. Purported mechanisms for the development of microatelectasis include infrequent, small sighs and rapid and shallow breathing.[5] The real impact of diffuse microatelectasis in NMDs has been put into question.[31] On high-resolution computed tomography, diffuse microatelectasis was found in only 2 of 14 patients with NMDs who had a 30% decrease in lung compliance.[31]

IMPAIRED GAS EXCHANGE: INEFFECTIVE COUGH/BRONCHOPNEUMONIA

Ineffective cough is a common cause of poor airway clearance and bronchopneumonia in patients with NMDs. Ineffective cough can result from an impairment of inspiratory, expiratory, and bulbar muscles or from a combination of the three.[1]

Inspiratory muscle weakness decreases the effectiveness of cough because the inhaled volume preceding the expulsive phase of cough is smaller. Smaller inhaled volume limits the increase in length (and thus in force output) of the expiratory muscles during the expulsive phase of cough. Expiratory muscle weakness and bulbar dysfunction decrease the effectiveness of cough because of impairment in cough-induced dynamic airway compression, leading to a reduction in the velocity of airflow. Dysfunction of the bulbar muscles can also impair cough through involuntary closure of the vocal cords during rapid exhalation.[1] Moreover, bulbar dysfunction predisposes to aspiration of secretions and foreign material into the airway. Bulbar muscle impairment occurs in several NMDs including ALS, post-polio syndrome, botulism, myasthenia, Parkinson's disease and tick paralysis.[1] Infants and young children with NMDs and bulbar impairment are at particular risk of secretion-associated airway obstruction mainly due to the smaller airway size, greater compliance of the airways and the chest wall, ineffective collateral ventilation and smaller elastic recoil pressure.[32]

IMPAIRED GAS EXCHANGE: DECREASED CARDIAC FUNCTION

In patients with NMDs and decreased cardiac function, impaired gas exchange can result from pulmonary congestion/alveolar flooding and pleural effusions. The combination of impaired gas exchange and decreased mixed venous O_2 content – caused by increased peripheral O_2 extraction – can contribute to hypoxaemia in patients with NMDs and decreased cardiac function.[3]

DIAGNOSIS

Early identification of bulbar, inspiratory and expiratory muscle impairment is critical to reduce excess morbidity and premature mortality in patients affected by NMDs.[1,33] It would seem biologically plausible to perform respiratory muscle testing less often in patients with slowly progressive NMDs (e.g. myotonic dystrophy, Duchenne's muscular dystrophy) and more often in patients with rapidly progressive NMDs (e.g. ALS), and even more often in hospitalised patients who have an evolving neuromuscular disorder (e.g. Guillain–Barré syndrome, botulism). Unfortunately, for most NMDs, it remains unclear how often respiratory muscle testing should be performed or when ventilatory support should be initiated. Although testing for muscle weakness is feasible, clinicians should always be on alert to identify signs and symptoms of subacute or chronic respiratory failure and muscle impairment in NMD patients (Table 39.2).

Diagnosis: Bulbar muscle impairment

In patients with NMDs, early bulbar muscle impairment is commonly unrecognised. A high level of suspicion and clinical observation are the primary means to assess these patients. Common signs of incipient bulbar dysfunction are summarised in Table 39.2. Oral accumulation of saliva often results from impaired swallowing (pseudo-sialorrhea) rather than true hyperproduction. Early consultation with an experienced speech pathologist can give objective quantification of the complex and coordinated actions of speech and swallowing. These patients seldom profit from pharmacological treatment of their underlying NMD to substantially improve speech and/or swallowing yet, they may still benefit from learning personalized functional compensations taught by a knowledgeable speech-language pathologist.

Table 39.2 Signs and symptoms of muscle impairment and subacute/chronic respiratory failure in patients with NMDs

Affected muscle group	Sign and symptom
Bulbar muscles (mouth, pharynx, palate, tongue and larynx)	Nasal tonality of the voice
	Slow speech/dysarthria
	Pseudo-sialorrhea
	Impaired gag reflex
	Dysphagia
	Cough after swallow
Inspiratory/ expiratory muscles	Exertional dyspnoea
	Tachypnoea
	Staccato speech
	Increased cervical muscle recruitment
	Paradoxical breathing/orthopnoea
	Sleep disruption/morning headache
	Nocturnal hypoxia/hypopnoea
	Obstructive sleep apnoea
	Central and pseudo-central sleep apnoea
	Weak cough

Diagnosis: Inspiratory muscle impairment

Signs of respiratory muscle weakness in NMDs may be limited to tachypnea, inability to finish long sentences (staccato speech) or list numbers from 1 to 20 without pausing to take a breath (Table 39.2). Complaints of nonrefreshing sleep and frequent nocturnal awakenings should be considered warning signs of imminent neuromuscular respiratory failure. Unfortunately, all these findings are nonspecific. A more objective assessment of inspiratory muscle impairment in NMDs consist in recording maximal inspiratory airway pressure (MIP), sniff pressure and, less often, maximal transdiaphragmatic inspiratory pressure (Pdimax) and transdiaphragmatic twitch pressure (Pditw) elicited by phrenic nerve stimulation.[1]

Measurements of MIP during forceful inhalation against an occluded airway reflect global inspiratory muscle strength.[5] In general, a MIP < -70 cmH_2O for women and < -100 cmH_2O for men exclude clinically significant muscle weakness. Global inspiratory muscle strength can also be quantified by recording nasal pressures during a sniff manoeuvre (SNIP). In general, a SNIP < -50 cmH_2O for women and < -60 cmH_2O for men exclude clinically significant weakness (Table 39.3).[34]

Table 39.3 Respiratory compromise due to NMDs causing respiratory muscle weakness

Finding	Compromise
Pressures	
MIP < -34 cmH_2O	Sleep disorder breathing
MIP < -20 cmH_2O	Inability to ventilate adequately
SNIP < 32% predicted	Hypercarbic respiratory insufficiency
MEP < 40 cmH_2O	Impaired cough, inability to clear secretions
Twitch gastric pressure < 7 cmH_2O	Impaired cough, inability to clear secretions
Vital capacity	
<30 mL/kg	Impaired cough/sleep disorder breathing
<20 mL/kg	Inability to sigh or prevent atelectasis
<10 mL/kg	Inability to ventilate adequately
Bulbar weakness/ paralysis	Inability to protect the airway and to avoid aspiration

Note: The large variability pressures and volumes associated with clinical compromise limit usefulness/generalisability of specific thresholds of pressures and volumes (see text for details).

Abbreviations: MIP, maximal inspiratory airway pressure; MEP, maximal expiratory airway pressure; SNIR, sniff nasal inspiratory pressure.

In patients who are unable or unwilling to make voluntary efforts, Pditw elicited by phrenic nerve stimulation has been used to objectively assess inspiratory muscle impairment. Phrenic nerve stimulation can be achieved with either electrical or magnetic stimulators,[35] although the latter are easier to use in mechanically ventilated patients (Figure 39.1).[29,36,37] In healthy subjects, magnetic stimulation elicits twitch pressures that average 31 to 39 cmH_2O.[38] In patients with severe chronic obstructive pulmonary disease, twitch pressures average 19 to 20 cmH_2O.[39,40] The amplitude Pditw in patients recovering from an episode of acute respiratory failure is about one-third of that recorded in healthy subjects (Figure 39.2).[28,29,36,37] This marked reduction in twitch pressure[28,36,37] indicates the presence of respiratory muscle weakness in most of these patients. Purported mechanisms of respiratory muscle weakness in critically ill patients include critical illness neuropathy and myopathy (Table 39.4).

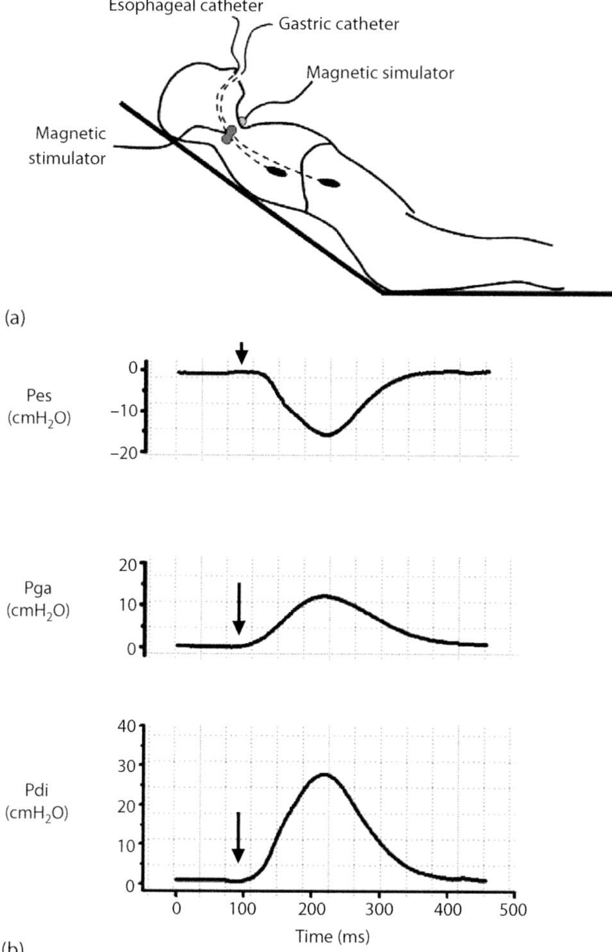

Figure 39.1 Recording of transdiaphragmatic twitch pressure. **(a)** An esophageal and a gastric balloon are passed through the nares. Magnetic stimulation of the phrenic nerves elicits diaphragmatic contraction. **(b)** Continuous recordings of esophageal (Pes) and gastric pressures (Pga) and transdiaphragmatic pressure (Pdi)—calculated by subtracting Pes from Pga. Phrenic nerve stimulation (arrows) results in contraction of the diaphragm with consequent fall in intrathoracic pressure (negative defection of Pes) and rise in intraabdominal pressure (positive deflection of Pga). These swings in pressure are responsible for the transdiaphragmatic twitch pressure. The smaller the transdiaphragmatic twitch pressure, the smaller the force generation capacity of the diaphragm. (Reproduced with permission from Laghi F. Hypoventilation and respiratory muscle dysfunction. In: Parillo JE and Dellinger RP, editors. *Critical Care Medicine: Principles of Diagnosis and Management in the Adult.* St Louis: Mosby, Inc. 3rd edition.)

Diaphragm fluoroscopy has been used to assess diaphragm function. Unfortunately, this test can be unreliable in the presence of global weakness, in patients who do not cooperate and in patients with bilateral diaphragm paralysis.[1] In contrast to fluoroscopy, diaphragmatic ultrasonography is a promising non-invasive method to assess diaphragmatic function in the outpatient and inpatients settings – including the evaluation of post-operative patients and ICU patients (Figure 39.3).[41–44] For instance, in the outpatient setting, diaphragmatic thickness at a functional residual capacity of less than 2 mm combined with a less than 20% increase in thickness during inspiration to total lung capacity can descriminate between a chronically paralysed and normal diaphragm.[45]

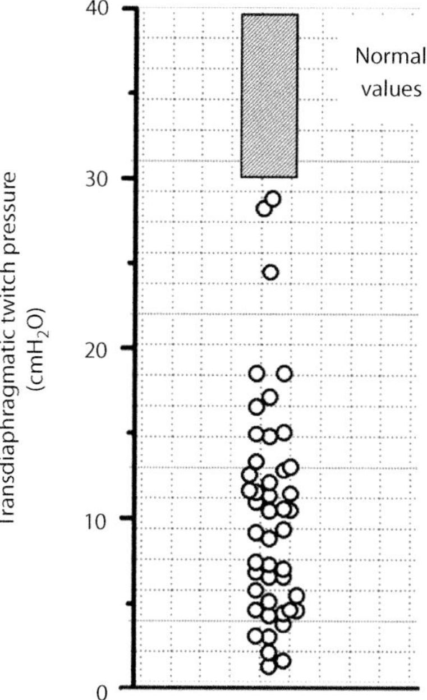

Figure 39.2 Transdiaphragmatic twitch pressure recorded in mechanically ventilated patients recovering from an episode of acute respiratory failure. Box represents range of transdiaphragmatic twitch pressures recorded in healthy subjects. Most mechanically ventilated patients had evidence of diaphragmatic weakness. (Modified from Laghi F. *Respir Care Clin N Am* 2005;11:173–199.)

Table 39.4 Characteristics of acute and subacute paralysis

	Guillain–Barré	Critical illness polyneuropathy	Critical illness myopathy	Spinal cord lesion	Poliomyelitis	Tick paralysis	Botulism
Progression	Days to weeks	Days to weeks	Days to weeks	Slow or immediate	Days to weeks	Hours to days	Days
Evolution of motor deficit	Usually ascending	Generalised	Generalised	Focal	Asymmetric	Ascending	Descending
Fever	Uncommon	Commonly present	Uncommon	Absent	Present	Uncommon	Absent
Meningeal signs	Uncommon	Absent	Absent	Absent	Present	Absent	Absent
Ataxia	Uncommon	Absent	Absent	Sometimes present	Absent	Present	Absent
Tendon reflexes	Absent	Reduced or absent	Reduced or absent	Variable	Absent	Absent	Reduced or absent
Babinski sign	Absent	Absent	Absent	Present	Absent	Absent	Absent
Sensory deficit	Mild	Mild	Absent	Present	Absent	Absent	Absent
CSF: protein	High	–	Normal	Normal or high	High	Normal	–
CSF: white cells (per mm^3)	<10	–	–	Variable	>10	<10	–
Recovery time	Weeks to months or no recovery	Weeks to months or no recovery	Weeks to months or no recovery	Variable according to etiology	Months to years or no recovery	<24 hours (North America),[a] >2 weeks (Australia)[a]	Weeks to months

Source: Laghi F, Tobin MJ. *Am J Respir Crit Care Med.* 2003;168(1):10–48.
Abbreviation: CSF, cerebrospinal fluid.
[a] After tick removal.

In critically ill patients, diaphragmatic dysfunction had been assessed via sequential ultrasonographic measurements of muscle thickness at the zone of apposition and of diaphragmatic excursions during tidal breathing.[45] In an investigation of 107 patients, Goligher et al.[46] reported that during the first week of mechanical ventilation, diaphragm thickness decreased by more than 10% in nearly half of the patients and it remained unchanged or increased in the remaining half. Loss of thickness was associated with less diaphragm shortening. This finding raises the possibility that loss of diaphragm thickness could be mechanistically linked to a reduction in diaphragm activation while receiving mechanical ventilator support. Of note, the investigators reported no appreciable outcome differences across these three groups of patients.

Despite these intriguing results, the use of ultrasonography to assess diaphragmatic function in the ICU has potential limitations. For example, ICU studies do not normalise for respiratory drive and mechanical load on the diaphragm – crucial determinants of muscle shortening.

Diagnosis: Expiratory muscle impairment

Measurement in gastric pressure following electrical or magnetic stimulation of the abdominal wall muscles (while patients relax at end-exhalation) – or twitch gastric pressure (Pgatw) – provides a selective and quantitative measure of expiratory muscle function.[47] In healthy subjects, Kyroussis and coworkers[48] reported that the mean (±SD) value of Pgatw was 24 ± 5 cmH_2O.[48] In patients with ALS, an effective cough is unlikely when Pgatw is less than 7 cmH_2O.[49] Using this technique, Ward et al.[50] concluded that impaired cortical modulation – and not intrinsic expiratory muscle weakness (normal Pgatw) – is responsible for ineffective cough following an hemispheric stroke.[50]

Diagnosis: Tests of inspiratory and expiratory muscle impairment

Generation of a VC manoeuvre, which is a maximal expiratory effort from total lung capacity requires maximal voluntary recruitment of the inspiratory muscles, followed by

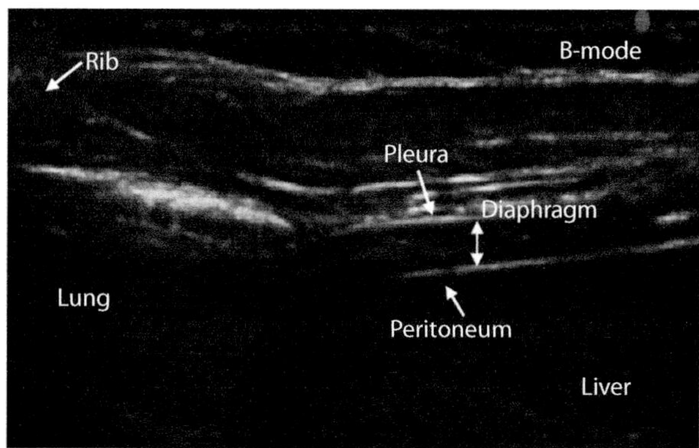

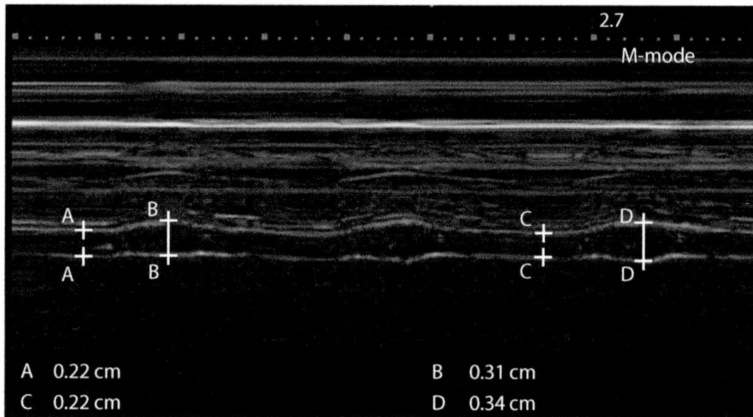

Figure 39.3 Ultrasound of right hemidiaphragm at zone of apposition in a healthy volunteer. (Upper panel) Bidimensional ultrasound (B-mode) image. The diaphragm next to the zone of apposition is displayed between the pleural and peritoneal line (right portion of the figure). As the diaphragm peels off the zone of apposition, it dives into the abdomen to then disappear. Cranial to the diaphragm (left portion of the upper panel) is the lung. (Lower panel) Motion-mode (M-mode) image: Recordings obtained during tidal breathing. The diaphragmatic thickness at end exhalation for the first (AA) and the third breath (CC) was 2.2 mm in both instances. The corresponding thickness during inhalation was 3.1 mm for the first breath (BB) and 3.4 mm (DD) for the third breath.

maximal voluntary recruitment of the expiratory muscles. This means that the test is affected by impairments of the inspiratory and/or expiratory muscles. VC in healthy adults is approximately 50 to 60 mL/kg. VC < 30 mL/kg is associated with a weak cough, impaired elimination of secretions and development of macro atelectasis.[51] Serial measurements that demonstrate a decline in VC to less than 15 to 20 mL/kg suggest an increased likelihood that ventilator assistance will be necessary. Ventilatory failure with need for mechanical ventilation occurs at a VC of around 10 to 15 mL/kg or 1 L.[51]

Maximal expiratory pressure (MEP) is the airway pressure recorded during a maximal effort at total lung capacity using a bedside manometer fitted with a mouthpiece. Normal values for MEP are approximately 100 cmH_2O for women and approximately 150 cmH_2O for men. When the MEP is <40 cmH_2O, cough is unlikely to be effective. Because of the voluntary nature of the manoeuvre, great caution has to be taken in interpreting low MEP values. For instance, Man and coworkers[52] reported that among 171 patients with suspected respiratory muscle dysfunction and MEP values below the lower 95% confidence interval recorded in healthy volunteers, 72 patients (42%) had normal expiratory muscle strength. (A sharp whistle from total lung capacity is an alternative method to assess MEP)[53] Measurements of the MEP/MIP ratio have been proposed as a tool to evaluate the relative impairment of inspiratory and expiratory muscles.[54]

The most widely user-friendly tool used to measure cough effectiveness is the peak cough expiratory flow (PCEF) meter device. PCEFs > 160 L/min are needed to clear secretions, and clinicians recommend using cough assist devices when PCEF is <270 L/min.[55] Among patients with ALS, those with a mean PCEF > 337 L/min have a greater chance of being alive at 18 months than those with a smaller PCEF.[55]

Diagnosis: Sleep studies

Polysomnographic studies are recommended in selected patients with suspected nocturnal hypoventilation (Table 39.2).[56] Hypopnoeas predominate in the early stage of an NMD.[20] As the respiratory muscle weakness progresses, clear, short-lasting hypopnoeas tend to be replaced by more prolonged episodes of hypoventilation that are not captured by the apnoea–hypopnoea score.[20] Accordingly, apnoea–hypopnoea scores can underestimate the effect of nocturnal hypoventilation on quality of life or functional status.[57] Sleep disruption in patients with NMDs may also result from an inability to change position during sleep, muscle twitches and leg jerks.[5]

Diagnosis: Arterial blood gas and electrolytes

Monitoring arterial blood gas – even in rapidly progressive NMDs such as ALS or Guillain–Barré syndrome – can give a false sense of security because gas exchange can be largely maintained despite severe respiratory muscle impairment.[58,59] In ALS, patients with a VC < 50% predicted and a MIP or MEP < 25% predicted are not necessarily hypercapnic,[58,60] making blood gas monitoring poorly reliable in the follow-up. This is true until the last months of life, at which point patients may show respiratory acidosis[61] and a precipitous fall in serum chloride (an indirect marker of respiratory acidosis).[5]

Transcutaneous capnography ($TcCO_2$) has been used as a means to detect hypoventilation on NMD.[62,63] In a retrospective study of 55 patients with various NMDs, Ogna et al.[64] reported that residual nocturnal hypoventilation following institution of mechanical ventilation ($TcCO_2$ > 49 mmHg during ≥10% of monitoring time), but not residual nocturnal hypoxaemia (SpO_2 < 90% during ≥10% of the total recording time), was associated with a higher risk of ICU admission and mortality in patients with NMDs.[64] (For an additional discussion on the diagnostic approach of NMDs and ventilatory failure, please see Chapter 37.)

FUTURE RESEARCH/CONCLUSION

Respiratory failure occurs with numerous NMDs. Severe impairment of respiratory muscle function may be recognised early in the disease process, as in the case of bilateral diaphragmatic paralysis, or it may go unrecognised until hypercapnic respiratory failure develops, as in the case of Duchenne's muscular dystrophy. NMDs involving the respiratory muscles often lead to breathing disturbances during sleep and pulmonary aspiration. Dyspnoea may not develop until respiratory impairment is far advanced because activity sufficient to induce dyspnoea is limited by associated weakness of the limb muscles. Accordingly, a high level of suspicion is necessary to recognise the presence of respiratory muscle impairment and allow the institution of specific therapies. While the understanding of the pathophysiologic mechanisms of respiratory failure in NMDs has greatly improved during the last four decades, the type of diagnostic tests to be employed in the identification of patients at risk of respiratory failure and the frequency with which these tests should be obtained remains elusive. Future research must focus on the development of disease-specific diagnostic strategies that will accurately monitor disease progression and identification of impending respiratory failure in patients with NMDs.

ACKNOWLEDGEMENT

Supported by a Merit Review Grant from the Veterans Administration Research Service.

REFERENCES

1. Laghi F, Tobin MJ. Disorders of the respiratory muscles. *Am J Respir Crit Care Med.* 2003;168(1):10–48.
2. Howard RS. Respiratory failure because of neuromuscular disease. *Curr Opin Neurol.* 2016;29(5): 592–601.
3. Laghi F, Tobin MJ. Indications for mechanical ventilation. In: Tobin MJ, editor. *Principles and Practice of Mechanical Ventilation.* 3rd edition. New York: McGraw-Hill Co., 2013:101–35.
4. Poussel M, Thil C, Kaminsky P et al. Lack of correlation between the ventilatory response to CO_2 and lung function impairment in myotonic dystrophy patients: Evidence for a dysregulation at central level. *Neuromuscul Disord.* 2015;25(5):403–8.
5. Laghi F, Shaikh H, Gungor G. Pathophysiology of respiratory failure in neuromuscular diseases. In: Elliott M, Nava S, Schoenhofer B, editors. *Non-Invasive Ventilation and Weaning: Principles and Practice.* 1st edition. London: Hodder Arnold, 2010:331–9.
6. Michelet P, Carreira S, Demoule A et al. Effects of acute respiratory and metabolic acidosis on diaphragm muscle obtained from rats. *Anesthesiology.* 2015;122(4):876–3.
7. Jaber S, Jung B, Sebbane M et al. Alteration of the piglet diaphragm contractility in vivo and its recovery after acute hypercapnia. *Anesthesiology.* 2008;108(4):651–8.
8. Sassoon CS, Gruer SE, Sieck GC. Temporal relationships of ventilatory failure, pump failure, and diaphragm fatigue. *J Appl Physiol.* 1996;81(1): 238–45.
9. Blatter JA, Finder JD. Perioperative respiratory management of pediatric patients with neuromuscular disease. *Paediatr Anaesth.* 2013;23(9):770–6.
10. Engel-Hoek L, Van AN, De Swart BJ et al. Quantitative ultrasound of the tongue and submental muscles in children and young adults. *Muscle Nerve.* 2012; 46(1):31–7.
11. Cabrera SM, Rabinstein AA. Causes and outcomes of acute neuromuscular respiratory failure. *Arch Neurol.* 2010;67(9):1089–94.
12. McCool FD, Tzelepis GE. Dysfunction of the diaphragm. *N Engl J Med.* 2012;366(10):932–42.
13. Podnar S. Nosology of idiopathic phrenic neuropathies. *J Neurol.* 2015;262(3):558–62.
14. Schoenhofer B, Koehler D, Polkey MI. Influence of immersion in water on muscle function and breathing pattern in patients with severe diaphragm weakness. *Chest.* 2004;125(6):2069–74.

15. Laghi F, Shaikh HS, Morales D et al. Diaphragmatic neuromechanical coupling and mechanisms of hypercapnia during inspiratory loading. *Respir Physiol Neurobiol.* 2014;198:32–41.
16. Bauman KA, Kurili A, Schmidt SL et al. Home-based overnight transcutaneous capnography/pulse oximetry for diagnosing nocturnal hypoventilation associated with neuromuscular disorders. *Arch Phys Med Rehabil.* 2013;94(1):46–52.
17. Bersanini C, Khirani S, Ramirez A et al. Nocturnal hypoxaemia and hypercapnia in children with neuromuscular disorders. *Eur Respir J.* 2012;39(5):1206–12.
18. Aboussouan LS. Sleep-disordered breathing in neuromuscular disease. *Am J Respir Crit Care Med.* 2015;191(9):979–89.
19. Brooks PL, Peever JH. Identification of the transmitter and receptor mechanisms responsible for REM sleep paralysis. *J Neurosci.* 2012;32(29):9785–95.
20. Ragette R, Mellies U, Schwake C et al. Patterns and predictors of sleep disordered breathing in primary myopathies. *Thorax.* 2002;57(8):724–8.
21. Esteban A, Anzueto A, Frutos F et al. Characteristics and outcomes in adult patients receiving mechanical ventilation: A 28-day international study. *JAMA.* 2002;287(3):345–55.
22. Jolley SE, Bunnell A, Hough CL. Intensive care unit acquired weakness. *Chest.* 2016;150:1129–40.
23. Petrof BJ, Hussain SN. Ventilator-induced diaphragmatic dysfunction: What have we learned? *Curr Opin Crit Care.* 2016;22(1):67–72.
24. Jaber S, Petrof BJ, Jung B et al. Rapidly progressive diaphragmatic weakness and injury during mechanical ventilation in humans. *Am J Respir Crit Care Med.* 2011;183(3):364–71.
25. Hooijman PE, Beishuizen A, Witt CC et al. Diaphragm muscle fiber weakness and ubiquitin-proteasome activation in critically ill patients. *Am J Respir Crit Care Med.* 2015;191(10):1126–38.
26. Laghi F, Sassoon CS. Weakness in critically ill: captain of the men of death or sign of disease severity? *Am J Respir Crit Care Med.* 2017;195:7–9.
27. Dres M, Dube BP, Mayaux J et al. Coexistence and impact of limb muscle and diaphragm weakness at time of liberation from mechanical ventilation in medical ICU patients. *Am J Respir Crit Care Med.* 2017;195:57–66.
28. Supinski GS, Westgate P, Callahan LA. Correlation of maximal inspiratory pressure to transdiaphragmatic twitch pressure in intensive care unit patients. *Crit Care.* 2016;20:77.
29. Laghi F, Cattapan SE, Jubran A et al. Is weaning failure caused by low-frequency fatigue of the diaphragm? *Am J Respir Crit Care Med.* 2003;167(2):120–7.
30. McNally EM, Goldstein JA. Interplay between heart and skeletal muscle disease in heart failure: The 2011 George E. Brown Memorial Lecture. *Circ Res.* 2012;110(5):749–54.
31. Estenne M, Gevenois PA, Kinnear W et al. Lung volume restriction in patients with chronic respiratory muscle weakness: The role of microatelectasis. *Thorax.* 1993;48(7):698–701.
32. Panitch HB. Respiratory issues in the management of children with neuromuscular disease. *Respir Care.* 2006;51(8):885–93.
33. Bourke SC, Tomlinson M, Williams TL et al. Effects of non-invasive ventilation on survival and quality of life in patients with amyotrophic lateral sclerosis: A randomised controlled trial. *Lancet Neurol.* 2006;5(2):140–7.
34. Uldry C, Fitting JW. Maximal values of sniff nasal inspiratory pressure in healthy subjects. *Thorax.* 1995;50(4):371–5.
35. Laghi F, D'Alfonso N, Tobin MJ. A paper on the pace of recovery from diaphragmatic fatigue and its unexpected dividends. *Intensive Care Med.* 2014;40(9):1220–6.
36. Cattapan SE, Laghi F, Tobin MJ. Can diaphragmatic contractility be assessed by airway twitch pressure in mechanically ventilated patients? *Thorax.* 2003;58(1):58–62.
37. Watson AC, Hughes PD, Louise HM et al. Measurement of twitch transdiaphragmatic, esophageal, and endotracheal tube pressure with bilateral anterolateral magnetic phrenic nerve stimulation in patients in the intensive care unit. *Crit Care Med.* 2001;29(7):1325–31.
38. Tobin MJ, Laghi F. Monitoring respiratory muscle function. In: Tobin MJ, editor. *Principles and Practice of Intensive Care Monitoring.* 1st edition. New York: McGraw-Hill Co., 1998:497–544.
39. Polkey MI, Kyroussis D, Hamnegard CH et al. Diaphragm strength in chronic obstructive pulmonary disease. *Am J Respir Crit Care Med.* 1996;154(5):1310–7.
40. Laghi F, Jubran A, Topeli A et al. Effect of lung volume reduction surgery on diaphragmatic neuromechanical coupling at 2 years. *Chest.* 2004;125(6):2188–95.
41. Matamis D, Soilemezi E, Tsagourias M et al. Sonographic evaluation of the diaphragm in critically ill patients. Technique and clinical applications. *Intensive Care Med.* 2013;39(5):801–10.
42. Goligher EC, Laghi F, Detsky ME et al. Measuring diaphragm thickness with ultrasound in mechanically ventilated patients: Feasibility, reproducibility and validity. *Intensive Care Med.* 2015;41(4):642–9.

43. Zambon M, Beccaria P, Matsuno J et al. Mechanical ventilation and diaphragmatic atrophy in critically ill patients: An ultrasound study. *Crit Care Med.* 2016;44(7):1347–52.
44. Zambon M, Greco M, Bocchino S et al. Assessment of diaphragmatic dysfunction in the critically ill patient with ultrasound: A systematic review. *Intensive Care Med.* 2017;43:29–38.
45. Gottesman E, McCool FD. Ultrasound evaluation of the paralyzed diaphragm. *Am J Respir Crit Care Med.* 1997;155(5):1570–4.
46. Goligher EC, Fan E, Herridge MS et al. Evolution of diaphragm thickness during mechanical ventilation. Impact of inspiratory effort. *Am J Respir Crit Care Med.* 2015;192(9):1080–8.
47. Man WD, Moxham J, Polkey MI. Magnetic stimulation for the measurement of respiratory and skeletal muscle function. *Eur Respir J.* 2004;24(5):846–60.
48. Kyroussis D, Mills GH, Polkey MI et al. Abdominal muscle fatigue after maximal ventilation in humans. *J Appl Physiol.* 1996;81(4):1477–83.
49. Polkey MI, Lyall RA, Green M et al. Expiratory muscle function in amyotrophic lateral sclerosis. *Am J Respir Crit Care Med.* 1998;158(3):734–41.
50. Ward K, Seymour J, Steier J et al. Acute ischaemic hemispheric stroke is associated with impairment of reflex in addition to voluntary cough. *Eur Respir J.* 2010;36(6):1383–90.
51. O'Donohue WJ, Jr., Baker JP, Bell GM et al. Respiratory failure in neuromuscular disease. Management in a respiratory intensive care unit. *JAMA.* 1976;235(7):733–35.
52. Man WD, Kyroussis D, Fleming TA et al. Cough gastric pressure and maximum expiratory mouth pressure in humans. *Am J Respir Crit Care Med.* 2003;168(6):714–7.
53. Chetta A, Harris ML, Lyall RA et al. Whistle mouth pressure as test of expiratory muscle strength. *Eur Respir J.* 2001;17(4):688–95.
54. Fregonezi G, Azevedo IG, Resqueti VR et al. Muscle impairment in neuromuscular disease using an expiratory/inspiratory pressure ratio. *Respir Care.* 2015;60(4):533–9.
55. Miller RG, Jackson CE, Kasarskis EJ et al. Practice parameter update: The care of the patient with amyotrophic lateral sclerosis: Drug, nutritional, and respiratory therapies (an evidence-based review): Report of the Quality Standards Subcommittee of the American Academy of Neurology. *Neurology.* 2009;73(15):1218–26.
56. Berry RB, Chediak A, Brown LK et al. Best clinical practices for the sleep center adjustment of noninvasive positive pressure ventilation (NPPV) in stable chronic alveolar hypoventilation syndromes. *J Clin Sleep Med.* 2010;6(5):491–509.
57. Bourke SC, Shaw PJ, Gibson GJ. Respiratory function vs sleep-disordered breathing as predictors of QOL in ALS. *Neurology.* 2001;57(11):2040–4.
58. Lyall RA, Donaldson N, Polkey MI et al. Respiratory muscle strength and ventilatory failure in amyotrophic lateral sclerosis. *Brain.* 2001;124(Pt 10):2000–13.
59. Vitacca M, Clini E, Facchetti D et al. Breathing pattern and respiratory mechanics in patients with amyotrophic lateral sclerosis. *Eur Respir J.* 1997;10(7):1614–21.
60. Stambler N, Charatan M, Cedarbaum JM. Prognostic indicators of survival in ALS. ALS CNTF Treatment Study Group. *Neurology.* 1998;50(1):66–72.
61. Cabrera SM, Rabinstein AA. Usefulness of pulmonary function tests and blood gases in acute neuromuscular respiratory failure. *Eur J Neurol.* 2012;19(3):452–6.
62. Nardi J, Prigent H, Adala A et al. Nocturnal oximetry and transcutaneous carbon dioxide in home-ventilated neuromuscular patients. *Respir Care.* 2012;57(9):1425–30.
63. Paiva R, Krivec U, Aubertin G et al. Carbon dioxide monitoring during long-term noninvasive respiratory support in children. *Intensive Care Med.* 2009;35(6):1068–74.
64. Ogna A, Nardi J, Prigent H et al. Prognostic value of initial assessment of residual hypoventilation using nocturnal capnography in mechanically ventilated neuromuscular patients: A 5-year follow-up study. *Front Med (Lausanne).* 2016;3:40.

40

Slowly progressive neuromuscular diseases

VIKRAM A. PADMANABHAN AND JOSHUA O. BENDITT

INTRODUCTION

A wide variety of neuromuscular disorders can result in progressive dysfunction of the ventilatory muscles that can result in respiratory failure, pneumonia and even death. Breathing disorders are recognised as the leading cause of mortality in neuromuscular disease.[1] Neuromuscular disease can affect any part of the neurologic system, from the central nervous system to the peripheral nervous system as well as the muscles, leading to impairment of respiratory system function. In this chapter, we will focus on a number of different conditions that affect the respiratory system in a slowly progressive manner. We will review the pathophysiology and data pertinent to respiratory function if available.

As respiratory dysfunction is the leading cause of morbidity and death in this population, respiratory interventions can be instituted to prevent complications and prolong life in individuals with neuromuscular disease.[2,3] Thus, we have found it very useful to take a 'respiratory care'-centred approach to the patient with respiratory muscle weakness from any cause.[4] We and others[4–6] have divided the respiratory system into three main areas of potential dysfunction (Figure 40.1):

1. Ventilatory function determined predominantly by the inspiratory muscles
2. Swallowing and airway protection determined by glottic muscles
3. Cough function determined by inspiratory, expiratory and glottic function[7]

With respiratory therapist assistance, simple testing can be performed at each clinic visit. This systematic and objective approach can ensure that no potential problems are missed and progression of respiratory dysfunction is followed (Table 40.1). Specific therapies for ventilatory failure, cough insufficiency and swallowing issues can be employed and are detailed in other chapters.

SPECIFIC DISEASES

Although there are a large number of neurologic diseases that can affect the respiratory system, we will focus on the following disease processes during the rest of the chapter in large part because not a great deal of data is available on respiratory issues pertaining to many of the disorders. General principles of management are, fortunately, similar for all neuromuscular disorders affecting the respiratory system.

- Spinal muscular atrophy
- Myasthenia gravis
- Post-polio syndrome
- Myotonic dystrophy
- Glycogen storage disease
- Congenital myopathies
- Mitochondrial myopathy

SPINAL MUSCULAR ATROPHY

Definition and pathophysiology

Spinal muscular atrophy (SMA) is the leading genetic cause of infant death. SMA is an autosomal recessive disease that results from a defect in the survival motor neuron 1 (SMN1) gene. The incidence of SMA is about 1 in 10,000 live births[8] and has a carrier frequency of 1 in 50.[9,10] Genetic testing can now diagnose about 95% of the patients.[11] The defective gene results in degeneration of motor neurons in the spinal cord, which results in hypotonia ('floppy baby'), muscle weakness and wasting of voluntary muscles. The weakness is proximal and lower extremity predominant. Tongue fasciculations and bulbar muscle involvement can occur, particularly in SMA Type 1. Depending on the severity of disease and age of presentation, SMA has been divided into four categories, SMA 1–4. Treatment is centred on supportive care and respiratory support; however, there has been recent excitement with the possibility of SMN gene therapy.[10]

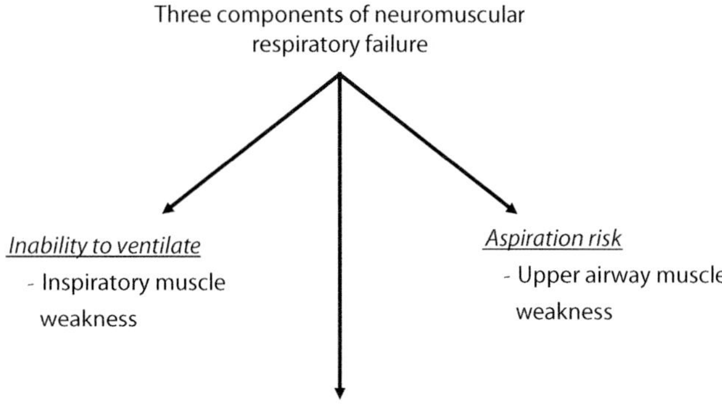

Figure 40.1 The three components of neuromuscular respiratory failure.

Table 40.1 Potential clinic measures for respiratory system function

Ventilatory Function
• Vital capacity
• Maximal inspiratory pressure
• Sniff nasal inspiratory pressure
• CO_2
• End-tidal
• Arterial
• Transcutaneous
• Cough function
• Peak cough expiratory flow
• Maximal expiratory pressure
• Swallowing function
• Historical data
• Observed barium study
• Endoscopic evaluation

SMA Type 1 (Werdnig–Hoffman) is the most common (50%) and severe presentation of the disease.[12] Diagnosed within the first 6 months of life, individuals have profound hypotonia, weak cry and weak neck flexors. Respiratory failure and death occurs within 2 years if respiratory interventions such as non-invasive or invasive ventilation are not employed.[11]

SMA Type 2, or intermediate SMA, is diagnosed between ages 6 and 18 months of age. Individuals are able to sit but not stand unsupported. The phenotypic presentation is less severe and individuals can survive into the third decade of life and beyond, sometimes without respiratory intervention.[11]

SMA Type 3 (Kugelberg–Welander disease) presents at or after 18 months of age. Individuals have an abnormal gait but a normal life expectancy. Adult-onset SMA has been labelled SMA Type 4 and includes a very mild disease that rarely requires respiratory intervention (often diagnosed incidentally after post-operative respiratory failure).[13,14]

Respiratory clinical issues

In this discussion, we will focus on SMA Types 1 and 2 as the most severe respiratory impairment occurs there. The diaphragm is relatively spared in comparison to the intercostal muscles, which results in paradoxical movement of the chest wall during respiration, with inward movement of the rib cage and outward movement of the diaphragm. The chest wall in the first year of life is compliant, which results in the development of a bell-shaped configuration of the chest wall with pectus excavatum that results from this muscular imbalance.

The physiologic result of this chest wall and muscle problem is as follows:

1. Chest wall and lung underdevelopment
2. Impaired cough resulting in poor clearance of lower airway secretions
3. Recurrent infections that can exacerbate muscle weakness
4. Hypoventilation during sleep[14]

Without respiratory intervention, there is a progression of respiratory failure beginning with the aforementioned anatomic changes that often lead to recurrent respiratory infections, nocturnal hypoventilation and ultimately full-time respiratory failure and death if untreated.[15,16]

A Consensus Statement for Standard of Care in Spinal Muscular Atrophy has been developed to aid in standardizing clinical care and also to make uniform study protocols.[14] With selected prenatal screening, SMA Types 1 and 2 have exciting therapeutic possibilities that must be delivered early such as gene therapy; however, these therapies are not generally available at this time. The Italian SMA Family Association has published management recommendations for the respiratory involvement with SMA.[10]

Respiratory management

Respiratory assessment for SMA is recommended according to the severity of the disease, starting with SMA Type 1 ('non-sitters'). Formal measurement of pulmonary function including vital capacity, maximal inspiratory and maximal expiratory pressures may be impossible; thus, the most useful evaluation of overall respiratory function may be that of direct visualisation of cough function and airway clearance. Evaluation should include observation of breathing, observation of cough function and evaluation of gas exchange that includes measurement of pulse oximetry, and CO_2 evaluation via end-tidal or transcutaneous methods.[14] The physical exam alone can provide very valuable information as to the requirement for airway clearance, which is the area of greatest weakness for those with SMA. Elevated respiratory rate, cyanosis or pallor, paradoxical breathing and/or intercostal muscle retractions may be indicators of respiratory insufficiency. A pulse oximetry reading of 94% or less suggests that augmentative airway clearance efforts should be undertaken. Overnight chart recording of pulse oximetry can be helpful in identifying sleep-disordered breathing. It was also suggested that end-tidal and transcutaneous CO_2 monitoring as well as home sleep monitoring may be helpful in assessing sleep-disordered breathing, but their utility has not been studied, and if doubt exists, a full polysomnogram should be obtained to look for treatable sleep-disordered breathing. If recurrent respiratory infections are noted despite adequate cough therapy, then a swallowing assessment should be undertaken. A baseline chest x-ray was suggested for comparison during the likely occurrence of an infection. It is suggested that formal clinic evaluation occurs every 3 to 6 months, more frequently warranted by symptoms at home.[17]

For SMA Type 2 ('sitters'), respiratory evaluation should continue to focus on the physical examination. As these patients can participate with pulmonary function tests, formal pulmonary function testing can be obtained. Formal evaluation for kyphoscoliosis should be obtained as this is a potentially treatable condition. If vital capacity can be obtained reliably, this can be followed serially (those with FVC > 60% predicted are at very low risk for nocturnal hypoventilation, whereas those with FVC < 50% predicted have high rates of pulmonary complications).

Bilevel ventilation may not be sufficient to provide adequate ventilatory support and/or mobility and, hence, mouthpiece ventilation can be considered.[18]

For those who are able to walk (SMA Types 3 and 4), physical exam continues to be important but greater emphasis falls on routine pulmonary function evaluation, which can be obtained more easily due to greater cooperation with greater age. Other evaluation should be directed by clinical symptoms and indications. As it is highly prevalent in this population, there should be a low threshold for obtaining a diagnostic polysomnogram to assess for sleep-disordered breathing.[17]

Airway clearance is of critical importance. A variety of interventions are available including chest physiotherapy, postural drainage and mechanically assisted cough devices such as the mechanical insufflator–exsufflator (MIE) (CoughAssist; Respironics, Murrysville, Pennsylvania). This can be required up to every few hours or more during an acute episode and is suggested on a daily basis in more severely affected individuals. A home-based protocol (MIE, followed by chest percussion, followed by postural drainage and MIE) has been developed and resulted in decreased incidence of respiratory infections and hospitalisations.[11] Those with SMA Types 3 and 4 rarely need cough assistance, most often following operative intervention or significant respiratory illness only.

The individual with SMA Type 1 may need immediate ventilatory support in the neonatal period. It is now possible with small paediatric interfaces to initiate non-invasive positive pressure ventilation (NPPV).

The benefits for NPPV for children with SMA Type 1 include the potential for ventilatory support without a surgical intervention,[19] amelioration of the chest wall deformity and improvement in lung development[20,21] and potentially lung function. The long-term goals for NPPV in SMA, as in other neuromuscular diseases, are amelioration of sleep quality, quality of life and avoidance of surgical interventions.[22] Complications of NPPV include those related to prolonged use (>16 hours/day) including skin irritation and breakdown and distortion of the midface (midface hypoplasia).[23] Gastric distention and emesis can also occur if gas insufflates the stomach, resulting in aspiration, pneumonia and possibly death.[11] As NPPV is not always effective, the options of invasive (tracheostomy) ventilation versus palliative care need to be discussed with each family individually and carefully, particularly for those individuals with SMA Type 1.

Invasive ventilation is generally not required chronically for SMA Type 2,[24] although for both SMA Type 2 and SMA Type 1, an acute lower respiratory tract infection can lead to a situation where non-invasive methodologies are unsuccessful. Intubation until improvement in secretion management and oxygenation occurs can provide a bridge to further non-invasive management.

Patients with SMA Types 3 and 4 rarely need non-invasive ventilatory support, other than in instances of perioperative care or if they develop sleep apnoea with ageing.[11]

Patients with SMA Types 1 and 2 are at risk of respiratory complications during any procedure requiring anaesthesia. Thus, a multidisciplinary team including a pulmonologist, respiratory therapist, rehabilitation medicine specialist and nutritionist should be employed in the pre- and post-operative period (Figure 40.2). Less invasive procedures, if at all possible (use of conscious sedation with NPPV rather than general anaesthesia and mechanical ventilation), should be considered.

MYASTHENIA GRAVIS

Pathophysiology

Although myasthenia gravis (MG) is not necessarily a progressive disease, we have included it here because it is the most common disease affecting neuromuscular junction transmission. MG is an autoimmune disease characterised by a post-synaptic antibody-mediated immune attack directed at acetylcholine receptors and/or receptor-associated proteins in the postsynaptic membrane of the neuromuscular junction. It causes weakness of many muscle groups including the respiratory, ocular and bulbar muscles. The Osserman classification is commonly used to functionally and regionally grade MG (Table 40.2). The respiratory muscles are particularly susceptible to fatigue during the severe, potentially life-threatening exacerbations known as myasthenic crises. Acute treatment of myasthenic crisis focuses on rapid initiation of immunomodulatory therapies including intravenous immunoglobulin (IVIG),

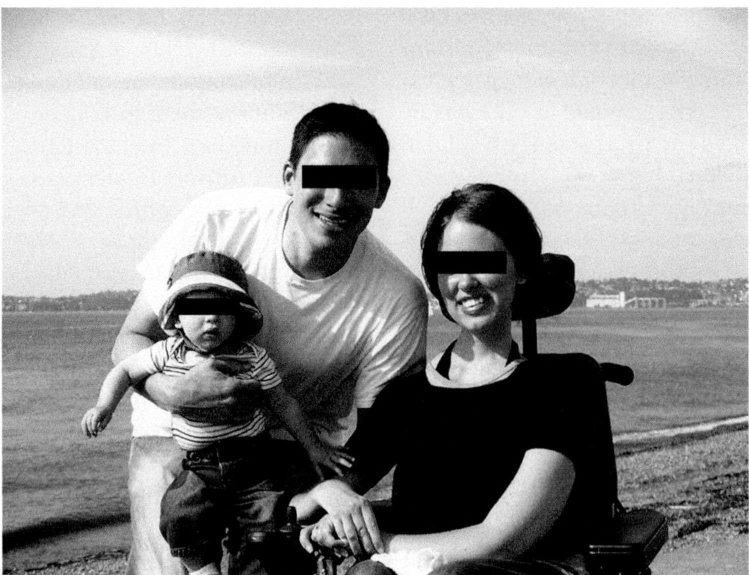

Figure 40.2 Female patient with spinal muscular atrophy type 2, who successfully completed a pregnancy and delivered a healthy infant with non-invasive ventilatory support.

Table 40.2 Osserman classification in myasthenia gravis

0	Asymptomatic
1	Ocular signs and symptoms – focal disease
2	Mild generalised weakness– subclassified as mild (IIa) or moderate (IIb)
3	Moderate generalised weakness, bulbar dysfunction, or both
4	Severe generalised weakness, respiratory dysfunction, or both

plasmapheresis and corticosteroid therapy.[25,26] As previously discussed, a 'respiratory care'-centred approach allows support of the patient, allowing time for therapy of the underlying myasthenia to be effective.

About 20% of MG patients are found to have a thymoma and, thus, all patients with newly diagnosed MG require a chest CT. Removal of the thymoma may result in amelioration of the myasthenia symptoms.

Respiratory clinical issues

Respiratory insufficiency can result from bulbar, inspiratory and inspiratory muscle weakness. Upper airway compromise can lead to aspiration and dysphagia. Loss of upper airway tone can lead to obstruction and loss of adequate ventilation. Weakness of inspiratory muscles can lead to hypoventilation, atelectasis and hypoxaemia. Finally, expiratory muscle weakness can lead to poor cough function. Thus, the decision to intubate for ventilatory insufficiency and inability to protect the airway is vital. In myasthenic crisis, absolute indications for intubation include cardiac or respiratory arrest, altered mental status, shock, arrhythmias, blood–gas alterations and bulbar dysfunction with confirmed aspiration. Much more difficult is the decision to intubate when such strict criteria are not met. Objective criteria have been proposed for elective intubation in myasthenic crisis. These include a vital capacity of less than <15 mL/kg ideal body weight; a maximal inspiratory pressure <30 cmH_2O and maximal expiratory pressure <40 cmH_2O have also been used. Physical examination signs to assess for include rapid shallow breathing, tachycardia, weak cough, staccato speech, accessory muscle use, abdominal muscle paradox and cough after swallowing.[23] A very high index of suspicion must be maintained and early rather than late intervention is certainly preferable. As above, prompt institution of immunomodulatory therapy is critical and is discussed in detail in the Association of British Neurologist's MG management guidelines.[27]

Respiratory management

In carefully selected patients, NPPV can be employed during a myasthenic crisis. Seneviratne et al.[28] studied 60 episodes of myasthenic crisis retrospectively in 52 patients. Bilevel ventilation was the initial method of ventilatory support in 24 episodes, and endotracheal intubation was performed in 36 episodes. In 14 episodes treated using BiPAP, intubation was avoided. The mean duration of BiPAP in these patients was 4.3 days. The only predictor of BiPAP failure (i.e. requirement for intubation) was a $PaCO_2$ level exceeding 45 mmHg on BiPAP initiation ($p = 0.04$). There were no differences in patient demographics or in baseline respiratory variables and arterial gases between the groups of episodes initially treated using NPPV versus endotracheal intubation. The mean ventilation duration was 10.4 days. The intensive care unit and hospital lengths of stay statistically significantly increased with ventilation duration ($p < 0.001$ for both). The only variable associated with decreased ventilation was the initial use of NPPV. In the patient with bulbar involvement, extra care should be employed when using NPPV, as there is a risk of aspiration.

POST-POLIO SYNDROME (PPS)

Definition and pathophysiology

In the developed world, acute poliomyelitis has essentially been eradicated. The ravages of this disease can resurface in patients with a distant history of acute poliomyelitis. The post-polio syndrome is defined as new weakness, which has developed in survivors of the polio epidemics of the mid-twentieth century.[25,26] Generally accepted criteria for the PPS include the following:

1. Confirmed history of polio
2. Partial or near-complete recovery after acute episode
3. Period of 15 or more years of neurologic and function stability
4. Onset of new neurogenic weakness
5. Two or more of the following symptoms: fatigue, new muscle or joint pain, muscle atrophy, new weakness in previously unaffected muscles, functional loss or cold intolerance
6. No other medical explanation found[29]

The prevalence of PPS is unknown and will vary greatly depending on the criteria used to define the syndrome. If patients are asked whether they have a new symptom related to previous polio, prevalence is reported at 50% or higher.[30] If new onset weakness is included as an identifying criterion, the prevalence may drop to as low as 20%–30% of overall polio survivors. The prevalence of PPS worldwide has been reported to occur from between 15% and 80% of individuals surveyed.[31] Most recently, an Italian case-control study revealed that about 42% of acute poliomyelitis survivors developed PPS, assessed by the European diagnostic criteria. Risks associated with the development of PPS included female gender, presence of respiratory disturbance at the onset of acute poliomyelitis and use of orthoses during the recovery period.[32]

There is no known treatment of PPS, except for supportive care, some of which is discussed below. Supportive respiratory care, as discussed below, and orthoses are paramount. Prednisone, amantadine, coenzyme Q and pyridostigmine have all been tried to no avail.[33] A recent Cochrane review revealed lamotrigine, IVIG and muscle strength training as interventions that may hold promise but require further rigorous investigation.[34]

Electromyography may be of assistance in assessing individuals with suspected post-polio syndrome in (1) showing the typical lower motor neuron involvement, (2) assessing the extent of neuronal involvement, (3) excluding other causes of new weakness such as entrapment syndromes and (4) assessing other possible concomitant neuromuscular disease.[29] It should be noted that EMG cannot differentiate findings related to the original polio injury from PPS.

Muscle biopsy is probably not useful in the evaluation of PPS as the findings are non-specific and can be seen in patients with both the absence and presence of findings of new weakness in a particular muscle group.[35]

Clinical respiratory issues

Reduced pulmonary function due to respiratory muscle weakness and chest wall deformity can occur in patients with PPS.[36] In one of the earlier and larger studies of pulmonary function in patients with PPS, Dean et al.[37] performed a cross-sectional study of 74 patients with a distant history of polio. These were subjects recruited by advertisement and were not using any respiratory aids. There was a fairly wide spread of normal and abnormal vital capacity, with the most striking finding a very significant reduction in maximal expiratory pressure. Factors associated with a decrease in pulmonary function included ventilator support at the onset of polio and age of onset of polio between ages 10 and 35.

In addition, in those individuals with shortness of breath present, pulmonary function tended to be lower. The authors suggested all patients with a history of polio, particularly with ventilatory support at the time of initial presentation and onset after age 10, should undergo careful screening for late respiratory effects of polio (neuromuscular pulmonary function tests, peak cough flow assessment, end-tidal CO_2 measurement, diagnostic polysomnogram and consultation with a neuromuscular neurologist to rule out other neurologic disorders).

Respiratory management

Individuals with PPS or a history of polio have a high incidence of sleep-disordered breathing.[38,39] Low forced vital capacity, chest wall restriction, ventilatory support during the initial bout of polio and current symptoms of sleep-disordered breathing such as daytime hypersomnolence and morning headaches are all predictors for likely sleep-disordered breathing. A high index of suspicion should be maintained when evaluating these individuals and, thus, there should be a low threshold to obtaining a diagnostic polysomnogram.

Diurnal ventilatory insufficiency will be present in some individuals with polio (either from the time of the original polio infection or due to PPS) such that full-time ventilation is required. Frank ventilatory failure can be triggered by a respiratory tract infection that results in increased work of breathing and an inability to maintain adequate blood gas homeostasis. In the modern era, a number of methodologies have been employed including tracheostomy ventilation, full-time mask ventilation, and mouthpiece ventilation (Figure 40.3). It is quite possible to support individuals with late-onset effects of polio with non-invasive methodologies.

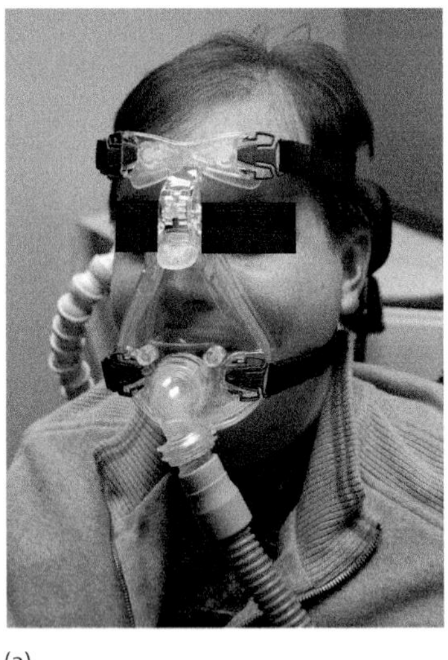
(a)

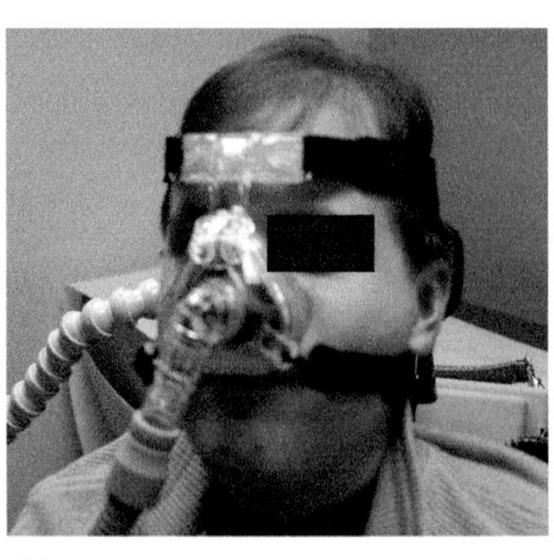
(b)

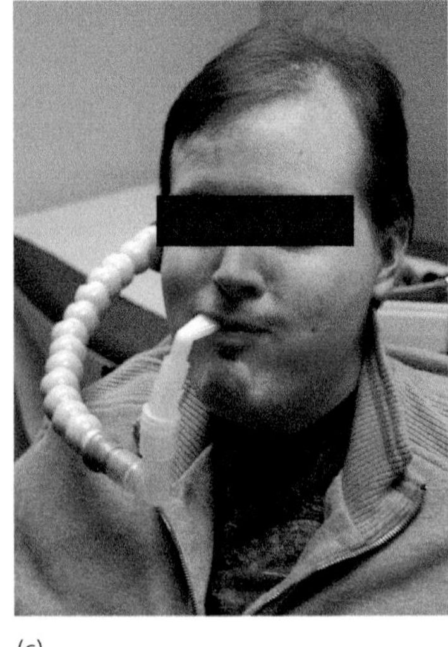
(c)

Figure 40.3 Typical interfaces for non-invasive ventilation. **(a)** Full facemask. **(b)** Nasal mask. **(c)** Mouthpiece interface for daytime ventilation.

MYOTONIC DYSTROPHY

Definition and pathophysiology

Myotonic dystrophy (MD) is the most frequently inherited neuromuscular disease with an estimated frequency worldwide of 2.1 to 14.3 in 100,000 births.[40] MD is an autosomal dominant disorder that is genetically heterogeneous with variable phenotypic expression. There are two major classifications including DM1, formerly known as Steinert's disease, and DM2, a milder disease form. In addition to neuromuscular weakness, MD is associated with cardiac conduction abnormalities, cataracts, infertility, insulin resistance, developmental delay, hypersomnolence and a unique avoidant personality.[41] Based on the age of clinical onset, DM1 can be classified as congenital, classical or minimal. Congenital DM1 presents at birth or within the first year of life as a severe form. In the classical form, the most common type, symptoms develop between the second and fourth decade with slow progression over time. Minimal DM1 is characterised by the development of mild symptoms after 50 years of age. DM2 is an adult-onset disease.

The biochemical basis for the systemic effects of MD is the unstable expansion of the DNA trinucleotide CTG.[36] The number of trinucleotide repeats is proportional to the severity of disease and inversely proportional to the age of onset.[42] The cause of muscle weakness and wasting is not yet known. A characteristic phenotypic feature of skeletal muscle weakness is facial muscle weakness in DM1, which is mild and occurs later in DM2. Oropharyngeal muscle weakness can result in dysphagia and dysarthria. Limb weakness is associated with weakness of the thigh, hip flexor and extensor muscles. Inability to release hand grip from a handshake is a classic myotonic phenomena. Cardiac abnormalities include both conduction disturbances and structural defects. Cardiac complications are the most common cause of death.[43,44]

In the adult patient, treatment is primarily supportive. However, in a mouse model, a genome editing technology was used to correct the dystophin gene in the germ line of DM mice. Phenotypic rescue was seen in most mice. Although far from clinical reality, this technology shows promise for a viable treatment for MD.[45,46]

Respiratory clinical issues

Respiratory muscle weakness is common in DM1, resulting in variable restrictive pulmonary impairment and alveolar hypoventilation. Increased trinucleotide repeats (CTG) has been associated with earlier onset of ventilator failure.[47] In congenital DM1, infants develop respiratory failure requiring continuous ventilation within the first year of life. Infants who survive the first year can develop improved motor function but are at a higher risk for cardiorespiratory mortality. In the classical form of DM1, restrictive pulmonary impairment can be mild to moderate, requiring nocturnal ventilatory support. Rarely, continuous ventilation is required in DM1. Oropharyngeal muscle weakness can result in dysphagia, aspiration and obstructive sleep apnoea. Sleep-disordered breathing and nocturnal hypoxaemia are common in MD. The severity of nocturnal hypoxaemia has been associated with the degree of obesity. Daytime hypercapnoea has also been observed and worsens with sleep. Polysomnography studies of MD patients with daytime hypersomnolence have identified both obstructive and central sleep apnoea. In one study, the majority of patients showed periodic breathing patterns indicating a central auto-regulatory dysfunction. Interestingly, this is likely attributable to a deficiency in orexin, a signaling protein in the hypothalamus that mediates sleepiness.[48] The incidence of sudden death in MD is associated with ventricular arrhythmias, and nocturnal hypoxaemia secondary to sleep-disordered breathing is a significant risk factor for cardiac arrhythmia.

Respiratory clinical management

Serial pulmonary function testing to assess respiratory muscle strength is recommended in patients with MD. Vital capacity testing and static mouth pressure testing have been commonly used to assess neuromuscular respiratory function.[49] The predominance of sleep-disordered breathing in this population should prompt the clinician to screen the patient for symptoms of sleep-disordered breathing.[50,51] Periodic evaluation using nocturnal oximetry studies can identify the need for polysomnography before the onset of overt symptoms. Polysomnography reveals upper airway obstructions and resultant apnoeas, central sleep apnoea, and hypoventilation. Transcutaneous CO_2 monitoring during polysomnography is recommended.[52,53] Most patients will have a combined obstructive and central sleep-disordered breathing affected by restrictive pulmonary impairment. These patients will require non-invasive bilevel pressure support ventilation with a spontaneous/timed backup rate to adequately support nocturnal ventilation. Nocturnal bilevel pressure ventilation has been associated with sustained improved ventilation and with improved survival.[54,55] Bilevel pressure titration with polysomnography monitoring may be necessary to determine the most supportive pressure regimen for nocturnal ventilation. Persistent hypersomnolence may remain unchanged despite compliance with nocturnal bilevel ventilation given the orexin deficiency and resultant maladaptive hypothalamic sleep drive.[56] Respiratory muscle aids including cough augmentation therapy may also be required for patients with weak cough strength secondary to restrictive pulmonary impairment. Peak expiratory cough flow, a measure of cough strength, should be done to serially evaluate cough effectiveness. MIE can be used to support cough clearance in myotonic patients with inadequate cough strength. Myotonic patients with severe oropharyngeal muscle weakness may develop chronic upper airway airflow restriction, aspiration or difficulty with NPPV tolerance. A tracheostomy may be indicated in order to better support these patients when aspiration is present or NPPV is not tolerated.

NPPV has been associated with improved survival; however, there are limitations in the use of this therapy due to the characteristic facial muscle weakness in this patient population. This limits the ability to successfully apply positive pressure mask ventilation. Cognitive impairment and the characteristic avoidant or laissez-faire personality have also been associated with a significant limitation in the patient's compliance to the nightly use of positive pressure mask ventilation.[57]

GLYCOGEN STORAGE DISEASE

Definition and pathophysiology

Glycogen is the stored form of glucose reserves that provides an energy substrate during periods of high energy expenditure or when glucose availability is low. Disorders that result in the abnormal storage of glycogen are identified as glycogen storage diseases. There are a number of genetic mutations in the synthesis of proteins involved in glycogen synthesis, degradation and regulation that can result in the abnormal storage of glycogen.[58] Glycogen storage diseases commonly manifest as muscle atrophy, muscle cramps, exercise intolerance, fatigue and progressive muscle weakness. A number of glycogen metabolism defects that result in the abnormal storage of glycogen have been classified. Lysosomal acid maltase deficiency, or Pompe disease, is the most common glycogen storage disease type that has been found to affect respiratory function the most. The incidence of Pompe disease is estimated to be between 1 in 40,000 and 1 in 600,000 depending on geographic and ethnic factors. Pompe disease has been classified as infantile, juvenile and adult forms depending on the age of onset. Infants are severely affected with cardiomegaly, hepatosplenomegaly, mental retardation and severe myopathy and generally do not survive past the age of 2 as a result of hypertrophic cardiomyopathy.[59] The childhood and adult forms are milder with slower progression. In these forms, skeletal muscle weakness is the primary symptom with progressive proximal weakness in the limb-girdle distribution.[60] Respiratory muscle weakness occurs in both forms, and in adults, respiratory insufficiency can be the first sign.

Pompe disease is an autosomal recessive disorder that results from a deficiency of the glycogen degrading lysosomal enzyme acid alpha-glucosidase (GAA). Symptom expression and disease severity are dependent on the amount of residual GAA activity.[61]

Respiratory issues

Unlike most other neuromuscular diseases where limb weakness usually occurs before respiratory involvement, respiratory insufficiency can be one of the first indications of the disease.[62,63] Diaphragmatic weakness is the predominant contributing factor, and weakness in the inspiratory muscles of the chest can also contribute to respiratory insufficiency.[61] Upper airway weakness can also contribute to sleep-disordered breathing and can be either independent of or more affected by inspiratory muscle weakness.[64] Chronic nocturnal hypoventilation can produce symptoms of hypercarbia including restlessness, frequent awakenings, nocturia, vivid nightmares, morning headaches and poor sleep quality. Progressive inspiratory muscle weakness can also affect cough strength by limiting the inspiratory volume necessary to produce an adequate peak expiratory cough flow in order to clear pulmonary secretions. In Pompe disease where respiratory involvement is often the primary limitation, outward symptoms may not be apparent to the clinician.[65] Acute respiratory failure, which is a common presentation, is most often precipitated by aspiration or acute respiratory infection in the face of cough insufficiency and hypoventilation.[61,64]

Respiratory clinical management

Patients who are diagnosed with Pompe disease before an acute respiratory event should be immediately referred for a neuromuscular respiratory assessment to evaluate their respiratory status and thereafter undergo serial respiratory assessment to monitor their respiratory status.[64,66,67] Upright and supine FVC spirometry and maximum inspiratory and expiratory pressure testing should be done to determine the degree of diaphragmatic weakness and global respiratory muscle weakness.[68] Peak cough flow testing should also be done to assess cough strength.[69] Diaphragmatic and upper airway muscle weakness should prompt the clinician to screen for symptoms of sleep-disordered breathing and a referral for diagnostic polysomnography testing should be made for any indication of symptoms.[61] NPPV has been shown to support nocturnal ventilation and improve the longevity of Pompe patients.[64,70] A spontaneous/timed mode of bilevel pressure support is necessary to support severe diaphragmatic limited ventilation during REM sleep. Cough insufficiency may be augmented by either manual or mechanical cough augmentation.[71] Manual hyperinflation combined with abdominal thrust has been shown to augment limited cough strength. MIE has also been shown to augment cough in patients who do not experience significant bulbar symptoms.

Anticipatory respiratory care should be practiced as progressive weakness will lead to respiratory failure. Premature death can occur when the eventual need for bilevel ventilation or mouthpiece ventilation is not adequately anticipated and discussed with the patient and their family.[72] Alglucosidase alpha enzyme replacement therapy is available and has efficacy data for the juvenile/adult form. Enzyme replacement therapy has shown preservation and reversal of cardiac muscle damage, improved overall survival and vital capacity preservation. Gene therapy is currently actively being investigated.[73]

CONGENITAL MYOPATHIES

Congenital myopathies are muscle disorders that are caused by genetic abnormalities of muscle development.[74] These disorders are present at birth, though symptoms may not develop until later in infancy or childhood, and in rare cases in adults. The most common disorders with respiratory involvement include nemaline myopathy, centronuclear (myotubular) myopathy and multicore myopathy. Congenital myopathies share many clinical features including hypotonia, primarily proximal muscle weakness, decreased tendon reflexes and skeletal deformities associated with developmental muscle weakness. Pathologic examination of muscle biopsy allows distinction among the congenital myopathies, although, when suspected, genetic testing can confirm the diagnosis as well. Recently, the American Academy of Neurology has published guidelines for the management of congenital myopathies, focused on the multidisciplinary, anticipatory care of the patient.[75]

NEMALINE MYOPATHY

Definition and pathophysiology

Nemaline myopathy is characterised by threadlike bodies in the longitudinal sections of muscle tissue. This disease has been classified into three forms based on the onset of clinical presentation including mild to severe infantile, moderate congenital (classic) and adult-onset forms.[76] In the severe infantile form, there is severe generalised weakness and hyptonia of the facial, bulbar and respiratory muscles.[77] In the milder infantile, congenital and adult forms, symptoms are less severe and progressive. Nemaline myopathy results from mutations in genes encoding for several different protein components in the thin filaments of skeletal muscle.[78]

Respiratory clinical issues

In the severe infantile disease form, marked respiratory muscle weakness and bulbar dysfunction generally result in respiratory failure and death within the first year, although prolonged survival with improvement has been reported.[79] In the milder congenital and adult forms, diaphragmatic weakness appears to be the primary restrictive respiratory limitation. In addition, nemaline myopathy has also been associated with impairment of the central respiratory drive during REM sleep.[80] A discrepancy between the rate of deterioration in motor function and the development of respiratory impairment has also been reported.[81,82]

CENTRONUCLEAR (MYOTUBULAR) MYOPATHY

Definition

Centronuclear myopathy is a clinically and genetically variable disorder with characteristic large nuclei located in the centre of muscle fibres that resemble myotubes, the early foetal muscle fibres. There are two primary clinical presentations. The more common milder form consisting of both autosomal dominant and autosomal recessive sub-forms consists of relatively mild skeletal muscle weakness and hypotonia that can be present in the newborn or have a later onset and slow progression. The more severe X-linked form presents in males at birth. Infants present with marked skeletal muscle weakness, hypotonia and bulbar dysfunction.[83] Respiratory muscle weakness leads to early respiratory failure.[84] In the autosomal dominant and recessive forms, the distribution of weakness is predominantly proximal. Facial weakness and ocular abnormalities including ophthalmoplegia and ptosis are variable depending on the form.[85]

PATHOPHYSIOLOGY

Mutations responsible for the X-linked form are in the gene encoding for myotubularin, a protein required for muscle cell differentiation.[86] In general, the autosomal dominant form has been associated with later onset and milder course, whereas the autosomal recessive form is generally intermediate in respect to onset and course.[87] An animal model has been developed and will hopefully lead to more research regarding targeted therapies.[88]

Respiratory clinical issues

In the X-linked severe form, marked respiratory muscle weakness results in early respiratory failure and only continuous mechanical ventilation can support survival.[89] In the autosomal recessive form, respiratory impairment can be mild to severe and associated cardiomyopathy has been reported.[90] While the more mild autosomal dominant form generally does not have cardiorespiratory involvement, earlier-onset cases may develop restrictive respiratory impairment.[91]

MULTICORE MYOPATHY

Definition

Multicore myopathy is characterised by the multifocal myofibrillar degeneration that is smaller in size and number as compared to larger central core degeneration. Type I fibres are predominantly affected.[92] Autosomal dominant and recessive patterns of inheritance as well as sporadic occurrence have been found. Multicore myopathy had previously been recognised as primarily infantile and benign with relatively non-progressive, mostly proximal weakness, hypotonia and hyporeflexia.[93] Clinical features include facial and respiratory muscle weakness, joint contractures, chest deformities and scoliosis. There have been reports of adult-onset cases with respiratory involvement and cardiomyopathy.[94,95] Paraspinal contractures can produce a characteristic scoliosis pattern described as the side-sliding spine.[96]

Pathophysiology

The pathophysiology of multicore myopathy is not well understood. Mitochondrial depletion and mitochondrial, myofibrillar function are thought to have a predominant effect on skeletal muscle weakness.

Respiratory clinical issues

In multicore myopathy, the intercostal muscles have been found to be affected more than the diaphragm in patients with respiratory involvement.[97] Paraspinal muscle contracture with resulting scoliosis-induced chest wall restriction has also been reported.[96] Nocturnal hypoventilation progressing to respiratory failure has been reported in adolescent and adult patients.[96]

Respiratory management of congenital myopathies

The severity of the respective disease form will affect the course of respiratory management. The more severe infantile disease forms will most often require either continuous or nocturnal mechanical ventilation via tracheostomy.[89] In general, earlier-onset forms may develop more severe respiratory impairment, whereas later-onset forms tend to have lesser cardiorespiratory involvement. Respiratory assessment should include upright and supine vital capacity testing, static mouth pressures to assess inspiratory and expiratory muscle strength[64] and peak cough flow. Arterial blood gas testing, end-tidal CO_2 and transcutaneous CO_2 testing can be used to monitor for developing hypercapnic respiratory failure.[64,98] A serial assessment for symptoms of sleep-disordered breathing should also be included. Polysomnography testing combined is indicated for any suspicion of sleep-disordered breathing.[82,99] Non-invasive mask ventilation has been shown to successfully support nocturnal hypoventilation in congenital myopathies with respiratory insufficiency.[100,101] Polysomnography with bilevel pressure titration should be done in order to determine the most effective bilevel pressure support and backup rate regimen.[99]

MITOCHONDRIAL MYOPATHY

Definition and pathophysiology

Mitochondria are cellular organelles responsible for oxidative phosphorylation, which produces ATP, the energy substrate for metabolic function. Defects in the process of oxidative phosphorylation that affects skeletal muscle alone or in conjunction with central nervous system disease are identified as mitochondrial myopathy. Myopathy can occur alone or as a part of a multi-system disease. Clinical manifestations of myopathy can include myalgia, exercise intolerance, proximal muscle weakness, external ophthalmoplegia and facioscapulohumeral syndrome. The diagnosis of mitochondrial myopathy is based on muscle biopsy showing morphological abnormalities in muscle mitochondria. Skeletal muscle and brain tissue are selectively affected by mitochondrial dysfunction as a result of the high energy demand of these tissues.

Respiratory clinical issues

Respiratory failure has been reported in adults with mitochondrial disease either as an acute event sometimes associated with respiratory infection or as a chronic recurrent problem.[102,103] Respiratory muscle weakness has been identified on spirometry testing and diaphragmatic paralysis has been reported. Impaired ventilatory response to hypercapnoea and hypoxia has also been reported.[104] There have been case reports of sleep apnoea associated with mitochondrial disease. Muscle weakness and phrenic nerve involvement may also contribute to sleep apnoea. Respiratory arrest during sleep has also been reported.[105]

Respiratory management

A neuromuscular respiratory assessment should be included with regular clinical evaluation. The patient should be screened for symptoms of sleep-disordered breathing since sleep apnoea has been associated with a decreased ventilatory drive. Patients with symptoms of sleep-disordered breathing should be considered for polysomnography testing, and a titration study to adjust non-invasive ventilation may be helpful.

SUMMARY

In summary, there are a wide variety of neuromuscular disorders that can all affect respiratory function. Neuromuscular disease requires a systematic clinical approach, focusing on ventilatory dysfunction, glottic dysfunction and cough dysfunction.[106] Careful screening for symptoms, evaluation of respiratory function at clinic visits and a high index of suspicion for respiratory issues and symptoms of sleep-disordered breathing are key in providing the best level of care for patients with neuromuscular disease. Non-invasive methodologies for ventilatory and cough support are widely available and should be offered to appropriate patients. Early referral to a multidisciplinary team-based approach is also beneficial.

REFERENCES

1. Bergofsky EH. Respiratory failure in disorders of the thoracic cage. *Am Rev Respir Dis*. 1979;119:643–69.
2. Bourke SC, Tomlinson M, Williams TL et al. Effects of non-invasive ventilation on survival and quality of life in patients with amyotrophic lateral sclerosis: A randomised controlled trial. *Lancet Neurol*. 2006;5:140–7.
3. Simonds AK, Muntoni F, Heather S, Fielding S. Impact of nasal ventilation on survival in hypercapnic Duchenne muscular dystrophy. *Thorax*. 1998;53:949–52.
4. Benditt JO. The neuromuscular respiratory system: Physiology, pathophysiology, and a respiratory care approach to patients. *Respir Care*. 2006;51:829–37; discussion 37–9.
5. Bach JR. *Nonivasive Mechanical Ventilation*. 1st edition. Philadelphia: Hanley and Belfus, 2002.
6. Perrin C, Unterborn JN, Ambrosio CD, Hill NS. Pulmonary complications of chronic neuromuscular diseases and their management. *Muscle Nerve*. 2004;29:5–27.
7. Leith DE, Butler JP, Sneddon SL et al. In: Macklem PT, Mead J, eds. *Handbook of Physiology: The Respiratory System Volume III Mechanics of Breathing, Part 2*. Bethesda: American Physiologic Society; 1990:315–36.
8. Koul R, Al Futaisi A, Chacko A et al. Clinical and genetic study of spinal muscular atrophies in Oman. *J Child Neurol*. 2007;22:1227–30.
9. Lunn MR, Wang CH. Spinal muscular atrophy. *Lancet*. 2008;371:2120–33.
10. Kolb SJ, Kissel JT. Spinal muscular atrophy: A timely review. *Arch Neurol*. 2011;68:979–84.
11. Schroth MK. Special considerations in the respiratory management of spinal muscular atrophy. *Pediatrics*. 2009;123 Suppl 4:S245–9.
12. Markowitz JA, Tinkle MB, Fischbeck KH. Spinal muscular atrophy in the neonate. *J Obstet Gynecol Neonatal Nurs*. 2004;33:12–20.
13. Russman BS. Spinal muscular atrophy: Clinical classification and disease heterogeneity. *J Child Neurol*. 2007;22:946–51.
14. Wang CH, Finkel RS, Bertini ES et al. Consensus statement for standard of care in spinal muscular atrophy. *J Child Neurol*. 2007;22:1027–49.
15. Mellies U, Dohna-Schwake C, Stehling F, Voit T. Sleep disordered breathing in spinal muscular atrophy. *Neuromuscul Disord*. 2004;14:797–803.
16. Mellies U, Ragette R, Dohna Schwake C et al. Long-term noninvasive ventilation in children and adolescents with neuromuscular disorders. *Eur Respir J*. 2003;22:631–6.
17. Sansone VA, Racca F, Ottonello G et al. 1st Italian SMA Family Association Consensus Meeting: Management and recommendations for respiratory involvement in spinal muscular atrophy (SMA) types I–III, Rome, Italy, 30–31 January 2015. *Neuromuscul Disord*. 2015;25:979–89.
18. Ward K, Ford V, Ashcroft H, Parker R. Intermittent daytime mouthpiece ventilation successfully augments nocturnal non-invasive ventilation, controlling ventilatory failure and maintaining patient independence. *BMJ Case Rep*. 2015;2015.
19. Oskoui M, Levy G, Garland CJ et al. The changing natural history of spinal muscular atrophy type 1. *Neurology*. 2007;69:1931–6.
20. Bach JR, Bianchi C. Prevention of pectus excavatum for children with spinal muscular atrophy type 1. *Am J Phys Med Rehabil*. 2003;82:815–9.
21. Perez A, Mulot R, Vardon G et al. Thoracoabdominal pattern of breathing in neuromuscular disorders. *Chest*. 1996;110:454–61.
22. Bach JR, Baird JS, Plosky D et al. Spinal muscular atrophy type 1: management and outcomes. *Pediatr Pulmonol*. 2002;34:16–22.

23. Houston K, Buschang PH, Iannaccone ST, Seale NS. Craniofacial morphology of spinal muscular atrophy. *Pediatr Res.* 1994;36:265–9.
24. Bach JR, Niranjan V, Weaver B. Spinal muscular atrophy type 1: A noninvasive respiratory management approach. *Chest.* 2000;117:1100–5.
25. Gajdos P, Chevret S, Toyka K. Intravenous immunoglobulin for myasthenia gravis. *Cochrane Database Syst Rev.* 2008:CD002277.
26. Qureshi AI, Choudhry MA, Akbar MS et al. Plasma exchange versus intravenous immunoglobulin treatment in myasthenic crisis. *Neurology.* 1999;52:629–32.
27. Sussman J, Farrugia ME, Maddison P et al. Myasthenia gravis: Association of British Neurologists' management guidelines. *Pract Neurol.* 2015;15:199–206.
28. Seneviratne J, Mandrekar J, Wijdicks EF, Rabinstein AA. Noninvasive ventilation in myasthenic crisis. *Arch Neurol.* 2008;65:54–8.
29. Farbu E, Gilhus NE, Barnes MP et al. EFNS guideline on diagnosis and management of post-polio syndrome. Report of an EFNS task force. *Eur J Neurol.* 2006;13:795–801.
30. Bruno RL. Post-polio sequelae: Research and treatment in the second decade. *Orthopedics.* 1991;14:1169–70.
31. Farbu E, Rekand T, Gilhus NE. Post-polio syndrome and total health status in a prospective hospital study. *Eur J Neurol.* 2003;10:407–13.
32. Bertolasi L, Acler M, dall'Ora E et al. Risk factors for post-polio syndrome among an Italian population: A case–control study. *Neurol Sci.* 2012;33:1271–5.
33. Farbu E. Update on current and emerging treatment options for post-polio syndrome. *Ther Clin Risk Manag.* 2010;6:307–13.
34. Koopman FS, Beelen A, Gilhus NE et al. Treatment for postpolio syndrome. *Cochrane Database Syst Rev.* 2015;5:CD007818.
35. Jubelt B, Cashman NR. Neurological manifestations of the post-polio syndrome. *Crit Rev Neurobiol.* 1987;3:199–220.
36. Kidd D, Howard RS, Williams AJ et al. Late functional deterioration following paralytic poliomyelitis. *QJM.* 1997;90:189–96.
37. Dean E, Ross J, Road JD et al. Pulmonary function in individuals with a history of poliomyelitis. *Chest.* 1991;100:118–23.
38. Bergholtz B, Mollestad SO, Refsum H. [Post-polio respiratory failure. New manifestations of a forgotten disease]. *Tidsskr Nor Laegeforen:* 1988;108:2474–5.
39. Howard RS, Wiles CM, Spencer GT. The late sequelae of poliomyelitis. *Q J Med.* 1988;66:219–32.
40. Mathieu J, Allard P, Potvin L et al. A 10-year study of mortality in a cohort of patients with myotonic dystrophy. *Neurology.* 1999;52:1658–62.
41. Delaporte C. Personality patterns in patients with myotonic dystrophy. *Arch Neurol.* 1998;55:635–40.
42. Brook JD, McCurrach ME, Harley HG et al. Molecular basis of myotonic dystrophy: Expansion of a trinucleotide (CTG) repeat at the 3′ end of a transcript encoding a protein kinase family member. *Cell.* 1992;69:385.
43. Finsterer J, Stollberger C, Maeztu C. Sudden cardiac death in neuromuscular disorders. *Int J Cardiol.* 2016;203:508–15.
44. Lau JK, Sy RW, Corbett A, Kritharides L. Myotonic dystrophy and the heart: A systematic review of evaluation and management. *Int J Cardiol.* 2015;184:600–8.
45. Long C, McAnally JR, Shelton JM et al. Prevention of muscular dystrophy in mice by CRISPR/Cas9-mediated editing of germline DNA. *Science.* 2014;345:1184–8.
46. Turner C, Hilton-Jones D. Myotonic dystrophy: Diagnosis, management and new therapies. *Curr Opin Neurol.* 2014;27:599–606.
47. Monteiro L, Souza-Machado A, Valderramas S, Melo A. The effect of levodopa on pulmonary function in Parkinson's disease: A systematic review and meta-analysis. *Clin Ther.* 2012;34:1049–55.
48. Ciafaloni E, Mignot E, Sansone V et al. The hypocretin neurotransmission system in myotonic dystrophy type 1. *Neurology.* 2008;70:226–30.
49. Griggs RC, Donohoe KM. The recognition and management of respiratory insufficiency in neuromuscular disease. *J Chronic Dis.* 1982;35:497–500.
50. Cirignotta F, Mondini S, Zucconi M et al. Sleep-related breathing impairment in myotonic dystrophy. *J Neurol.* 1987;235:80–5.
51. Gilmartin JJ, Cooper BG, Griffiths CJ et al. Breathing during sleep in patients with myotonic dystrophy and non-myotonic respiratory muscle weakness. *Q J Med.* 1991;78:21–31.
52. Finnimore AJ, Jackson RV, Morton A, Lynch E. Sleep hypoxia in myotonic dystrophy and its correlation with awake respiratory function. *Thorax.* 1994;49:66–70.
53. Kumar SP, Sword D, Petty RK et al. Assessment of sleep studies in myotonic dystrophy. *Chron Respir Dis.* 2007;4:15–8.
54. Nitz J, Burke B. A study of the facilitation of respiration in myotonic dystrophy. *Physiother Res Int.* 2002;7:228–38.
55. Nugent AM, Smith IE, Shneerson JM. Domiciliary-assisted ventilation in patients with myotonic dystrophy. *Chest.* 2002;121:459–64.
56. Dauvilliers YA, Laberge L. Myotonic dystrophy type 1, daytime sleepiness and REM sleep dysregulation. *Sleep Med Rev.* 2012;16:539–45.
57. Gamez J, Calzada M, Cervera C, Sampol G. Non-compliance of domiciliary ventilatory treatment in patients with myotonic dystrophy. *Neurologia.* 2000;15:371.

58. Nakajima H, Raben N, Hamaguchi T, Yamasaki T. Phosphofructokinase deficiency; past, present and future. *Curr Mol Med.* 2002;2:197–212.
59. Kishnani PS, Hwu WL, Mandel H et al. A retrospective, multinational, multicenter study on the natural history of infantile-onset Pompe disease. *J Pediatr.* 2006;148:671–6.
60. Engel AG. Acid maltase deficiency in adults: studies in four cases of a syndrome which may mimic muscular dystrophy or other myopathies. *Brain.* 1970;93:599–616.
61. Kishnani PS, Steiner RD, Bali D et al. Pompe disease diagnosis and management guideline. *Genet Med.* 2006;8:267–88.
62. Rosenow EC, 3rd, Engel AG. Acid maltase deficiency in adults presenting as respiratory failure. *Am J Med.* 1978;64:485–91.
63. Keunen RW, Lambregts PC, Op de Coul AA, Joosten EM. Respiratory failure as initial symptom of acid maltase deficiency. *J Neurol Neurosurg Psychiatry.* 1984;47:549–52.
64. Mellies U, Dohna-Schwake C, Voit T. Respiratory function assessment and intervention in neuromuscular disorders. *Curr Opin Neurol.* 2005;18:543–7.
65. Fuller DD, ElMallah MK, Smith BK et al. The respiratory neuromuscular system in Pompe disease. *Respir Physiol Neurobiol.* 2013;189:241–9.
66. Pellegrini N, Laforet P, Orlikowski D et al. Respiratory insufficiency and limb muscle weakness in adults with Pompe's disease. *Eur Respir J.* 2005;26:1024–31.
67. Santamaria F, Montella S, Mirra V et al. Respiratory manifestations in patients with inherited metabolic diseases. *Eur Respir Rev.* 2013;22:437–53.
68. Fromageot C, Lofaso F, Annane D et al. Supine fall in lung volumes in the assessment of diaphragmatic weakness in neuromuscular disorders. *Arch Phys Med Rehabil.* 2001;82:123–8.
69. Dohna-Schwake C, Ragette R, Teschler H et al. Predictors of severe chest infections in pediatric neuromuscular disorders. *Neuromuscul Disord.* 2006;16:325–8.
70. Mellies U, Stehling F, Dohna-Schwake C et al. Respiratory failure in Pompe disease: Treatment with noninvasive ventilation. *Neurology.* 2005;64:1465–7.
71. Trebbia G, Lacombe M, Fermanian C et al. Cough determinants in patients with neuromuscular disease. *Respir Physiol Neurobiol.* 2005;146:291–300.
72. Cupler EJ, Berger KI, Leshner RT et al. Consensus treatment recommendations for late-onset Pompe disease. *Muscle Nerve.* 2012;45:319–33.
73. Kishnani PS, Beckemeyer AA. New therapeutic approaches for Pompe disease: Enzyme replacement therapy and beyond. *Pediatr Endocrinol Rev.* 2014;12 Suppl 1:114–24.
74. Sarnat HB. Myotubular myopathy: Arrest of morphogenesis of myofibres associated with persistence of fetal vimentin and desmin. Four cases compared with fetal and neonatal muscle. *Can J Neurol Sci.* 1990;17:109–23.
75. Kang PB, Morrison L, Iannaccone ST et al. Evidence-based guideline summary: Evaluation, diagnosis, and management of congenital muscular dystrophy: Report of the Guideline Development Subcommittee of the American Academy of Neurology and the Practice Issues Review Panel of the American Association of Neuromuscular & Electrodiagnostic Medicine. *Neurology.* 2015;84:1369–78.
76. Martinez BA, Lake BD. Childhood nemaline myopathy: A review of clinical presentation in relation to prognosis. *Dev Med Child Neurol.* 1987;29:815–20.
77. Sarnat HB. New insights into the pathogenesis of congenital myopathies. *J Child Neurol.* 1994;9:193–201.
78. Sanoudou D, Beggs AH. Clinical and genetic heterogeneity in nemaline myopathy—A disease of skeletal muscle thin filaments. *Trends Mol Med.* 2001; 7:362–8.
79. Banwell BL, Singh NC, Ramsay DA. Prolonged survival in neonatal nemaline rod myopathy. *Pediatr Neurol.* 1994;10:335–7.
80. Riley DJ, Santiago TV, Daniele RP et al. Blunted respiratory drive in congenital myopathy. *Am J Med.* 1977;63:459–66.
81. Sasaki M, Yoneyama H, Nonaka I. Respiratory muscle involvement in nemaline myopathy. *Pediatr Neurol.* 1990;6:425–7.
82. Kudou M KY et al. Two cases of nemaline myopathy diagnosed after episodes of respiratory failure. *Nihon Kokyuki Gassai Zasshi.* 2006;44:474–8.
83. Oldfors A, Kyllerman M, Wahlstrom J et al. X-linked myotubular myopathy: Clinical and pathological findings in a family. *Clin Genet.* 1989;36:5–14.
84. Braga SE, Gerber A, Meier C et al. Severe neonatal asphyxia due to X-linked centronuclear myopathy. *Eur J Pediatr.* 1990;150:132–5.
85. Jeannet PY, Bassez G, Eymard B et al. Clinical and histologic findings in autosomal centronuclear myopathy. *Neurology.* 2004;62:1484–90.
86. Blondeau F, Laporte J, Bodin S et al. Myotubularin, a phosphatase deficient in myotubular myopathy, acts on phosphatidylinositol 3-kinase and phosphatidylinositol 3-phosphate pathway. *Hum Mol Genet.* 2000;9:2223–9.
87. Wallgren-Pettersson C CA, Samson F, Fardequ M et al. The myotubular myopathies: Differential diagnosis of the X-linked recessive, autosomal dominant and autosomal recessive forms and present state of DNA studies. *J Med Genet.* 1995;32:673–9.
88. Goddard MA, Mack DL, Czerniecki SM et al. Muscle pathology, limb strength, walking gait, respiratory function and neurological impairment establish

disease progression in the p.N155K canine model of X-linked myotubular myopathy. *Ann Transl Med.* 2015;3:262.

89. Herman GE, Finegold M, Zhao W et al. Medical complications in long-term survivors with X-linked myotubular myopathy. *J Pediatr.* 1999;134:206–14.
90. Verhiest W, Brucher JM, Goddeeris P et al. Familial centronuclear myopathy associated with 'cardiomyopathy'. *Br Heart J.* 1976;38:504–9.
91. Bitoun M, Bevilacqua JA, Prudhon B et al. Dynamin 2 mutations cause sporadic centronuclear myopathy with neonatal onset. *Ann Neurol.* 2007;62:666–70.
92. Gardner-Medwin D. *Neuromuscular Disorders in Infance and Childhood.* Edinburgh: Churchill-Livingston, 1994.
93. Penegyres PK, Kakulas BA. The natural history of minicore–multicore myopathy. *Muscle Nerve.* 1991;14:411–5.
94. Shuaib A, Martin JM, Mitchell LB, Brownell AK. Multicore myopathy: Not always a benign entity. *Can J Neurol Sci.* 1988;15:10–4.
95. Magliocco AM, Mitchell LB, Brownell AK, Lester WM. Dilated cardiomyopathy in multicore myopathy. *Am J Cardiol.* 1989;63:150–1.
96. Rowe PW, Eagle M, Pollitt C et al. Multicore myopathy: Respiratory failure and paraspinal muscle contractures are important complications. *Dev Med Child Neurol.* 2000;42:340–3.
97. Rimmer KP, Whitelaw WA. The respiratory muscles in multicore myopathy. *Am Rev Respir Dis.* 1993;148:227–31.
98. Kotterba S, Patzold T, Malin JP et al. Respiratory monitoring in neuromuscular disease—Capnography as an additional tool? *Clin Neurol Neurosurg.* 2001;103:87–91.
99. Sasaki M, Takeda M, Kobayashi K, Nonaka I. Respiratory failure in nemaline myopathy. *Pediatr Neurol.* 1997;16:344–6.
100. Bielen P, Sliwinski P, Kaminski D, Zielinski J. [Respiratory failure during the course of congenital myopathy effectively treated with nocturnal noninvasive nasal positive pressure ventilation]. *Pneumonol Alergol Pol.* 2000;68:151–5.
101. Shahrizaila N, Lim WS, Robson DK et al. Tubular aggregate myopathy presenting with acute type II respiratory failure and severe orthopnoea. *Thorax.* 2006;61:89–90.
102. Barohn RJ, Clanton T, Sahenk Z, Mendell JR. Recurrent respiratory insufficiency and depressed ventilatory drive complicating mitochondrial myopathies. *Neurology.* 1990;40:103–6.
103. Kim GW, Kim SM, Sunwoo IN, Chi JG. Two cases of mitochondrial myopathy with predominant respiratory dysfunction. *Yonsei Med J.* 1991;32:184–9.
104. Carroll JE, Zwillich C, Weil JV, Brooke MH. Depressed ventilatory response in oculocraniosomatic neuromuscular disease. *Neurology.* 1976;26:140–6.
105. Tatsumi C, Takahashi M, Yorifuji S et al. Mitochondrial encephalomyopathy, ataxia, and sleep apnea. *Neurology.* 1987;37:1429–30.
106. Benditt JO, Boitano LJ. Pulmonary issues in patients with chronic neuromuscular disease. *Am J Respir Crit Care Med.* 2013;187:1046–55.

41

Amyotrophic lateral sclerosis

STEPHEN C. BOURKE AND JOHN STEER

INTRODUCTION

Amyotrophic lateral sclerosis (ALS) is a progressive neurological disease of unknown cause characterised by degeneration of upper and lower motor neurones. The broader term 'motor neurone disease' (MND) is sometimes used to include conditions limited to either the spinal motor neurones (spinal muscular atrophy) or the upper motor neurones (primary lateral sclerosis), but both variants usually progress to involve upper and lower motor neurones. In effect, the terms ALS and MND are synonymous. It is mainly a disease of late middle age, with median onset around 60 years, a slight male predominance[1] and an incidence of ~2.5/100,000.[2,3] Patterns at presentation include predominant involvement of limb, trunk, bulbar or respiratory muscles. The condition is relentlessly progressive, with median survival from symptom onset of about 3 years and death usually due to respiratory failure secondary to respiratory muscle weakness (RMW). However, the rate of progression varies, with ~8% of patients surviving more than 10 years from diagnosis.[1] About 10% of patients develop fronto-temporal dementia, which is associated with bulbar onset, older age, poor compliance with NIV and percutaneous endoscopic gastrostomy (PEG) feeding and shorter survival.[4] Milder degrees of cognitive dysfunction are more common.

Respiratory involvement

Respiratory muscle function is a strong predictor of quality of life (QoL)[5] and survival.[6] Weakness of respiratory muscles, predominantly those involved with inspiration, causes hypoventilation. This initially occurs during sleep and is most marked during REM sleep when, normally, ventilation is almost entirely dependent on the diaphragm. Possibly as an adaptation to this vulnerability, individuals with severe diaphragmatic weakness may show reduced or even absent REM sleep.[7] Central and obstructive apnoeas and hypopnoeas, frequent arousals and reduced sleep efficiency are common. With progression of muscle weakness, hypoventilation persists when awake and type 2 respiratory failure develops. Weakness of bulbar muscles impairs phonation, swallowing and airway protection, thereby increasing the risk of aspiration. An effective cough requires adequate force and coordination of inspiratory, expiratory and bulbar muscles.

The rate of decline of respiratory function is variable.[8] Although the initial rate of decline of VC is alinear,[9] once weakness is at least moderate, this becomes approximately rectilinear, typically 2.4% to 4.1% of predicted vital capacity (VC) per month.[8,10,11]

Respiratory features are strong predictors of survival: unsurprisingly, people with respiratory onset disease have a worse outlook than other phenotypes[1] and are more likely to present in extremis before the diagnosis has been made. VC, actual and estimated decline in VC, maximum pressures and nocturnal hypoxaemia all convey prognostic information.[1,12–15] Hypercapnia is an ominous prognostic feature, and raised serum bicarbonate and low chloride concentrations (which accompany chronic respiratory acidosis) also predict shorter survival. Other adverse predictive variables include poor nutritional status, older age, executive dysfunction, bulbar onset and a shorter time interval between initial symptoms and diagnosis.[1,15–17] The ALS Prognostic index risk stratifies patients based on site of disease onset, rate of deterioration in the Revised ALS Functional Rating Scale and presence of executive dysfunction.[17]

ASSESSING RESPIRATORY MUSCLE FUNCTION

Symptoms and signs

At presentation, less than 20% of patients are aware of respiratory symptoms, although RMW is demonstrable in most if assessed.[8] The symptoms of RMW depend on the severity of weakness and pattern of muscles involved. Exertional breathlessness is a late feature, particularly when mobility is restricted. Orthopnoea indicates moderate or severe diaphragmatic weakness and is the best predictor of benefit

Table 41.1 Symptoms and signs of respiratory muscle weakness

Direct symptoms of RMW	Sleep-disordered breathing	Hypercapnia	Signs on clinical examination
Orthopnoea	Frequent wakenings	Morning headaches	Tachypnoea
Exertional breathlessness	Nocturia	Drowsiness	Weak cough/sniff
Sputum retention*	Unrefreshing sleep	Confusion	Abdominal paradox
Recurrent LRTI*	Daytime sleepiness	Hallucinations	Central cyanosis
Weak cough*	Poor concentration and memory	Fatigue	Signs of hypercapnia
	Irritability and depression	Poor appetite	
Notes: Orthopnoea is the best predictor of NIV benefit. *Consider cough augmentation	*Notes:* Sleep disruption is common, but may be due to problems other than RMW.	*Notes:* If hypercapnia confirmed, refer urgently for NIV.	*Notes:* Typically evident only when RMW is already severe.

from, and adherence to, NIV.[18] However, orthopnoea is not universal in RMW: intercostal weakness causes breathlessness when upright (platypnoea); and in combined diaphragmatic and intercostal weakness, patients may be most comfortable semi-recumbent. In addition, patients with severe bulbar impairment may confuse the sensation of choking on lying flat with orthopnoea. Weakness of inspiratory, expiratory and bulbar muscles contributes to weak cough, poor sputum clearance and recurrent lower respiratory tract infections (LRTIs).

In people with RMW, breathing is further compromised during sleep by loss of wakefulness drive to breathe, the mechanical disadvantage of lying flat and REM-related suppression of intercostal and accessory muscles. Symptoms related to sleep disruption and nocturnal hypoventilation (Table 41.1) are common. However, sleep-related symptoms are not specific to RMW, as sleep may be disturbed by other factors, such as choking on secretions, pain or anxiety and depression. As RMW progresses, daytime hypercapnia ensues. Symptoms include headaches (typically worse in the morning), muscle twitching, drowsiness and fatigue. Progressive respiratory failure and sleep disruption may contribute to cognitive dysfunction and although irreversible cognitive impairment is well recognised in ALS, when the impairment is due to RMW, it may improve with ventilatory support.

Non-specific signs on clinical examination of RMW include tachypnoea, accessory muscle use, reduced chest expansion and a weak cough or sniff. Abdominal paradox (inward movement of abdomen on inspiration) signals diaphragmatic weakness. Central cyanosis and signs of hypercapnia (e.g. peripheral vasodilation, bounding pulse, asterixis) are late features.

Tests of respiratory muscle function

RMW reduces VC and may increase residual volume (RV), while total lung capacity can remain within the normal range despite fairly severe weakness.[19] The reduction of VC is due to loss of inspiratory and expiratory force and a reduction in pulmonary compliance.[20] A fall in VC in the supine posture is an index of the severity of diaphragmatic weakness.[21] Compared to sitting VC, supine VC is a better index of diaphragmatic function, but it is difficult to perform when mobility is restricted.

Respiratory muscle function is assessed more directly by measurements of maximal pressures including maximum inspiratory and expiratory pressure measured at the mouth (MIP, MEP) or during a forceful sniff (sniff nasal inspiratory pressure – SNIP). Pressure measurements are more sensitive for detecting the earlier stages of RMW, whilst VC falls significantly only with moderate or severe weakness.[22] VC performed sitting may span the normal range at initiation of NIV in symptomatic patients. SNIP is the best predictor of daytime hypercapnia (Figure 41.1),[23] but MIP may be more reliable when RMW is severe.[24] Typically, but not universally, patients find SNIP easier to perform than MIP: both tests should be performed and the better of the two accepted. Invasive measurements such as transdiaphragmatic pressure offer limited advantages[23] and are impracticable for routine clinical use. Respiratory and/or bulbar muscle weakness reduces peak cough flow (PCF), which can be measured to identify patients with potential problems clearing secretions (see below).

True respiratory muscle strength is often underestimated in patients with severe bulbar impairment due to difficulties performing volitional respiratory function tests.[23,25] This cannot be overcome by using an adapted face mask, suggesting that it is not simply due to air leak. In such patients, emphasis should be placed on measures of gas exchange: if oxygen saturations (SpO_2) when breathing room air are ≤94% if there is no coexistent chronic lung disease, or ≤92% if there is coexistent chronic lung disease, then arterial blood gases should be measured. Hypoventilation and impairment of gas exchange initially occur during sleep; nocturnal oximetry and transcutaneous carbon dioxide recording are more sensitive than daytime measures.[23]

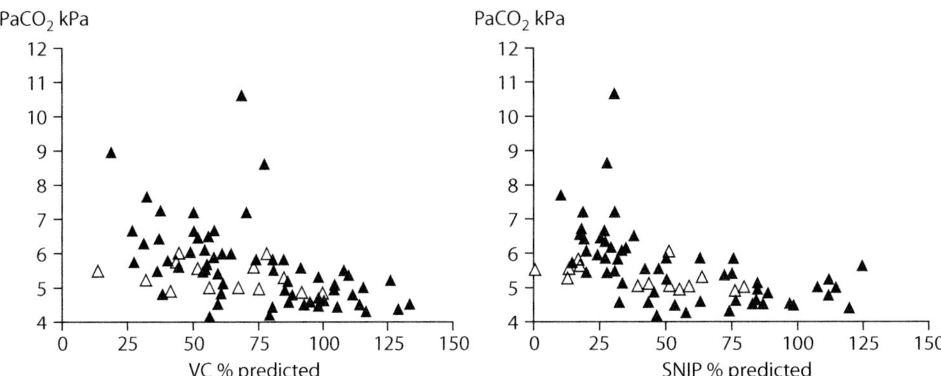

Figure 41.1 Relations of arterial $PaCO_2$ to (left) vital capacity (VC) and (right) sniff nasal inspiratory pressure (SNIP), both expressed as percentage of predicted values. Open symbols represent patients with predominant bulbar features. (Reproduced from Lyall RA et al. *Brain*. 2001;124:2000–13. With permission.)

Monitoring nocturnal oximetry in patients without severe bulbar impairment adds little information regarding prognosis or timing of NIV, and therefore, for these patients, volitional testing and assessment of symptoms are usually sufficient. For patients with prominent sleep-related symptoms, a limited sleep study will assess sleep-disordered breathing, whilst full polysomnography provides additional information on sleep architecture. Ideally such tests should be performed in the patients' home.

LUNG VOLUME RECRUITMENT AND AIRWAY CLEARANCE

RMW may cause atelectasis, which impairs lung compliance and gas exchange. Changes are typically most pronounced in the lower lobes, particularly when the diaphragm is weak. Bulbar impairment increases the risk of aspiration, whilst respiratory and bulbar muscle weakness, singly or in combination, reduce cough effectiveness and airway clearance. This increases the risk of, and delays recovery from, LRTIs and pneumonia. During acute infections, including simple upper respiratory tract infections,[26] muscle function is further compromised. Patients should be asked about their ability to cough and clear secretions at review. PCF is a simple measure that should be assessed alongside symptoms to guide the introduction of lung volume recruitment (LVR) and other cough augmentation techniques: if PCF < 270 L/min, introduce and use during respiratory infections or sedation; if PCF < 160 L/min, encourage regular adherence.[27]

LVR refers to techniques that maximally inflate the lungs. It helps to prevent atelectasis and improves airway secretion clearance and lung compliance.[20] The simplest approach is breath stacking, which involves taking three to five successive breaths in without expiration, repeating the cycle three times. Breath stacking is more effective when assisted by the use of a volume recruitment bag with a one-way valve and mask, or provided bulbar and facial muscle function is preserved, a mouthpiece. If the patient has a ventilator, this may be used to assist LVR (particularly if volume cycled). Following LVR, airway clearance can be further improved by huffing thoraco-abdominal thrusts timed with a cough effort (avoid after meals) and use of a mechanical insufflator–exsufflator (MI-E). MI-E may be combined with thoraco-abdominal thrusts and achieves a higher PCF than alternative techniques,[28] but it is less effective if bulbar function is severely impaired.[29] MI-E can be applied through an endotracheal or tracheostomy tube, offering better airway clearance than deep suctioning. More recent devices include an oscillatory pressure wave during inspiration and expiration, and automatic cycling to exsufflation, triggered by cough effort. MI-E and assisted breath stacking have been compared in a small randomised controlled trial (RCT).[30] Assisted breath stacking showed a trend for fewer LRTIs than MI-E at <1% of the cost. MI-E showed a trend towards shorter symptom duration and lower risk of hospitalisation, but of concern is shorter survival (MI-E 266 days, breath stacking 535 days; $p = 0.105$), particularly if bulbar function was severely impaired. Unfortunately imbalance arose following randomisation; baseline PCF was lower in the MI-E arm. In the absence of a definitive trial, breath stacking should be used first line. MI-E should be considered if breath stacking proves ineffective, particularly during respiratory infections and hospitalisation,[31] but should be used with caution if bulbar function is severely impaired.

USE OF NIV

NIV and survival

In early non-randomised studies of NIV, intolerance was associated with shorter survival from the onset of respiratory insufficiency.[32–34] The results of these studies are, however, inconclusive, as factors that influence tolerance of NIV, particularly bulbar function, may also independently affect survival, while non-concordance with NIV might also imply non-concordance with other aspects of care. A subsequent RCT confirmed that NIV improves survival in subjects with normal, or at most moderately impaired, bulbar function.[25] The trial was inclusive; no patients were

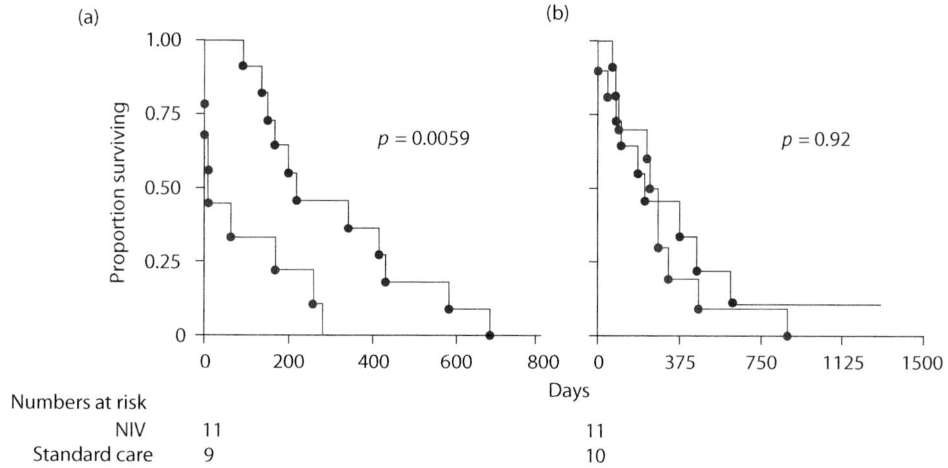

Figure 41.2 Survival from randomisation in an RCT of NIV (blue) compared to no ventilation (red) in patients with normal or only moderately impaired bulbar function **(a)**, and with severe bulbar impairment **(b)**. (Modified from Bourke SC et al. *Lancet Neurol.* 2006;5:140–147. With permission.)

excluded on the basis of bulbar function, level of disability, social support or views on life-prolonging therapy. Initially, 92 patients were enrolled and assessed every 2 months. Those who developed orthopnoea with $P_I$max < 60% predicted (of whom 20 were normocapnic) or symptomatic hypercapnia within the time frame of the study were randomised to receive NIV ($n = 22$) or standard care ($n = 19$). In patients with normal or only moderately impaired bulbar function, NIV increased median survival by 205 days ($p < 0.006$), with improvements in, and maintenance of, QoL for most of this period. Although patients with severe bulbar impairment showed no survival benefit, some QoL indices improved (Figure 41.2).

In the pilot study preceding this RCT, survival following initiation of NIV was substantially longer (512 days).[18] Similar variations in survival are reported across other cohorts. In addition to differences in recognised prognostic indices, other factors likely to be of importance include patients' views on life prolonging therapy, motivation and social support.

Effect of NIV on QoL, cognitive function and carers

In a progressive and debilitating condition such as ALS, it is important that interventions that improve survival do not prolong suffering, but rather extend life with symptom control and QoL that are acceptable to the patient. Several prospective cohort studies[18,35] and non-randomized controlled trials[34,36,37] have shown sustained improvements in QoL with NIV, but none included a contemporaneous and equivalent control group. The largest improvements were seen in domains assessing sleep-related problems and mental health. Of importance, normocapnic subjects with orthopnoea showed similar improvements to those with hypercapnia or nocturnal oxygen desaturation, and reliance on the latter as essential criteria for initiating NIV may deprive many patients of benefit.[18] The QoL benefits associated with NIV in these studies were confirmed in an RCT.[25] Compared to controls, subjects with normal or only moderately impaired bulbar function showed sustained benefit in all domains of the SF-36 (except physical function), CRQ and SAQLI. Even in subjects with severe bulbar impairment, the CRQ dyspnoea domain and some domains of the SAQLI improved. Following initiation of NIV, improvements in some aspects of cognitive function have been reported,[38] although in a subsequent study only a favourable trend was seen.[34] At the end of life, improvement in patient comfort and anxiety has been reported.[39]

Comparison of the strain, anxiety, depression and QoL of carers of ALS patients receiving NIV and a control group of carers of patients with similar disability but without RMW showed no differences in caregiver strain, although the SF-36 energy vitality domain was lower at 12 months in the NIV carers' group.[34] These results compare favourably with the greater burden experienced by carers of patients receiving tracheostomy ventilation.[40,41]

Effect of NIV on respiratory function and sleep

Studies comparing subjects who use NIV and those who refuse NIV or are intolerant of it have shown a slower decline of VC in the former.[18,33] Following initiation of NIV, the rate of decline in VC, MIP, MEP and SNIP is slower.[42] In hypercapnic patients receiving nocturnal NIV, pulmonary gas exchange improves during both the period of assisted ventilation and spontaneous breathing, with progressive benefit over weeks and months following initiation of NIV. The sustained reduction in $PaCO_2$ probably results mainly from 'unloading' CO_2 during the period of assisted ventilation, thus reversing the associated chronic respiratory acidosis and increasing the ventilatory stimulus during daytime spontaneous ventilation.[43] A small increase in lung compliance, possibly due to reversal of atelectasis, has been reported after a session of treatment with NIV.[20]

In patients with good bulbar function, NIV improves nocturnal gas exchange and sleep architecture, including sleep efficiency, REM sleep and arousal frequency, whilst those with bulbar dysfunction show a limited improvement in gas exchange.[44]

Influence of bulbar impairment

Severe bulbar impairment is associated with poor adherence to NIV[18,25,32,45] and less effective ventilation. However, patients with bulbar impairment may survive longer if they tolerate NIV.[32] Early initiation of NIV in patients with bulbar disease has been advocated to improve adherence. However, one cohort study showed that in the bulbar subgroup, NIV tolerance was associated with better survival only in those who were hypercapnic at initiation.[46]

Some cohort studies have reported good outcomes with bulbar *onset* disease treated with NIV,[33,47] but bulbar function at *initiation of NIV* is more relevant. Further confounding factors in cohort studies are that patients with bulbar impairment perform volitional respiratory function tests poorly,[23] and the sensation of choking on lying flat may be confused with orthopnoea due to RMW. Consequently, in such patients, NIV may be initiated at a time when their true respiratory muscle strength is better than assumed, which may explain the apparent survival advantage. This conclusion is supported by the results of our RCT[25]: compared to subjects with better bulbar function, those with severe bulbar impairment had apparently similar VC, $P_I$max and SNIP, but lower $PaCO_2$ at randomisation and, in the control arm, survived longer (better bulbar function = 11 days, severe bulbar impairment = 261 days). Among ventilated patients, survival was similar in those with and without severe bulbar impairment (216 and 222 days, respectively). In cohort studies lacking the benefit of an unselected control group, it is understandable how similar results may be misinterpreted. In a large cohort,[42] use of NIV was associated with longer survival from symptom onset in bulbar patients (NIV = 32.61 months; no NIV = 13.57 months). Surprisingly, the apparent benefit was greater than in other phenotypes, and persisted after adjustment for differences in age at onset, gender, riluzole and PEG use. However, the median time from symptom onset to initiation of NIV was 24.5 months, substantially longer than overall survival in those not receiving NIV. Consequently, use of NIV cannot explain the larger part of the observed survival difference.

Tracheostomy ventilation

Worldwide, long-term ventilatory support via tracheostomy is generally used much less frequently than NIV in ALS,[42,48–50] with the notable exception of Japan.[51] This may reflect concern that home care is more difficult; it may commit the patient to institutional care and can lead to ventilator entrapment, potentially with the patient totally unable to communicate. Survival from initiation of tracheostomy ventilation varies greatly between cohorts; in one study in which the diagnosis of ALS had not been established prior to ventilation in 71% of patients, median survival was 2.8 months,[52] whilst more recent cohorts cite 21–56.8 months.[41,53,54] Older age at initiation and institutional care are associated with shorter survival. Compared to NIV, patients receiving tracheostomy ventilation survive longer, particularly if bulbar function is poor,[41] but they are less likely to be cared for at home.[55] QoL has been reported to be similar to patients receiving NIV.[56] An earlier study showed this was the case if care was provided in the patients' home, whilst institutional care was associated with significantly worse QoL. In contrast to NIV,[34] tracheostomy ventilation provided in the patients' home is associated with greater carer burden.[40,41] Additional advantages of NIV are that speech and swallowing are better preserved, natural airway defences are not compromised, ventilator entrapment is less of an issue, and there probably are psychological benefits, such as a feeling of better control. Patients who have experienced both NIV and tracheostomy ventilation usually prefer the former.[57] With careful attention to control of sialorrhoea, selection of interfaces and cough augmentation, NIV can be used to support patients virtually 24/7. Consequently, tracheostomy ventilation should generally be considered only for patients with severe bulbar impairment or those who are intolerant of, or failing on, NIV.

Diaphragmatic pacing

Compared to phrenic nerve stimulation, insertion of the NeurRx RA/4 diaphragmatic pacing (DP) system is less invasive. Electrodes are fitted into the underside of the diaphragm laparoscopically, and the procedure is safe and well tolerated. Use of the device in ALS was granted FDA approval on humanitarian grounds in 2011, based on a comparison of survival in a selected subset of patients who underwent insertion of the device (n = 84) and matched controls receiving NIV within a separate retrospective study (n = 43). DP was associated with a survival advantage from diagnosis of 16.1 months, and from NIV of 9 months. Subsequently, a UK RCT (DiPALS) showed that the median survival from randomisation was 11.0 months in the DP and NIV arm, compared to 22.5 months with NIV alone (p = 0.01; Figure 41.3).[58] The trial was stopped early by the Data Monitoring and Ethics Committee. Of note, the excess deaths in the DP arm were not due to procedural complications or differences in NIV use. An interim analysis of a French RCT of DP in ALS (RespiStimALS) confirmed a similar excess mortality in the DP arm, and this trial was also stopped. At randomisation, patients had less respiratory compromise (VC 60%–85%). Importantly, control patients underwent insertion of the DP system and sham pacing, and therefore the excess deaths appear to be related to DP rather than a direct or indirect effect of the operative procedure.

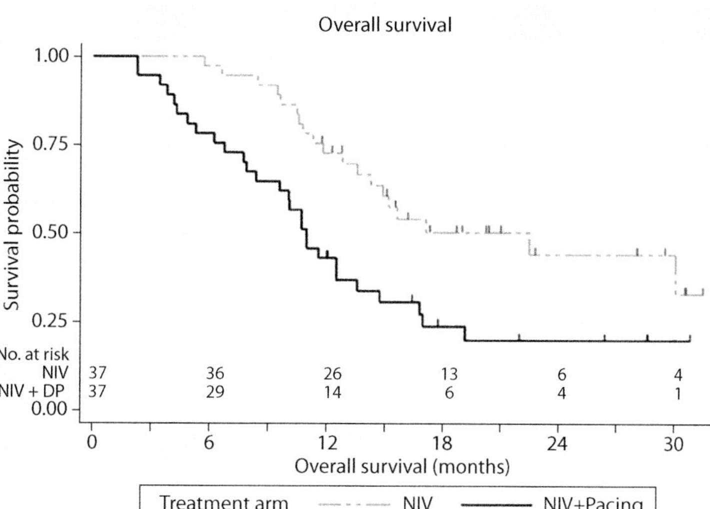

Figure 41.3 Survival following randomisation in an RCT of NIV compared to NIV and DP. (Reproduced from DiPALS. DiPals Writing Committee, *Lancet Neurol.* 2015;14:883–92.)

CLINICAL APPLICATION OF NIV IN ALS

Indications and timing

NIV should be considered in all patients with ALS and respiratory insufficiency. The decision to initiate treatment should take account of the patient's views on potentially life-prolonging therapy, where s/he wishes to be cared for, the level of caregiver and social support and factors likely to influence adherence to, and benefit from, NIV (including age, nutritional status and upper limb, bulbar and cognitive function). There is no legal or ethical difference between not initiating NIV and discontinuing NIV when a competent patient no longer wishes to continue treatment. Furthermore, valid advance directives to refuse treatment stipulating a patient's wishes in the event they become no longer competent should be respected. Consequently, patients should be reassured that they can discontinue ventilation at a time of their choosing, and will not become trapped on NIV against their wishes.

The optimum time to start treatment is unclear. Most studies have included several criteria for initiation of NIV, but few have compared different criteria. One small prospective study compared five different criteria: orthopnoea, sleep-related symptoms, apnoea–hypopnoea index (AHI) >10, nocturnal oxygen desaturation and daytime hypercapnia.[18] Orthopnoea (even in normocapnic subjects) was associated with a large improvement in QoL and good adherence to NIV. Nocturnal desaturation and daytime hypercapnia were also associated with good results, but reliance on these alone would have excluded several patients with orthopnoea who benefited. Sleep-related symptoms were sensitive, but less specific, predictors of benefit, and AHI > 10 was unhelpful. The rate of disease progression varies greatly in ALS, and survival following the development of orthopnoea or daytime hypercapnia may be short, possibly only a few weeks.[25] This highlights the importance of close monitoring of respiratory muscle function as well as symptoms and lends support to earlier initiation of NIV, particularly in patients with rapidly progressive disease and better bulbar function.

In a retrospective cohort study,[59] survival from symptom onset was better in patients with a VC ≥ 65% predicted at initiation of NIV than those with VC < 65%. However, time from symptom onset (weakness of any muscle group) to initiation of NIV was similar in both arms, and therefore the rate of disease progression was clearly different, which may explain the difference in mortality. In a separate study, patients who only achieved good adherence to NIV with effective control of hypoventilation after 6 months showed similar survival to those achieving this within 1 month. This suggests that earlier initiation of NIV may not confer a substantial survival advantage. However, this does not preclude other advantages such as improved symptom control and QoL. The term 'early NIV' normally refers to use in patients with minimal or no symptoms, but with confirmed RMW, and its role is even less clear. A French RCT comparing early and standard initiation of NIV was closed due to poor recruitment.[60] Of concern, in Duchenne muscular dystrophy, an RCT surprisingly showed higher mortality in the early NIV arm.[61]

Regular formal assessment of respiratory symptoms and function reduces the likelihood of emergency intubation, increases the proportion of patients treated with NIV and, in patients with preserved bulbar function, improves survival.[46] Measurement of $P_I$max[6] and SNIP[14] should be included in routine monitoring every 2–3 months.[31]

Current UK guidance recommends urgent (within 1 week) referral for NIV if daytime hypercapnia ($PaCO_2$ > 6kPa) is present, and consideration of referral for NIV:

if VC < 50% predicted alone or VC < 80% and symptoms or signs of RMW are present; if SNIP or MIP < 40 cm H_2O alone, or if symptoms and signs of RMW and SNIP < 65 cm H_2O in men or <55 cm H_2O in women; or if SNIP or MIP decline by over 10 cm H_2O in 3 months. A trial of NIV is also recommended if there is evidence of significant nocturnal hypoventilation.[31] The EFNS guideline on the clinical management of ALS[62] acknowledges the lack of evidence in this area and recommends that NIV should be considered if at least one symptom or sign of RMW is present in combination with at least one abnormal respiratory function test (VC < 80%, SNIP < 40 c mH_2O, $P_I$max < 60 cm H_2O, significant nocturnal desaturation, or morning $PaCO_2$ > 45 mmHg).

On current evidence, the authors recommend routine assessment of relevant symptoms (Table 41.1), bulbar and respiratory muscle function every 2–3 months. Advised functional tests and indications for referral for NIV are shown in Table 41.2. In particular, we highlight that hypercapnia warrants urgent referral, regardless of bulbar function. In patients with severe bulbar impairment, volitional tests of respiratory function are unreliable; in the presence of symptoms, if daytime $PaCO_2$ is normal, NIV should be considered if there is evidence of nocturnal hypoventilation. When NIV is poorly tolerated despite careful introduction, either tracheostomy ventilation or alternative palliation may be more appropriate. Patients without severe bulbar impairment should be offered NIV without further investigation if orthopnoea and evidence of RMW are present. NIV is intrusive and adherence to treatment may be poor and later treatment may be compromised if introduced too early. However, earlier introduction of NIV should be considered in patients showing a rapid decline in respiratory muscle strength. In one study, the best predictor of daytime hypercapnia was SNIP < 32% predicted.[23] To allow time to initiate NIV, we suggest considering NIV once the better of SNIP and MIP < 40% predicted or there is a rapid decline in respiratory muscle strength, even if symptoms are mild. Difficulty clearing secretions, frequent respiratory tract infections, weak cough and PCF should also be routinely assessed, and LVR/cough augmentation techniques introduced if indicated (see above).

Outcome of acute presentation in respiratory failure

Acute or acute on chronic respiratory failure may be triggered by mucus plugging, upper[26] or LRTIs, pneumonia, uncontrolled oxygen therapy,[63] sedative drugs or abdominal distension. Virtually all survivors require long-term ventilatory support.[52,64] In patients without severe bulbar impairment, NIV offers significant advantages over invasive ventilation even in the acute setting, including lower mortality, fewer treatment failures, shorter ITU stay and fewer complications.[64,65] Mechanical cough assistance may help clearance of secretions and avoid the need for minitracheostomy.[66] Mucolytics, such as N-acetylcisteine 1–2 g nebulised 4 hourly, may be helpful.

Patients with ALS may present with acute respiratory failure before the diagnosis is clear,[61] but in those with an established diagnosis, this should usually be avoidable by regular monitoring. Ventilatory support and alternative palliative therapies should be openly discussed with patients at an early stage. Advance directives should be drawn up and

Table 41.2 Criteria for NIV referral

Method of assessment	Without severe bulbar impairment		With severe bulbar impairment	
	Test result	Symptoms	Test result	Symptoms
Vital capacity	(F)VC <50% predicted	Refer even if asymptomatic	Volitional tests of respiratory function unreliable.	Orthopnoea may be confused with the sensation of choking on lying flat.
	(F)VC <80% predicted	Symptoms of RMW[a]		
Respiratory muscle strength	SNIP or MIP < 40 cm H_2O	Refer even if asymptomatic	Perform ABG if SpO_2 < 95% on air.	
	SNIP or MIP < 65 cm H_2O for men	Symptoms of RMW[a]		
	SNIP or MIP < 55 cm H_2O for women	Symptoms of RMW[a]		
Nocturnal hypoventilation	SpO_2 <90% for >5% of night	Refer even if asymptomatic	SpO_2 <90% for >5% of night	
	$P_{TC}CO_2$ >6.5kPa		$P_{TC}CO_2$ >6.5kPa	
Urgent referral	Daytime hypercapnia	Refer even if asymptomatic	Daytime hypercapnia	Refer even if asymptomatic

Note: ABG – arterial blood gas; MIP – maximal inspiratory pressure; $P_{TC}CO_2$ – transcutaneous PCO_2; RMW – respiratory muscle weakness; SNIP – sniff nasal inspiratory pressure; SpO_2 – peripheral arterial oxygen saturation.

[a] Symptoms of RMW include: orthopnoea, exertional breathlessness, weak cough, weak sniff, recurrent LRTIs, morning headache and drowsiness. Less specific symptoms include: disturbed sleep, unrefreshing sleep, nightmares, daytime sleepiness, poor concentration/memory, fatigue, poor appetite.

respected, and effective palliative therapy offered instead of ventilation when appropriate. Communication is better preserved with NIV than with invasive ventilation, which is of particular importance in the acute setting when patients present *in extremis* and their views on long-term ventilation are unclear. If such patients are invasively ventilated initially (often reflecting the inexperience of the receiving team or to facilitate transfer between units), they can usually be extubated and weaned onto NIV subsequently.

TECHNICAL ASPECTS OF NIV IN ALS

The general technical aspects of NIV are covered in Part 1 of this volume. Certain aspects more specific to ALS warrant particular mention.

Interface

A suitable and comfortable interface is essential, and a wide selection of interfaces from various manufacturers should be available. Careful interface selection, combined with education on fitting and removal for the patient, their family and carers, is vital. Custom-made masks may be considered for individual patients if it is difficult to obtain a good seal with standard interfaces. Mouth leak is particularly common with bulbo-facial weakness. In our experience, most patients prefer an oronasal interface to a nasal mask and chin strap. Both oronasal masks with nasal pillows and a total face mask avoid contact with the nasal bridge, which is particularly helpful if local skin problems arise. When using an oronasal mask, it is important to ensure that the patient can remove it in an emergency or, at the very least, raise an alarm quickly. This may entail customising headgear (e.g. rip cord) and fitting an alarm system, which the patient can easily activate. Those needing intermittent ventilatory support during the daytime may prefer to use a mouthpiece, provided bulbar and facial muscle function is adequate. A lip seal can be added to reduce problems with mouth leak. Patients with poor upper limb function can retain independence in daytime ventilation if provided with a mouth-piece supported within easy reach, use of which automatically activates the ventilator. Secure mask ventilation is still required overnight. Anecdotally, appropriate provision of such systems markedly improves adherence to NIV.

Saliva

Bulbar impairment causes difficulty swallowing, with consequent pooling of saliva, choking episodes and drooling. Education on safe swallowing techniques, frequent swallowing, attention to posture and use of suction are helpful. Pooling of watery saliva, combined with impaired airway protection, is particularly problematic when the patient requires NIV as saliva is easily blown into the trachea. This may trigger coughing bouts, contribute to LRTIs and reduce tolerance of NIV. Measures to reduce the volume and increase the viscosity of the saliva include drugs (e.g. glycopyrronium), injection of botulinum toxin into the salivary glands[67] and irradiation of the salivary glands.[68]

In some patients, thick viscous saliva results from dehydration, mouth breathing or over-treatment of excessive thin saliva. Ensuring adequate fluid intake, avoiding dairy products and drinking fruit juice, particularly pineapple and papaya, may help. Mucolytics, such as carbocisteine, and artificial saliva should be considered if the problem persists. If the patient is using NIV, an oronasal mask to prevent mouth-leak and the addition of a heated humidifier should be considered.

Gastrostomy tube placement

In ALS, difficulty swallowing, breathlessness during eating, difficulty feeding and loss of independence may contribute to nutritional depletion. Placement of a gastrostomy tube should be considered if, despite conservative measures, the patient is failing to maintain adequate intake (BMI < 18.5 or 10% weight loss), has great difficulty swallowing such that eating is tiring, or has an unsafe swallow with frequent episodes of aspiration and LRTIs. In cohort studies, patients fed via gastrostomy tubes survive longer than those who decline[69] or are fed via a nasogastric tube.

The traditional approach of PEG tube placement under conscious sedation is associated with a higher complication rate in patients with VC < 50%.[69,70] Early placement of a PEG tube should be considered in patients with rapidly declining respiratory function. In patients with serious respiratory compromise (VC < 50%, $P_I$max or/SNIP < 40% predicted, daytime or nocturnal hypercapnia), radiologically guided insertion of a gastrostomy (RIG) tube may be safer than PEG[71] as sedation is not required, NIV is more easily provided during the procedure, and the patient does not have to lie completely supine. However RIG tubes are smaller and more susceptible to dislodgement, and successful PEG insertion has been described, with avoidance of sedation[72] or use of NIV during the procedure.[73] When NIV is used, air leak may necessitate substantial increases in pressure support and FiO_2. Alternatively, the patient may be briefly intubated and ventilated during PEG insertion and then extubated onto NIV. The approach in individual centres will be strongly influenced by local experience and skill. Regardless of the technique employed, the 30 day mortality is higher than the mortality during the procedure.[70] Diaphragmatic splinting and post-procedure pneumonia contribute to the complication rate; careful post-procedure care is essential.

REFERENCES

1. Louwerse ES, Visser CE, Bossuyt PMM, Weverling GJ. Amyotrophic lateral sclerosis: Mortality risk during the course of the disease and prognostic factors. *J Neurol Sci.* 1997;152:s10–s17.

2. Bourke SC, Williams TL, Bullock RE et al. Non-invasive ventilation in motor neuron disease: Current UK practice. *Amyotroph Lateral Scler Other Motor Neuron Disord.* 2002;3:145–149.
3. Chio A, Logroscino G, Traynor BJ et al. Global epidemiology of amyotrophic lateral sclerosis: A systematic review of the published literature. *Neuroepidemiology.* 2013;41:118–130.
4. Olney RK, Murphy J, Forshew D et al. The effects of executive and behavioral dysfunction on the course of ALS. *Neurology.* 2005;65:1774–1777.
5. Bourke SC, Shaw PJ, Gibson GJ. Respiratory function vs sleep-disordered breathing as predictors of QOL in ALS. *Neurology.* 2001;57:2040–2044.
6. Gay PC, Westbrook PR, Daube JR et al. Effects of alterations in pulmonary function and sleep variables on survival in patients with amyotrophic lateral sclerosis. *Mayo Clin Proc.* 1991;66:686–694.
7. Arnulf I, Similowski T, Salachas F et al. Sleep disorders and diaphragmatic function in patients with amyotrophic lateral sclerosis. *Am J Respir Crit Care Med.* 2000;161:849–856.
8. Schiffman PL, Belsh JM. Pulmonary function at diagnosis of amyotrophic lateral sclerosis. Rate of deterioration. *Chest.* 1993;103:508–513.
9. Fallat RJ, Jewitt B, Bass M et al. Spirometry in amyotrophic lateral sclerosis. *Arch Neurol.* 1979;36:74–80.
10. Fitting J-W, Paillex R, Hirt L, Aebischer P, Schluep M. Sniff nasal pressure: A sensitive respiratory test to assess progression of amyotrophic lateral sclerosis. *Ann Neurol.* 1999;46:887–893.
11. Vender RL, Mauger D, Walsh S et al. Respiratory systems abnormalities and clinical milestones for patients with amyotrophic lateral sclerosis with emphasis upon survival. *Amyotroph Lateral Scler.* 2007;8:36–41.
12. Armon C, Graves MC, Moses D et al. Linear estimates of disease progression predict survival in patients with amyotrophic lateral sclerosis. *Muscle Nerve.* 2000;23:874–882.
13. Desport JC, Preux PM, Truong TC et al. Nutritional status is a prognostic factor for survival in ALS patients. *Neurology.* 1999;53:1059–1059.
14. Morgan RK, McNally S, Alexander M et al. Use of Sniff nasal-inspiratory force to predict survival in amyotrophic lateral sclerosis. *Am J Respir Crit Care Med.* 2005;171:269–274.
15. Stambler N, Charatan M, Cedarbaum JM. Prognostic indicators of survival in ALS. *Neurology.* 1998;50:66–72.
16. Tysnes O, Vollset SE, Larsen JP, Aarli JA. Prognostic factors and survival in amyotrophic lateral sclerosis. *Neuroepidemiology.* 1994;13:226–235.
17. Elamin M, Bede P, Montuschi A et al. Predicting prognosis in amyotrophic lateral sclerosis: A simple algorithm. *J Neurol.* 2015;262:1447–1454.
18. Bourke SC, Bullock RE, Williams TL et al. Noninvasive ventilation in ALS: Indications and effect on quality of life. *Neurology.* 2003;61:171–177.
19. Serisier DE, Mastaglia FL, Gibson GJ. Respiratory muscle function and ventilatory control I in patients with motor neurone disease II in patients with myotonic dystrophy. *QJM.* 1982;51:205–226.
20. Lechtzin N, Shade D, Clawson L, Wiener CM. Supramaximal inflation improves lung compliance in subjects with amyotrophic lateral sclerosis. *Chest.* 2006;129:1322–1329.
21. Lechtzin N, Wiener CM, Shade DM et al. Spirometry in the supine position improves the detection of diaphragmatic weakness in patients with amyotrophic lateral sclerosis. *Chest.* 2002;121:436–442.
22. De Troyer A, Borenstein S, Cordier R. Analysis of lung volume restriction in patients with respiratory muscle weakness. *Thorax.* 1980;35:603–610.
23. Lyall RA, Donaldson N, Polkey MI et al. Respiratory muscle strength and ventilatory failure in amyotrophic lateral sclerosis. *Brain.* 2001;124:2000–13.
24. Hart N, Polkey MI, Sharshar T et al. Limitations of sniff nasal pressure in patients with severe neuromuscular weakness. *J Neurol Neurosurg Psychiatr.* 2003;74:1685–1687.
25. Bourke SC, Tomlinson M, Williams TL et al. Effects of non-invasive ventilation on survival and quality of life in patients with amyotrophic lateral sclerosis: A randomised controlled trial. *Lancet Neurol.* 2006;5:140–147.
26. Poponick JM, Jacobs I, Supinski G, DiMarco AF. Effect of upper respiratory tract infection in patients with neuromuscular disease. *Am J Respir Crit Care Med.* 1997;156:659–664.
27. Bach JR. Amyotrophic lateral sclerosis: Prolongation of life by noninvasive respiratory aids. *Chest.* 2002;122:92–98.
28. Chatwin M, Ross E, Hart N et al. Cough augmentation with mechanical insufflation/exsufflation in patients with neuromuscular weakness. *Eur Respir J.* 2003;21:502–508.
29. Sancho J, Servera E, Diaz J, Marin J. Efficacy of mechanical insufflation-exsufflation in medically stable patients with amyotrophic lateral sclerosis. *Chest.* 2004;125:1400–1405.
30. Rafiq MK, Bradburn M, Proctor AR et al. A preliminary randomized trial of the mechanical insufflator-exsufflator versus breath-stacking technique in patients with amyotrophic lateral sclerosis. *Amyotroph Lateral Scler Frontotemporal Degener.* 2015;16:448–455.
31. National Clinical Guideline Centre (UK). Motor Neurone Disease: Assessment and Management [Internet]. London: National Institute for Health and Care Excellence (UK); 2016 [cited 2016 Jun 13].

(National Institute for Health and Care Excellence: Clinical Guidelines). Available from http://www.ncbi.nlm.nih.gov/books/NBK349620/
32. Aboussouan LS, Khan SU, Meeker DP et al. Effect of noninvasive positive-pressure ventilation on survival in amyotrophic lateral sclerosis. *Ann Intern Med.* 1997;127:450–453.
33. Kleopa KA, Sherman M, Neal B et al. Bipap improves survival and rate of pulmonary function decline in patients with ALS. *J Neurol Sci.* 1999;164:82–88.
34. Mustfa N, Walsh E, Bryant V et al. The effect of noninvasive ventilation on ALS patients and their caregivers. *Neurology.* 2006;66:1211–1217.
35. Aboussouan LS, Khan SU, Banerjee M et al. Objective measures of the efficacy of noninvasive positive-pressure ventilation in amyotrophic lateral sclerosis. *Muscle Nerve.* 2001;24:403–409.
36. Lyall RA, Donaldson N, Fleming T et al. A prospective study of quality of life in ALS patients treated with noninvasive ventilation. *Neurology.* 2001;57:153–156.
37. Pinto AC, Evangelista T, Carvalho M de et al. Respiratory assistance with a non-invasive ventilator (Bipap) in MND/ALS patients: Survival rates in a controlled trial. *J Neurol Sci.* 1995;129:19–26.
38. Newsom-Davis IC, Lyall RA, Leigh PN et al. The effect of non-invasive positive pressure ventilation (NIPPV) on cognitive function in amyotrophic lateral sclerosis (ALS): A prospective study. *J Neurol Neurosurg Psychiatr.* 2001;71:482–487.
39. Baxter SK, Baird WO, Thompson S et al. The use of non-invasive ventilation at end of life in patients with motor neurone disease: A qualitative exploration of family carer and health professional experiences. *Palliat Med.* 2013;27:516–523.
40. Gelinas DF, O'Connor P, Miller RG. Quality of life for ventilator-dependent ALS patients and their caregivers. *J Neurol Sci.* 1998;160:S134–S136.
41. Marchese S, Coco DL, Coco AL. Outcome and attitudes toward home tracheostomy ventilation of consecutive patients: A 10-year experience. *Respir Med.* 2008;102:430–436.
42. Berlowitz DJ, Howard ME, Fiore JF et al. Identifying who will benefit from non-invasive ventilation in amyotrophic lateral sclerosis/motor neurone disease in a clinical cohort. *J Neurol Neurosurg Psychiatr.* 2016;87:280–6.
43. Annane D, Quera-Salva MA, Lofaso F et al. Mechanisms underlying effects of nocturnal ventilation on daytime blood gases in neuromuscular diseases. *Eur Respir J.* 1999;13:157–162.
44. Vrijsen B, Buyse B, Belge C et al. Noninvasive ventilation improves sleep in amyotrophic lateral sclerosis: A prospective polysomnographic study. *J Clin Sleep Med.* 2015;11:559–566.
45. Lo Coco D, Marchese S, Pesco MC et al. Noninvasive positive-pressure ventilation in ALS Predictors of tolerance and survival. *Neurology.* 2006;67:761–765.
46. Farrero E, Prats E, Povedano M et al. Survival in amyotrophic lateral sclerosis with home mechanical ventilation: The impact of systematic respiratory assessment and bulbar involvement. *Chest.* 2005;127:2132–2138.
47. Peysson S, Vandenberghe N, Philit F et al. Factors predicting survival following noninvasive ventilation in amyotrophic lateral sclerosis. *Eur Neurol.* 2008;59:164–171.
48. O'Neill CL, Williams TL, Peel ET et al. Non-invasive ventilation in motor neuron disease: An update of current UK practice. *J Neurol Neurosurg Psychiatr.* 2012;83:371–376.
49. Lechtzin N, Wiener CM, Clawson L et al. Use of noninvasive ventilation in patients with amyotrophic lateral sclerosis. *Amyotroph Lateral Scler Other Motor Neuron Disord.* 2004;5:9–15.
50. Ritsma BR, Berger MJ, Charland DA et al. NIPPV: Prevalence, approach and barriers to use at Canadian ALS centres. *Can J Neurol Sci.* 2010;37:54–60.
51. Tagami M, Kimura F, Nakajima H et al. Tracheostomy and invasive ventilation in Japanese ALS patients: Decision-making and survival analysis: 1990–2010. *J Neurol Sci.* 2014;344:158–164.
52. Bradley MD, Orrell RW, Clarke J et al. Outcome of ventilatory support for acute respiratory failure in motor neurone disease. *J Neurol Neurosurg Psychiatr.* 2002;72:752–756.
53. Vianello A, Arcaro G, Palmieri A et al. Survival and quality of life after tracheostomy for acute respiratory failure in patients with amyotrophic lateral sclerosis. *J Crit Care.* 2011;26(3):329.e7–329.e14.
54. Dreyer P, Lorenzen CK, Schou L, Felding M. Survival in ALS with home mechanical ventilation non-invasively and invasively: A 15-year cohort study in west Denmark. *Amyotroph Lateral Scler Frontotemporal Degener.* 2014;15(1):62–67.
55. Cazzolli PA, Oppenheimer EA. Home mechanical ventilation for amyotrophic lateral sclerosis: Nasal compared to tracheostomy-intermittent positive pressure ventilation. *J Neurol Sci.* 1996;139:123–128.
56. Rousseau M-C, Pietra S, Blaya J, Catala A. Quality of life of ALS and LIS patients with and without invasive mechanical ventilation. *J Neurol.* 2011;258:1801–1804.
57. Bach JR. A comparison of long-term ventilatory support alternatives from the perspective of the patient and care giver. *Chest.* 1993;104:1702–1706.
58. DiPals Writing Committee. Safety and efficacy of diaphragm pacing in patients with respiratory insufficiency due to amyotrophic lateral sclerosis (DiPALS): A multicentre, open-label, randomised controlled trial. *Lancet Neurol.* 2015;14:883-92.

59. Lechtzin N, Scott Y, Busse AM et al. Early use of non-invasive ventilation prolongs survival in subjects with ALS. *Amyotroph Lateral Scler.* 2007;8: 185–188.
60. Perez T, Salachas F. Early nasal ventilation in amyotrophic latéral sclerosis: Impact on survival and quality of life (the VNP-SLA study). *Rev Mal Respir.* 2003;20:589–98.
61. Raphael J-C, Chevret S, Chastang C, Bouvet F. Randomised trial of preventive nasal ventilation in Duchenne muscular dystrophy. *Lancet.* 1994;343:1600–1604.
62. EFNS Task Force on Diagnosis and Management of Amyotrophic Lateral Sclerosis, Andersen PM, Abrahams S, Borasio GD, de Carvalho M, Chio A et al. EFNS guidelines on the clinical management of amyotrophic lateral sclerosis (MALS)—Revised report of an EFNS task force. *Eur J Neurol. 2012*;19:360–75.
63. Gay PC, Edmonds LC. Severe hypercapnia after low-flow oxygen therapy in patients with neuromuscular disease and diaphragmatic dysfunction. *Mayo Clin Proc.* 1995;70:327–330.
64. Servera E, Sancho J, Zafra MJ et al. Alternatives to endotracheal intubation for patients with neuromuscular diseases. *Am J Phys Med Rehabil.* 2005;84:851–857.
65. Vianello A, Bevilacqua M, Arcaro G et al. Non-invasive ventilatory approach to treatment of acute respiratory failure in neuromuscular disorders. A comparison with endotracheal intubation. *Intensive Care Med.* 2000;26:384–390.
66. Vianello A, Corrado A, Arcaro G et al. Mechanical insufflation–exsufflation improves outcomes for neuromuscular disease patients with respiratory tract infections. *Am J Phys Med Rehabil.* 2005;84:83–88.
67. Jackson CE, Gronseth G, Rosenfeld J et al. Randomized double-blind study of botulinum toxin type B for sialorrhea in ALS patients. *Muscle Nerve.* 2009;39:137–143.
68. Neppelberg E, Haugen DF, Thorsen L, Tysnes O-B. Radiotherapy reduces sialorrhea in amyotrophic lateral sclerosis. *Eur J Neurol.* 2007;14:1373–1377.
69. Mazzini L, Corra T, Zaccala M et al. Percutaneous endoscopic gastrostomy and enteral nutrition in amyotrophic lateral sclerosis. *J Neurol.* 1995;242:695–698.
70. Kasarskis EJ, Scarlata D, Hill R et al. A retrospective study of percutaneous endoscopic gastrostomy in ALS patients during the BDNF and CNTF trials. *J Neurol Sci.* 1999;169:118–125.
71. Stavroulakis T, Walsh T, Shaw PJ, McDermott CJ. Gastrostomy use in motor neurone disease (MND): A review, meta-analysis and survey of current practice. *Amyotroph Lateral Scler Front Degener.* 2013;14:96–104.
72. Sarfaty M, Nefussy B, Gross D et al. Outcome of percutaneous endoscopic gastrostomy insertion in patients with amyotrophic lateral sclerosis in relation to respiratory dysfunction. *Amyotroph Lateral Scler Front Degener.* 2013;14:528–32.
73. Sancho J, Servera E, Chiner E et al. Noninvasive respiratory muscle aids during PEG placement in ALS patients with severe ventilatory impairment. *J Neurol Sci.* 2010;297:55–9.

42

Duchenne muscular dystrophy

ANITA K. SIMONDS

INTRODUCTION

Duchenne muscular dystrophy (DMD) is important to the field of non-invasive ventilation (NIV) for several notable reasons. Rideau,[1] one of the pioneers of NIV, first explored nasal delivery in this group in the 1980s, and DMD has become the exemplar for a progressive neuromuscular condition in which management of the respiratory consequences has a marked effect of survival. This is quite different from NIV use in chest wall disease or post-tuberculous lung disease where the precipitating cause is static although the pathophysiological decline has become a vicious cycle. Furthermore, use of NIV in DMD has been a stepping stone to its application in older patients with acquired neuromuscular disease, for example, amyotrophic lateral sclerosis/motor neurone disease, and extension into younger paediatric groups with inherited neuromuscular and neurological conditions.

PATHOPHYSIOLOGY

DMD is due to deficiency of the sarcolemmal related protein, dystrophin. The dystrophin gene on the X chromosome is huge, being the largest gene described in humans so far. Its genomic sequence makes up about 1.5% of the human genome. The size of the dystrophin gene makes it more liable to mutations, most of which affect the muscle isoform leading to DMD or Becker muscular dystrophy (BMD).[2,3] There are several other isoforms of the gene that are expressed in the brain or cardiac muscle. Dystrophin is a rod-shaped protein that, at a cellular level, interacts at the sarcolemma with integral membrane proteins (dystroglycans, syntrophin and dystrobrevin complexes) to form the dystrophin–glycoprotein complex. The key role of this complex is to stabilise the sarcolemma and protect muscle fibres from contraction-related damage. This may explain why while dystrophin has been shown to be absent even by the second trimester in affected fetuses, the cumulative consequences of mechanical damage do not become evident until the child is several years old. As there is no evidence of the disease or muscular weakness at birth, strictly speaking, DMD is not a congenital muscular dystrophy.

Deletions in the gene occur in about 60%–65% of DMD and BMD patients, duplications are rarer and range from 5% to 15%. Although deletions can arise anywhere in the dystrophin gene, the two commonest deletion 'hotspots' are in the central part of the gene and toward the end. Interestingly, there is no relationship whatsoever between the size of the deletion and phenotypic impact; for example, very large deletions that involve up to 50% of the gene may result in mild Becker variants. The phenotype depends instead on whether the deletion or duplication affects the reading frame of the dystrophin gene. As described by Muntoni et al.,[3] mutations that maintain the reading frame (in-frame) tend to result in abnormal but partly functional dystrophin. If the deletion or duplication disrupts the reading frame (frame-shift), unstable RNA results, leading to the production of virtually undetectable levels of abnormal protein.[3] It is thought that dystropin levels of 30%–60% are needed to preserve muscle strength.

The brain and retina are also affected by lack of dystrophin. Results are somewhat variable, however, and can range from very occasional severe retardation to less severe effects. The overall IQ in DMD is about 1 standard deviation below the mean and there is some evidence of preferential effect on verbal memory. However, there is no evidence that intellectual impairment is progressive or correlated with the severity or duration of the muscle disease. There are a few rare mutations that cause cardiac muscle involvement alone (X-linked cardiomyopathy). Cardiac involvement in typical DMD is discussed below.

CLINICAL COURSE

Clinically, the consequences of DMD are first seen in early childhood: 50% of DMD children do not walk until 18 months and 25% are only walking by the age of 2 years.[4] Parents are often alerted by a waddling gait, tendency to fall and pseudohypertrophy of calf muscles. About 20% of cases are diagnosed by the age of 2 years and 75% by 4 years, but phenotypically there is wide variation.[5] On average, patients required a wheelchair for mobility by the age of 10–12 years, but the introduction of steroid therapy and walking orthoses have extended the period individuals can remain ambulant. This is important as about 50% of DMD cases develop a scoliosis and progression of spinal curvature is associated with increasing muscle weakness and the adolescent growth spurt. If steroid therapy reduces the decline in muscle strength, there will be less overlap with growth spurt, and scoliosis (and impact on chest wall restriction) should be less marked. For example, in one non-randomised study[6] of boys matched for age and pulmonary function at baseline, a scoliosis of >20° occurred in 67% of the control group but only 17% of the steroid (deflazacort)-treated group. These factors may feed into better peak lung function and ultimately better survival, although there have been no definitive randomised controlled trials of steroid therapy. The distribution of muscle involvement in DMD is relatively characteristic. Overall, lower limbs are affected more than upper limbs and proximal muscles more than distal groups. Preferential involvement of the sternomastoids, latissimus dorsi, glutei and quadriceps is usually seen. Inspiratory and expiratory muscles are usually similarly affected (unlike spinal muscular atrophy where early expiratory muscle weakness may be seen). Facial, buccal, sphincter and swallowing muscles are only involved late in the course of the disease. Indeed, old textbooks report that swallowing muscles are 'never affected', but this was the case before ventilatory support had produced long-term survival and late complications (see below). Progression in muscle weakness is not linear, and there may be periods of apparent arrest in the course of the disease. Once individuals are using wheelchairs full-time, contractures of the hips, knees and elbows can occur with a talipes equinovarus, and typical frog-leg posture. The evolution of lung function changes in DMD falls into three stages.[7] In the first stage, during the first decade or so, forced vital capacity (FVC) increases as predicted; in the second phase, lung volumes plateau as inspiratory muscle weakness scoliosis becomes manifest; and in the final phase, FVC initially falls slowly and then may decline by as much as 250 mL/year. Peak vital capacity in the absence of ventilatory support is a prognostic factor in that a peak vital capacity of less than 1.2 L was associated with average age of death at 15.3 years and those with a peak vital capacity in excess of 1.7 L survived to an average of 21 years. With ventilatory support, it is now possible to support individuals with an unrecordably low VC for many years, but peak vital capacity is still likely to be a prognostic marker and indicates whether NIV is likely to be needed sooner rather than later. Assessment with sleep studies is important as the first signs of ventilatory compromise are seen during sleep. Rapid eye movement (REM)–related hypoventilation tends to occur when vital capacity is less than 60% predicted and hypoventilation progresses to non-REM sleep and ultimately daytime ventilatory failure[8] unless that pathophysiological sequence is addressed (see below). The clinical course is frequently punctuated by chest infections due to weakness of inspiratory muscles and reduced cough efficacy due to decreased expiratory muscle strength. Cardiac involvement takes the form of conduction defects or left ventricular disease. A cardiomyopathy may involve the right ventricle, but since the advent of effective respiratory support, cor pulmonale is unheard of. There is no correlation between extent of cardiomyopathy and limb muscle weakness in young children. Nigro et al.[9] found preclinical evidence of cardiac disease in 25% DMD under the age of 6 years and almost 60% between the ages of 6 and 10 years. Clinically apparent cardiac involvement in this series was present in all patients by the age of 18 years and 72% of the patients were symptomatic. Although not conclusively demonstrated, NIV may alter the course of cardiomyopathy as fewer patients seem to be symptomatic in current cohorts, although this may reflect early use of angiotensin-converting enzyme (ACE) inhibitor drugs[10] and beta-blockers.

EVIDENCE BASE FOR NIV

The outlook for DMD patients without ventilatory support is very poor. With an FVC of less than 1 L, the 5-year survival is 8%.[11] In the 1970s and 1980s, DMD patients were treated with tracheostomy ventilation, although it is difficult to compare results with studies done today. While there has been no randomised controlled study of NIV in DMD, Vianello et al.[12] compared the 2-year course in hypercapnic patients who received NIV and those who did not. All NIV recipients survived, whereas 4/5 who did not receive NIV died. In a single-centre cohort treated with NIV, once they had become hypercapnic during the day, 1-year and 5-year survival rates were 85% and 73%, respectively.[13] This compares with an earlier trial[14] in which asymptomatic patients with vital capacity between 20% and 50% predicted were randomised to NIV or a control group in order to see whether NIV halted the decline in lung function. The results showed no impact on lung function; moreover, there were excess deaths in the NIV group. This trial has been criticised on the grounds that cardiological function was significantly worse in the NIV limb, families were given no advice about use of NIV or other techniques for secretion clearance and families in the control group were also aware that NIV was available should respiratory problems occur, and so they might have sought help earlier. Furthermore, patients did not undergo sleep studies, so it is unclear whether sleep-disordered breathing was present, although it would be expected in at least a proportion with vital capacity in the 20%–50% range. Even taking into account these factors, there are no good grounds to recommend NIV as preventive therapy in asymptomatic DMD boys with no evidence of nocturnal hypoventilation.

To clarify this point, another randomised controlled trial[15] explored use of NIV at an intermediate stage, that is, in patients with nocturnal hypoventilation but daytime normocapnia. Subjects were mixed and did not solely comprise those with DMD. However, results in the control

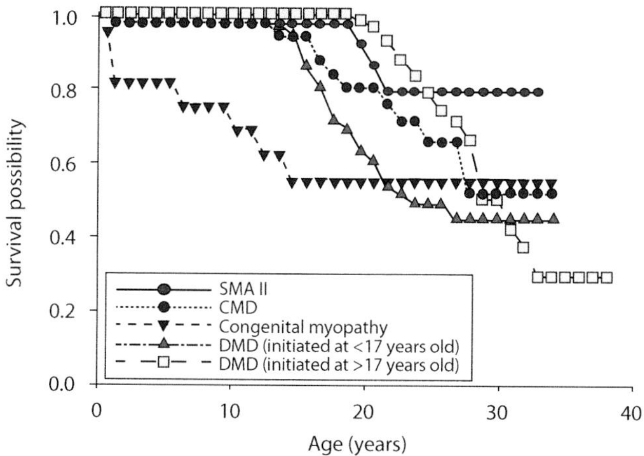

Figure 42.1 Survival probability in patients with DMD using NIV compared to other neuromuscular disorders (spinal muscular atrophy type II, SMA II, and congenital muscular dystrophy, CMD). (From Chatwin M et al. *PLoS One.* 2015; doi:10.1371/journal.pone.0125839.)

(non-NIV) group showed that virtually all patients who had nocturnal hypoventilation became hypercapnic within the following 12–24 months. Nocturnal blood gas tensions and quality of life measures improved in the group randomised to NIV, but deteriorated in controls. This provides evidence that the best time to introduce NIV is at the stage of symptomatic nocturnal hypoventilation. Eagle et al.[16] have shown the impact of NIV on successive cohorts of DMD patients.

A more recent survival study[17] examining the long-term impact of NIV in childhood and transition to adulthood showed longer trends in survival. Not surprisingly, prognosis is less good in those Duchenne patients who started on NIV at age less than 17 years (a more severely affected group) than those older than 17 years (Figure 42.1). Around a third of the total cohort (n = 151) are living into their 30s and above.

QUALITY OF LIFE

Kohler et al.[18] evaluated health-related quality of life in DMD patients using the Medical Outcome Survey Short Form 36. While physical function was reduced with age as expected, domains representing general and mental health, emotional health, social function and pain were not reduced and were near values in populations without chronic illness. Despite a greater reduction in pulmonary function and activities of daily living, individuals receiving NIV had similar health-related quality of life scores to those who did not need ventilator support. In addition, Bach and team[19] have shown consistently that life satisfaction in DMD is rated as good and may be underestimated by observers, but there can be major psychosocial pressures on parents and siblings. These are often exacerbated by frustrations over practical issues such as housing, transportation, seating, electric beds and availability of caregivers (see burden of care below). It is always important to keep a focus on the family as well as the patient. Getting the ventilator settings right is but a small part of the overall care plan.

Titration of ventilator settings

Most teams titrate ventilator settings to overnight monitoring. Oximetry and transcutaneous carbon dioxide monitoring are helpful. Leaks often fragment sleep by causing arousals. More detailed polysomnography studies are required if problems cannot be solved by simpler monitoring or symptoms persist despite apparent good overnight control of ventilation. Ramsay et al.[20] evaluated the effects of patient–ventilator asynchrony (assessed using monitoring of parasternal muscle electromyogram) on overnight arterial blood gas control with NIV in a group with NMD. While triggering and cycling asynchronies were common, these were not a determinant of ineffective ventilation, although effects on sleep quality may be more subtle.

TECHNICAL CONSIDERATIONS

Ventilators

Early studies used volume ventilators in the main, but more recently, pressure support ventilation has been widely used in neuromuscular groups.[21] In truth, neuromuscular patients are relatively easy to ventilate; however, expiratory positive airway pressure (EPAP) in bilevel devices may be helpful in reducing tendency to upper airway collapse, recruiting functional residual capacity and dealing with atelectasis. Increasing EPAP, say, from 5 to 7 cmH_2O, may be helpful in these situations, especially when atelectasis complicates an acute chest infection.[22] Bilevel NIV use may also improve cardiac function by offloading the left ventricle, but this effect is difficult to separate out from improvement in PaO_2 and PCO_2 that is also likely to occur.

Volume ventilators have the advantage in that they can be used to help the patient breath stack but applying serial tidal volume insufflations. However, this function can also be achieved by using an Ambu bag with one-way valve or cough insufflator–exsufflator (see Chapter 70).

Patients with neuromuscular disease can be prone to gastric bloating, which can be reduced by adjusting sleeping position or decreasing IPAP level. Usually, bilevel ventilators are less likely to provoke gastric bloating than volume ventilators. Importantly, most Duchenne patients wish to get out and about during the day. Ventilators must be suitable to fit beneath a wheelchair and have long-term battery power. Battery power is also crucial as patients become more dependent on ventilation to manage risks such as power failures/disruptions in power supplies and practicalities such as the transfer of patients on NIV, for example, to hospital or between hospital wards.

New ventilator modes

Newer ventilatory modes that combine a delivered target volume with bilevel positive pressure are now available, for example, AVAPS (average volume assured pressure support) and IVAPS (intelligent volume assured pressure support).

While these may have some advantages in selected cases over standard pressure support – for example, one study showed shorter stage 1 sleep on IVAPS, suggesting that patients fell asleep quicker,[23] and another showed better adherence[24] – there is no evidence that these combination modes should supersede standard practice.

Interfaces

There are a number of important considerations when choosing interfaces. Leaks can be problematical because of facial characteristics and inability to close the mouth due to weakness or jaw contractures. Furthermore, to retain independence where possible, neuromuscular patients wish to place their own mask. This is often not possible in Duchenne patients as upper limb strength is lost. If a full face mask is used and the patient cannot remove it himself, there is a theoretical risk of inhalation if the patient vomits, although in practice, this seems rare and choices should be made balancing the risk of aspiration against consequences of leaks and inadequate ventilation.

Decision making should also be recorded in the patient's notes. Use of a mask may also limit the patient's ability to communicate and so consideration should be given to additional means of communication such as a buzzer at night.

Daytime NIV

Oral delivery of NIV in neuromuscular disease has a long track record.[19] Toussaint et al.[25] have explored the use of mouthpiece NIV during the day, having established this in patients already on nocturnal NIV but in whom uncontrolled hypercapnia is occurring during the day due to progression of disease. This is simply assessed by daytime transcutaneous carbon dioxide measurements. Initially, PCO_2 control and symptom relief can be achieved by short top-ups of NIV in the day, for example, an hour after lunch or coming home from college in the evening. If that is not sufficient, then NIV via a mouthpiece (supported with a headstand) can be helpful, provided the individual has neck power to turn to access the mouthpiece as needed.

The Belgian group[25] showed that mouthpiece ventilation in their cohort was introduced on average 4.1 to 2.5 years after initiation of nocturnal NIV, and 1-, 3-, 5- and 7-year survival rates from initiation were 88%, 77%, 58% and 51%, respectively. Symptoms resolved, and in six out of seven patients, swallowing function also improved. Increasing daytime NIV is often required once vital capacity drops below around 400 mL.

Tracheostomy ventilation

The proportion of DMD patients receiving non-invasive and invasive ventilation varies considerably from country to country. The main indications for tracheostomy ventilation are listed in Box 42.1. There have been comparisons of pulmonary morbidity in DMD groups on tracheostomy invasive positive pressure support (T-IPPV) and NIV showing less pulmonary morbidity and hospitalisations than in those on NIV.[26] These comparisons are fraught in that groups may not be comparable.

BOX 42.1: Indications for tracheostomy ventilation in DMD

- Swallowing dysfunction with recurrent aspiration
- Failure to thrive using NIV
- Intractable upper airway or interface problems
- Failure to wean after acute episode of respiratory decompensation
- Patient preference

However, Soudon et al.[27] showed worse morbidity in the full-time tracheostomy ventilated group (mucus hypersecretions and tracheal injury), although nutritional supplementation was needed more frequently in the NIV group, who were younger. In many centres now, most DMD patients are on NIV with T-IPPV reserved for those with swallowing issues that cannot be resolved with a combination of NIV, cough assistance and gastrostomy (PEG) feeding. The care package for those with a tracheostomy is inevitably more complex[28] and there is a risk of other complications such as tracheal haemorrhage. In a small but comprehensive study of DMD patients on 24-hour non-invasive ventilatory support, McKim et al.[29] showed this to be a safe alternative to tracheostomy ventilation with a median survival of 5.7 years (range, 0.17 to 12 years).

TRANSITIONAL CARE

Transition from paediatric to adult care is an important issue for DMD patients as problems with sleep-disordered breathing are likely to be developing in the mid-teenage years. Ideally, paediatric and adult care can be carried out in the same institution, but if not, a gradual planned handover helps both the boys and their parents and is likely to reduce unplanned admissions. Paediatric care is often more multidisciplinary than adult care and so exact team plans may be difficult to replicate. However, cardiology, respiratory, physiotherapy, occupational therapy and nutritional support are vital. Neurological input is helpful and new orthopaedic issues may arise (see below). Psychological support for the family needs to meet individual requirements, with the young Duchenne patient gradually encouraged to assume an increasing role in decision making. Social networking will inevitably play an increasing role.

LONG-TERM FINDINGS

Complications

With improved survival and reduced respiratory morbidity and mortality, the natural history of DMD has changed with many living into their late 20s and 30s.[16,17,30,31] More young men now die of cardiomyopathy. Cardiosurveillance should occur twice yearly from diagnosis, and then from the age of 10 years once a year with echo and electrocardiography (ECG), together with 24-hour monitoring if required.[32] In many protocols, an ACE inhibitor is added once left ventricular fractional shortening falls below 28% and a beta-blocker is then added to stabilise the heart rate.[32,33] Up-titration of cardiac medication should be pursued in accordance with echocardiography results, bearing in mind that hypotensive effects may be more marked in DMD. Brain natriuretic peptide (BNP) measurement may be helpful and useful to assess any left ventricular contribution to decompensation at the time of chest infections.

Osteoporosis may add to orthopaedic problems, particularly in young men who have received steroid therapy, and vitamin D levels should be regularly assessed. In young patients in their late 20s and 30s we have seen an increased incidence of bowel pseudo-obstruction exacerbated by weakness of abdominal muscles to expel bowel motions, and renal/urinary calculi and urinary retention. It is not clear in these patients whether there is an additional smooth muscle involvement. Most patients can tolerate surgery with careful specialist management and use of NIV in the perioperative period. There is a consensus document[34] on perioperative care, which is essential reading for teams managing these patients. A list of complications in older DMD patients is given in Box 42.2.

SUPPORTIVE CARE, PALLIATION OF SYMPTOMS AND PROGRESSIVE CARE PLANS

Although survival has been extended, ultimately, most DMD patients become ventilator dependent for most of the day and night by their late 20s or 30s. Orthopaedic and back pain and worsening cardiomyopathy require comprehensive treatment and symptom relief, and more frequent chest infections can complicate the course. Symptom palliation is key and of course there is no contraindication to pain relief including opiates for severe discomfort as ventilator settings can be adjusted to control PCO_2. Muscle pain and nerve root pain may be helped by a range of drugs including baclofen and pregabalin. In our experience, most DMD patients wish to have full supportive measures when resuscitation choices are discussed until a very late stage, but this is of course an individual decision. All young men should be invited to take part in decision making at an age and emotionally appropriate time. When providing information about outcomes and choice, it is important to provide written information for patients to take away and digest, as verbal memory problems may limit understanding and recollection of discussions. When individuals with DMD are admitted to a hospital that has few such patients and limited experience with DMD, it is vital to liaise with specialist centres and transfer must be carried out if required to reduce any tendency to nihilism.

Standards of care

There are consensus documenents[32,33,35–37] for the respiratory and wider multidisciplinary management of DMD children and adults, but in practice, care including respiratory support for DMD patients is variable. Parents and families are not always informed about ventilatory options and discussion may occur too late,[38] increasing the risk of uncontrolled decompensation.

As the natural history is clear, it should be possible to plan the timing of initiation of therapy around the patient and family.[15] In selected stable patients, outpatient initiation

BOX 42.2: Complications in long-term DMD survivors

System	Complication	Management
Bowel	Pseudo-obstruction, volvulus	May settle with conservative measures or require surgical intervention
Joints	Back, hip, shoulder and large joint pain, worsening contractures	Analgesia, palliative care, orthotics, supportive wheelchair seat mould, orthopaedic surgical advice
Bone	Fractures, osteoporosis	Check vitamin D level and supplement as needed, bone surveillance
Renal/urinary	Renal and bladder calculi	Urological advice
Vascular	Deep venous thrombosis, vascular insufficiency lower limbs	Doppler studies and anticoaguation as required
Cardiology	Cardiomyopathy inevitable, but beware tachy-bradyarrhythmias	Cardiosurveillance – regular echocardiogram and 24-hour (or more detailed) ECG monitoring
Mood	Anxiety, depression	Regular assessment and psychological input and therapy as required

of NIV may be as effective as inpatient initiation and more convenient for families.[39] In one UK report,[40] 67% of parents rated their local medical care as poor to really poor, and 68% of parents did not feel well informed – although this varied considerably from region to region, and in some areas, patients and families were content with care. This variability probably represents care provision elsewhere in Europe. It is clear that in a complex and evolving condition such as DMD, NIV is one part of the management, and a multidisciplinary, informed, shared care approach is vital.[32,36]

NEW THERAPEUTIC APPROACHES IN DMD

These approaches can be classified for ease into four main groups: gene therapy, drugs, cell therapy and mutation specific (Box 42.3). Delivery of the dystrophin gene is limited by its large size, but animal trials are progressing in the delivery of microdystrophin. Drug therapy included anti-inflammatory medication (e.g. steroids), antifibrotic agents (e.g. idebenone), vasodilators and those that increase muscle mass (e.g. myostatin inhibitors or the myotstain receptor drug Acceleron) or agents that upregulate utrophin. Cell therapy approaches include stem cell therapy with myoblasts or mesangioblasts, but targeting of these cells to muscles throughout the body is problematical. Mutation-specific trials will only work in subsets of DMD patients, and the areas of interest are exon-skipping and stop codon intervention.[41] Several of the most relevant recent human trials in these areas are considered below.

BOX 42.3: New therapeutic possibilities in DMD

Option	Comment
Gene therapy	For example, via viral vector. Dystropin is a very large gene; therefore, animal work on microdystrophin delivery – at early stage
Anti-inflammatory agents	Prednisolone, deflazacort
Antifibrotic agent	Idebenone
Vasodilators and agents affecting muscle mass	Myostatin inhibitors
Cell therapy	Stem cell injections; myoblasts, mesangiobalsts, autologous bone marrow cells. Difficult to target to all muscles, work at early stage
Upregulation of other proteins	Utropin
Mutation specific: exon skipping and stop codon drugs	Stop codon: e.g., Ataluren Exon skipping antisense oligoncleotides: e.g., Eteplirsen

Idebenone: As indicated above, steroid therapy can slow the decline in muscle strength in DMD and increase duration of ambulation, but side effects are common and responses are variable. Buyse et al.[42] examined the efficacy of idebenone in a double-blind randomised controlled study ('Delos' trial) in DMD patients aged 10–18 years using a primary endpoint of peak expiratory flow rate. Idebenone is a strong antifibrotic antioxidant, which inhibits lipid peroxidation and stimulates mitochondrial and cellular energy production. The authors found that idebenone reduced the fall in peak expiratory flow (PEF) compared to the placebo group at 1 year. Favourable trends were also seen in FVC and FEV1. A post hoc analysis[43] showed more bronchopulmonary adverse events and greater cumulative use of antibiotics in the placebo arm, indicating that small pulmonary function gains with idebenone were translated into clinical benefit. However, these results were most pronounced in those with more advanced lung disease, and it is not clear whether physiotherapy management was standardised or the need for ventilatory support was assessed.

Stop codon gene modification: Ataluren is a small-molecule drug that is used to suppress stop codons in patients with nonsense mutations. Safety and tolerability were confirmed in a phase IIa study in which an increase in dystrophin of 11.1% and a decrease in creatinine kinase was seen. In a phase 2b study,[44] an increase in the 6-min walking test marginally above the minimally clinically important difference of 30 m was found. This has led to European Medicines Agency (EMA) conditional approval and National Institute for Clinical Excellence approval of Ataluren in the United Kingdom for use in DMD children with a nonsense mutation who are over the age of 5 years and remain ambulant.

Exon skipping drugs (antisense oligonucleotides) can restore frame-shifting mutations back into frame and therefore rescue dystrophin production. Eteplirsen has shown small benefits on disease progression[45] and is going through an accelerated Food and Drug Administration (FDA) approval process, but recently, another antisense drug, Drisapersen, failed FDA approval and has been withdrawn due to safety concerns.[46]

It is important to note that these gene modifiers are only suitable for individuals with specific mutations and have been evaluated in young ambulant children before the development of ventilatory insufficiency, over relatively short periods of time. Improvements in exercise tolerance are so far small, and the long-term impact on respiratory muscle strength is unclear. It is likely that ventilatory support for older patients will be required for the foreseeable future, and continued in conjunction with emerging therapies.

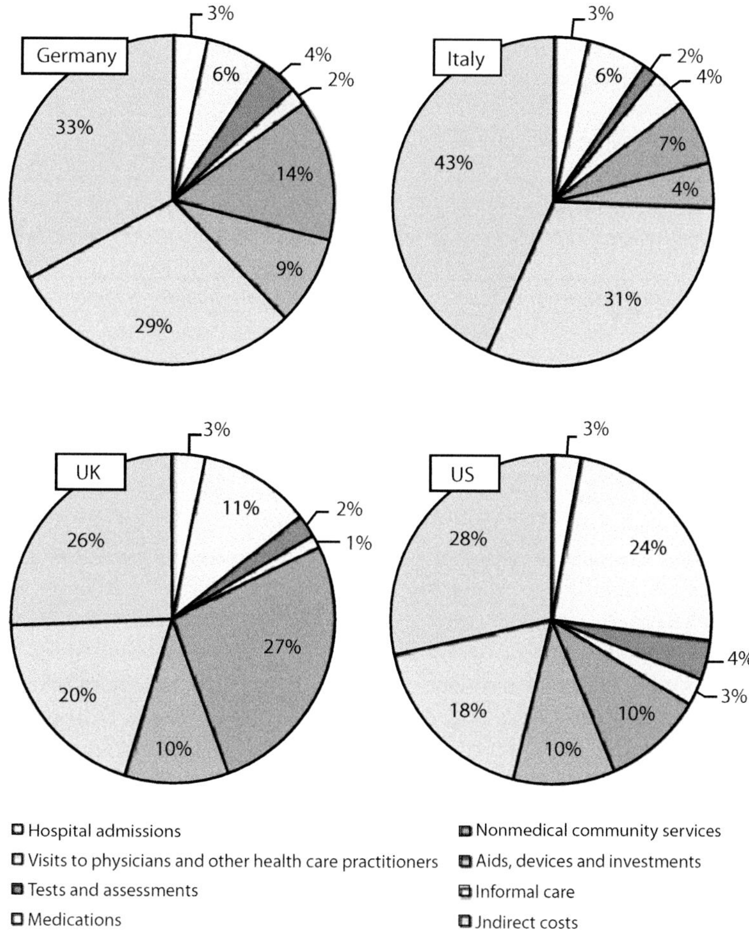

Figure 42.2 Components of estimated annual cost of DMD in Germany, Italy, UK and the United States. (From Landfeldt et al. *Neurology.* 2014;83:529–36.)

Social considerations

The economic burden of DMD has been considered in an international cross-sectional study comparing patient groups in Germany, Italy, the United Kingdom and the United States (n = 770)[47] via the TREAT-MD registry. A range of age groups was included, and ventilation was supported in 24%–41% of patients. A breakdown of annual costs across the four countries is shown in Figure 42.2. Mean per-patient annual direct cost was estimated to be between 23,920 and 54,270 US dollars, which represents a multiple of 7–16 times the mean per-capita expenditure. Indirect and informal costs were high at between 18% and 43% of total costs. Not surprisingly, the majority of caregivers were mothers of patients and overall participation in the workforce of patients was low at <4%, while between 27% and 49% of caregivers had stopped working, or had reduced working hours because of care responsibilities. This work excludes costs of newer therapeutic drugs.

Of course, early curative or disease-modifying therapies, although expensive to develop, could significantly reduce downstream costs. These burdens and costs also relate to the patients and caregivers participating in trials of emerging therapies. Peay et al.[48] assessed priorities and preferences in these groups when taking part in trials. She found that caregivers were prepared to accept serious risks to their affected children when balanced against non-curative treatment that slows or stops muscle weakness, in the absence of increase in survival. Further work in this area should inform the benefit–risk assessments of regulatory authorities (FDA and EMA), clinical trialists and ethics committees, and importantly enhance patient and family engagement in the advocacy process.

REFERENCES

1. Rideau Y, Janoski LW, Grellet G. Respiratory function in the muscular dystrophies. *Muscle Nerve.* 1981;4:155–64.
2. Mercuri E, Muntoni F. Muscular dystrophies. *Lancet.* 2013;381:845–60.
3. Muntoni F, Torelli S, Ferlini A. Dystrophin and mutations: One gene, several proteins, multiple phenotypes. *Lancet Neurol.* 2003;2:731–8.

4. Emery AEH. Duchenne muscular dystrophy or Meryon's disease. In: Emery AEH, editor. *The Muscular Dystrophies*. 1st edition. Oxford: Oxford University Press, 2001:55–71.
5. Desguerre D, Christov C, Mayer M et al. Clinical heterogeneity of Duchenne muscular dystrophy (DMD): Definition by sub-phenotypes and predictive criteria by long term follow-up. *PLoS One*. 2009;4:e4347.
6. Alman BA, Raza SN, Biggar WDB. Steroid treatment and the development of scoliosis in males with Duchenne Muscular Dystrophy. *J Bone Joint Surg*. 2004;86:519–24.
7. Baydur A, Gilgoff I, Prentice W et al. Decline in respiratory function and experience with long term assisted ventilation in advanced Duchenne's muscular dystrophy. *Chest*. 1990;97:884–9.
8. Ragette R, Mellies U, Schwake C et al. Patterns and predictors of sleep disordered breathing in primary myopathies. *Thorax*. 2002;57:724–8.
9. Nigro G, Coni LI, Politano L, Bain RJI. The incidemce and evolution of cardiomyopthy in Duchenne muscular dystrophy. *Int J Cardiol*. 1990;26:271–7.
10. Duboc D, Meaune C, Lerebours G et al. Effect of perindopril on the onset and progression of left ventricular dysfunction in Duchenne muscular dystrophy. *J Am Coll Cardiol*. 2005;45:855–7.
11. Phillips MF, Smith PE, Carroll N et al. Nocturnal oxygenation and prognosis in Duchenne muscular dystrophy. *Am J Respir Crit Care Med*. 1999; 160:198–202.
12. Vianello A, Bevilacqua M, Salvador V et al. Long-term nasal intermittent positive pressure ventilation in advanced Duchenne's Muscular Dystrophy. *Chest*. 1994;105:445–8.
13. Simonds A.K, Muntoni F, Heather S, Fielding S. Impact of nasal ventilation on survival in hypercapnic Duchenne muscular dystrophy. *Thorax*. 1998;53:949–52.
14. Raphael J-C, Chevret S, Chastang C et al. A prospective multicentre study of home mechanical ventilation in Duchenne de Boulogne muscular dystrophy. *Eur Respir Rev*. 1992;2:312–6.
15. Ward SA, Chatwin M, Heather S, Simonds AK. Randomised controlled trial of non-invasive ventilation (NIV) for nocturnal hypoventilation in neuromuscular and chest wall disease patients with daytime normocapnia. *Thorax*. 2005;60:1019–24.
16. Eagle M, Baudouin S, Chandler C et al. Survival in Duchenne muscular dystrophy: Improvements in life expectancy since 1967 and the impact of home nocturnal ventilation. *Neuromusc Disord*. 2002;12:926–9.
17. Chatwin M, Tan LB, Bush A et al. Long term non-invasive ventilation in children: Impact on survival and transition to adult care. *PLoS One*. 2015; doi:10.1371/journal.pone.0125839.
18. Kohler M, Clarenbach CF, Boni L et al. Quality of life, physical disability, and respiratory impairment in Duchenne muscular dystrophy. *Am J Resp Crit Care Med*. 2005;172:1032–6.
19. Bach JR, Campagnolo DI, Hoeman S. Life satisfaction of individuals with Duchenne muscular dystrophy using long-term mechanical ventilatory support. *Am J Phys Med Rehabil*. 1991;70:129–35.
20. Ramsay M, Mandal S, Suh E-S et al. Parasternal electromyography to determine the relationship between patient–ventilator asynchrony and nocturnal gas exchange during home mechanical ventilation set-up. *Thorax*. 2015; doi:10.1136/thoraxjnl-2015-206944.
21. Lloyd-Owen SJ, Donaldson GC, Ambrosino N et al. Patterns of home mechanical use in Europe: Results from the Eurovent survey. *Eur Respir J*. 2005;25:1025–31.
22. Simonds AK. Patient with acute hypercapnic respiratory failure and neuromuscular or chest wall disease. In: Simonds AK, editor. *ERS Practical Handbook of Noninvasive Ventilation*. 1st edition. Sheffield: ERS Publications, 2015:49–55.
23. Jaye J, Chatwin M, Dayer M et al. Autotitrating versus standard noninvasive ventilation: A randomised crossover trial. *Eur Respir J*. 2009;33:566–73.
24. Kelly JL, Jaye J, Pickersgill RE et al. Randomized trial of 'intelligent' autotitrating ventilation versus standard pressure support non-invasive ventilation: Impact on adherence and physiological measures. *Respirology*. 2014;19:596–603.
25. Toussaint M, Steens M, Wasteels G, Soudon P. Diurnal ventilation via mouthpiece: Survival in end-stage Duchenne patients. *Eur Respir J*. 2006;28:549–55.
26. Bach JR, Ishikawa Y, Kim H. Prevention of pulmonary morbidity for patients with Duchenne muscular dystrophy. *Chest*. 1998;112:1024–8.
27. Soudon P, Steens M, Toussaint M. A comparison on invasive versus noninvasive fulltime mechanical ventilation in Duchenne muscular dystrophy. *Chronic Resp Dis*. 2008;5:87–93.
28. Simonds AK. Discharging the ventilator-dependent patient and the home ventilatory care network. In: Simonds AK, editor. *Non-invasive Respiratory Support. A Practical Handbook*. 3rd edition. London: Edward Arnold, 2007:229–48.
29. McKim DA, Griller N, LeBlanc C, Woolnough A. Twenty-four hour noninvasive ventilation in Duchenne muscular dystrophy: A safe alternative to tracheostomy. *Can Resp J*. 2013;e5–e9.
30. Jeppesen J, Green A, Steffensen BF, Rahbek J. The Duchenne muscular dystrophy population in Denmark, 1977–2001: Prevalence, incidence and survival in relation to the introduction of ventilator use. *Neuromusc Disord*. 2003; 13:804–12.

31. Chatwin M, Tan H-L, Bush A et al. Long term non-invasive ventilation in children: Impact on survival and transition to adult care. *PLoS One.* 2015; doi:10.1371/journal.pone.0125839.
32. Bushby K, Bourke J, Bullock R et al. The multidisciplinary management of Duchenne muscuar dystrophy. *Curr Paediatr.* 2005;15:292–300.
33. Bushby K, Finkel R, Case LE et al. Diagnosis and management of Duchenne muscular dystophy, part 1 diagnosis, pharmacological and pyschosocial management. *Lancet Neurol.* 2010;9:77–93.
34. Birnkrant DJ, Panitch HB, Benditt JO et al. American College of Chest Physicians Consensus Statement on the Respiratory and related management of patients with Duchenne muscular dystrophy undergoing anesthesia or sedation. *Chest.* 2007;132:1977–86.
35. Finder J, Birnkrant D, Carl J et al. ATS Consensus Statement: Respiratory care of the patient with Duchenne muscular dystrophy. *Am J Resp Crit Care Med.* 2004;170:456–65.
36. Bushby K, Finkel R, Birnkrant DJ et al. Diagnosis and management of Duchenne muscular dystrophy, part 2: Implementation of multidisciplinary care. *Lancet Neurol.* 2010;9:177–89.
37. Road J, McKim DA, Avendana M et al. Home Mechanical Ventilation. A Canadian Thoracic Society Clinical Practice Guideline. *Canadian Respiratory Society* 2011.
38. Kinali M, Manzur AY, Gibson BE et al. UK Physicians' attitudes and practices of long term non-invasive ventilation of children with Duchenne muscular dystrophy. *Ped Rehabil.* 2006;9:351–64.
39. Chatwin M, Nickol AH, Morrell MJ et al. Randomised trial of inpatient versus outpatient initiation of home mechanical ventilation in patients with nocturnal hypoventilation. *Respir Med.* 2008;102:1528–35.
40. Action Duchenne. Duchenne Families Standards of Care Consultations. 2009.
41. Hoffman EP, Bronson A, Levin AA et al. Restoring dystrophin expression in Duchenne muscular dystrophy muscle. Progress in exon skipping and stop codon read through. *Am J Pathol.* 2011;179:12–22.
42. Buyse G, Voit T, Schara U et al. Efficiency of idebenone on respiratory function in patients with Duchenne muscular dystrophy not using glucocorticoids (DELOS): A double blind randomised placebo-controlled phase 3 trial. *Lancet.* 2015;385:1748–57.
43. McDonald CM, Meier T, Voit T et al. Idebenone reduces respiratory complications in patients with Duchenne muscular dystrophy. *Neuromusc Disord.* 2016; http://dx.doi.org/10.1016/j.nmd.2016.05.008.
44. Bushby K, Finkel R, Wong B et al. Ataluren treatment of patients with nonsense mutation dystrophinopathy. *Muscle Nerve.* 2014;50:477–87.
45. Mendell JR, Goemans N, Lowes LP et al. Longitudinal effect of eteplirsen versus historical control on ambulation in Duchenne muscular dystrophy. *Ann Neurol.* 2016;79:257–71.
46. Voit T, Topaloglu H, Straub V et al. Safety and efficacy of drisapersen for the treatment of Duchenne muscular dystrophy (DEMAND II): An exploratory, randomised, placebo-controlled phase 2 study. *Lancet Neurol.* 2014;13:987–96.
47. Landfeldt E, Lindgren P, Bell CF et al. The burden of Duchenne muscular dystrophy. *Neurology.* 2014;83:529–36.
48. Peay H, Hollin I, Fischer R, Bridges JFP. A commuity-engaged appraoch to quantifying caregiver preferences for the benefits and risks of emerging therapies for Duchenne muscular dystrophy. *Clin Therapeutics* 2014;36:624–37.

43

Central sleep apnoea

SHAHROKH JAVAHERI AND MARK W. ELLIOTT

KEY MESSAGES

- Central sleep apnoea (CSA) is a heterogeneous condition with a number of very different causes.
- The mechanism depends on the cause.
- There are a number of patterns, the most distinctive of which is the crescendo–decrescendo pattern, unique to heart failure.
- Patients with 'idiopathic' CSA should be investigated for the presence of asymptomatic cardio- and cerebrovascular disease.
- There are little data from randomised clinical trials to inform treatment but usually requires positive pressure ventilation.

INTRODUCTION

Central sleep apnoea (CSA) occurs in association with a number of conditions[1] (Table 43.1), but no matter what the cause, the failure of respiratory rhythmogenesis is the neurophysiological basis. This results in the loss of activation of inspiratory pump muscles and cessation of oronasal airflow into the lungs. Polygraphically, oronasal airflow is best measured by a combination of a pressure probe and a temperature-sensitive probe. Classifying an apnoea accurately as central requires that both probes and thoraco-abdominal excursions be flat for at least 10 s or longer.

Central apnoea may occur during normal sleep, but the number of such events is limited. Under normal circumstances, these events occur with sleep onset, after an arousal and sometimes during rapid eye movement (REM) sleep (these events are referred to as physiological CSA), and discussion of the mechanisms of this is beyond the scope of this review but is discussed elsewhere.[1]

There are many causes of CSA. Table 43.1 shows the various physiological and pathological conditions associated with CSA.[1] These disorders are classified by aetiology and/or according to arterial PCO_2 (hypercapnic and hypocapnic). Arbitrarily, to be considered abnormal, the central apnoea index (CAI) should be ≥5 per hour of sleep. In heart failure, the most common cause of CSA in the general population, we arbitrarily chose an apnoea–hypopnoea index (AHI) of ≥15 per hour of sleep as the threshold,[2–4] and this was followed by other investigators.[5,6] However, in a later study, lower thresholds of AHI were found to be associated with excess mortality,[7] suggesting that in the presence of CVD, perhaps low AHI values are clinically significant. In this study, hypopnoeas were included in the index, acknowledging the difficulty in accurately differentiating central from obstructive hypopnoeas.

NON-HYPERCAPNIC CSA (EUCAPNIC–HYPOCAPNIC)

These disorders are characterised by (a) an awake steady-state $PaCO_2$, which is either within the range of, or less than, the normal value (<36 mmHg at sea level), and (b) increased hypercapnic and hypoxic ventilatory responses. Heart failure is the classic example of this and is discussed in detail in previous publications[8] and in Chapter 37. However, in heart failure, the pattern of breathing is unique in that the breathing cycle has long crescendo–decrescendo arms (Figure 43.1). This is due to the long arterial circulation time, a pathophysiological feature of heart failure. This breathing pattern is known as Cheyne–Stokes breathing (CSB), even though it was first described, almost four decades earlier, by a surgeon named John Hunter[8] and we have therefore used the abbreviation HCSB.

Table 43.1 Central sleep apnoea

Physiologic CSA
1. Sleep-onset
2. Post-arousal/post-sigh
3. Phasic REM sleep

I. Non-hypercapnic CSA (hypocapnic/eucapnic)
1. Heart failure
2. Idiopathic
3. Idiopathic pulmonary arterial hypertension
4. High altitude
5. Hyperventilation syndrome

II. Hypercapnic/eucapnic CSA
1. Opioids
2. Alveolar hypoventilation with normal pulmonary function
   a. Congenital and primary
   b. Brainstem and spinal cord disorders (encephalitis; tumour; infracts, cervical cordotomy; anterior cervical spinal artery syndrome)
3. Neuromuscular disorders
   a. Muscular disorders (myotonic and Duchenne dystrophies, acid maltase deficiency)
   b. Neuromuscular junction disorders (myasthenia gravis)
   c. Spinal cord/peripheral nerve disorders (amyotrophic lateral sclerosis; multiple sclerosis, polio)
   d. Spinal cord injury

III. CSA associated with central nervous system and cervical spinal cord injury

IV. CSA associated with asymptomatic cardio-/cerebrovascular pathology
1. Left ventricular systolic dysfunction
2. Left ventricular diastolic dysfunction
3. Carotid artery stenosis
4. Silent central nervous system disorders

V. CSA associated with endocrine disorders
1. Acromegaly
2. Hypothyroidism

VI. Treatment-emergent CSA (TECSA; complex CSA)
1. Post-tracheostomy
2. Post-tonsillectomy
3. Therapy with CPAP
4. Therapy with oral appliances
5. Therapy with Provent
6. Maxillomandibular surgery

Source: Modified from Javaheri S, Dempsey JA. *Compr Physiol.* 2013;3(1):141–63.

Abbreviations: REM, rapid eye movement; CSA, central sleep apnoea; OSA, obstructive sleep apnoea.

CSA in atrial fibrillation

Atrial fibrillation (AF) is the most common sustained rhythm disorder, affecting 33 million individuals worldwide. It is associated with an increased risk of cardiovascular complications, including cerebral and systemic embolisation, heart failure, hospitalisation, excess mortality, impaired quality of life and increased healthcare costs.[9] AF is associated with both obstructive sleep apnoea (OSA) and CSA.[8] The association with CSA has been best documented in AF in association with heart failure with reduced ejection fraction (HFrEF). In one study of 100 patients with HFrEF, 80% of those with AF had CSA.[4] However, in another study of 150 patients with AF and normal LVEF, CSA was observed in 31% of the patients.[10] Interestingly, though cycle length and circulation time were not reported, CSA occurred on a background of HCSB, suggesting that circulation time was increased, most probably because of excess intrathoracic blood pool due to increased left atrial pressure and size, and pulmonary congestion.

The prevalence of AF is also high in patients with so-called idiopathic CSA. Leung and colleagues[11] reported a prevalence of 27% in 60 consecutive patients with idiopathic CSA. In contrast to increased circulation time in the AF associated with left ventricular systolic or diastolic dysfunction noted above,[4,10] circulation time in AF associated with idiopathic CSA is not prolonged.

The mechanisms of the association between AF with CSA remain to be fully elucidated. AF is commonly associated with increased mean left atrial and pulmonary capillary pressure, which precipitates periodic breathing and CSA. In chronically instrumented naturally sleeping dogs, increasing left atrial pressure (by inflating a balloon in the left atrium) resulted in CSA.[12] CSA developed because of narrowing of PCO_2 reserve, the difference between the eupneoic and apneoic threshold for PCO_2. In a study of 25 patients with HFrEF (ejection fraction <35%) who had CSA, Calvin and colleagues[13] reported that increased left atrial volume index calculated from echocardiography was associated with heightened CO_2 chemosensitivity and greater frequency of CSA. The investigators suggested that this index may be useful to guide referral for polysomnography for detection of CSA in patients with HFrEF. It is emphasised that increased CO_2 response is an important component of the loop gain underlying periodic breathing in HFrEF.[14] Therefore, the mechanisms linking AF to CSA appear to relate to increased left atrial pressure[12] and size both in HF with reduced[13] and preserved ejection fraction.[10]

It is also hypothesised that CSA may be a cause of both incident AF and heart failure. In a study of 842 older men (average age, 75 years) enrolled in the multicentre Outcomes of Sleep Disorders in Older Men Study, who underwent polysmography and were followed for an average of 6.5 years, those with CSA were 2.58 times more likely to develop AF than those without.[15] Adjustments were made for established risk factors of AF including age, race, body mass index, cholesterol and various cardiovascular

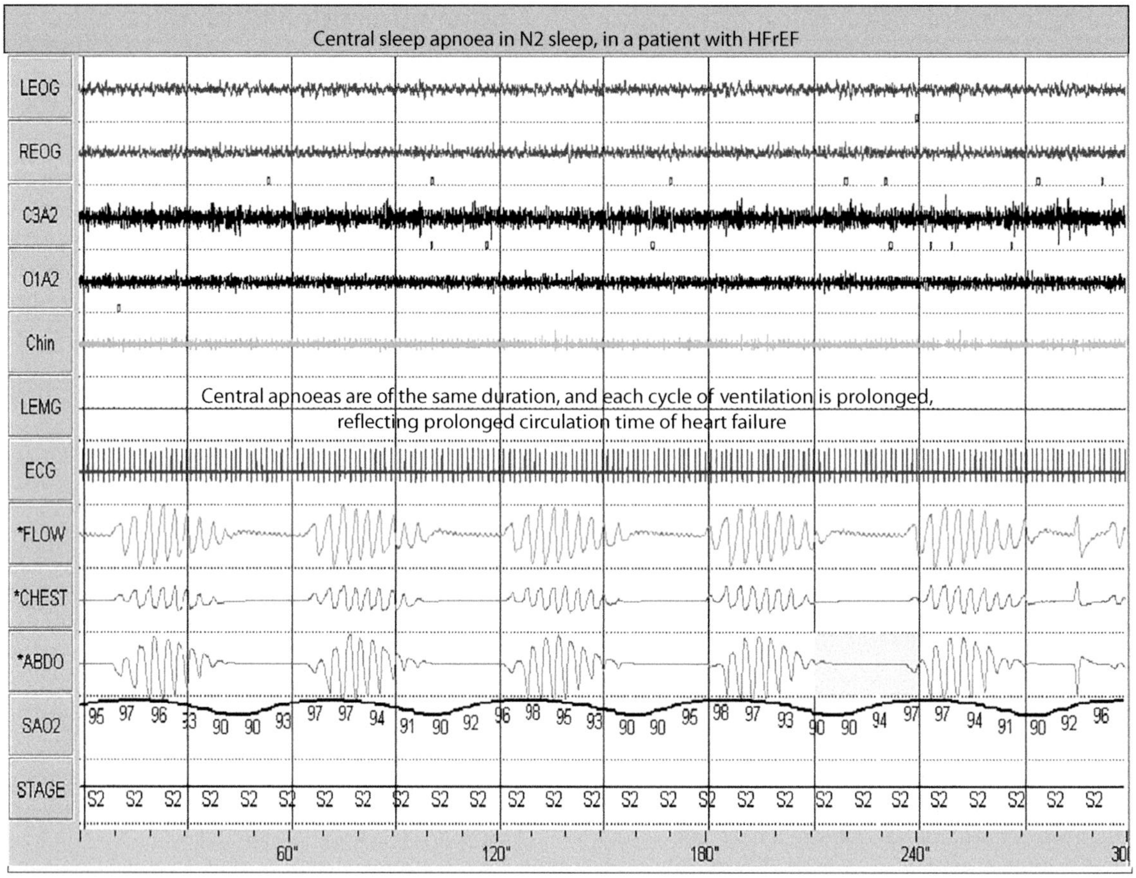

Figure 43.1 A 5-min epoch of periodic breathing with CSA in N2 non-REM sleep, in a patient with heart failure and reduced ejection fraction. The pattern first observed by Dr Hunter and several years later by Dr Cheyne and Dr Stokes (Hunter–Cheyne–Stokes breathing). Respiratory tracings show gradual reduction in amplitude ending in a central apnoea. Out of apnoea, there is gradual rise in respiratory excursions. Note that the rhythm is atrial fibrillation, the most common variable associated with HCSB in the setting of HFrEF. From top to bottom: EOG, electrooculogram; EEG, electroencephalogram; EKG, electrocardiogram; naso-oral airflow; RC, ribcage; ABD, abdominal wall movement; SaO_2, arterial oxyhaemoglobin saturation. The signals of respiration are not proportional. (Modified from Javaheri S, Dempsey JA. *Compr Physiol.* 2013;3(1):141–63.)

diseases. In another related long-term prospective study of 2865 community-dwelling older men who underwent baseline polysomnography and followed for a mean of 7.3 years, elevated CAI/HCSB was significantly associated with increased risk of decompensated heart failure and/or development of clinical heart failure.[16] This latter study provides evidence that CSA/HCSB is not necessarily the consequence of severe left ventricular dysfunction as thought previously. Such individuals with CSA/HCSB probably suffered from clinically unrecognised left ventricular dysfunction that, in time, led to overt heart failure.

CSA in pacemaker recipients

Cardiovascular diseases leading to pacemaker implantations are suspected of being associated with a high rate of undiagnosed sleep apnoea. In a Multicentre European study, Garrigue et al.[17] enrolled 98 consecutive pacemaker implanted patients not known to have sleep apnoea in a polysomnographic study to determine the presence and phenotype of sleep-disordered breathing (SDB) in this population. Twenty-nine per cent were paced for dilated cardiomyopathy, 34% for high-degree atrioventricular block and 37% for sinus node disease. Using an AHI ≥ 15/hour of sleep as the threshold, respectively, 44%, 50% and 40% of the patients had moderate to severe SDB. Most patients were diagnosed to have OSA, with about 5% having predominantly CSA. In this study, most SDB events were hypopnoeas and were mostly classified as obstructive, a confounding issue regarding the true prevalence of OAHI (obstructive AHI) versus CAHI (central AHI). However, even taking this into account, the prevalence of CSA is high in this population, relative to the very low prevalence in the general population.

IDIOPATHIC CSA

Idiopathic CSA is a relatively rare disorder with a poorly understood pathophysiology and natural history. In a population study of 741 men, aged 20 years and older, prevalence of CSA was 0.4% with higher prevalence in the oldest age group (1.1%) and less frequently in the middle age group (0.4%).[18] The prevalence of central apnoeas is even less in women than in men. Polysomnographically, there are many central apnoeas followed by arousals. Importantly, there are several differences between the pattern of breathing in idiopathic CSA[19,20] compared to CSA/HCSB:

1. The pattern is not waxing and waning as in HCSB but rather central apnoea is followed by abrupt hyperventilation and arousal.
2. The arousal typically occurs at the end of the central apnoea, in contrast to CSA/HCSB when arousal occurs at the peak of hyperventilation.
3. The cycle period is shorter, by about 20 seconds, than in CSA/HCSB.

Clinically, patients with idiopathic CSA are commonly older males. They may complain of frequent awakenings, restless sleep, insomnia and daytime somnolence or fatigue, all consequences of excessive arousals. Sleep fragmentation may favour instability of ventilatory control, arousal-induced hyperventilation may lower PCO_2 below the apneoic threshold for PCO_2, and as soon as sleep resumes, the apneoic threshold is exposed and central apnoea occurs.

There are a number of asymptomatic pathological conditions that could cause CSA (see the 'CSA in asymptomatic cardio-/cerebrovascular pathology' section). Because these pathological conditions have not usually been ruled out in the so-called idiopathic cases of CSA, the question of how 'idiopathic' it is remains unanswered. These pathological conditions could be associated with an increased ventilatory response to carbon dioxide, which has been known to be associated with idiopathic CSA. The augmented response facilitates ventilatory control instability while asleep.[14] When presented with CSA, in the absence of a known cause, carotid ultrasound, echocardiography or cardiac magnetic resonance imaging (MRI), and brain imaging should be considered to rule out these other conditions.[15,16]

Treatment of idiopathic CSA

The underlying cause needs to be investigated and, if appropriate, treated. Acetazolamide, a respiratory stimulant, could be used to treat CSA itself. A double-blind placebo-controlled trial has shown the efficacy of acetazolamide in attenuating CSA in patients with HFrEF.[21] Two open non-randomised studies[22,23] show similar results in idiopathic CSA as well. The mechanism of action of acetazolamide in alleviating CSA of various aetiologies is due to induction of metabolic acidosis and consequent hyperventilation. The latter decreases the plant gain, an important component of the loop gain, making it difficult for CSA to occur[24] (Figure 43.2). However, the increased hypercapnic ventilatory response (the other component of the loop gain) caused by acetazolamide counteracts, to a degree, the full therapeutic effect of the decreased plant gain.[25] In a case report, bilevel positive airway pressure resulted in worsening of central apnoea, presumably by lowering the prevailing PCO_2 below the apneoic threshold;[26] we generally do not recommend the use of bilevel devices for treatment of hypocapnic CSA, whatever the aetiology. New-generation adaptive servo ventilators,[27,28] however, should in theory be effective, but there are little data in this patient group.

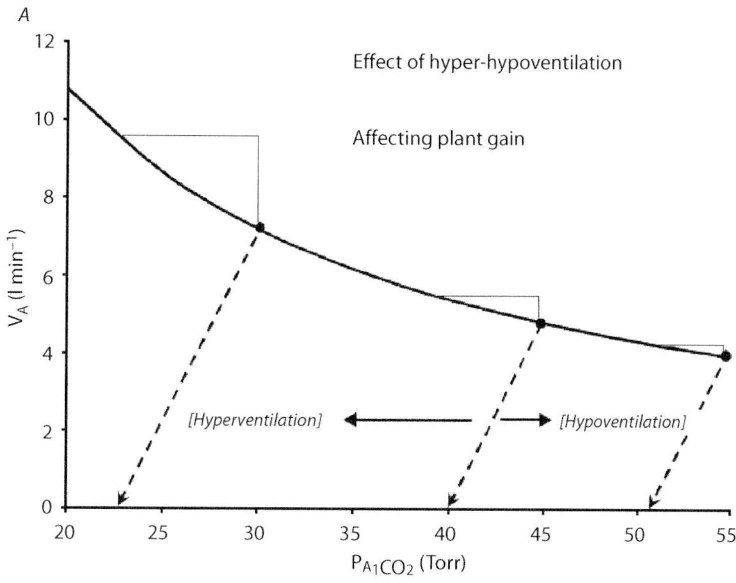

Figure 43.2 Concept of plant gain. The figure depicts the isometabolic hyperbola showing the relationship between alveolar ventilation VA and alveolar PCO_2 ($PaCO_2$) at stable constant CO_2 production. If $PACO_2$ is low, a greater transient increase in ventilation is required to lower it below the apnoeic threshold than it would be when PCO_2 is not low. (Modified from Javaheri S, Dempsey JA. *Compr Physiol.* 2013;3(1):141–63.)

IDIOPATHIC PULMONARY ARTERIAL HYPERTENSION

There is a bidirectional relation between pulmonary hypertension and SDB. OSA is a known cause of pulmonary hypertension, mostly mild in nature,[29] and SDB may also be a consequence of idiopathic pulmonary arterial hypertension.[30,31] In one of these studies, CSA/HCSB was observed in a quarter of patients who had the most severe central haemodynamics and a long circulation time. This suggests that severe right ventricular dysfunction, in the absence of obvious structural left ventricular dysfunction, could lead to CSA/HCSB. Expert consensus recommends polysomnography for all patients with pulmonary hypertension.[32]

Treatment

In two randomised, placebo-controlled, double-blind crossover trials,[33,34] treatment with nocturnal oxygen (3 L/min) for 1 week significantly improved 6-min walk distance and had favourable electrocardiographic effects when compared to sham therapy (room air, 3 L/min from a concentrator). In one patient with idiopathic pulmonary arterial hypertension, CSA was eliminated after lung transplantation. In another case report, use of bilevel positive airway pressure therapy was associated with death, though cause and effect cannot be proven.

HIGH ALTITUDE

Annually, millions of people travel to high altitude, and when at or above 2500–3000 m, CSA is invariable.[35] High altitude–induced CSA is due to hypoxic stimulation of carotid bodies narrowing the PCO_2 reserve. As expected, inhalation of supplemental oxygen[36] ameliorates periodic breathing at high altitude. Acetazolamide used orally also improves high altitude–induced CSA[35] and is prescribed to be taken 1 or 2 days ahead of a sojourn to prevent or attenuate periodic breathing and mountain sickness. We also prescribe acetazolamide for patients with OSA travelling to high altitudes, as in these patients, while on continuous positive airway pressure (CPAP), CSA emerges.[37,38]

HYPERCAPNIC CSA

By definition, in these disorders, there is sustained hypercapnia. However, frequently, $PaCO_2$ may be within the upper range of normal, as we observed in few patients on chronic opioids who had arterial blood gas measurements.[39] It should also be noted that in a number of hypercapnic disorders in this category, including congenital central hypoventilation syndrome and idiopathic alveolar hypoventilation, hypoventilation rather than frequent central apnoeas is the prominent sleep/breathing disorder.

1. There are important adverse pathophysiological alterations that specifically occur during sleep and are shared in this group of disorders, independent of the cause. Normally, with sleep onset, and removal of the wakefulness drive to breathe, ventilation decreases. This small reduction in ventilation may result in profound hypercapnia. This phenomenon is dictated by the hyperbolic relation of PCO_2 with alveolar ventilation.[40] Accordingly, when arterial PCO_2 is elevated, a small reduction in ventilation increases PCO_2 considerably (increased plant gain), resulting in acute acidosis on the one hand and a considerable equal drop in PaO_2 on the other. This effect is most pronounced in REM sleep. The increase in plant gain imposed by the ventilation curve at elevated PCO_2 levels dictates that when ventilation increases slightly, for example, with an arousal from sleep, a considerable drop in PCO_2 occurs. Consequently, if PCO_2 decreases below the apneoic threshold,[41] a central apnoea or long expiratory pause occurs, which is sustained until PCO_2 rises above the apnoeic threshold for PCO_2.
2. Central apnoea may occur in REM sleep in neuromuscular disorders involving the diaphragm, which is the only inspiratory thoracic pump muscle normally active during REM sleep (pseudo CSA). Therefore, in these disorders, in REM sleep, with intercostal muscle atonia, airflow ceases and thoracoabdominal tracings mimic central apnoea.
3. In conditions involving automatic pathways of breathing (such as cervical) or anterior cervical spinal artery syndrome,[42] the wakefulness drive to breathe may provide adequate respiratory drive to breathe while awake, but as it is absent while asleep, profound hypercapnia and hypoxaemia ensue (Ondine's curse).
4. Last but not least, in neuromuscular disorders involving cranial nerves compromising upper airway muscles, obstructive disordered breathing becomes manifest. These and other effects of sleep in neuromuscular disorders are discussed elsewhere[43] and therefore are not considered here.

OPIOIDS

While awake, ventilatory depression, characterised by a reduction in tidal volume and breathing rate, is a well-known adverse effect of opioids.[44,45] However, the profound ventilatory depression of opioids during sleep became unmasked only when polysomnography was performed on patients using opioids for chronic pain.[46] Ventilatory depression in the form of CSA was reported in a number of studies,[39,47] even with buprenorphine.[48] Opioids may cause CSA via their inhibitory effect on opioid-μ receptors in the pre-Botzinger complex.[49,50] The proof that opioids cause CSA in humans has come from case reports in which patients were studied before and after withdrawal of opioids.[51–53]

The SDB in patients taking opioids is quite distinct from that seen in heart failure (compare Figures 43.1 and 43.3). Cluster breathing is a common pattern, characterised by

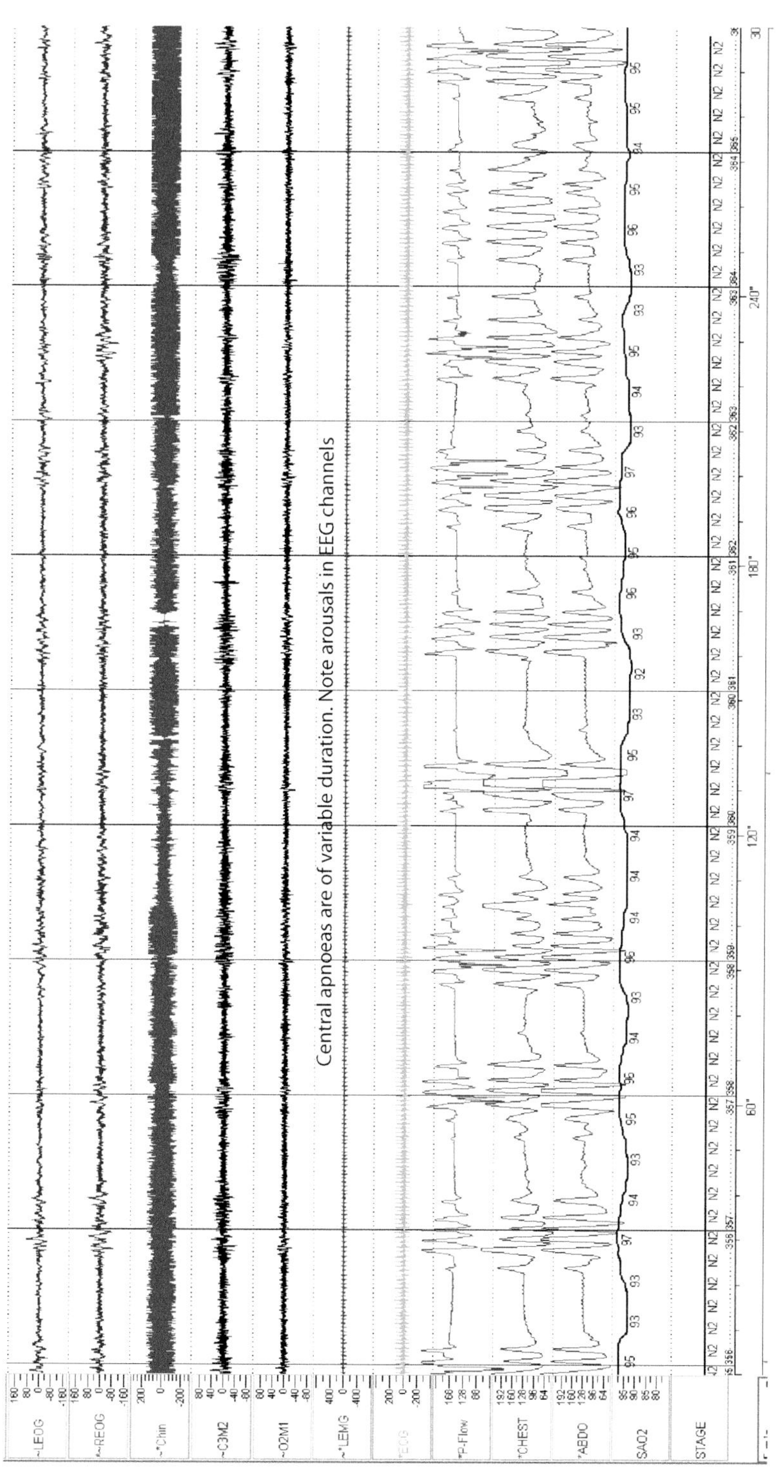

Figure 43.3 A 5-min epoch of a polysomnogram of a patient on chronic opioids. The tracings are the same as in Figure 43.1. Note the differences in the pattern of breathing between this patient and the patient with heart failure in Figure 43.1. The central apnoeas are of different duration. In addition, obstructive apnoeas and hypopnoeas and apnoeas also present. Note that out of apnoea, there are at times very large breaths. (Modified from Javaheri S, Patel S. *J Clin Sleep Med.* 2017;18:829–33.)

cycles of deep breaths in which the amplitude of the tidal volume is relatively stable, interspersed with central apnoeas of variable duration (Figure 43.3). The other pattern is ataxic breathing characterised by variable amplitude in tidal volume and breathing rate (Figure 43.3). In contrast to heart failure in which central apnoeas are quite regular and of the same duration, opioid-induced central apnoeas are of various durations, and the crescendo–decrescendo pattern is invariably absent. However, one shared polysomnographic finding is that in both, central apnoeas primarily occur in non-REM sleep and are rarely observed in REM sleep.

Treatment of CSA due to opioids is best achieved by discontinuation of the drugs; unfortunately, this is usually very difficult. Bilevel ventilation devices, with an appropriate backup rate or adaptive servo ventilation (ASV), are generally effective to attenuate or eliminate CSA, as well as obstructive events.[28,39] CPAP is generally ineffective.[39] Ampekines, a group of drugs with an affinity for glutaminergic receptors, are promising,[54] but randomised controlled trials are lacking.

CSA ASSOCIATED WITH CENTRAL NERVOUS SYSTEM AND SPINAL CORD INJURY

A variety of central nervous system disorders including stroke, transient ischaemic attack, Parkinson's disease and other neurodegenerative disorders are associated with SDB. Here, we concentrate on stroke, which has a bidirectional relation with SDB. OSA is a known potential cause of stroke.[55] Conversely, stroke could be a cause of both OSA and CSA. In a meta-analysis[56] of 2343 patients with stroke or transient ischaemic attack, 38% had an AHI of more than 20 per hour, with CSA accounting for 7% of the disorders. In most patients, however, CSA resolves with time,[57] perhaps as inflammation and oedema subside. If CSA persists, there may be another underlying cause such as left ventricular dysfunction,[58] carotid artery stenosis or atrial fibrillation (see idiopathic CSA above). However, if, due to stroke, structural changes, such as gliosis, occur in the centres controlling breathing, CSA may persist. When left ventricular systolic dysfunction is the cause of post-stroke CSA, the pattern of breathing is similar to HCSB, though this has also been reported in three patients with stroke with normal left ventricular ejection fraction;[59] however, diastolic dysfunction, which could be a potential reason for CSA, was not evaluated in these patients.

Treatment

Supplemental nasal oxygen and theophylline have proved effective in the treatment of stroke-related CSA.[60,61] In a retrospective study involving 15 post-acute ischemic stroke patients with CSA, Brill et al. reported that CPAP and bilevel devices were unsatisfactory and patients were switched to ASV. With ASV, AHI decreased significantly from 47 to 9/hour ($p = 0.001$). The mean nightly use of ASV was 5.4 ± 2.4 hours at 3 months after the initiation of treatment, and this was maintained at 6 months.[62]

SDB IN CHRONIC SPINAL CORD INJURY

Multiple studies from different countries have shown a high prevalence of OSA in patients with spinal cord injury (SCI) ranging from 27% to 62%.[63–65] Severe OSA may develop only a few days after the injury, having been absent in the first few days.[66] At the same time, a high prevalence of CSA has been described in a group of 26 consecutive patients with cervical and thoracic SCI, though concomitant therapy with opioids may have been a factor in some.[67] The mechanisms of CSA in the remaining patients is unexplained. Whether SDB contributes to the morbidity and mortality of patients with SCI remains to be determined.

CSA IN ASYMPTOMATIC CARDIO-/CEREBROVASCULAR PATHOLOGY

Predominant CSA pattern, or a CAI ≥ 5/hour, may be observed in polysomnography of individuals referred for a sleep study but not necessarily suspected of having CSA. This unexpected finding may occur in a number of pathological cardiovascular conditions in individuals not known to have symptoms of a cardiovascular pathology. These include (Table 43.1) carotid artery stenosis,[68,69] asymptomatic left ventricular dysfunction[70] and silent intracranial pathological conditions.[71,72] Rupprecht et al.[68] performed polysomnography in 59 such subjects and found that 19 (39%) of 49 with extracranial (none of the 10 with intracranial) carotid artery stenosis had CSA. In patients with occult left ventricular systolic dysfunction, an estimated 55% of patients have moderate to severe CSA, defined by an AHI ≥ 15/hour of sleep.[70] This prevalence is similar to that of patients with symptomatic heart failure and reduced ejection fraction.[4,5] A lower prevalence of CSA (4%) has been reported in subjects with asymptomatic left ventricular dysfunction. CSA may also be present in asymptomatic individuals with underlying left ventricular structural alterations found in cardiac MRI. In the Multi-Ethnic Study of Atherosclerosis, 1412 participants underwent both overnight polysomnography and cardiac MRI. Twenty-seven (2%) individuals had CSA defined by CAHI ≥ 5/hour of sleep, or presence of HCSB. In the adjusted multivariate linear regression models, presence of CSA was significantly associated with elevated left ventricular mass/volume ratio signifying concentric remodeling.[73]

It is also conceivable that CSA could be caused by silent cerebral ischemia.[71] In a prospective population-based study of 394 stroke-free elderly subjects who underwent polysomnography and were followed for 6 years, 20 ischaemic strokes occurred. The event-free survival was lowest in the highest CAI group, an association independent of any other vascular risks. The investigators suggested that CSA could be a marker of silent brain ischaemia involving central nervous system respiratory mechanisms.

CSA IN ENDOCRINE DISORDERS

Acromegaly is the most common endocrine disorder causing CSA. Grunstein and colleagues[74] performed polysomnography in 53 patients with acromegaly, 33 of whom had been referred because of symptoms of OSA. Surprisingly, 14 (33%) had predominantly CSA. Patients with CSA had higher insulin-like growth factor 1 and growth hormone levels, indicating that the degree of hypersecretion was associated with the presence but not the severity of CSA. The investigators reported that patients with CSA had augmented hypercapnic ventilatory response, which increases the loop gain, increasing the likelihood of developing CSA. Furthermore, patients with acromegaly may suffer from cardiac dysfunction, which could be another reason for a high prevalence of CSA in these patients. Treatment of acromegaly with octreotide decreases CSA and also OSA.[75]

TREATMENT-EMERGENT CSA (TECSA) (COMPLEX SLEEP APNOEA)

Historically, complex CSA came to light when OSA patients were treated with CPAP and central apnoeas emerged. However, it is probably best to refer to this condition as TECSA as it describes the condition more accurately. While considered to be a new concept, TESCA was first reported many years ago by a group of investigators,[76] in OSA patients who underwent tracheostomy. In these patients, post-tracheostomy, OSA was eliminated but CSA emerged, though with time, these events disappeared spontaneously. TESCA has also been reported after other non-positive pressure therapies of OSA such as after tonsillectomy, with nasal expiratory positive airway device (Provent),[77] after surgical relief of nasal obstruction in OSA,[78] maxillomandibular surgery[79] and after treatment with an oral appliance.[80,81] However, the most common association has been with CPAP.

The current estimated prevalence of CPAP-emergent CSA is about 5% to 20%.[82–87] In our study,[82] which included 1286 consecutive OSA patients who had undergone full-night attended polysomnography followed by two full-night attended CPAP titration studies (the first immediately after diagnosis and the second a few weeks later), the average prevalence over a 1-year period was 6.5%. Two studies from Japan show a similar prevalence.[86,87]

Multiple mechanisms may work hand in hand in the development of CPAP-emergent CSA[82] including severity of OSA and increased chemosensitivity,[88,89] similar to patients with systolic heart failure.[4] Increased loop gain is a major reason to promote breathing instability during sleep. Importantly, it has been shown that after long-term use of CPAP, CO_2 chemosensitiviy decreases,[89] and this could be the reason for resolution of CPAP-emergent CSA with time, as demonstrated in our study.[82] These data indicate that the increased chemosensitivity is acquired and perhaps related to exposure to intermittent hypoxaemia associated with severe OSA.[90]

Management of CPAP-emergent CSA

CSA resolves with continued use of CPAP in most patients[82] consistent with early studies of OSA patients who underwent tracheostomy.[91,92] ASV has been used to treat CPAP-emergent CSA. Morgenthaler et al.[93] tested the hypothesis that ASV devices are superior to CPAP from the standpoint of residual AHI. In a randomised controlled trial of 66 OSA patients with CPAP-emergent CSA, at 3 months, residual AHI was 4.7 ± 8.1 (central, 1.1 ± 3.7) in the ASV arm and 14.1 ± 21 (central, 8.8 ± 16.3, $p < 0.001$) in the CPAP arm. In the accompanying editorial,[94] we have questioned the clinical implications of these findings as the secondary outcomes of the trial including PAP adherence, sleepiness, quality of life and feeling refreshed were all the same in the ASV group as compared to CPAP.

CONCLUSIONS

Central apnoeas occur in many pathophysiological conditions. Depending on the cause or mechanism, central apnoeas may not be clinically significant. In contrast, in some disorders, central apnoeas result in pathophysiological consequences. Under such circumstances, diagnosis and treatment of CSA may improve quality of life, morbidity and perhaps mortality. Overall, however, much less is known about the clinical significance of CSA than OSA.

REFERENCES

1. Javaheri S, Dempsey JA. Central sleep apnea. *Compr Physiol.* 2013;3(1):141–63.
2. Javaheri S, Parker TJ, Wexler L et al. Occult sleep-disordered breathing in stable congestive heart failure. *Ann Intern Med.* 1995;122(7):487–92.
3. Javaheri S, Parker TJ, Liming JD et al. Sleep apnea in 81 ambulatory male patients with stable heart failure. Types and their prevalences, consequences, and presentations. *Circulation.* 1998;97(21):2154–9.
4. Javaheri S. Sleep disorders in systolic heart failure: A prospective study of 100 male patients. The final report. *Int J Cardiol.* 2006;106(1):21–8.
5. Sin DD, Fitzgerald F, Parker JD et al. Risk factors for central and obstructive sleep apnea in 450 men and women with congestive heart failure. *Am J Respir Crit Care Med.* 1999;160(4):1101–6.
6. Oldenburg O, Wellmann B, Buchholz A et al. Nocturnal hypoxaemia is associated with increased mortality in stable heart failure patients. *Eur Heart J.* 2016;37(21):1695–703.
7. Javaheri S, Shukla R, Zeigler H, Wexler L. Central sleep apnea, right ventricular dysfunction, and low diastolic blood pressure are predictors of mortality in systolic heart failure. *J Am Coll Cardiol.* 2007;49(20):2028–34.

8. Javaheri S, Barbe F, Campos-Rodriguez F et al. Sleep apnea: Types, mechanisms, and clinical cardiovascular consequences. *J Am Coll Cardiol.* 2017;69(7):841–58.
9. Chugh SS, Havmoeller R, Narayanan K et al. Worldwide epidemiology of atrial fibrillation: A Global Burden of Disease 2010 Study. *Circulation.* 2014;129(8):837–47.
10. Bitter T, Langer C, Vogt J et al. Sleep-disordered breathing in patients with atrial fibrillation and normal systolic left ventricular function. *Dtsch Arztebl Int.* 2009;106(10):164–70.
11. Leung RS, Huber MA, Rogge T et al. Association between atrial fibrillation and central sleep apnea. *Sleep.* 2005;28(12):1543–6.
12. Chenuel BJ, Smith CA, Skatrud JB et al. Increased propensity for apnea in response to acute elevations in left atrial pressure during sleep in the dog. *J Appl Physiol (1985).* 2006;101(1):76–83.
13. Calvin AD, Somers VK, Johnson BD et al. Left atrial size, chemosensitivity, and central sleep apnea in heart failure. *Chest.* 2014;146(1):96–103.
14. Javaheri S. A mechanism of central sleep apnea in patients with heart failure. *N Engl J Med.* 1999;341(13):949–54.
15. May AM, Blackwell T, Stone PH et al. Central sleep-disordered breathing predicts incident atrial fibrillation in older men. *Am J Respir Crit Care Med.* 2016;193(7):783–91.
16. Javaheri S, Blackwell T, Ancoli-Israel S et al. Sleep-disordered breathing and incident heart failure in older men. *Am J Respir Crit Care Med.* 2016;193(5):561–8.
17. Garrigue S, Pepin JL, Defaye P et al. High prevalence of sleep apnea syndrome in patients with long-term pacing: The European Multicenter Polysomnographic Study. *Circulation.* 2007;115(13):1703–9.
18. Bixler EO, Vgontzas AN, Ten Have T et al. Effects of age on sleep apnea in men: I. Prevalence and severity. *Am J Respir Crit Care Med.* 1998;157(1):144–8.
19. Xie A, Rutherford R, Rankin F et al. Hypocapnia and increased ventilatory responsiveness in patients with idiopathic central sleep apnea. *Am J Respir Crit Care Med.* 1995;152(6 Pt 1):1950–5.
20. Xie A, Wong B, Phillipson EA et al. Interaction of hyperventilation and arousal in the pathogenesis of idiopathic central sleep apnea. *Am J Respir Crit Care Med.* 1994;150(2):489–95.
21. Javaheri S. Acetazolamide improves central sleep apnea in heart failure: A double-blind, prospective study. *Am J Respir Crit Care Med.* 2006;173(2):234–7.
22. White DP, Zwillich CW, Pickett CK et al. Central sleep apnea. Improvement with acetazolamide therapy. *Arch Intern Med.* 1982;142(10):1816–9.
23. DeBacker WA, Verbraecken J, Willemen M et al. Central apnea index decreases after prolonged treatment with acetazolamide. *Am J Respir Crit Care Med.* 1995;151(1):87–91.
24. Nakayama H, Smith CA, Rodman JR et al. Effect of ventilatory drive on carbon dioxide sensitivity below eupnea during sleep. *Am J Respir Crit Care Med.* 2002;165(9):1251–60.
25. Javaheri S, Sands SA, Edwards BA. Acetazolamide attenuates Hunter–Cheyne–Stokes breathing but augments the hypercapnic ventilatory response in patients with heart failure. *Ann Am Thorac Soc.* 2014;11(1):80–6.
26. Hommura F, Nishimura M, Oguri M et al. Continuous versus bilevel positive airway pressure in a patient with idiopathic central sleep apnea. *Am J Respir Crit Care Med.* 1997;155(4):1482–5.
27. Javaheri S, Brown LK, Randerath WJ. Positive airway pressure therapy with adaptive servoventilation: Part 1: operational algorithms. *Chest.* 2014;146(2):514–23.
28. Javaheri S, Brown LK, Randerath WJ. Clinical applications of adaptive servoventilation devices: Part 2. *Chest.* 2014;146(3):858–68.
29. Javaheri S, Javaheri S, Javaheri A. Sleep apnea, heart failure, and pulmonary hypertension. *Curr Heart Fail Rep.* 2013;10(4):315–20.
30. Ulrich S, Fischler M, Speich R, Bloch KE. Sleep-related breathing disorders in patients with pulmonary hypertension. *Chest.* 2008;133(6):1375–80.
31. Schulz R, Baseler G, Ghofrani HA et al. Nocturnal periodic breathing in primary pulmonary hypertension. *Eur Respir J.* 2002;19(4):658–63.
32. McLaughlin VV, Archer SL, Badesch DB et al. ACCF/AHA 2009 expert consensus document on pulmonary hypertension a report of the American College of Cardiology Foundation Task Force on Expert Consensus Documents and the American Heart Association developed in collaboration with the American College of Chest Physicians; American Thoracic Society, Inc.; and the Pulmonary Hypertension Association. *J Am Coll Cardiol.* 2009;53(17):1573–619.
33. Ulrich S, Keusch S, Hildenbrand FF et al. Effect of nocturnal oxygen and acetazolamide on exercise performance in patients with pre-capillary pulmonary hypertension and sleep-disturbed breathing: Randomized, double-blind, cross-over trial. *Eur Heart J.* 2015;36(10):615–23.
34. Schumacher DS, Muller-Mottet S, Hasler ED et al. Effect of oxygen and acetazolamide on nocturnal cardiac conduction, repolarization, and arrhythmias in precapillary pulmonary hypertension and sleep-disturbed breathing. *Chest.* 2014;146(5):1226–36.
35. Caravita S, Faini A, Lombardi C et al. Sex and acetazolamide effects on chemoreflex and periodic breathing during sleep at altitude. *Chest.* 2015;147(1):120–31.
36. Lahiri S, Maret K, Sherpa MG. Dependence of high altitude sleep apnea on ventilatory sensitivity to hypoxia. *Respir Physiol.* 1983;52(3):281–301.

37. Nussbaumer-Ochsner Y, Schuepfer N, Ulrich S, Bloch KE. Exacerbation of sleep apnoea by frequent central events in patients with the obstructive sleep apnoea syndrome at altitude: A randomised trial. *Thorax*. 2010;65(5):429–35.
38. Nussbaumer-Ochsner Y, Latshang TD, Ulrich S et al. Patients with obstructive sleep apnea syndrome benefit from acetazolamide during an altitude sojourn: A randomized, placebo-controlled, double-blind trial. *Chest*. 2012;141(1):131–8.
39. Javaheri S, Harris N, Howard J, Chung E. Adaptive servoventilation for treatment of opioid-associated central sleep apnea. *J Clin Sleep Med*. 2014;10(6): 637–43.
40. Sinha P, Fauvel NJ, Singh S, Soni N. Ventilatory ratio: A simple bedside measure of ventilation. *Br J Anaesth*. 2009;102(5):692–7.
41. Boden AG, Harris MC, Parkes MJ. Apneic threshold for CO_2 in the anesthetized rat: Fundamental properties under steady-state conditions. *J Appl Physiol (1985)*. 1998;85(3):898–907.
42. Manconi M, Mondini S, Fabiani A et al. Anterior spinal artery syndrome complicated by the ondine curse. *Arch Neurol*. 2003;60(12):1787–90.
43. Aboussouan LS. Sleep-disordered breathing in neuromuscular disease. *Am J Respir Crit Care Med*. 2015;191(9):979–89.
44. Santiago TV, Edelman NH. Opioids and breathing. *J Appl Physiol (1985)*. 1985;59(6):1675–85.
45. Weil JV, McCullough RE, Kline JS, Sodal IE. Diminished ventilatory response to hypoxia and hypercapnia after morphine in normal man. *N Engl J Med*. 1975;292(21):1103–6.
46. Arora N, Cao M, Javaheri S. Opioids, sedatives, and sleep hypoventilation. *Sleep Med Clin*. 2014;9(3):391–8.
47. Farney RJ, Walker JM, Cloward TV, Rhondeau S. Sleep-disordered breathing associated with long-term opioid therapy. *Chest*. 2003;123(2):632–9.
48. Farney RJ, McDonald AM, Boyle KM et al. Sleep disordered breathing in patients receiving therapy with buprenorphine/naloxone. *Eur Respir J*. 2013;42(2):394–403.
49. Feldman JL, Del Negro CA. Looking for inspiration: New perspectives on respiratory rhythm. *Nat Rev Neurosci*. 2006;7(3):232–42.
50. Montandon G, Qin W, Liu H et al. PreBotzinger complex neurokinin-1 receptor-expressing neurons mediate opioid-induced respiratory depression. *J Neurosci*. 2011;31(4):1292–301.
51. Davis MJ, Livingston M, Scharf SM. Reversal of central sleep apnea following discontinuation of opioids. *J Clin Sleep Med*. 2012;8(5):579–80.
52. Ramar K. Reversal of sleep-disordered breathing with opioid withdrawal. *Pain Pract*. 2009;9(5):394–8.
53. Javaheri S, Patel S. Opioids cause central and complex sleep apnea in humans: Reversal with discontinuation: A plea for detoxification. *J Clin Sleep Med*. 2017;13:829–33.
54. Javaheri S, Germany R, Greer JJ. Novel therapies for the treatment of central sleep apnea. *Sleep Med Clin*. 2016;11(2):227–39.
55. Yaggi HK, Concato J, Kernan WN et al. Obstructive sleep apnea as a risk factor for stroke and death. *N Engl J Med*. 2005;353(19):2034–41.
56. Johnson KG, Johnson DC. Frequency of sleep apnea in stroke and TIA patients: A meta-analysis. *J Clin Sleep Med*. 2010;6(2):131–7.
57. Parra O, Arboix A, Bechich S et al. Time course of sleep-related breathing disorders in first-ever stroke or transient ischemic attack. *Am J Respir Crit Care Med*. 2000;161(2 Pt 1):375–80.
58. Nopmaneejumruslers C, Kaneko Y, Hajek V et al. Cheyne–Stokes respiration in stroke: Relationship to hypocapnia and occult cardiac dysfunction. *Am J Respir Crit Care Med*. 2005;171(9):1048–52.
59. Hermann DM, Siccoli M, Kirov P et al. Central periodic breathing during sleep in acute ischemic stroke. *Stroke*. 2007;38(3):1082–4.
60. Hermann DM, Bassetti CL. Sleep apnea and other sleep–wake disorders in stroke. *Curr Treat Options Neurol*. 2003;5(3):241–9.
61. Nachtmann A, Siebler M, Rose G et al. Cheyne–Stokes respiration in ischemic stroke. *Neurology*. 1995;45(4):820–1.
62. Brill AK, Rosti R, Hefti JP et al. Adaptive servo-ventilation as treatment of persistent central sleep apnea in post-acute ischemic stroke patients. *Sleep Med*. 2014;15(11):1309–13.
63. Leduc BE, Dagher JH, Mayer P et al. Estimated prevalence of obstructive sleep apnea-hypopnea syndrome after cervical cord injury. *Arch Phys Med Rehabil*. 2007;88(3):333–7.
64. Short DJ, Stradling JR, Williams SJ. Prevalence of sleep apnoea in patients over 40 years of age with spinal cord lesions. *J Neurol Neurosurg Psychiatry*. 1992;55(11):1032–6.
65. McEvoy RD, Mykytyn I, Sajkov D et al. Sleep apnoea in patients with quadriplegia. *Thorax*. 1995;50(6):613–9.
66. Berlowitz DJ, Brown DJ, Campbell DA, Pierce RJ. A longitudinal evaluation of sleep and breathing in the first year after cervical spinal cord injury. *Arch Phys Med Rehabil*. 2005;86(6):1193–9.
67. Sankari A, Bascom A, Oomman S, Badr MS. Sleep disordered breathing in chronic spinal cord injury. *J Clin Sleep Med*. 2014;10(1):65–72.
68. Rupprecht S, Hoyer D, Hagemann G et al. Central sleep apnea indicates autonomic dysfunction in asymptomatic carotid stenosis: A potential marker of cerebrovascular and cardiovascular risk. *Sleep*. 2010;33(3):327–33.

69. Ehrhardt J, Schwab M, Finn S et al. Sleep apnea and asymptomatic carotid stenosis: A complex interaction. *Chest.* 2015;147(4):1029–36.
70. Lanfranchi PA, Somers VK, Braghiroli A et al. Central sleep apnea in left ventricular dysfunction: Prevalence and implications for arrhythmic risk. *Circulation.* 2003;107(5):727–32.
71. Munoz R, Duran-Cantolla J, Martinez-Vila E et al. Central sleep apnea is associated with increased risk of ischemic stroke in the elderly. *Acta Neurol Scand.* 2012;126(3):183–8.
72. Garcia-Sanchez A, Fernandez-Navarro I, Garcia-Rio F. Central apneas and REM sleep behavior disorder as an initial presentation of multiple system atrophy. *J Clin Sleep Med.* 2016;12(2):267–70.
73. Javaheri S, Sharma RK, Bluemke DA, Redline S. Association between central sleep apnea and left ventricular structure: The Multi-Ethnic Study of Atherosclerosis. *J Sleep Res.* 2017;26:477–80.
74. Grunstein RR, Ho KY, Berthon-Jones M et al. Central sleep apnea is associated with increased ventilatory response to carbon dioxide and hypersecretion of growth hormone in patients with acromegaly. *Am J Respir Crit Care Med.* 1994;150(2):496–502.
75. Grunstein RR, Ho KK, Sullivan CE. Effect of octreotide, a somatostatin analog, on sleep apnea in patients with acromegaly. *Ann Intern Med.* 1994;121(7):478–83.
76. Fletcher EC. Recurrence of sleep apnea syndrome following tracheostomy. A shift from obstructive to central apnea. *Chest.* 1989;96(1):205–9.
77. Chopra A, Das P, Ramar K et al. Complex sleep apnea associated with use of nasal expiratory positive airway (nEPAP) device. *J Clin Sleep Med.* 2014;10(5):577–9.
78. Goldstein C, Kuzniar TJ. The emergence of central sleep apnea after surgical relief of nasal obstruction in obstructive sleep apnea. *J Clin Sleep Med.* 2012;8(3):321–2.
79. Corcoran S, Mysliwiec V, Niven AS, Fallah D. Development of central sleep apnea after maxillofacial surgery for obstructive sleep apnea. *J Clin Sleep Med.* 2009;5(2):151–3.
80. Avidan AY, Guilleminault C, Robinson A. The development of central sleep apnea with an oral appliance. *Sleep Med.* 2006;7(2):187–91.
81. Kuzniar TJ, Kovacevic-Ristanovic R, Freedom T. Complex sleep apnea unmasked by the use of a mandibular advancement device. *Sleep Breath.* 2011;15(2):249–52.
82. Javaheri S, Smith J, Chung E. The prevalence and natural history of complex sleep apnea. *J Clin Sleep Med.* 2009;5(3):205–11.
83. Morgenthaler TI, Kagramanov V, Hanak V, Decker PA. Complex sleep apnea syndrome: Is it a unique clinical syndrome? *Sleep.* 2006;29(9):1203–9.
84. Dernaika T, Tawk M, Nazir S et al. The significance and outcome of continuous positive airway pressure-related central sleep apnea during split-night sleep studies. *Chest.* 2007;132(1):81–7.
85. Lehman S, Antic NA, Thompson C et al. Central sleep apnea on commencement of continuous positive airway pressure in patients with a primary diagnosis of obstructive sleep apnea-hypopnea. *J Clin Sleep Med.* 2007;3(5):462–6.
86. Endo Y, Suzuki M, Inoue Y et al. Prevalence of complex sleep apnea among Japanese patients with sleep apnea syndrome. *Tohoku J Exp Med.* 2008;215(4):349–54.
87. Yaegashi H, Fujimoto K, Abe H et al. Characteristics of Japanese patients with complex sleep apnea syndrome: A retrospective comparison with obstructive sleep apnea syndrome. *Intern Med.* 2009;48(6):427–32.
88. Younes M, Ostrowski M, Thompson W et al. Chemical control stability in patients with obstructive sleep apnea. *Am J Respir Crit Care Med.* 2001;163(5):1181–90.
89. Salloum A, Rowley JA, Mateika JH et al. Increased propensity for central apnea in patients with obstructive sleep apnea: Effect of nasal continuous positive airway pressure. *Am J Respir Crit Care Med.* 2010;181(2):189–93.
90. Pialoux V, Hanly PJ, Foster GE et al. Effects of exposure to intermittent hypoxia on oxidative stress and acute hypoxic ventilatory response in humans. *Am J Respir Crit Care Med.* 2009;180(10):1002–9.
91. Coccagna G, Mantovani M, Brignani F et al. Tracheostomy in hypersomnia with periodic breathing. *Bull Physiopathol Respir (Nancy).* 1972;8(5):1217–27.
92. Guilleminault C, Simmons FB, Motta J et al. Obstructive sleep apnea syndrome and tracheostomy. Long-term follow-up experience. *Arch Intern Med.* 1981;141(8):985–8.
93. Morgenthaler TI, Kuzniar TJ, Wolfe LF et al. The complex sleep apnea resolution study: A prospective randomized controlled trial of continuous positive airway pressure versus adaptive servoventilation therapy. *Sleep.* 2014;37(5):927–34.
94. Orr J, Javaheri S, Malhotra A. Comparative effectiveness research in complex sleep apnea. *Sleep.* 2014;37(5):833–4.

44

Mouthpiece ventilation for daytime ventilatory support

MIGUEL R. GONÇALVES AND TIAGO PINTO

HISTORICAL INTRODUCTION

Before 1953, non-invasive ventilation (NIV) referred to the use of body ventilators such as the iron lung. Despite their success for continuous ventilatory support, tracheostomy mechanical ventilation (TMV) became the standard for ventilatory support after the 1952 Danish polio epidemic, for which few iron lungs were available. Because TMV freed patients from iron lungs to be mobilised in wheelchairs and facilitated airway secretion management for many, this spread to other European countries and to the United States.[1,2]

Then, in 1953, Dr John Affeldt wrote, 'some of our physical therapists, in struggling with [iron lung] patients, noticed that they could simply take the positive pressure attachment, apply a small plastic mouthpiece…, and allow that to hang in the patient's mouth... We even had one patient who has no breathing ability who has fallen asleep and been adequately ventilated by this procedure, so that it appears to work very well, and I think does away with a lot of complications of difficulty of using [invasive] positive pressure. You just hang it by the patients and they grip it with their lips, when they want it, and when they don't want it, they let go of it. It is just too simple'.[3]

Patients who were using body ventilators around the clock began using mouthpiece non-invasive intermittent positive pressure ventilation (IPPV) during daytime hours. Many then used mouthpiece NIV around the clock, refusing to return to body ventilators for sleep. Losing the mouthpiece during sleep could have meant death. The advent of the Bennett Lipseal (Philips-Respironics International Inc., Murrysville, Pennsylvania) in 1968 prevented this by securing the mouthpiece and diminishing oral air leakage. This permitted the use of NIV for up to full continuous non-invasive ventilatory support (CNVS) as an alternative to TMV.

In 1956, the Harris Thompson portable 28-lb Bantam positive pressure ventilator became available. The next year, it was noted, 'if a patient is going to be left a respirator cripple with a very low VC, a tracheotomy may be a great disadvantage. It is very difficult to get rid of a tracheotomy tube when the VC is only 500 or 600 mL and there is no power of coughing, whereas, as we all know, a patient who has been treated in a respirator (body ventilator) from the first can survive and get out of all mechanical devices with a VC of that figure'.[4] Thus, it was recognised that TMV could result in greater ventilator dependence because of deconditioning, tube-induced secretions, hyperventilation by bypassing upper airway afferents and, possibly, other factors.[5]

Mouthpiece/lip seal NIV was reported to have been used for up to CNVS by 257 patients, most of whom were cared for by Goldwater Memorial Hospital in the United States from 1968 through 1987.[6]

Mechanisms by which daytime NIV can improve the clinical picture include relieving symptoms; resting the respiratory muscles and decreasing metabolic demand; increasing tidal volumes and relieving hypercapnia; resetting chemoreceptors; opening atelectatic areas; maintaining airway patency; improving ventilation/perfusion matching; maintaining lung and chest wall range of motion and compliance; improving cough flows and airway clearance; and, most importantly, assisting, supporting and substituting for respiratory muscle function. Nighttime bilevel positive airway pressure (PAP) only may not adequately achieve these goals and cannot provide CNVS. Nocturnal NIV at full ventilatory support settings is typically spontaneously extended into daytime hours and eventually around the clock, thereby averting hospitalisations for respiratory failure and tracheostomy tubes, and has been used by some patients for up to 58 years. The use of daytime mouthpiece NIV was described in 16 articles and its use for up to CNVS was described in 10 different articles in patients with neuromuscular disorders.[7]

INDICATIONS AND PROTOCOLS FOR DAYTIME MOUTHPIECE VENTILATION

Mouthpiece ventilation (MPV) is the most important method of daytime ventilatory support for patients who need ventilatory support continuously and following extubation of patients who are unable to breathe autonomously.[8] Most commonly, simple, flexed mouthpieces are grabbed by the patient's lips and teeth for deep insufflations as needed. Some patients keep the mouthpiece between their teeth all day, but most of the patients prefer to have the mouthpiece held near the mouth and get ventilatory support intermittently (Figure 44.1). The ventilator is set for large tidal volumes, often 1000 to 2000 mL. The patient grabs the mouthpiece with the mouth, thereby supplementing or substituting for inadequate autonomous breath volumes. The patient varies the volume of air taken from ventilator cycle to ventilator cycle and breath to breath to vary tidal volume, speech volume and cough flows, as well as to air stack to fully expand the lungs to maintain lung and chest wall compliance.[6]

To use MPV effectively and conveniently, adequate neck rotation and oral motor function are necessary to grab the mouthpiece and receive IPPV without insufflation leakage. To prevent the latter, the soft palate must move posteriocaudally to seal off the nasopharynx. In addition, the patient must open the glottis and vocal cords, dilate the hypopharynx and maintain airway patency to receive the air. These normally reflex movements may require a few minutes to relearn for patients who have been receiving IPPV via an indwelling tube, especially one with an inflated cuff, because reflex abduction of the hypopharynx and glottis is lost during invasive ventilation. Often patients are thought to have tracheal stenosis or other reasons for upper airway obstruction before they learn to re-open the glottis to permit MPV. MPV users can avoid nasal leakage by having their nostrils clipped or plugged by cotton. Covering the nostrils was found to be needed for 5 of 163 MPV users with little or no breathing tolerance.[6]

Along with the improvement of ventilator performance,[9] there is room for improvement in practical equipment such as mouthpieces and their fixation systems. Few supports are commercially available, in contrast with nasal and oronasal interfaces, with some hundred available models. However, nowadays, some mouthpiece support arms are available (Figure 44.2). Furthermore, mouthpieces are made of a single rigid part, requiring to be precisely installed with respect to the patient position, with the risk of ventilation loss if the patient moves the head.[10] As an additional problem, their shapes prevent them to be kept in the mouth during speech and may cause orthodontic problems in the long term.

There are various types of mouthpiece for MPV.[11] Angled mouthpieces are the most commonly used, because they are the easiest for the patient to grab and

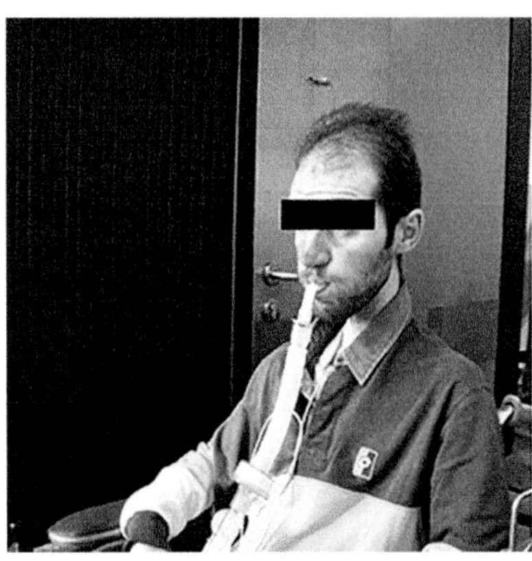
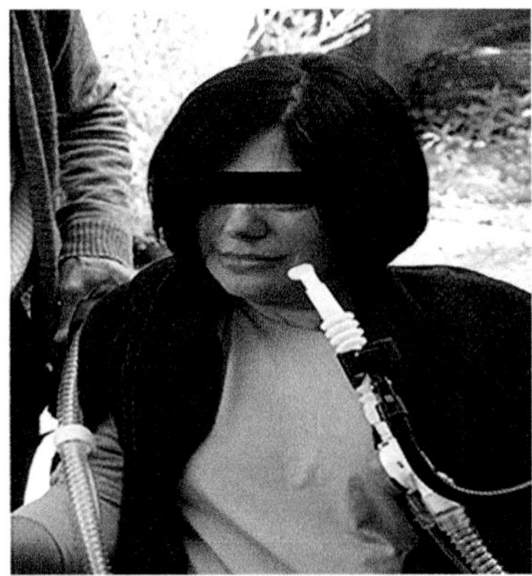

Figure 44.1 A 34-year-old DMD patient using MPV between his teeth all day and a 42-year-old SMA type 2 woman that prefers to have the mouthpiece held near the mouth and get ventilatory support intermittently.

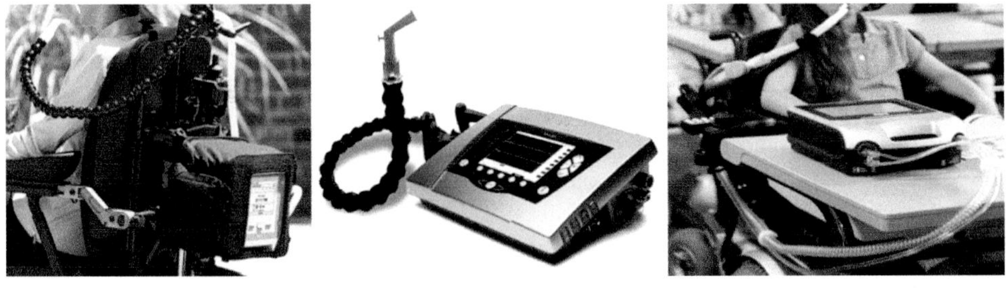

Figure 44.2 Mouthpiece support arms available in the market. From left to right: Philips Respironics Ventilator and Support Arm, Breas Ventilator and Support Arm and ResMed Ventilator and Support Arm.

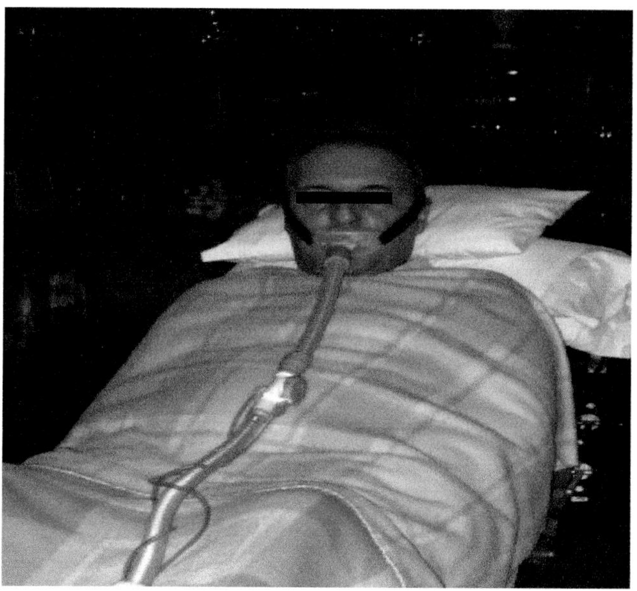

Figure 44.3 Patient with ALS using MPV through a Lipseal for sleep.

there are rigid angled mouthpiece (15 and 22 mm), flexible and straw mouthpiece.[12] Recent data show measurable differences in the ventilation's performances comparing the interfaces for MPV, according to the differences in their resistive characteristics. These differences seem to have a minor relevance for the clinical practice in most settings but should be systematically checked when the hydraulic characteristics of the ventilator circuit are modified.[10]

When using MPV during sleep, a Lipseal retention system with two cloth straps with Velcro closures is strongly recommended (Figure 44.3).

The Lipseal can provide an essentially closed system of non-invasive ventilatory support delivered during sleep with little insufflation leakage out of the mouth and with virtually no risk of the mouthpiece falling out of the mouth. A strapless lipseal system called the Oracle is also now available. Yet another newly available lipseal is made of transparent silicon. It has no intra-oral mouthpiece but a similar strap retention system (Masque Buccal, Metamed, France).

In the complete (24 hour/day) ventilator-dependent patient, daytime ventilation with angled mouthpiece in association with nocturnal NIV with a nasal or oronasal interface or mouthpiece with Lipseal retention has been reported to offer a better quality of life.[13]

ADVANTAGES, DISADVANTAGES AND SIDE EFFECTS OF VENTILATION WITH MOUTHPIECE

The most significant advantage compared to a nasal or oronasal interface is that mouthpiece produces less interference with speech, better appearance and absence of claustrophobia. Another significant advantage of MPV is that it permits air stacking[14] and also allows the patient to be able to perform glossopharyngeal breathing (GPB) in case of sudden failure of the ventilator or accidental disconnection from the ventilator,[15,16] which is not possible with tracheostomy.

A major disadvantage is the difficulty of use at night;[17] other issues include air leak from the mouth or nose.[18] In some patients, the mouthpiece may cause gastric distension, increased salivation and sometimes vomiting.[11] The failure of MPV and/or NIV is seen: if patients are not cooperative, or more often, in the presence of a severe bulbar spastic dysfunction and in patients unable to protect the upper airway.[19–21]

CHOICE OF VENTILATOR, MODES, ALARMS AND SETTINGS FOR MPV

Modes

With MPV, any mode of ventilation including the pressure assisted, pressure support or bilevel positive airway ventilation mode could be used with several ventilator circuits (single-limb circuit with expiratory valve up to single limb with an intentional leak).[22,23] Pressure modes are usually not used because of the high airflow that the devices continue to deliver when the patient is disconnected from the circuit and they also do not permit air stacking.[24–27] The volume cycled ventilation with single-limb circuit is usually performed using portable ventilators in volume assisted/controlled mode (ACV)[28] and appears the most suitable and efficient because the flow provided is slow and steady; it also permits the patient to air stack.[26,29,30]

Alarms

The low-pressure alarm will need to be set to minimum or where possible set to off. The apnoea alarm should also be set to off when possible or set to the maximum time.[24,27,31] In the new ventilators that have a specific MPV feature on ACV mode, it is possible to set a positive expiratory pressure (EPAP or PEEP) to 0 cmH_2O. In other home volume cycled ventilators, the low-pressure alarm cannot be turned off; therefore, it is necessary to set up a PEEP (often 2 cmH_2O) that, due to the resistance to the airflow created from the angle of the mouthpiece, assures the necessary back pressure that is adequate to prevent low-pressure alarm sounding.[9,24]

Eight life-support ventilators were recently tested, aiming to use MPV by minimising nuisance alarms and measure the bias flow exiting from the distal part of the circuit during disconnection from MPV when the end-expiratory pressure was set to zero. Because of these results, the operators are aware of the possibility of using

MPV with the majority of the tested ventilators. A correct combination of tidal volume and inspiratory time avoided activation of the low-pressure alarm when the user was disconnected from the circuit.[32]

Settings

Volume-cycled modes allow the patient to choose at every inspiration the amount of air, which they want to inhale, adjusting the seal with the lips on the mouthpiece. A tidal volume between 700 and 1500 mL for adult patients ensures adequate ventilation and permits the patient to take a deeper breath to speak, shout or cough.[27,31]

Recently, new ventilatory modes specially dedicated for MPV has been developed (MPV—Philips Respironics, Pittsburgh Murrysville and Breas, Mölnlycke, Sweden), with a dedicated arm and circuit without an active or passive expiratory valve allowing the patient to exhale outside the mouthpiece. Dedicated MPV settings have been reported to be safe and comfortable and facilitate the setting of alarms.[24] Nevertheless, recent data show large differences in the capacity of different life-support ventilators to deal with the rapid change in respiratory load features that characterise MPV, which can be further accentuated according to the choice of ventilator settings. Furthermore, the newly developed MPV modes allow a better performance of ventilators only in some definite situations. This has practical consequences, since the choice of the ventilator to be used for MPV in a specific patient should also contemplate the advantages and limitations of each machine, which depend on the prescribed ventilator mode.[33]

Moreover, these recent ventilator modes have a system of triggering dedicated for its purpose, which improve its use, by delivering the air only when the patients connect to the mouthpiece with their lips. This feature has been tested with good results in selected patients and is commonly known as 'kiss trigger'.[9] The patient activates the breath by putting the mouth on the mouthpiece and creating a small negative pressure in the circuit by sipping or inhaling from the mouthpiece (Figure 44.4). Indeed, the negative pressure generated by a sip is much higher than that generated by a maximum static inspiratory pressure and can explain why a patient with advanced neuromuscular disease (NMD) is able to activate the trigger without any inspiratory effort after a sip manoeuvre.[23] The following is an example of an MPV setting to be used for daytime ventilatory support in a patient with NMD:

- Mode—ACV MPV
- Vt—1000 to 1500 mL
- PEEP—0 cmH_2O
- RR—0 bpm (or a backup rate of 12 to 16 bpm if too weak to trigger)
- Insp. time—1.3 s

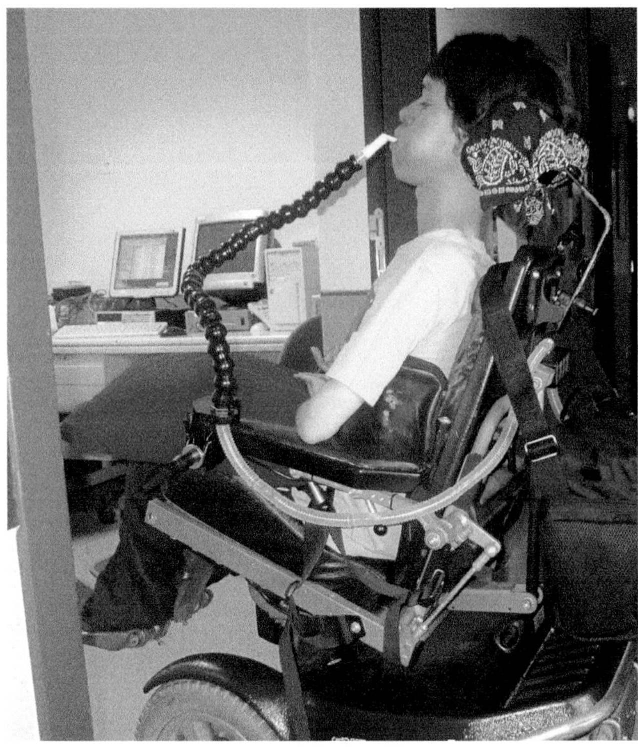

Figure 44.4 A 24-year-old DMD patient using MPV with the 'kiss trigger' system.

MOUTHPIECE VENTILATORY SUPPORT TO FACILITATE AMBULATION

Severe restrictive ventilatory patients often avoid exercise or are encouraged to walk using supplemental oxygen (O_2).[34] However, O_2 administration can ameliorate dyspnoea but augment hypercapnia and the myriad of symptoms and cardiovascular sequelae caused by severe hypercapnia.[35–37] The role of NIV to improve exercise tolerance and functional tasks, such as walking, is not clear in patients with severe restrictive ventilatory syndromes and daytime ventilatory dependence. Using MPV during a 6-min walking test (6MWT) significantly increases the walking distance, ambulation time and initial and final SpO_2 and decreases dyspnoea sensation in this patient population (Figure 44.5). The potential action mechanism of MPV during 6MWT that allowed the increase in the distance walked and ambulation time may be related to higher tidal volume and the reduction of dyspnoea. One remarkable effect of MPV during exercise was the significant improvement of the initial and final SpO_2 during the 6MWT, when compared with the same test performed in spontaneous breathing. Another positive effect of MPV is that it helps some patients achieve any significant walking distance and improves exercise tolerance for the more mildly affected ventilator-dependent patients. This fact may also improve exercise tolerance and motivate many of such patients to use MPV in their daily life activities and allow the patients to perform their other daily life activities without respiratory discomfort or symptoms.

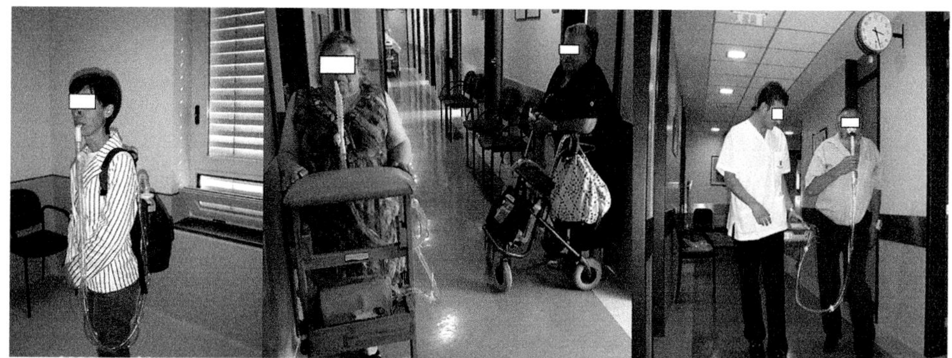

Figure 44.5 Patients using MPV during walking. From left to right: patient with a ventilator in a backpack, patient using a ventilator with a rollator and a patient that has a person that carries the ventilator for him.

CONCLUSION

Some authors still acknowledge tracheostomy as the most effective and secure form of continuous ventilatory support. However, there are studies showing that survival is significantly longer and there are fewer reported complications with NIV[38] compared to a variety of other strategies. As noted above, a randomised controlled trial with NIV and tracheostomy is neither feasible nor ethical. CNVS is a safe and acceptable alternative to ventilation by tracheostomy.[17,25] There is actually a widespread consensus that the NIV is preferable to tracheostomy during the early stages of early ventilatory failure in patients with NMD,[5,39–41] but its long-term effectiveness when ventilatory dependence progresses remains a controversy. The side effects of tracheostomy are well known: dysphagia, decreased or loss of vocalisation, the inability to perform air stacking and GPB. Patients suffering from severe NMD, in whom nocturnal NIV alone becomes insufficient, should have a trial of NIV with a mouthpiece for daytime use.[7,38,41,42]

REFERENCES

1. Bach JR, Barrow SE, Goncalves M. A historical perspective on expiratory muscle AIDS and their impact on home care. *Am J Phys Med Rehabil.* 2013;92(10):930–941.
2. Bach J. A historical perspective on the use of non-invasive ventilatory support alternatives. *Am Rev Respir Dis.* 1996(22):161–81.
3. Round Table Conference on Poliomyelitis Equipment, Roosevelt Hotel, White Plaines, New York City *National Foundation for Infantile Paralysis-March of Dimes, Inc.* May 1953.
4. Bach J. The history of mechancial ventilation and respiratory muscle aids. In: Bach JR, editor. *Non-invasive Mechanical Ventilation.* Philadephia, Hanley & Belfus, 2002:45–72.
5. Bach JR. Update and perspectives on noninvasive respiratory muscle aids. Part 1: The inspiratory aids. *Chest.* 1994;105(4):1230–40.
6. Bach JR, Alba AS, Saporito LR. Intermittent positive pressure ventilation via the mouth as an alternative to tracheostomy for 257 ventilator users. *Chest.* 1993;103(1):174–82.
7. Bach JR, Goncalves MR, Hon A et al. Changing trends in the management of end-stage neuromuscular respiratory muscle failure: Recommendations of an international consensus. *Am J Phys Med Rehabil.* 2013;92(3):267–77.
8. Bach JR, Goncalves MR, Hamdani I, Winck JC. Extubation of patients with neuromuscular weakness: A new management paradigm. *Chest.* 2010;137(5):1033–9.
9. Khirani S, Ramirez A, Delord V et al. Evaluation of ventilators for mouthpiece ventilation in neuromuscular disease. *Respir Care.* 2014;59(9):1329–37.
10. Ogna A, Prigent H, Falaize L et al. Bench evaluation of commercially available and newly developed interfaces for mouthpiece ventilation. *Clin Respir J.* 2016.
11. Nava S, Navalesi P, Gregoretti C. Interfaces and humidification for noninvasive mechanical ventilation. *Respir Care.* 2009;54(1):71–84.
12. Nicolini A, Santo M, Ferrari-Bravo M, Barlascini C. Open-mouthpiece ventilation versus nasal mask ventilation in subjects with COPD exacerbation and mild to moderate acidosis: A randomized trial. *Respir Care.* 2014;59(12):1825–31.
13. Bach JR. A comparison of long-term ventilatory support alternatives from the perspective of the patient and care giver. *Chest.* 1993;104(6):1702–6.
14. Bach JR. Amyotrophic lateral sclerosis: Predictors for prolongation of life by noninvasive respiratory aids. *Arch Phys Med Rehabil.* 1995;76(9):828–32.
15. Sferrazza Papa GF, Di Marco F, Akoumianaki E, Brochard L. Recent advances in interfaces for non-invasive ventilation: From bench studies to practical issues. *Minerva Anestesiol.* 2012;78(10):1146–53.
16. Dean S, Bach JR. The use of noninvasive respiratory muscle aids in the management of patients with progressive neuromuscular diseases. *Respir Care Clin N Am.* 1996;2(2):223–40.

17. Benditt JO. Full-time noninvasive ventilation: Possible and desirable. *Respir Care.* 2006;51(9): 1005–12; discussion 1005–12.
18. Hess DR. The growing role of noninvasive ventilation in patients requiring prolonged mechanical ventilation. *Respir Care.* 2012;57(6):900–918; discussion 918–920.
19. Vandenberghe N, Vallet AE, Petitjean T et al. Absence of airway secretion accumulation predicts tolerance of noninvasive ventilation in subjects with amyotrophic lateral sclerosis. *Respir Care.* 2013;58(9):1424–32.
20. Farrero E, Prats E, Povedano M et al. Survival in amyotrophic lateral sclerosis with home mechanical ventilation: The impact of systematic respiratory assessment and bulbar involvement. *Chest.* 2005;127(6):2132–8.
21. Bourke SC, Bullock RE, Williams TL et al. Noninvasive ventilation in ALS: Indications and effect on quality of life. *Neurology.* 2003;61(2):171–7.
22. Bach JR, Goncalves MR, Hon A et al. Changing trends in the management of end-stage neuromuscular respiratory muscle failure: Recommendations of an international consensus. *Am J Phys Med Rehabil.* 2013;92:267–77.
23. Toussaint M, Steens M, Wasteels G, Soudon P. Diurnal ventilation via mouthpiece: Survival in end-stage Duchenne patients. *Eur Respir J.* 2006;28:549–55.
24. Garuti G, Nicolini A, Grecchi B et al. Open circuit mouthpiece ventilation: Concise clinical review. *Rev Port Pneumol.* 2014;20(4):211–8.
25. Heritier Barras AC, Adler D, Iancu Ferfoglia R et al. Is tracheostomy still an option in amyotrophic lateral sclerosis? Reflections of a multidisciplinary work group. *Swiss Med Weekly.* 2013;143:w13830.
26. Ambrosino N, Carpene N, Gherardi M. Chronic respiratory care for neuromuscular diseases in adults. *Eur Respir J.* 2009;34(2):444–51.
27. Boitano LJ, Benditt JO. An evaluation of home volume ventilators that support open-circuit mouthpiece ventilation. *Respir Care.* 2005; 50(11):1457–61.
28. Bach JR. Management of post-polio respiratory sequelae. *Ann N Y Acad Sci.* 1995;753:96–102.
29. Boitano LJ. Equipment options for cough augmentation, ventilation, and noninvasive interfaces in neuromuscular respiratory management. *Pediatrics.* 2009;123 Suppl 4:S226–30.
30. Soudon P, Steens M, Toussaint M. A comparison of invasive versus noninvasive full-time mechanical ventilation in Duchenne muscular dystrophy. *Chron Respir Dis.* 2008;5(2):87–93.
31. Hess DR. Noninvasive ventilation in neuromuscular disease: Equipment and application. *Respir Care.* 2006;51(8):896–911; discussion 892–911.
32. Carlucci A, Mattei A, Rossi V et al. Ventilator settings to avoid nuisance alarms during mouthpiece ventilation. *Respir Care.* 2016;61(4):462–7.
33. Ogna A, Prigent H, Falaize L et al. Accuracy of tidal volume delivered by home mechanical ventilation during mouthpiece ventilation: A bench evaluation. *Chron Respir Dis.* 2016.
34. Schonhofer B, Zimmermann C, Abramek P et al. Non-invasive mechanical ventilation improves walking distance but not quadriceps strength in chronic respiratory failure. *Respir Med.* 2003;97(7):818–24.
35. Mokhlesi B, Tulaimat A, Parthasarathy S. Oxygen for obesity hypoventilation syndrome: A double-edged sword? *Chest.* 2011;139:975–7.
36. Meecham Jones D, Paul E, Bell J, Wedzicha J. Ambulatory oxygen therapy in stable kyphoscoliosis. *Eur Respir J.* 1995;8:819–23.
37. Kirshblum SC, Bach JR. Walker modification for ventilator-assisted individuals. Case report. *Am J Phys Med Rehabil.* 1992;71(5):304–6.
38. McKim DA, Griller N, LeBlanc C et al. Twenty-four hour noninvasive ventilation in Duchenne muscular dystrophy: A safe alternative to tracheostomy. *Can Respir J.* 2013;20(1):e5–9.
39. Fauroux B, Khirani S. Neuromuscular disease and respiratory physiology in children: Putting lung function into perspective. *Respirology.* 2014;19(6):782–91.
40. Toussaint M, Chatwin M, Soudon P. Mechanical ventilation in Duchenne patients with chronic respiratory insufficiency: Clinical implications of 20 years published experience. *Chron Respir Dis.* 2007;4(3):167–77.
41. Toussaint M, Steens M, Wasteels G, Soudon P. Diurnal ventilation via mouthpiece: Survival in end-stage Duchenne patients. *Eur Respir J.* 2006;28(3):549–55.
42. Pinto T, Chatwin M, Banfi P et al. Mouthpiece ventilation and complementary techniques in patients with neuromuscular disease: A brief clinical review and update. *Chron Respir Dis.* 2017;14:187–93.

PART 9

Chest wall deformity

45 Scoliosis 426
William J. M. Kinnear

45

Scoliosis

WILLIAM J. M. KINNEAR

INTRODUCTION

The bony structure of the spinal column reminds us that we are segmental organisms. In our quadripedal ancestors, the spine was suspended between the shoulder and pelvic girdles. Adopting an upright posture has brought us many advantages, but we pay a price in that the spine no longer hangs in the configuration for which it evolved: a column of blocks stacked on top of each other is inherently unstable.

When we assumed our current upright posture, we maintained the spinal curvature of our ancestors. Forward curvature of the spine, convex when viewed from behind, is called kyphosis (Figure 45.1). A gentle kyphosis appears to make the spine more stable: loss of this curvature is a predictor of the likelihood of developing the rotational deformity of scoliosis.[1] Thoracic kyphosis is normally associated with lumbar lordosis (concave, when viewed from behind).

In quadripeds, the scope for rotational distortion of the spine is limited: since all four limbs touch the ground, the pelvic and shoulder girdles remain in alignment. This corrective mechanism is lost in bipeds, and the spine is vulnerable to rotational deformity. This rotation is called scoliosis. (The term *kyphoscoliosis* is sometimes used, but it is probably better to try and distinguish kyphosis and scoliosis, since their effects on breathing tend to be different.) If you look at the spinous processes on the x-ray of a patient with mild scoliosis, you can see how the vertebrae twist around at the apex of the deformity, emphasising that this is a rotational problem and not just lateral curvature.

Cervical and lumbar spinal deformities have little effect on the mechanics of respiration. If the thoracic spine is involved, the rib cage is inevitably distorted. In mild cases, the effects may only be cosmetic, but more severe disruption of the normal configuration of the ribs constrains their movement. On the concave side of the curve, the ribs are crushed together, whereas on the convex side, they are splayed apart, although they must still join together anteriorly onto the sternum (Figure 45.2).

Although scoliosis is a rotational deformity, its severity is often assessed by measuring the angulation in a two-dimensional plane, in this case the coronal (as opposed to the sagittal angulation of kyphosis). To do this, we need a frontal x-ray of the spine, on which we calculate the Cobb angle.[2] Draw a line along the upper and lower bony margins of the two vertebrae at the top and bottom of the curved segment – this is more accurate than trying to draw a line through the middle of the vertebra. Cobb realised that drawing two lines at right angles to these lines allows you to measure the angle of curvature (Figure 45.3). (This was particularly useful on hard copies of x-rays, where the Cobb angle could be measured alongside the spine on the edge of the plate, rather than overlying the image itself.) Respiratory failure is uncommon if the angle of spinal curvature is less than 100° (i.e. approximately a right angle).

If the spine is curved, the affected person will try to get their head back into vertical alignment by developing a compensatory curve in the unaffected segments. If you look carefully at a patient with scoliosis, you will notice that their head is not centred over their pelvis (Figure 45.4). If the primary abnormality is lumbar, the thoracic curve that develops in compensation is rarely severe enough to compromise gas exchange.

Scoliosis causes loss of vertical height. Another clinical clue to the presence of scoliosis is the length of a patient's arms compared to the height of their trunk (Figure 45.4). Arm span is similar to vertical height, a trick we use to estimate what the height would be without the spinal curvature when calculating predicted lung function parameters for a patient with scoliosis.[3]

On the convex side of the spinal curvature, the ribs are splayed apart. This may form a 'rib hump', which is a cosmetic issue for the patient, sometimes corrected by costoplasty. On the concave side, the ribs are crowded together, and there may be discomfort where the lower ribs rub against the iliac crest. The more vertebral bodies in the curve, the more severe the effects on respiration.

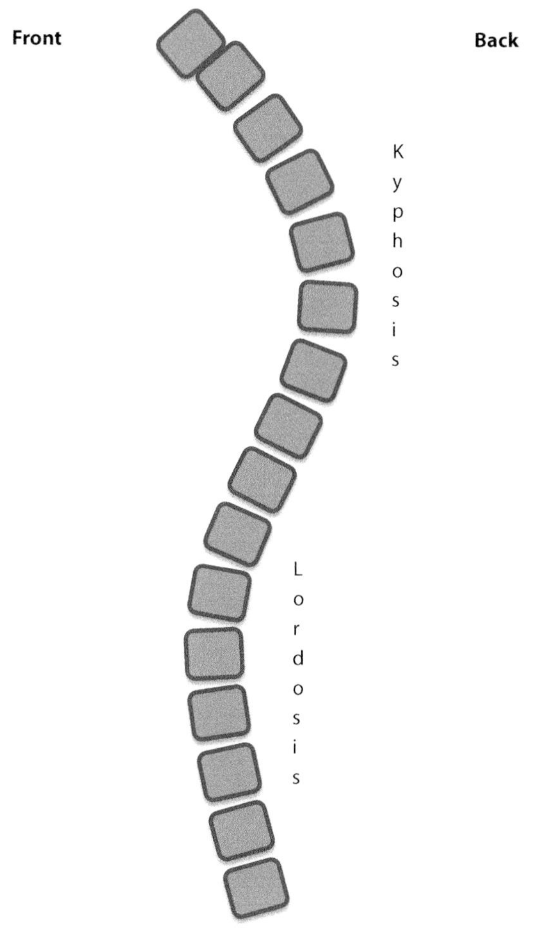

Figure 45.1 Diagrammatic saggital view of thoraco-lumbar spine. Convexity (as seen from the back) is termed kyphosis; concavity is called lordosis.

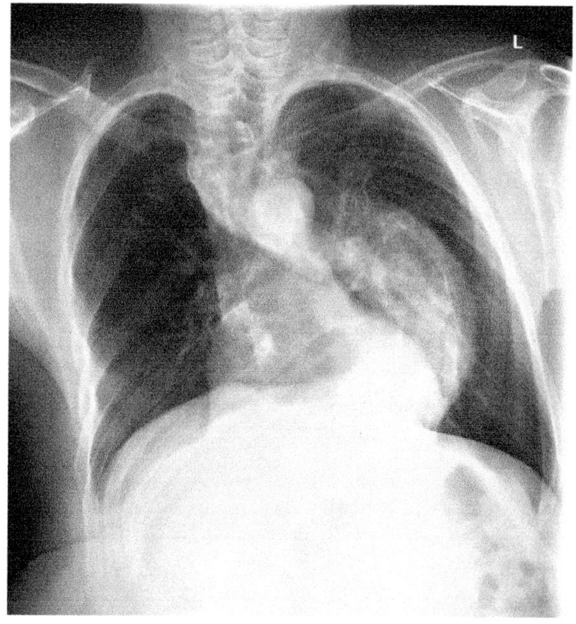

Figure 45.2 Chest x-ray of a patient with thoracic scoliosis. Note the narrow gaps between the ribs posteriorly in the left upper zone, compared with the wider gaps on the right.

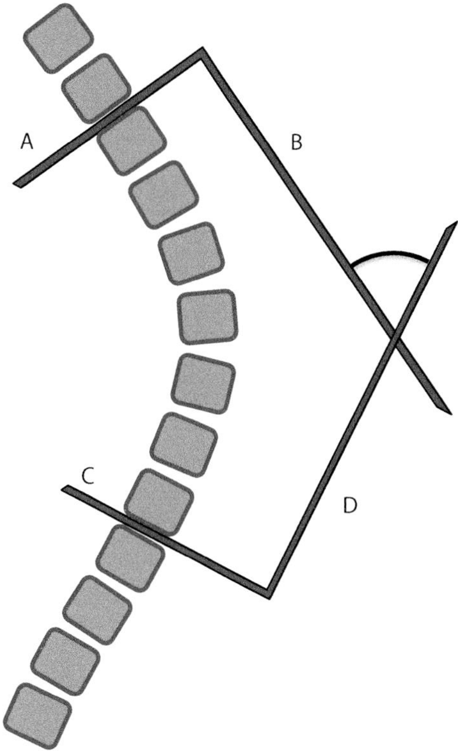

Figure 45.3 To measure the Cobb angle, draw a line extending along the top of the vertebra just above the start of the curve (A). Then, draw a line at a right angle to this (B). Draw a line along the top of the vertebra just below the curvature (C). Draw another line (D) at right angles to line C. Measure the angle where line D crosses line B, indicated by the arc in this figure. This is the Cobb angle. This is exactly the same angle you would get if you drew lines through the middle of the vertebrae at the upper and lower ends of the curve, but in practice, it is easier to draw a line along the bony upper margin of the vertebra rather than the middle. Measuring the Cobb angle alongside the spine is clearer than drawing lines directly over the bony vertebral bodies.

Most cases of scoliosis are idiopathic (Box 45.1). Rarely, congenital absence of one-half of the vertebra or fusion of adjacent vertebrae will lead to a scoliosis (Figure 45.5). These congenital curves are important in that the full complement of alveoli do not develop in the lung on the concave side of the curve. An echocardiogram should be performed to look for associated cardiac defects.

Familial aggregation of idiopathic scoliosis implies a genetic component to the disease, but other factors affecting bone growth, muscles, nerves, collagen, blood vessels, ligaments and so on are likely to be involved. Much work remains to be done to elucidate the genetics of this disease. For reasons that are not clear, adolescent idiopathic scoliosis is more common in females, with curvature convex to the left. Screening programmes have been put in place to detect asymptomatic scoliosis, with a view to intervening before the curve progresses too far, but their value is much

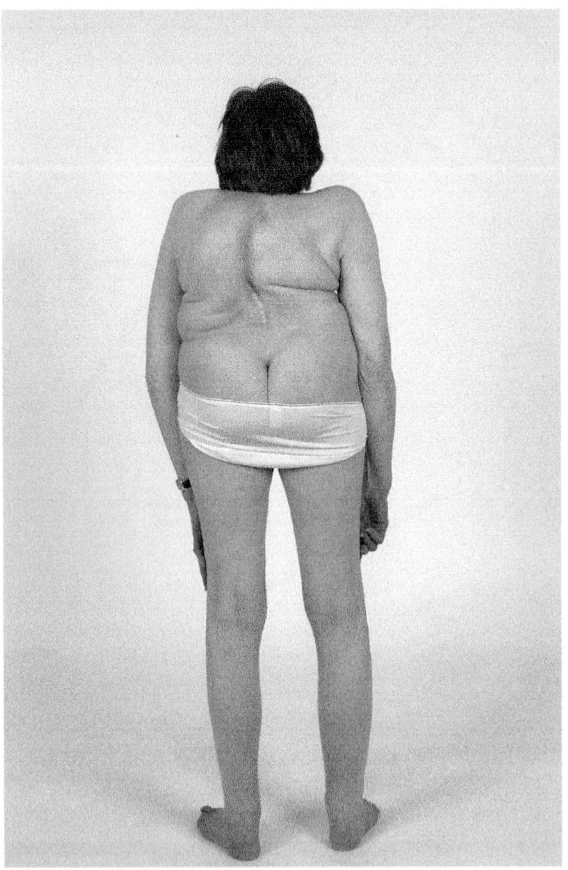

Figure 45.4 Thoracic scoliosis: note the rib hump, how the person's head is not centred over the pelvis, and how long the arms are compared with the trunk.

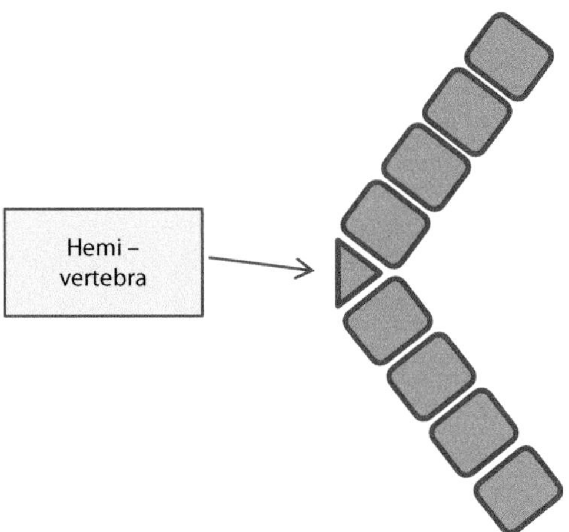

Figure 45.5 Embryologically, each side of the vertebra forms by fusion of mesodermal plates from two adjacent segments, which then fuse with the corresponding tissue from the opposite side. The commonest congenital vertebral abnormality is for this process to fail on one side, which results in a triangular hemi-vertebra. Other congenital abnormalities, such as bony bars between vertebrae, result from failure of segmentation. These abnormalities inevitably produce a scoliosis.

BOX 45.1: Classification of scoliosis

- Congenital (vertebral abnormalities, myelomeningocele)
- Neuromuscular
- Idiopathic
- Connective tissue diseases (Marfan's syndrome, osteogenesis imperfecta)
- Neurofibromatosis
- Vertebral destruction (infection, trauma, tumour, radiation, etc.)
- Thoracoplasty

debated. Look carefully for clinical features of an underlying skeletal condition in all patients with scoliosis.

Scoliosis in neuromuscular disorders

The spine is flanked by two large groups of muscles – the paraspinal muscles. The stabilizing influence of these muscles is illustrated by the fact that patients with diseases such as muscular dystrophy develop scoliosis. When the paraspinal muscles on one side are weak – for example, when affected by poliomyelitis – spinal deformity is very common. These curves are sometimes referred to as 'paralytic' scoliosis. The muscle weakness may not become apparent until limb muscles become affected, sometimes many years later. Keep the possibility of an underlying neuromuscular aetiology in mind whenever you review a patient with 'idiopathic' scoliosis.

Tuberculosis

In the days prior to anti-tuberculous chemotherapy, thoracoplasty was performed as a means of collapsing upper lobe cavities. Several ribs were removed, sometimes under local anaesthesia. Scoliosis usually developed subsequently, because of loss of the stabilizing effect of the ribs on the spine. These patients always had severe pulmonary tuberculosis (TB), inevitably leaving them with fibrosis and bronchiectasis. They often had other procedures such as phrenic nerve crush or artificial pneumothorax. The aetiology of hypercapnic respiratory failure as a late complication involves several different influences on the work of breathing and capacity of the respiratory muscles. In many published series, these patients are referred to as 'sequelae of tuberculosis' rather than 'thoracoplasty'. For simplicity, I will use the term 'post-TB'.

PATHOPHYSIOLOGY

Ventilation

As we have noted, scoliosis causes the ribs on the concave side of the curve to be crushed together. On the convex side, the ribs are splayed apart (Figure 45.2). As a consequence, ventilation is uneven.[4–6] If you look carefully at a patient with severe

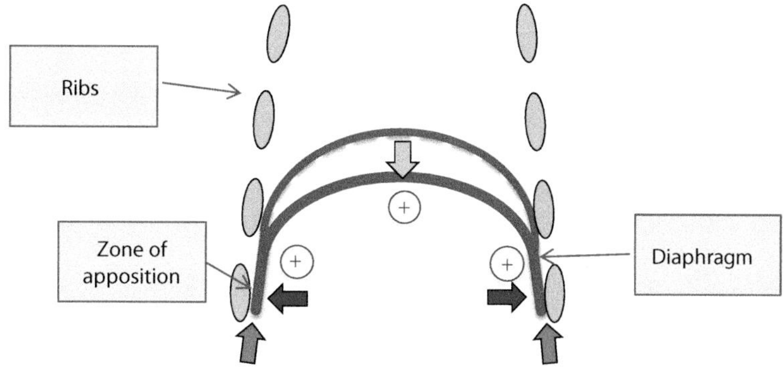

Figure 45.6 Diagrammatic representation of a coronal cross section through a normal thorax. The diaphragm (in red) is attached to the lower ribs and spine, with a central dome ascending into the chest. When the diaphragm contracts, the insertional force on the lower ribs tends to pull them upward (green arrows). Descent of the diaphragm when it contracts creates a positive pressure underneath it; where the diaphragm is closely apposed to the ribs, this positive pressure pushes them outward (blue arrows).

CLINICAL SCENARIO 1: EXTRA-PULMONARY RESTRICTION AND CHEST WALL DEFORMITY OF UNKNOWN AETIOLOGY

A 52-year-old male is admitted with hypercapnic respiratory failure. His chest x-ray shows a small left hemithorax, with a lot of pleural shadowing on that side. His spine is curved, concave to the left. He says that he was treated for a lung abscess as a teenager. How should he be managed?

Most long-term home non-invasive ventilation (NIV) services will have a few older patients who have slipped into ventilatory failure as a result of a combination of lung scarring and chest wall deformity, the exact cause of which is unclear. Thoracic imaging shows asymmetrical pleural scarring, with scoliosis and some rib cage distortion on the side of the more severely affected lung. Often the patient will recount a long spell in hospital in their youth, perhaps with a lung abscess or empyema, or some serious chest trauma. Many will have had some sort of thoracic surgical intervention. They will usually be very clear that they had repeatedly tested negative for TB.

They should be managed in the same way as patients with scoliosis, that is, nocturnal NIV for life. Many will also need supplementary oxygen, reflecting the underlying lung scarring.

scoliosis, when they breathe in, there may well be parts of the rib cage that move in rather than out; this paradoxical motion wastes the inspiratory force generated by the respiratory muscles. Post-TB patients may also have paradoxical motion of the segment of the rib cage where their ribs were removed.

An important function of the normal diaphragm is to inflate the lower part of the rib cage. This is achieved as a consequence of the 'zone of apposition', where the diaphragm lies closely up against the lower ribs. When the diaphragm contracts, the insertional force tends to pull the ribs cranially. These lower ribs are also exposed to the positive pressure that is generated underneath the diaphragm when it contracts, pushing them outward (Figure 45.6). In scoliosis, the normal insertion of the dome of the diaphragm into the lower ribs is distorted, with flattening of the hemi-diaphragms similar to that seen in severe chronic obstructive pulmonary disease (COPD) (Figure 45.7). When the diaphragm contracts in this alignment, the insertional force pulls the lower rib cage inward. There is also no zone of apposition, so the ribs are influenced by negative intrathoracic pressure (rather than the positive sub-diaphragmatic abdominal pressure when the diaphragm is its normal configuration as a dome), which also causes the ribs to move inward (Figure 45.8). Interestingly, this paradoxical inward

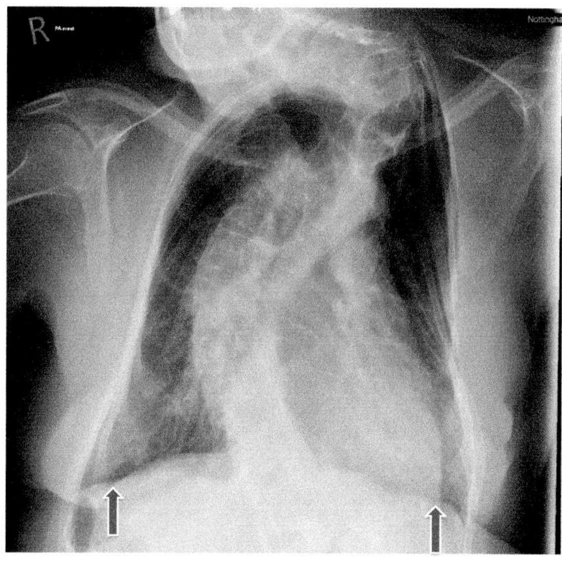

Figure 45.7 Chest x-ray of a subject with scoliosis, demonstrating flattening of the diaphragms. As a consequence, there is no zone of apposition (see Figure 45.6).

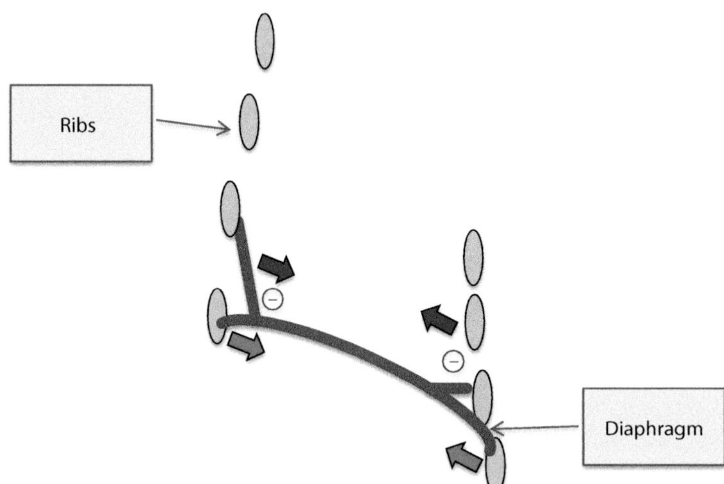

Figure 45.8 Diagrammatic representation of a coronal cross section through the thorax of a subject with scoliosis. Distortion of the rib cage changes the orientation of the diaphragm such that it is more flattened and there is no zone of apposition. The insertional force when the diaphragm contracts now pulls the ribs inward (green arrows). Moreover, the lack of a zone of apposition means that the lower rib cage is exposed to negative intrathoracic pressure, rather than the positive abdominal pressure, which also pulls it inward. The result of these two forces is paradoxical inward motion of the lower rib cage during inspiration.

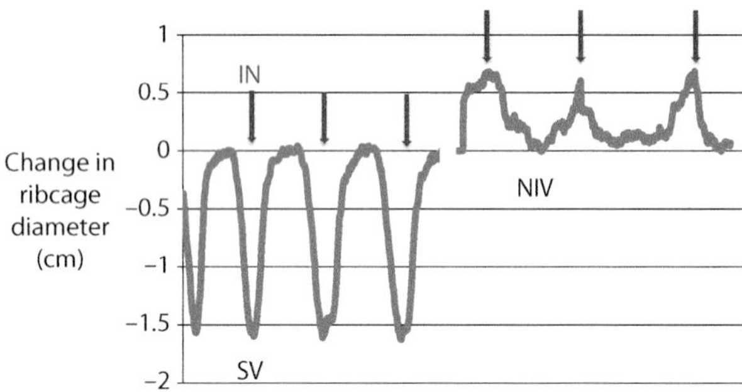

Figure 45.9 In these recordings, linearised magnetometers have been used to record the lateral diameter of the lower rib cage in a patient with scoliosis. Zero is taken as the resting end-expiratory diameter. During spontaneous inspiration (indicated by red arrows), the diameter of the rib cage reduces; that is, the ribs move inward. When NIV is commenced, in the right-hand sample of the recording, normal motion is restored with the rib cage increasing in diameter during inspiration. NIV induces relaxation of respiratory muscles, so the abolition of the paradoxical motion by NIV implies that the cause was diaphragmatic contraction (see Figures 45.6 and 45.8).

motion of the rib cage during inspiration is corrected during NIV,[7] when the predominant force is the positive pressure within the whole thorax (Figure 45.9).

Perfusion

On the convex side of the spinal curvature, the lungs are overdistended. The pulmonary vascular tree is also stretched, which reduces the size of the vessels. On the concave side, the vessels are less affected, so ventilation–perfusion imbalance is inevitable.[4–6,8] Ventilation–perfusion matching is worse the more severe the spinal curvature (and the lower the vital capacity) and deteriorates with age.[9] As a result, hypoxia with pulmonary hypertension and right heart failure are common in adults with severe scoliosis.

Right heart failure may be exacerbated by chronic nocturnal hypoxia.[10] Schonhofer et al.[11] documented a mean fall in pulmonary artery pressure of 8.5 mmHg in patients with scoliosis or post-TB after a year of nocturnal NIV, without any significant change in lung volumes. Mean overnight oxygen saturation increased from 72.5% to 90.5%. It is impossible to work out whether the pulmonary hypertension that persists in many patients despite nocturnal NIV is related to distortion of the pulmonary vascular tree or reflects irreversible damage from repeated episodes of nocturnal hypoxia over many years (see ‘Sleep’ section below).

Pulmonary hypertension, combined with distortion of the shape of the heart when it is stretched over the spinal deformity, may result in a patent foramen ovale. While rare, this should always be considered when a patient with scoliosis is found to be hypoxaemic.[12]

Compliance

Clearly, distorted ribs will be more difficult to expand, so the compliance of the chest wall will be reduced in scoliosis. Compliance is the increase in volume for a set amount of applied inflation pressure. A stiff chest wall will show a smaller increase in size for any given pressure, compared to a more compliant chest wall. The compliance of the whole respiratory system can be measured by observing the increase in volume when positive pressure is applied to the airway (or negative pressure around the outside

CLINICAL SCENARIO 2: PERSISTENT HYPOXAEMIA IN SCOLIOSIS

A 44-year-old female with congenital thoracic scoliosis has been commenced on home-NIV, which has improved her sleep and corrected her daytime hypercapnia. In the outpatient clinic 6 months later, her PaO_2 remains low at 6.3 kPa while breathing air, but her $PaCO_2$ is normal. Overnight studies show a mean oxygen saturation of 83% with a normal transcutaneous CO_2 throughout the night. There are no clinical signs of right heart failure. Does she need further investigation or supplementary oxygen?

Hypoxaemia is common in scoliosis, usually caused by ventilation–perfusion mismatching. The normal $PaCO_2$ excludes hypoventilation as the cause of her hypoxaemia, so there is no need to adjust her NIV settings. It would be prudent to perform an echocardiogram to look for a patent foramen ovale, which will also pick up whether there is any suggestion of right ventricular hypertrophy.

There is no evidence-base for long-term supplementary oxygen in patients with diseases other than COPD, and there is no lower limit below which hypoxaemia must be corrected. In the absence of right heart strain, if she is sleeping well, then it is reasonable to leave her without supplementary oxygen. In practice, many patients with a mean SpO_2 of less than 85% will find their way onto supplementary oxygen. They may need careful explanation that this is perfectly safe when they are using NIV, having previously been told that they should resist being given oxygen as it could be dangerous for them.

of the chest, for example, in an iron lung), but of course this reflects the compliance of the lungs as well as the rib cage. Alternatively, you could inflate the lungs by a known amount – let us say half a litre – and get the subject to relax onto an occluded mouthpiece; the pressure measured at the mouthpiece is called the elastic recoil pressure, which again includes the pressure from the rib cage and the lungs as they try to deflate back to their normal resting volume. You will gather that it is quite difficult to measure the compliance of the rib cage, because of the need to measure lung compliance as well (which requires an estimate of pleural pressure, such as oesophageal pressure) and to ensure that none of the respiratory muscles are contracting when the pressure measurements are made. Most of the data on rib cage compliance in scoliosis come from patients undergoing spinal surgery under general anaesthesia.

The application of expiratory positive airway pressure (EPAP) during NIV increases the end-expiratory lung volume. In long-term ventilator users, who tend to be good at relaxing their respiratory muscles and allowing the ventilator to do all the work of breathing, this effect can be used to estimate the passive mechanical properties of the respiratory system. Normal values for compliance (the rib cage and lungs combined) are in the region of 100 mL/cmH_2O. Data from patients with scoliosis studied during NIV yield values of around 30 mL/cmH_2O.[13] This should be borne in mind when choosing inflation pressures (Figure 45.10).

It may not be immediately obvious why the compliance of the lungs should be reduced in scoliosis.[14] In congenital scoliosis, the total number of alveoli is less than normal, so the lungs will be less compliant. In addition, chronic under-expansion may lead to changes in the elastic properties of the lung. Inflation to larger lung volumes – as happens with NIV – should help correct these changes. This hypothesis is supported by the observation that 5 min of positive pressure

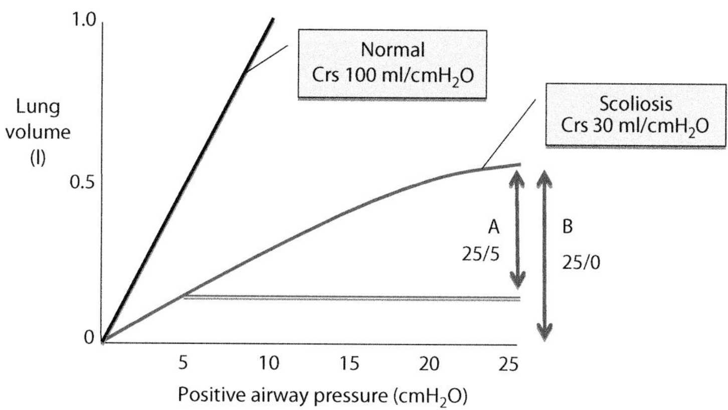

Figure 45.10 Pressure–volume curve of the respiratory system (lungs and chest wall combined) in normality and scoliosis. Compliance, that is, the increase in volume produced by any given increase in airway pressure, is lower in scoliosis. The red arrow marked 'A' indicates the change in volume (tidal volume) with bilevel NIV using an inspiratory positive airway pressure (IPAP) of 25 cmH_2O and an EPAP of 5 cmH_2O. The larger tidal volume produced with no EPAP but the same IPAP is shown by arrow 'B'. The difference between these two tidal volumes reflects the slope of the pressure–volume curve, that is, the compliance.

breathing in patients with scoliosis resulted in an increase in lung compliance.[15]

Resistance

Airway calibre is proportional to lung volume. Patients with scoliosis breathe at low lung volumes, so their airway resistance is high[16] and they may be flow-limited toward the end of expiration.[17] The trachea and major bronchi are sometimes distorted in severe scoliosis, with the spine pressing on the airways.[18,19] This kinking improves when the spinal curvature is corrected.

The ANTADIR series[20] found that airflow obstruction is an independent predictor for the development of hypercapnic respiratory failure in post-TB and scoliotic patients. While much of this may be post-tuberculous endobronchial scarring or volume-related changes in airway calibre, the possibility of concomitant asthma or COPD should not be overlooked. Consider a trial of bronchodilator therapy in scoliotic and post-TB patients if they have audible wheeze or obstructive spirometry.

Work of breathing

The work of breathing in scoliosis at rest is high and related to the extent of restriction.[8,9] Most of this is caused by low compliance rather than increased resistance. In order to keep the work of breathing as low as possible, the person increases their respiratory rate and keeps their tidal volumes low.[21] If they need to increase ventilation, for example, on exercise or if they become unwell, they are forced to increase their tidal volume. At this point of their compliance curve, much more pressure is required to produce any change in volume, with the result that the work of breathing increases rapidly.

RESPIRATORY MUSCLE STRENGTH

Contraction of the inspiratory muscles moves the rib cage to produce lung expansion. When the ribs are distorted, the mechanical coupling of the respiratory muscles is disrupted, so the force they exert is less efficient in producing movement of the rib cage. Similarly, the diaphragm is displaced from its normal position and is less effective at displacing the abdominal contents in order to inflate the lungs. Indeed, you may see paradoxical inward motion of some parts of the rib cage during inspiration in patients with scoliosis – another indicator of the mechanical inefficiency of the respiratory muscles, whereby work is wasted on moving the chest wall without producing ventilation (Figures 45.8 and 45.9).

Many studies have documented low respiratory muscle strength in scoliosis.[14,22–27] After starting NIV, maximum inspiratory pressures (MIPs) are often considerably better. This improvement, in the absence of any significant change in the size or shape of the rib cage, is consistent with the hypothesis that the muscles are weakened by the work they have to do to expand the stiff rib cage. Hypoxia and hypercapnia impair muscle contraction, but there is no consistent relationship between changes in arterial blood gases and the improvement in maximum mouth pressures. The most likely explanation for improvement in these volitional measures of strength after NIV is that the subjects are more awake, feel better and try harder at the tests.

Respiratory muscle fatigue

Thus, the respiratory muscles are less effective than normal, but are faced with increased work. Accessory muscles are recruited to help.[14] With each breath, if the force needed to produce an adequate tidal volume starts to approach the maximum available force, then the inspiratory muscles will become fatigued. This may happen insidiously as the chest becomes stiffer and age-related changes weaken the muscles, or acutely when an event such as an infection increases the work of breathing or the ventilation that must be achieved to maintain normal gas exchange.

Some evidence for the existence of respiratory muscle fatigue in scoliosis comes from observations of the effects of NIV. Schonhofer et al.[28] documented an improvement in respiratory muscle endurance after 3 months of nocturnal NIV. The threshold load against which the inspiratory muscles had to work was set at 33% of baseline MIP; this represented only 22% of MIP after NIV, on account of an increase from 43 to 66 cmH_2O, so the endurance task was not strictly comparable. Nevertheless, the improvement in endurance time was substantial and likely to represent a real improvement in their resistance to fatigue.

Respiratory drive

In mild scoliosis, the drive to breathe may be greater than normal in order to maintain normal ventilation, but in more severe cases, ventilatory drive is usually reduced.[9] In measuring the ventilatory output in response to elevation of carbon dioxide levels, the drive to breathe might be normal but mechanical factors prevent the patient from increasing tidal volume. This is overcome by looking at the pressure generated when the airway is occluded briefly—one-tenth of a second, hence the term P0.1.

Impaired ventilatory drive could be a protective strategy, allowing the arterial carbon dioxide to rise in order to protect the respiratory muscles if they are in danger of becoming fatigued. This implies a reduction in alveolar ventilation to a level that the muscles may be able to sustain. In addition, a rise in arterial carbon dioxide levels increases the back pressure, driving carbon dioxide out of the bloodstream into the air, which is to be exhaled; hence, overall carbon dioxide elimination from the body is increased.

Bicarbonate accumulates in patients with chronic hypercapnic respiratory failure. This larger pool of buffer blunts any change in pH with any further increases in carbon dioxide, which means that the ventilatory response to carbon dioxide is impaired. Possibly the most likely explanation for the blunted respiratory drive in scoliosis is that it is the consequence of sleep deprivation and repeated periods of hypoventilation at night. Improvement in the ventilatory response to carbon dioxide is a fairly consistent finding after NIV, even in the absence of any change in chest wall mechanics or respiratory muscle strength.[28–30]

CLINICAL SCENARIO 3: MILD DIURNAL HYPERCAPNIA IN SCOLIOSIS

A 64-year-old female under regular follow-up in the outpatient clinic is found to have a $PaCO_2$ of 6.8 kPa. She is breathless with an elevated jugular venous pressure but no ankle oedema. Her vital capacity is 0.9 L. She commences nocturnal NIV but over many months struggles to use it for more than an hour, despite using different interfaces, ventilator modes and settings. At subsequent clinic visits, her $PaCO_2$ remains mildly elevated, between 6.5 and 7.5 kPa. Should she persevere with NIV?

Experience from neuromuscular disease suggests that once the $PaCO_2$ is elevated, progression to life-threatening severe respiratory failure is almost inevitable unless the patient starts NIV. Most patients with scoliosis behave similarly, but there seems to be a small group with mild hypercapnia who remain stable. They repeatedly try NIV, but never get used to it and seem to manage well without it. They should be kept under regular follow-up. Provided their arterial blood gases remain stable, after a while, the interval between visits can be extended to a year.

Sleep

Sleep is associated with a reduction in ventilation and ventilatory drive, and elevation of arterial carbon dioxide levels. In scoliosis, rapid eye movement (REM) sleep seems to be the most vulnerable period[10,31–35] (Figure 45.11). Central hypoventilation and periodic breathing are the most common abnormalities. Apnoeas are usually central, although obstructive episodes have been described.[31]

During REM sleep, breathing is less regular and tidal volumes fall. The intercostal and accessory muscles are inhibited in this phase of sleep, and the diaphragm alone may be incapable of maintaining adequate alveolar ventilation. Loss of intercostal tone will reduce functional residual capacity; since there is less oxygen within the lungs to act as a buffer, any episodes of hypoventilation will have a more profound effect on arterial oxygen saturation.

The vulnerability of this group of patients to problems during sleep is emphasized by studies of NIV withdrawal. Hill et al.[36] reported the effects of withdrawing nocturnal NIV from patients with chronic hypercapnic respiratory failure. Of the six patients studied, two had scoliosis and two had a thoracoplasty. The intention was to stop NIV for 2 weeks, but only two patients managed this because of sleep disturbance and recurrence of their daytime symptoms, associated with deterioration in nocturnal gas exchange. Masa et al.[33] investigated the effect of withdrawing NIV for 15 days in five patients with scoliosis or post-TB. During REM sleep, gas exchange was much worse than it had been when they were on NIV, with disruption of their sleep pattern.

CLINICAL SCENARIO 4: ASYMPTOMATIC NOCTURNAL HYPOXIA

Overnight oximetry in patients with severe scoliosis is almost always abnormal. Hypoxia during REM sleep is highly likely. Provided the patient is not repeatedly woken up during the night, they will feel refreshed on wakening and not suffer from daytime tiredness. It is always worth just checking diurnal arterial blood gases, but provided these are normal, there is no need to start NIV. At an annual outpatient review, check for symptoms of sleep disturbance and have a low threshold for repeating the overnight oximetry.

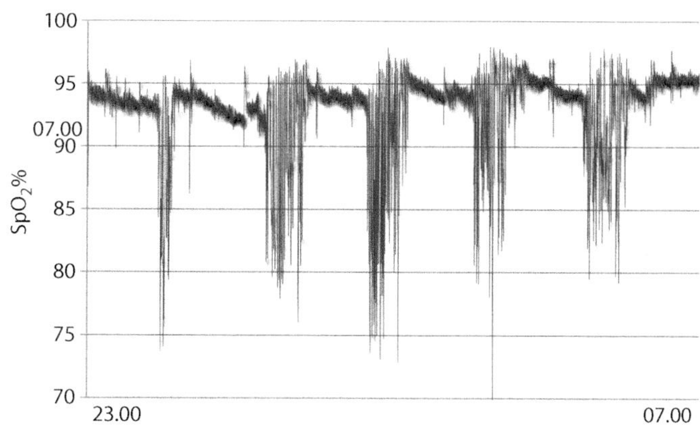

Figure 45.11 Overnight oximetry in a subject with scoliosis, showing episodes of hypoxia suggestive of desaturation during REM sleep.

Respiratory effects of spinal surgery for scoliosis

Surgical correction of spinal curvature may be undertaken for cosmetic appearances. In muscular dystrophy, stabilisation of the spine may be necessary for maintenance of posture, but the effect on lung function is often disappointing.[37,38] In idiopathic scoliosis, good quality evidence on the respiratory consequences of spinal surgery is sparse. Overall, it seems that any improvement in the mechanics of respiration is likely to be small, and surgery should not be undertaken for this reason alone. A period of halo traction pre-operatively may help identify those patients whose curvature can be improved, with concomitant increase in vital capacity.[39] Spinal surgery is a major undertaking with a significant mortality,[40] although this may change with refinement of surgical techniques. The post-operative use of NIV will be considered below.

Scoliosis and the risk of hypercapnic respiratory failure

On the basis of the pathophysiology we have considered and the evidence of large observational studies,[8,41–43] patients with scoliosis who have the features listed in Box 45.2 should be considered at greater risk of developing ventilatory failure.

BOX 45.2: Risk factors for respiratory failure in scoliosis

- The thoracic spine is involved.
- The curvature was present before the age of 5 years.
- The angle of curvature is greater than 90°.
- The vital capacity is less than 50 per cent of predicted.
- The spine has never been surgically stabilised.
- The scoliosis is secondary to neuromuscular weakness (including poliomyelitis).
- There is additional lung disease such as asthma or COPD.

This may help you identify patients who need to be kept under regular review. In addition to measuring vital capacity, you should have a low threshold for measuring arterial blood gases and assessing gas exchange overnight.

Post-TB

These patients are almost invariably hypoxic, on account of their extensive pulmonary scarring.[44,45] The work of breathing is high, and the mechanical efficiency of the chest wall is impaired as a consequence of removal of ribs. The capacity of the inspiratory muscles may be impaired by phrenic nerve crush or avulsion. On this basis, it seems reasonable to suggest that they might develop respiratory muscle fatigue, which NIV could relieve. Although detailed studies are lacking, REM sleep is likely to be a vulnerable period for this group of patients, for exactly the same reasons as for those with scoliosis.

EVIDENCE BASE

Early trials

In 1988, Ellis et al.[46] reported a study of seven patients with scoliosis who were in hypercapnic respiratory failure. Two improved on continuous positive airway pressure, but the remaining five needed NIV. Traditional volume-controlled ventilators designed for home use were fitted to customised nasal masks. Abnormal gas exchange during sleep was corrected, accompanied by improvement in sleep quality. After 3 months of NIV, daytime blood gases and MIP were also better. This new technique was soon taken up by centres around the world that historically had provided ventilatory support via a tracheostomy or older non-invasive techniques such as external negative pressure ventilation or rocking beds. Bach and Alba[47] included five patients with scoliosis in a mixed group of 52 patients transferring to NIV from other methods of ventilatory support, in whom it was shown to be effective in maintaining normal gas exchange. In Bach's centre and many others, this signalled a rapid drift away from the use of tracheostomy.

Zaccaria et al.[48] reported their experience with 17 scoliotic patients. The more severely compromised patients were managed with a tracheostomy, whereas the remainder were managed with NIV. They noted similar improvements in gas exchange in both groups, suggesting that they were equally effective. Leger et al.[49] reported reduction in hospitalisation and improvement in blood gases in 105 scoliotic and 80 post-TB patients. Three years after starting NIV, survival was 76% for the post-TB and scoliosis groups. The survival of patients with scoliosis secondary to poliomyelitis was noted to be just as good as for idiopathic scoliosis. Pehrsson et al.[50] included 13 patients with scoliosis and 5 post-TB in a survey of patients on home mechanical ventilation, in which they found good psychosocial functioning and mental well-being, despite severe physical limitations.

Jackson et al.[51] followed 32 post-TB patients who were treated with different methods of NIV. The 5-year survival was 74%. Arterial blood gases improved in the first few days of NIV, but with little further improvement subsequently. Slowly deteriorating arterial blood gases were associated with worsening right heart failure and a poor prognosis.

Wider experience

As the size of the reported series became larger, confidence grew in NIV as an effective long-term treatment. Simonds and Elliott[52] reported 5-year survival of 79% for scoliosis (n = 47), 100% for polio (n = 30) and 94% for post-TB (n = 20). As other groups had noted, arterial blood gases improved in the months after starting NIV and remained stable thereafter.

In 1996, Chailleux et al.[20] reported the French ANTADIR experience of more than 26,000 patients using oxygen or ventilators at home. NIV was associated with increased survival, particularly for scoliosis compared to post-TB. Ferris et al.[53] noted improvement in gas exchange and vital capacity in 17 patients with scoliosis commencing NIV. In 2005, Lloyd-Owen et al.[54] reported the results of the Eurovent study, in which approximately a third of patients had thoracic deformity as the aetiology of their ventilatory failure.

Mechanisms

MECHANICS

Once it was clear that NIV was effective, attention turned to how it worked. Some studies showed an increase in vital capacity,[53,55] but the majority of reports demonstrated little change. The consistent improvement in gas exchange is unlikely to be explained by changes in the mechanics of the lungs or rib cage.

MUSCLES

Respiratory muscle strength often improves with NIV. The study of Schonhofer et al.[28] showing improved respiratory muscle endurance is consistent with the hypothesis that NIV rests the respiratory muscles and allows them to recover from respiratory muscle fatigue. Gonzalez et al.[56] undertook a prospective study of 16 patients with scoliosis who were treated with NIV for 3 years. Vital capacity and inspiratory muscle strength increased, with the result that the duty cycle of the inspiratory muscles moved away from the critical fatigue threshold. The possibility remains that the improvement in respiratory drive seen with NIV (see below) is only possible because the respiratory muscles regain the capacity to do the work necessary to maintain normal alveolar ventilation.

DRIVE

NIV leads to an improvement in ventilatory drive. Dellborg et al.[29] showed improvement in the ventilator response to hypercapnia after 9 months of NIV in patients with alveolar ventilation from a variety of causes, including four with scoliosis. The magnitude of improvement correlated with changes in daytime and overnight carbon dioxide levels. Nickol et al.[30] included eight patients with scoliosis in a study of the mechanism of improvement of respiratory failure with NIV. After 3 months, this subgroup showed similar improvement in $PaCO_2$ and hypercapnic respiratory drive to the patients with neuromuscular problems.

Increased ventilatory drive is likely to be a pivotal mechanism for the longer-term changes seen with NIV. The changes in drive seem to correlate well with improved gas exchange, both during NIV and while breathing spontaneously. It is unclear whether the improvement in gas exchange causes the increase in drive, or the other way around.

SLEEP

Gas exchange is undoubtedly worse during sleep in scoliosis and is corrected by NIV. Masa et al.[34] included seven scoliotic and one post-TB patient in a study of 21 patients with nocturnal hypoventilation. Gas exchange was much worse in REM sleep, and these abnormalities were corrected more effectively by NIV than supplementary oxygen. Schonhofer and Kohler[35] studied 11 patients with scoliosis, of which four were post-TB. Polysomnography showed improvement in sleep architecture. On the other hand, Buyse et al.[55] failed to show much change in sleep architecture with NIV in their patients, despite improvement in gas exchange. Bach et al.[57] studied seven patients with scoliosis (one secondary to pleuroparietal TB) who had been using NIV at night for 3 months or more. Symptoms, hospitalisation rates, daytime $PaCO_2$ and overnight oxygenation improved, but again polysomnographic sleep parameters were not significantly different.

Further light on the relevance of sleep comes from a study by Schonhofer et al.[58] comparing nocturnal with diurnal NIV. Seventeen patients were included in each group, six with scoliosis and seven post-TB. In both groups, gas exchange during the day and overnight improved and sleep studies showed an improvement in sleep architecture even with daytime NIV.

In summary, improving alveolar ventilation using NIV leads to recovery of respiratory drive. This leads to increased ventilation when breathing spontaneously, which can only be maintained because the respiratory muscles are in better shape than they were before NIV was started. Sleeping better probably helps, but is not pivotal.

CLINICAL APPLICATIONS

Hypercapnic respiratory failure

An elevated daytime $PaCO_2$ in a scoliotic or post-TB patient almost always means they have passed a critical point whereby their respiratory muscles are too fatigued to maintain normal alveolar ventilation. NIV should be started soon, since a small further reduction in alveolar ventilation will result in a disproportionately large – and potentially dangerous – rise in $PaCO_2$. If the daytime $PaCO_2$ has risen during an acute illness and returned to normal, it is usually appropriate to discuss starting NIV anyway: the transient elevation in $PaCO_2$ implies very little reserve, and the likelihood of needing NIV within a year is very high.

Nocturnal hypoventilation

Patients who hypoventilate during the daytime will always be worse at night. During the progression toward diurnal respiratory failure, there will be a stage where they are normocapnic during the day, but hypoventilate at night. Periods of oxygen desaturation are seen commonly when performing screening sleep studies on patients with scoliosis who have no symptoms of nocturnal hypoventilation. More detailed monitoring will reveal that these periods occur in REM sleep and are associated with a rise in $PaCO_2$. These episodes may be truly asymptomatic, but it is important to question the patient carefully – the classical morning headaches are much less common than vaguer symptoms such as poor appetite, lethargy, tiredness and so on. Masa et al.[33] noted that their patients considered themselves asymptomatic but reported that they felt a lot better on NIV.

Ward et al.[59] reported a prospective trial of elective NIV versus a wait-and-watch approach in 26 patients with nocturnal hypoventilation but normal daytime arterial blood gases. Most of the patients had neuromuscular problems but small numbers of patients with scoliosis were included in each group. The main conclusion of the study was that patients with asymptomatic nocturnal hypoventilation are likely to need NIV within the following 2 years. It is difficult to know how well this applies to the scoliotic subgroup: the authors of the paper themselves noted that nocturnal hypoventilation may evolve more slowly than in neuromuscular patients.

Daytime NIV

Schonhofer et al.[58] suggested that daytime NIV is as effective as nocturnal use. Clearly, it is less intrusive for the patients to use NIV at night, but if they are unable to sleep with the ventilator on – as sometimes happens – then daytime use is an alternative. There will be a time on NIV below which it is ineffective, but even a few hours is probably better than nothing. Highcock et al.[60] studied daytime NIV to see if this improved exercise capacity on a treadmill in scoliosis, but it appears to be ineffective in this regard. An hour or two of NIV in the middle of the day may be beneficial for a patient using nocturnal NIV who finds they are struggling to last all day breathing spontaneously. Whether this works by resting the respiratory muscles or altering the mechanics of the lungs and/or chest wall is not known.

Post-operative (spinal surgery)

It can often be anticipated that a patient with scoliosis undergoing spinal surgery is likely to need ventilatory support for a few days post-operatively. Traditionally, this has involved an elective tracheostomy, but NIV may be an alternative in selected patients. Given that the surgery is almost always planned well in advance, the opportunity should be taken to get the patient accustomed to NIV pre-operatively. This improves the chances of avoiding a tracheostomy post-operatively, since the patient has had time to become accustomed to the mask and ventilator.

Pregnancy

Pregnancy places a mechanical and metabolic burden on someone with scoliosis. This may necessitate the implementation of NIV in the third trimester, possibly continuing for some time post-partum. Respiratory function should return to the pre-pregnancy level.[61]

TECHNICAL CONSIDERATIONS

Mode

Bilevel pressure support ventilators, commonly used to treat hypercapnic respiratory failure in acute exacerbations of COPD, are not ideal for correcting hypoventilation in scoliosis. Given their wide availability, they can be used when patients present acutely,[34,36] but as soon as possible, the patient should be transferred onto a ventilator that has a 'control' mode.

The aim of NIV in scoliosis is to provide adequate alveolar ventilation, resting the respiratory muscles and normalising arterial blood gases. This is achieved by using a control mode of ventilation, whereby the patient is not required to trigger the ventilator on or off. This can be thought of as 'providing' rather than 'supporting' ventilation. Pressure- or volume-targeted modes can be used, although the former are used much more commonly these days. Volume control remains an option for patients in whom normalisation of gas exchange is problematical.

Schonhofer et al.[62] studied a group of 30 patients with chronic ventilatory failure which included four with scoliosis and eight post-TB. After 1 month of volume-controlled NIV, respiratory rate, $PaCO_2$, P0.1, P0.1/MIP, MIP and VT had all improved. When switched to pressure-controlled NIV, some patients deteriorated, only to recover when they returned to the volume-controlled mode. These patients were slightly more hypoxic and more hypercapnic before treatment, but it was not possible to predict at the outset which mode would suit which patient. In practice, pressure-controlled NIV is likely to be the first choice, but the option of changing to volume controlled should be borne in mind if the patient does not improve after a month or so.

Tuggey and Elliott[63] compared pressure- and volume-targeted NIV in 13 patients with chest wall deformity. There was no difference in efficacy between the two modes. The authors noted that patients would settle for a low backup rate, even when this compromised nocturnal ventilation. Leakage was the main cause of persisting hypoventilation in both groups.

Pressure

We have already noted that the compliance of the chest wall is low in patients with scoliosis, so they need high pressures to inflate their chest. This pressure is likely to be at least 25 cmH_2O, and this should be the starting pressure for pressure-targeted modes. If a bilevel pressure ventilator is used, the expiratory pressure should be kept as low as possible (Figure 45.10).

Rate

Patients with scoliosis will allow their respiratory rate to drop during sleep, even if this means that they do not maintain adequate alveolar ventilation. For this reason, the backup rate should be set fairly high.

It is vital for the patient to coordinate with the ventilator during NIV. Patients with scoliosis may breathe at rates of 30 or more breaths per minute. Start with a rate similar to their spontaneous rate; as they get used to NIV, their rate may slow down a little, and you can reduce the backup rate accordingly. For most patients with scoliosis, the range will be 15–20 breaths per minute, but occasionally, you will need to leave them with a higher rate in order to maintain coordination with the ventilator.

Inspiratory time

In order to minimise the peak pressure that the inspiratory muscles have to develop, patients with scoliosis may prolong their inspiratory time. An inspiratory/expiratory ratio of 1:1 or even higher may be necessary for full inflation of the chest. In the majority of patients, expiration is not a problem, so they tolerate short expiratory times without becoming hyperinflated.

Rise time

In ventilators with the facility to adjust this parameter, rise time should be set initially to match the patient's own spontaneous breathing pattern. Further adjustments should be guided by how comfortable the patient feels on the ventilator.

Oxygen

Ventilation–perfusion imbalance can cause persistent hypoxia in scoliosis. Asymptomatic desaturation in REM sleep is quite common in patients with scoliosis on NIV, but if right heart failure does not resolve despite correction of nocturnal hypoventilation, then it seems reasonable to add in supplementary oxygen, aiming for a mean oxygen saturation of greater than 90%.

FUTURE RESEARCH

The aetiology of scoliosis seems likely to be multifactorial, but more research is needed to identify the genetic factors involved and their interaction with environmental influences. As surgical techniques are refined and become less invasive, there will be a need for studies to review the effect of correcting the deformity on lung function. More sophisticated imaging techniques may allow us to study the physiology of respiration in real time, for example, how ventilation and perfusion are distributed in the lungs of patients, and whether NIV has an effect on this.

While there seems little doubt that the respiratory muscles develop fatigue, more studies are needed on how they adapt to changes in their operational length – because of distortion of the rib cage – and increased workload. Allowing arterial carbon dioxide levels to rise may be a protective mechanism to prevent irreversible damage in respiratory muscles in the face of a load/capacity ratio that is unsustainable. This hypothesis is supported by the recovery of drive when NIV is started, but serial studies of the hypercapnic ventilatory response as patients with scoliosis approach respiratory failure would be interesting.

SUMMARY

Patients with a scoliosis are at risk of hypercapnic respiratory failure if

- The thoracic spine is involved
- The curvature was present before the age of 5 years
- The angle of curvature is greater than 90°
- The vital capacity is less than 50% of predicted
- The spine has never been surgically stabilized
- The scoliosis is secondary to neuromuscular weakness (including poliomyelitis)
- There is additional lung disease such as asthma or COPD

If the daytime $PaCO_2$ is elevated in a patient with scoliosis, they need to start nocturnal NIV and stay on it indefinitely.

NIV parameters in a patient with scoliosis should be as follows:

- Pressure control mode (i.e. the patient triggers neither the start nor the end of inspiration)
- Inspiratory positive airway pressure (IPAP) of at least 25 cmH_2O
- Lowest EPAP possible if bilevel circuit is used
- Respiratory rate and inspiratory time approximately the same as the patient's spontaneous breathing pattern

REFERENCES

1. Kearon C, Viviani GR, Kirkley A. Factors determining pulmonary function in adolescent idiopathic thoracic scoliosis. *Am Rev Respir Dis.* 1993;148: 288–94.
2. Cobb JR. Outline for the study of scoliosis. *Instr Course Lect.* 1948;5:261–75.
3. Hepper NGG, Black LF, Fowler WS. Relationship of lung volume to height and arm span in normal subjects and in patients with spinal deformity. *Am Rev Respir Dis.* 1965;91:356–62.
4. Giordano A, Fuso L, Calcagni ML et al. Evaluation of pulmonary ventilation and diaphragmatic movement in idiopathic scoliosis using radioaerosol ventilation scintigraphy. *Nucl Med Commun.* 1997;18:105–11.

5. Secker-Walker Rh, Ho JE, Gill IS. Observations on regional ventilation and perfusion in kyphoscoliosis. *Respiration*. 1979;38:194–203.
6. Redding G, Song K, Inscore S et al. Lung function asymmetry in children with congenital and infantile scoliosis. *Spine*. 2008;8:639–44.
7. Kinnear W, Sovani M, Khanna A et al. Correction of paradoxical ribcage motion in scoliosis by non-invasive ventilation. *Spine*. 2018 (in press).
8. Bergofsky EH, Turino GM, Fishman AP. Cardiorespiratory failure in kyphoscoliosis. *Medicine (Baltimore)*. 1959;38:263–317.
9. Kafer ER. Idiopathic scoliosis. Gas exchange and the age dependence of arterial blood gases. *J Clin Invest*. 1976;58:825–33.
10. Mezon BL, West P, Israels J et al. Sleep breathing abnormalities in kyphoscoliosis. *Am Rev Respir Dis*. 1980;122:617–21.
11. Schonhofer B, Barchfeld T, Wenzel M et al. Long term effects of non-invasive mechanical ventilation on pulmonary haemodynamics in patients with chronic respiratory failure. *Thorax*. 2001;56:524–8.
12. Herry I, Iung B, Piechaud JY et al. Cardiac causes of hypoxaemia in a kyphoscoliotic patient. *Eur Resp J*. 1999;14:1433–4.
13. Kinnear W, Watson L, Smith P et al. Effect of expiratory positive airway pressure on tidal volume during non-invasive ventilation. *Chronic Respir Dis*. 2016;14:105–9.
14. Estenne M, Derom E, De Troyer A. Neck and abdominal muscle activity in patients with severe thoracic scoliosis. *Am J Respir Crit Care Med*. 1998;158:452–7.
15. Sinha R, Bergovsky EH. Prolonged alteration of lung mechanics in kyphoscoliosis by positive pressure hyperinflation. *Am Rev Respir Dis*. 1972;106:47–57.
16. van Noord JA, Cauberghs M, Van de Woestijne KP et al. Total respiratory resistance and reactance in ankylosing spondylitis and kyphoscoliosis. *Eur Resp J*. 1991;4:945–51.
17. Bjure J, Grimby G, Kasalicky J et al. Respiratory impairment and airway closure in patients with untreated idiopathic scoliosis. *Thorax*. 1970;25:451–6.
18. McPhail GL, Howells SA, Boesch RP et al. Obstructive lung disease is common in children with syndromic and congenital scoliosis: A preliminary study. *J Ped Orth*. 2013;33:781–5.
19. De Torres Garcia I, de Cabo Moreno P, Ramirez AMG. Extrinsic bronchial obstruction caused by scoliosis. *Spine*. 2013;38:E840–3.
20. Chailleux E, Fauroux B, Binet F et al. Predictors of survival in patients receiving domiciliary oxygen therapy or mechanical ventilation. A 10-year analysis of ANTADIR observatory. *Chest*. 1996;109:741–9.
21. Ramonatxo M, Milic-Emili J, Prefaut C. Breathing pattern and load compensatory responses in young scoliotic patients. *Eur Resp J*. 1988;1:421–7.
22. Jones RS, Kennedy JD, Hasham F et al. Mechanical inefficiency of the thoracic cage in scoliosis. *Thorax*. 1981;36:456–61.
23. Cook CD, Barrie H, DeForest SA et al. Lung volumes, mechanics of respiration and respiratory muscle strength in scoliosis. *Pediatrics*. 1960;25:766–74.
24. Smyth RJ, Chapman KR, Wright TA et al. Pulmonary function in adolescents with mild idiopathic scoliosis. *Thorax*. 1984;39:901–4.
25. Lisboa C, Moreni R, Fava M et al. Inspiratory muscle function in patients with severe kyphoscoliosis. *Am Rev Respir Dis*. 1985;132:48–52.
26. Szeinberg A, Canny GJ, Rashed N et al. Forced vital capacity and maximal respiratory pressures in patients with mild and moderate scoliosis. *Pediatr Pulmonol*. 1988;4:8–12.
27. Cooper DM, Rojas JV, Mellins RB et al. Respiratory mechanics in adolescents with idiopathic scoliosis. *Am Rev Respir Dis*. 1984;130:16–22.
28. Schonhofer B, Wallstein S, Wiese C et al. Noninvasive mechanical ventilation improves endurance performance in patients with chronic respiratory failure due to thoracic restriction. *Chest*. 2001;119:1371–8.
29. Dellborg C, Olofson J, Hamnegard C-H et al. Ventilatory response to CO_2 re-breathing before and after nocturnal nasal intermittent positive pressure ventilation in patients with chronic alveolar hypoventilation. *Respir Med*. 2000;94:1154–60.
30. Nickol AH, Hart N, Hopkinson NS et al. Mechanisms of improvement of respiratory failure in patients with restrictive thoracic disease treated with non-invasive ventilation. *Thorax*. 2005;60:754–60.
31. Guilleminault C, Kurland G, Winkle R et al. Severe kyphosis, breathing and sleep. *Chest*. 1982;79:626–30.
32. Sawicka EH, Branthwaite MA. Respiration during sleep in kyphoscoliosis. *Thorax*. 1987;42:801–8.
33. Masa JF, Sénchez de Cos Escuin J, Disdier Vicente C et al. Nasal intermittent positive pressure ventilation. Analysis of its withdrawal. *Chest*. 1995;107:382–8.
34. Masa JF, Celli B, Riesco JA et al. Noninvasive positive pressure ventilation and not oxygen may prevent overt ventilatory failure in patients with chest wall diseases. *Chest*. 1997;112:207–13.
35. Schonhofer B, Kohler D. Effect of non-invasive mechanical ventilation on sleep and nocturnal ventilation in patients with chronic respiratory failure. *Thorax*. 2000;55:308–13.
36. Hill NS, Eveloff SE, Carlisle CC et al. Efficacy of nocturnal nasal ventilation in patients with restrictive thoracic disease. *Am Rev Respir Dis*. 1992;145:365–71.

37. Larsson E-LC, Aaro SI, Normelli HCM et al. Long-term follow-up of functioning after spinal surgery in patients with neuromuscular scoliosis. *Spine*. 2005;30:2145–52.
38. Kennedy JD, Staples AJ, Brook PD et al. Effect of spinal surgery on lung function in Duchenne muscular dystrophy. *Thorax*. 1995;50:1173–8.
39. Swank SM, Winter RB, Moe JH. Scoliosis and cor pulmonale. *Spine*. 1982;7:343–54.
40. Rizzi PE, Winter RB, Lonstein JE et al. Adult spinal deformity and respiratory failure. Surgical results in 35 patients. *Spine*. 1997;22:2517–31.
41. Branthwaite MA. Cardiorespiratory consequences of unfused idiopathic scoliosis. *Chest*. 1986;80:360–9.
42. Pehrsson K, Bake B, Larsson S et al. Lung function in adult idiopathic scoliosis: A 20 year follow up. *Thorax*. 1991;46:474–8.
43. Pehrsson K, Nachemson A, Olofson J et al. Respiratory failure in scoliosis and other thoracic deformities. A survey of patients with home oxygen or ventilator therapy in Sweden. *Spine*. 1992;17:714–18.
44. Phillips MS, Kinnear WJ, Shneerson JM. Late sequelae of pulmonary tuberculosis treated by thoracoplasty. *Thorax*. 1987;42:445–51.
45. Phillips MS, Miller MR, Kinnear WJ et al. Importance of airflow obstruction after thoracoplasty. *Thorax*. 1987;42:348–52.
46. Ellis ER, Grunstein RR, Chan S et al. Noninvasive ventilatory support during sleep improves respiratory failure in kyphoscoliosis. *Chest*. 1988;94:811–5.
47. Bach JR, Alba AS. Management of chronic alveolar hypoventilation by nasal ventilation. *Chest*. 1990;97:52–7.
48. Zaccaria S, Zaccaria E, Zanaboni S et al. Home mechanical ventilation in kyphoscoliosis. Monaldi *Arch Chest Dis*. 1993;48:161–4.
49. Leger P, Bedicam JM, Conrnette A et al. Nasal intermittent positive pressure ventilation. Long-term follow-up in patients with severe chronic respiratory insufficiency. *Chest*. 1994;105:100–5.
50. Pehrsson K, Olofson J, Larsson S et al. Quality of life of patients treated by home mechanical ventilation due to restrictive disorders. *Resp Med*. 1994;88:21–6.
51. Jackson M, Smith I, King M et al. Long term domiciliary assisted ventilation for respiratory failure following thoracoplasty. *Thorax*. 1994;49:915–9.
52. Simonds AK, Elliott MW. Outcome of domiciliary nasal intermittent positive pressure ventilation in restrictive and obstructive disorders. *Thorax*. 1995;50:604–9.
53. Ferris G, Severa-Pieras E, Vergara P et al. Kyphoscoliosis ventilatory insufficiency: Noninvasive management outcomes. *Am J Phys Med Rehab*. 2000;79:24–9.
54. Lloyd-Owen SJ, Donaldson GC, Ambrosino N et al. Patterns of home mechanical ventilation use in Europe: Results of the Eurovent survey. *Eur Resp J*. 2005;25:1025–31.
55. Buyse B, Meersseman W, Demedts M. Treatment of chronic respiratory failure in kyphoscoliosis: Oxygen or ventilation? *Eur Resp J*. 2003;22:525–8.
56. Gonzalez C, Ferris G, Diaz J et al. Kyphoscoliotic ventilatory insufficiency. Effects of long-term intermittent positive-pressure ventilation. *Chest*. 2003;124:857–62.
57. Bach JR, Robert D, Leger P et al. Sleep fragmentation in kyphoscoliotic individuals with alveolar hypoventilation treated by NIPPV. *Chest*. 1995;107:1552–8.
58. Schonhofer B, Geibel M, Sonneborn M et al. Daytime mechanical ventilation in chronic respiratory insufficiency. *Eur Resp J*. 1997;10:2840–6.
59. Ward S, Chatwin M, Heather S et al. Randomised controlled trial of non-invasive ventilation (NIV) for nocturnal hypoventilation in neuromuscular and chest wall disease patients with daytime normocapnia. *Thorax*. 2005;60:1019–24.
60. Highcock MP, Smith IE, Shneerson JM. The effect of noninvasive intermittent positive-pressure ventilation during exercise in severe scoliosis. *Chest*. 2002;121:1555–60.
61. Kahler CM, Hogl B, Habeler R et al. Management of respiratory deterioration in a pregnant patient with severe kyphoscoliosis by non-invasive positive pressure ventilation. *Wiener Klinische Wochenschrift*. 2002;114:874–7.
62. Schonhofer B, Sonneborn M, Haidl P et al. Comparison of two different modes for non-invasive mechanical ventilation in chronic respiratory failure: Volume versus pressure controlled device. *Eur Resp J*. 1997;10:184–91.
63. Tuggey JM, Elliott MW. Randomised crossover study of pressure and volume non-invasive ventilation in chest wall deformity. *Thorax*. 2005;60:859–64.

PART 10

Obesity

46 Pathophysiology of respiratory failure in obesity 441
Francesco Fanfulla
47 Acute non-invasive ventilation in obesity-related respiratory failure 452
Patrick B. Murphy and Nicholas Hart
48 Non-invasive ventilation in acute and chronic respiratory failure due to obesity 457
Juan Fernando Masa, Isabel Utrabo and Francisco Javier Gómez de Terreros

46

Pathophysiology of respiratory failure in obesity

FRANCESCO FANFULLA

INTRODUCTION

Obesity is one of the biggest public health problems and is now considered a worldwide epidemic. A huge number of subjects, nearly 1.5 billion adults, are estimated to be overweight, whereas 400 million adults are obese.[1] Obesity has considerable effects on morbidity and mortality. The term *metabolic syndrome* was introduced to describe the cluster of abdominal obesity with hypertension, dyslipidaemia and impaired insulin resistance; this problem affects 20%–30% of the total population in the European region.[2] The burden of disease attributable to a high body mass index (BMI) among adults in the European region amounted to more than 1 million deaths and about 12 million life-years of ill health (disability-adjusted life years) in 2000.[3] Data from the Framingham study in the United States showed that obesity reduces life expectancy: obesity at the age of 40 years led to a reduction in life expectancy of 7 years in women and 6 years in men.[4] Two recent different meta-analyses including 239 and 230 perspective studies, respectively, demonstrated that overweight and obesity are associated with increased risk of all-cause mortality and that this relationship is strong and positive in every global region of the world.[5,6]

THE EFFECTS OF OBESITY ON RESPIRATORY PHYSIOLOGY

Obesity has been demonstrated to lead to alterations in all components of respiratory physiology: mechanical properties of the respiratory system, airway resistance, control of breathing, gas exchange, work of breathing and so on. These effects are summarised in Table 46.1.

The number and severity of the respiratory alterations vary considerably among patients. Numerous factors may contribute to an individual's clinical and physiological status, including age, severity of obesity, distribution of fat, fertility status in females, smoking, physical activity, control of breathing, sleep-disordered breathing, sleep restrictions, medications and comorbid conditions.

Many years ago, Naimark and Cherniak reported a decrease, of as much as two-thirds of normal values, in total respiratory system compliance in obese subjects.[7] In a study performed on sedated, paralysed, postoperative, morbidly obese patients, Pelosi et al. found that, compared to normal subjects, the obese patients had a lower respiratory system compliance, caused by decreases in both lung and chest wall compliance, higher lung resistance with marked increases in airway and lung resistance and a smaller functional residual capacity (FRC).[8] In another similar physiological study, Pelosi et al. found that obese patients had marked alterations of the mechanical properties of the respiratory system, largely explained by a reduction in lung volumes due to the excessive unopposed intra-abdominal pressure. The average static volume–pressure curves of the total respiratory system indicated an overall higher elastance in obese subjects and the presence of an 'inflection point' at a pressure between 5 and 15 cmH_2O, after which the volume increased linearly with pressure.[9] They found that, in normal subjects, the elastance did not change with increasing volume, whereas in obese patients, it dropped sharply along the inflection point and, subsequently, remained constant.

The effect of the increasing respiratory load on the breathing pattern has been first investigated by Sampson and Grassino. They found that obese subjects presented normal inspiratory and expiratory flow rates, duty cycles and minute ventilation. The maintenance of mean inspiratory flow was strictly dependent on augmentation of neuromuscular drive expressed as $P_{0.1}$ (pressure at mouth measured in the first 100 ms of occluded inspiration) that, in turn, was strongly positively correlated with the degree of obesity. Furthermore, they observed that the diaphragm's volume generating function in obese subjects is reduced with prevalent rib cage expansion during tidal volume and the persistence of diaphragmatic activity during early expiration to attenuate the rate of expiratory flow.[10]

Table 46.1 Main respiratory function alterations in obesity

Respiratory physiology	Impairment due to obesity
Respiratory mechanics	Decreased total respiratory system compliance
	Increased airway resistance
Lung volumes	Mild to moderate reduction. Variable changes in residual volume
Gas exchange	Reduced PaO_2
	Increased A-a gradient
	Increased $PaCO_2$
Work of breathing	Increased work of breathing
	Increased oxygen cost of breathing

Several studies investigating the relationship between body weight and various spirometric indices showed that increased body weight decreases lung volumes.[11–13] Lung function impairment and metabolic syndrome have been associated with an increased risk of cardiovascular disease and premature death.[14,15] In a large-scale population-based study, a positive relationship was found between lung function impairment and metabolic syndrome; this was mainly due to abdominal obesity and was independent of major cardiovascular risk factors, including BMI.[16]

Jones et al. found an inverse linear relationship between BMI and vital capacity and total lung capacity.[17] The most dramatic effects of BMI were seen for FRC and expiratory reserve volume: they decreased exponentially with increasing BMI, so that morbid obesity resulted in patients breathing near their residual volume.

In normal subjects, there is a reduction in FRC and an increase in airflow resistance when the supine posture is adopted; most of the reduction in FRC is related to gravitational effects of the abdominal contents, so that the diaphragm takes a more expiratory position. In contrast, in obese subjects, there is no supine decrease in FRC or total lung capacity, as recently demonstrated by Watson and Pride.[18] The mechanism of this different pattern of postural changes in lung volumes in obese subjects is not understood, but it has a favourable effect of restricting increases in inspiratory work of breathing and deterioration in gas exchange during tidal breathing when supine.

The effects of longitudinal changes of BMI on spirometric indices and diffusion capacity of the lung were investigated in the general population by Bottai et al. in an 8-year follow-up survey.[19] The authors evaluated the effects of weight changes over time in a group of 1426 adults aged >24 years and found that lung function loss tended to be greater among those who, at baseline, reported higher BMI values: the loss was greater in males. The detrimental effect of gaining weight might be reversible in many adults since those whose BMI decreased over time had an improvement in lung function. Similar results were recently reported in a cohort of young adults in New Zealand followed for 6 years. Increase of adiposity over time was associated with impairment in lung function across a broad range of static and dynamic lung volumes, independently of the distribution of body fat. A relevant finding of this study is the association between increases in adiposity and a decline in the FEV1/FVC ratio in women, indicating a possible differential effect of adiposity on airway function between the sexes.[20]

Expiratory flow rate could decrease in non-smoker obese individuals.[21] Maximal expiratory flow rates decrease progressively with decreasing lung volume, so that breathing at a low lung volume is associated with a reduction in expiratory flow reserve, which can further diminish in the presence of airway obstruction. This phenomenon is more likely to occur with the subject in the supine position. Tidal expiratory flow limitation (EFL) promotes dynamic hyperinflation with a concurrent increase in work of breathing due to the presence of intrinsic positive end-expiratory pressure (PEEPi): inspiratory muscles are loaded not only by decreased compliance of the total respiratory system but also by the presence of PEEPi.[22] Steier et al. confirmed that obese subjects have a markedly increased neural respiratory drive, two to three times that of non-obese subjects, assessed by measurement of respiratory pressure and electromyogram (EMG) of the diaphragm and extradiaphragmatic respiratory muscles.[23] Moving from sitting to supine position, obese subjects showed an increase in oesophageal pressure swings as well as an increase in EMG activity of diaphragm (EMGdi), and some of them developed PEEPi when supine. The application of CPAP in the supine position abolished the PEEPi and the level of EMGdi or inspiratory pressure swings (Figure 46.1).

Several studies performed in normal subjects have demonstrated that there is a straight relationship between body weight and arterial oxygen concentration.[24,25] BMI is one of the main factors explaining the variability of arterial oxygen tension in the reference equation for PaO_2 proposed by Cerveri et al.[25] The physiological basis of this finding is not well understood. Ulmer et al. demonstrated a great variation in lung ventilation/perfusion ratio, according to BMI[26]: higher BMI is associated with increasing mismatch between ventilation and perfusion, and lower value of PaO_2. Holley et al. found, in a group of obese subjects, a significant ventilation/perfusion ratio alteration, consisting in a prevalent perfusion in lower zones of the lung where ventilation was considerably reduced.[27] Yamane et al. demonstrated that hypoxia in obese subjects in the supine position is caused primarily by insufficient gas exchange in the regions of the lung, linked to the inferior pulmonary veins.[28] They found an inverse relationship between BMI and PO_2 in the inferior pulmonary veins, suggesting a possible subclinical manifestation of obesity-related respiratory insufficiency. The authors attributed these findings in part to the regional alveolar V/Q mismatch caused by the closure of dependent airways within the range of tidal breathing[29] and in part to alveolar hypoventilation.

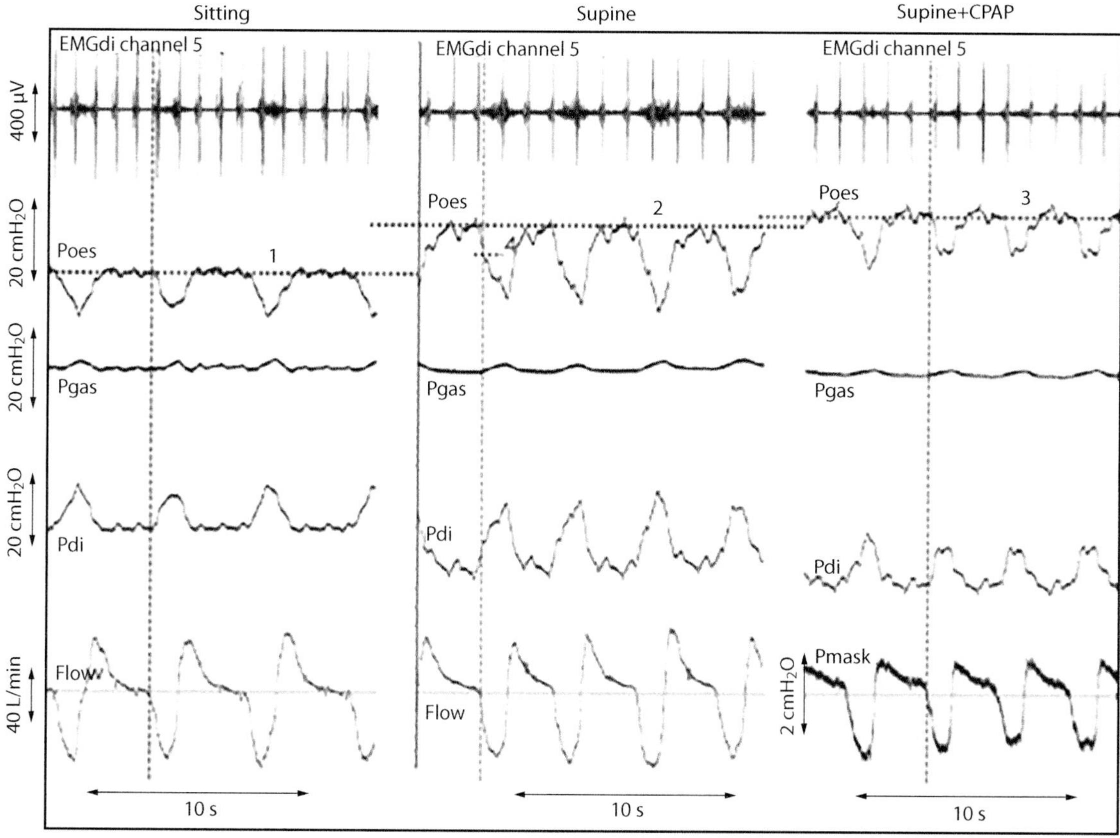

Figure 46.1 Resting breathing in an obese seated (left), supine without (middle) and with (right) CPAP. The change in end-expiratory oesophageal baseline pressure is reflected by the horizontal dotted lines (nos. 1–3). There is intrinsic PEEP of approximately 6 cmH_2O. The right panel shows the same patient supine breathing with CPAP of 6 cmH_2O. Neural respiratory drive to the diaphragm increases when changing posture from sitting to supine and decreases with CPAP; intrinsic PEEP is offset with CPAP, and pressure swings of Poes and Pdi are smaller. EMGdi, electromyogram of the diagram (Channel 5 records the biggest EMG signal, as described in the method section); Poes, oesophageal pressure; Pgas, gastric pressure; Pdi, transdiaphragmatic pressure (Pdi = Pgas − Poes); PEEPi, intrinsic PEEP; EMGdi in μV, all pressures in cmH_2O, flow in L/min. (Reproduced with permission from Steier J et al. *Thorax*. 2009;64:719–25.)

Sleep-disordered breathing: Obstructive sleep apnoea syndrome and obesity hypoventilation syndrome

Sleep is associated with normal changes in many physiological functions, including respiration. The relevant differences in comparison with wakefulness regard control of breathing, airflow resistance, ventilatory response to increased load, activity of respiratory muscles and body position. Obesity is a condition associated with a high prevalence of sleep-disordered breathing that, untreated, leads to daytime hypoxia and chronic respiratory failure. The two most important diseases associated with obesity are obstructive sleep apnoea (OSA) and obesity hypoventilation syndrome (OHS). The mechanisms by which obesity may lead to chronic hypoxaemia and hypercapnia are summarised in Figure 46.2.

OSA is defined as the repetitive collapse of the upper airways during sleep, occurring more than five times per hour of sleep. Intermittent hypoxaemia, hypercapnia and large negative intrathoracic pressure swings, associated with arousals and sleep fragmentation, are typical findings of this syndrome.[30] Obesity seems to explains only 30%–50% of the variance in the apnoea–hypopnoea index, with a prevalent effect in patients aged <60 years.[31] Obesity may predispose to OSA by accumulation of fat around the neck, resulting in increased extraluminal pressure and a propensity to upper airway collapse or in a modification of the geometry of the airways. Abdominal obesity, through its negative effects on lung volumes, determines a reduction in longitudinal traction predisposing to upper airway collapse. Finally, changes in body weight in patients with OSA are associated with changes in the severity of the syndrome. Data from the Wisconsin sleep cohort suggest that weight gain has a greater effect on OSA than an equivalent weight loss: a 20% increase in weight was associated with a 70% increase in AHI, whereas a 20% reduction in weight was associated with a 48% decrease in AHI.[32] The development of respiratory failure in patients with OSA is still a matter of discussion.[33]

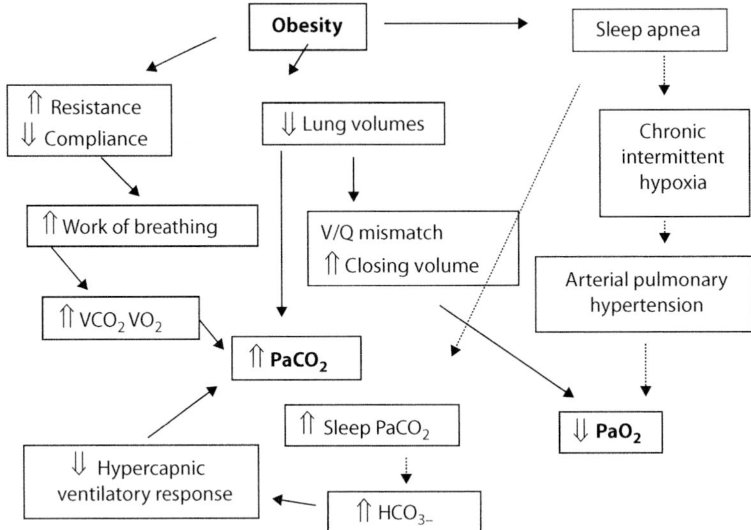

Figure 46.2 Mechanisms by which obesity may lead to chronic hypoxaemia and hypercapnia. Dashed lines represent modifications induced directly by OSA.

The development of daytime hypoxaemia has been attributed to pre-existing lung disease such as chronic obstructive pulmonary disease, so that airway obstruction and lung hyperinflation were considered to have major roles in determining the lower values of PaO_2.[34] Fanfulla et al. demonstrated that OSA patients, in the absence of lung comorbidity, had lower values of PaO_2 than those expected on the basis of age.[35] The main factor responsible for this reduction in daytime PaO_2 was the degree of nocturnal hypoxia.

The term *OHS* has been used with different meanings over time in the literature. The new diagnostic criteria included in the third International Classification of Sleep disorders are reported in Table 46.2.[36]

Generally, the respiratory alteration during sleep consists in a picture of severe OSA (≈90% of patients with OHS), while the remaining cases have severe, prolonged sleep hypoventilation with rare episodes of obstructive apnoea/hypopnoea (<5 events per hour of sleep). Few data are available about the prevalence of OHS in the general population. The prevalence in patients attending sleep laboratories or admitted to hospital ranges from 11% to 38%.[37]

The mechanisms leading to chronic carbon dioxide retention in obese patients are not completely understood. It is known that the clinical and functional disorders in patients with OHS are generally more severe than those in patients with the same degree of obesity but with OSA. At this point, it is not clear whether OHS is the final step in the natural clinical history of OSA, as postulated by Lugaresi et al. many years ago or whether OHS is a separate clinical entity with a specific pathophysiology.[38] Indeed, although the likelihood of developing diurnal hypercapnia increases as BMI rises, weight alone does not explain the presence of hypercapnia.[39] As mentioned above, in patients with OHS, the respiratory

Table 46.2 Diagnostic criteria for OHS

Criteria A–C must be met	
A	Presence of hypoventilation during wakefulness ($PaCO_2$ > 45 mmHg) as measured by arterial PCO_2, end-tidal PCO_2 or transcutaneous PCO_2
B	Presence of obesity (BMI > 30 kg/m^2; >95th percentile for age and sex for children)
C	Hypoventilation is not primarily due to lung parenchymal or airway disease, pulmonary vascular pathology, chest wall disorder (other than mass loading from obesity), medication use, neurologic disorder, muscle weakness or a known congenital or idiopathic central alveolar

Note: 1. PSG shows worsening of hypoventilation during sleep if $PaCO_2$ or non-invasive estimate of the $PaCO_2$ is measured; 2. OSA is often present and, in such cases, a diagnosis of both OSA and OHS should be made; 3. Arterial oxygen desaturation is usually present but is not required for the diagnosis.

function impairment is usually enhanced, causing a two- to threefold increase in the work of breathing compared to that in lean subjects.[8,9] Similarly, global oxygen consumption (V_{O2}) is increased in obesity, as reported by Kress et al.,[40] who measured V_{O2} during spontaneous breathing in morbidly obese patients immediately before the scheduled gastric bypass surgery and again during mechanical ventilation to determine the effects of morbid obesity on oxygen consumption dedicated to respiratory muscle work. They found that morbid obesity is associated with a substantial increase in V_{O2} dedicated to respiratory muscle work during quiet breathing when compared to that in normal control patients. This increase in energy expenditure could represent a limited ventilatory reserve that may predispose such patients to respiratory failure during acute pulmonary or systemic illnesses.

The presence of altered control of breathing in patients with OHS is a matter of concern. Several studies reported abnormalities in ventilatory control of patients with OHS.[41–43] Other studies found that the respiratory drive of obese eucapnic patients was increased in order to compensate for the respiratory system changes associated with obesity,[44] whereas obese patients who developed hypoventilation while awake did not show this augmented drive.[45] On the other hand, Leech et al. documented that the great majority of a group of patients with OHS were able to normalise $PaCO_2$ during voluntary hyperventilation.[46]

The occurrence of a reduced ventilatory response to increased mechanical load and/or carbon dioxide (CO_2) level is considered by many authors to be an acquired phenomenon, since most patients show improvements in ventilatory responsiveness after appropriate treatment.[47,48] A mutual relationship between OHS and sleep-induced upper airway obstruction[49] has been proposed by several investigators on the basis of various considerations: the great majority of OHS patients still have severe OSA, the clinical presentation of OHS with and without OSA is identical and a high proportion of patients with OHS with pure sleep hypoventilation at presentation go on to develop OSA once daytime hypercapnia improves with nocturnal ventilation.[50]

The mechanism by which OSA could cause chronic hypercapnia during wakefulness has been intensively investigated.[45,51–53] Berger et al. demonstrated that minute ventilation during sleep is not reduced (and is, indeed, sometimes increased) in those OSA patients with daytime hypercapnia because of the marked hyperventilation at the end of each apnoea/hypopnoea event (inter-critical period).[51] Minute ventilation during the inter-critical period is strictly related to CO_2 loading during the obstructive event[52] (Figure 46.3). Berger et al. demonstrated the presence of a strong inverse relationship between the post-event ventilatory response slope (the ratio between the ventilatory response and CO_2 loading during the event) and chronic awake arterial PCO_2 ($r = 0.90$, $p < 0.001$), suggesting that this mechanism is impaired in patients with chronic hypercapnia. Patients may fail to eliminate CO_2 completely during the post-apnoeic period when the ratio between the duration of the obstructive event and the hyperventilation period is higher than 3:1. In this case, the washout of CO_2 loaded during the apnoea/hypopnoea may not be complete, leading to progressive CO_2 retention during sleep.[53] Norman et al. identified bicarbonate retention compensating for the acute rise in CO_2, as well as the inability to unload the increased CO_2 and bicarbonate during wakefulness, as important mechanisms that would further blunt respiratory drive and promote awake hypercapnia. A raised level of serum bicarbonate is a typical clinical finding in patients with OHS.[45]

Areas of future research

The role of leptin in the development of chronic hypoventilation is a much debated issue.[54–57] Obese subjects usually have higher circulating levels of leptin than normal subjects; further increases have been found in patients with OSA and OHS.[54–58]

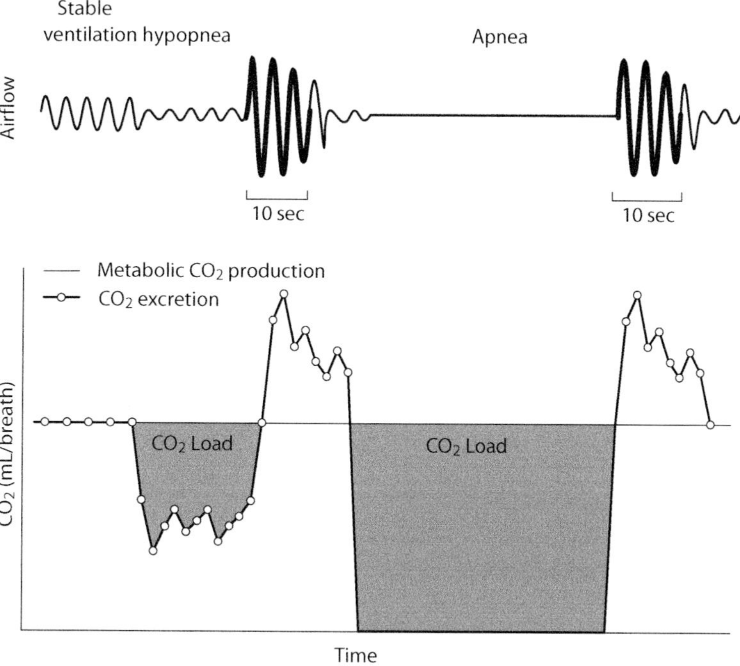

Figure 46.3 Diagram depicting CO_2 loading and unloading during respiratory events. Dark shaded areas represent CO_2 loading due to reduced CO_2 excretion during obstructive events. Light shaded areas represent CO_2 unloading due to compensatory hyperventilation between events. (Reproduced with permission from Berger KI et al. *J Appl Physiol.* 2000;88:257–64.)

Generally, leptin is considered as a respiratory stimulant. O'Donnell et al. demonstrated that leptin activates the central nervous system to compensate for the adipose load on the respiratory system and upper airway structure.[55] In this way, one can assume that obese subjects may develop hypoventilation as a consequence of reduced leptin action in the brain.[56] Experimental studies demonstrated that leptin-deficient (ob/ob) mice have an impaired ventilator response to hypercapnia that was improved after systemic or subcutaneous leptin administration.[57] Another physiological study performed in rats showed that acute systemic leptin infusion evoked a long-lasting respiratory motor output, expressed as phrenic nerve discharge, persisting over 1 hour after the infusion termination.[59] Similarly, Polotsky et al. showed that, in ob/ob mice, the administration of leptin may improve upper airway obstruction and sleep hypoventilation.[60]

A possible explanation of the conflicting data from human and animal models is that the increased leptin levels in humans are necessary to maintain adequate minute ventilation as a consequence of the increased ventilatory load.[54] In contrast, Campo et al. found an association between higher serum leptin levels and reductions in baseline respiratory drive and chemoresponsiveness to CO_2 in obese subjects, but it has yet to be established whether this is linked to the development of daytime chronic hypercapnia.[61] However, in the presence of so-called 'leptin resistance', this compensatory mechanism would be lost and hypercapnia during wakefulness could emerge.[55] The term *leptin resistance* has been introduced to describe the failure of elevated circulating leptin to reduce common obesity. The resistance may be the consequence of an inability of leptin to target specific sites within the brain (the so-called 'peripheral resistance') or the consequence of an impaired cellular response in specific brain areas (the 'central resistance'). Peripheral resistance seems to be associated to an impaired transport of serum leptin across the blood–brain barrier, resulting in insufficient level within the brain[62,63] (Figure 46.4). Two mechanisms have been proposed: high serum leptin levels may partially saturate the transporter (inability to upregulate the transporter) and there should be a defect in the transporter itself.

Central resistance is characterised by reduced responses to intra-brain administered leptin: the nature of blunted response varies according to the different areas of brain specifically stimulated. The mechanism involved in the central resistance are far to be understood. Available data have highlighted a possible role of leptin receptors, particularly the soluble isoform.[63,64] The leptin in the cerebrospinal fluid, expressed as percentage of plasma leptin, declines with increasing BMI, consistently with a saturable transport mechanism.[64]

Leptin participates in different regulation pathways in the central nervous system: it is involved in the appetite, sympathetic activity, blood pressure and thermogenesis regulation.[65]

The mechanisms and pathways activated by leptin to facilitate breathing are still not completely understood. Direct administration of leptin into the fourth ventricle and the nucleus of the tract solitaries increases the hypercapnic ventilatory response.[66] However, data on the effect of leptin on chemosensitive neurons of retrotrapezoid nucleus are conflicting. Micro-injections of leptin for three consecutive days into the rostral ventrolateral medulla increased baseline minute ventilation and ventilatory response to hypercapnia in ob/ob mice.[67] On the other hand, acute exposure to leptin did not change the activity of retrotrapezoid nucleus in the brainstem of rats. These data may indicate that leptin should stimulate non-chemosensitive neurons involved in the chemoreflex pathway: presence of leptin receptors has been demonstrated in the neurons of rostral ventrolateral medulla or Botzinger complex.[68]

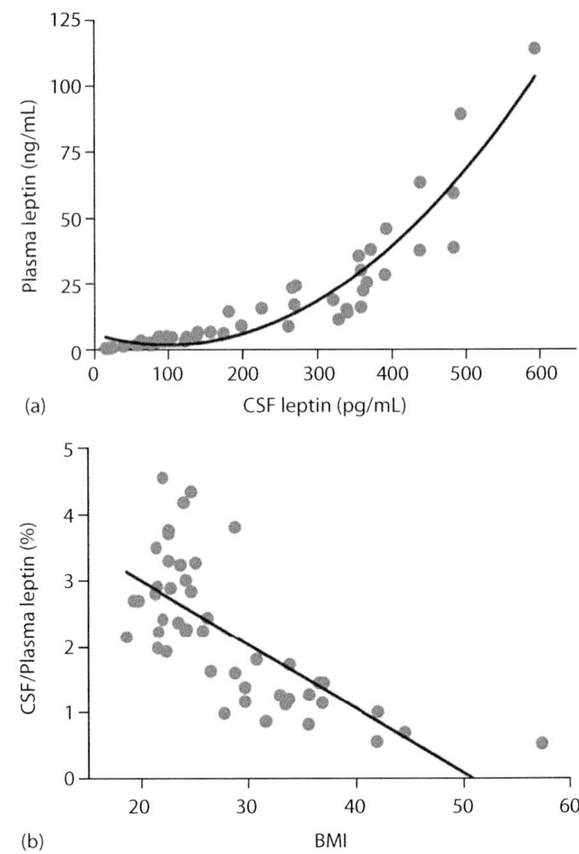

Figure 46.4 Correlation between cerebro-spinal fluid (CSF) and plasma leptin level **(a)** and between body mass index (BMI) and CSF/leptin ratio (expressed as %, **(b)**. (Reproduced with permission from Page-Wilson G et al. *Am J Physiol Endocrinol Meta.* 2015;309:E458–65.)

Leptin may contribute to chemoreflex through an hypothalamic circuit involving the proopiomelanocortin and α-melanocyte-stimulating hormone pathway that, in turn, activates the melanocortin 3 and 4 receptors. The inhibition of this pathway, which could be obtained with different experimental protocols, induces a reduction in minute ventilation and ventilatory response to CO_2, particularly during non–rapid eye movement (NREM) sleep.[68]

The hypothalamic pathway exerts important and specific effects on control of upper airway patency, as recently demonstrated by Yao et al. (Figure 46.5).[69] The activation of this

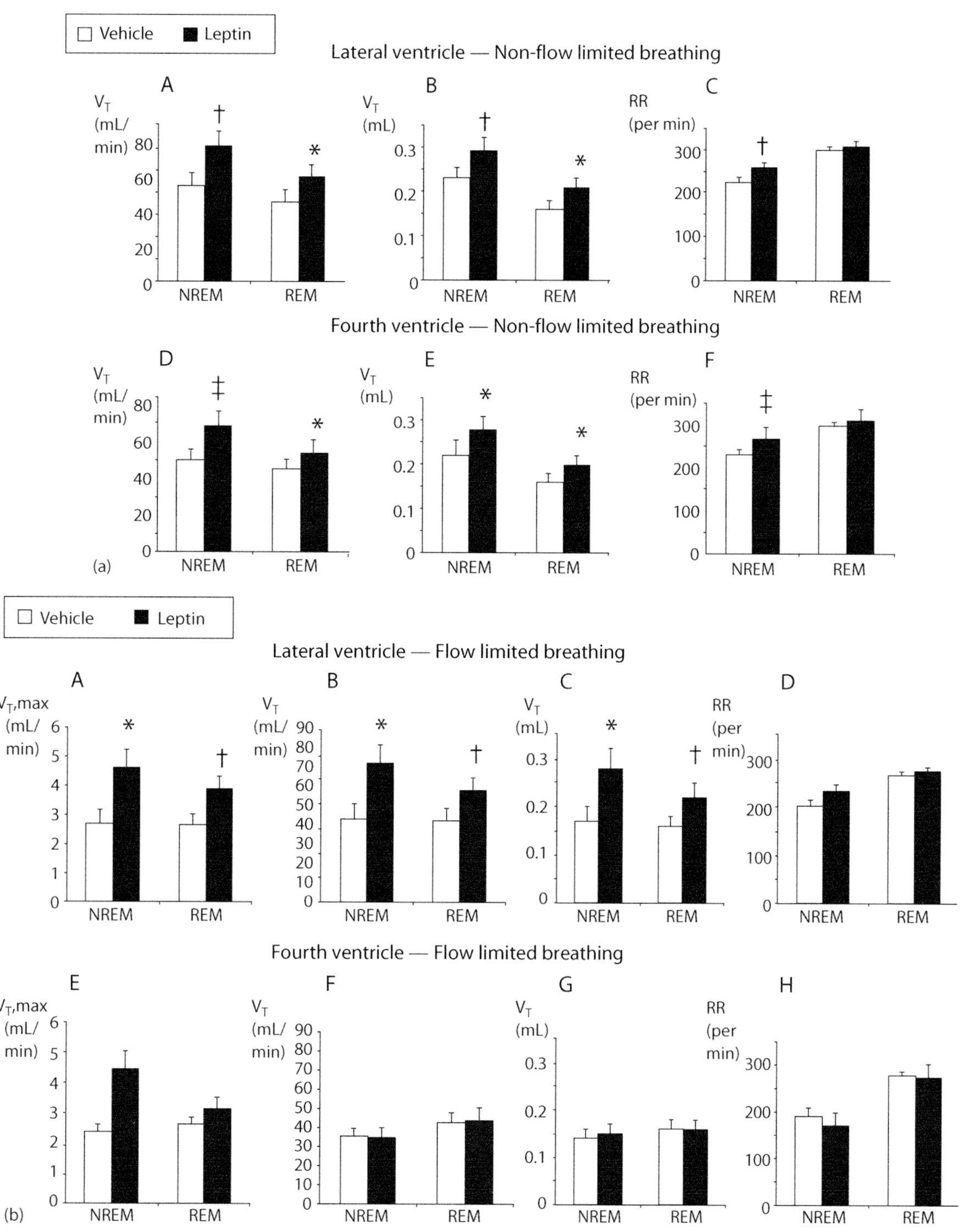

Figure 46.5 **(a)** The effects of intracerebroventricular administration of leptin or vehicle on minute ventilation (VE), tidal volume (VT), and respiratory rate (RR) during non–flow-limited breathing in non–rapid eye movement (NREM) and rapid eye movement (REM) sleep. (A–C) Lateral ventricle administration. (D–F) Fourth ventricle administration. *$p < 0.05$, $^{\dagger}p < 0.01$ and $^{\ddagger}p < 0.001$, respectively, for the effect of leptin. **(b)** The effects of intracerebroventricular administration of leptin or vehicle on the maximal inspiratory flow (Vmax), minute ventilation (V_E), tidal volume (V_T), and respiratory rate (RR) during flow-limited breathing in nonrapid eye movement (NREM), and rapid eye movement (REM) sleep. (A–D) Lateral ventricle administration. (E–H) Fourth ventricle administration. * and $^{\dagger}p < 0.05$ and <0.01, respectively, for the effect of leptin. (Reproduced with permission from Yao et al. *Sleep*. 2016;39:1097–1106.)

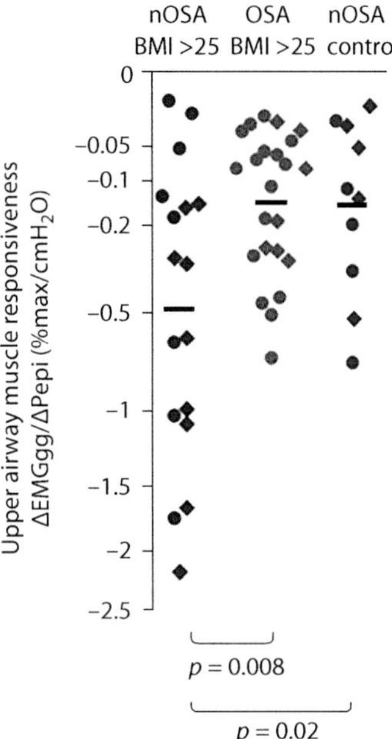

Figure 46.6 Physiologic differences between overweight/obese nonapnoeic individuals (nOSA BMI >25), overweight/obese patients with OSA (OSA BMI >25) and normal-weight control subjects (nOSA control). Upper airway dilator muscles are markedly more responsive in overweight/obese nOSA compared with both overweight/obese OSA and normal-weight control subjects. Responsiveness is defined as the genioglossus electromyogram (EMGgg) response to negative epiglottic pressure, ΔEMGgg/ΔPepi (EMGgg is reported relative to maximum achievable activity). Data were square root transformed before statistical analysis to achieve normally distributed data and are plotted on a square root scale. (Reproduced with permission from Sands SA et al. *Am J Respir Crit Care Med.* 2014;190:930–7.)

pathway may be the physiological mechanism explaining the enhanced response of upper airway dilator muscles that protect some overweight or obese individuals from OSA (Figure 46.6).[70]

In clinical practice, there is a great variability in respiratory impairment in individual patients, ranging from small changes in lung volumes to severe acute-on-chronic respiratory failure needing admission to an intensive care unit. The source of this variability is far from having been identified since most of the studies that have generated data were cross-sectional or characterised by small sample sizes. Recent studies have led to an increasing awareness of the importance of the hypothalamus in maintaining normal breathing by means of the activity of orexin neurons.[71–73] Williams et al. demonstrated in mice that acidification increases intrinsic excitability of orexin neurons, whereas alkalinisation depresses it, suggesting a new mechanism of controlling breathing comparable to that of the classical chemosensory neurons of the brainstem.[71] Deng et al. showed that orexin knock-out mice had a blunted hypercapnic chemoreflex that was partially restored after supplementation of orexins; similarly, the hypercapnic chemoreflex was reduced in wild-type mice after injection of an orexin antagonist.[74]

Data obtained in humans are quite different. Han et al., comparing the hypoxic and hypercapnic ventilatory response in patients with type 1 narcolepsy and in controls, found only a depressed hypoxic responsiveness in patients.[75] However, the lower hypoxic responsiveness was a result of DQB10602 HLA (human leukocyte antigen) status rather than a clinical feature of narcolepsy: a similar blunted responsiveness to hypoxia was also observed in normal subjects positive to HLA status.

Exposure to hypoxia elicits ventilatory acclimatisation and different forms of respiratory plasticity through various mechanisms, predominantly related to type of hypoxic stimulus (continuous or intermittent).[76–79] Chronic hypoxia usually induces long-term facilitation or progressive augmentation through mechanisms involving the peripheral carotid body chemoreceptors, whereas intermittent hypoxia acts on the brainstem and spinal cord. Long-term facilitation is a form of neuronal plasticity characterised by a progressive increase in respiratory output during the normoxic periods that separate hypoxic episodes and by a sustained elevation in respiratory activity for up to 90 min after exposure to hypoxia. How these mechanisms are involved in the pathogenesis of chronic respiratory failure remains to be clarified. Mateika et al. demonstrated an inverse correlation between the ventilatory response to hypoxia/hypercapnia and the severity of apnoea in individuals with OSA. Chronic intermittent hypoxia may have a differential effect on this response, initially causing an enhancement but later leading to depression.[80] Extracellular ATP signalling seems to play a role in ventilatory control, mediating both peripheral and central chemosensory transduction in response to changes in arterial levels of oxygen and CO_2.[80] Recently, the specific role of AMP-activated protein kinase (AMPK) in the cellular processes responsible for the ventilatory adjustments to variation in oxygen demand and supply has been clarified. Mahmoud et al. demonstrated that AMPK deficiency leads to respiratory depression during hypoxia, characterised by hypoventilation and apnoea, despite a regular activity of carotid body.[81]

REFERENCES

1. The WHO Global Infobase. 2007. Accessed at: www.who.int/infobas/report.aspx
2. The challenge of obesity in the WHO European Region and the strategies for response: Summary. Branca F, Nikogosian H and Lobstein T, editors.
3. James WPT; Jackson-Leach R, Ni Mhurchu C et al. Overweight and obesity (high body mass index). In: Ezzati M, Lopez AD, Rodgers A, Murray CJL, editors. *Comparative Quantification of Health Risks: Global and Regional Burden of Disease Attribution to Selected Major Risk Factors*. Chapter 8, Vol. 1. Geneva: World Health Organization, 2004:497–596 (http://www.who.int/publications/cra/en).

4. Peeters A, Barendregt JJ, Willekens F et al. Obesity in adulthood and its consequences for life expectancy: A life-table analysis. *Ann Intern Med.* 2003;138:24–32.
5. The Global BMI Mortality Collaboration body-mass index and all-cause mortality: Individual-participant-data meta-analysis of 239 prospective studies in four continents. *Lancet.* 2016;388:776–86.
6. Aune D, Sen A, Prasad M et al. BMI and all cause mortality: Systematic review and non-linear dose-response meta-analysis of 230 cohort studies with 3.74 million deaths among 30.3 million participants. *BMJ.* 2016;353:i2156 http://dx.doi.org/10.1136/bmj.i2156.
7. Naimark A, Cherniack RM. Compliance of the respiratory system and its components in health and obesity. *J Appl Physiol.* 1960;15:377–82.
8. Pelosi P, Croci M, Ravagnan I et al. Total respiratory system, lung, and chest wall mechanics in sedated-paralyzed postoperative morbidly obese patients. *Chest.* 1996;109:144–51.
9. Pelosi P, Croci I, Ravagnan I et al. Respiratory system mechanics in sedated, paralyzed morbidly obese patients. *J Appl Physiol.* 1997;82:811–8.
10. Sampson MG, Grassino AE. Load compensation in obese patients during quiet tidal breathing. *J Appl Physiol Respir Environ Exerc Physiol.* 1983;55(4):1269–76.
11. Ray CS, Sue DY, Bray G et al. Effects of obesity on respiratory function. *Am Rev Respir Dis.* 1983;128:501–6.
12. Collins LC, Hoberty PG, Walker JF et al. The effect of body fat distributions on pulmonary function tests. *Chest.* 1995;107:1298–1302.
13. Lazarus R, Sparrow D, Weiss ST. Effects of obesity and fat distribution on ventilatory function. *Chest.* 1997;111:891–8.
14. Young RP, Hopkins R, Eaton TE. Forced expiratory volume in one second: Not just a lung function test but a marker of premature death from all causes. *Eur Respir J.* 2007;30:616–22.
15. Lakka HM, Laaksonen DE, Lakka TA et al. The metabolic syndrome and total and cardiovascular disease mortality in middle-aged men. *JAMA.* 2002;288:2709–16.
16. Leone N, Courbon D, Thomas F et al. Lung function impairment and metabolic syndrome. *AJRCCM.* 2009;179:509–16.
17. Jones RL, Nzekwu MMU. The effects of body mass index on lung volumes. *Chest.* 2006;130:827–33.
18. Watson RA, Pride NB. Postural changes in lung volumes and respiratory resistance in subjects with obesity. *J Appl Physiol.* 2005;98:512–7.
19. Bottai M, Pistelli F, Di Pede F et al. Longitudinal changes of body mass index, spirometry and diffusion in a general population. *Eur Respir J.* 2002;20:665–73.
20. Sutherland TJT, McLachlan CR, Sears MR et al. The relationship between body fat and respiratory function in young adults. *Eur Respir J.* 2016;48:734–47.
21. Rubinstein I, Zamel N, DuBarry L et al. Airflow limitation in morbidly obese, nonsmoking men. *Ann Intern Med.* 1990;112:828–32.
22. Pankow W, Podszus T, Gutheil T et al. Expiratory flow limitation and intrinsic positive end-expiratory pressure in obesity. *J Appl Physiol.* 1998;85:1236–43.
23. Steier J, Jolley CJ, Seymour J et al. Neural respiratory drive in obesity. *Thorax.* 2009;64:719–25.
24. Hardie JA, Vollmer WM, Buist AS et al. Reference values for arterial blood gases in the elderly. *Chest.* 2004;125:2053–60.
25. Cerveri I, Zoia MC, Fanfulla F et al. Reference values of arterial oxygen tension in the middle-aged and elderly. *Am J Respir Crit Care Med.* 1995;152:934–41.
26. Ulmer WT, Reichel G. Untersuchungen uber die Altersabhangigkeit der aleolaren und arteriellen Sauerstoff-und Kohlensauredrucke. *Klein Wochenschr.* 1963;41:1–6.
27. Holley HS, Milic-Emili J, Becklake MR, Bates DV. Regional distribution of pulmonary ventilation and perfusion in obesity. *J Clin Invest.* 1967;46:475–81.
28. Yamane T, Date T, Tokuda M et al. Hypoxemia in inferior pulmonary veins in supine position is dependent on obesity. *Am J Respir Crit Care Med.* 2008;178:295–98.
29. Farebrother MJB, McHardy GJR, Munro JF. Relationship between pulmonary gas exchange and closing volume before and after substantial weight loss in obese subjects. *BMJ.* 1974;3:391–3.
30. American Academy of Sleep Medicine. *International Classification of Sleep Disorders, 2nd edition. Diagnostic and Coding Manual.* Westchester, Illinois: American Academy of Sleep Medicine, 2005.
31. Young T, Peppard PE, Taheri S. Excess weight and sleep-disordered breathing. *J Appl Physiol.* 2005;99:1592–9.
32. Peppard PE, Young T, Palta M et al. Longitudinal study of moderate weight change and sleep-disordered breathing. *JAMA.* 2000;284:3015–21.
33. Sajkov D, McEvoy RD. Obstructive sleep apnea and pulmonary hypertension. *Prog Cardiovasc Dis.* 2009;51:363–70.
34. Weitzenblum E, Krieger J, Appril M et al. Daytime pulmonary hypertension in patients with obstructive sleep apnea syndrome. *Am Rev Respir Dis.* 1988;138:345–9.
35. Fanfulla F, Grassi M, Taurino AE et al. The relationship of daytime hypoxemia and nocturnal hypoxia in obstructive sleep apnea syndrome. *Sleep.* 2008;31:249–55.
36. American Academy of Sleep Medicine. *International Classification of Sleep Disorders, 3rd edition.* Darien, Illinois: American Academy of Sleep Medicine, 2014.
37. Piper A. Obesity hypoventilation syndrome. *Chest.* 2016;149(3):856–68.

38. Lugaresi E, Cirignotta F, Gerardi R, Montagna P. Snoring and sleep apnea: Natural history of heavy snorers disease. In: Guilleminault C, Partinen M, editors. *Obstructive Sleep Apnea Syndrome*. New York: Raven Press, 1990:25–36.
39. Mokhlesi B, Krygher MH, Grunstein RR. Assessment and management of patients with obesity hypoventilation syndrome. *Proc Am Thorac Soc.* 2008;5:218–25.
40. Kress JP, Pohlman AS, Alverdy J, Hall JB. The impact of morbid obesity on oxygen cost of breathing (O_{2RESP}) at rest. *Am J Respir Crit Care Med.* 1999;160:883–6.
41. Sampson MG, Grassino A. Neuromechanical properties in obese patients during carbon dioxide rebreathing. *Am J Med.* 1983;75:81–90.
42. Lopata M, Onal E. Mass loading, sleep apnea, and the pathogenesis of obesity hypoventilation. *Am Rev Respir Dis.* 1982;126:640–5.
43. Chouri-Pontarollo N, Borel JC, Tamisier R et al. Impaired objective daytime vigilance in obesity-hypoventilation syndrome: Impact of noninvasive ventilation. *Chest.* 2007;131:148–55.
44. Burki NK, Baker RW. Ventilatory regulation in eucapnic morbid obesity. *Am Rev Respir Dis.* 1984;129:538–43.
45. Norman RG, Goldring RM, Clain JM et al. Transition from acute to chronic hypercapnia in patients with periodic breathing: Predictions from a computer model. *J Appl Physiol.* 2006;100:1733–41.
46. Leech J, Onal E, Aronson R, Lopata M. Voluntary hyperventilation in obesity hypoventilation. *Chest.* 1991;100:1334–8.
47. Jokic R, Zintel T, Sridhar G et al. Ventilatory responses to hypercapnia and hypoxia in relatives of patients with the obesity hypoventilation syndrome. *Thorax.* 2000;55:940–5.
48. Redolfi S, Corda L, La Piana G et al. Long-term noninvasive ventilation increases chemosensitivity and leptin in obesity-hypoventilation syndrome. *Respir Med.* 2007;101:1191–5.
49. Akashiba T, Akahoshi T, Kawahara S et al. Clinical characteristics of obesity-hypoventilation syndrome in Japan: A multi-center study. *Intern Med.* 2006;45:1121–5.
50. De Miguel Diez J, De Lucas Ramos P, Perez Parra JJ et al. Analysis of withdrawal from noninvasive mechanical ventilation in patients with obesity-hypoventilation syndrome. Medium term results. *Arch Bronconeumol.* 2003;39:292–7.
51. Berger KI, Ayappa I, Sorkin IB et al. CO_2 homeostasis during periodic breathing in obstructive sleep apnea. *J Appl Physiol.* 2000;88:257–64.
52. Berger KI, Ayappa I, Sorkin IB et al. Postevent ventilation as a function of CO_2 load during respiratory events in obstructive sleep apnea. *J Appl Physiol.* 2002;93:917–24.
53. Ayappa I, Berger KI, Norman RG et al. Hypercapnia and ventilatory periodicity in obstructive sleep apnea syndrome. *Am J Respir Crit Care Med.* 2002;166:1112–5.
54. O'Donnell CP, Tankersley CG, Polotsky VP et al. Leptin, obesity, and respiratory function. *Respir Physiol.* 2000;119:163–70.
55. O'Donnell CP, Schaub CD, Haines AS et al. Leptin prevents respiratory depression in obesity. *Am J Respir Crit Care Med.* 1999;159:1477–84.
56. Phipps PR, Starritt E, Caterson I et al. Association of serum leptin with hypoventilation in human obesity. *Thorax.* 2002;57:75–6.
57. Shimura R, Tatsumi K, Nakamura A et al. Fat accumulation, leptin, and hypercapnia in obstructive sleep apnea-hypopnea syndrome. *Chest.* 2005;127:543–9.
58. Malli F, Papaioannou AI, Gourgoulinais KI, Daniil Z. The role of leptin in the respiratory system: An overview. *Respir Res.* 2010;111:152.
59. Chang Z, Ballou E, Jiao W et al. Systemic leptin produces a long-lasting increase in respiratory motor output in rats. *Front Physiol.* 2013;4:16.
60. Polotsky M, Elsayed-Ahmed AS, Pichard L et al. Effects of leptin and obesity on upper airway function. *J Appl Physiol.* 2012;112:1637–43.
61. Campo A, Fuhbeck G, Zulueta JJ et al. Hyperleptinaemia, respiratory drive and hypercapnic response in obese patients. *Eur Respir J.* 2007;30:223–31.
62. Caro JF, Kolaczynski JW, Nyce MR et al. Decreased cerebrospinal-fluid/serum leptin ratio in obesity: A possible mechanism for leptin resistance. *Lancet.* 1996;348:159–61.
63. Banks WA, DiPalma CR, Farrell CI. Impaired transport of leptin across the blood–brain barrier in obesity. *Peptides.* 1999;20:1341–5.
64. Page-Wilson G, Meece K, White A et al. Proopiomelanocortin, agouti-related protein and leptin in human cerebrospinal fluid: Correlations with body weight and adiposity. *Am J Physiol Endocrinol Meta.* 2015;309:E458–65.
65. Bassi M, Werner LF, Zoccal DB et al. Control of respiratory and cardiovascular functions by leptin. *Life Sciences.* 2015;125:25–31.
66. Inyushkina EM, Merkulova N, Inyushkin A. Mechanism of the respiratory activity of leptin at the level of the solitary tract nucleus. *Neurosci Behav Physiol.* 2010;40:707–13.
67. Bassi M, Furuya WI, Menani JV et al. Leptin into the ventrolateral medulla facilitates chemorespiratory response in leptin deficient (ob/ob) mice. *Acta Physiol.* 2014;211:240–8.
68. Bassi M, Furuya W, Zoccal DB et al. Facilitation of breathing by leptin effects in the central nervous system. *J Physiol.* 2016;594:1617–25.

69. Yao Q, Pho H, Kirkness et al. Localizing effects of leptin on upper airway and respiratory control during sleep. *Sleep.* 2016;39:1097–1106.
70. Sands SA, Eckert DJ, Jordan AS et al. Enhanced upper-airway muscle responsiveness is a distinct feature of overweight/obese individuals without sleep apnea. *Am J Respir Crit Care Med.* 2014; 190:930–7.
71. Williams RH, Jensen LT, Verkhratsky A et al. Control of hypothalamic orexin neurons by acid and CO_2. *PNAS.* 2007;107:10685–90.
72. Willie JT, Chemelli RM, Sinton CM, Yanagisawa M. To eat or to sleep? Orexin in the regulation of feeding and wakefulness. *Ann Rev Neurosci.* 2001;24:429–58.
73. Young JK, Wu M, Manaye KF et al. Orexin stimulates breathing via medullary and spinal pathways. *J Appl Physiol.* 2005;98:1387–95.
74. Deng BS, Nakamura A, Zhang W et al. Contribution of orexin in hypercapnic chemoreflex: Evidence from genetic and pharmacological disruption and supplementation in mice. *J Appl Physiol.* 2007;103:1772–9.
75. Han F, Mignot E, Wei YC et al. Ventilatory chemoresponsiveness, narcolepsy-cataplexy and human leukocyte antigen DQB1*0602 status. *Eur Respir J.* 2010;36:577–83.
76. Mateika JH, Narwani G. Intermittent hypoxia and respiratory plasticity in humans and other animals: Does exposure to intermittent hypoxia promote or mitigate sleep apnoea? *Exp Physiol.* 2009;94:279–96.
77. Wilkerson JER, MacFarlane PM, Hoffman MS, Mitchell GS. Respiratory plasticity following intermittent hypoxia: Roles of protein phosphatases and reactive oxygen species. *Biochem Soc Trans.* 2007;35:1269–72.
78. MacFarlane PM, Mitchell GS. Respiratory long-term facilitation following intermittent hypoxia requires reactive oxygen species formation. *Neuroscience.* 2008;152:189–97.
79. Mateika JH, Ellythy M. Chemoreflex control of ventilation is altered during wakefulness in humans with OSA. *Respir Physiol Neurobiol.* 2003;138:45–57.
80. Ackland GL, Kasymov V, Gourine AV. Physiological and pathophysiological roles of extracellular ATP in chemosensory control of breathing. *Biochem Soc Trans.* 2007;35:1264–8.
81. Mahmoud AD, Lewis S, Juričić L et al. AMP-activated protein kinase deficiency blocks the hypoxic ventilatory response and thus precipitates hypoventilation and apnea. *Am J Respir Crit Care Med.* 2016;193:1032–43.

47

Acute non-invasive ventilation in obesity-related respiratory failure

PATRICK B. MURPHY AND NICHOLAS HART

KEY MESSAGES

- Acute obesity-related respiratory failure is an increasingly common clinical presentation but remains to be under- or misdiagnosed.
- The majority of patients with acute obesity-related respiratory failure can be managed with non-invasive ventilation with invasive ventilation reserved for those with multiorgan failure.
- Following an episode of acute obesity-related respiratory failure, patients should be referred on for assessment by a specialist service for consideration of domiciliary non-invasive ventilation.

INTRODUCTION

Non-invasive ventilation (NIV) is a standard treatment in the management of both acute and acute-on-chronic respiratory failure.[1] Whilst the best evidence for NIV remains in its application in acute hypercapnic exacerbations of chronic obstructive pulmonary disease (COPD), its role has expanded to include acute respiratory failure complicating postextubation failure and immunosuppression.[2–5] In addition, and reflecting the general population trends of rising rates of obesity, NIV has become an important treatment in the management of acute respiratory failure associated with obesity.[6,7] This treatment approach has been used to accommodate the increasing prevalence of obesity-related respiratory failure in unselected acute medical patients admitted to hospital.[8] The detection of obesity-related respiratory failure has been complicated by the limited self-reporting of chronic symptoms and poor self-perception of symptom burden of the patient cohort,[9] leading to the underdiagnosis of the condition during the initial assessment in the emergency department.[8] Consequently, there should be a low clinical threshold for assessing for hypercapnia with either an arterial blood gas sample or a derived value from a venous sample.[10] The latter can sometime be considered, as there is an acknowledged anxiety and discomfort associated with arterial sampling, which may dissuade patients from subsequent testing.[11] The use of transcutaneous carbon dioxide ($tcCO_2$) measurement also offers a painless technique that has a lower technical skill requirement and can be utilised to assess for hypercapnia in the acutely unwell patient.[12,13]

PATHOPHYSIOLOGY OF OBESITY-RELATED RESPIRATORY FAILURE

The underlying mechanisms of obesity-related respiratory failure are covered elsewhere in this book (Chapter 10), and it is only revised in brief here. In essence, obesity contributes to respiratory failure with effects on the respiratory muscle load capacity–drive relationship, which is exacerbated at times of acute illness. Whilst acute obesity-related respiratory failure has been reported to confer a poor outcome,[14,15] when other associated comorbidities have been accounted for, obesity confers a potential advantage in patients with acute respiratory failure managed in the critical care environment.[16] The reasons for this obesity paradox are not fully elucidated but may include the ability to deliver lung protective ventilation more successfully as the driving pressure is moderated by the increased respiratory muscle load resulting in a reduction in transpulmonary pressure. In addition, the beneficial outcome is probably the consequence of the greater nursing and therapy care that has to be provided to the obese critically ill patient.

Load

Obesity increases the respiratory muscle load not only by directly decreasing the compliance of the respiratory system as a consequence of the physical load of fat mass on the chest wall, but also by adversely effecting pulmonary mechanics with increased threshold load produced by increased intra-abdominal pressure and intrinsic positive end-expiratory pressure.[17–19] Furthermore, the respiratory load is increased due to upper airway resistance, both seated and supine, in patients with chronic obesity-related respiratory failure even during wakefulness.[20] Acute decompensation can be the consequence of generalised and specific pulmonary infection which leads to fluid overload as a result of decompensated right heart failure ('acute cor pulmonale'), which further adds to the respiratory muscle loading.

Capacity

Respiratory muscle capacity is normal in eucapnic obesity, but may be normal or reduced in patients with obesity-related chronic hypercapnia.[21] Respiratory muscle function can be further impaired during an acute decompensation due to hypoxia, hypercapnia and acidosis contributing to further hypoventilation and worsening of the clinical picture.

Neural respiratory drive

There is a reduction in neural respiratory drive in patients with ventilatory failure associated with obesity. Indeed, there is a blunting of the hypercapnic ventilatory response, which renders patients less able to deal with the extra demand posed by acute infection or other additional stresses placed on the respiratory system.[21] Furthermore, the injudicious use of oxygen therapy can contribute to worsening hypoventilation and respiratory acidosis.[22] Consideration must be given to the level of ventilatory support, which may need to be further increased overnight to manage the associated fall in minute ventilation associated with changes in body position and sleep stage.[23]

CAUSE OF ACUTE DECOMPENSATION

Obesity has a high prevalence in the general population and may therefore complicate the clinical presentation of a range of respiratory pathologies, which can lead to ventilatory failure. It is important to not only manage any acute decompensation with ventilatory support but also investigate the underlying cause of the ventilatory failure. Data are currently limited in assisting the clinician, and so a comprehensive clinical assessment should be undertaken, including a detailed medical history and physical examination, which should in turn drive the choice of further investigations. It must be remembered that many investigations may be directly affected by the degree of obesity, rendering interpretation challenging (Figure 47.1). Particular attention should be focused on the clinical features of cor pulmonale, respiratory infection and uncontrolled blood glucose levels with associated skin infection, which commonly contribute to, and are indeed common features of, multimorbidity obesity syndrome. Although obstructive sleep apnoea (OSA) may complicate COPD,[24] adding a further complexity to the ventilatory management, many obese patients have erroneous diagnosis of COPD, which should be confirmed or excluded with appropriate clinical assessment and investigations.[25] The few data available suggest that respiratory infection, fluid overload and untreated sleep-disordered breathing are the most common causes for decompensation in obesity-related respiratory failure.[7]

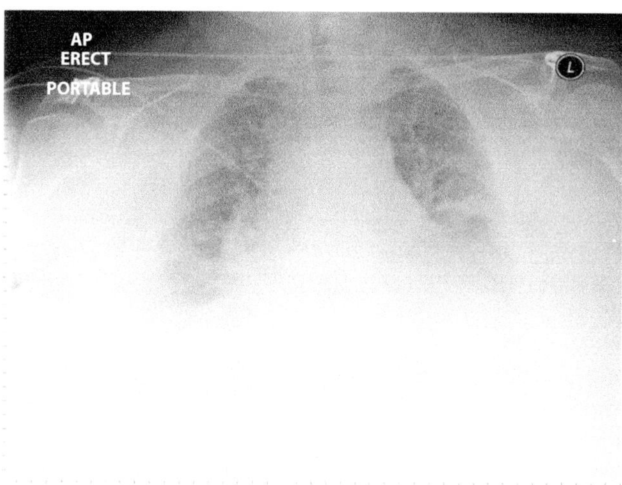

Figure 47.1 Chest radiograph of an obese patient highlighting the difficulties interpreting investigations that may be influenced by body habitus.

MANAGEMENT OF ACUTE OR ACUTE ON CHRONIC OBESITY-RELATED RESPIRATORY FAILURE

As outlined earlier, the underlying cause of the acute decompensation must be sought and appropriately managed. Patients should be established on NIV by a skilled multidisciplinary team with an appropriate level of cardiorespiratory monitoring. It is essential that an appropriate skill mix and educational level is maintained by the staff administering NIV and that this is provided within identified clinical areas to allow the consolidation of skills and the audit of the outcomes.[26–28] The level and type of monitoring should be scaled to the patient's clinical state but as a minimum should include continuous monitoring of oxygen saturation of pulsatile haemoglobin (SpO_2). Unstable and acclimatising patients should be considered for $tcCO_2$ monitoring,[29] and invasive arterial monitoring should be reserved for the most severely unwell and, in particular, those with multiorgan failure as a consequence of, for example, sepsis.

The choice of interface significantly affects patient tolerance. An oronasal mask should be used as first line in all patients with obesity-related respiratory failure. Nasal or total facemasks can be considered for those patients not tolerating standard interfaces, but may have disadvantages of triggering and leak problems. Initial NIV settings should support ventilation, but the pressures delivered must be assessed with respect to the comfort of the patient so as to enhance patient adherence. Over the first hour of therapy, the NIV settings should be optimised to ensure reduction in work of breathing with a focus on improving patient comfort. Common problems encountered in clinical practice that can affect the delivery of NIV in acute obesity-related respiratory failure along with possible remedial actions are outlined in Table 47.1. Expiratory positive airway pressure (EPAP) should be set to abolish upper airway obstruction, in particular, during sleep. Inspiratory positive airway pressure (IPAP) should be set sufficiently above EPAP to allow adequate chest expansion and tidal volume. A backup rate, set just below resting tidal rate, usually on the order of 12–14 breaths per minute, and appropriate inspiratory time, set at 1.2–1.4 s, should also be set to provide adequate ventilatory support overnight. There are few data to support the use of a volume-targeted mode in the acute setting, and thus this mode should be reserved for those familiar with their use and limitations.[30] Patients will frequently require supplementary oxygen during the acute episode, and this should be entrained at the lowest flow rate, which maintains SpO_2 level in the target range of 88%–92%, following treatment of upper airway obstruction with EPAP and increasing tidal volume with an adequate level of IPAP. The initial NIV prescription should be reviewed after the first hour to ensure physiological improvement with the optimisation of settings to ensure therapeutic efficacy and patient comfort. Although the data are limited, the response rate to NIV appears to be superior in obesity hypoventilation syndrome patients compared to those with COPD.[7] A management algorithm for acute obesity-related respiratory failure is provided in Figure 47.1.

Patients who deteriorate following initial improvement with NIV have a poor outcome,[31] and appropriate escalation decisions should be made in advance to decide if intubation and mechanical ventilation are appropriate strategies. This decision may influence the location of delivery of NIV therapy, as a critical care unit with access to rapid intubation may be appropriate for patients deemed at high risk of NIV failure but appropriate for escalation to invasive ventilation. Furthermore, the presence of OSA and obesity are associated with a difficult airway,[32] and therefore, appropriate risk assessment should be made prior to NIV initiation to ensure that appropriately skilled staff and equipment are available should the need for intubation arise. There are a number of factors which may identify patients at risk of failure of NIV, in particular, the super-obese with a body mass index greater than 60 kg/m^2 and those with poor adherence to domiciliary continuous positive airway pressure (CPAP) therapy.[33] NIV should be applied for as long as possible during the first 24–48 hours with daytime comfort breaks for medication as well as oral nutrition and hydration. As patients respond to therapy, NIV can be gradually withdrawn during the day and applied at night only to control sleep-disordered breathing.

Table 47.1 Common clinical issues affecting NIV delivery and possible solutions

Clinical problem	Potential solution
Agitation or poor patient tolerance	Ensure patient education on need and response for NIV Check and refit NIV interface Reduce pressures and retitrate as tolerance is improved Consider sedation (e.g., remifentanil)
Mask leak	Check and refit NIV interface Consider reduction in pressures if ventilation maintained
Snoring	Increase EPAP
Persistent hypoxia (aim SpO_2 88%–92%)	In the following order: Ensure adequate ventilation (chest wall expansion, appropriate Vt delivered [if measured], improving hypercapnia etc.) prior to entraining additional oxygen Check oxygen inlet (higher FiO_2 achieved if delivered after rather than before intentional leak)
No reduction in hypercapnia	Check and refit NIV interface to minimise mask leak Ensure adequate EPAP to maintain upper airway patency Ensure adequate pressure support to delivery chest wall expansion Optimise FiO_2 to ensure not over oxygenating

POST-ACUTE MANAGEMENT

Whilst there may be further improvement in patients' sleep-disordered breathing and physiology following an acute episode, once clinically stable, patients can frequently be safely discharged home without overnight respiratory support and indeed return for an outpatient sleep study. However, the practicalities may often make an assessment of sleep-disordered breathing more appropriate at the end of the acute admission, and this approach ensures that patients have optimal long-term therapy instituted prior to discharge.

CONCLUSION

Obesity-related respiratory failure is frequently undiagnosed and, even when detected, is often managed suboptimally. Clinicians should maintain a high index of suspicion of acute, and acute-on-chronic, respiratory failure in obese patients presenting to acute medical services. Once acute respiratory failure is diagnosed, acute management should be initiated to reverse the cause of decompensation and control hypoventilation. NIV should be administered in an appropriate environment by a specialised multidisciplinary team with adequate experience and support from critical care. Assessment should include a clinical review to determine the need for long-term home NIV therapy prior to patient discharge.

REFERENCES

1. Chandra D, Stamm JA, Taylor B et al. Outcomes of noninvasive ventilation for acute exacerbations of chronic obstructive pulmonary disease in the United States, 1998–2008. *Am J Respir Crit Care Med.* 2012 15;185:152–9.
2. Bott J, Carroll MP, Conway JH et al. Randomised controlled trial of nasal ventilation in acute ventilatory failure due to chronic obstructive airways disease. *Lancet.* 1993;341:1555–7.
3. Vital FM, Ladeira MT, Atallah AN. Non-invasive positive pressure ventilation (CPAP or bilevel NPPV) for cardiogenic pulmonary oedema. *Cochrane Database Syst Rev.* 2013;5:CD005351.
4. Burns KE, Adhikari NK, Keenan SP, Meade MO. Noninvasive positive pressure ventilation as a weaning strategy for intubated adults with respiratory failure. *Cochrane Database Syst Rev.* 2010:CD004127.
5. Antonelli M, Conti G, Bufi M et al. Noninvasive ventilation for treatment of acute respiratory failure in patients undergoing solid organ transplantation: A randomized trial. *JAMA.* 2000;283:235–41.
6. Ng M, Fleming T, Robinson M et al. Global, regional, and national prevalence of overweight and obesity in children and adults during 1980–2013: A systematic analysis for the Global Burden of Disease Study 2013. *Lancet.* 2014;384:766–81.
7. Carrillo A, Ferrer M, Gonzalez-Diaz G et al. Noninvasive ventilation in acute hypercapnic respiratory failure caused by obesity hypoventilation syndrome and chronic obstructive pulmonary disease. *Am J Respir Crit Care Med.* 2012;186: 1279–85.
8. Nowbar S, Burkart KM, Gonzales R et al. Obesity-associated hypoventilation in hospitalized patients: Prevalence, effects, and outcome. *Am J Med.* 2004;116:1–7.
9. Murphy PB, Davidson C, Hind MD et al. Volume targeted versus pressure support non-invasive ventilation in patients with super obesity and chronic respiratory failure: A randomised controlled trial. *Thorax.* 2012;67:727–34.
10. McKeever TM, Hearson G, Housley G et al. Using venous blood gas analysis in the assessment of COPD exacerbations: A prospective cohort study. *Thorax.* 2016;71:210–5.
11. Patout M, Lamia B, Lhuillier E et al. A randomized controlled trial on the effect of needle gauge on the pain and anxiety experienced during radial arterial puncture. *PLoS One.* 2015;10:e0139432.
12. Delerme S, Montout V, Goulet H et al. Concordance between transcutaneous and arterial measurements of carbon dioxide in an ED. *Am J Emerg Med.* 2012;30:1872–6.
13. Bobbia X, Claret PG, Palmier L et al. Erratum: Concordance and limits between transcutaneous and arterial carbon dioxide pressure in emergency department patients with acute respiratory failure: A single-center, prospective, and observational study. *Scand J Trauma Resusc Emerg Med.* 2015;23:77.
14. Miller A, Granada M. In-hospital mortality in the Pickwickian syndrome. *Am J Med.* 1974;56:144–50.
15. Marik PE, Desai H. Characteristics of patients with the 'malignant obesity hypoventilation syndrome' admitted to an ICU. *J Intensive Care Med.* 2013;28: 124–30.
16. Anzueto A, Frutos-Vivar F, Esteban A et al. Influence of body mass index on outcome of the mechanically ventilated patients. *Thorax.* 2011;66:66–73.
17. Steier J, Jolley CJ, Seymour J et al. Neural respiratory drive in obesity. *Thorax.* 2009;64:719–25.
18. Sharp JT, Henry JP, Sweany SK et al. The total work of breathing in normal and obese men. *J Clin Invest.* 1964;43:728–39.
19. Steier J, Lunt A, Hart N et al. Observational study of the effect of obesity on lung volumes. *Thorax.* 2014;69:752–9.
20. Lin CC, Wu KM, Chou CS, Liaw SF. Oral airway resistance during wakefulness in eucapnic and hypercapnic sleep apnea syndrome. *Respir Physiol Neurobiol.* 2004;139:215–24.
21. Sampson MG, Grassino K. Neuromechanical properties in obese patients during carbon dioxide rebreathing. *Am J Med.* 1983;75:81–90.

22. Hollier CA, Harmer AR, Maxwell LJ et al. Moderate concentrations of supplemental oxygen worsen hypercapnia in obesity hypoventilation syndrome: A randomised crossover study. *Thorax*. 2014; 69:346–53.
23. Becker HF, Piper AJ, Flynn WE et al. Breathing during sleep in patients with nocturnal desaturation. *Am J Respir Crit Care Med*. 1999;159:112–8.
24. Sanders MH, Newman AB, Haggerty CL et al. Sleep and sleep-disordered breathing in adults with predominantly mild obstructive airway disease. *Am J Respir Crit Care Med*. 2003;167:7–14.
25. Marik PE. The malignant obesity hypoventilation syndrome (MOHS). *Obes Rev*. 2012;13:902–9.
26. Elliott MW, Confalonieri M, Nava S. Where to perform noninvasive ventilation? *Eur Respir J*. 2002;19:1159–66.
27. Ballard E, McDonnell L, Keilty S et al. Survey of knowledge of health care professionals managing patients with acute hypercapnic exacerbation of COPD requiring non-invasive ventilation. *Thorax*. 2007;62:A90.
28. Davidson AC, Banham S, Elliott M et al. BTS/ICS guideline for the ventilatory management of acute hypercapnic respiratory failure in adults. *Thorax*. 2016;71 2:ii1–35.
29. Storre JH, Magnet FS, Dreher M, Windisch W. Transcutaneous monitoring as a replacement for arterial PCO_2 monitoring during nocturnal non-invasive ventilation. *Respir Med*. 2011;105:143–50.
30. Briones Claudett KH, Briones Claudett M, Chung Sang Wong M et al. Noninvasive mechanical ventilation with average volume assured pressure support (AVAPS) in patients with chronic obstructive pulmonary disease and hypercapnic encephalopathy. *BMC Pulm Med*. 2013;13:12.
31. Lemyze M, Taufour P, Duhamel A et al. Determinants of noninvasive ventilation success or failure in morbidly obese patients in acute respiratory failure. *PLoS One*. 2014;9:e97563.
32. Chung SA, Yuan H, Chung F. A systemic review of obstructive sleep apnea and its implications for anesthesiologists. *Anesth Analg*. 2008 Nov;107:1543–63.
33. Duarte AG, Justino E, Bigler T, Grady J. Outcomes of morbidly obese patients requiring mechanical ventilation for acute respiratory failure. *Crit Care Med*. 2007;35:732–7.

48

Non-invasive ventilation in acute and chronic respiratory failure due to obesity

JUAN FERNANDO MASA, ISABEL UTRABO AND FRANCISCO JAVIER GÓMEZ DE TERREROS

INTRODUCTION

Non-invasive ventilation (NIV) is a recognised therapy for several chronic diseases that results in nocturnal and daytime hypoventilations, especially neuromuscular diseases and conditions that cause the restriction of the chest wall such as obesity hypoventilation syndrome (OHS). It is also approved for the treatment of acute respiratory diseases such as chronic obstructive pulmonary disease (COPD), but there is lower evidence on the efficacy of NIV during similar episodes in OHS.

Obesity is a major public health problem, and rates are continuing to increase,[1] associated with a high risk of morbidity and mortality.[2,3] Obesity compromises waking respiratory function, primarily in the supine position. This difficulty and the tendency for decreased ventilation in normal sleep physiology, hypotonia of the intercostals muscles and lower lung volume can lead to nocturnal oxyhaemoglobin desaturation and hypercapnia. Moreover, the accumulation of fat in the lateral parts of the pharynx intensifies extraluminal pressure and can modify the geometry of the upper airway, facilitating collapse[4] (apnoeas and hypopnoeas). These mechanisms can lead to daytime hypercapnic respiratory failure. It is called obesity hypoventilation syndrome when this daytime hypercapnia is associated with a body mass index (BMI) of over 30 kg/m^2.

The therapeutic mechanisms resulting in nocturnal and daytime gas exchange improvement in patients with restrictive chest wall diseases (e.g. kyphoscoliosis) treated with NIV are not completely understood. Since OHS can generate mechanical difficulties and nocturnal hypoventilation similar to kyphoscoliosis, NIV may be effective in OHS. The first effective positive airway pressure (PAP) treatment for OHS, used in a small series of patients, was continuous positive airway pressure (CPAP) in 1982[5] and intermittent positive pressure ventilation in 1992,[6] both used non-invasively.

The aim of this chapter is to review the role of PAP, NIV (intermittent positive pressure ventilation) and CPAP in OHS, in particular, the mechanisms that produce improvement, the available evidence, clinical applications, technical considerations and future research.

PATHOPHYSIOLOGY (POTENTIAL MECHANISMS FOR IMPROVEMENT WITH PAP)

Chronic failure

The mechanisms by which diurnal hypercapnia improves with PAP are complex and not entirely understood. The principal mechanisms implicated are abnormal respiratory mechanics (including respiratory muscle dysfunction), central responses to hypercapnia and/or neurohormonal dysfunction (leptin resistance), and sleep-disordered breathing (Figure 48.1).

RESPIRATORY MECHANICS

Mechanical alterations in the respiratory system produced by the obesity component of OHS can result in respiratory muscle dysfunction[7] and, potentially, daytime hypercapnia. NIV can reduce inspiratory muscular activity,[8] and consequently, it could decrease mechanical load, favouring greater muscular efficacy after NIV treatment (during the day). CPAP may decrease the mechanical load, avoiding upper airway repetitive obstructions.

The evidence of improvement in vital capacity and lung volume with long-term NIV is contradictory. Several studies[9–11] have shown no change in lung volumes or forced vital capacity in OHS after effective treatment with NIV therapy. On the other hand, two other studies in patients with OHS[12,13] have reported significant improvement in vital capacity and expiratory reserve volume after NIV therapy.

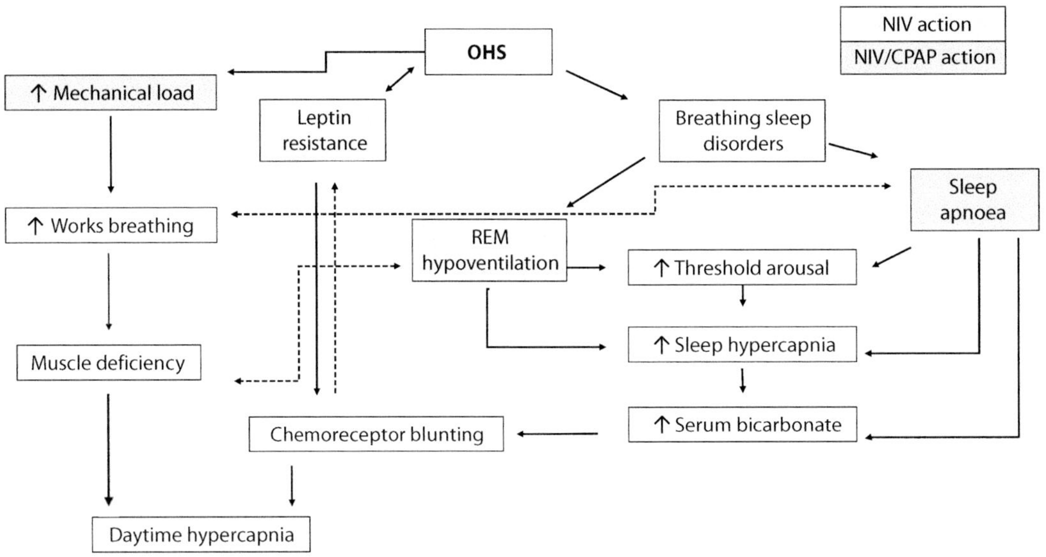

Figure 48.1 Potential mechanisms to achieve improvement with NIV or CPAP. Daytime hypercapnia in OHS can result in an increase in mechanical respiratory load, central leptin resistance, breathing sleep disorders or a combination of all of them. CPAP prevents nocturnal obstructive events and consequently decreases sleep hypercapnia, serum bicarbonate and chemoreceptor blunting. It can alleviate breathing effort as well, and NIV can resolve sleep apnoeas and nocturnal hypoventilation caused by non-apnoeic episodes. In addition, NIV decreases breathing effort and may produce improvement in respiratory drive, decreasing central leptin resistance. REM, rapid eye movement; NIV, non-invasive ventilation; OHS, obesity hypoventilation syndrome; CPAP, continuous positive airway pressure.

BREATHING CONTROL

The altered response to hypercapnia observed in OHS[11] can improve with NIV treatment,[11,13] suggesting that central chemosensitivity recovery could result in daytime normocapnia. However, this change cannot be caused by a direct effect on the neural drive, but it can be the consequence of NIV acting to improve other mechanisms (mechanical, neurohormonal dysfunction and sleep-disordered breathing improvement).

The hormone leptin, produced by fat cells, is implicated in appetite reduction and may act on the nervous system to increase ventilation.[14] In humans, leptin deficiency in obesity is extremely rare, and instead, higher serum levels are detected. High leptin levels increase ventilation, and that is the reason why the majority of severely obese patients do not develop hypercapnia, but there is another group that develops awake hypoventilation. These observations suggest that patients with OHS might be resistant to leptin or maybe have a central leptin resistance.[15–17] The level of serum leptin decreases to normal limits in patients with obstructive sleep apnoea (OSA) treated with CPAP,[18] but it is assumed that apnoeas and hypopnoeas are the cause of elevated leptin levels rather than being the result of them.[19] Leptinaemia also decreases with NIV treatment[20] as does daytime hypercapnia, and some studies have shown a correlation between leptinaemia and a reduction in the hypercapnic ventilatory response.[21] Nevertheless, a study[22] reported contradictory results – leptin increased with NIV. Therefore, the role of leptin in how NIV treatment achieves improvement is still unclear.

SLEEP

Nocturnal hypoventilation is the confluent factor of all sleep-breathing disorders. Although OHS can exist without sleep apnoea, approximately 90% of OHS patients have sleep apnoea.[9,23] Despite the correction of nocturnal obstructive events with CPAP in patients with OHS, daytime $PaCO_2$ does not return to normal values in all cases. Several studies have emphasised that the CPAP response may depend on the predominance of nocturnal obstructive events.[24,25] Thus, if the time with apnoeas is a high proportion of total sleep time, CPAP can be effective in reverting daytime $PaCO_2$.[26] NIV can prevent obstructive events and reduce hypoventilation during sleep (including rapid eye movement [REM] sleep). Both NIV and CPAP should decrease nocturnal hypercapnia, leading to lower daytime serum bicarbonate and consequently less blunting of the central carbon dioxide response.[27] Because most of the mechanisms that improve with NIV are interrelated, the combined action of all (or the majority) of them is the most reasonable explanation to understand the action of NIV in OHS (Figure 48.1).

Acute failure

Limited information is available about the efficacy and mechanisms by which NIV produces improvement in an acute setting. Probably they are not very different from those mentioned earlier, although decreasing breathing effort by reducing the load on respiratory muscles and opening microatelectasis, as well as improvement of central chemosensitivity, may be the most important factors.[28]

EVIDENCE BASE

Chronic failure

Weight loss is the ideal treatment for OHS. It can improve respiratory failure, pulmonary hypertension and sleep disorders.[29] However, it is difficult to achieve and maintain significant weight loss in these patients. Limited long-term data are available about the efficacy of bariatric surgery in OHS,[30] and it is not an alternative for most patients because of significant morbidity and mortality.[31] Moderate weight loss can also improve $PaCO_2$, although this outcome has not been confirmed over the long term.[29]

Currently, NIV and CPAP are extensively used worldwide. Clinical series have reported improvement in symptoms, arterial blood gases and sleep disorders with these treatments (Table 48.1). As mentioned earlier, improvement in spirometry, lung volumes and chemosensitivity to carbon dioxide were reported in some studies but not in others. In non-controlled longitudinal studies, decreases in days of hospital admission have been observed.[10,32,33] There are no controlled trials assessing mortality, and decreased mortality was only observed in a series of treated patients when compared with other studies in which they were not treated.[34] Only one clinical series reported higher mortality in treated patients compared with patients who rejected treatment.[9]

CPAP treatment is able to prevent nocturnal obstructive events in patients with OHS, but nocturnal and daytime $PaCO_2$ do not revert to normal values in all cases. A controlled study[35] compared the impact of overnight CPAP titration in 23 patients with OHS and 23 patients with eucapnic OSA who were matched for BMI, apnoea hypopnoea index (AHI) and lung function. Forty-three per cent of patients with OHS had refractory hypoxaemia during CPAP titration. From this and other studies,[35–39] non-responding patients to CPAP treatment appeared to have more obesity, higher $PaCO_2$ and lower PaO_2 and nocturnal oxygen saturation (SaO_2) than responding patients.

At the present time, there are three randomised controlled studies that compare different treatments in OHS. One compares CPAP to NIV,[40] other NIV to conservative measures,[41] and more recently, the first results of the largest clinical trial (Pickwick study) done in this topic that includes the three most extended treatment modalities (life style modification, CPAP and NIV) have been published.[42]

The first of the randomised trials compared the short-term efficacy of NIV and CPAP treatments in 36 OHS patients, selected for their favourable response to an initial night of CPAP treatment.[40] From 45 eligible patients, nine (20%) did not achieve acceptable improvement with CPAP based on the following criteria: SaO_2 remaining below 80% continuously (>10 min) in the absence of apnoeas; acute increase in transcutaneous $PaCO_2$ during REM sleep (>10 mm Hg); or increase in afternoon to morning $PaCO_2$of >10 mm Hg in patients with an awake $PaCO_2$ > 55 mm Hg. After three months, daytime sleepiness, $PaCO_2$ and polysomnographic improvements were similar in both CPAP and NIV groups.

In a second trial, also in the short term, NIV was compared to conservative measures in 35 newly diagnosed OHS patients with mild hypercapnia.[41] In this investigation, arterial blood gases and polysomnographic variables as well as the glucidic and lipidic metabolism and the inflammatory profile were analysed. The NIV group had a significant reduction in diurnal $PaCO_2$ and bicarbonate and an increase in pH. The treatment with NIV, as could be expected, was associated with a huge improvement in all sleep variables analysed, sleep architecture; mean oxygen SaO_2; time spent with oxygen SaO2 under 90%; and AHI, with a positive and significant correlation between mean SaO_2 during sleep and daytime arterial blood gases. In contrast, no change was observed in any of the metabolic and inflammatory parameters studied. In this chapter, the patients had a lower BMI and were less hypercapnic than subjects included in others trials.[40,42]

The first results from the Pickwick study to determine the efficacy of NIV, CPAP and lifestyle modification in OHS are available.[42] This is a very ambitious project, still ongoing, that intends to provide the necessary evidence to answer which is the best choice in OHS treatment.[43] The first publication includes 221 OHS patients with severe OSA randomised in three groups: NIV, CPAP and lifestyle counselling. Polysomnographic data, arterial blood gases, spirometry, 6 min walking distance test and quality of life questionnaires were performed at baseline and after two months. $PaCO_2$ improved with each of the three treatments, but the improvement was greater with NIV with a significant difference only relative to the conservative measures group. In the CPAP group, the $PaCO_2$ reduction was dependent on treatment compliance. NIV and CPAP decreased bicarbonate blood levels, but after adjusting by baseline values, only the NIV achieves statistical significance compared to the control group. Sleep variables markedly improved with NIV and CPAP without differences between these treatments. Only in the NIV group, increments in forced vital capacity (FVC), forced expiratory volume in one second (FEV1) and 6 min walking test values were found. In this Pickwick study, 86 OHS patients without severe OSA were randomised and treated for 2 months either with NIV or lifestyle modifications.[44] After 2 months of treatment, $PaCO_2$ and serum bicarbonate significantly improved in the NIV group compared to the control group. The impact of these treatments in the long term and its influence in hospital resource utilisation, cardiovascular and all-cause morbidity and mortality as well as the cost-effectiveness are still unknown.

In one study, obese patients with nocturnal hypoventilation but without daytime hypercapnia were treated first with oxygen and then with NIV. Oxygen increased transcutaneous $PaCO_2$ during sleep compared with NIV.[45] However, no randomised studies have been carried out to show the efficacy of long-term oxygen therapy in OHS or oxygen therapy together with weight loss. In addition, oxygen treatment has not been compared with CPAP or NIV in OHS. While oxygen therapy is commonly supplemented to NIV in patients with persistent hypoxaemia, there are no available data about the long-term benefits or clear deleterious effect of this procedure.

Table 48.1 Main publications on efficacy of NIV and CPAP in chronic hypercapnic respiratory failure

Author, year	Patients	Study type	Intervention	Duration	Clinical improvement	Respiratory function improvement	Sleep disorder improvement	Hospitalisation and mortality reduction
Sullivan et al.,[5] 1983	2	Case reports	CPAP	1–3 months	Oedema, EDS; mental function	PaO_2, $PaCO_2$	SDB, $SatO_2$	
Piper et al.,[39] 1994	13	Retrospective	NIV	3 months		PaO_2, $PaCO_2$	$PaCO_2tc$	
Berg et al.,[32] 2001	20	Retrospective	NI–CPAP	2 years			SDB, $SatO_2$	Hospital days
Hida et al.,[46] 2003	26	Before/after	CPAP	3 months	EDS, QoL			
Piper et al.,[40] 2008	36	RCT	NIV vs. CPAP	3 months	Similar EDS; NIV: better sleep quality	Similar $PaCO_2$ and $SatO_2$		
Chouri-Pontarollo et al.,[11] 2007	15	Before/after	NIV	5 months	EDS, objective vigilance	$PaCO_2$	Sleep architecture, SDB, $SatO_2$	
Masa et al.,[10] 2001	22	Before/after	NIV	4 months	EDS, headache, oedema, dyspnoea, mental function	PaO_2, $PaCO_2$		Hospital days
Berger et al.,[24] 2001	23	Before/after	NIV–CPAP	4 days–7 years		$PaCO_2$		
De Lucas-Ramos et al.,[13] 2004	13	Before/after	NIV	12 months		PaO_2, $PaCO_2$, FVC, CO_2 chemosensitivity		
Pérez de Llano et al.,[9] 2005	20	Retrospective	NIV–CPAP	7 years	EDS, dyspnoea	PaO_2, $PaCO_2$		Higher mortality in rejected NIV

(Continued)

Table 48.1 (Continued) Main publications on efficacy of NIV and CPAP in chronic hypercapnic respiratory failure

Author, year	Patients	Study type	Intervention	Duration	Clinical improvement	Respiratory function improvement	Sleep disorder improvement	Hospitalisation and mortality reduction
Storre et al.,[47] 2006	10	RCT	NIV vs. AVAPS	1.5 months	Sleep quality, QoL	$PaCO_2$ with AVAPS	Sleep architecture, SDB, $SatO_2$ with both treatments. $PaCO_2$tc with AVAPS	
Redolfi et al.,[22] 2007	6	Before/after	NIV	6–20 months		PaO_2, $PaCO_2$, CO_2 chemosensitivity		
Budweiser et al.,[34] 2007	126	Retrospective	NIV	10 year		PaO_2, $PaCO_2$ FEV_1, IVC, TLC, RV/TLC		Mortality
Heinemann et al.,[12] 2007	35	Before/after	NIV	12–24 months		PaO_2, $PaCO_2$, VC, TLC, RV/TLC		
Janssens et al.,[33] 2003	71	Retrospective	NIV	7 year		PaO_2, $PaCO_2$		Hospital days, mortality
Borel et al.,[41] 2012	35	RCT	NIV vs. conservative measures	1 months		$PaCO_2$, HCO_3, TLC	Sleep architecture, SDB, $SatO_2$	
Masa et al.,[42] 2015	221	RCT	NIV vs. CPAP vs. lifestyle modification	3 months	ESS, FOSQ, VAWS	$PaCO_2$, HCO_3, FEV1, 6-MWD	Sleep architecture, SDB, $SatO_2$	
Masa et al.,[44] 2016	86 (OHS without OSA)	RCT	NIV vs. CPAP vs. lifestyle modification	3 months	ESS, mental component SF-36, VAWS	$PaCO_2$, HCO_3	Arousal index, SDB, $SatO_2$	

Note: QoL, quality of life; TLC, total lung capacity; RV, residual volume; RCT, randomised controlled trial; EDS, excessive daytime sleepiness; ESS, Epworth Sleepiness Scale; FOSQ, Functional Outcomes Sleep Questionnaire; VAWS, Visual Analogical Well-being Scale; IVC, inspiratory vital capacity; SDB, sleep disordered breathing.

Table 48.2 Main publications on efficacy of NIV and CPAP in acute hypercapnic respiratory failure

Author, year	Patients	Study type	Intervention	Clinical improvement	Respiratory function improvement	Intubations and mortality
Shivaram et al.,[48] 1993	6	Before/after	CPAP	Mental function	PH, PaO_2, $PaCO_2$	No intubations, 1 patient died
Pérez de Llano et al.,[9] 2005	34	Retrospective	NIV–CPAP		PH, PaO_2, $PaCO_2$	No intubations, 1 patient died
Ortega et al.,[49] 2006	17	Before/after	NIV		PH, $PaCO_2$	No intubations or deaths
Duarte et al.,[50] 2007	33	Retrospective	NIV–CPAP		PH, $PaCO_2$	36% intubated, 5 patients died
Carrillo et al.,[51] 2012	173	Prospective	NIV	RR, HR, Glasgow coma score	PH, $PaCO_2$, PaO_2/FiO_2	4% intubated, 6% NIV failure, 1% ICU mortality, 6% hospital mortality

Note: RR, respiratory rate; HR, heart rate.

Acute failure

Acute respiratory failure due to obesity has been increasing over the past few years.[52] To our knowledge, there are no randomised controlled trials comparing NIV to CPAP or oxygen, and probably, there will be none due to ethical issues. Little published information is available about the efficacy of NIV and CPAP in acute hypercapnic respiratory failure in OHS (Table 48.2). In published studies, NIV was more frequently used than CPAP, and improvement in pH and $PaCO_2$ was the norm. Apparently, the number of intubations and deaths was low. One study showed lower mortality with NIV than with invasive ventilation (23.5% and 15%, respectively),[41] and the other studies, already mentioned earlier, reported lower mortality in patients treated with NIV compared to those who refused it (3% with NIV and 57% without it).[9] A large prospective study included 173 patients with OHS and 543 patients with COPD admitted in an intensive care unit with acute hypercapnic respiratory failure and treated with NIV with the same protocol and compared the outcomes between these groups. There were no differences in NIV failure, but $PaCO_2$ at discharge, readmissions and hospital mortality were higher in the COPD group.[51] Factors associated to NIV failure or death in OHS with acute hypercapnic respiratory failure have been multiple organ failure and pneumonia.[53]

CLINICAL APPLICATIONS

Non-invasive ventilation or continuous positive airway pressure

As mentioned earlier, NIV (pressure or volume limited) and CPAP have a role in OHS treatment. Nocturnal hypoventilation can be effectively improved with CPAP in between 47% and 80% of the OHS patients[28,45,46] and diurnal $PaCO_2$ reduced or restored (to normal values).[45] However, in clinical practice, the selection of patients for one or the other treatment is not clearly established, but conceptually, CPAP should not be an effective treatment for patients with OHS and without significant OSA. According to the new data available, NIV and CPAP are effective treatments with similar medium-term results in patients with OHS and severe OSA with some functional advantages for NIV. It is possible to select patients based on an initial response to a night of CPAP treatment, as has been previously done.[47] Therefore, if CPAP prevents obstructive events and maintains adequate oxygenation and ventilation, CPAP could be a good choice for long-term treatment, and NIV should be used if this is not the case. However, some non-controlled studies and one randomised controlled trial have shown that NIV may be more strongly indicated than CPAP in patients with a predominance of hypoventilation over obstructive events during sleep, higher obesity, higher $PaCO_2$ and lower PaO_2 while awake.[27,30,35–38,42,46,54] Therefore, a more refined selection of patients for NIV or CPAP treatment could also be used until more long-term information becomes available. Patients with a large number of apnoeas and, consequently, high sleep time in apnoea can very probably respond to CPAP[29] (see section on 'Pathophysiology'). On the other hand, in patients without a significant number of apnoeas, their nocturnal hypoventilation could depend on other mechanisms (i.e. obesity); then NIV should be preferable (Figure 48.2).

In patients with acute hypercapnic respiratory failure, NIV should be the first choice, due to an apparently higher efficacy and the severity of respiratory failure and, because, probably OSA is not the only cause of the acute respiratory failure of these patients. In addition, the diagnosis of severe OSA may be unknown in this moment.

Length of treatment

Unless drastic weight loss occurs, NIV or CPAP treatments seem indefinitely necessary. NIV is well tolerated in the long term, and 5-year survival has been reported to be of 77.3%.[55] However, long-term randomised control trial comparing the efficacy of NIV and CPAP is absent.

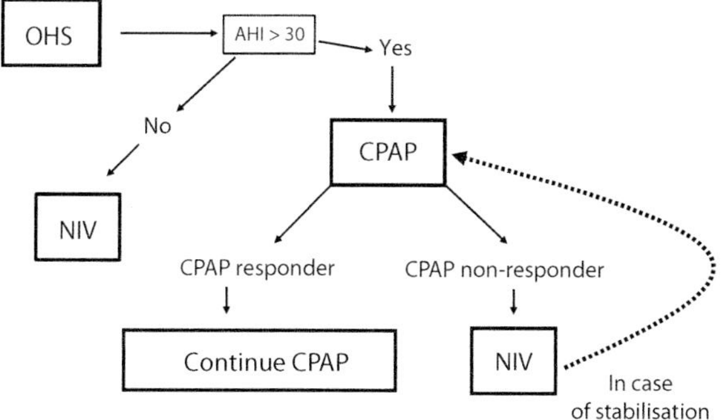

Figure 48.2 Recommended treatment election. Patients with OHS and significant sleep apnoea should be initially treated with CPAP. If relevant nocturnal or daytime hypoventilations remain with CPAP (non-responding patients), NIV should be the best treatment option. Once appropriate improvement in nocturnal and daytime hypoventilation has been achieved for a long time, patients may be, optionally, treated again with CPAP. Patients with OHS but without significant sleep apnoea should be directly treated with NIV. NIV, non-invasive ventilation; OHS, obesity hypoventilation syndrome; CPAP, continuous positive airway pressure; and AIH, apnoea hypopnoea index.

Some patients effectively treated with NIV can be switched to CPAP or even discontinue treatment for a period. Some clinical series[6,37,38,54] have reported that patients who are non-responders to CPAP treatment (daytime hypercapnia unresolved), but who are effectively treated with NIV for several weeks, could return to CPAP for long periods without the reappearance of daytime hypercapnic respiratory failure (Figure 48.2). In a prospective study,[25] 24 patients effectively treated with NIV were switched to CPAP. In 13 patients (54%), oxygen desaturation persisted after the elimination of apnoeas and hypopnoeas, and they were returned to NIV. The remaining patients continued with CPAP, maintaining slightly better daytime $PaCO_2$ and oxygenation (daytime and nocturnal) than the OHS group treated with NIV.

In another prospective study,[56] 12 OHS patients successfully treated with NIV for 1 year were required to cease the treatment for 3 months. They had diurnal and nocturnal $PaO_2 \geq 60$ mm Hg and $PaCO_2 \leq 45$ mm Hg as well as nocturnal $SaO_2 \geq 90\%$ for more than 70% of the night. After the withdrawal period, daytime and nocturnal pH, PaO_2 and $PaCO_2$ were similar to the previous period. Although these patients would probably show worse blood gas measurements with greater withdrawal time, this study suggests the possibility of discontinuing NIV for short (weekend) or intermediate (vacation) periods in some patients who desire it.

When to treat

The standard indication is to treat obese patients (BMI > 30 kg/m²) with daytime hypercapnia ($PaCO_2$ > 45 mm Hg) and without other potential causes of hypercapnia such as severe obstructive or restrictive pulmonary disease (significant kyphoscoliosis or neuromuscular diseases), severe hypothyroidism or other central hypoventilation syndromes.[29]

However, some patients with obesity have relevant nocturnal hypoventilation and secondary clinical symptoms without daytime hypercapnia. This situation could be considered in an early phase of OHS, at least in some individuals, resulting in daytime hypercapnia after a progressive increase of bicarbonate (Figure 48.1). A nonrandomised study, mentioned earlier,[45] compared the efficacy of sequential treatments with oxygen and NIV in a group of 11 patients with obesity who had nocturnal hypoventilation without daytime respiratory failure or relevant apnoeic episodes during sleep. Only NIV improved all clinical symptoms and nocturnal $PaCO_2$, maintaining a level of oxygenation similar to oxygen therapy. The early initiation of NIV treatment can improve clinical symptoms and possibly prevent the development of OHS.

Finally, obese patients with daytime $PaCO_2$ close to the upper normal limit (45 mmHg) and bicarbonate of ≥27 mmol/L could also be considered mild OHS patients and treated with PAP.[41,57,58]

Additional oxygen therapy

As mentioned, supplementing NIV with oxygen is common and the rule in acute failure. Chronic oxygen treatment is used in approximately 25% of OHS patients,[9,12,58] although the necessity of oxygen therapy can decrease after weeks or months of NIV use.[9,58] The goal should be to maintain the SaO_2 > 90% during the night when NIV cannot achieve this alone, although no studies have demonstrated that this approach provides additional benefits or deleterious effects for patients.

Follow-up

There are no standard recommendations for carrying out follow-up of OHS patients treated with NIV. However, follow-up is essential to verify the efficacy of treatment and to ensure proper adherence and compliance. A study has shown that improvement in clinical symptoms and blood gases depends on adherence to NIV. Accordingly, daytime $PaCO_2$ decreased 1.84 mm Hg per hour of real daily use.[58] A recent study has shown that the efficacy of the CPAP was more related to treatment compliance than to the case of NIV treatment in OHS patients with severe OSA.[42] Long-term efficacy and treatment compliance monitoring (or telemonitoring) is necessary.

TECHNICAL CONSIDERATIONS

There are no widely accepted and implemented recommendations for the technical application of NIV in OHS, and this can lead to the assumption that there are no treatment differences with other restrictive chest wall diseases. However, some considerations must be highlighted, since patients with OHS have high impedance in the respiratory system, especially when extremely obese, and 90% of them have a significant number of apnoeas and hypopnoeas.

Setting and titration

CONTINUOUS POSITIVE AIRWAY PRESSURE

CPAP was the first described PAP modality for the treatment of OHS. The CPAP level is positively correlated with BMI.[59] Therefore, the pressure used for OHS treatment is usually higher than that used for patients with OSA (without daytime hypercapnia). Moreover, OSA severity is higher in OHS also leading to higher CPAP level. The mean pressure required in some studies was about 14 cm H_2O.[35,40]

Determining optimal CPAP in OSA patients is well understood.[60] For OHS, in some studies,[35,40] pressure was increased once obstructive events were eliminated to improve nocturnal oxygen desaturation (Figure 48.3). However, it is not clear if this process has benefits for nocturnal or daytime hypercapnic respiratory failure.

Today, auto-CPAP titration is a common procedure to achieve optimal CPAP in OSA patients.[61] Since most studies of efficacy of autotitration excluded patients with OHS, the efficacy of these devices is unknown in these patients. Conventional polysomnographic CPAP titration is required for OHS patients until more information becomes.

NON-INVASIVE VENTILATION

The first studies testing the efficacy of NIV in OHS mainly used volume limited ventilators.[10,39] There are no studies comparing the two types of ventilators (pressure and volume) in OHS, although a study including patients with chronic respiratory failure showed similar efficacy between the two.[62] At present, the use of pressure limited ventilators (or hybrid ventilators with pressure modes) is the rule in daily clinical practice. Bi-level pressure support is the most frequently employed mode.

Inspiratory positive air pressure (IPAP) can be high, and the average is frequently around 18–20 cm H_2O.[33,40] The level of expiratory positive air pressure (EPAP) or CPAP can vary depending on the presence and severity of OSA (see the following). Although a fixed respiratory rate is not required in this ventilation mode (pressure support), some studies used a security rate of 12–15 breaths/min instead of spontaneous bi-level ventilation to assure a respiratory rate during sleep.[42] Although this setting could introduce asynchronies, Contal et al.[63] demonstrated that low or high levels of backup rates reduce the number of central and mixed respiratory events.

Recent ventilators offer the possibility of estimating the expiratory tidal volume and responding by adjusting the IPAP to maintain ventilation. This mode, called average volume-assured pressure support (AVAPS) or target volume, is supposed to maintain adequate ventilation during

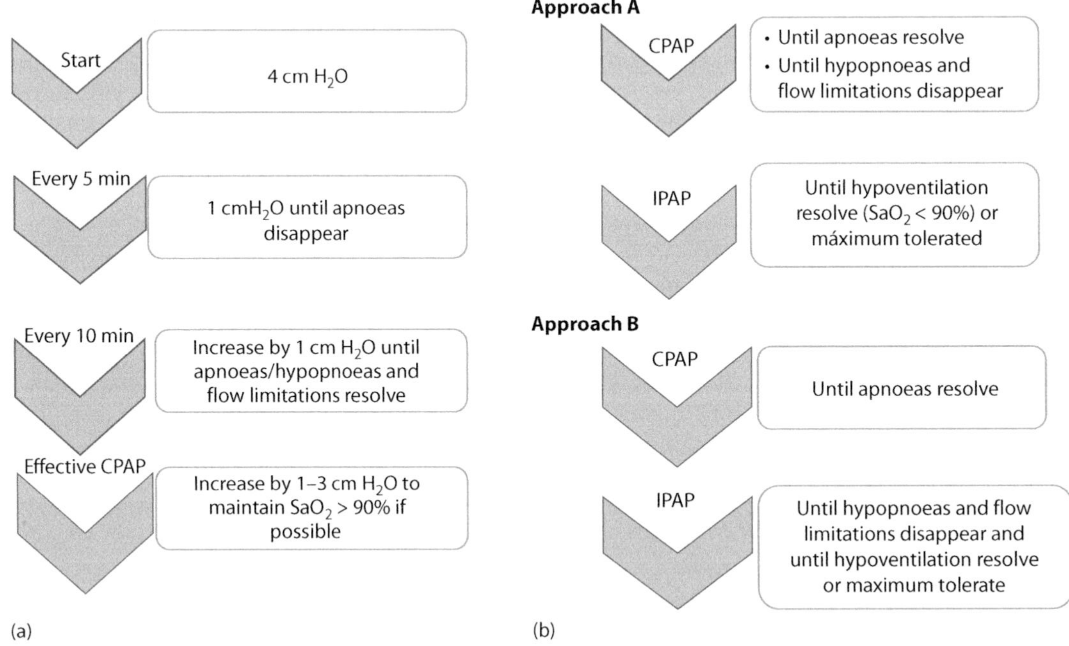

Figure 48.3 CPAP and NIV titration in OHS. **(a)** CPAP titration: starting at 4 cm H_2O, the technician increases CPAP by 1 cm H_2O every 5 min until the apnoeas resolve and then increases pressure by 1 cm H_2O every 10 min until hypopnoeas and flow limitation resolve. Finally, CPAP is increased by 1–3 cm H_2O to maintain SaO_2 > 90% or until the limit of tolerance is reached. **(b)** NIV titration: in approach A, CPAP is as it is used earlier to prevent apnoeas hypopnoeas and flow limitations, and then IPAP is increased to maintain SaO_2 > 90%; in approach B, CPAP is as it used earlier to resolve apnoeas, and then IPAP is increased to prevent hypopnoeas and flow limitations and to maintain SaO_2 > 90% or until the limit of tolerance is reached. CPAP, continuous positive airway pressure; NIV, non-invasive ventilation, OHS: obesity hypoventilation syndrome; IPAP, inspiratory positive airway pressure.

the changes in pulmonary mechanics that occur throughout sleep. Storre et al.[47] compared bi-level pressure support with AVAPS in a randomised crossover trial. Ten patients with OHS who did not respond to CPAP treatment were included. Six weeks of therapy with AVAPS achieved greater improvement in nocturnal and daytime $PaCO_2$ than bi-level pressure support. However, changes in sleep quality and quality of life were similar between the two ventilation modes. Janssens et al.[64] compared bi-level with usual settings with AVAPS in a group of 12 patients in two consecutive nights, and they found that although volume targeting improved the control of nocturnal hypoventilation, the sleep fragmentation and impaired subjective sleep quality increased. More recently, in a single-blind randomised trial, Murphy et al.[65] compared this mode with pressure support (PS) during 3 months in 50 super-obese patients, studying daytime $PaCO_2$ as a main outcome, and they concluded that fixed bilevel PS is as effective as AVAPS. Therefore, until more data arose, AVAPS may be beneficial in OHS patients without super-obesity.

A study in patients with OHS[66] observed frequent patient–ventilator asynchronies, which degraded sleep quality. More studies are necessary to confirm this observation, if these asynchronies result in other deleterious effects and, above all, if the correction of them prevents the problem.

Classically, treatment with NIV in OHS has not been nocturnally titrated. However, most patients with OHS have concurrent sleep apnoea, requiring at least EPAP adjustment. Furthermore, IPAP can prevent hypopnoeas and hypoventilation, depending on the level of pressure used. Therefore, arguments for performing titration during sleep in OHS are similar to those for OSA. Two approaches using polysomnography (PSG) have been recommended (Figure 48.3): conventional titration of EPAP (CPAP) as it is used in OSA and IPAP used to improve nocturnal desaturation ($SaO_2 > 90\%$)[40,67,68]; in the second approach, EPAP could be used to prevent apnoeas (static obstruction) and IPAP to prevent hypopnoeas (dynamic obstruction) and improve nocturnal desaturation (hypoventilation).[42,69] This last method can result in lower EPAP and similar IPAP, which would be more comfortable for the patient, potentially improving adherence and compliance.

On the other hand, a European group (SomnoNIV) used a more simplified device than PSG to adjust NIV.[70] Moreover, some recent ventilatory modes can 'automatically' adjust NIV.[71] Future studies are necessary to determine the optimal NIV titration.

When acute respiratory failure is present, the main objective is to reverse respiratory acidosis as soon as possible. In this circumstance, no titrated ventilation setting is advisable. High EPAP pressure (12–14 cm H_2O) can prevent obstructive events during sleep. If this level of EPAP is poorly tolerated, intermediate pressure (7–9 cm H_2O) can prevent apnoeas, and additional IPAP completes the treatment of obstructive events (hypopnoeas). Relatively high IPAP pressure (18–20 cm H_2O) or even higher is initially recommended, primarily in extreme obesity. Daytime $PaCO_2$ and nocturnal SaO_2 (and transcutaneous $PaCO_2$) should help adjust EPAP and IPAP. If repetitive, continuing decreases in SaO_2 are observed, EPAP should be increased, and if persistent desaturation (or persistent elevations of transcutaneous $PaCO_2$) occurs, IPAP should be increased.[28] A preset safety respiratory rate could be more recommendable in acute than in chronic respiratory failure. Alternative ventilation modes such as AVAPS, pressure control or volume control ventilation can be considered.

Treatment time

Most patients with chronic failure only need nocturnal NIV to obtain dramatic improvement. In patients with extreme obesity and residual daytime hypercapnia, one option is to extend treatment to the daytime, although there is no formal evidence for the effectiveness of this regimen in OHS. In acute respiratory failure, ventilation time must be maximised during the first 12–24 hours, with some brief interruptions, because expected pH improvement should occur in the first hours of therapy.[28]

Interfaces

The most extensive experience in long-term treatment for chronic failure is the use of nasal masks. Nevertheless, as with other diseases treated using PAP, switching to another kind of mask or nasal prongs can be beneficial if there is a justifiable cause (e.g. important oral leakage might indicate a switch to an oronasal mask).[72] In one study,[73] some masks with a high intentional leak could impede efficient IPAP when the intentional leak increases. More recent ventilators seem to avoid this problem, and they can be used in acute respiratory failure.

FUTURE RESEARCH

Obesity hypoventilation syndrome is a relatively recent indication for NIV,[74] but today, it is probably the most frequent illness requiring long-term treatment in the developed world. Despite extensive use, the level of evidence about its efficacy is intermediate or low, and future research must focus on the following topics.

Long-term efficacy

A recent large randomised study has confirmed the previous finding of greater medium-term NIV efficacy related to lifestyle modification[42,44] and similar efficacy to CPAP, although NIV reported some respiratory functional advantages. Randomised controlled studies must demonstrate long-term efficacy in respiratory function, polysomnographic parameters and quality of life improvements as well as more relevant outcomes such as arterial and pulmonary hypertension, incidence of cardiovascular events, days of hospitalisation and survival. In addition, the benefit of adding oxygen to NIV to improve residual desaturation should be clarified.

Pathogenesis

The treatment effect makes exploring causality possible. In this way, the role of sleep apnoea or leptin in the genesis of daytime hypercapnia can be investigated in CPAP responders and non-responders.

Prophylactic treatment

NIV is indicated for symptomatic nocturnal hypoventilation based on a clinical series.[62] Nocturnal hypoventilation may be the principal factor leading to daytime hypercapnia. It remains to be demonstrated whether early initiation of NIV (for nocturnal hypoventilation without daytime hypercapnia) can prevent the development of daytime hypercapnia.

Technical considerations

The optimal NIV settings, ventilatory modes, NIV titration and long-term monitoring for OHS are not well established. Future research and consensus should focus on standardising these procedures.

REFERENCES

1. Wang Y, Beydoun MA. The obesity epidemic in the United States-gender, age, socio-economic, racial/ethnic, and geographic characteristics: A systematic review and meta-regression analysis. *Epidemiol Rev.* 2007;29:6–28.
2. World Health Organization. *Obesity: Preventing and managing the global epidemic – Report of a WHO consultation on obesity.* Geneva: World Health Organization 1998:1–276.
3. Zhang C, Rexrode KM, Van Dam RM. Abdominal obesity and the risk of all-cause, cardiovascular and cancer mortality: Sixteen years of follow-up in US women. *Circulation.* 2008;17:1658–67.
4. Crummy F, Piper AJ, Naughton MT. Obesity and the lung: 2. Obesity and sleep-disordered breathing. *Thorax* 2008;63:738–46.
5. Sullivan CE, Berthon-Jones M, Issa FG. Remission of severe obesity-hypoventilation syndrome after short-term treatment during sleep with nasal continuous positive airway pressure. *Am Rev Respir Dis.* 1983;128:177–81.
6. Waldhorn RE. Nocturnal nasal intermittent positive pressure ventilation with bi-level positive airway pressure (BiPAP) in respiratory failure. *Chest.* 1992;101:516–21.
7. Kress JP, Pohlman AS, Alverdy J. The impact of morbid obesity on oxygen cost of breathing (VO2(RESP)) at rest. *Am J Respir Crit Care Med.* 1999;160:883–6.
8. Pankow W, Hijjeh N, Schüttler F. Influence of noninvasive positive pressure ventilation on inspiratory muscle activity in obese subjects. *Eur Respir J.* 1997;10:2847–52.
9. Pérez de Llano LA, Golpe R, Ortiz Piquer M. Short-term and long-term effects of nasal intermittent positive pressure ventilation in patients with obesity-hypoventilation syndrome. *Chest.* 2005;128:587–94.
10. Masa JF, Celli BR, Riesco JA. The obesity hypoventilation syndrome can be treated with noninvasive mechanical ventilation. *Chest.* 2001;119:1102–7.
11. Chouri-Pontarollo N, Borel JC, Tamisier R. Impaired objective daytime vigilance in obesity-hypoventilation syndrome: Impact of noninvasive ventilation. *Chest.* 2007;131:148–55.
12. Heinemann F, Budweiser S, Dobroschke J. Non-invasive positive pressure ventilation improves lung volumes in the obesity hypoventilation syndrome. *Respir Med.* 2007;101:1229–35.
13. De Lucas-Ramos P, de Miguel-Díez J, Santacruz-Siminiani A. Benefits at 1 year of nocturnal intermittent positive pressure ventilation in patients with obesity-hypoventilation syndrome. *Respir Med.* 2004;98:961–7.
14. O'Donnell CP, Schaub CD, Haines AS. Leptin prevents respiratory depression in obesity. *Am J Respir Crit Care Med.* 1999;159:1477–84.
15. Atwood CW. Sleep-related hypoventilation: The envolving of role of leptin. *Chest.* 2005;128:1079–81.
16. Lin CK, Lin CC. Work of breathing and respiratory drive in obesity. *Respirology.* 2012;17:402–11.
17. Malli F, Papaioannou AI. The role of the leptin in the respiratory system: An overview. *Respir Res.* 2010;11:1–16.
18. Ip MSM, Lam KSL, Ho C. Serum leptin and vascular risk factors in obstructive sleep apnea. *Chest.* 2000;118:580–6.
19. Fitzpatrick M. Leptin and the obesity hypoventilation syndrome: A leap of faith? *Thorax.* 2002;57:1–2.
20. Yee, BJ, Cheung J, Phipps P. Treatment of obesity hypoventilation syndrome and serum leptin. *Respiration.* 2006;73:209–12.
21. Campo A, Freihbeck G, Zueta JJ. Hypercapnic response in obese patients. *Eur Respir J.* 2007;30:223–31.
22. Redolfi S, Corda L, La Piana G. Long-term noninvasive ventilation increases chemosensitivity and leptin in obesity-hypoventilation syndrome. *Respir Med.* 2007;101:1191–5.
23. Kessler R, Chaovat A, Schinkewitch P. The obesity-hypoventilation syndrome revisited: A prospective study of 34 consecutive cases. *Chest.* 2001;120:369–76.
24. Berger KI, Ayappa I, Chatramontri B. Obesity hypoventilation syndrome as a spectrum of respiratory disturbances during sleep. *Chest.* 2001;120:1231–8.
25. Pérez de Llano LA, Golpe R, Ortiz Piquer M. Clinical heterogeneity among patients with obesity hypoventilation syndrome: Therapeutic implications. *Respiration.* 2008;75:34–9.

26. Ayappa I, Berger KI, Norman RG. Hypercapnia and ventilatory periodicity in obstructive sleep apnea syndrome. *Am J Respir Crit Care Med.* 2002;166:1112–5.
27. Mokhlesi B, Tulaimat A, Faibursowitsch I. Obesity hypoventilation syndrome: Prevalence and predictors in patients with obstructive sleep apnea. *Sleep Breath.* 2007;11:117–24.
28. Lee WY, Mokhlesi B. Diagnosis and management of obesity hypoventilation syndrome in the ICU. *Crit Care Clin.* 2008;24:533–49.
29. Olson AL, Zwillich C. The obesity hypoventilation syndrome. *Am J Med.* 2005;118:948–56.
30. Martí-Valeri C, Sabaté A, Masdevall C. Improvement of associated respiratory problems in morbidly obese patients after open roux-en-y gastric bypass. *Obes Surg.* 2007;17:1102–10.
31. Surgeman HJ, Fairman RP, Sood RK. Long-term effects of gastric surgery for treating respiratory insufficiency of obesity. *Am J Clin Nutr.* 1992;55:5975–6015.
32. Berg G, Delaive K, Manfreda J. The use of health-care resources in obesity-hypoventilation syndrome. *Chest.* 2001;120:377–83.
33. Janssens JP, Derivaz S, Breitenstein E. Changing patterns in long-term noninvasive ventilation: A 7 year prospective study in the Geneva lake area. *Chest.* 2003;123:67–79.
34. Budweiser S, Riedl SG, Jörres RA. Mortality and prognostic factors in patients with obesity-hypoventilation syndrome undergoing non-invasive ventilation. *J Intern Med.* 2007;261:375–83.
35. Banerjee D, Yee BJ, Piper AJ. Obesity hypoventilation syndrome: Hypoxemia during continuous positive airway pressure. *Chest.* 2007;131:1678–84.
36. Resta O, Guido P, Picca V. Prescription of nCPAP and nBIPAP in obstructive sleep apnoea syndrome: Italian experience in 105 subjects. A prospective two centre study. *Respir Med.* 1998;92:820–7.
37. Rabec C, Merati M, Baudouin N. Management of obesity and respiratory insufficiency: The value of dual-level pressure nasal ventilation. *Rev Mal Respir.* 1998;15:269–78.
38. Schäfer H, Ewig S, Hasper E. Failure of CPAP therapy in obstructive sleep apnoea syndrome: Predictive factors and treatment with bilevel-positive airway pressure. *Respir Med.* 1998;92:208–15.
39. Piper AJ, Sullivan CE. Effects of short-term NIPPV in the treatment of patients with severe obstructive sleep apnea and hypercapnia. *Chest.* 1994;105:434–40.
40. Piper AJ, Wang D, Yee BJ. Randomised trial of CPAP vs bilevel support in the treatment of obesity hypoventilation syndrome without severe nocturnal desaturation. *Thorax.* 2008;63:395–401.
41. Borel JC, Tamisier R, Gonzalez-Bermejo J. Noninvasive ventilation in mild obesity hypoventilation syndrome: A randomized controlled trial. *Chest.* 2012;141:692–702.
42. Masa JF, Corral J, Alonso ML. Efficacy of different treatment alternatives for obesity hypoventilation syndrome: Pickwick study. *Am J Respir Crit Care Med.* 2015;192:86–95.
43. López-Jiménez MJ, Masa JF, Corral J et al. Mid- and long-term efficacy of non-invasive ventilation in obesity hypoventilation syndrome: The Pickwick's study. *Arch Bronconeumol.* 2016;52:158–65.
44. Masa JF, Corral J, Caballero C. Noninvasive ventilation in obesity hypoventilation syndrome without severe sleep apnea. *Thorax.* 2016 Jul 12. pii: Thoraxjnl-2016-208501. doi: 10.1136/thoraxjnl-2016-208501. In press.
45. Masa JF, Celli BR, Riesco JA. Noninvasive positive pressure ventilation and not oxygen may prevent overt ventilatory failure in patients with chest wall diseases. *Chest.* 1997;112:207–13.
46. Hida W, Okabe S, Tatsumi K. Nasal continuous positive airway pressure improves quality of life in obesity hypoventilation syndrome. *Sleep Breath.* 2003;7:3–12.
47. Storre JH, Seuthe B, Fiechter R. Average volume-assured pressure support in obesity hypoventilation: A randomized crossover trial. *Chest.* 2006;130:815–21.
48. Shivaram U, Cash ME, Beal A. Nasal continuous positive airway pressure in decompensated hypercapnic respiratory failure as a complication of sleep apnea. *Chest.* 1993;104:770–4.
49. Ortega A, Peces-Barba G, Fernández I. Evolution of patients with chronic obstructive pulmonary disease, obesity hypoventilation syndrome or congestive heart failure in a respiratory monitoring unit. *Arch Bronconeumol.* 2006;42:423–9.
50. Duarte AG, Justino E, Bigler T. Outcomes of morbidly obese patients requiring mechanical ventilation for acute respiratory failure. *Crit Care Med.* 2007;35:732–7.
51. Carrillo A, Ferrer M, Gonzalez-Diaz G. Noninvasive ventilation in acute hypercapnic respiratory failure caused by obesity hypoventilation syndrome and chronic obstructive pulmonary disease. *Am J Respir Crit Care Med.* 2012;186:1279–85.
52. Gacouin A, Jouneau S, Letheulle J. Trend in prevalence and prognosis in subjects with acute chronic respiratory failure treated with noninvasive and/or invasive ventilation. *Respir Care.* 2015;60:10–8.
53. Lemyze M, Taufour P, Duhamel A. Determinants of noninvasive ventilation success or failure in morbidly obese patients in acute respiratory failure. *Plos One* 2014;9:e97563.
54. Smith IE, King MA, Siklos PW. Treatment of ventilatory failure in the Prader–Willi syndrome. *Eur Respir J.* 1998;11:1150–2.
55. Priou P, Hamel JF, Person C et al. Long-term outcome of noninvasive positive pressure ventilation for obesity hypoventilation syndrome. *Chest.* 2010 Jul;138:84–90.

56. De Miguel J, De Lucas P, Pérez JJ. Analysis of withdrawal from noninvasive mechanical ventilation in patients with obesity-hypoventilation syndrome: Medium term results. *Arch Bronconeumol* 2003;9:292–7.
57. Pepin JL, Borel JC, Janssens JP. Obesity hypoventilation syndrome: An underdiagnosed and untreated condition. *Am J Respir Crit Care Med.* 2012;186:1205–7.
58. Mokhlesi B, Tulaimat A, Evans AT. Impact of adherence with positive airway pressure therapy on hypercapnia in obstructive sleep apnea. *J Clin Sleep Med.* 2006;2:57–62.
59. Miljeteig H, Hoffstein V. Determinants of continuous positive airway pressure level for treatment of obstructive sleep apnea. *Am Rev Respir Dis.* 1993;147:1526–30.
60. Kushida CA, Chediak A, Berry RB. Positive airway pressure titration task force: American Academy of Sleep Medicine clinical guidelines for the manual titration of positive airway pressure in patients with obstructive sleep apnea. *J Clin Sleep Med.* 2008;4:157–71.
61. Masa JF, Jiménez A, Durán J. Alternative methods of titrating continuous positive airway pressure: A large multicenter study. *Am J Respir Crit Care Med.* 2004;170:1218–24.
62. Schönhofer B, Sonneborn M, Haidl P et al. Comparison of two different modes for noninvasive mechanical ventilation in chronic respiratory failure: Volume versus pressure controlled device. *Eur Respir J.* 1997;10:184–91.
63. Contal O, Adler D, Borel JC. Impact of different backup respiratory rates on the efficacy of non-invasive positive pressure ventilation in obesity hypoventilation syndrome: A randomized trial. *Chest.* 2013,143:37–46.
64. Janssens JP, Metzger M, Sforza E. Impact of volume targeting on efficacy of bi-level non-invasive ventilation and sleep in obesity-hypoventilation. *Respir Med.* 2009;103:165–72.
65. Murphy PB, Davidson C, Hind MD. Volume targeted versus pressure support non-invasive ventilation in patients with super obesity and chronic respiratory failure: A randomized controlled trial. *Thorax.* 2012;67:727–34.
66. Guo YF, Sforza E, Janssens JP. Respiratory patterns during sleep in obesity-hypoventilation patients treated with nocturnal pressure support: A preliminary report. *Chest.* 2007;131:1090–9.
67. Mokhlesi B, Tulaimat A. Recent advances in obesity hypoventilation syndrome. *Chest.* 2007;132:1322–36.
68. Berry RB, Chediak A, Brown LK et al. Best clinical practices for the sleep center adjustment of non-invasive positive pressure ventilation (NPPV) in stable chronic alveolar hypoventilation syndromes. *J Clin Sleep Med.* 2010;6:491–509.
69. Sanders MH, Kern N. Obstructive sleep apnea treated by independently adjusted inspiratory and expiratory positive airway pressures via nasal mask: Physiologic and clinical implications. *Chest.* 1990;98:317–24.
70. Gonzalez-Bermejo J, Perrin C, Janssens JP et al. Proposal for a systematic analysis of polygraphy or polysomnography for identifying and scoring abnormal events occurring during non-invasive ventilation. *Thorax.* 2012 Jun;67:546–52.
71. Jaye J, Chatwin M, Dayer M et al. Autotitrating versus standard noninvasive ventilation: A randomised cross-over trial. *Eur Respir J.* 2009;33:566–71.
72. Elliott MW. The interface: Crucial for successful non-invasive ventilation. *EurRespir J.* 2004;23:7–8.
73. Borel JC, Sabil A, Janssens JP. Intentional leaks in industrial masks have a significant impact on efficacy of bilevel noninvasive ventilation: A bench test study. *Chest.* 2009;135:669–77.
74. Clinical indications for non-invasive positive pressure ventilation in chronic respiratory failure due to restrictive lung disease COPD, and nocturnal hypoventilation – A consensus conference report. *Chest.* 1999;116:521–34.

PART 11

Other conditions

49 Bronchiectasis and adult cystic fibrosis 470
Sean Duffy, Frederic Jaffe and Gerard J. Criner

50 Non-invasive ventilation in highly infectious conditions: Lessons from severe acute respiratory syndrome 474
David S. C. Hui

51 NIV in cancer patients 481
Raffaele Scala, Uberto Maccari, Giuseppina Ciarleglio, Valentina Granese and Chiara Madioni

52 Non-invasive ventilation in the elderly 487
Erwan L'Her and Corinne Troadec-L'Her

53 Post-surgery non-invasive ventilation 496
Maria Laura Vega and Stefano Nava

54 Trauma 504
Umberto Lucangelo, Massimo Ferluga and Matteo Segat

55 Spinal cord injuries 509
Sven Hirschfeld

49

Bronchiectasis and adult cystic fibrosis

SEAN DUFFY, FREDERIC JAFFE AND GERARD J. CRINER

INTRODUCTION

Bronchiectasis is defined as the pathological dilatation of the airways characterised by computed tomography findings of a bronchus with larger diameter than the accompanying blood vessel or a bronchus that does not taper as it approaches the periphery of the chest.[1] The resultant clinical symptoms include increased sputum production, recurrent lung infections and progressive lung damage, which can mirror symptoms of cystic fibrosis (CF).[1]

CF is a recessively inherited, life-limiting disease that affects over 70,000 people worldwide. It most commonly affects the Caucasian population, but is also found in Hispanics and Native Americans, along with people of African and Asian descent. Due to recent advances in pharmacology and other therapeutics, the median survival in CF patients is 40.7 years as of 2013, an increase from 33.4 years in 2001.[2]

This chapter discusses the pathophysiology of CF and bronchiectasis, the indications and evidence base for the use of non-invasive positive pressure ventilation (NIV) for acute and chronic respiratory failure in CF and bronchiectasis and technical considerations in the use of NIV.

PATHOPHYSIOLOGY

CF is the result of a gene mutation in the cystic fibrosis transmembrane conductance regulator (CFTR) gene which causes a defect in sodium and chloride transport across the respiratory epithelial cell membrane.[3,4] The CFTR has been shown to be a cyclic adenosine monophosphate-mediated and protein kinase A-regulated protein that transports chloride across the cell membrane.[3] The result of this impaired ion transport is dehydration of the airway surface, which leads to disruption of the ciliary function and ineffective mucous clearance.[5,6] Disruption in mucous clearance results in ductal dilatation of the airways and bacterial colonisation. In turn, the affected airways attract neutrophils, which release elastase and reactive oxygen species, which cause damage to surrounding cells. Neutrophils then undergo apoptosis, causing further accumulation of thick debris.[3–5] Non-CF bronchiectasis is thought to occur due to a similar cycle of neutrophil inflammation, structural damage to the airway, impaired mucous clearance and bacterial colonisation.[1] The inciting disease or event often remains unclear in non-CF bronchiectasis, but may include autoimmune diseases, foreign body obstruction, infection and immune deficiency.[1]

Clinically, CF is characterised by progressively worsening lung function along with periodic exacerbations of acutely increased respiratory symptoms such as cough, increased sputum production, dyspnoea and chest pain.[4,7] Exacerbations are most commonly attributed to viral respiratory tract infections and clonal expansion of pre-existing bacteria.[6] Additional aetiologies include mucous plugging and atelectasis, which may result from splinting and poor cough due to post-surgical or traumatic pain.[8,9] When atelectasis develops, ventilation–perfusion (V/Q) mismatch ensues, causing hypoxaemia, reduced functional residual capacity (FRC) and increased work of breathing (WOB).[9] Exacerbations are associated with accelerated lung function decline in CF patients and increased mortality.[6] Progressive lung disease and respiratory failure is the cause of death in over 80% of patients with CF.[7]

NIV has been used as one mechanism to combat the progressive respiratory failure of CF and bronchiectasis. NIV provides positive pressure during inhalation and exhalation. During inhalation, positive pressure is meant to increase tidal volume and reduce the workload of respiratory muscles. During exhalation, the aim of positive pressure is to maintain airway patency and reduce atelectasis, thereby improving V/Q matching. The goal of NIV therapy in CF patients is to increase FRC while decreasing atelectasis and resistance, resulting in improved airway compliance and V/Q matching.[9] NIV acts as an alternative to endotracheal intubation and allows patients to remain in the ambulatory setting or on a general ward rather than an intensive care unit (ICU).[10] NIV also limits use of sedating medications and enables the patient to continue eating by mouth as well as to communicate and participate in physical therapy.[9,10]

EVIDENCE-BASED USE OF NIV IN ACUTE RESPIRATORY FAILURE

NIV can be used to quickly improve the clinical status of patients with bronchiectasis in acute respiratory failure. A Cochrane review demonstrated that NIV has been shown to improve sputum clearance and can improve gas exchange parameters in patients with CF and respiratory failure.[11] Additionally, Piper et al.[12] performed a case series study showing that patients with CF complicated by hypercapnia had improved levels of partial pressure of CO_2 (pCO_2), improved respiratory muscle strength and subjective improvement in daily and nocturnal symptoms within days of initiation of nocturnal NIV.

In non-CF bronchiectasis, a retrospective review showed that nocturnal NIV stabilised previously increasing levels of hypercapnia and resulted in fewer days in the hospital over a 1-year period.[13] Furthermore, the British Thoracic Society recommendations state that patients with a pH < 7.35 may benefit from NIV; however, increased secretions may be prohibitive during acute exacerbation.[14] The improved gas exchange fostered by NIV may play a role in the improvement in respiratory muscle strength in patients with respiratory acidosis as shown in a study on the effect of pCO_2 on the diaphragm.[15] Chest physiotherapy has been a mainstay of treatment in patients with CF and non-CF bronchiectasis, and recent studies have evaluated the efficacy of NIV compared to that of standard chest physiotherapy.[16,17] Holland et al.[17] showed that NIV improved inspiratory muscle function and oxygen saturation when compared with standard chest physiotherapy. In addition, patients tend to have subjective improvements in fatigue and ease of expectoration with NIV.[16]

EVIDENCE-BASED USE OF NIV IN CHRONIC RESPIRATORY FAILURE

The major cause of hypoxaemia in CF remains V/Q mismatch as a result of chronic progressive lung disease, although hypoventilation also plays a role. Other factors including kyphosis, respiratory muscle weakness, central nervous system (CNS) depression and sleep-disordered breathing (SDB) contribute to the development of chronic hypoventilation.

Adults with CF have a high prevalence of osteoporosis and kyphosis. Bone disease in CF is a multifactorial disorder resulting from poor nutrition, vitamin D deficiency, chronic glucocorticoid administration and increased inflammation.[18] On average, adult CF patients have a two-fold greater risk of fracture and a significantly abnormal kyphosis angle when compared to healthy age-matched peers.[19] Kyphosis decreases chest wall compliance and causes inefficient coupling of the chest wall and respiratory muscles. This abnormality may result in reduced respiratory muscle strength, increased WOB and a restrictive lung defect.[20] Moreover, CF patients are often treated with opiates for chronic pain, which can reduce the CNS respiratory drive.[21]

The combination of these factors puts patients at risk for chronic hypoventilation. Young et al.[22] studied the impact of nocturnal NIV on the quality of life of CF patients with daytime hypercapnia. The results showed significant improvements in exercise capacity via the shuttle walk test, subjective dyspnoea, chest symptoms and nocturnal hypercapnia after 6 weeks of nocturnal NIV.[22] Additionally, Flight et al.[23] reviewed the effect of NIV on lung function in 47 patients with advanced CF. This study showed that NIV was associated with the stabilisation of lung function in this patient population.[23] Faroux et al.[24] followed CF patients for 1 year on NIV and found similar stabilisation when patients were compared with matched controls. Despite the recent increase in positive evidence, no guidelines for the use of NIV in CF patients currently exist. A survey of accredited CF centres in France showed that 7.6% of adult patients were being treated with NIV.[25] In this survey, most of the adult centres used a partial pressure of carbon dioxide in arterial blood (P_aCO_2) cut-off of 45 mmHg for initiation of NIV in stable CF patients and adjusted ventilation settings based on arterial blood gas measures. Interestingly, sleep study results did not tend to be a major factor in the initiation of NIV. The therapy was well tolerated with an adherence rate of 70%–80%.[25]

In non-CF bronchiectasis, patients also develop hypoxaemia as a result of V/Q mismatch, which may progress to hypercapnia due to hypoventilation.[26] Despite similar pathophysiologic mechanisms, when compared with NIV in CF, there are fewer studies and more conflicting data. For instance, Gacouin et al.[13] retrospectively reviewed 16 patients with bronchiectasis and chronic, progressively worsening hypercapnic respiratory failure and showed stabilisation of gas exchange with up to 2 years of therapy.[13] The study also showed good compliance, benefits in quality of life, daytime activity level and Forced expiratory volume in 1 second (FEV_1) stabilisation.[13] However, another study, done in the United Kingdom, revealed that less than 20% of patients with bronchiectasis were likely to continue using NIV at 2 years after initiation.[27]

Other investigators have analysed the effect of NIV on hospitalisation in addition to blood gas parameters.[28,29] Leger et al.[29] studied 25 patients treated with NIV for bronchiectasis and found no significant effect on gas exchange or hospitalisation rate. Benhamou et al.[28] retrospectively compared treatment with NIV to long-term oxygen therapy in 14 patients with severe bronchiectasis.[28] This study revealed no difference in survival or P_aCO_2 over time, but did show an improvement in oxygenation when NIV with oxygen therapy was compared to oxygen therapy alone. In addition, there was a trend towards reduced days in the hospital for patients treated with NIV.[28]

TECHNICAL CONSIDERATIONS

In some cases, long-term compliance with NIV therapy can be difficult to achieve.[29] Common adverse reactions included mouth dryness, skin irritation of the nose, gastric distension and bloating and mirrored those of other disease processes.[29] Other considerations include disruption of family life and the absence of a clear subjective benefit.[25]

Some have proposed periodically repositioning the mask or placing a bio-occlusive dressing to combat skin irritation. Along with upright patient positioning and titration to the lowest effective inspiratory pressure, periodic decompression can be performed to relieve gastric distension that may arise due to NIV.[9]

INITIATION AND WEANING OF NIV

In most studies of NIV in CF and bronchiectasis, inspiratory pressures are initially set at low values and titrated upwards slowly.[9] Young et al.[22] used polysomnography to titrate settings, increasing inspiratory positive airway pressure (IPAP) by 2 cm H_2O and expiratory positive airway pressure (EPAP) by 1 cm H_2O until goals were met. The mean IPAP in this study was 12 cm H_2O, and the mean EPAP was 5 cm H_2O.[22] In the French survey, most adult centres favoured pressure control setting and adjust based on arterial blood gas measurements.[25]

Weaning patients from NIV can be done once clinical stability is achieved. One method of weaning is to initiate NIV-free periods which can be progressively lengthened if stability is maintained without NIV or strictly nocturnal NIV. Another method is to slowly reduce the inspiratory pressure while maintaining stability until a trial off NIV can be attempted.[9]

ADDITIONAL THERAPEUTIC STRATEGIES AND IDEAS FOR FUTURE RESEARCH

The treatment of non-CF bronchiectasis is focused on managing symptoms and prevention and treatment of exacerbations. Exacerbations in this group are thought to be caused by an insult to the lung due to a pathogen or irritant which causes an increase in lung inflammation.[14] A common method of prevention includes treating with macrolides three times per week, which has shown some efficacy in reducing exacerbations. This effect is likely due to the anti-inflammatory effect of macrolide therapy.[30] Conventional therapy for exacerbations consists of treatment with broad-spectrum antibiotics to include coverage for *Haemophilus influenzae*, *Pseudomonas aeruginosa* and staph species; mucous clearance techniques; and occasional positive pressure ventilation.[30]

In patients with CF, maintenance therapies include chest physiotherapy, antibiotic prophylaxis, inhaled medications and nutritional supplementation. Recently, ivacaftor, a CFTR gene potentiator, has emerged as an important therapeutic agent in CF. This medication was shown to improve lung function, exacerbation rate and symptom scores in patients with CF who were 12 or older and had a G551D mutation.[31] Antibiotic therapies including inhaled tobramycin and chronic macrolide therapy have shown positive results with respect to exacerbation rates and change in FEV_1 from baseline.[32,33] Mucolytics also play a role in therapy. Specifically, nebulised dornase alfa and hypertonic saline have been used to improve expectoration and mucociliary clearance in patients with CF.[34,35] Both of these therapies have shown a beneficial effect on lung function over time in the CF population.[34,36] A great deal of progress has been made in the treatment of these diseases due to recent advances. However, much of the therapeutic approach in these patients is based on small, retrospective reviews comparing single therapies against one another. Future research should focus on the benefits of combined therapies in larger randomised trials.

CONCLUSION

NIV may benefit patients with CF and non-CF bronchiectasis by reversing hypoxaemia and hypercapnia in the short term during exacerbation. In addition, NIV may be helpful as a chronic therapy in this population to stabilise long-term gas exchange abnormalities. For this reason, NIV may be viable as a stabilising therapy for patients with severe disease, who are awaiting lung transplantation.[10,37]

REFERENCES

1. McShane PJ, Naureckas E, Tino G, Strek ME. Non-cystic fibrosis bronchiectasis. *American Journal of Respiratory and Critical Care Medicine*. 2013;188:647–56.
2. Cystic Fibrosis Foundation. *Annual data report*. Bethesda, MD: Cystic Fibrosis Foundation; 2014.
3. Rowe SM, Miller S, Sorscher EJ. Mechanisms of disease: Cystic fibrosis. *NEJM*. 2005;352:1992–2001.
4. Gibson RL, Burns JL, Ramsey BW. Pathophysiology and management of pulmonary infections in cystic fibrosis. *Am J Respir Crit Care Med*. 2003;168:918–31.
5. Randell SH, Boucher RC. Effective mucous clearance is essential for respiratory health. *Am J Respir Cell Mol Biol*. 2006;35:20–8.
6. Goss CH, Burns JL. Exacerbations in cystic fibrosis: 1. Epidemiology and pathogenesis. *Thorax*. 2007; 62:360–7.
7. Flume PA, Mogayzel Jr PJ, Robinson KA et al. Cystic fibrosis pulmonary guidelines: Treatment of pulmonary exacerbations. *Am J Respir Crit Care Med*. 2009;180:802–8.
8. Smyth A, Elborn JS. Exacerbations in cystic fibrosis: 3. Management. *Thorax*. 2008;63:180–4.
9. Sprague K, Graff G, Tobias JD. Noninvasive ventilation in respiratory failure due to cystic fibrosis. *South Med J*. 2000;93:954–61.

10. Madden BP, Kariyawasam H, Siddiqi AJ et al. Noninvasive ventilation in cystic fibrosis patients with acute or chronic respiratory failure. *Eur Respir J.* 2002;19:310–3.
11. Moran F, Bradley JM, Piper AJ. Non-invasive ventilation for cystic fibrosis. *Cochrane Database Syst Rev.* 2009;1:CD002769.
12. Piper AJ, Parker S, Torzillo PJ et al. Nocturnal nasal IPPV stabilizes patients with cystic fibrosis and hypercapnic respiratory failure. *Chest.* 1992;102:846–50.
13. Gacouin A, Desrues B, Lena H et al. Long-term nasal intermittent positive pressure ventilation (NIV) in sixteen consecutive patients with bronchiectasis: A retrospective study. *Eur Respir J.* 1996;9:1246–50.
14. Chang AB, Dilton B. Exacerbations in cystic fibrosis: 4: Non-cystic fibrosis bronchiectasis. *Thorax.* 2008;63:269–76.
15. Juan G, Calverley P, Talamo C et al. Effect of carbon dioxide on diaphragm function in human beings. *N Engl J Med.* 1984;310:874–9.
16. Faroux B, Boule M, Lofaso F et al. Chest physiotherapy in cystic fibrosis: Improved tolerance with nasal pressure support ventilation. *Pediatrics.* 1999;103:E32.
17. Holland AE, Denehy L, Ntoumenopoulos G et al. Non-invasive ventilation assists chest physiotherapy in adults with acute exacerbations of cystic fibrosis. *Thorax.* 2003;58:880–4.
18. Stalvey MS, Clines GA. Cystic fibrosis-related bone disease: Insights into a growing problem. *Curr Opin Endocrinol Diabetes Obes.* 2013;20:547–52.
19. Aris RM, Renner JB, Winders AD et al. Increased rate of fractures and severe kyphosis: Sequelae of living into adulthood with cystic fibrosis. *Ann Intern Med.* 1998;128:186–93.
20. Fishman AP, Elias JA, Fishman JA et al., eds. *Fishman's Pulmonary Diseases and Disorders*, 4th ed. Vol. 1. New York: McGraw-Hill; 2008.
21. Festini F, Ballarin S, Codamo T et al. Prevalence of pain in adults with cystic fibrosis. *J Cyst Fibros.* 2004;5:51–7.
22. Young AC, Wilson JW, Kotsimbos et al. Randomised placebo controlled trial of non-invasive ventilation for hypercapnia in cystic fibrosis. *Thorax.* 2008;63:72–7.
23. Flight WG, Shaw J, Johnson et al. Long-term non-invasive ventilation in cystic fibrosis – Experience over two decades. *J Cyst Fibros.* 2012;11:187–92.
24. Faroux B, Le Roux E, Ravilly S et al. Long-term non-invasive ventilation in patients with cystic fibrosis. *Respiration.* 2008;72:168–74.
25. Faroux B, Burgel PR, Boelle PY et al. Practice of non-invasive ventilation for cystic fibrosis: A nationwide survey in France. *Respir Care.* 2008;53:1482–9.
26. Wedzicha JA, Muir JF. Noninvasive ventilation in chronic obstructive pulmonary disease, bronchiectasis and cystic fibrosis. *Eur Respir J.* 2002;30:777–84.
27. Simonds AK, Elliott MW. Outcome of domiciliary nasal intermittent positive pressure ventilation in restrictive and obstructive disorders. *Thorax.* 1995;50:604–9.
28. Benhamou D, Muir JF, Raspaud C et al. Long-term efficacy of home nasal mask ventilation in patients with diffuse bronchiectasis and severe chronic respiratory failure. *Chest.* 1997;112:1259–66.
29. Leger P, Bedicam JM, Cornette A et al. Nasal intermittent positive pressure ventilation: Long term follow-up in patients with severe chronic respiratory insufficiency. *Chest.* 1994;105:100–5.
30. Wong C, Jayaram L, Karalus N et al. Azithromycin for prevention of exacerbations in non-cystic fibrosis bronchiectasis (EMBRACE): A randomised, double-blind, placebo-controlled trial. *Lancet.* 2012;380:660e7.
31. Ramsey B, Davies J, McElvaney NG et al. A CFTR potentiator in patients with cystic fibrosis and the *G551D* mutation. *NEJM.* 2011;365;1663–72.
32. Saiman L, Marshall BC, Mayer-Hamblett NM et al. Azithromycin in patients with cystic fibrosis chronically infected with *Pseudomonas aeruginosa*: A randomized controlled trial. *JAMA* 2003;290:1749–56.
33. Ramsey BW, Pepe MS, Quan JM et al. Intermittent administration of inhaled tobramycin in patients with cystic fibrosis. *NEJM.* 1999;340:23–30.
34. McCoy K, Hamilton S, Johnson C. Effects of 12-week administration of dornase alfa in patients with advanced cystic fibrosis lung disease. *Chest.* 1996;110:889–95.
35. Kellett F, Redfern J, Niven RM. Evaluation of nebulised hypertonic saline (7%) as an adjunct to physiotherapy in patients with stable bronchiectasis. *Respir Med.* 2005;99:27–31.
36. Elkins MR, Robinson M, Rose BR et al. A controlled trial of long-term inhaled hypertonic saline in patients with cystic fibrosis. *NEJM.* 2006; 354;229–40.
37. Hodson ME, Madden BO, Steven MH et al. Non-invasive mechanical ventilation for cystic fibrosis patients: A potential bridge to transplantation. *Eur Respir J.* 1991;4:524–7.

50

Non-invasive ventilation in highly infectious conditions: Lessons from severe acute respiratory syndrome

DAVID S. C. HUI

KEY LEARNING POINTS

- Non-invasive ventilation may play a supportive role for early acute respiratory distress syndrome/acute lung injury as a bridge to invasive mechanical ventilation in severe acute respiratory syndrome and other emerging respiratory infections.
- It is important to exclude pneumothorax before starting non-invasive ventilation and look for pneumothorax if there are signs of deterioration during non-invasive ventilation.
- Non-invasive ventilation is performed to reduce the risk of cross infection.
- It is particularly important to ensure good mask seal and minimize leakage during non-invasive ventilation.
- Non-invasive ventilation should be started with low inflation pressures.
- Healthcare workers should take precautions when managing all patients with community-acquired pneumonia of unknown aetiology that is complicated by respiratory failure.

INTRODUCTION

The rapid emergence of severe acute respiratory syndrome (SARS) in 2003 caught the medical profession by surprise and posed an enormous threat to international health and economies.[1–4] By the end of the epidemic in July 2003, 8096 probable cases were reported in 29 countries and regions, with a mortality of 774 (9.6%).[5] A novel coronavirus (CoV) was responsible for SARS[6]; the genome sequence of the SARS-CoV was not closely related to any of the previously characterised coronaviruses.[7] SARS reemerged at small scales in late 2003 and early 2004 in South China after the resumption of wild animal trading activities in markets.[8,9] A virus very similar to SARS-CoV has been discovered in Chinese horseshoe bats, bat SARS-CoV,[10] and data suggest that bats are natural reservoirs of SARS-like CoV.[11]

SARS appears to spread by close person-to-person contact via droplet transmission or fomites.[12] The high infectivity of this viral illness is shown by the fact that 138 patients (many of whom were healthcare workers) were hospitalised with SARS within 2 weeks as a result of exposure to one index patient, who was admitted with community-acquired pneumonia (CAP) to a general medical ward at the Prince of Wales Hospital in Hong Kong.[1,13] This super-spreading event was thought to be related to the use of a nebulised bronchodilator for its mucociliary clearance effect to the index case, together with overcrowding and poor ventilation in the hospital ward.[1,13] In addition, there was evidence to suggest that SARS might have spread by airborne transmission in a major community outbreak in a private residential complex in Hong Kong.[14] There are additional data in support of SARS having the potential of being converted from droplet to airborne transmission.[15,16] Two polymerase chain reaction (PCR)-positive air samples were obtained from a room occupied by a patient with SARS in Canada, indicating the presence of the virus in the air of the room and the possibility of airborne droplet transmission.[15] These data emphasise the need for adequate respiratory protection in addition to strict contact and droplet precautions when managing patients with pneumonia due to highly infectious diseases.

CLINICAL FEATURES

The estimated mean incubation period of SARS was 4.6 days (95% confidence interval [CI] 3.8–5.8 days), whereas the mean time from symptom onset to hospitalisation varied between 2 and 8 days, decreasing over the course of the epidemic. The mean time from onset to death was 23.7 days (CI 22.0–25.3 days), whereas the mean time from onset to discharge was 26.5 days (CI 25.8–27.2 days).[17] The major clinical features on presentation include persistent fever, chills/rigor, myalgia, dry cough, headache, malaise and dyspnoea. Sputum production, sore throat, coryza, nausea and vomiting, dizziness and diarrhoea are relatively less common features.[1,12,18]

The clinical course of SARS generally follows a typical pattern:[19] phase 1 (viral replication) is associated with increasing viral load and clinically characterised by fever, myalgia and other systemic symptoms that generally improve after a few days; phase 2 (immunopathological injury) is characterised by recurrence of fever, hypoxaemia and radiological progression of pneumonia with falls in viral load. The high morbidity of SARS was highlighted by the observation that even when there was only 12% of total lung field involved by consolidation on chest radiographs, 50% of patients would require supplemental oxygen to maintain satisfactory oxygenation above 90%.[20] About 20% of patients would progress into acute respiratory distress syndrome (ARDS), necessitating invasive ventilatory support.[19] Peiris et al.[19] have shown progressive decrease in rates of viral shedding from the nasopharynx, stool and urine from day 10 to day 21 after symptom onset in 20 patients who had serial measurements with RT-PCR. Thus, clinical worsening during phase 2 is most likely the result of immune-mediated lung injury due to an overexuberant host response and cannot be explained by uncontrolled viral replication.[19]

The route of entry for SARS-CoV in humans is through the respiratory tract mainly by droplet transmission. Once infection can be established, the mechanisms by which SARS-CoV causes disease can be separated into direct lytic effects on host cells and indirect consequences resulting from the host immune response. While, clinically, SARS is characterised by a pronounced systemic illness, the pathology of SARS, as revealed from fatal cases, was mainly confined to the lungs where diffuse alveolar damage was the most prominent feature. Multinucleated syncytial giant cells, although characteristic, are rarely seen. In cases without secondary infection, a remarkable lack of immune response was observed at this late terminal stage. Apart from those related to end-stage multiorgan failure, the pathology of gastrointestinal tract, urinary system, liver and other organ systems were unremarkable.[21–23] Lungs and the intestinal tract are the only two organ systems that support a high level of SARS-CoV replication.[24]

When epidemiologically evaluating, high-risk patients with CAP and no immediate alternative diagnosis and a low absolute neutrophil count on presentation, along with poor responses after 72 hours of antibiotic treatment, may raise the index of suspicion for SARS.[25]

EVIDENCE BASE FOR USE OF NON-INVASIVE VENTILATION

Several uncontrolled studies have shown that single-circuit non-invasive positive pressure ventilation (NIV) might provide life-saving treatment for patients in respiratory failure as a result of SARS infection.[26–28] Among 120 patients meeting clinical criteria for SARS, who were admitted to a hospital for infectious diseases in Beijing, 25% of patients (30/120) had experienced acute respiratory failure (ARF) at 10.7 ± 3.8 days after the onset of SARS. Of interest, 16 of these patients (53%) exhibited hypercapnia ($PaCO_2 >$ 45 mm Hg), and 10 hypercapnic events occurred within 1 week of admission. NIV was instituted in 28 patients; one was intolerant of NIV. In the remaining 27 patients, NIV was initiated 1.2 ± 1.6 days after ARF onset. An hour of NIV therapy led to significant increases in PaO_2 and PaO_2/fraction of inspired oxygen (FiO_2) and a decrease in respiratory rate ($p < 0.01$). Endotracheal intubation was required in a third of the patients (9 of 27) who initially had a favourable response to NIV. Pulmonary barotrauma was noted in 7 of all 120 patients (5.8%) and in 6 of those (22%) on NIV. The overall fatality rate at 13 weeks was 6.7% (8/120), but it was higher (26.7%) in those needing NIV. No caregiver contracted SARS. The authors concluded that NIV was a feasible and appropriate treatment for ARF occurring as a result of SARS infection.[26]

In another study, NIV was applied via oronasal masks to 20 SARS patients without chronic obstructive pulmonary disease who developed severe hypoxaemic respiratory failure in a hospital ward environment in Hong Kong with efficient room air exchange, (>8 air changes/hour following urgent installation of powerful window exhaust fans), stringent infection control measures with airborne precautions and full personal protective equipment (PPE) and addition of a viral–bacterial filter to the exhalation port of the NIV device (Figure 50.1). The mean age was 51.4 years, and the mean acute physiology and chronic health evaluation II score was 5.35. SARS-CoV serology was positive in 95% of patients (19 of 20 patients). NIV was started 9.6 days (mean) from symptom onset, and the mean duration of NIV usage was 84.3 hours. Endotracheal intubation was avoided in 14 patients (70%), in whom the length of intensive care unit (ICU) stay was shorter (3.1 days vs. 21.3 days, $p < 0.001$), and the chest radiograph score within 24 hours of NIV was lower (15.1 vs. 22.5, $p = 0.005$) compared with intubated patients. The avoidance of intubation was predicted by a marked reduction in respiratory rate (−9.2 versus

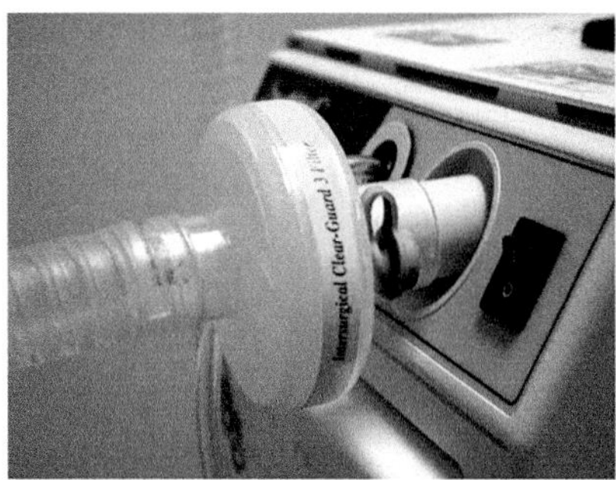

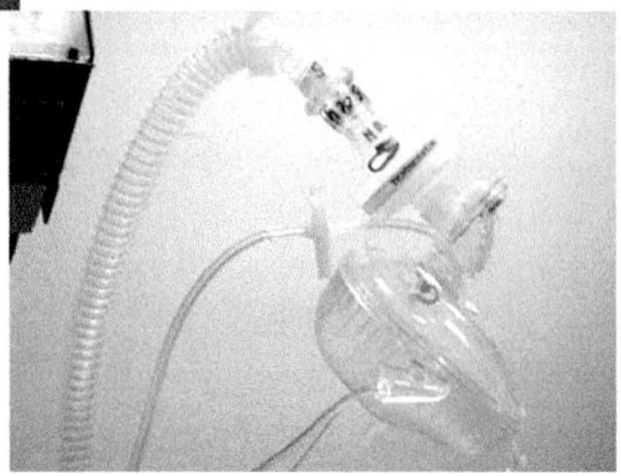

Figure 50.1 A viral-bacterial filter was inserted between the expiratory port and the NIV device, and another on the exhalation outlet of the ventilator during SARS outbreak in 2003.

4.0 breaths/min) and supplemental oxygen requirement (−3.1 vs. −0.2 L/min) within 24 hours of NIV when comparing patients who improved and those who failed NIV and subsequently required intubation. Complications were few and reversible. There were no clinical infections among the 105 healthcare workers caring for the patients receiving NIV. NIV appeared effective in the treatment of ARF in the patients with SARS who were studied, and its use was safe for healthcare workers in this single-centre study.[27]

A retrospective analysis was conducted on all respiratory failure patients identified from the Hong Kong Hospital Authority SARS Database. Intubation rate, mortality and secondary outcome of a hospital utilising NIV under standard infection control conditions (NIV hospital) were compared against 13 hospitals using solely invasive mechanical ventilation (IMV hospitals). Both hospital groups had comparable demographics and clinical profiles, but the NIV hospital (42 patients) had higher lactate dehydrogenase ratio and worse radiographic score on admission and ribavirin–corticosteroid commencement. Compared with IMV hospitals (451 patients), the NIV hospital had lower adjusted odds ratios (ORs) for intubation (0.36, 95% CI 0.164–0.791, $p = 0.011$) and death (0.235, 95% CI 0.077–0.716, $p = 0.011$), and improved earlier after pulsed systemic corticosteroid rescue. There were no instances of transmission of SARS among healthcare workers due to the use of NIV. Compared with IMV, NIV as initial ventilatory support for ARF in the presence of SARS appeared to be associated with reduced intubation need and mortality in this study.[28]

IMPLICATIONS FOR HEALTHCARE WORKERS

During the global outbreak of SARS, 13%–26% of patients developed ARDS, necessitating invasive ventilatory support at a time of reaching very high viral load, and thus, healthcare workers were particularly prone to infection while caring for their patients.[1,18,19] The relative risk of developing SARS was 13-fold for healthcare workers in Toronto who were involved in performing intubation of SARS patients compared with those who were not, whereas NIV was not associated with a statistically significant risk for the healthcare workers (1/6 exposed healthcare workers versus 2/28 non-exposed, risk ratio: 2.33, $p = 0.5$).[29] This was probably because tracheal suctioning was not generally performed for patients ventilated with NIV, and the study sample size was small.[29] However, a retrospective study by Xiao et al.[30] described NIV exposure as being associated with clinical SARS infection in two healthcare workers in Guangzhou, China.

A major case control study involving 124 medical wards in 26 hospitals in Guangzhou and Hong Kong has

Table 50.1 Independent risk factors of super-spreading nosocomial outbreaks of SARS

- Minimum distance between beds <1 m (OR 6.98, 95% CI 1.68–28.75, $p = 0.008$)
- Washing or changing facilities for staff (OR 0.12, 95% CI 0.02–0.97, $p = 0.05$)
- Performance of resuscitation (OR 3.81, 95% CI 1.04–13.87, $p = 0.04$)
- Staff working while experiencing symptoms (OR 10.55, 95% CI 2.28–48.87, $p = 0.003$)
- SARS patients requiring oxygen therapy (OR 4.30, 95% CI 1.00–18.43, $p = 0.05$)
- SARS patients requiring NIV (OR 11.82, 95% CI 1.97–70.80, $p = 0.007$)

Source: Xiao Z et al., *Clin Infect Dis*, 44, 1017–1025, 2007.

identified NIV as one of six independent risk factors of super-spreading nosocomial outbreaks of SARS (Table 50.1).[31] A systematic review has shown that four aerosol-generating procedures would increase the risk of the nosocomial transmission of SARS to healthcare workers including tracheal intubation, NIV, tracheotomy and manual ventilation before intubation.[32] The use of nebulisers should also be avoided.

NIV should be commenced under infection control measures as listed in Table 50.2 for patients with SARS if nasal oxygen above 5 L/min fails to maintain target SpO_2 at 93%–96%. NIV is delivered from a positive airway pressure system with independent inspired (IPAP) and expired positive air pressures (EPAP).[33] IPAP is adjusted to achieve respiratory rates below 25 breaths per minute and exhaled tidal volumes above 6 mL/kg. EPAP is adjusted to achieve target oxygenation with minimum carbon dioxide rebreathing. Criteria for intubation are intolerance to NIV, patient fatigue or when supplemental oxygen at 12 L/min fails to maintain at least 93% SpO_2 while on NIV.[28]

Table 50.2 Infection control precautions in the ICU

a. Staff education and PPE
   1. Limit opportunities for exposure: limit aerosol-generating procedures and limit number of healthcare workers present
   2. Effective use of time during patient contact
   3. How to 'gown up' and 'gown down' without contamination
   4. Emphasis on the importance of vigilance and adherence to all infection control measures in addition to monitoring own health
   5. Particulate respirator for airborne and surgical mask for droplet precautions
   6. Contact precautions: disposable gloves, gown and cap
   7. Eye protection with non-reusable goggles and face shield
   8. Powered air purification respirators if available may be used when performing high-risk procedures
   9. Pens, paper, other personal items and medical records should not be allowed into or removed from the room
   10. Immediate removal of grossly contaminated PPE and showering in nearby facility
b. Environment/equipment and transport
   1. Conform to Centers for Disease Control and Prevention recommendation for environmental control of tuberculosis: Minimum six air changes (ACHs) per hour. Where feasible, increase to 12 ACH or recirculate air through high-efficiency particulate air filter.
   2. Preferred: Negative pressure isolation rooms with antechambers, with doors closed at all times.
   3. Equipment should not be shared among patients.
   4. Use alcohol-based hand and equipment disinfectants.
   5. Gloves, gowns, masks and disposal units should be readily available.
   6. Carefully and frequently clean surfaces with disposable cloths and alcohol-based detergents.
   7. Discard all masks, circuits, filters and headsets immediately and safely after use according to routine infection control procedures. The routine exterior cleaning of ventilators and replacement of external filters should be sufficient to stop the spread of infection if ventilators are used on other NIV patients. Complete decontamination may be considered before ventilators are used for patients without infections such as H1N1.
   8. Use video camera equipment or windows to monitor patients.
   9. Avoid patient transport where possible: Balance risks and benefits of investigations which necessitate patient transport.
c. Special precautions for ICU
   1. Place the viral–bacterial filter in the expiratory port of the bag-valve mask.
   2. Use two filters per ventilator: between the expiratory port and the ventilator and another on the exhalation outlet of the ventilator.
   3. Use double circuit tubes via full facemasks or helmets (or special filters for non-rebreathing devices).
   4. Minimise leaks during application of NIV.
   5. Closed system in-line suctioning of endotracheal/tracheostomy tubes.
   6. A heat and moisture exchanger (HME) is preferred to a heated humidifier: Careful handling of contaminated HME is required.
   7. A scavenger system for the exhalation port of the ventilator is optional if negative pressure with high ACH (>12/hour) is achieved.

Source: Yam LY et al., *Chin Med J (Engl)*, 118, 1413–21, 2005; Yam LY et al., *Respirology*, 8, S31–5, 2003; Conti G et al., On the role of non-invasive ventilation (NIV) to treat patients during the H1N1 influenza pandemic. *ERS & ESICM*, 2009.

TECHNICAL CONSIDERATIONS

Healthcare workers should take precautions when managing all patients with CAP of unknown aetiology that is complicated by respiratory failure. Experimental studies based on a sophisticated human patient simulator (HPS) and laser visualisation technique have shown that the maximum exhaled air particle dispersion distances from patients receiving oxygen via Hudson mask and NIV via the ResMed Ultra Mirage mask were 0.4 m and 0.5 m, respectively, along the exhalation port.[34,35] Another study showed that the maximum exhaled air dispersion distance from the Respironics ComfortFull 2 mask was 0.95 m at a predictable direction from the exhalation diffuser perpendicular to the patient, whereas leakage through the Respironics Image 3 mask, connected to the whisper swivel exhalation port, was much more extensive and diffuse.[36] The whisper swivel is an efficient exhalation device to prevent carbon dioxide rebreathing, but it would not be advisable to use such an exhalation port in managing patients with a febrile respiratory illness of unknown aetiology, especially in the setting of highly infectious conditions such as SARS with high human-to-human transmission potential, for fear of causing major nosocomial infection. It is also important to avoid the use of higher IPAP, which could lead to the wider distribution of exhaled air and substantial room contamination.[36] Following the outbreak of SARS and emergence of the influenza A(H1N1)pdm09 infection, it has been recommended that when NIV is required for patients with acute hypoxemic respiratory failure due to severe acute respiratory infections, infection control measures such as the use of helmets or full facemasks and double circuit tubes and addition of viral–bacterial filters be considered (Table 50.3).[37,38] However, during NIV via a helmet on the HPS programmed in mild lung injury, exhaled air leaked through the neck–helmet interface with a radial distance of 150–230 mm when IPAP was increased from 12 to 20 cm H_2O, respectively, while keeping the expiratory pressure at 10 cm H_2O, whereas a helmet with a good seal around the neck could prevent such leakage. In contrast, when NIV via a total facemask was applied on the HPS programmed in mild lung injury, air leaked through the exhalation port to 618 and 812 mm when inspiratory pressure was increased from 10 to 18 cm H_2O, respectively, with the expiratory pressure at 5 cm H_2O.[39] These data have important clinical implications in preventing any future nosocomial outbreaks of SARS and other highly infectious conditions such as tuberculosis, pandemic influenza and Middle East respiratory syndrome (MERS).

NIV should be applied in severe CAP only if there is adequate protection for healthcare workers, because of the potential risk of transmission via deliberate or accidental mask interface leakage and flow compensation causing dispersion of contaminated aerosols.[36,37] In patients with respiratory failure receiving NIV via nasal masks, air leakage through the mouth or other routes besides the exhalation valve can occur.[40] In clinical practice, pressure necrosis often develops at the skin around the nasal bridge if the mask is tightly applied for a prolonged period. Many patients loosen the mask strap to relieve discomfort, and air leakage from the nasal bridge is definitely a potential source for the transmission of viral infection.[36] Careful mask fitting is important for the successful and safe application of NIV.[40] The addition of a viral–bacterial filter to the breathing system of NIV between the mask and the exhalation port[26–28] or using a dual circuit NIV may reduce the risk of the nosocomial transmission of viral infection (Table 50.3).[36–38] However, the use of viral–bacterial filters is sometimes difficult due to frequent blockage by moist secretions.[26–28]

In view of the observation that higher ventilator pressures result in a wider dispersion of exhaled air and a higher concentration of air leakage,[36,37] it is advisable to start NIV with low IPAP level (8–10 cm H_2O) and gradually increase as necessary, instead of starting high and titrating downwards if the patient is intolerant.[41] SARS-related ARF readily responds to low positive pressures of CPAP of 4–10 cm H_2O or IPAP of <10 cm H_2O and EPAP of 4–6 cm H_2O.[33] Higher pressures should be avoided because of the common finding of spontaneous pneumomediastinum and pneumothorax in SARS.[1,18–20]

Table 50.3 Infection control recommendations by the European Society of Intensive Care Medicine and European Respiratory Society for the use of NIV in patients infected with influenza A(H1N1)pdm09

- In general, the prudent isolation of the patient and protective measures for care providers and other patients are the keys to limit disease transmission.
- Use double circuit tubes (or special filters for non-rebreathing devices).
- Minimise leaks.
- Use full facemasks or helmets.
- Avoid heated humidification.
- Protect hospital personnel with standard measures (i.e. wearing gloves, washing hands, use of masks 'negative pressure' rooms).
- Discard all masks, circuits, filters and headsets immediately and safely after use according to routine infection control procedures. The routine exterior cleaning of ventilators and replacement of external filters should be sufficient to stop the spread of infection if ventilators are used on other NIV patients with H1N1. Complete decontamination may be considered before ventilators are used for patients without H1N1.

Source: Conti G et al., On the role of non-invasive ventilation (NIV) to treat patients during the H1N1 influenza pandemic. *ERS & ESICM*, 2009.

The World Health Organization (WHO) interim guidelines on the prevention and control of acute respiratory diseases in healthcare has included NIV among those aerosol-generating procedures in which there is possible increased risk of respiratory pathogen transmission. In addition to maintaining contact, droplet and standard precautions among healthcare workers when providing routine care to such patients, the WHO recommends full PPE for the healthcare worker, covering the torso, arms, eyes, nose and mouth, and this should include long-sleeved gown, single-use gloves and eye protection and wearing a particulate respirator such as an N95 mask or equivalent as the minimum level of respiratory protection. NIV should be provided in an adequately ventilated single room, and the addition of an expiratory port with a viral–bacterial filter can reduce aerosol emission.[42]

FUTURE RESEARCH

Emerging infectious diseases such as SARS, MERS and influenza are highly infectious conditions with significant morbidity and mortality. NIV has been applied to some patients with severe influenza A(H7N9) infection[43] and MERS,[44] but the majority of patients eventually required IMV. Several groups have applied NIV to patients hospitalised with influenza A(H1N1)pdm09 and acute hypoxemic respiratory failure with variable success.[45–47] NIV may play a limited supportive role for early ARDS/acute lung injury as a bridge to IMV in SARS and other emerging respiratory infections, although it is contraindicated in critically ill patients with multiorgan failure and haemodynamic instability.[36] However, as the application of NIV may disperse potentially infected aerosols,[35–39] further research is needed to examine the exhaled air dispersion distances during the application of NIV via different mask interfaces so that healthcare providers can better protect themselves within dangerous distances when managing patients in ARF due to highly infectious diseases. In addition, more research is needed in the technical improvement of the different NIV masks/viral–bacterial filters and in the engineering design of a safe hospital ward environment in order to prevent the nosocomial transmission of these infections. Advances in knowledge will facilitate the management of ARF due to any future SARS outbreaks, emergence/mutation of other SARS-like cluster of circulating CoVs in bat populations[48] and other emerging infectious diseases such as pandemic influenza and MERS.[49]

REFERENCES

1. Lee N, Hui DS, Wu A et al. A major outbreak of severe acute respiratory syndrome in Hong Kong. *N Engl J Med.* 2003;348:1986–94.
2. Hsu LY, Lee CC, Green JA et al. Severe acute respiratory syndrome in Singapore: Clinical features of index patient and initial contacts. *Emerg Infect Dis.* 2003;9:713–17.
3. Booth CM, Matukas LM, Tomlinson GA et al. Clinical features and short-term outcomes of 144 patients with SARS in the greater Toronto area. *JAMA.* 2003; 289:2801–9.
4. Twu SJ, Chen TJ, Chen CJ et al. Control measures for severe acute respiratory syndrome (SARS) in Taiwan. *Emerg Infect Dis.* 2003;9:718–20.
5. World Health Organization (WHO). Summary of probable SARS cases with onset of illness from 1 November to 31 July 2003. Available at: http://www.who.int/csr/sars/country/table2004_04_21/en/ (last update 31 December 2003) (accessed 10 January 2016.).
6. Peiris JS, Lai ST, Poon LL et al. Coronavirus as a possible cause of severe acute respiratory syndrome. *Lancet.* 2003;361:1319–25.
7. Marra MA, Jones SJ, Astell CR et al. The genome sequence of the SARS-associated coronavirus. *Science.* 2003;300:1399–404.
8. Wang M, Yan M, Xu H et al. SARS-CoV infection in a restaurant from palm civet. *Emerg Infect Dis.* 2005;11:1860–5.
9. Che XY, Di B, Zhao GP et al. A patient with asymptomatic severe acute respiratory syndrome (SARS) and antigenemia from the 2003–2004 community outbreak of SARS in Guangzhou, China. *Clin Infect Dis.* 2006;43:e1–5.
10. Lau SK, Woo PC, Li KS et al. Severe acute respiratory syndrome coronavirus-like virus in Chinese horseshoe bats. *Proc Natl Acad Sci USA.* 2005;102:14040–5.
11. Li W, Shi Z, Yu M et al. Bats are natural reservoirs of SARS-like coronaviruses. *Science.* 2005;310:676–9.
12. Peiris JS, Yuen KY, Osterhaus AD et al. The severe acute respiratory syndrome. *N Engl J Med.* 2003;349:2431–41.
13. Wong RS, Hui DS. Index patient and SARS outbreak in Hong Kong. *Emerg Infect Dis.* 2004;10:339–41.
14. Yu IT, Li Y, Wong TW et al. Evidence of airborne transmission of the severe acute respiratory syndrome virus. *N Engl J Med.* 2004;350:1731–9.
15. Booth TF, Kournikakis B, Bastien N et al. Detection of airborne severe acute respiratory syndrome (SARS) coronavirus and environmental contamination in SARS outbreak units. *J Infect Dis.* 2005;191:1472–7.
16. Yu IT, Wong TW, Chiu YL et al. Temporal–spatial analysis of severe acute respiratory syndrome among hospital inpatients. *Clin Infect Dis.* 2005;40:1237–43.
17. Leung GM, Hedley AJ, Ho LM et al. The epidemiology of severe acute respiratory syndrome in the 2003 Hong Kong epidemic: An analysis of all 1755 patients. *Ann Intern Med.* 2004;141:662–73.
18. Hui DS, Wong PC, Wang C. Severe acute respiratory syndrome: Clinical features and diagnosis. *Respirology.* 2003;8:S20–4.
19. Peiris JS, Chu CM, Cheng VC et al. Clinical progression and viral load in a community outbreak of coronavirus-associated SARS pneumonia: A prospective study. *Lancet.* 2003;361:1767–72.

20. Hui DS, Wong KT, Antonio GE et al. Severe acute respiratory syndrome (SARS): Correlation of clinical outcome and radiological features. *Radiology.* 2004;233:579–85.
21. Lo AW, Tang NL, To KF. How the SARS coronavirus causes disease: Host or organism? *J Pathol.* 2006;208:142–51.
22. Ng WF, To KF, Lam WW et al. The comparative pathology of severe acute respiratory syndrome and avian influenza A subtype H5N1 – A review. *Hum Pathol.* 2006;37:381–90.
23. Gu J, Korteweg C. Pathology and pathogenesis of severe acute respiratory syndrome. *Am J Pathol.* 2007;170:1136–47.
24. To KF, Tong JH, Chan PK et al. Tissue and cellular tropisms of the coronavirus associated with severe acute respiratory syndrome-an in-situ hybridization study of fatal cases. *J Pathol.* 2004;202:157–63.
25. Lee N, Rainer TH, Ip M et al. Role of laboratory variables in differentiating SARS-coronavirus from other causes of community-acquired pneumonia within the first 72 hrs of hospitalization. *Eur J Clin Microbiol Infect Dis.* 2006;25:765–72.
26. Han F, Jiang YY, Zheng JH et al. Noninvasive positive pressure ventilation treatment for acute respiratory failure in SARS. *Sleep Breath.* 2004;8:97–106.
27. Cheung TM, Yam LY, So LK et al. Effectiveness of noninvasive positive pressure ventilation in the treatment of acute respiratory failure in severe acute respiratory syndrome. *Chest.* 2004;126:845–50.
28. Yam LY, Chan AY, Cheung TM et al. Hong Kong Hospital Authority SARS Collaborative Group (HASCOG): Non-invasive versus invasive mechanical ventilation for respiratory failure in severe acute respiratory syndrome. *Chin Med J (Engl).* 2005; 118:1413–21.
29. Fowler RA, Guest CB, Lapinsky SE et al. Transmission of severe acute respiratory syndrome during intubation and mechanical ventilation. *Am J Respir Crit Care Med.* 2004;169:1198–202.
30. Xiao Z, Li Y, Chen RC et al. A retrospective study of 78 patients with severe acute respiratory syndrome. *Chin Med J.* 2003; 116: 805–10.
31. Yu IT, Xie ZH, Tsoi KK et al. Why did outbreaks of severe acute respiratory syndrome occur in some hospital wards but not in others? *Clin Infect Dis.* 2007;44:1017–25.
32. Tran K, Cimon K, Severn M et al. Aerosol generating procedures and risk of transmission of acute respiratory infections to healthcare workers: A systematic review. *PLoS One.* 2012;7:e35797.
33. Yam LY, Chen RC, Zhong NS. SARS: Ventilatory and intensive care. *Respirology.* 2003;8:S31–5.
34. Hui DS, Hall SD, Chan MT et al. Exhaled air dispersion during oxygen delivery via a simple oxygen mask. *Chest.* 2007;132:540–6.
35. Hui DS, Hall SD, Chan MT et al. Non-invasive positive pressure ventilation: An experimental model to assess air and particle dispersion. *Chest.* 2006;130:730–40.
36. Hui DS, Chow BK, Ng SS et al. Exhaled air dispersion distances during noninvasive ventilation via different respironics face masks. *Chest.* 2009;136:998–1005.
37. Hui DS, Sung JJ. Editorial: Treatment of severe acute respiratory syndrome. *Chest.* 2004;126:670–4.
38. Conti G, Larrsson A, Nava S, Navalesi P. On the role of non-invasive ventilation (NIV) to treat patients during the H1N1 influenza pandemic. European Respiratory Society (ERS) & European Society of Intensive Care Medicine (ESICM), 2009. http://dev.ersnet.org/uploads/Document/63/WEB_CHEMIN_5410_1258624143.pdf (accessed on 25 April 2014).
39. Hui DS, Chow BK, Lo T et al. Exhaled air dispersion during noninvasive ventilation via helmets and a total facemask. *Chest.* 2015;147:1336–43.
40. Hill NS, Carlisle C, Kramer NR. Effect of a nonrebreathing exhalation valve on long-term nasal ventilation using a bilevel device. *Chest.* 2002;122:84–91.
41. Meduri GU, Turner RE, Abou-Shala N et al. Noninvasive positive pressure ventilation via face mask: First-line intervention in patients with acute hypercapnic and hypoxemic respiratory failure. *Chest.* 1996;109:179–93.
42. WHO. Infection and control of epidemic- and pandemic-prone acute respiratory diseases in health care: WHO Interim Guidelines. Geneva: World Health Organization, 2007. Available at: www.who.int/csr/resources/publications/WHO CD_EPR_2007_6/en/ (accessed 1 June 2016).
43. Gao HN, Lu HZ, Cao B et al. Clinical findings in 111 cases of influenza A (H7N9) virus infection. *N Engl J Med.* 2013;368(24):2277–85.
44. Arabi YM, Arifi AA, Balkhy HH et al. Clinical course and outcomes of critically ill patients with Middle East respiratory syndrome coronavirus infection. *Ann Intern Med.* 2014;160:389–97.
45. Masclans JR, Pérez M, Almirall J et al. H1N1 GTEI/SEMICYUC Investigators: Early non-invasive ventilation treatment for severe influenza pneumonia. *Clin Microbiol Infect.* 2013;19:249–56.
46. Brink M, Hagberg L, Larsson A, Gedeborg R. Respiratory support during the influenza A (H1N1) pandemic flu in Sweden. *Acta Anaesthesiol Scand.* 2012;56:976–86.
47. Nicolini A, Tonveronachi E, Navalesi P et al. Effectiveness and predictors of success of noninvasive ventilation during H1N1 pandemics: A multicenter study. *Minerva Anestesiol.* 2012;78:1333–40.
48. Menachery VD, Yount BL Jr, Debbink K et al. A SARS-like cluster of circulating bat coronaviruses shows potential for human emergence. *Nat Med.* 2015;21:1508–13.
49. Zumla A, Hui DS, Perlman S. Middle East respiratory syndrome. *Lancet.* 2015;386:995–1007.

51

NIV in cancer patients

RAFFAELE SCALA, UBERTO MACCARI, GIUSEPPINA CIARLEGLIO, VALENTINA GRANESE AND CHIARA MADIONI

BACKGROUND

Acute respiratory failure (ARF) is the most frequent and challenging complication in cancer as it occurs in up to 40%–50% of patients with solid tumours, haematological malignancies and bone marrow transplantation recipients.[1–8] Mechanical ventilation was required in 44%–69% of cancer patients admitted to the intensive care unit (ICU).[4–8]

The severity of the patient's condition and the institution of invasive mechanical ventilation (IMV) are independently associated with hospital mortality at ICU admission.[1,3–8] The mortality of mechanically ventilated cancer patients remains high, but it has significantly decreased over the past two decades from 80% to 90% in the 1980s to 65%–75% in the 1990s and less than 50% in specialised centres.[3,7,9–11] Whereas mechanical ventilation has been 'traditionally' considered as a futile therapy in cancer patients, most commentaries nowadays advocate no limitations in the use of ventilatory support at the earliest phases of malignancies with high chances of extended disease-free survival.[12,13]

The improved outcome in mechanically ventilated cancer patients could be attributed to (1) better and earlier referral to ICU with the exclusion of patients with poor functional status or those wishing no life-prolonging treatment; (2) better management of septic complications with the implementation of sepsis 'bundle' ICU protocols; and (3) a closer cooperation between oncohaematologists and intensivists.[11,14] Among all, non-invasive ventilation (NIV) has been considered crucial for the 'turning point' in the mortality of critically ill malignant patients as it averts IMV-associated life-threatening complications, such as ventilator-associated pneumonia.[15]

This chapter will focus on the use of NIV as a means to treat ARF in adult cancer patients, summarising the current evidence and providing recommendations for selection of patients, including those with do-not-intubate orders (DNIs); the still controversial usefulness of NIV as 'palliation' in terminal neoplastic patients will be reported too.

PATHOPHYSIOLOGY OF NIV IN CANCER

ARF in malignancies could develop as a consequence of both, isolated or combined, 'pump' and 'lung failure' according to different aethiopathogenetic mechanisms, such as direct pulmonary involvement, opportunistic infection, therapy-induced pulmonary toxicity, pulmonary embolism, post-operative complications and diffuse alveolar haemorrhage.[13,16,17] Additionally, ARF may be caused by exacerbations of comorbid illness as chronic obstructive pulmonary disease (COPD) or congestive cardiac failure.[13,18]

The primary approach in hypoxaemic patients is to raise alveolar oxygen content by increasing the inspired fraction of oxygen (FiO_2); more profound hypoxaemia can be reversed by pushing up alveolar oxygen pressure and inducing alveolar recruitment with either continuous positive airway pressure (CPAP) or bilevel airway positive pressure (e.g. NIV).[15] Furthermore, CPAP and NIV are effective in cardiogenic pulmonary oedema thanks to their favourable hemodynamic effects.[15] Correcting hypercarbia requires increasing alveolar ventilation and unloading respiratory muscles by means of NIV.[15]

While mechanical ventilation supports the failing respiratory system, the aetiology of ARF should be aggressively investigated to guide therapy and estimate prognosis. The relationship between aetiology and outcome is determined by the availability of effective therapies and by the speed at which the underlying disease may be reversed. Some aetiologies such as haematological malignancies, bacterial sepsis or cardiogenic pulmonary oedema carry a better prognosis than others, such as invasive fungal disease or direct pulmonary involvement by solid tumours.[4,6,7,17–19] Being able to identify the aetiology of ARF is associated with a better outcome, as mortality is higher in patients without a clear diagnosis.[4,13,17]

The use of NIV for cancer patients with ARF could be classified into three categories: (1) NIV as 'life support' without limitations of life-sustaining treatments; (2) NIV as 'ceiling ventilation' for patients refusing endotracheal intubation; and (3) NIV as 'palliation' for patients wishing to receive only comfort measures (e.g. relief of dyspnoea).[20,21]

CLINICAL USE OF NIV IN CANCER

The evidence about the usefulness of NIV in cancer patients consists of five randomised controlled trials (RCTs),[22–26] as well as a larger set of observational studies. The clinical use of NIV in patients without and with limitations of escalating treatments will be analysed separately.

NIV in patients without limitations of care

Non-palliative NIV has been investigated in four RCTs[22–25] and mainly focused on haematological malignancies, two of them showing favourable and two unfavourable findings.

In the first French RCT, Hilbert et al.[22] compared the effectiveness of the addition of NIV to standard medical therapy in a heterogeneous population of 52 immunocompromised patients (30 of them having haematological malignancies) with pulmonary infiltrates, fever and moderate acute respiratory distress syndrome (ARDS) (PaO_2/FiO_2 between 100 and 200). The rates of intubation (46% vs. 77%; $p = 0.03$) and of serious complications (13% vs. 21%; $p = 0.02$), as well as ICU (38% vs. 69%; $p = 0.03$) and hospital mortality (50% vs. 81%; $p = 0.02$), were significantly reduced in NIV compared to control group. This advantage with NIV was demonstrated only in haematological malignancies.

In the subsequent Italian RTC, Squadrone et al.[23] compared the effects of early CPAP delivered with helmet plus oxygen therapy versus only oxygen therapy in 40 patients with leucopenia and mild ARDS (PaO_2/FiO_2 between 200 and 300) in the absence of infectious causes. The study was performed in the ward under the supervision of an emergency ICU team. CPAP reduced to 0.25 (95% confidence interval: 0.10–0.62), the relative risk of developing more severe ARF needing ICU admission for invasive or non-invasive ventilatory support. Compared to the control group, the CPAP group showed lower incidence of pulmonary (25% vs. 65%; $p = 0.025$) and systemic infections (10% vs. 65%; $p = 0.001$), fewer ICU admissions (4 vs. 16 patients; $p = 0.0002$) and lower intubation (10% vs. 70%; $p = 0.0001$) and mortality rate (25% vs. 85%; $p = 0.0004$).

In a German RCT, Wermke et al.[24] evaluated the impact of the adjunct of NIV to oxygen therapy in 86 patients undergoing allogeneic haematopoietic stem cell transplantation (HSCT) at the initial phase of ARDS (PaO_2/FiO_2 between 250 and 300) in the haematological ward. Although early ARF treatment with NIV was associated with a non-significant decreased rate of failure to achieve sufficient oxygenation (24% vs. 39%; $p = 0.17$), neither ICU admission rate nor need for intubation or survival parameters were significantly improved by NIV. Unfortunately, the study has several drawbacks (e.g. use of NIV as 'rescue' in 16 out of 17 patients worsening with oxygen; insufficient sample size; poor life expectancy of patients undergoing HSCT after several relapses).[14,17]

Recently, in a large multicenter French RCT, Lemiale et al.[25] investigated whether early NIV adjunct to only oxygen therapy improved survival in 374 critically immunocompromised ill patients (317 with malignancies), who were admitted in ICU for moderate ARDS (PaO_2/FiO_2 between 100 and 200). Compared to oxygen, NIV did not reduce the day 28 all-cause mortality (24.1% vs. 27.3%). There were no differences on ICU-acquired infections, duration of mechanical ventilation and lengths of ICU and hospital stays. Unfortunately, the study has several limitations, such as lower than expected mortality rate with oxygen therapy, higher proportion of patients receiving high-flow nasal oxygen therapy (HFNO) in control group and undefined criteria for intubation.

Due to the heterogeneity of their design and their several methodological biases, results of the observational studies dealing with NIV in acute cancer patients should be cautiously taken. Several studies compared patients treated with either NIV or IMV as the initial mode of ventilatory support.[4,5,9,10,27–32] NIV was provided to 4%–59% of patients,[6,33–38] and intubation averted in 30%–90% of cases.[9,31,34] In most but not all studies,[9,27] NIV compared to IMV was associated with better survival, but only a few studies corrected this for differences in the severity of illness. The inclusion of sicker patients may have biased the results against IMV patients. In some reports, intubation following NIV failure was the independent predictor of mortality.[4,33,38] However, in non-RCT studies, criteria for intubation are usually not reported,[5,9,33] and some patients were intubated for less than 48 hours, probably for not-ARF reasons (e.g. interventional procedures).[30] The association between initial ventilatory support and outcome may have also been confounded by the case mix of the population, as higher chances of NIV success are expected in cancer patients with hypercapnic ARF due to the decompensation of chronic cardiopulmonary disease compared to those experiencing de novo hypoxaemic ARF.[15] Moreover, in non-RCTs, the time lag to ICU referral is variable. In a large observational study[36] involving 1302 subjects with haematological malignancies, NIV was started in the advanced course of ARF (i.e. $PaO_2/FiO_2 < 200$) in three quarters of cases. Since a longer delay to start NIV predicts an unsuccessful ventilation, this issue may explain the high failure rates in some non-RCTs.[30]

The actual evidence suggests potential benefits from a trial of 'prophylactic' CPAP or NIV in the early phases of ARF (i.e. $PaO_2/FiO_2 > 200$) in cancer patients without multiple organ dysfunctions.[17,23] Intubation should not be delayed as poor outcome is associated with late NIV failure.[30] Hence, in selected subjects at high-risk of NIV failure, IMV could be the preferable first-line ventilatory support.[4,30,33,39] The failure of NIV was associated with delay in initiating ventilation, severe hypoxaemia (i.e. $PaO_2/FiO_2 < 200$), extrapulmonary organ failure (i.e. need for vasopressors and renal replacement therapy) and increasing respiratory rate under NIV.[30,33] Moreover, a NIV trial is likely to fail when the underlying cause of ARF is unknown or not rapidly reversible.[4,28] Like for non-cancer patients, NIV should be avoided in the presence of absolute contraindications (i.e. respiratory arrest, cardiovascular instability, inability to protect airway, vomiting).[15] Conversely, excessive secretions, recent upper gastrointestinal or airway surgery and altered consciousness related to hypercapnic encephaloptahy are considered relative contraindications (Figure 51.1).[13,15,16,40,41]

Aside from patient characteristics, the success of NIV may depend upon the appropriate choice of ventilators, modes of NIV and patient–ventilator interfaces. In mildly hypoxaemic cancer patients, CPAP delivered with helmet could be a better tolerated and cheaper alternative to facemask NIV.[42]

The strategy based on the early application of NIV outside the ICU is still debated. In fact, starting NIV in the ward may be risky because a delayed admission in ICU of patients failing NIV may worsen their outcome. The favourable findings of the Italian RCT may be explained by a long experience in using a simple technology (i.e. CPAP) in the ward under the strict supervision of an ICU team.[23]

Recently, HFNO has been increasingly applied to treat different patterns of hypoxaemic ARF, including those occurring in cancer patients, due to its advantages over conventional oxygen therapy (e.g. delivery of high FiO_2, adequate humidification, patient comfort, provision of low positive end-expiratory pressure values).[43] Consequently, HFNO could be proposed as either a preventive or alternative or integrative treatment of NIV in cancer patients with milder degrees of hypoxaemia.

NIV in patients with limitations of care

An increasing amount of published data has described the use of NIV in ARF patients who refused intubation.[44–48] Whereas a subgroup of DNI patients with advanced cancer experienced 85% failure of NIV in one report,[44] other studies described the successful reversal of ARF and ICU survival in more than half of DNI cancer patients.[46,48] In a multicenter observational study performed on 780 patients (a quarter of them affected by cancer) admitted in ICU, Azoulay et al.[48] demonstrated that NIV used as 'ceiling treatment' was not associated with increased anxiety, depression or stress among both patients and relatives, compared to NIV used without treatment-limitation decisions. Of note, 'ceiling NIV' should be withdrawn, and palliative care has to be intensified if NIV fails and/or is not tolerated any longer.[20,21]

In patients with terminal malignancy who do not want any form of life-prolonging therapy, 'palliative' NIV could be considered only if it improves dyspnoea, provides time to come to terms with death as well as allows to get their personal affairs in order.[20,21] The more controversial point is whether the benefit of NIV in palliating dyspnoea may be outweighed by the discomfort and limited communication induced by the facemask.[20,21] Few studies reported that NIV is feasible and reduced dyspnoea in advanced cancer patients with ARF.[26,49] In a multicentre RCT on palliative NIV performed in 200 advanced solid cancer patients, Nava et al.[26] showed that compared to only oxygen therapy, the adjunct of NIV was more effective in reducing dyspnoea

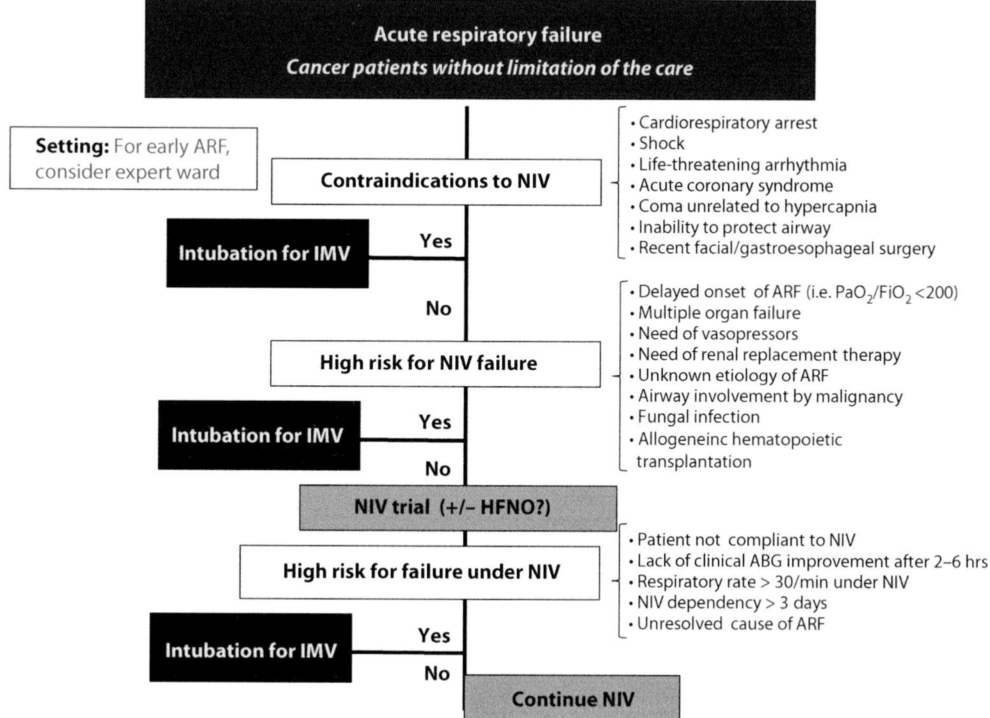

Figure 51.1 Flow chart depicting the use of NIV in cancer patients with ARF without limitation of care. ABG, arterial blood gases.

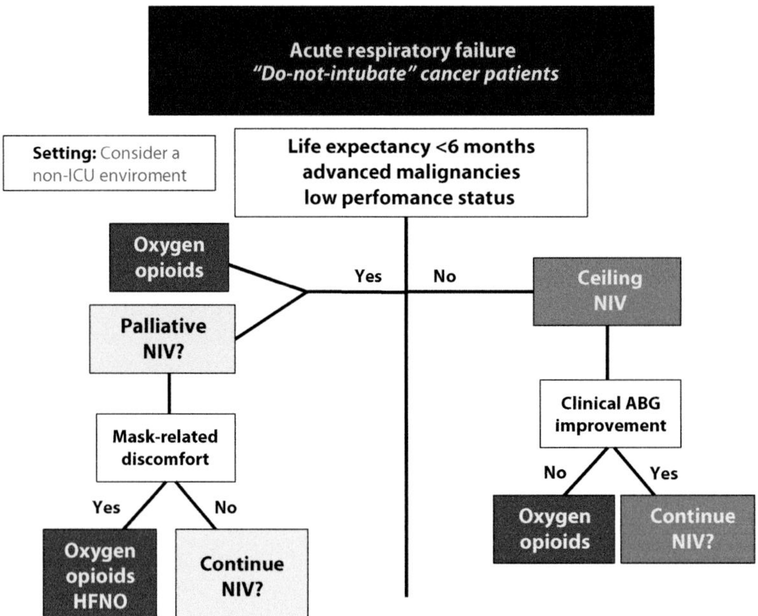

Figure 51.2 Flow chart depicting the use of NIV in cancer patients with ARF who refuse intubation. ABG, arterial blood gases.

and the amount of the needed doses of opiates and their side effects (e.g. depressed sensorium). This may mean a better capability of communication for the patient at the end of life, with a good control of symptoms.

In this context, palliative HFNO is likely to be a good alternative to NIV as shown by a preliminary RCT performed in 30 hospitalised patients with advanced cancer, which demonstrated that HFNO was as effective as NIV in relieving dyspnoea and improving physiologic parameters (Figure 51.2).[50]

CHAPTER SUMMARY

ARF is the most frequent reason for ICU admission in cancer patients; most of them require mechanical ventilation. The substantial drop in the mortality of mechanically ventilated cancer patients over the last four decades has strongly mitigated the nihilistic behaviour of physicians against the ventilatory support in cancer. The large application of NIV has contributed to improve the prognosis of cancer complicated by ARF. Nevertheless, mortality still remains high especially in patients with severe hypoxaemia, extrapulmonary complications and unknown cause of ARF and in those who fail NIV. The majority of the published data, mostly consisting of observational studies, shows drawbacks, mainly due to methodological aspects that limit the reliability of their findings. The actual evidence suggests benefits from a trial of prophylactic CPAP or NIV in the early ARF (i.e. $PaO_2/FiO_2 > 200$) in cancer patients without multiple organ dysfunctions. Intubation should not be delayed as poor hospital survival is associated with late NIV failure. The option of starting early CPAP/NIV in the ward to reduce ICU admission is still controversial. Recent data suggested the feasibility of NIV as palliation in terminally ill cancer patients. HFNO is a new promising option both for treating mildly hypoxaemic patients as an alternative of integrative support with NIV and for palliation in terminally ill cancer patients.

REFERENCES

1. Groeger JS, Lemeshow S, Price K et al. Multicenter outcome study of cancer patients admitted to the intensive care unit: A probability of mortality model. *J Clin Oncol.* 1998;16:761–70.
2. Maschmeyer G, Bertschat FL, Moesta KT et al. Outcome analysis of 189 consecutive cancer patients referred to the intensive care unit as emergencies during a 2-year period. *Eur J Cancer.* 2003;39:783–92.
3. Taccone F, Artigas A, Sprung C et al. Characteristics and outcomes of cancer patients in European ICUs. *Crit Care.* 2009;13:R15.
4. Azoulay E, Thiéry G, Chevret S et al. The prognosis of acute respiratory failure in critically ill cancer patients. *Medicine.* 2004;83:360–70.
5. Lecuyer L, Chevret S, Guidet B et al. Case volume and mortality in haematological patients with acute respiratory failure. *Eur Respir J.* 2008;32:74–54.
6. Soares M, Salluh J, Spector N et al. Characteristics and outcomes of cancer patients requiring mechanical ventilatory support for >24 hours. *Crit Care Med.* 2005;33:520–6.
7. Benoit D, Vandewoude K, Decruyenaere J et al. Outcome and early prognostic indicators in patients with a hematologic malignancy admitted to the intensive care unit for life-threatening complication. *Crit Care Med.* 2003;31:104–12.

8. Chaoui D, Legrand O, Roche N et al. Incidence and prognostic value of respiratory events in acute leukemia. *Leukemia.* 2004;18:670–5.
9. Depuydt PO, Benoit DD, Vandewoude KH et al. Outcome in noninvasively and invasively ventilated hematologic patients with acute respiratory failure. *Chest.* 2004;126:1299–306.
10. Azoulay E, Alberti C, Bornstain C et al. Improved survival in cancer patients requiring mechanical ventilatory support: Impact of noninvasive mechanical ventilatory support. *Crit Care Med.* 2001; 29:519–25.
11. Adam AK, Soubani AO. Outcome and prognostic factors of lung cancer patients admitted to the medical intensive care unit. *Eur Respir J.* 2008;31:47–53.
12. Azoulay E, Afessa A. The intensive support of patients with malignancy: Do everything that can be done. *Intensive Care Med.* 2006;32:3–5.
13. Soares M, Pieter O, Depuydt PO et al. Mechanical ventilation in cancer patients: Clinical characteristics and outcomes. *Crit Care Clin.* 2010;26:41–58.
14. Pene F, Percheron S, Lemiale V et al. Temporal changes in management and outcome of septic shock in patients with malignancies in the intensive care unit. *Crit Care Med.* 2008;36:690–6.
15. Nava S, Hill N. Non-invasive ventilation in acute respiratory failure. *Lancet.* 2009;374:250–9.
16. Squadrone V, Ferreyra G, Ranieri VM. Non-invasive ventilation in patients with hematologic malignancy: A new prospective. *Minerva Anestesiol.* 2015;81:1118–26.
17. Pastores SM, Voigt LP. Acute respiratory failure in the patient with cancer: Diagnostic and management strategies. *Crit Care Clin.* 2010;26: 21–40.
18. Benoit D, Depuydt P, Peleman A et al. Documented and clinically suspected bacterial infection precipitating intensive care unit admission in patients with hematological malignancy: Impact on outcome. *Intensive Care Med.* 2005;31:934–42.
19. Benoit D, Depuydt P, Vandewoude K et al. Outcome in severely ill patients with hematological malignancies who received intravenous chemotherapy in the intensive care unit. *Intensive Care Med.* 2006;32:93–9.
20. Scala R, Nava S. NIV and palliative care. *Eur Respir Mon.* 2008;41:287–306.
21. Curtis JR, Cook DJ, Sinuff T et al. Non-invasive positive pressure ventilation in critical and palliative care settings: Understanding the goals of therapy. *Crit Care Med.* 2007;35:932–9.
22. Hilbert G, Gruson D, Vargas D et al. Noninvasive ventilation in immunosuppressed patients with pulmonary infiltrates, fever, and acute respiratory failure. *N Engl J Med.* 2001;344:481–7.
23. Squadrone V, Massaia M, Bruno B et al. Early CPAP prevents evolution of acute lung injury in patients with hematologic malignancy. *Intensive Care Med.* 2010;36:1666–74.
24. Wermke M, Schiemanck S, Höffken G et al. Respiratory failure in patients undergoing allogeneic hematopoietic SCT – A randomized trial on early non-invasive ventilation based on standard care hematology wards. *Bone Marrow Transplant.* 2012;47:574–80.
25. Lemiale V, Mokart D, Resche-Rigon M et al. Effect of noninvasive ventilation vs oxygen therapy on mortality among immunocompromised patients with acute respiratory failure: A randomized clinical trial. *JAMA.* 2015;314:1711–9.
26. Nava S, Ferrer M, Esquinas A et al. Palliative use of non-invasive ventilation in end-of-life patients with solid tumours: A randomised feasibility trial. *Lancet Oncol.* 2013;14:219–27.
27. Depuydt PO, Benoit DD, Roosens CD. The impact of the initial ventilatory strategy on survival in hematological patients with acute hypoxemic respiratory failure. *J Crit Care.* 2010;25:30–6.
28. Rabbat A, Chaoui D, Montani D et al. Prognosis of patients with acute myeloid *Leukemia.* admitted to intensive care. *Br J Haematol.* 2005;29:350–57.
29. Rabitsch W, Staudinger T, Locker G et al. Respiratory failure after stem cell transplantation: Improved outcome with non-invasive ventilation. *Leuk Lymphoma.* 2005;46:1151–7.
30. Adda M, Coquet I, Darmon M et al. Predictors of noninvasive ventilation failure in patients with hematologic malignancy and acute respiratory failure. *Crit Care Med.* 2008;36:2766–72.
31. Tognet E, Mercatello A, Coronel B et al. Treatment of acute respiratory failure with non-invasive positive pressure ventilation in haematological patients. *Clin Intensive Care.* 1994;5:282–8.
32. Conti G, Marino P, Cogliati A et al. Noninvasive ventilation for the treatment of acute respiratory failure in patients with hematologic malignancies: A pilot study. *Intensive Care Med.* 1998;24:1283–8.
33. Molina R, Bernal T, Borges M et al. Ventilatory support in critically ill hematology patients with respiratory failure. *Crit Care.* 2012;16:R133.
34. Müller AM, Gazzana MB, Silva DR. Outcomes for patients with lung cancer admitted to intensive care units. *Rev Bras Ter Intensiva.* 2013;25:12–16.
35. Azevedo LC, Caruso P, Silva UV et al. Outcomes for patients with cancer admitted to the ICU requiring ventilatory support: Results from a prospective multicenter study. *Chest.* 2014;146:257–66.
36. Gristina GR, Antonelli M, Conti G et al. Noninvasive versus invasive ventilation for acute respiratory failure in patients with hematologic malignancies: A 5-year multicenter observational survey. *Crit Care Med.* 2011;39:2232–9.

37. Lemiale V, Lambert J, Canet E et al. Identifying cancer subjects with acute respiratory failure at high risk for intubation and mechanical ventilation. *Respir Care.* 2014;59:1517–23.
38. Ferreira JC, Medeiros P Jr, Rego FM et al. Risk factors for noninvasive ventilation failure in cancer patients in the intensive care unit: A retrospective cohort study. *J Crit Care.* 2015;30:1003–7.
39. Meert AP, Berghmans T, Markiewicz E et al. Invasive mechanical ventilation in cancer patients. Prior non invasive ventilation is a poor prognostic factor. *J BUON* 2011;16:160–5.
40. Ozyilmaz E, Ugurlu AO, Nava S. Timing of non-invasive ventilation failure: Causes, risk factors, and potential remedies. *BMC Pulm Med.* 2014;14:19.
41. Scala R. Non-invasive ventilation in acute respiratory failure with altered consciousness syndrome: A bargain or an hazard? *Minerva Anestesiol.* 2013;79:1291–9.
42. Principi T, Pantanetti S, Catani F et al. Noninvasive continuous positive airway pressure delivered by helmet in hematological malignancy patients with hypoxemic acute respiratory failure. *Intensive Care Med.* 2004;30:147–50.
43. Roca O, Hernández G, Díaz-Lobato S et al. Current evidence for the effectiveness of heated and humidified high flow nasal cannula supportive therapy in adult patients with respiratory failure. *Crit Care.* 2016;28;20:10.
44. Schettino G, Altobelli N, Kacmarek R. Noninvasive positive pressure ventilation reverses acute respiratory failure in select 'do-not-intubate' patients. *Crit Care Med.* 2005;33:1976–82.
45. Levy M, Tanios M, Nelson D et al. Outcomes of patients with do-not-intubate orders treated with noninvasive ventilation. *Crit Care Med.* 2004;32:2002–7.
46. Meert A, Berghmans T, Hardy M et al. Non-invasive ventilation for cancer patients with life-supporting techniques limitation. *Support Care Cancer.* 2006;14:167–71.
47. Fernandez R, Baigorri F, Artigas A. Noninvasive ventilation in patients with 'do-not-intubate' orders: Medium-term efficacy depends critically on patient selection. *Intensive Care Med.* 2007;33:350–4.
48. Azoulay E, Kouatchet A, Jaber S et al. Noninvasive mechanical ventilation in patients having declined tracheal intubation. *Intensive Care Med.* 2013;39:292–301.
49. Cuomo A, Delmastro M, Ceriana P et al. Noninvasive mechanical ventilation as a palliative treatment of acute respiratory failure in patients with end-stage solid cancer. *Palliat Med.* 2004;18:602–10.
50. Hui D, Morgado M, Chisholm G et al. High-flow oxygen and bilevel positive airway pressure for persistent dyspnea in patients with advanced cancer: A phase II randomized trial. *J Pain Symptom Manage.* 2013;46:463–73.

52

Non-invasive ventilation in the elderly

ERWAN L'HER AND CORINNE TROADEC-L'HER

INTRODUCTION

Non-invasive positive pressure ventilation (NIV) reduces endotracheal intubation (ETI) and mortality in adult patients with various causes of acute respiratory failure (ARF).[1,2] However, most patients included within the randomised controlled trials were deemed to undergo invasive mechanical ventilation if necessary, and few of them were identified as 'elderly'. One could therefore argue that such beneficial results cannot be transferred to such a specific population, even if others could point to the fact that age by itself does not confer specific pathological patterns.

Until recently, there have been a number of studies examining the invasive mechanical ventilation of elderly patients within an intensive care unit (ICU), but only a few about NIV administration. Considering this argumentation, the use of NIV in the very old age (>75 years) was given a favourable level 4 of evidence (*case series and poor quality cohorts and case-control studies*) in a systematic review of the literature.[3]

There is also an increased interest in the use of NIV for patients who have declined invasive life support measures.[4] However, the utility of NIV in patients with ARF who have declined intubation and resuscitation[5,6] or those who have chosen comfort measures only is rather controversial.[7] While NIV can reverse non-terminal ARF, it may be considered inappropriate when patients have elected to limit life support near the end of their lives. Nevertheless, NIV may benefit some patients who have chosen a *do-not-resuscitate* (DNR) status, and such indication could be considered as recommended with a favourable level 2 of evidence (*homogeneous cohort studies analysis or low-quality randomised controlled trials*).[3] In such patients, beyond mortality and ICU length of stay, outcomes such as functional status and health-related quality of life have assumed greater importance.[8]

The purpose of this chapter is to review the potential uses of NIV in elderly patients and to provide clinicians details about the indications and determinants of success. It will also discuss about NIV endpoints and response to failure in this specific population.

PATHOPHYSIOLOGY

Definition of elderly

Most industrialised countries have accepted the chronological age of 65 years as a definition of *elderly*. Although there are commonly used definitions of *old age*, there is no general agreement on the age at which a person really becomes old.[9] It is important to stress that the common use of a calendar age to mark the threshold of old age assumes equivalence between chronological and biological age, yet it is also generally accepted that these two are not necessarily synonymous. Other authors have focused on the age of 80, considering that octogenarians, compared to others, are more likely to have impaired functional status before they develop critical illness, and they have relatively short remaining life spans even without a critical illness.[10,11]

Whatever the chosen threshold for the definition of *elderly*, the assessment of patients' vulnerability is certainly of importance. *Vulnerable elderlies* could be defined as persons aged 65 and older, who are at increased risk of functional decline or death within 2 years.[12] These people are likely to have already been confronted with aggressive life-sustaining care, which makes the discussion more crucial. Indeed, many of these patients will die despite ICU admission, raising questions about whether critical care services could have unnecessarily prolonged their dying experience or caused harm to their family and relatives.

Epidemiology of ageing population

The oldest sector of the population is growing worldwide,[13] and population ageing is accelerating since 2011, when the first baby boom cohort had reached the age of 65 years. The fastest growing age cohort is made up of those aged

≥80 years, increasing at an estimated 3.8% per year and projected to represent one-fifth of all older persons by 2050.[14]

A study performed by Rockwood et al.[15] in the early 1990s established that patients 65 years and older were already accounting for 26%–51% of all ICU admissions.[15] The number of ventilated patients was expected to increase by a 31%-fold in 2010 in some regions,[16] a fact that is daily observed in our units.

Clinical impact of comorbidities in elderly patients

Older age is associated with higher prevalence of chronic illness and functional impairment, contributing to an increased rate of hospitalisation. The coexistence of cardiac and respiratory diseases in elderly patients admitted for acute respiratory distress strengthens the difficulty of the aetiological/pathogenical diagnosis.[17,18] In a study of 122 patients admitted for a presumed cardiac decompensation, the initial diagnosis of cardiogenic pulmonary oedema (CPE) was confirmed in only 29% of cases. Chronic obstructive pulmonary disease (COPD) or underlying obesity was considered responsible for 42% of 'false diagnoses'.[19] In a study of 11,000 patients hospitalised for cardiogenic pulmonary oedema, 54% of patients were aged over 70 years, and 24% were suffering from an associated chronic lung disease.[20] This difficult diagnosis and the frequent coexistence of multiple pathologies means that clinical NIV application in elderly patients will often be initiated for a symptomatic diagnosis (i.e. hypercarbic vs. pure hypoxaemic ARF), rather than for a precise specific diagnosis.

Patients' prognosis and preferences

In most industrial countries, the dying experience has largely become a hospital experience, with one in five of these deaths occurring in the ICU.[21,22] Little attention has been paid to the quality of care that vulnerable elders receive, and previous studies exploring the association of age and ICU outcome have yielded conflicting results. A few studies conclude that age is not a predictor,[23,24] while others conclude that increasing age is associated with increased ICU short-term mortality.[25–27]

When questioned, most people would prefer to die at home,[28,29] and most elderly patients, when provided with a choice, would prefer a less aggressive treatment plan than a technologically supported, institutionalised death.[30]

A contrario, evidence suggests that clinicians sometimes underestimate the degree of intervention desired by older patients.[31] In fact, there exists a complex relationship among physiologic impairment, functional status, quality of life (QOL), commenting on the discordance between decreased functional status and perceived QOL. This may be due to changes in individuals' expectations or perceptions, as a result of changing internal standards and patients' conceptualisation of health-related QOL.[8] Unhealthy or frail elderlies frequently express preferences for a longer life under compromised health conditions more frequently than do healthy responders.[32]

Nevertheless, in a study of hospitalised elderly patients in the United States, 70% reported that their baseline QOL was fair or poor, and most wanted comfort measures as opposed to life-prolonging treatments.[33] Nevertheless, 54% of these patients were admitted to ICUs. In another study, at least half of seriously ill patients reported pain, and many died after unwanted prolongation of their dying process in an ICU.[34]

Such considerations must be put forward when considering NIV initiation in an elderly patient, especially when the patient is unconscious or demented and cannot provide agreement to care.

CLINICAL APPLICATION

NIV has become a standard for the treatment of ARF and is used in different acute care settings.[35,36] In a prospective cohort of 1019 patients requiring ventilator support over a 2-year period, 376 (37%) of them received NIV, among whom 163 (16%) were considered as elderlies.[37] These patients were depicted to more frequently receive NIV with DNR orders than younger patients (40% vs. 8%). The 6-month survival rate was 49% in elderlies and 33% for DNR patients. Of the survivors at 6 months, 13.5% were still living at home, with an overall satisfactory functional status.

In elderlies, NIV should be considered for similar indications as in younger patients, even if clinical diagnosis may often be more imprecise and the main goal to be somewhat different.

Acute hypercapnic exacerbation of chronic pulmonary disease

During the acute exacerbation of COPD, NIV reduces the rates of ETI, mortality and hospital length of stay.[1,38,39] Its specific use in an elderly population has rarely been studied, and it is not known with a high level of evidence whether elderly patients gain similar benefits.

In a retrospective study of over 7.5 million admissions for acute exacerbations of COPD, over a 10 years period, a more than 4-fold increase in the use of NIV was depicted. Thirty-seven percent of patients were over 75 years, of whom 9% were equal or over 85 years. NIV use in these categories represented 30% of all attempts and approximately 25% of survivors after treatment, with and without the need for subsequent transition to invasive mechanical ventilation.[40] These data confirm that this population is of importance and that it may require a more specific focus.

Benhamou et al.[41] first reported the results of NIV in 30 elderly patients with hypercapnic respiratory failure, but only 20 of whom had COPD. Treatment failure was 40% in this study, probably because only 68% of patients had COPD. In a prospective cohort of 36 patients aged 65 years or above hospitalised for an ARF related to COPD, Balami et al. investigated the impact of NIV.[42] The staff were fully trained in the administration of NIV, and two beds with high-dependency facilities for the administration of NIV were specifically available within the unit. The mean age of patients was 77.4 years, compared to a mean of 60 years in most randomised studies. Patients' condition was severe, with a pre-NIV pH value of 7.23 ± 0.07 and a $PaCO_2$ of 80 ± 21 mm Hg. For all patients, a decision that NIV was to be the ceiling of treatment has been made prior to its initiation. An overall 79% success rate was observed, and all patients who failed NIV died (25%). In a retrospective cohort of 127 elderly hypercapnic COPD exacerbations, NIV treatment was also considered successful in 78.3% of cases.[43] Cumulative delirium was present in 38% of cases, and almost 28% were concomitantly disabled and demented. Four patients (3.4%) were intubated and 21 other patients (18.3%) were considered for subsequent treatment limitation; all these 25 patients died within the hospital. The authors concluded that although high, mortality in elderly patients under NIV was probably not worse than that in younger patients and that the success rate was high. Moreover, they also indicated that NIV was generally well tolerated. Finally, a recent randomised controlled trial including 82 elderly patients with preexisting chronic pulmonary disease demonstrated that the rate for meeting the ETI criteria was lower in the group treated by NIV, compared to standard medical treatment (7.3% vs. 63.5%, respectively; $p < 0.001$).[44]

Cardiogenic pulmonary oedema

NIV is beneficial during CPE, in the absence of acute coronary ischaemia.[45–49] It reduces the risk for intubation (−52%; relative risk [RR] 0.48, 95% confidence interval [CI] 0.25–0.92) and in-hospital mortality (−20%; RR 0.8, 95% CI 0.58–1.10), without difference between bi-level pressure support ventilation or continuous positive airway pressure (CPAP).[49]

However, in a prospective randomised study dedicated to the treatment of CPE in a specific population of 89 consecutive elderly patients (≥75 years) admitted to emergency departments with an ARF related to CPE, L'Her et al.[50] evaluated the clinical efficacy of CPAP versus standard medical treatment. The mean age of the patients was 86 years. Within 1 hour, CPAP led to decreased respiratory rate and improved oxygenation compared to baseline, whereas no differences were observed within the standard treatment group. Early 48-hour mortality was 7% in the CPAP group, compared with 24% in the standard treatment group (p = 0.017); however, no sustained benefits were observed during the overall hospital stay, probably because of therapeutic limitations or the exacerbations of comorbidities during the subsequent hospital stay. Although early clinical improvement is a worthy goal by itself, these beneficial results must however be tempered by a lack of sustained benefit. A meaningful benefit should include both a decrease in mortality and morbidity, whereas a short-term mortality benefit that is ultimately erased by the time of discharge could just be considered as a way of delaying the inevitable.

As demonstrated in the Three Interventions in Cardiogenic Pulmonary Oedema (3CPO) study,[51] bi-level pressure support ventilation seems to be associated with a more rapid and better oxygenation than CPAP,[49] which may favour its use in such a population, where comfort improvement is mandatory.

NIV in palliative care

The concept of palliative NIV applies to its use in case of ARF with DNR orders or when patients have refused ETI but cannot spontaneously breathe. Patients may therefore present severe ARF symptoms, respiratory acidosis and/or haemodynamic failure, all these conditions being well known as failure criteria for NIV. In these conditions, NIV may be less effective than ETI, but it will at least aim to alleviate ARF symptoms or provide specific benefits.

NIV FOR PATIENTS WHO REFUSE ENDOTRACHEAL INTUBATION OR WITH DNR ORDERS

In most NIV trials, if the treatment failed, the standard therapy was intubation and mechanical ventilation. Although NIV is a widely accepted treatment for some patients with ARF, the use of NIV in the vulnerable elderly, who may have decided to forego ETI, is controversial.[52] Given its high success rate in the previously developed indications, NIV appears to be an attractive option to support patients with respiratory failure who refuse intubation. It should therefore be used as the treatment ceiling. Unfortunately, some authors also pointed out the fact that many physicians were considering NIV to be a routine therapeutic option for patients who have explicitly requested that mechanical ventilation not be implemented in the event of severe or life-threatening medical illness.[53] This is compounded by the additional observation that patients in such condition may frequently require either chemical or physical restraints to tolerate this intervention, inducing major ethical concerns.

In a prospective observational study about the use of NIV in COPD patients who refused ETI, a 1-year survival of ~30% was recorded in COPD patients with the DNR code, who developed acute hypercapnic respiratory failure requiring NIV. The majority of survivors developed another life-threatening event in the following year.[54]

NIV IN PALLIATIVE CARE

Some authors have suggested that NIV should be used in palliative care patients on a trial basis, to help alleviate respiratory distress and attempt to provide some additional time to finalise personal affairs.[55] In such a situation, NIV may lessen dyspnoea and tachypnea, preserve patient autonomy and permit eating and verbal communication, thus improving patients' comfort. But the realistic aspect of such a therapy in terms of palliative measure has also been questioned. Some authors have suggested that it should be inappropriate to use NIV because it is still a form of artificial life support, whatever the type of interface, and that it may therefore cause discomfort while only prolonging the dying process.[56] The answer to that question clearly depends on how the clinician defines palliation for a specific patient. If the goal is patient comfort during an inevitable and untreatable dying process, then not only is NIV of dubious value – but it should also be contraindicated. It will only prolong a dying process that is expected and anticipated. However, if the goal is to aggressively treat the palliative patient who has a predetermined stop order (i.e. therapeutic limitation such as 'no intubation and/or mechanical ventilation'), NIV may be of some value as a palliative treatment, to reduce the discomfort of dyspnoea, with no expectation of coincidental prolongation of life.

Several different situations might be individualised, the common denominator being the DNR order for all patients: (1) palliative care but curative approach, to avoid intubation in a good NIV indication; (2) palliative but curative approach, to withdraw ETI; and (3) palliative and non-curative approach, with the sole sake to improve ARF symptoms and give time to the patient and their family.

Situation (1) is not different from standard NIV practice. Situation (2) is driven by results depicting that a non-invasive weaning has been demonstrated to decrease death, weaning failure, pneumonia and length of stay in the hospital and ICU, without increase in the reintubation rate, especially for COPD patients.[57] Situation (3) will aim to provide patients the best level of comfort, i.e. lessening as much as possible ARF symptoms, NIV only being used as a medical adjuvant. Despite differences in between these approaches, the evaluation of the NIV impact on ARF symptoms is prominent. It will be mandatory to provide a suitable medical treatment for dyspnoea and tachypnea (opioids and/or benzodiazepins) and to stop NIV when failure occurs.

TECHNICAL CONSIDERATIONS

Concerning the technical aspects of NIV in the elderly, a very few specificities arise compared with a younger population. An empirical therapeutic algorithm for NIV consideration in the elderly can be drawn, even if it mainly relies on clinical experience and general ethical concerns, rather than on scientific evidences (Figure 52.1).

One may also question the fact that most published studies have been performed in the ICU setting, while the vast majority of elderly patients may nowadays be ventilated in the emergency ward, which induces several logistic problems after a first successful NIV trial (should it be continued and where should the patient be transferred?), especially in the case of DNR and/or palliative care.

Should NIV be initiated?

Elderly patients without chronic disabilities should be treated with NIV regardless of their age. However, the use of NIV as the treatment ceiling should always be discussed on an individual basis, taking into account various data and patient's will.

If the patient comfort is maintained and families are supported, a time-limited trial of treatment for elderly with chronic critical illness may sometimes be appropriate. However, the continuation of treatment in the chronic phase of critical illness should never be driven by default, i.e. in the absence of conscious medical decisions that are informed by effective communication and taking into account the patient's goals, preferences and values.[58] It will always be necessary to weigh the benefits and burdens of treatment and to reevaluate this balance as the clinical situation evolves. In ideal circumstances, the patient would directly participate in this process, but the reality of both acute and chronic critical illnesses is that decisional capacity is typically lacking.

Take into account patients' and relatives' wills

Many clinicians seem to be interpreting a DNI order as an order permitting all forms of treatment except intubation. But is NIV any different from ETI in a practical sense? Except for the presence of a foreign body in the trachea, NIV is essentially the same, in that it uses hardware to achieve an end-stage therapeutic advantage not possible with more conservative methods. Patient preferences regarding end-of-life treatment are usually unknown.[59] In such situations, family caregivers' wills play a major role. Neither a proxy nor another advance directive is a perfect alternative, but both may help illuminate decision making from the patient's perspective. Physicians therefore frequently consult relatives regarding the appropriateness of treatment intervention, despite data suggesting that the consulted relatives find this emotionally stressful and do not consistently make decisions that accurately reflect their relative's wishes.[60,61]

What should be the intensity of care?

Although ICU resources and intensive treatments are often denied to elderly patients, it is clear that age as such is a poor predictor of medical outcome. When confronted with extended mechanical ventilation and associated care, a significant proportion of elderly patients would accept this care only for an improved prognosis.[62] However, among patients with chronic critical illness admitted to the ICU, severe brain dysfunction and delirium is highly prevalent.[63] If elderly patients with a potential critical illness are questioned about end-of-life decisions, up to 41% choose to limit certain life-sustaining therapies including cardiopulmonary resuscitation, ventilation and ICU admission.[64,65]

Critical care decision making is an imprecise process. It takes time to see whether therapy works. The institution of aggressive care gives the patient the benefit of the doubt, but an aggressive approach increases the possibility of dependence on life support.[66] Accordingly, it soon became necessary to ponder limiting a critical care plan when a point of diminishing returns was reached.[67] Without limits, 'the

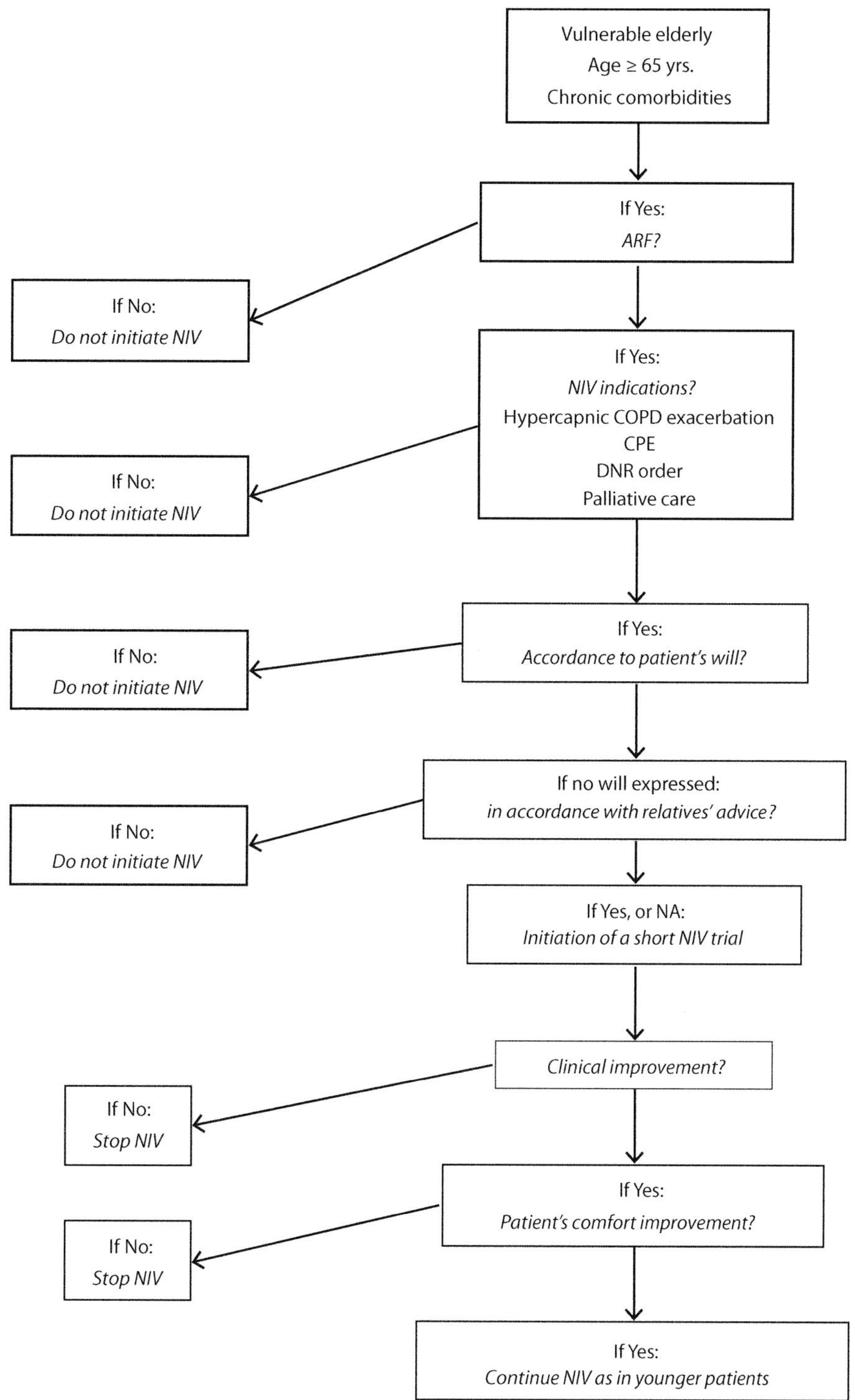

Figure 52.1 Therapeutic algorithm for NIV consideration in elderly. This algorithm relies on clinical experience and general ethical concerns, rather than on scientific evidence. Without chronic disabilities, patients should be treated with NIV regardless of their age. In elderly patients with chronic disabilities, a time-limited trial of treatment may be appropriate. The use of NIV should always be discussed on an individual basis, taking into account various data and patient's will. In most cases, NIV should be used as the treatment ceiling.

potential for warehousing warm cadavers looms large'.[68] That care plan will lead 'to another population, one composed of patients who were left not alive (in the sense of being capable of enjoying life) and not able to die (because technology temporarily arrested a disease process but did not reverse it)'.[69]

The use of NIV has been conceptualised in three categories by the Society of Critical Care Medicine Noninvasive Positive Pressure Ventilation Task Force.[52] This scheme, which must also take into account patients' specific characteristics and nuances, allows to provide clinicians with a conceptual framework that may help not only to proportionate care and determine goals and determinants of success, but also to set NIV endpoints and response to failure and to discuss about the ideal location of NIV initiation (Table 52.1). This scheme does not specifically fit to elderly patients, but may be applied to institute proportionate care in all vulnerable patients that may require NIV initiation.

Briefly, Category 1 patients are patients for which life support without pressure limits have to be applied. In these patients, response to NIV failure will require intubation and mechanical ventilation. These patients may be treated not only within ICUs, but also in some specific step-down or acute care units with appropriate monitoring and trained personnel. Category 3 patients are patients for which solely comfort measures are to be applied. In these patients, NIV should be initiated outside the ICU, in specific beds with appropriately trained personnel. NIV failure should be considered if patients are not more comfortable or becomes unable to communicate. Response to failure should be to palliate symptoms without NIV. Category 2 is a mismatch of both categories, but in which the goal should be to restore patients' health without using ETI and without causing unacceptable discomfort.

Interfaces

No specific difference has to be drawn concerning these items. NIV tolerance has been shown to be a major

Table 52.1 Three-category approach for the use of non-invasive ventilation in ARF

	Category 1	Category 2	Category 3
Definition	Life support without limits	Life support with preset limits (do-not-intubate)	Comfort measures only
Primary goals of care	• Assist ventilation and/or oxygenation • Alleviate dyspnoea • Achieve comfort • Reduce risk of intubation • Reduce risk of mortality • Avoid intubation	• Include same as category 1 except intubation • In some cases, to prolong life for specific purposes (e.g. arrival of family member)	• Palliation of symptoms (relief of dyspnoea)
Goals to communicate with patient and family	• To restore health and use intubation if necessary	• To restore health without using intubation and without unacceptable discomfort	• To maximise comfort • To minimise adverse effects of opiates
Determinants of success	• Improved oxygenation and/or ventilation • Tolerance of NIV with minimal discomfort (outweighed by benefit)	• Improved oxygenation and/or ventilation • Tolerance of NIV with minimal discomfort (outweighed by benefit)	• Improved symptoms • Tolerance of NIV
Endpoints	• Unassisted ventilation • NIV intolerance	• Unassisted ventilation • NIV intolerance	• Patient is not more comfortable • Patient wants NIV to be stopped • Patient becomes unable to communicate
Response to failure	• Intubation and mechanical ventilation	• Change to comfort measures and palliate symptoms only	• Palliate symptoms without NIV
Likely location of NIV	• ICU • Possible in step-down units or acute care beds with appropriate monitoring and training	• ICU in some cases • Step-down units or acute care beds with appropriate monitoring and training	• Not in the ICU • Acute care beds • Should also be possible in hospice if trained personnel is available

Source: Society of Critical Care Medicine Palliative Noninvasive Positive Pressure Ventilation Task Force; Curtis JR et al., *Crit Care Med*, 35, 932–9, 2007.

Note: ICU, intensive care unit; NIV, non-invasive positive pressure. The use of NIV has been conceptualised in three categories by the Society of Critical Care Medicine Palliative Noninvasive Positive Pressure Ventilation Task Force.[52] This table is only an abstract of the original table and the reader should both refer to the original table and article that describe in more details the subsequent categories. Clinicians may take into account this conceptual framework while dealing with vulnerable elderlies with ARF, but they might also consider several variables, nuances and specific characteristics of every individual, either patients or relatives.

determinant of success in general.[70] The vulnerability of elderly patients, combined with the fact that NIV will often be considered as the ceiling of treatment, may enhance the necessity to help patients tolerate as much as possible the interfaces. One should therefore focus on more comfortable masks, promote rotation of masks to modify pressure points over the patient's face and mainly use intermittent sessions.

CONCLUSION

Despite few literature references, NIV seems to be as efficient in elderly patients as in younger ones. Moreover, it should be offered as an alternative to patients considered to be poor candidates for intubation and those with DNR orders. However, much more than in younger patients, the need for a proportionate care is crucial. NIV should be used as the treatment ceiling in most elderly patients, especially the vulnerable ones.

Patients' preferences regarding end-of-life treatment are generally unknown, whereas most patients are unconscious and/or demented on admission, which makes such a discussion difficult in emergency. Relatives' opinion will therefore be the only possibility to appreciate patients' preference regarding the intensity of treatment, but they may not be available at the moment of the decision. NIV goals should never be to unnecessarily prolong life, but rather to restore health as much as possible and, if not possible, at least to relieve dyspnoea. Physicians should be able to face NIV failure and to cease treatment if the patient is not more comfortable having NIV, if he or she wants NIV to be stopped, or if he or she becomes unable to communicate.

REFERENCES

1. Keenan SP, Sinuff T, Cook DJ et al. Which patients with acute exacerbation of chronic obstructive pulmonary disease benefit from noninvasive positive-pressure ventilation? A systematic review of the literature. *Ann Intern Med.* 2003;138:861–70.
2. Masip J, Roque M, Sanchez B et al. Noninvasive ventilation in acute cardiogenic pulmonary edema: Systematic review and metaanalysis. *JAMA.* 2005;294:3124–30.
3. Nava S, Hill N. Non-invasive ventilation in acute respiratory failure. *Lancet.* 2009;374:250–9.
4. Sinuff T, Cook DJ, Keenan SP et al. Noninvasive ventilation for acute respiratory failure near the end of life. *Crit Care Med.* 2008;36:789–94.
5. Clarke DE, Vaughan L, Raffin TA. Noninvasive positive pressure ventilation for patients with terminal respiratory failure: The ethical and economic costs of delaying the inevitable are too great. *Am J Crit Care.* 1994;3:4–5.
6. Evans TW, Albert RK, Non-invasive positive pressure ventilation in acute respiratory failure. *Am J Respir Crit Care Med.* 2001;163:283–91.
7. Crippen DW, Whetstine LM. Noninvasive ventilation and palliative care: Unfolding the promise. *Crit Care Med.* 2004;32:881–2.
8. Henessy D, Juzwishin K, Yergens D et al. Outcomes of elderly survivors of intensive care. A review of the literature. *Chest.* 2005;127:1764–74.
9. Roebuck J. When does old age begin? The evolution of the English definition. *J Soc Hist.* 1979;12:416–28.
10. Campion EW, Mulley AG, Goldstein RL et al. Medical intensive care for the elderly: A study of current use, costs, and outcomes. *J Am Med Assoc.* 1981;246:2052–6.
11. Bo M, Massaia M, Raspo S et al. Predictive factors of in hospital mortality in older patients admitted to a medical intensive care unit. *J Am Geriatr Soc.* 2003;51:529–33.
12. Wenger NS, Solomon DS, Roth CP et al. The quality of medical care provided to vulnerable community-dwelling older patients. *Ann Intern Med.* 2003;139: 740–7.
13. Anonymous. *World population ageing: 1950–2050.* New York: Department of Economic and Social Affairs PD; 2001.
14. Population Division, Department of Economic and Social Affairs. United Nations: World population ageing 1950–2050. Available at http://www.un.org /esa/population/publications/worldageing19502050 (access 11 March 2018).
15. Rockwood K, Noseworthy TW, Gibney RT et al. One year outcomes of elderly and young patients admitted to intensive care units. *Crit Care Med.* 1993;21:687–91.
16. Needham DM, Bronskill SE, Sibbald WJ et al. Mechanical ventilation in Ontario, 1992–2000: Incidence, survival, and hospital bed utilization of noncardiac surgery adult patients. *Crit Care Med.* 2004;32:1504–9.
17. Owen A, Cox S. Diagnosis of heart failure in elderly patients in primary care. *Eur J Heart Fail.* 2001;3:79–81.
18. Caruana L, Petrie MC, Davie AP, McMurray JJ. Do patients with suspected heart failure and preserved left ventricular systolic function suffer from 'diastolic heart failure' or from misdiagnosis? A prospective descriptive study. *BMJ.* 2000;321: 215–8.
19. Cowie MR, Struthers AD, Wood DA et al. Value of natriuretic peptides in assessment of patients with possible new heart failure in primary care. *Lancet.* 1997;350:1349–53.
20. Cleland JG, Cohen-Solal A, Aguilar JC et al. Management of heart failure in primary care (the IMPROVEMENT of heart failure programme): An international survey. *Lancet.* 2002;360:1631–9.
21. Heyland DK, Lavery JV, Tranmer JE et al. Dying in Canada: Is it an institutionalized, technologically supported experience? *J Palliat Care.* 2000;16:S10–6.

22. Cook D, Rocker G, Marshall J et al. Withdrawal of mechanical ventilation in anticipation of death in the intensive care unit. *N Engl J Med.* 2003;349:1123–32.
23. Torres OH, Francia E, Longobardi V et al. Short and long term outcomes of older patients in intermediate care unit. *Intensive Care Med.* 2006;32:1052–9.
24. Somme D, Maillet J-M, Gisselbrecht M et al. Critically ill old and the oldest-old patients in intensive care: Short- and long-term outcomes. *Intensive Care Med* 2003;29:2137–43.
25. Martin GS, Mannino DM, Moss M. The effect of age on the development and outcome of adult sepsis. *Crit Care Med* 2006;34:15–21.
26. Boumendil A, Aegerter P, Guidet B, CUB-Rea Network. Treatment intensity and outcome of patients aged 80 and older in intensive care units: A multicentre matched-cohort study. *J Am Geriatr Soc* 2005;53:88–93.
27. Campion EW, Muley AG, Goldstein RL et al. Medical intensive care for the elderly: A study of current use, costs, and outcomes. *JAMA.* 1981;246:2052–6.
28. Townsend J, Frank AO, Fermont D et al. Terminal cancer care and patients' preference for place of death: A prospective study. *BMJ.* 1990;301:415–7.
29. Stajduhar KI, Allan DE, Cohen SR, Heyland DK. Preferences for location of death of seriously ill hospitalized patients: Perspectives from Canadian patients and their family caregivers. *Palliat Med.* 2008;22:85–8.
30. Lynn J, Teno JM, Phillips RS et al. Perceptions by family members of the dying experiences of older and seriously ill patients: SUPPORT Investigators. *Ann Intern Med.* 1997;126:97–106.
31. Hakim RB, Teno JM, Harrell FE Jr et al. Factors associated with do-not-resuscitate orders: Patients' preferences, prognoses, and judgments: SUPPORT Investigators: Study to understand prognoses and preferences for outcome and risks of treatment. *Ann Intern Med.* 1996;125:284–93.
32. Winter L, Lawton MP, Ruckdeschel K. Preferences for prolonging life: A prospect theory approach. *Int J Aging Hum Dev.* 2003;56:155–70.
33. Somogyi-Zalud E, Zhong Z, Hamel MB, Lynn J. The use of life-sustaining treatments in hospitalized persons aged 80 and older. *J Am Geratr Soc.* 2002;50:930–4.
34. SUPPORT Investigators. A controlled trial to improve care for seriously ill hospitalized patients. *JAMA.* 1995;274:1591–8.
35. Mehta S, Hill NS. Noninvasive ventilation. *Am J Respir Crit Care Med.* 2001;163:540–77.
36. Demoule A, Girou E, Richard JC et al. Increased use of noninvasive ventilation in French intensive care units. *Intensive Care Med.* 2006;32:1747–55.
37. Schortgen F, Follin A, Piccari L et al. Results of noninvasive ventilation in very old patients. *Ann Intensive Care.* 2012;2:5.
38. Peter JV, Moran JL, Phillips-Hughes J et al. Noninvasive ventilation in acute respiratory failure: A meta-analysis update. *Crit Care Med.* 2002;30:555–62.
39. Lightowler JV, Wedzicha JA, Elliott MW, Ram FS. Non-invasive positive pressure ventilation to treat respiratory failure resulting from exacerbations of chronic obstructive pulmonary disease: Cochrane systematic review and meta-analysis. *BMJ.* 2003;326:185.
40. Chandra D, Stamm JA, Taylor B et al. Outcomes of noninvasive ventilation for acute exacerbations of chronic obstructive pulmonary disease in the United States, 1998–2008. *Am J Respir Crit Care Med.* 2012;185:152–9.
41. Benhamou D, Girault C, Faure C et al. Nasal mask ventilation in acute respiratory failure: Experience in elderly patients. *Chest.* 1992;102:912–7.
42. Balami JS, Packham SM, Gosney MA. Non-invasive ventilation for respiratory failure due to acute exacerbations of chronic obstructive pulmonary disease in older patients. *Age Ageing.* 2006;35:78–9.
43. Rozzini R, Sabatini T, Trabucchi M. Non-invasive ventilation for respiratory failure in elderly patients. *Age Ageing.* 2006;35:546–7.
44. Nava S, Grassi M, Fanfulla F et al. Non-invasive ventilation in elderly patients with acute hypercapnic respiratory failure: A randomised controlled trial. *Age Ageing.* 2011;40:444–50.
45. Vital FM, Saconato H, Ladeira MT et al. Non-invasive positive pressure ventilation (CPAP or bilevel NPPV) for cardiogenic pulmonary edema. *Cochrane Database Syst Rev.* 2008;3: CD005351.
46. Collins SP, Mielniczuk LM, Whittingham HA et al. The use of noninvasive ventilation in emergency department patients with acute cardiogenic pulmonary edema: A systematic review. *Ann Emerg Med.* 2006;48:260–9.
47. Winck JC, Azevedo LF, Costa-Pereira A et al. Efficacy and safety of non-invasive ventilation in the treatment of acute cardiogenic pulmonary edema – A systematic review and meta-analysis. *Crit Care.* 2006;10:R69.
48. Masip J, Roque M, Sánchez B et al. Noninvasive ventilation in acute cardiogenic pulmonary edema: Systematic review and meta-analysis. *JAMA.* 2005;294:3124–30.
49. Mariani J, Macchia A, Belziti C et al. Noninvasive ventilation in acute cardiogenic pulmonary edema: A meta-analysis of randomized controlled trials. *J Cardiac Fail.* 2011;17:850–9.

50. L'Her E, Duquesne F, Girou E et al. Noninvasive continuous positive airway pressure in elderly cardiogenic pulmonary edema patients. *Intensive Care Med.* 2004;30:882–8.
51. Gray A, Goodacre S, Newby DE et al. Noninvasive ventilation in acute cardiogenic pulmonary edema. *N Engl J Med.* 2008;359:142–51.
52. Curtis JR, Cook DJ, Sinuff T et al. Noninvasive positive pressure ventilation in critical and palliative care settings: Understanding the goals of therapy. *Crit Care Med.* 2007;35:932–9.
53. Crausman RS. The ethics of bilevel positive airway pressure. *Chest.* 1998;113:258.
54. Chu CM, Chan VL, Wong IW et al. Noninvasive ventilation in patients with acute hypercapnic exacerbation of chronic obstructive pulmonary disease who refused endotracheal intubation. *Crit Care Med.* 2004;32:372–7.
55. Freichels TA. Palliative ventilatory support: Use of noninvasive positive pressure ventilation in terminal respiratory insufficiency. *Am J Crit Care.* 1994;3:6–10.
56. Clarke DE, Vaughan L, Raffin TA. Noninvasive positive pressure ventilation for patients with terminal respiratory failure: The ethical and economic costs of delaying the inevitable are too great. *Am J Crit Care.* 1994;3:4–5.
57. Burns KEA, Meade MO, Premji A, Adhikari NKJ. Noninvasive positive-pressure ventilation as a weaning strategy for intubated adults with respiratory failure. *Cochrane Database Syst Rev.* 2013;12:CD004127.
58. Camhi SL, Mercado AF, Morrison RS et al. Deciding in the dark: Advance directives and continuation of treatment in chronic critical illness. *Crit Care Med.* 2009;37:919–25.
59. Wunsch H, Harrison DA, Harvey S, Rowan K. End-of-life decisions: A cohort study of the withdrawal of all active treatment in intensive care units in the United Kingdom. *Intensive Care Med.* 2005;6:823–31.
60. Azoulay E, Pochard F, Kentish-Barnes N, and the FAMIREA Study Group. Risk of post-traumatic stress symptoms in family members of intensive care unit patients. *Am J Respir Crit Care Med.* 2005;171:987–94.
61. Emmanuel EJ, Emmanuel LL. Proxy decision making for incompetent patients: An ethical and empirical analysis. *JAMA.* 1992;267:2067–71.
62. Lloyd CB, Nietert PJ, Silvestri GA. Intensive care decision making in the seriously ill and elderly. *Crit Care Med.* 2004;32:649–54.
63. Nelson JE, Tandon N, Mercado AF et al. Brain dysfunction: Another burden for the chronically critically ill. *Arch Intern Med.* 2006;166:1993–9.
64. Reilly BM, Magnussen CR, Ross J et al. Can we talk? Inpatient discussions about advance directives in a community hospital: Attending physicians' attitudes, their inpatients' wishes, and reported experience. *Arch Intern Med.* 1994;154:2299–308.
65. Essebag V, Cantarovich M, Crelinsten G. Routine advance directive and organ donation questioning on admission to hospital. *Ann R Coll Phys Surg Canada.* 2002;35:225–31.
66. Crippen D. Terminally weaning awake patients from life sustaining mechanical ventilation: The critical care physician's role in comfort measures during the dying process. *Clin Intensive Care.* 1992;3:206–12.
67. Schneiderman LJ, Gilmer T, Teetzel HD. Impact of ethics consultations in the intensive care setting: A randomized, controlled trial. *Crit Care Med.* 2000;28:3920–4.
68. Crippen DW, Whetstine LM. Noninvasive ventilation and palliative care: Unfolding the promise. *Crit Care Med.* 2004;32:881–2.
69. Danis M, Federman D, Fins JJ et al. Incorporating palliative care into critical care education: Principles, challenges, and opportunities. *Crit Care Med.* 1999;27:2005–13.
70. Carlucci A, Richard JC, Wysocki M et al. Noninvasive versus conventional mechanical ventilation. An epidemiologic survey. *Am J Respir Crit Care Med.* 2001;163:874–80.

53

Post-surgery non-invasive ventilation

MARIA LAURA VEGA AND STEFANO NAVA

KEY MESSAGES

- Post-operative pulmonary complications following surgery are common and associated with increased morbidity and mortality and hospital length of stay.
- Few randomised controlled trials have been performed to assess the efficacy of non-invasive ventilation (NIV) both as a preventing tool to avoid overt acute respiratory failure and as a curative treatment for acute respiratory failure.
- The preventing role of NIV is still not fully elucidated.
- The use of NIV as a curative tool is particularly indicated in patients showing hypoxia after major abdominal or thoracic surgery.
- Before the initiation of NIV, surgical complications (anastomosis leakage, intra-abdominal sepsis etc.) should be treated and possibly eliminated.

INTRODUCTION

Post-operative pulmonary complications following surgery are common and associated with increased morbidity and mortality and hospital length of stay.[1,2] Hypoxaemia and/or acute respiratory failure (ARF) mainly develop following abdominal and/or thoracic surgery.[1–3] Anaesthesia, pain and surgery (more so as the site of the surgery approaches the diaphragm) induce alterations in respiratory function: hypoxaemia, reduced pulmonary volume and atelectasis,[4] associated with a restrictive syndrome and diaphragm dysfunction.[5] These alterations of respiratory function occur early after surgery and are most often transient. The major objectives are, first, to prevent the occurrence of post-operative complications and, second, if ARF does occur, to ensure oxygen administration and carbon dioxide removal while avoiding intubation.[1,4] Non-invasive ventilation (NIV) does not require an artificial airway (endotracheal tube or tracheostomy), and its use is well established for ARF prevention (prophylactic treatment) and treatment of ARF to avoid reintubation (curative treatment). Studies demonstrate that patient-related risk factors, such as chronic obstructive pulmonary disease, age older than 60 years, American Society of Anesthesiologists class of II or higher, obesity, functional dependence and congestive heart failure increase the risk for post-operative pulmonary complications.[1–4]

This chapter aims to review the main respiratory alterations induced by surgery and anaesthesia to justify using post-operative NIV and to present the results of studies on preventive and curative NIV in a surgical context.

SURGERY AND ANAESTHESIA-INDUCED RESPIRATORY ALTERATIONS AND RATIONALE FOR POST-OPERATIVE NON-INVASIVE VENTILATION USE

Major changes in respiratory function occur in all patients after anaesthesia and surgical incisions, especially on the thorax and upper abdomen. The main pathophysiological mechanisms of post-surgical ARF are shunt and changes in ventilation/perfusion ratio, generated during the surgical anaesthetics, where 90% of patients undergoing general anaesthesia suffer from the collapse of 20% of their alveoli. The manipulation, the trauma to the lung and high FiO_2 levels used, leads to a decrease in functional residual capacity and impaired ventilation/perfusion.[6,7] In addition, perioperative-related modifications of the ventilatory system may be aggravated by other factors such as excessive perioperative vascular loading,[8] transfusion-related acute lung injury, inflammation and aspiration. Another variable that directly affects this mechanism is pain, resulting in a rapid and shallow breathing pattern that changes lung volumes, so it is crucially important to implement a protocol for pain management in these cases.[9] Moreover, sedatives and neuromuscular blocking agents, used during anaesthesia, affect the upper and lower airways and the respiratory muscles, causing dysfunction and incoordination, thus resulting in an increased work of breathing (WOB).[10] Diaphragmatic function should also be evaluated as it is often found as a post-operative dysfunction.[11,12]

The expected benefit of NIV would be to partially compensate for the affected respiratory function by reducing the WOB, by improving alveolar ventilation associated with increased gas exchange, by reducing left ventricular afterload with an increase in cardiac output and by reducing atelectasis.[13]

CONTINUOUS POSITIVE AIRWAY PRESSURE AND BI-LEVEL POSITIVE AIRWAY PRESSURE

Two types of NIV are commonly used: continuous positive airway pressure (CPAP) and bi-level positive airway pressure (BiLevel), which refers to the combinations of pressure support ventilation (PSV) with positive end expiratory pressure (PEEP).

The way to administer positive pressure is through a multiprocessed ventilator, a continuous flow equipment or Boussignac CPAP (flow accelerator + Boussignac valve). When choosing a device, the characteristics of the patient and the resources available in the unit must be analysed, since there is no evidence that shows the superiority of one over another.

Non-invasive ventilation application

Post-operative NIV can be applied in two ways. The first is a 'prophylactic' application in order to prevent post-operative ARF, and the second consists of a 'curative' application, in order to alleviate respiratory failure.

When analysing patients according to the *equation of motion* ($P_{RS} = E_{RS} \times Vt + R_{aw} \times Flow + PEEP_{tot}$, where RS represents the respiratory system, P is the pressure, E is the elastance, Vt is the tidal volume and R is the resistance), the increase in the elastic load (E) due to loss of the distensibility of the RS and the increase in the resistive load (R) due to the collapse of the small airway become manifested.[14] The use of CPAP/PEEP efficiently counteracts the increased loads, stabilising the upper airway, avoiding alveolar cyclic collapse (atelectrauma), increasing CRF and consequently compliance.[14] If another level of pressure (PSV/inspiratory positive air pressure [IPAP]) is added to PEEP, it is also possible to unload the respiratory muscles, vitally important in patients with increased ventilatory demand during the post-operative period.

Setting up NIV and duration of trial

CPAP of 7–10 cm H_2O are required to keep tracheal pressure positive during the entire respiratory cycle. In PSV/PEEP, patient comfort and interface acceptance may be improved by starting with PEEP alone and then slowly increasing the PSV level. We recommend starting with a PSV of 3–5 cm H_2O making increments to achieve a 6–10 mL/kg expiratory tidal volume.[15] PEEP is started at 3–5 cm H_2O and increased as needed to improve oxygenation without adverse haemodynamic effects. The insufflation pressure (PSV/PEEP) applied should be less than 25 cm H_2O. These setting recommendations are based solely on clinical experience without any formal data to support the superiority of one technique over another.[16]

Evidence to guide the duration of a NIV trial is lacking, so the recommendations are largely based on practitioner experience. In the post-operative area, we recommend 'sequential' use, wherein periods of use alternate with lengthy ventilator-free periods, and total daily use range between 3 and 12 hours, depending on the type of application (curative or prophylactic use). In our practice,[9] during the first 24 hours, for the majority of the patients, NIV is applied for approximately 30–45 minutes at 2- to 4-hour intervals (prophylactic), depending on the patient's clinical condition. Some patients are treated during the initial period with NIV for 60–90 minutes at 2- to 3-hour intervals (range: 8–2 hours/day; curative). Between the periods of NIV, the patients breathe through a Venturi mask or high-flow cannula.[17,18] The length of NIV cycles is progressively reduced and NIV is completely withdrawn.

Cardiovascular effects that occur on patients under positive pressure are complex. The reduction of venous return and left ventricular afterload is the main variable to be monitored. The decrease in venous return will depend on the decrease of the right ventricular preload, while the decrease of the afterload imposed on the left ventricle will be directly related to the decrease in pulmonary vascular resistance. Anyway, haemodynamic complications caused by the application of NIV are not reported.

Interfaces

To date, there is no evidence to support the use of a particular interface in the surgical context. Therefore, practitioners should try different mask sizes and types in an effort to enhance patient comfort, considering mask dead space and the patient's breathing pattern.[11,12,19,20]

Contraindications and limitations

Patient cooperation without deteriorating mental status, absence of haemodynamic instability and ability to protect airways are crucial to the application and the success of NIV. The relative and absolute contraindications of NIV use are given in Box 53.1.

BOX 53.1: Contraindications for the use of post-operative NIV

Absolute contraindications
- Cardiac or respiratory arrest
- Multiple organ failure
- Severe agitation or encephalopathy
- Copious secretions
- Uncontrolled vomiting
- Inability to protect airway
- Severe upper gastrointestinal bleeding or haemoptysis
- Immediate endotracheal intubation necessary (except for preoxygenation NIV)
- Facial trauma
- Haemodynamic instability or unstable cardiac arrhythmia

Relative contraindications
- Mildly decreased level of consciousness
- Progressive severe respiratory failure
- Uncooperative patient who cannot be calmed or comforted

Problems related to digestive tubes and their relationship with NIV

Upper digestive tract stitching necessitates great prudence with the use of early post-operative NIV. Historically, NIV was contraindicated in cases of upper gastrointestinal tract anastomoses. In fact, there is a risk of intradigestive air insufflation when high insufflation pressures are applied (PSV+ PEEP > 25 cm H_2O).[10]

RESULTS OF THE USE OF NON-INVASIVE VENTILATION WITH PREVENTIVE OR CURATIVE INTENT IN DIFFERENT TYPES OF SURGERY (TABLE 53.1)[21–33]

Cardiac surgery

Restrictive syndrome following cardiac surgery is generally less severe than that observed after thoracic or abdominal surgery. However, the incidence of diaphragm dysfunction is higher.[3]

PREVENTIVE NIV

Early studies mainly compared CPAP to standard treatment (oxygen/physiotherapy). Most of them reported improved oxygenation and ventilation parameters. None of these studies found any reduction in the incidence of atelectasis in the groups treated by CPAP, except for Jousela et al.[34] and Gust et al.,[35] who obtained a reduction in extravascular lung water when NIV was applied. Matte et al.,[21] in a study including 96 patients, evaluated 'preventive' NIV in the first 2 days following surgery. Various strategies were compared in three randomised groups. The first group received 1 hour of bi-level NIV every 3 hours with an average assistance level of 12 cm H_2O of PSV and 5 cm H_2O of PEEP. The second group received a 1-hour session of CPAP at 5 cm H_2O every 3 hours, and a third group had 20 min of incentive spirometry every 2 hours. Using NIV, whether with one or two pressure levels, improves oxygenation. However, the incidence of atelectasis was similar (12%–15%) in all three groups.[21] Pasquina et al.[22] compared the effect of systematic application of a 30-min trial of 5 cm H_2O CPAP with NIV (PSV 10/PEEP 5) in two groups of 75 patients. The PSV/PEEP group improved radiological scores (i.e. less marked atelectasis) on standard chest X-ray. There was no significant difference in oxygenation parameters.[22] Zarbock et al.[23] reported, in a prospective randomised study, which included 500 patients, the effect of prophylactic nasal CPAP of 10 cm H_2O for at least 6 hours per day following surgery in comparison to standard treatment including 10 min of intermittent nasal CPAP at 10 cm H_2O every 4 hours. In the study group, CPAP improved arterial oxygenation, reduced the incidence of pneumonia and reintubation rate and reduced the ICU readmission rate. The author refers to the pressure values applied in previous studies, defining them as insufficient to reach the maximum potential of this treatment and proposes an efficient positive pressure level of 10 cm of water. On the other hand, no differences in mortality or length of stay were reported.[36]

CURATIVE NIV

In a trial published in 2007, authors evaluated 57 patients with ARF and increased WOB during the post-operative period. NIV was applied avoiding reintubation rates in more than 50% of the patients. The initial IPAP was 10 cm H_2O, adjustable in order to reach 5–7 mL/kg of exhaled volume and PEEP of 5 cm of water, also adjustable, until reaching a SaO_2 equal or greater than 95% with a FiO_2 of 0.6. The remaining 45% of the patients were reintubated because of the progression of the respiratory failure, haemodynamic instability and deterioration of consciousness. The latter group presented higher cardiac comorbidities, high respiratory rates and lack of improvement in oxygenation during the first hour of NIV.[37] Additionally, in a retrospective analysis, 425 patients with ventilatory failure during the post-operative period of cardiac surgery were studied. One hundred twenty-five patients required immediate reconnection to invasive mechanical ventilation (IMV), 264 received CPAP and 36 were treated with BiLevel; 25.8% of the patients in the CPAP group needed reintubation, while 22.2% in the BiLevel group. Reported mortality was 8.8%, 4.2% and 5.6%, for the immediate reintubated patients, the CPAP and BiLevel group, respectively. In this analysis, patients treated with NIV also had fewer hospital stay and ICU stay. García Delgado[38] retrospectively analysed data from 1225 cardiac surgeries, concluding that obese patients with a BMI > 30 and those with lobar atelectasis are those who most benefit by the application of NIV. The authors described these variables as success factors.

Table 53.1 Main studies on post-surgery NIV classified by type of surgery and date

Authors	Year	Type of surgery	Study design	Indication	Patients	NIV mode and main settings	Interface	Results	Success rate of NIV (%)
Gust et al.[8]	1996	Cardiac	Physiological	Preventive	$n = 75$; 3 groups	SB; CPAP; PSV + PEEP	Facial CPAP Nasal PSV + PEEP	Extravascular lung water decrease	NA
Matte et al.[21]	2000	Cardiac	Physiological	Preventive	$n = 96$; 3 groups	SB; CPAP + 5; PSV + 12 – PEEP + 5	Facial	Oxygenation and lung volumes improvement	NA
Pasquina et al.[22]	2004	Cardiac	Physiological	Preventive	$n = 150$; 2 groups	CPAP + 5; PSV + 10 – PEEP + 5	Facial	Atelectasis decrease	100
Zarbock et al.[23]	2009	Cardiac	Prospective, randomised	Preventive	$n = 500$	CPAP	Nasal	Oxygenation improvement, reduced the incidence of pulmonary complications and reduced readmission rate to ICU	99
International Consensus Conferences in Intensive Care Medicine[16]	1997	Pulmonary	Physiological	Preventive	$n = 20$; 2 groups	SB; PSV + 10 – PEEP + 5	Nasal	Oxygenation improvement	NA
Rocco et al.[24]	2001	Pulmonary (transplant)	Retrospective, observational	Curative	$n = 21$	PSV + 14 – PEEP + 5	Facial	Feasibility, safety, oxygenation improvement	86
Auriant et al.[25]	2001	Pulmonary	Prospective, randomised	Curative	$n = 48$; 2 groups	SB; PSV + 9 – PEEP + 4	Nasal	Intubation and mortality decrease	79
Lefebvre et al.[26]	2009	Pulmonary	Retrospective, observational	Curative	$n = 89$	CPAP and/or NIV	Facial or nasal	Feasibility, safety, oxygenation improvement	85

(Continued)

Table 53.1 (Continued) Main studies on post-surgery NIV classified by type of surgery and date

Authors	Year	Type of surgery	Study design	Indication	Patients	NIV mode and main settings	Interface	Results	Success rate of NIV (%)
Stock et al.[27]	1985	Abdominal (cholecystectomy)	Physiological	Preventive	n = 65; 2 groups	SB; CPAP + 8	Facial	Atelectasis decrease, FRC improvement	NA
Joris et al.[28]	1997	Abdominal (obsess-gastroplasty)	Physiological	Preventive	n = 33; 3 groups	SB; PSV + 8 – PEEP + 5; PSV + 12 – PEEP + 5	Nasal	Oxygenation and lung volume improvement	NA
Kindgen-Miles et al.[29]	2000	Thoracoabdominal	Prospective, observational	Curative	n = 20	CPAP + 10	Nasal	Oxygenation improvement	90
Antonelli et al.[30]	2000	Thoracoabdominal (liver transplant, renal, lung)	Prospective, randomised	Curative	n = 40; 2 groups	SB; PSV + 15 PEEP + 6	Facial	Intubation and mortality decrease	80
Kindgen-Miles et al.[39]	2005	Thoracoabdominal	Prospective, randomised	Preventive	n = 50; 2 groups	SB; CPAP + 10	Nasal	Oxygenation improvement, hospital stay decrease	96
Jaber et al.[13]	2005	Abdominal	Prospective, observational	Curative	n = 72	PSV + 14 – PEEP + 6	Facial	Feasibility, safety, oxygenation improvement	66
Squadrone et al.[31]	2005	Abdominal	Prospective, randomised	Curative	n = 209; 2 groups	SB; CPAP + 7.5	Facial and helmet	Intubation and sepsis decrease	99
Michelet et al.[32]	2009	Abdominal and thoracic (oesophagectomy)	Retrospective, Case mix	Curative	n = 72; 2 groups	SB; PSV + 13-PEEP + 5	Facial	Lower intubation, ARDS rate and lower ICU stay	75
Wallet et al.[33]	2009	Abdominal	Prospective, observational	Curative	n = 72	SB; PSV + 15 – PEEP + 6	Facial	Feasibility, safety, oxygenation improvement	58

Note: CPAP, continuous positive airway pressure; ICU, intensive care unit; NA, not applied; PEEP, positive end-expiratory pressure; PSV, pressure support ventilation; SB, spontaneous breathing.

Thoracic surgery

Respiratory complications following thoracic surgery are similar to those reported in cardiac surgery. Unlike heart surgery, pulmonary sutures can lead to air leakage or fistulas, or immunosuppression in transplanted patients, in which NIV plays a relevant role.

PREVENTIVE NIV

In a physiological study, International Consensus Conferences in Intensive Care Medicine[16] studied the effects of a 1-hour NIV trial after pulmonary resection; NIV improved oxygenation without increasing leaks around thoracic drains compared with a control group who did not receive NIV.[16] Parke et al.[17] reported a prospective randomised clinical trial on the benefits of NIV administered pre- and post-operatively. Patients were required to follow standard treatment with or without NIV for 7 days at home before the surgery and 3 days post-operatively. In this study, 2 hours after surgery, oxygenation and lung volume values were significantly better in the NIV group.[17] Moreover, hospital stay was significantly longer in the control group. This first prospective randomised study has shown that the prophylactic use of NIV pre- and post-operatively significantly reduces pulmonary dysfunction after lung resection.[17]

CURATIVE NIV

Rocco et al.[24] described their experience of NIV in 21 patients who developed ARF after lung transplantation. In this case, BiLevel was able to avoid reintubation in 18 patients. Within the group that progressed to reintubation, the main causes were acute respiratory distress syndrome (ARDS) and pneumonia. In a prospective randomised study including 24 patients in each group, Auriant et al.[25] showed the efficiency of nasal NIV in ARF after lung resection. NIV was delivered using a single circuit ventilator (plus physiotherapic treatment) compared with standard treatment (oxygen–physiotherapy–bronchodilators). The former reduced the need for IMV (21% vs. 50%) and mortality (13% vs. 38%). Lefebvre et al.[26] confirmed in an observational prospective survey the feasibility and efficacy of early NIV in ARF following lung resection where the overall success rate of NIV was 85%.

Abdominal surgery

The risk of post-operative hypoxaemia increases as the surgical region gets closer to the diaphragm. Endotracheal intubation and IMV may be necessary in 8%–10% of these patients. Respiratory changes are in the first few hours after surgery, so oxygenation and ventilation have to be effectively provided in the early post-operative period.

PREVENTIVE NIV

Hypoxaemia complicates the recovery of 30%–50% of patients after abdominal surgery. Warner[3] showed that applying CPAP in patients having cholecystectomy by laparotomy led to a significant reduction in the incidence of atelectasis compared with treatment by incentive spirometry. After bariatric surgery (gastroplasty), Joris et al.[28] demonstrated a significant reduction of the occurrence of restrictive syndrome and significant improvement in oxygenation with NIV applied in the first post-operative 24 hours. Compared with the control group, forced vital capacity significantly improved only with a moderately high PSV level (12 cm H_2O). This finding remains important today, given the sharp increase in the rate of obesity surgery.[34] In a non-controlled study,[40] Boussignac CPAP of 10 cm H_2O improved blood oxygenation compared to standard treatment in 19 morbidly obese patients scheduled for elective open gastric bypass. In the study by Joris et al.,[28] which investigated the efficiency of post-operative nasal BiLevel in morbidly obese patients who had undergone gastroplasty, authors showed that the effect of expired positive air pressure 4 cm H_2O and IPAP 12 cm H_2O on blood gas was maintained despite the treatment being interrupted. They conclude that the prophylactic use of BiLevel can be beneficial in patients at high risk with regard to the development of pulmonary complications.

Compared to respiratory therapy (incentive spirometry or coughing and deep breathing), the periodic application of CPAP after extubation and continued in the post-operative period was associated with significantly higher arterial oxygenation, a quicker recovery of lung volumes and a lower rate of atelectasis.[27,41,42]

CURATIVE NIV

Patients with post-operative ARF have been included with other types of patients in studies evaluating NIV to treat ARF of multiple causes.[16] In these studies, no comparison has been made between patients with ARF resulting from medical causes and those with post-operative ARF, probably because of the heterogeneity and small numbers of patients included. Varon et al.[43] reported the feasibility of NIV in post-operative ARF in cancer patients (25 gastrointestinal, 15 urogenital, 6 lung). Intubation was avoided in 70% of patients.[21] Kindgen-Milles et al.,[29] in a non-controlled prospective study, showed that CPAP rapidly improved oxygenation and avoided intubation in 18 of 20 patients treated after abdominal and/or thoracic surgery. Jaber et al.[15] reported, in an observational study, their experience over a 2-year period using NIV in 72 patients with severe ARF after gastrointestinal surgery. In this prospective trial, intubation was avoided in 66% of patients. More severe initial hypoxaemia and lower improvement of PaO_2 after NIV were predictive of NIV failure. Jaber's results were confirmed in a recent study that included patients who developed ARF after abdominal surgery, whereby intubation was avoided in 58% of the patients.[33]

In a controlled randomised trial in organ transplant recipients with hypoxaemic ARF, Antonelli et al.[30] showed that NIV reduced the rate of intubation, the incidence of fatal complications and ICU mortality compared with oxygen treatment alone. More recently, Michelet et al.[32] compared the efficacy of NIV with conventional treatment in 36 patients who developed post-operative ARF after planned oesophagectomy. Authors showed that the use of NIV was associated with a lower intubation rate, a lower incidence of ARDS and a reduction in UCI length of stay.

A large Italian study[31] was stopped early due to reduction in intubation related to CPAP therapy in hypoxaemic patients after abdominal surgery. This randomised study included 209 patients in two groups: one group received CPAP of 7.5 cm H_2O and a control group received oxygen via a Venturi mask. The PaO_2/FiO_2 was higher in the patients treated with CPAP. Moreover, patients receiving CPAP had significantly lower ICU length of stay and infection rates compared with the control group.

CONCLUSION

Regardless of the presence of complications, thoracic and/or abdominal surgery necessarily and profoundly alters the respiratory system for long periods. IMV may be responsible for increased morbidity. During the past decade, NIV has proven to be an effective strategy to reduce intubation rates, nosocomial infections, ICU and hospital lengths of stay and morbidity and mortality in patients with either hypercapnic or non-hypercapnic ARF. However, before the initiation of NIV in patients with post-operative ARF, surgical complications (anastomosis leakage, intra-abdominal sepsis etc.) should be treated and eliminated. Then, if the patient is cooperative and able to protect their airway, NIV can be initiated with due regard to safety procedures and contraindications. The application of post-operative NIV by a trained and experienced intensive care unit team, with careful patient selection, should optimise patient outcomes.

REFERENCES

1. Qaseem A, Snow V, Fitterman N et al. Risk assessment for and strategies to reduce perioperative pulmonary complications for patients undergoing noncardiothoracic surgery: A guideline from the American College of Physicians. *Ann Intern Med.* 2006;144:575–80.
2. Smetana G. Preoperative pulmonary evaluation. *N Engl J Med.* 1999;340:937–45.
3. Warner M. Preventing postoperative pulmonary complications: The role of the anesthesiologist. *Anesthesiology.* 2000;92:1467–72.
4. Duggan M, Kavanagh BP. Pulmonary atelectasis: A pathogenic perioperative entity. *Anesthesiology.* 2005;102:838–54.
5. Simonneau G, Vivien A, Sartene R et al. Diaphragm dysfunction induced by upper abdominal surgery: Role of postoperative pain. *Am Rev Respir Dis.* 1983;128:899–903.
6. Magnusson L. New concepts of atelectasis during general anaesthesia. *Brit J Anaesth.* 2003;91:61–72.
7. Hedenstierna G. Alveolar collapse and closure of airways: Regular effects of anaesthesia. *Clin Physiol Funct Imaging.* 2003;23:123–9.
8. Gust R, Gottschalk A, Schmidt H et al. Effects of continuous (CPAP) and bi-level positive airway pressure (BiPAP) on extravascular lung water after extubation of the trachea in patients following coronary artery bypass grafting. *Intensive Care Med.* 1996;22:1345–50.
9. Pasquina P, Merlani P, Granier J, Ricou B. Continuous positive airway pressure versus noninvasive pressure support ventilation to treat atelectasis after cardiac surgery. *Anesth Analg.* 2004;99:1001–8.
10. Sasaki N, Meyer M, Eikermann M. Postoperative respiratory muscle dysfunction. *Anesthesiology.* 2013;118:961–78.
11. Vassilakopoulos T, Mastora Z, Katsaounou P et al. Contribution of pain to inspiratory muscle dysfunction after upper abdominal surgery: A randomized controlled trial. *Am J Respir Crit Care Med.* 2000; 161:1372–5.
12. Ford G, Whitelaw W, Rosenal T et al. Diaphragm function after upper abdominal surgery in humans 1–3. *Am Rev Respir Dis.* 1983;127:431–6.
13. Jaber S, Gallix B, Sebbane M et al. Noninvasive ventilation improves alveolar recruitment in postoperative patients with acute respiratory failure: A CT-scan study. *Intensive Care Med.* 2005;S148.
14. Prinianakis G, Klimathianaki M, Georgopoulos D. Physiological rationale of noninvasive mechanical ventilation use in acute respiratory failure. *Eur Respir Monogr.* 2008;41:3–23.
15. Jaber S, Delay J, Sebbane M et al. Outcomes of patients with acute respiratory failure after abdominal surgery treated with noninvasive positive-pressure ventilation. *Chest.* 2005;128:2688–95.
16. International Consensus Conferences in Intensive Care Medicine. Noninvasive positive pressure ventilation in acute respiratory failure. *Am J Respir Crit Care Med.* 2001;163:283–91.
17. Parke R, McGuinness S, Dixon R, Jull A. Open-label, phase II study of routine high-flow nasal oxygen therapy in cardiac surgical patients. *Br J Anaesth.* 2013;111.6:925–31.
18. Stéphan F, Barrucand B, Petit P et al. High-flow nasal oxygen vs noninvasive positive airway pressure in hypoxemic patients after cardiothoracic surgery: A randomized clinical trial. *JAMA.* 2015;313:2331–9.
19. Antonelli M, Pennisi MA, Pelosi P et al. Noninvasive positive pressure ventilation using a helmet in patients with acute exacerbation of chronic obstructive pulmonary disease: A feasibility study. *Anesthesiology.* 2004;100:16–24.
20. Conti G, Cavaliere F, Costa R et al. Noninvasive positive pressure ventilation with different interfaces in patients with respiratory failure after abdominal surgery. A match-control study. *Respir Care.* 2007;52:1463–71.
21. Matte P, Jacquet M, Vandyck M et al. Effects of conventional physiotherapy, continuous positive airway pressure and non-invasive ventilatory support

with bilevel positive airway pressure after coronary artery bypass grafting. *Acta Anaesthesiol Scand.* 2000;44:75–81.

22. Pasquina P, Merlani P, Granier J et al. Continuous positive airway pressure versus noninvasive pressure support ventilation to treat atelectasis after cardiac surgery. *Anesth Analg.* 2004;99:1001–8.
23. Zarbock A, Mueller E, Netzer S et al. Prophylactic nasal continuous positive airway pressure following cardiac surgery protects from postoperative pulmonary complications: A prospective, randomized, controlled trial in 500 patients. *Chest.* 2009;135:1252–9.
24. Rocco M, Conti G, Antonelli M et al. Non-invasive pressure support ventilation in patients with acute respiratory failure after bilateral lung transplantation. *Intensive Care Med.* 2001;27:1622–6.
25. Auriant I, Jallot A, Hervé P et al. Noninvasive ventilation reduces mortality in acute respiratory failure following lung resection. *Am J Respir Crit Care Med.* 2001;164:1231–5.
26. Lefebvre A, Lorut C, Alifano M et al. Noninvasive ventilation for acute respiratory failure after lung resection. An observational study. *Intensive Care Med.* 2009;35:663–70.
27. Stock MC, Downs JB, Gauer PK et al. Prevention of postoperative pulmonary complications with CPAP, incentive spirometry, and conservative therapy. *Chest.* 1985;87:151–7.
28. Joris J, Sottiaux T, Chiche J et al. Effect of bi-level positive airway pressure (BiPAP) nasal ventilation on the postoperative pulmonary restrictive syndrome in obese patients undergoing gastroplasty. *Chest.* 1997;111:665–70.
29. Kindgen-Milles D, Buhl R, Gabriel A et al. Nasal continuous positive airway pressure: A method to avoid endotracheal reintubation in postoperative high-risk patients with severe nonhypercapnic oxygenation failure. *Chest.* 2000;117:1106–11.
30. Antonelli M, Conti G, Bufi M et al. Noninvasive ventilation for treatment of acute respiratory failure in patients undergoing solid organ transplantation: A randomized trial. *JAMA.* 2000;283:235–41.
31. Squadrone V, Coha M, Cerutti E et al. Continuous positive airway pressure for treatment of postoperative hypoxemia: A randomized controlled trial. *JAMA.* 2005;293:589–95.
32. Michelet P, D'Journo XB, Seinaye F et al. Noninvasive ventilation for treatment of postoperative respiratory failure after oesophagectomy. *Br J Surg.* 2009;96:54–60.
33. Wallet F, Scoeffler M, Reynaud M et al. Factors associated with noninvasive ventilation failure in postoperative acute respiratory insufficiency: An observational study. *Eur J Anaesthesiol* 2009 [Epub ahead of print].
34. Jousela I, Rasanen J, Verkkala K et al. Continuous positive airway pressure by mask in patients after coronary surgery. *Acta Anaesthesiol Scand.* 1994; 38:311–16.
35. Gust R, Gottschalk A, Schmidt H et al. Effects of continuous (CPAP) and bi-level positive airway pressure (BiPAP) on extravascular lung water after extubation of the trachea in patients following coronary artery bypass grafting. *Intensive Care Med.* 1996;22:1345–50.
36. Zarbock A. Prophylactic nasal continuous positive airway pressure following cardiac surgery protects from postoperative pulmonary complications. *Chest.* 2009;135:1252.
37. Coimbra V, Lara R, Flores É et al. Application of noninvasive ventilation in acute respiratory failure after cardiovascular surgery. *Arq Bras Cardiol.* 2007; 89:270–6.
38. García-Delgado M, Navarrete I, García-Palma M, Colmenero M. Postoperative respiratory failure after cardiac surgery: Use of noninvasive ventilation. *J Cardiothorc Vasc Anesth.* 2012;26:443–7.
39. Kindgen-Milles D, Müller E, Buhl R et al. Nasal-continuous positive airway pressure reduces pulmonary morbidity and length of hospital stay following thoracoabdominal aortic surgery. *Chest.* 2005 Aug;128(2):821–8.
40. Gaszynski T, Tokarz A, Piotrowski D, Machala W. Boussignac CPAP in the postoperative period in morbidly obese patients. *Obesity Surg.* 2007;17:452–6.
41. Lindner KH, Lotz P, Ahnefeld FW. Continuous positive airway pressure effect on functional residual capacity, vital capacity and its subdivisions. *Chest.* 1987;92:66–70.
42. Ricksten SE, Bengtsson A, Soderberg C et al. Effects of periodic positive airway pressure by mask on postoperative pulmonary function. *Chest.* 1986;89:774–81.
43. Varon J, Walsh G, Fromm RJ. Feasibility of noninvasive mechanical ventilation in the treatment of acute respiratory failure in postoperative cancer patients. *J Crit Care.* 1998;13:55–7.

54

Trauma

UMBERTO LUCANGELO, MASSIMO FERLUGA AND MATTEO SEGAT

INTRODUCTION

Blunt chest trauma is a frequent finding in multiple trauma patients, with an incidence during 2015 of approximately 31% in the National Italian Registry.[1] Chest injuries are associated with a mortality rate of up to 10%, and they are responsible for 25% of deaths in multiple trauma patients.[2] Road accidents are the principal cause of blunt chest trauma (68.7%), followed by high-energy falls (24.5%), with work accidents accounting for 18% of the entire incidence.

In trauma settings, tracheal intubation and intermittent positive pressure ventilation is the gold standard in the presence of inadequate oxygenation despite supplementary oxygen.[3] Tracheal intubation is associated with the risk of developing ventilator-associated pneumonia, so this procedure (and length of invasive mechanical ventilation) could add another risk factor for pulmonary complications. Therefore, in patients with pulmonary contusion, when gas exchange is not too severely compromised and when there are no severe lesions that could lead to alterations in consciousness or haemodynamic instability, tracheal intubation should be avoided. In fact, Antonelli et al.[4] demonstrated an increased incidence of pneumonia in intubated chest and abdominal trauma patients. These authors also observed that early intubation may reduce the incidence of early-onset pneumonia, as it guarantees the adequate ventilation of atelectatic lung areas and reduces bacterial translocation; on the other hand, intubation for more than 5 days has been associated with an increased risk of developing late-onset pneumonia.

Non-invasive ventilation (NIV) provides ventilatory support using a facemask or similar, and its use recently increased in emergency departments (EDs) and intensive care units (ICUs). The main indications for its use are acute respiratory failure (ARF) in patients with relapsing chronic obstructive pulmonary disease, acute cardiogenic pulmonary oedema, asthma and hypoxaemic respiratory failure and post-extubation respiratory failure.[5] Among the large number of publications on NIV, there is a growing interest for its application on trauma patients, and recently, different systematic reviews and meta-analysis have been pubblished.[6–8]

NIV was already used in 1945 in chest trauma patients combined with intercostal nerve block to improve gas exchanges.[9] Later, with innovations in the material used for endotracheal tubes and with the development of increasingly reliable ventilators, endotracheal intubation and mechanical ventilation became the first choice of treatment in patients with ARF of any origin. During the early 1980s, to avoid infectious complications caused by invasive ventilation, some authors suggested the use of continuous positive airway pressure (CPAP) as a conservative treatment in chest trauma patients,[10,11] and with ulterior technological development, non-invasive pressure support ventilation (PSV) proved to be comparably effective.[12,13] Nowadays, NIV is also used in prehospital settings for ARF, with the reduction of mortality and intubation rates.[14] Despite growing interest and studies, some societies do not recommend the use of NIV in trauma because of inadequate evidence.[15]

PATHOPHYSIOLOGY

Pulmonary parenchymal contusion is a common traumatic injury with described prevalence varying from 5% to 27% among trauma patients,[16,17] with a complication rate (pneumonia, respiratory failure and acute respiratory distress syndrome [ARDS]) that reach 50% and a mortality of 25%.[18] The extent of contusions has been associated with risk of developing ARDS[18,19] that can be in early-onset forms (within 48 hours), due to haemorrhagic shock and capillary oedema, or in late-onset forms, associated with pneumonia or multiple organ failure.[20]

The initial lung injury is generated via different mechanisms. The bursting effect of the shock wave at the interface between two media of different density can result in the disruption of the alveolus ('spalling effect'), while different acceleration rates of alveolar and heavier hilar tissues can determine a stripping between those two. Also, interaction with the thoracic cage can cause damage (for example, because of direct laceration or compression).[17]

Bleeding and lung oedema result from this condition, which lead to alveolar collapse; pleural effusion; either reactive or caused by associated pleural lesion; and consolidation of the injured regions. This causes decreased lung compliance and altered ventilation/perfusion ratio, due to arteriovenous shunt through the non-ventilated lung. From a clinical viewpoint, patients present with dyspnoea, tachypnoea and hypoxia. Furthermore, the reduced clearance of mucus despite its increased production and shallow breathing caused by pain and increased elastic load may encourage the development of atelectasis and bacterial super-infection.

The early changes may not be visible on chest X-ray until 4–6 hours after the incident; afterwards, the exam generally shows irregular infiltrates or inhomogeneous opacities, caused by alveolar haemorrhage and oedema often localised near rib, sternal or clavicular fractures. The best modality for the diagnosis and staging of pulmonary contusion is chest computed tomography (CT); in a study by Miller and colleagues, patients with a contusion that is >20% of the total lung volume on chest CT were four times more likely to develop ARDS.[19] In the absence of a progressive reduction of oedema and haemorrhage, pneumonia may develop in 5%–50% of pulmonary contusion cases, and if there is a coexisting flail chest, the incidence may reach 85%.

As previously described, endotracheal intubation is indicated in chest trauma patients with ARF, airway obstruction, severely compromised awareness and Glasgow Coma Scale score lower than 8 and with severe haemodynamic instability.[3] However, it must be pointed out that if there is no indication, such as in the absence of severe respiratory failure, tracheal intubation does not improve the prognosis of trauma patients.[21] In fact, using an endotracheal tube makes the tracheal portion above the cuff a constant reservoir for bacteria and germs that may easily migrate into the distal airways. In addition, intubation could further alter the already impaired mucociliary clearance, decreasing the patient's capacity to remove bronchial secretions.

The effects of the application of positive pressure through non-invasive devices have been widely studied. Positive pressure determines an increased functional residual capacity by reopening the collapsed alveoli; an improvement in gas exchange by reducing the arteriovenous shunt; a decrease in respiratory rate and an increase in tidal volume, leaving the minute volume unchanged. The reduced work of breathing leads to an increase in PaO_2 and $PaCO_2$ and, at the same time, a decrease in pH. In flail chest patients, NIV dramatically reduces the severity of the paradoxical motion, helping the intercostal muscles to contract during inspiration.[22]

EVIDENCE BASE

Important studies on the use of NIV in the treatment of trauma patients were conducted in the 1980s and 1990s. After a retrospective study showed shorter hospital stay in patients treated with CPAP and epidural analgesia versus mechanical ventilation,[13] Hurst et al.[11] treated 33 patients with CPAP with different levels of pressure, and only two patients needed tracheal intubation.[11] The first randomised controlled trial (RCT) was done by Bolliger and Van Eeden,[23] who compared patients treated with CPAP and regional analgesia with patients who had been intubated and treated with intravenous analgesia; the results were in favour of the first group, with a significantly reduced length of ICU stay and incidence of pneumonia. An important confounding factor of this study was that the intubated patients had a higher injury severity score than the NIV patients.[23] Gregoretti et al.[12] and Beltrame et al.[13] proved the effectiveness of NIV using PSV in chest trauma patients in two clinical studies. In the first study, NIV showed comparable effects to invasive ventilation in terms of gas exchange and spirometric values, whereas the second study retrospectively examined 46 patients who had been admitted to the ICU with spontaneous breathing and had undergone NIV for ARF; 33 of them were successfully weaned and maintained spontaneous breathing.

Following these findings, in the British Thoracic Society recommendations concerning the use of NIV published in 2002, the use of NIV was recommended, although supported by low evidence, in trauma patients who remained hypoxaemic despite adequate analgesia and high oxygen concentrations. Due to the risk of developing or worsening of a pneumothorax, the application of NIV or CPAP in chest trauma patients required intensive monitoring, which was only possible in an ICU.[24] In the same year, in a retrospective study, Vidhani et al.[25] founded a favourable outcome in trauma patients non-invasively treated with either CPAP or bi-level positive airways pressure (BiPAP), although they recommended not to delay tracheal intubation in patients who did not respond to NIV treatment.

Other authors proposed NIV as a strategy to avoid intubation, comparing it with high-flow oxygen therapy for respiratory failure: Ferrer and Torres[5] founded a reduction in intubation rate and ICU mortality in patients with acute hypoxaemic respiratory failure.[5] Based on this finding, a recent study focused on trauma patients, using BiPAP in the intervention group and high-flow oxygen in the control group. The study was prematurely stopped for the much higher incidence of intubation in the control group, and a shorter hospital stay was observed in NIV patients. The risk of establishing a pneumothorax after treatment was not significantly greater with NIV.[26]

Systematic reviews and meta-analysis about this topic were recently published, but as outlined by Duggal et al.,[7] there is a great clinical heterogeneity among studies, regarding the period of intervention, selection criteria and control groups.[7] If NIV is compared with all other strategies, it shows a protective effect,[6] but this effect is minor if we consider only RCT,[8] although with shorter ICU and hospital length of stay.

Despite studies suggesting a positive effect of NIV, strong evidence is still lacking, due to the limited number of studies with different methodologies. For this reason, there is no uniform consensus among different societies to recommend use of NIV in trauma patients.[15]

CLINICAL APPLICATIONS

Concerning the possible clinical applications of CPAP, it may be used outside the ICU, beginning with out-of-hospital first aid,[14] and in the emergency settings, where chest trauma patients with multiple rib fractures and no major head trauma or other severe lesions that may compromise cooperation or state awareness might benefit from the positive pressure generated by a facemask and high-flow oxygen. In this case, the possible presence of a pneumothorax must be borne in mind, which, in the absence of chest drainage, might be worsened by extrinsic positive pressure. Hence, if there is suspicion of a pneumothorax, or if after the application of CPAP, the application of the respiratory and haemodynamic functions are progressively compromised, this technique must be immediately abandoned.

In the ICU, patients may be treated by NIV, thus reducing the need for intubation.[13] In this case, the use of a ventilator with the same level of pressure support and the same positive end-expiratory pressure that would have been used during invasive ventilation is suggested. If the patient needs tracheal intubation, once admitted to the ICU and after undergoing adequate monitoring, early extubation and maintenance of gas exchange by NIV prevents the onset of injured airway bacterial suprainfection and favours lung reexpansion.[12]

Adequate pain control is of paramount importance: according to the patient's specific problems, this can be achieved with different techniques. An interesting approach is the one proposed by Michelet and Boussen,[27] who consider the different phases of thoracic trauma management. In the prehospital setting, intravenous opioids and ketamine can be used, the latter guaranteeing the respiratory drive and more stable haemodynamic. Morphine is the most used opioid, but fentanyl or sufentanyl could also be used.[28] In the ED, if possible, opioid administration can be switched to patient controlled analgesia, while considering a regional technique, which should be used whenever possible for ICU patients with thoracic trauma. Thoracic epidural analgesia is indicated for bilateral costal fractures, but coagulation disorders, vertebral fractures or haemodynamic instability are important contraindications. In this case, paravertebral block associated with systemic analgesia could be used, and for unilateral fractures, it could be the technique of choice. If fractures involve less than four ribs, intercostal nerve block could also be considered.[27]

The patient must be correctly instructed on bronchial secretion removal; patients must be invited to repeatedly cough, and they must be able to remove the mask to allow expectoration. For the same reason, respiratory physiokinesitherapy must be started as soon as possible.

The most important contraindications to NIV in trauma patients are confused or clouded consciousness, haemodynamic instability, craniofacial trauma, inability to cough or expectorate and undrained pneumothorax.

Trauma patients may also have the usual complications associated with NIV, particularly, gastric distension and spontaneous pneumothorax, when the latter is not already present. If there is pneumomediastinum, caution is mandatory, because positive pressure could worsen it, and tracheal–bronchial lesions or oesophageal perforation[29] have to be ruled out.

In addition, particular care must be paid to possible non-invasive treatment failure, either due to the patient's intolerance or to the positive pressure, or because of the underlying disease. In all cases, tracheal intubation must never be delayed, as it has been demonstrated that patients in whom invasive ventilation is delayed had a worse outcome.[25,30]

TECHNICAL CONSIDERATIONS

For NIV administration in chest trauma patients, facemasks as well as nasal masks have been successfully used. There are no data or reports about the use of a helmet in trauma patients, and it does not seem to be indicated.

With regard to the method of NIV administration, high-flow CPAP is used, which only requires dedicated flow meters that are easy to use in an emergency setting, as well as ventilators that use modalities increasingly dedicated to this ventilation technique. These ventilators are able to compensate for possible leaks and to improve patient–ventilator interaction. In fact, in patients with pulmonary contusion, ventilation modalities such as bi-level or PSV have now become much more common than CPAP, and superiority of the former has been hypothesized.[31] Not only do these two types of assisted ventilation prevent injured lung region atelectasis (and this is also ensured by CPAP), but they also permit the recruitment of perfused but non-ventilated lung regions to reduce the shunt and to improve gas exchange. Furthermore, the support provided by the ventilator significantly reduces inspiratory muscle work and, at the same time, alleviates patient's pain.

An appropriate pressure support with adequate trigger threshold values and ventilator cycling are crucial for minimising patient–ventilator asynchrony. This phenomenon seems to be the main cause for the increased work of breathing and for NIV failure.[32] A possible cause is in the interface, to which the ventilator has to offer an adequate compensation.[33] In modern ventilators, the analysis of flow and pressure curves plays a key role in the early detection of asynchronies such as inefficient trigger, inadequate cycling or flow starvation.[34]

A recently introduced and diffusing method of ventilation is neurally adjusted ventilation assistance (NAVA), which uses a modified nasogastric tube to measure diaphragmatic electrical activity, improving patient–ventilator interaction and regulating the ventilation support according to the patient's actual need, thus promoting early extubation by helping the patient to progressively recover respiratory autonomy.[35] NAVA has been proven to dramatically reduce asynchronies during non-invasive ventilation.[36]

Airway humidification – essential in other lung diseases – is not suggested in non-invasively treated patients with pulmonary contusion, because it could delay alveolar oedema reabsorption. Blood gas analysis monitoring is also equally important, with the recommendation to draw blood 1 hour after each variation in the ventilatory parameters or in the fraction of inspiratory oxygen (FiO_2).

The favourable outcome that may be achieved with NIV is not free from side effects: in fact, the increase in intrathoracic pressure leads to an increase in central venous pressure, which compromises venous return, leading to reduced cardiac output. Hence, the importance of absolutely preventing hypovolaemia must be emphasised, because this is a condition that could possibly affect patients with pulmonary contusion, as they frequently undergo fluid restriction, while correct treatment is to maintain normovolaemia. It must also be remembered that NIV leads to an increase in intracranial pressure which lowers cerebral perfusion pressure; the latter is almost never clinically relevant, although attention must be paid to it when applying NIV to multiple trauma patients.

FUTURE RESEARCH

NIV represents an easy-to-learn and easy-to-apply technique, and intensivists should develop a good confidence with it to evaluate its use in trauma patients. As previously described, recent systematic reviews and meta-analysis confirm the potential role of NIV in trauma patients,[6] despite studies still being not enough uniform to give strong recommendations.[7] Only an increased use and a greater diffusion could lead to carrying out the necessary studies to have strong evidence concerning NIV.

REFERENCES

1. Registro Intraospedaliero Multiregionale Traumi Gravi. Available at http://www.cgsi.it/rit/home page2.htm.
2. Allen GS, Coates NE. Pulmonary contusion: A collective review. *Am Surg*. 1996;62:895–900.
3. American College of Surgeons. *Advanced trauma life support student course manual*. 9th ed. Chicago, IL: American College of Surgeons; 2012.
4. Antonelli M, Moro ML, Capelli O et al. Risk factors for early onset pneumonia in trauma patients. *Chest*. 1994;105:224–8.
5. Ferrer M, Torres A. Noninvasive ventilation for acute respiratory failure. *Curr Opin Crit Care*. 2015;21:1–6.
6. Chiumello D, Coppola S, Froio S et al. Noninvasive ventilation in chest trauma: Systematic review and meta-analysis. *Intensive Care Med*. 2013;39:1171–80.
7. Duggal A, Perez P, Golan E et al. Safety and efficacy of noninvasive ventilation in patients with blunt chest trauma: A systematic review. *Crit Care*. 2013; 17:R142.
8. Roberts S, Skinner D, Biccard B, Rodseth RN. The role of non-invasive ventilation in blunt chest trauma: Systematic review and meta-analysis. *Eur J Trauma Emerg Surg*. 2014;40:553–9.
9. Burford TH, Burbank B. Traumatic wet lung: Observations on certain physiologic fundamentals of thoracic trauma. *J Thorac Surg*. 1945;14:415–24.
10. Linton DM, Potgieter PD. Conservative management of blunt chest trauma. *S Afr Med J*. 1982;61:917–9.
11. Hurst JM, DeHaven CB, Branson RD. Use of CPAP mask as the sole mode of ventilatory support in trauma patients with mild to moderate respiratory insufficiency. *J Trauma*. 1985;25:1065–8.
12. Gregoretti C, Beltrame F, Lucangelo U et al. Physiologic evaluation of non-invasive pressure support ventilation in trauma patients with acute respiratory failure. *Intensive Care Med*. 1998;24: 785–90.
13. Beltrame F, Lucangelo U, Gregori D, Gregoretti C. Noninvasive positive pressure ventilation in trauma patients with acute respiratory failure. *Monaldi Arch Chest Dis*. 1999;54:109–14.
14. Pandor A, Thokala P, Goodacre S et al. Pre-hospital non-invasive ventilation for acute respiratory failure: A systematic review and cost-effectiveness evaluation. *Health Technol Assess (Rockv)*. 2015;19:1–8.
15. Keenan S, Sinuff T, Burns K et al. Clinical practice guidelines for the use of noninvasive positive-pressure ventilation and noninvasive continuous positive airway pressure in the acute care setting. *CMAJ*. 2011;183:E195–214.
16. Landeen C, Smith HL. Examination of pneumonia risks and risk levels in trauma patients with pulmonary contusion. *J Trauma Nurs*. 2014;21:41–9.
17. Cohn SM, Dubose JJ. Pulmonary contusion: An update on recent advances in clinical management. *World J Surg*. 2010;34:1959–70.
18. Becher RD, Colonna AL, Enniss TM et al. An innovative approach to predict the development of adult respiratory distress syndrome in patients with blunt trauma. *J Trauma Acute Care Surg*. 2012;73:1229–35.
19. Miller PR, Croce MA, Bee TK et al. ARDS after pulmonary contusion: Accurate measurement of contusion volume identifies high-risk patients. *J Trauma*. 2001;51:223–30.
20. Croce MA, Fabian TC, Davis KA, Gavin TJ. Early and late acute respiratory distress syndrome: Two distinct clinical entities. *J Trauma*. 1999;46:366–8.

21. Ruchholtz S, Waydhas C, Ose C et al. Prehospital intubation in severe thoracic trauma without respiratory insufficiency: A matched-pair analysis based on the Trauma Registry of the German Trauma Society. *J Trauma*. 2002;52:879–86.
22. Davignon K, Kwo J, Bigatello LM. Pathophysiology and management of the flail chest. *Minerva Anestesiol*. 2004;70:193–9.
23. Bolliger CT, Van Eeden SF. Treatment of multiple rib fractures: Randomized controlled trial comparing ventilatory with nonventilatory management. *Chest*. 1990;97:943–8.
24. British Thoracic Society Standards of Care Committee. Non-invasive ventilation in acute respiratory failure. *Thorax*. 2002;57:192–211.
25. Vidhani K, Kause J, Parr M. Should we follow ATLS® guidelines for the management of traumatic pulmonary contusion: The role of non-invasive ventilatory support. *Resuscitation*. 2002;52:265–8.
26. Hernandez G, Fernandez R, Lopez-Reina P et al. Noninvasive ventilation reduces intubation in chest trauma-related hypoxemia: A randomized clinical trial. *Chest*. 2010;137:74–80.
27. Michelet P, Boussen S. Case scenario-thoracic trauma. *Ann Fr Anesth Reanim*. 2013;32:504–9.
28. Beckers SK, Brokmann JC, Rossaint R. Airway and ventilator management in trauma patients. *Curr Opin Crit Care*. 2014;20:626–31.
29. Carrié C, Morel N, Delaunay F et al. Noninvasive ventilation in blunt chest trauma: Beware of missed esophageal injuries! *Intensive Care Med*. 2014;40:1055–6.
30. Esteban A, Frutos-Vivar F, Ferguson ND et al. Noninvasive positive-pressure ventilation for respiratory failure after extubation. *N Engl J Med*. 2004;350:2452–60.
31. Xirouchaki N, Kondoudaki E, Anastasaki M et al. Noninvasive bilevel positive pressure ventilation in patients with blunt thoracic trauma. *Respiration*. 2005;72:517–22.
32. Ozyilmaz E, Ugurlu AO, Nava S. Timing of noninvasive ventilation failure: Causes, risk factors, and potential remedies. *BMC Pulm Med*. 2014;14:19.
33. Hess DR. Patient–ventilator interaction during noninvasive ventilation. *Respir Care*. 2011;56:153–67.
34. Murias G, Lucangelo U, Blanch L. Patient-ventilator asynchrony. *Curr Opin Crit Care*. 2016;22:53–9.
35. Navalesi P, Costa R. New modes of mechanical ventilation: Proportional assist ventilation, neurally adjusted ventilatory assist, and fractal ventilation. *Curr Opin Crit Care*. 2003;9:51–8.
36. Sehgal IS, Dhooria S, Aggarwal AN et al. Asynchrony index in pressure support ventilation (PSV) versus neurally adjusted ventilator assist (NAVA) during non-invasive ventilation (NIV) for respiratory failure: Systematic review and meta-analysis. *Intensive Care Med*. 2016;42:1813–5.

55

Spinal cord injuries

SVEN HIRSCHFELD

INTRODUCTION AND EPIDEMIOLOGY

Worldwide, the average prevalence of spinal cord injury (SCI) is estimated to be 1:1000, and the mean incidence is proposed to be between 4 and 9 cases per 100,000 inhabitants per year. Numbers substantially vary for different parts of the world. The incidence of SCI in developing countries is verified with 25.5/million/year (95% confidence interval: 21.7–29.4/million/year) and ranges from 2.1 to 130.7/million/year.[1] Incidence data for industrialised countries are known and comparable only for regions in North America (39/million), Western Europe (15/million) and Australia (16/million).[2] The most common causes of traumatic SCI are traffic accidents, falls and results of violence, whereas the leading causes of non-traumatic SCI are degenerative causes or conditions, infections or tumours (developed countries) and, particularly, tuberculosis and HIV (developing countries).[3] The majority of people with traumatic SCI are males with a ratio of men to women of approximately 3:1, whereas in non-traumatic SCI genders are almost equally distributed. The distribution of para- and tetraplegia, previously dominated by paraplegic patients, is nowadays almost equal.

In high-income countries, the life expectancy of the general population has continuously increased over the last century and is associated with the risk of developing a tumour, an infection or a circulatory disorder.[4] These diseases might also lead to a SCI with the associated paralysis.

The mortality rate in the first phase after SCI is directly linked to the availability and quality of surgical, primary care and rehabilitation approaches. Life expectancy is in the end determined by the level of integration into a functional socioeconomic environment after initial treatment. Additionally, life expectancy is directly related to the availability of qualified medical care in an event of SCCI typical complications such as pressure ulcers or urological problems.[5]

Due to these circumstances, the incidence and age of temporary or permanently ventilated SCI patients have also dramatically increased over the last decade.[6] Nearly 10% of all SCI patients need at least temporary ventilation during initial treatment directly after the impairment. Six per cent from this group are in need of permanent artificial ventilation due to unsuccessful weaning attempts.[6] Older patients often have multiple comorbidities, which prolong the time of weaning as well as primary rehabilitation. The diagnostic procedures and individual therapy of respiratory dysfunctions are complex and can be adequately handled only by a multidisciplinary team. Life-long medical support for inpatient and out-of-hospital treatment, the correct application of non-invasive and invasive ventilation, proper adaptation of an appropriate weaning regime and the setup of long-term ventilation including the evaluation for implantation of an electrical diaphragm stimulator represent clinical challenges.

PATHOPHYSIOLOGY

Every SCI has an impact on the respiratory function. But whereas thoracic and lumbar lesions mainly affect the expiratory capacity, a cervical SCI (especially above the level C5) usually results in a severe impairment of both the inspiratory and expiratory functions. The paralysis of the muscles needed for inspiration, foremost the diaphragm muscle, leads to a significant loss of vital capacity (VC) and results in the dependency on partial or complete mechanical ventilation. In general, the rule applies that the more cranial the level of lesion is located, the more the respiratory pump is affected. Several factors contribute to this, including the following:

1. Decreased strength of respiratory muscles
2. Reduced compliance of lungs and thoracic wall
3. Chronic central hypoventilation
4. Changes of the patency and reactivity of the airways
5. Dyssynergies concerning the muscles of thorax and abdomen

Decreased strength of respiratory muscles

As a result of the weakness of inspiratory muscles, the VC, the tidal volume (TV) and the forced one-second capacity decrease in patients with a cervical SCI.[7] While patients try to maintain a sufficient minute volume, they automatically increase their respiratory rate. Additionally, the reduced stability of the thorax due to the partially or completely paralysed intercostal muscles leads to a paradoxical inspiration, which means that the thorax flattens during the inspiration.[8,9]

The reduced strength of expiratory muscles leads to a decrease of the end-expiratory reserve volume and, as a consequence, to an increase of the residual capacity. This, in turn, lowers the VC.[10,11] Another result of the weakness of expiratory muscles is a limited ability to cough with the associated reduction in peak cough flow. With peak cough flow less than 270 L/min, efficient coughing is not possible.[12] The measurement of peak cough flow with a peak-flow meter represents a simple and cheap method to objectively assess the ability for patients for sufficient coughing, which can be easily implemented into the clinical routine.

Reduced compliance of lungs and thoracic wall

The lung and thorax compliance is immediately impaired after the lesion in tetraplegic patients caused by decrease of the VC and changes of the surfactants due to respiration with low TVs.[13,14] The stiffening of the thorax and the spasticity of the intercostal muscles additionally contribute to the decrease of the compliance.[15–17]

Chronic central hypoventilation

The central control of respiration is affected in tetraplegic patients.[18] The underlying mechanisms have not been investigated. What we know is that breathing effort as a response to a hypercapnia is decreased and correlates with the blood pressure fluctuations caused by the spinal lesion.[18] Especially at night, breathing and sleep disorders may become more apparent[19] and, in the case of necessary complementary drug therapy, partially enhanced by side effects of centrally acting medication (such as pain and antispastic medication).

Changes of the patency and reactivity of the airways

A bronchial hyperreactivity often occurs after cervical SCI and is significantly associated with decreased airway calibre and consistency.[20] The hypoactivity of the disrupted sympathetic airway innervation in addition to a parasympathetic hyperactivity is assumed as a cause not only for the hyperreactivity but also for the increased production of bronchial secretion and bronchoconstriction.[20,21]

Dyssynergies of muscles of thorax and abdomen

The interaction between abdominal and thorax muscles is also impaired after cervical SCI. The increased compliance of the abdomen as a consequence of the loss of voluntary innervation of abdominal muscles results in a caudal shift of the diaphragm. The weight of the intraabdominal organs additionally contributes to a ventral and caudal shift. Therefore, the vertical diaphragmatic effectivity decreases, and position changes, such as mobilisation in a wheelchair, lead to a decrease of the TV and, accordingly, to a faster occurrence of dyspnoea.[22,23] Therefore, static and dynamic lung volumes are reduced as a direct consequence of the paralysis.

A long-term degradation of the lung function is often reported.[13,23,24] Additionally, smoking, persistent wheezing, overweight and the level of the lesion have a negative impact on both the TV in terms of significant reduction and lung function according to poor oxygenation.[25–27]

NON-INVASIVE OR INVASIVE VENTILATION MANAGEMENT

Basically SCI patients can be ventilated both ways. Which way is chosen fundamentally depends on the experience and the expertise of the attending clinicians. SCI patients, even with the same neurological level and similar preconditions, such as comorbidities, height and weight, could react differently when they need artificial or permanent ventilation.

Therefore, a precise instruction for a particular setting cannot be provided. The decision is rather made individually with the best of the clinician's knowledge and belief adapting the best possible form of ventilation. Clinical circumstances such as acute or chronic SCI, comorbidities, injuries and patient compliance will also influence the decision in accordance with existing guidelines.[28–30] Regarding such complex issues, specialised SCI centres offer best decision support.

Nevertheless, it is expedient to differentiate between patients with acute and chronic SCI. As previously said, patients with chronic SCI are usually more stable regarding vegetative, physical and psychological aspects.[31–33]

Acute SCI patient ventilation

According to the mentioned conditions, it seems clear that nearly 95% of all acute SCI patients with severe respiratory problems will be quickly intubated and near-term tracheotomised.[34] In the context of acute care of tetraplegic patients, a tracheostomy is often required to enable sufficient respiration. Tracheotomy may also be needed in case of prolonged respiratory insufficiency or if typical problems associated with the use of oropharyngeal or nasopharyngeal tubes appear. A tracheotomy can be done either by dilatation percutaneously (PT) or surgically as an open tracheostomy (OT). Further advantages of a tracheotomy are the early reduction or suspension of the analgosedation, resulting in an alert and compliant patient, who is able to participate in a SCI-specific therapy programme, consisting of, e.g. mobilisation into the wheelchair, phonation, eating during ventilation and weaning.

In general, a tracheostomy is recommended in tetraplegic patients with the following:

- Motor complete tetraplegia according to Asia Impairment Scales A and B[34]
- VC ≤ 500 mL
- Injury severity score > 32
- PAO_2/FIO_2 ratio < 300 for 3 days after initiation of ventilation[35]

Studies also demonstrated that an early tracheostomy (<10 days after the onset of paralysis) shortens both the duration of stay in an intensive care unit and the overall ventilation period (assuming that weaning was successful).[36] With regard to complication rates of both techniques (PT and OT), there is inconsistent evidence.[37,38] In the case of a permanently invasively ventilated patient, the current German Respiratory Society guideline 'non-invasive and invasive ventilation' recommends stable medical care for outpatient ventilation and, therefore, the placement of an epithelial open tracheostomy.[29] Regardless of the used technique, PT can be accepted only on rare occasions due to the tendency to shrink and the risk of malposition of the cannula.[29]

NIV ventilation, e.g. via oronasal or nasal approaches, is also possible[39] but often used only in the case of temporary ventilation in SCI patients with pneumonia or after a severe trauma. Stabile spontaneous breathing capacity during the daytime associated with, e.g. the need of nighttime artificial ventilation, is also a very common scenario. The following aspects often prevent an adequate NIV application:

- Insufficient spontaneous breathing capacity
- Lack of patient's compliance
- Lack of protective reflexes such as coughing and swallowing (aspiration hazard)
- Upper airway obstructions
- Repeated obstructions caused by excessive formation of mucus that cannot be controlled by both NIV and invasive intervention
- Pressure sores in the area surface of the mask[40]
- Severe aerophagy, especially with the consequence of minor diaphragm movement and/or higher risk of developing an ileus[41]

But even during the treatment of an acute SCI patient, NIV ventilation should be taken into account and, if possible, applied by an experienced clinician. If possible, the published advantages of NIV (avoiding of intubation and/or tracheostomy and their well-known potential complications, preservation of endogenous air filtering and humidification) could be exploited.[42]

Chronic SCI

In the case of a persistent ventilation situation for more than 12 hours a day, the majority of the tracheotomised SCI patients decide to keep their cannula even when an NIV via mask is possible.[38] The patient's reasons were as follows:

- Simplified mucus management in the absence of sufficient coughing (no acceptance of in-/exsufflators)
- Unrestricted use of face muscle functions (facial expression)
- Better ability to speak
- Being confined by the mask

At the very latest, since Bach et al.[39] have published the possibility of using mouthpiece ventilation in combination with other NIV facilities, this form of ventilation must be taken into account more than previously done before and, if possible, offered to the patient by competent practitioners.[39]

The most common use of NIV application in SCI centres is the ventilator support of SCI patient with signs of respiratory insufficiency during nighttime. NIV may be used as a long-term therapy to compensate the consequences of respiratory insufficiency including hypoventilation as well as obstructive and central apnoea. Further diagnostics in the form of polysomnographic assessments are recommended, if one or more of the following conditions are present:

- Arterial $paCO_2$ > 45 mmHg during daytime
- Hypoventilation at nighttime with constantly decreased oxygen saturation
- Constantly increased $paCO_2$ or $tcCO_2$ at night > 55 mmHG (during 1 min out of 10 min)
- Daytime sleepiness
- Lack of concentration during daytime

When ventilator support is necessary, hospitalisation in a specialised centre is recommended, particularly in patients with more severe impairments of the respiratory function. During this inpatient stay, individual and careful adaption of interfaces, respirators and ventilation modes should be accomplished.[29] This also includes the testing and prescription of in-/exsufflators and the amount of nursing while using mask and ventilator.[42] If finger and/or hand functions are not sufficient and the patient is using a full facemask, any complication during ventilation (e.g. ventilator dysfunction and tube disconnection) could lead to a life-threatening situation, because an active intervention of the patient (e.g. removal of the mask) is not possible. Therefore, the patient's homecare situation must be adjusted as necessary.

FURTHER SCI PATIENT PARTICULARITIES

Ventilation modes

Modern respirators offer at least two basic modes of operation, which are the mandatory and spontaneous ventilation modes. When in mandatory ventilation mode, the respirator controls and performs the breathing work completely or, in case of minimal residual respiratory function, complemented. While working in a complemented mode, important parameters (inspiration pressure, TV and ventilation frequency) are monitored and, if necessary, adjusted by the respirator at any time.

The spontaneous ventilation mode allows the patient to either completely breathe on his or her own or be supported by the respirator.[43] The two most important parameters in artificial ventilation are volume and pressure. With adaption of these two parameters, literally every available ventilation mode can be implemented. Just as the discussion over the optimal ventilation mode continues, so does the debate over the optimal control variable. Volume-controlled ventilation (VCV) offers the safety of a preset TV and minute ventilation but requires the clinician to appropriately set the inspiratory flow, flow waveform and inspiratory time. During VCV, airway pressure increases in response to reduced compliance or increased resistance and may increase the risk of ventilator-induced lung injury. Pressure-controlled ventilation (PCV), by design, limits the maximum airway pressure delivered to the lung, but may result in variable tidal and minute volumes. According to current recommendations, the target TV should range between 6 and 8 mL/kg body weight in patients with a normal body mass index (BMI).[44]

Most studies comparing the effects of VCV and PCV upon SCI patients were not well controlled or designed and offer little to our understanding of when and how to use each control variable in invasive ventilation.[28] Nevertheless, in SCI patients, PCV seems to be more advantageous for the prevention of atelectasis and for the potential compensation of volume loss (e.g. during phonation while ventilated with an unblocked cannula).

When choosing the ventilation mode for an individual patient, clinicians have to keep in mind that a spinal cord-injured patient is usually lung healthy, but suffers from an impairment of the respiratory pump. Patients with an SCI and associated severe pulmonary diseases have to be additionally treated according to the pneumological respiratory guidelines including carefully selected medication and adapted ventilation modes.

Tidal volumes

The aims of the artificially assisted ventilation in persons with SCI are as follows:

- Sufficient oxygenation with subjective well-being
- Prevention of forming atelectasis
- Enabling of phonation during ventilation

There are a few reports published about TVs between 900 and 1000 mL (sometimes even higher) applied in tetraplegics requiring invasive ventilation.[45] In case of ideal BMI, 10–15 mL/kg body weight is recommended during the acute phase.[46] In the presence of atelectasis, a slow increase of 20 mL/kg ideal body weight with a maximal pressure of 30 cm H_2O is described in order to minimise the risk of a barotrauma.[47] It was shown in a 10-year observational study that the risk for developing an atelectasis increases with lower TVs.[24] As a consequence, it is recommended to apply higher TVs for the successful treatment of atelectasis while reducing the breathing frequency to avoid chronic hyperventilation.[45]

On the basis of clinical experience with long-term ventilated tetraplegic patients with inserted unblocked tracheal cannula, six main advantages of using higher TVs were stated:[48]

- Improvement of ability to speak
- Prevention of atelectasis
- Enablement of alternating ventilation volumes without developing hypoxaemia
- Maintenance of pulmonary compliance
- Suppression of residual respiratory muscles activity due to low $paCO_2$ values
- Prevention of subjective dyspnoea during ventilation by achieving normal blood gas values

General observations of long-term ventilation with high TVs show that respiratory alkalosis associated with hypocapnia can be completely renal compensated for without pathological pH values. Theoretically, possible negative effects of hypocapnia, e.g. reduced cerebral blood flow caused by vasoconstriction and thereby increased susceptibility for cerebral seizures, were not observed in the long-term course.[49]

In principle, high TVs with hyperventilation also offer the risk of potassium loss and increased osteoporosis by chronic hypocapnia. The former has to be regularly verified and, if necessary, applied. Concerning osteoporosis, it should be noted that tetraplegia by itself is leading to an increased osteoporosis in the long-term course, to which many factors besides the hypocapnia contribute.[49]

In conclusion, according to the literature, the following recommendations can be given with regard to invasive (but also non-invasive[50]) long-term ventilation of lung-healthy persons with tetraplegia:

- Use of PCV modes with relatively high TVs starting with 10–12 mL/kg body weight (normal BMI assumed) and reduced breathing frequency depending on the clinical course. A maximal inspiratory ventilation pressure of 30 cm H_2O should not be exceeded. If necessary (e.g. in order to avoid atelectasis), TVs up to 15–20 mL/kg body weight could be applied.
- Although mentioned recommendations for parameters of ventilation such as inspiratory pressure or ventilation frequency exist, there is still the need to individually

adapt these parameters to each patient. These adaptations may vary because of thermal and/or circulatory dysregulations and due to changes in muscular or bronchial spasticity. They should be based on the application of an adequate monitoring including capnometry, also in the non-clinical follow-up.

- When tracheotomised, the use of a non-blocked or non-cuffed tracheal cannula on an individual basis for as long as possible for both the improvement of phonation and prevention of tracheal ulcers is recommended.

Special types of long-term ventilation

PHRENIC NERVE STIMULATORS

In case of spinal cord lesions above C3 resulting in long-term and permanent ventilation, a phrenic nerve stimulator (PNS) represents a serious therapeutic alternative. The PNS has been introduced in the mid-1960s for patients with severe respiratory insufficiency.[51] It has the advantage that the inhaled air is drawn into the lungs by the diaphragm under negative pressure, rather than being forced into the chest under positive pressure such as in positive pressure ventilation. This is physiologically more accurate and comfortable for the patient. Currently, there are two phrenic nerve stimulation systems commercially available which have a Communauté Européenne or Food and Drug Administration approval for routine clinical use: The first is the Atrostim Yukka® (Atrotech, Finland), and the second is the Avery System® (Avery Biomedical Devices, United States).

In both systems, electrodes are surgically implanted on both phrenic nerves in the mediastinum at the third to fourth intercostal space. Electrode leads are intracorporally attached to radio frequency-operated receivers. The receivers are supplied with energy and stimulation commands from an induction coil placed on the skin area over the implant. No transcutaneous cables are needed for these systems.

Contraindications for the implantation of a PNS system are severe cognitive restrictions, e.g. as a consequence of a head injury, a severe preexisting condition of the heart and/or lung or an unfavourable prognosis in the case of terminally ill patients. Intact lower neurons of both phrenic nerves and an intact diaphragm muscle are general prerequisites for the use of an electrical stimulation system including PNS; therefore, patients with damaged neurons, phrenic nerves or diaphragm could not be supplied.

Possible complications of an implantation, besides the general surgical risks, are damages of the phrenic nerve (with consecutive dysfunctions) and haemo- or pneumothoraces.

Patients using a PNS are at much lower risk of upper airway infections including ventilator-associated pneumonia, due to the reduction in suctioning, elimination of external humidifier and ventilator circuits and the potential, also temporary (e.g. with stoma buttons), removal of the tracheostomy tube in appropriate patients.[52–54] Some studies showed significantly lower pulmonary complication rates and lower mortality rates. PNS provides some other benefits such as normal breathing and speech patterns; ease of eating and drinking; and improved sense of smell, which result in an increased quality of life.[53–55] The external components of PNS systems are relatively small compared to the bulky tubing and batteries of mechanical ventilators, and therefore, they improve the patient's mobility. The silent operation of a PNS enhances the patient's ability to participate in social and educational environments. Long-term observation studies showed that the electrode thresholds do not change over a long time, proving that the systems are suitable for long-term ventilation over decades.[56] In contrast to external ventilators, no consumables are needed resulting in a financial payback period of only a few years.[53] More than 70% of all patients use the PNS for 24 hours/day. However, PNS 24 hours/day is recommended only for adults. For children and adolescents, a maximum of 12 hours/day is recommended, because the sufficient bony consolidation of the thorax must be ensured first.

DIAPHRAGM PACEMAKER

In more recent times, an alternative and more cost-efficient system for diaphragm pacing (DP), the semiinvasive NeurX® (Synapse Biomedical, United States), was introduced. With this system, hook electrodes are laparoscopically inserted into the diaphragm muscle, and electrode cables are percutaneously connected to an external stimulator.[57] The system has the advantage that only a minimally invasive, technically easier implantation procedure needs to be performed with lower general surgical risks and faster recreation. However, pneumothorax is also one described complication of implantation. In chronic use, care and careful inspection of the site, where the percutaneous leads pass the skin, needs to be regularly performed to avoid infections. Until now, sufficient data on associated infections are not available.

The contra-/indications of the DP system and the PNS are basically the same. At this point, it needs to be explicitly mentioned that although the DP system uses intramuscular electrodes, it is based on the stimulation of the phrenic nerves and its muscular endplates. Therefore, also in DP, a sufficient number of spinal motor neurons of both phrenic nerves need to be intact for successful application.

The DP system was also used in patients with amyotrophic lateral sclerosis (ALS) for temporary treatment of respiratory problems until a publication stated a higher mortality rate of the patients and therefore did not recommend the system as a routine treatment for this patient group.[58]

Nevertheless, permanent application over many years for 24 hours/day in patients with high SCI is described.[59] Some patients with preserved sensory functions complain about pain under stimulation, which is most likely caused by the relatively strong stimulation currents.[60]

Regarding both systems, magnetic resonance imaging (MRI) examinations could lead to nerve muscle damage and are therefore obsolete.

WEANING OF SCI PATIENTS

Even for specialised centres, the weaning of ventilated SCI patients is a challenge for many reasons especially because of recurrent pulmonary infections.[61] Besides this, vegetative dysfunctions such as hypotonia, bradycardia, autonomic dysreflexia or hypothermia represent additional complications during the weaning process.[31,32] The weaning process is usually prolonged and often interrupted[62,63]; therefore, the majority of the patients are ventilated via tracheostomy. But the following weaning procedure is also applicable to non-invasive ventilated patients. Published data concerning the length of this process range between 40 and 232 days. The rate of weaning failure is consistently reported to be in the range of 30%.[62]

Pathophysiology

The innervation and strength of the diaphragm muscle is mainly determining the VC of the lung.[64,65] The higher the patient's VC, the better the prognosis for a successful weaning.[66] The weaning process should not be initiated when the VC of a lung-healthy patient is below 1000 mL.[67] The aim during the weaning process is to systematically train the diaphragm muscle avoiding excessive fatigue of the muscle. Disregarding may lead to the extension of the weaning period or to failure of the weaning process.[67]

The diaphragm muscle is prone to a fast conversion from slow-fatiguing type 1 to fast-fatiguing type 2b fibres after paralysis. The training during the weaning reverts this paralysis-induced fibre transformation and leads to slower fatiguing muscle fibres.[68–72]

Confounding factors

From clinical experience, weaning should not be started or interrupted when at least one of the following confounding factors is present:

- Pneumonia
- Septicaemia
- Fever > 38.5°C
- Complete paralysis of the diaphragm muscle
- VC < 1000 mL
- Relevant autonomic dysreflexia
- Severe spasticity of relevant respiratory muscles
- Serious consuming pressure sores
- Constant heart rate > 140 beats per minute
- Constant breathing rate > 35/min
- Metabolic acidosis
- Inadequate mental status
- Anaesthesia

Execution of the weaning process

Weaning should be started in bed or wheelchair in a supine position at daytime (e.g. 8 am to 8 pm) and in IC units under the control of certain vital parameters. This includes breathing frequency, breathing volume (spirometry) and values of carbon dioxide (capnography). During nighttime, the convalescence of all respiratory muscles should be ensured by the correct setting of mandatory ventilation modes of the external respirator.[63]

During daytime every hour should consist of a spontaneous breathing (training) part and a ventilator (recovery) part. In clearly defined steps of 5–10 min, the training sessions (up to 12) are slowly increased day by day until the patient is spontaneously breathing for 12 hours without any ventilator support. If the patient is stable during daytime, the nighttime weaning can be initiated with increasing periods of spontaneous breathing, e.g. 1 hour/night.

During the whole discontinuous process, vital parameters of the patient including the present TV (spirometry) should be monitored and the weaning process interrupted, if aforementioned confounding factors evolve. The application of a standardised protocol is recommended.[73–75]

The supervision and adaption of the weaning process requires a highly trained staff to achieve a successful outcome. This knowledge is normally present only in specialised SCI centres. Therefore, a fast transfer of patients in need of artificial ventilation from conventional IC units to SCI centres is recommended by all SCI societies around the world to ensure an adequate weaning progress.[75]

SUMMARY

A high SCI above the fifth cervical level usually results in a neurogenic respiratory failure. Within the last 13 years, the number of these patients has quadrupled, and nearly 10% of all SCI patients need temporary or permanent ventilation as part of their initial treatment in the hospital. Six per cent from this group are in need of permanent artificial ventilation mainly via tracheostoma due to unsuccessful weaning attempts. In addition to the partial or complete diaphragm, insufficiency comorbidities such as reduced lung compliance, bronchial hyperreactivity, central dysregulations and prolonged age aggravate an adequate treatment. In the acute phase, early mobilisation, phonation despite ventilation and, if necessary, early tracheostomy are recommended and could minimise the risk of typical SCI acute complications such as pneumonia, thrombosis and bed rest-related pressure sores. Simultaneously, an experienced team has to provide the selection of the most appropriate ventilator with a suitable mode, a permanent reviewing of the vital parameters to detect weaning and NIV potential and, if possible, the initiation of the SCI-adapted weaning process. Even for specialised centres, the weaning of ventilated tetraplegic patients is a challenge for many reasons especially because of recurrent pulmonary vegetative dysfunctions such as hypotonia, bradycardia, autonomic dysreflexia or hypothermia.

Treatment during the chronic phase is marked by further adapting and supporting the patient with facilities and a constantly present specialised nursing team in view of the demission into handicapped-accessible domesticity. If possible, at this stage, the implantation of a diaphragm stimulator or adjusting a fitting conventional NIV could minimise the risk of suffering pneumonia, which is still the most common long-term complication. Studies on other long-term outcomes had shown that the first 2 years after demission recorded high mortality rates, because of the individual learning curve of the multiprofessional team. Subsequently, increasing survival rates accompanied with an acceptable quality of life were reported not least because of the proceeded training for house doctors, caregivers and family members.

For these mentioned reasons, SCI patients in need of ventilation should be transferred to centres specialising in the treatment of SCI at an early stage after onset of SCI. After acute treatment and SCI rehabilitation, they should be integrated into a SCI-specialised life-long aftercare system in order to prevent life-threatening complications. Therefore, recommendations have been published by various national societies worldwide for out-of-hospital ventilation. The led to the establishment of a general high standard of care, and treatment should be performed in accordance with those guidelines.

REFERENCES

1. Rahimi-Movaghar J, Sayyah MK et al. Epidemiology of traumatic spinal cord injury in developing countries: A systematic review. *Neuroepidemiology* 2013;41(2):65–85.
2. Cripps RA, Lee BB, Wing P et al. A global map for traumatic spinal cord injury epidemiology: Towards a living data repository for injury prevention. *Spinal Cord.* 2011 Apr; 49 (4):493–501.
3. New PW, Cripps RA, Bonne Lee B. Global maps of non-traumatic spinal cord injury epidemiology: Towards a living data repository. *Spinal Cord.* 2014 Feb; 52(2):97–109.
4. Thietje R, Kowald B, Hirschfeld S. Causes of death in SCI patients – A study of 102 cases. *Rehabilitation (Stuttg).* 2011;50(4):251–4.
5. DeVivo MJ, Chen Y. Trends in new injuries, prevalent cases, and aging with spinal cord injury. *Arch Phys Med Rehabil.* 2011;92(3):332–8.
6. Hirschfeld S, Exner G, Tiedemann S, Thietje R. Long term ventilation of SCI patients – Results and perspectives in 25 years of experience with clinical and out-of-hospital ventilation, SCI Center, BG-Klinikum Hamburg. *J Trauma Berufskrankheit.* 09/2010;12(3):177–181. DOI: 10.1007/s10039-010-1655-2, Springer-Verlag.
7. Mueller G, de Groot S, van der Woude LH et al. Prediction models and development of an easy to use open-access tool for measuring lung function of individuals with motor complete spinal cord injury. *J Rehabil Med.* 2012;44:642.
8. Linn WS, Spungen AM, Gong H et al. Forced vital capacity in two large outpatient populations with chronic spinal cord injury. *Spinal Cord.* 2001;39:263–8.
9. Linn WS, Adkins RH, Gong H, Waters RL. Pulmonary function in chronic spinal cord injury: A cross-sectional survey of 222 southern California adult outpatients. *Arch Phys Med Rehabil.* 2000;81:757–63.
10. De Troyer A, Estenne M. The expiratory muscles in tetraplegia. *Paraplegia.* 1991;29:359–63.
11. Fujiwara T, Hara Y, Chino N. Expiratory function in complete tetraplegics: Study of spirometry, maximal expiratory pressure, and muscle activity of pectoralis major and latissimus dorsi muscles. *Am J Phys Med Rehabil.* 1999;78:464–9.
12. Bach JR, Saporito LR. Criteria for extubation and tracheostomy tube removal for patients with ventilatory failure: A different approach to weaning. *Chest.* 1996;110:1566–71.
13. Tow AM, Graves DE, Carter RE. Vital capacity in tetraplegics twenty years and beyond. *Spinal Cord.* 2001;39:139–44.
14. Brown R, DiMarco AF, Hoit JD, Garshick E. Respiratory dysfunction and management in spinal cord injury. *Respir Care.* 2006;51:853.
15. Scanlon PD, Loring SH, Pichurko BM. Respiratory mechanics in acute quadriplegia: Lung and chest wall compliance and dimensional changes during respiratory maneuvers. *Am Rev Respir Dis.* 1989;139:615.
16. Goldmann JM, Williams SJ, Denison DM. The rib cage and abdominal components of respiratory system compliance in tetraplegic patients. *Eur Respir J.* 1988;1:242.
17. Estenne M, De Troyer A. The effects of tetraplegia on chest wall statics. *Am Rev Respir Dis.* 1986;134:121.
18. Manning HL, Brown R, Scharf SM. Ventilatory and blood pressure response to hypercapnia in quadriplegia. *Respir Physiol.* 1992;89:97.
19. Bergovsky EH. Mechanisms for respiratory insufficiency after spinal cord injury: A source of alveolar hypoventilation. *Ann Intern Med.* 1964;61:435.
20. Grimm DR, Chandy D, Almenoff PL. Airway hyperreactivity in subjects with tetraplegia is associated with reduced baseline airway caliber. *Chest.* 2000;118:1397.
21. Schilero GJ, Grimm DR, Baumann WA. Assessment of airway caliber and bronchodilator responsiveness in subjects with spinal cord injury. *Chest.* 2005;127:149.
22. Estenne M, De Troyer A. Mechanics of postural dependence of vital capacity in tetraplegic subjects. *Am Rev Respir Dis.* 1987;135:367.
23. Baydur A, Adkins RH, Milic-Emili J. Lung mechanics in individuals with spinal cord injury: Effects of injury level and posture. *J Appl Physiol.* 2001;90:405.
24. Postma K, Haisma JA, de Groot S et al. Changes in pulmonary function during the early years after inpatient rehabilitation in persons with spinal cord injury: A prospective cohort study. *Arch Phys Med Rehabil.* 2013;94:1540–6.

25. Linn WS, Spungen AM, Gong H Jr. Smoking and obstructive lung dysfunction in persons with chronic spinal cord injury. *Spinal Cord Med.* 2003;26:28.
26. Almenoff PL, Spunge AM, Lesser M, Baumann WA. Pulmonary function survey in spinal cord injury: Influences of smoking and level and completeness of injury. *Lung.* 1995;173:297.
27. Stolzmann KL, Gagnon DR, Brown R et al. Risk factors for chest illness in chronic spinal cord injury: A prospective study. *Am J Phys Med Rehabil.* 2010;89:576–83.
28. Mc Kim DA, Road J and the Canadian thoracic society home mechanical ventilation committee: Home mechanical ventilation: A canadian thoracic society clinical practice guideline. *Can Respir J.* 2011;18:197–215.
29. Windisch W, Brambring J, Budweiser S et al. Non-invasive and invasive mechanical ventilation for treatment of chronic respiratory failure S2 – Guideline. *Pneumologie.* 2010;64:207–40.
30. Westhoff M, Schönhofer B, Windisch W et al. *Non-invasive mechanical ventilation in acute respiratory failure: Clinical practice S3 guidelines on behalf of the German Society of Pneumology and Ventilatory Medicine. Pneumologie.* 2015;69(12):719–56. Epub 2015 Dec 9. German.
31. Popa C, Popa F, Grigorean VT et al. Vascular dysfunctions following spinal cord injury. *J Med Life.* 2010;3:275–85.
32. Krassioukov A. Autonomic function following cervical spinal cord injury. *Respir Physiol Neurobiol.* 2009;169:157–64.
33. Wu J, Zhao Z, Kumar A et al. Endoplasmic reticulum stress and disrupted neurogenesis in the brain are associated with cognitive impairment and depressive-like behavior after spinal cord injury. *J Neurotrauma.* 2016;33:1919–35.
34. Menaker J, Kufera JA, Glaser J et al. Admission AIS motor score predicting the need for tracheostomy after cervical spinal cord injury. *J Trauma Acute Care Surg.* 2013;75:629–34.
35. Leelapattana P, Fleming JC, Gurr KR et al. Predicting the need for tracheostomy in patients with cervical spinal cord injury. *J Trauma Acute Care Surg.* 2012;73:880–4.
36. Choi HJ, Paeng SH, Kim ST et al. The effectiveness of early tracheostomy (within at least 10 Days) in cervical spinal cord injury patients. *Korean Neurosurg Soc.* 2013;54:220–4.
37. Ladra J. Perkutane Verfahren nach Ciaglia und Griggs versus konventionelle Tracheotomie – Verfahren – Metaanalyse und Literaturvergleich. Dissertation Universität Köln, Köln, 2005.
38. Hirschfeld S, Jürgens N, Tiedemann S, Thietje R. Invasives Beatmungs- und Sekretmanagement bei hoher Tetraplegie: Kompendium Außerklinische Beatmung im Kindes- und Erwachsenenalter; Martin Bachmann, Bernd Schucher (Hrsg.), Kleanthes, Dresden, 2013;185–90, ISBN 978-3-942 622-12-7.
39. Bach, JR, Alba AS, Saporito BA. Intermittent positive pressure ventilation via the mouth as an alternative to tracheostomy for 257 ventilator users. *Chest.* 1993;103:174–82.
40. Bambi S, Peris A, Esquinas AM. Pressure ulcers caused by masks during noninvasive ventilation. *Am J Crit Care.* 2016;25:6.
41. Rodriguez GM. Bowel function after spinal cord injury. *Arch Phys Med Rehabil.* 2016;97:339–40.
42. Bach JR, Sinquee DM, Saporito LR, Botticello AL. Efficacy of mechanical insufflation and exsufflation in extubating unweanable subjects with restrictive pulmonary disorders. *Respir Care.* 2015;60:477–83.
43. Chatburn RL. Classification of ventilator modes: Update and proposal for implementation. *Respir Care.* 2007;52:301–23.
44. The Acute Respiratory Distress Syndrome Network. Ventilation with lower tidal volumes as compared with traditional tidal volumes for acute lung injury and the acute respiratory distress syndrome. *N Engl J Med.* 2000;342:1301–8.
45. Peterson WP, Barbalata L, Brooks CA et al. The effect of tidal volumes on the time to wean persons with high tetraplegia from ventilators. *Spinal Cord.* 1999;37:284–8.
46. Arora A, Flower O, Murray NP, Lee BB. Respiratory care of patients with cervical spinal cord injury: A review. *Crit Care Resusc.* 2012;14:64–73.
47. Vásquez RG, Sedes PR, Fariña MM et al. Respiratory management in the patient with spinal cord injury. *BioMedResearch Int.* 2013;2013:168757.
48. Watt JW, Fraser MJ. The effect of insufflation leaks in long-term ventilation: Waking and sleeping transcutaneous gas tensions in ventilator-dependent patients with an uncuffed tracheostomy tube. *Anaesthesia.* 1994;49:328–30.
49. Watt JW, Devine D. Does dead-space ventilation always alleviate hypocapnia? Long-term ventilation with plain tracheostomy tubes. *Anaesthesia.* 1995;50:688–91.
50. Bach JR. Continuous noninvasive ventilation for patients with neuromuscular disease and spinal cord injury. *Semin Respir Crit Care Med.* 2002;23:283–92.
51. Glenn WWL, Phelps ML. Diaphragm pacing by electrical stimulation of the phrenic nerve. *Neurosurgery.* 1985;17:974–84.
52. Bach JR, Bakshiyev R, Hon A. Noninvasive respiratory management for patients with spinal cord injury and neuromuscular disease. *Tanaffos.* 2012;11:7–11.
53. Hirschfeld S, Exner G, Luukkaala T, Baer GA. Mechanical ventilation or phrenic nerve stimulation for treatment of spinal cord injury-induced respiratory insufficiency. *Spinal Cord.* 2008;46:738–42.

54. Romero FJ, Gambarrutta C, Garcia-Forcada A et al. Long-term evaluation of phrenic nerve pacing for respiratory failure due to high cervical spinal cord injury. *Spinal Cord.* 2012;50:895–8.
55. Esclarin M, Bravo P, Arroyo O et al. Tracheostomy ventilation versus diaphragmatic pacemaker ventilation in high spinal cord injury. *Paraplegia.* 1994;32:687–93.
56. Hirschfeld S, Vieweg H, Schulz AP et al. Threshold currents of platinum electrodes used for functional electrical stimulation of the phrenic nerves for treatment of central apnea. *Pacing Clin Electrophysiol.* 2013;36:714–8.
57. Tedde ML, Onders RP, Teixeira MJ et al. Electric ventilation: Indications for and technical aspects of diaphragm pacing stimulation surgical implantation. *J Bras Pneumol.* 2012;38:566–72.
58. McDermott CJ, Shaw PJ, Cooper CL et al. Safety and efficacy of diaphragm pacing in patients with respiratory insufficiency due to amyotrophic lateral sclerosis (DiPALS): A multicentre, open-label, randomised controlled trial. *Lancet Neurol.* 2015;14:883–92.
59. Onders RP, Elmo MJ, Ignagni AR. Diaphragm stimulation system for tetraplegia in individuals injured during childhood or adolescence. *J Spinal Cord Med.* 2007;30:S25–9.
60. Morélot-Panzini C, Le Pimpec-Barthes F, Menegaux F et al. Referred shoulder pain (C4 dermatome) can adversely impact diaphragm pacing with intramuscular electrodes. *Eur Respir J.* 2015;45:1751–4.
61. Fromm B, Hundt G, Gerner HJ et al. Management of respiratory problems unique to high tetraplegia. *Spinal Cord.* 1999;37:239–44.
62. Chiodo AE, Scelza W, Forchheimer M. Predictors of ventilator weaning in individuals with high cervical spinal cord injury. *J Spinal Cord Med.* 2008;31:72–7.
63. Hirschfeld S, Tiedemann S, Jürgens N, Thietje R. Hohe Querschnittlähmung und invasive Beatmung – Besonderheiten im Weaning. *Med Review.* 2012;8:24–5.
64. McCool D, Ayas N, Brown R. Mechanical ventilation and disuse atrophy of the diaphragm. *N Engl J Med.* 2008;359:89.
65. Faulkner JA, Maxwell LC, Ruff GL et al. The diaphragm as a muscle: Contractile properties. *Am Rev Respir Dis.* 1979;119:89–92.
66. Kang SW, Shin JC, Park CI et al. Relationship between inspiratory muscle strength and cough capacity in cervical spinal cord injured patients. *Spinal Cord.* 2006;44:242–8.
67. Füssenich W1, Hirschfeld S1, Kowald B et al. Discontinuous ventilator weaning of patients with acute SCI *Spinal Cord.* 2018 Jan 16. doi: 10.1038/s41393-017-0055-x.
68. Mantilla CB, Seven YB, Zhan WZ et al. Diaphragm motor unit recruitment in rats. *Respir Physiol Neurobiol.* 2010;173:101–6.
69. Salmons S. Functional adaptation in skeletal muscle. *Trends Neurosci.* 1980;3:134–7.
70. Roussos CS, Macklem PT. Diaphragmatic fatigue in man. *J Appl Physiol.* 1977;43:189–97.
71. Edwards RHT. The diaphragm as a muscle: Mechanics underlying fatigue. *Am Rev Respir Dis.* 1979;119:81–4.
72. Walker DJ, Walterspacher S, Schlager D et al. Characteristics of diaphragmatic fatigue during exhaustive exercise until task failure. *Respir Physiol Neurobiol.* 2011;176:14–20.
73. Brown R, DiMarco AF, Hoit JD, Garshick E. Respiratory dysfunction and management in spinal cord injury. *Respir Care.* 2006;51:853–68;discussion 869–70.
74. Gutierrez CJ, Harrow J, Haines F. Using an evidence-based protocol to guide rehabilitation and weaning of ventilator-dependent cervical spinal cord injury patients. *J Rehabil Res Dev.* 2003;40:99–110.
75. Schönhofer B, Geiseler J, Dellweg D et al. S2k Guideline "prolonged Weaning". *Pneumologie* 2015; 69(10):595–607. doi: 10.1055/s-0034-1392809, Epub 2015 Oct 7.

PART 12

Paediatric ventilatory failure

56 Equipment and interfaces in children 519
Alessandro Amaddeo, Annick Frapin and Brigitte Fauroux
57 Chronic non-invasive ventilation for children 525
Alessandro Amaddeo, Annick Frapin and Brigitte Fauroux
58 Non-invasive positive pressure ventilation in children with acute respiratory failure 533
Giorgio Conti, Marco Piastra and Silvia Pulitanò

56

Equipment and interfaces in children

ALESSANDRO AMADDEO, ANNICK FRAPIN AND BRIGITTE FAUROUX

INTRODUCTION

Non-invasive ventilation (NIV) comprises (1) continuous positive airway pressure (CPAP), which utilises the delivery of a constant positive pressure in the airways aiming to maintain airway patency throughout the entire breathing cycle, and (2) biphasic positive airway pressure (BiPAP), which aims to assist the breathing of the patient by delivering a supplemental higher positive pressure during each inspiration.

NIV is increasingly used in children, in both the acute and the chronic settings. Indeed, acute or chronic respiratory failure of various origins may be improved or cured by means of NIV. NIV is recommended as a first-line therapy in the paediatric intensive care unit (PICU) for bronchiolitis,[1–4] acute respiratory exacerbations caused by neuromuscular disease or cystic fibrosis,[5–7] pneumonia,[8,9] acute chest syndrome due to sickle cell disease[10] and upper airway obstruction.[11,12] The number of children treated at home with long-term NIV for neuromuscular or lung disease, or various causes of upper airway obstruction, is also growing rapidly.[13–15] Respiratory mechanics and maxillofacial development differ in children compared to adults, which justifies age-adapted ventilators and interfaces. The setting of NIV, in the intensive care unit (ICU) or at home, will determine the type of ventilator and interface that can be used.

In this chapter, paediatric specificities, with the exception of the neonates, and ventilatory modes, ventilators and interfaces, in both the acute and the chronic settings, will be discussed.

PAEDIATRIC SPECIFICITIES

Respiratory pattern

Compared to adults, breathing pattern in children is characterised by a smaller tidal volume and a higher respiratory rate. In children, normal tidal volume is approximately 10 mL/kg, with a respiratory rate of approximately 40 breaths/min at rest at birth and 20 breaths/min at the age of 2 years. In case of respiratory failure, tidal volume decreases and respiratory rate increases. A ventilator should thus be able to deliver small tidal volumes with a relatively high frequency. Also, when a spontaneous BiPAP mode is used, the ventilator should be able to detect the onset of the patient's inspiratory effort (by means of a change in pressure or flow) and deliver a preset pressure or volume within a time delay compatible with the patient's respiratory rate. As such, an inspiratory trigger time delay exceeding 100 ms for young children is too long and inadequate because the patient may have terminated his or her inspiration before the delivery of the pressure or volume by the ventilator.[16] Similarly, in case of a spontaneous mode, the ventilator should be able to detect the onset of the termination of the inspiration in order to allow an adequate cycling of inspiration to expiration.

The respiratory effort, i.e. the negative intrathoracic pressure that the patient has to generate during inspiration, varies according to the underlying condition. This inspiratory effort may be high in the case of upper airway obstruction or lung disease such as cystic fibrosis,[11,12,17,18] but low in the case of a neuromuscular disease, because of the weakness of the respiratory muscles. It may be difficult for a ventilator to detect the onset of the inspiration in a patient who has a minimal inspiratory effort because the change in airway pressure or flow may be too small.[16] NIV may thus be challenging in young children having an 'extreme' breathing pattern because the ventilator needs to be able to detect minor changes in airway pressure or flow and capable of an adapted response within a tight time frame. Such requirements are further challenged by leaks, which are unavoidable during NIV. Leaks are the main cause of ineffective ventilation with persistent hypercapnia, patient–ventilator asynchrony and NIV failure.[19] The detrimental effects of leaks will be more pronounced in the youngest patients in whom the volume of leaks may represent a greater percentage of their tidal volume.

Maxillofacial specificities

The anatomy of the facial bones and the proportions between the facial elements differ in children compared to adults. The anatomy of the maxillofacial structures continuously changes during growth, which is particularly rapid during the first 2 years of life. Interfaces for NIV thus need to be specifically adapted to the facial anatomy and physiognomy of children. They need to be frequently changed, especially within the first months of life, because of the rapid growth of the facial structures. The anatomy of the skull differs also in children as compared to adults. A proportional simple reduction in size of a headgear designed for adults may not be suitable for children. Moreover, numerous children requiring NIV may have deformities of the face and the skull, such as children with craniofaciostenosis or mucopolysaccharidosis, which may require not only adapted interfaces but also headgears.

The soft tissue beneath the skin is thinner in children compared to adults. Children are thus at greater risk of skin injury than adults. Skin injury occurs as a consequence of pressure sores, which are defined as a lesion on any skin surface that occurs as a result of pressure. The principal causative factor is the application of localised pressure to an area of skin not adapted to the magnitude and duration of such external forces. Tissue damage will occur if both a critical pressure threshold and a critical time are exceeded. Because young children may need NIV during extended periods including nocturnal sleep and daytime naps, they are at increased risk of skin injury.[20]

Also of importance is the effect of repetitive loading on skin and bone tissue, which is the case during NIV. Facial growth predominantly occurs in an anterior and sagittal axes in children. NIV may hinder normal facial growth and cause facial deformity. Facial flattening and maxilla retrusion are commonly observed in children receiving long-term NIV and justify the prioritised choice of the interface having the least facial contact associated with a systematic evaluation and follow-up by a paediatric maxillofacial specialist before and during NIV.[20]

VENTILATORY MODES AND VENTILATORS FOR NIV IN CHILDREN

Ventilatory modes

The simplest mode is CPAP, which consists of the delivery of a constant positive airway pressure. The aim of CPAP is to maintain upper airway patency during the entire breathing cycle. This treatment represents the first line choice of severe upper obstructive events during sleep in children.[21–23] CPAP reduces the work of breathing in patients with flow limitation by overcoming the inspiratory threshold imposed by intrinsic positive end-expiratory pressure (PEEP). Thus, even if the main indication of CPAP is obstructive sleep apnoea (OSA), it is also advocated in obstructive lung disease, when intrinsic PEEP increases the work of breathing.[24,25] Whereas constant CPAP was the first and the simplest CPAP 'mode', other algorithms have been developed. Autotitrated CPAP is a mode during which the positive airway pressure is automatically adjusted between a minimal and a maximal airway pressure set by the prescriber, according to an analysis of the flow curve and airway resistance by the device software. More sophisticated modes, associating a moderate decrease in airway pressure at the onset of expiration, or a variable increase in the airway pressure during inspiration, are also available.[26] The few studies that have compared constant CPAP to more complex CPAP modes have not been able to demonstrate a superiority of these modes with regard to comfort or efficacy compared to constant CPAP.[27,28]

During BiPAP, a higher level of positive pressure is delivered during inspiration, by means of a volume- or pressure-targeted mode. During volume-targeted ventilation, the ventilator delivers a fixed volume during a given time span. Its advantage is the strict delivery of the preset volume. Its main disadvantage is that this mode is not able to adjust to the variable requirements of the patient, such as physiological changes in central drive, lung compliance and airway resistance during sleep. Moreover, compensation for unintentional leaks is not possible, which exposes the patient to the risk of an insufficient effective inspired volume in the presence of unintentional leaks.[29] This explains why this mode tends to be less used during the last years. Pressure support (PS) is a pressure-targeted mode during which each breath is triggered and terminated by the patient and supported by the ventilator; the patient can control his or her respiratory rate, inspiratory duration and tidal volume.[30] This explains the relative ease in adapting to, and the greater comfort and patient–ventilator synchrony of, this mode. In contrast to volume-targeted ventilation, tidal volume is not predetermined but depends on the level of PS, the inspiratory effort of the patient and the mechanical properties of the patient's respiratory system. A main advantage of this mode is its ability to compensate for unintentional leaks. During this mode, since there are no mandatory breaths, an in-built low frequency backup rate is used to prevent episodes of apnoea. Furthermore, because the breaths are triggered by the patient, the sensitivity of the trigger is crucial.[18] Because during PS, inspiratory muscle activity may influence respiratory frequency and tidal volume, this ventilatory mode is generally proposed in patients who can spontaneously breathe for substantial periods and mainly require nocturnal ventilation such as patients with lung disease.

Hybrid modes, also called 'volume targeting pressure ventilation' (VTPV), combine the characteristics of volume-targeted ventilation and pressure-targeted ventilation with the aim to overcome the previous limitations.[31] These modes provide a predetermined target volume (TV) while maintaining the physiological benefits of pressure-targeted ventilation. The ventilator measures or estimates each consecutive expired volume and automatically adjusts inspiratory pressure within a predeterminated range to ensure a stable TV. More recent devices also allow adding a variable backup rate. These devices automatically adjust both the inspiratory pressure level and the backup rate within a predefined range to achieve a target ventilation. These devices include also a 'learning' mode during which the ventilator 'copies' the patient's breathing pattern in order to determine an optimal target ventilation. Finally, the newest devices combine VTPV with an autoadjusted expiratory pressure level committed to maintain airway patency. Additionally, these devices provide an 'automatic' backup rate. By automatically adjusting the inspiratory pressure, the expiratory pressure and the backup rate, these devices are expected to provide a full automatic mode. There is currently no evidence for a clear benefit of these modes compared to conventional modes. Hence, even if they might give the impression of a better ventilatory control with the possibility of a 'fully automatic mode', which may simplify NIV, these modes should not be used as a first-line therapy. Further studies are thus needed to evaluate these modes and features and to establish if effective ventilation may be more easily obtained and therefore more cost-effective.

Neurally adjusted ventilatory assist (NAVA) is a mode that is exclusively available in the ICU.[31] During NAVA, the ventilator assist is not activated by a pneumatic trigger, but is rather synchronised with the diaphragm electrical activity (EAdi). The EAdi, recorded using a specific nasogastric tube equipped with electrodes, is a reliable and a very fast reflection of the respiratory drive. During NAVA, the ventilatory assist is triggered when EAdi exceeds a threshold (usually 0.5 μV). The proportionality factor 'NAVA level' permits to adapt the magnitude of respiratory unloading. Inspiratory support is interrupted when EAdi decreases below 70% of peak EAdi, with the maintenance of the sole PEEP. The major advantages of NAVA are a better synchronisation of the patient with the ventilator, a proportional assistance in response to the patient's drive and a ventilatory variability that is closer to a physiological variability. The most important limitation in long-term practice is that NAVA is currently available only with one ICU ventilator. NAVA is therefore available only in the ICU and not for home ventilation. However, large clinical trials are warranted to evaluate if this optimisation leads to improved clinical outcomes such as a greater NIV success rate or decreases in the duration of ventilatory assistance.

Ventilators for NIV in children

In the acute setting, ICU ventilators are used for NIV as most of these devices incorporate an NIV mode. However, compared to home ventilators, no study has validated or compared the efficacy of the different ICU ventilators for NIV.[16]

Numerous ventilators are available for home NIV. Constant CPAP is effective whatever the patient's age and can be efficiently performed with any CPAP device. However, as all CPAP devices have been designed for adult patients, manufacturers recommend a minimal weight, usually between 10 and 30 kg, for the use of complex CPAP modes. Moreover, the analysis of the in-built software of the ventilator is a simple way to monitor patient's compliance and variable ventilator parameters such as airway pressure and unintentional leaks. However, the sensitivity of the in-built software of CPAP devices is insufficient for infants, which limits the use of these data. Furthermore, most CPAP devices do not have a battery and/or alarms adapted for young children. The choice of the CPAP device will thus depend on the necessity of a humidification system, a battery, alarms and, of course, the weight and the cost of the ventilator.

Devices specifically designed for children and even infants, delivering volume, pressure, or combined modes, are now available. Important improvements have been made in trigger sensitivities, minimal volumes, backup rates and alarms, allowing the use of these devices in totally ventilator-dependent children or children with complex respiratory disorders.

INTERFACES FOR NIV IN CHILDREN

Numerous different types of interfaces are available for NIV in children (Table 56.1). Interfaces may cover the nose (nasal mask) (Figure 56.1), the nose and the mouth (nasobuccal mask), the face (total facemask) and exceptionally the mouth only (mouthpiece)[32,33] (Table 56.1). Nasal pillows (or prongs or cannulas) are minimal contact interfaces, which are available for school-aged children and are very well tolerated (Figure 56.2).[32] Interfaces can be vented, meaning that they incorporate intentional leaks to be used with a single circuit and a minimal positive expiratory pressure and non-vented masks, which can be used with a double circuit, a circuit with an expiratory valve and with or without a positive expiratory pressure. A minimal level of expiratory pressure is mandatory for vented masks, in order to allow the clearing of carbon dioxide during expiration.[34,35] The choice of the interface is determined by the patient's age, weight, facial anatomy, nasal permeability, presence of mouth breathing, ventilatory mode (requiring a vented or non-vented interface), comfort and tolerance with the interface and the patient's ability to remove the interface by him(her)self. The headgear is as important as the interface. Indeed, in case of an appropriate headgear, it will not be possible to deliver NIV to the child, even in the case of an appropriate interface. This is of major importance as numerous children requiring NIV have deformities of the skull (such as patients with craniofaciostenosis). Nasal masks and full facemasks are also now available for newborns and infants, which contribute to the rapid expansion of NIV use in this age group.[36] Nasal masks also allow the use of a pacifier in infants, which contributes to the better acceptance of NIV and the reduction of mouth leaks. An algorithm for the choice of an interface for children is presented in Figure 56.3.

The helmet has been shown to be a very effective interface but its high dead space and the risk of asphyxia in case of power failure or other technical problems restrict its use in the PICU (Figure 56.4).[37,38] Moreover, the quality of the

Table 56.1 Interfaces for NIV in children

Interface	Advantages	Disadvantages	Side effects
Nasal prongs	Small, light, no pressure sores	Not usable in case of mouth leaks	Nasal irritation
Nasal mask	Small volume; large choice	Not usable in case of mouth leaks	Pressure sores
Nasobuccal mask	Prevents mouth leaks	Large volume Risk of inhalation in case of gastro-oesophageal reflux Communication/vocalisation impairment Increased aerophagia	Pressure sores
Full facemask	Prevents mouth leaks	Large volume Risk of inhalation in case of gastro-oesophageal reflux Communication/vocalisation impairment Increased aerophagia	Pressure sores
Helmet	Prevents mouth leaks; no pressure sores	Large volume Risk of inhalation in case of gastro-oesophageal reflux Communication/vocalisation impairment Increased aerophagia Reserved for the ICU	Noise

Note: ICU, intensive care unit.

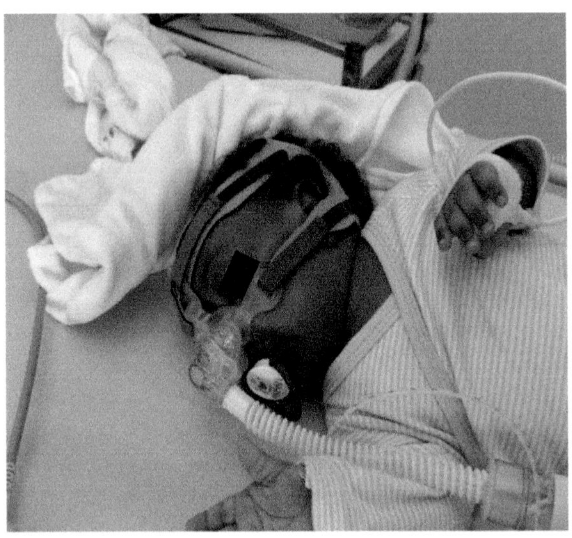

Figure 56.1 Nasal mask in an infant on home CPAP.

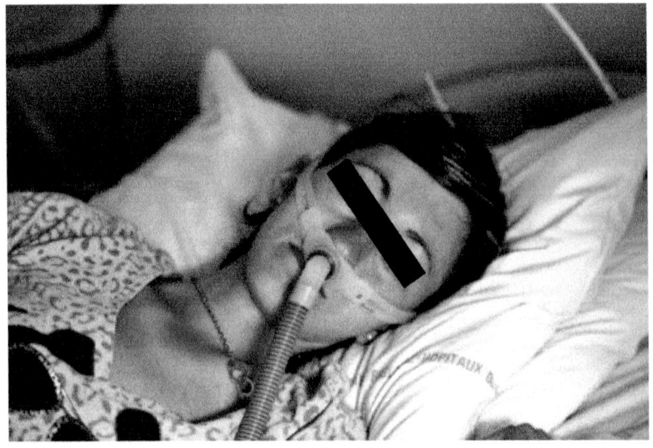

Figure 56.2 Nasal cannula in an adolescent.

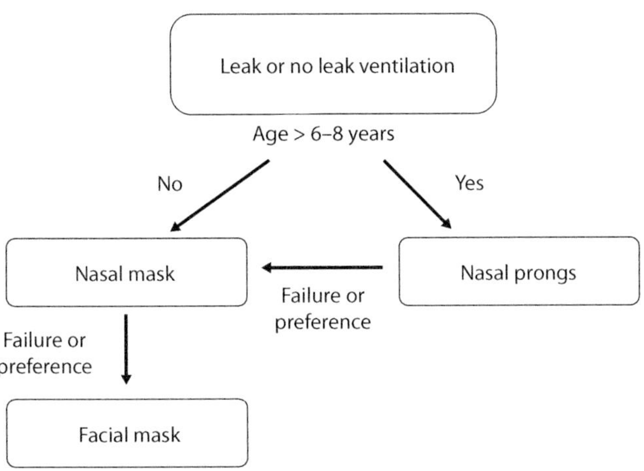

Figure 56.3 Algorithm for the choice of an interface for children.

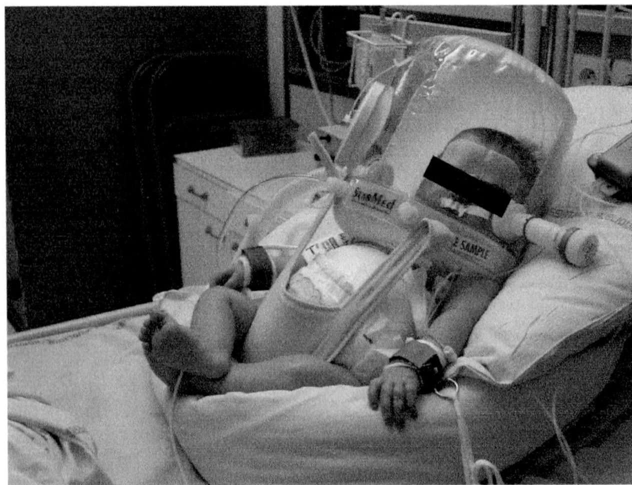

Figure 56.4 Helmet in an infant with bronchiolitis in the PICU.

ventilatory support may be less optimal with this interface compared to a facemask or a tracheal cannula.[39]

The interface represents a crucial determinant of the success of NIV. The patient will be unable to tolerate and accept NIV in case of facial discomfort, skin injury or significant air leaks. The evaluation of the short-term tolerance of the nasal mask is thus an essential component of NIV.[20,32]

CHAPTER SUMMARY

NIV is rapidly expanding in children, in both the acute and chronic settings. This increase in the use of NIV contrasts with the lack of validated initiating criteria and limited proven benefits. In children, NIV is characterised by a tremendous heterogeneity of the disorders, ages, prognosis and outcomes. Important improvements have been made in ventilators and interfaces. An important area of research will thus be to determine the optimal (and minimal) technical requirements for a ventilator for a specific condition or disease. Ergonomic characteristics, such as weight and autonomy, are also important aspects for home NIV, but the major contributor of NIV success remains the expertise of the paediatric team dealing with these patients.

REFERENCES

1. Pirret AM, Sherring CL, Tai JA et al. Local experience with the use of nasal bubble CPAP in infants with bronchiolitis admitted to a combined adult/paediatric intensive care unit. *Intensive Crit Care Nurs.* 2005; 21:314–9.
2. Shah PS, Ohlsson A, Shah JP. Continuous negative extrathoracic pressure or continuous positive airway pressure for acute hypoxemic respiratory failure in children. *Cochrane Database Syst Rev.* 2008;23:CD003699.
3. Javouhey E, Barats A, Richard N et al. Non-invasive ventilation as primary ventilatory support for infants with severe bronchiolitis. *Intensive Care Med.* 2008;34:1608–14.
4. Thia LP, McKenzie SA, Blyth TP et al. Randomised controlled trial of nasal continuous positive airways pressure (CPAP) in bronchiolitis. *Arch Dis Child.* 2008;93:45–7.
5. Ellafi M, Vinsonneau C, Coste J et al. One-year outcome after severe pulmonary exacerbation in adults with cystic fibrosis. *Am J Respir Crit Care Med.* 2005;171:158–64.
6. Sood N, Paradowski LJ, Yankaskas JR. Outcomes of intensive care unit care in adults with cystic fibrosis. *Am J Respir Crit Care Med* 2001;163:335–8.
7. Texereau J, Jamal D, Choukroun G et al. Determinants of mortality for adults with cystic fibrosis admitted in intensive care unit: A multicenter study. *Respir Res.* 2006;7:14–24.
8. Fortenberry JD, Del Toro J, Jefferson LS et al. Management of pediatric acute hypoxemic respiratory insufficiency with bilevel positive pressure (BiPAP) nasal mask ventilation. *Chest.* 1995;108:1059–64.
9. Padman R, Lawless S, Von Nessen S. Use of BiPAP by nasal mask in the treatment of respiratory insufficiency in pediatric patients: Preliminary investigation. *Pediatr Pulmonol.* 1994;17:119–23.
10. Essouri S, Durand P, Chevret L et al. Physiological effects of noninvasive positive ventilation during acute moderate hypercapnic respiratory insufficiency in children. *Intensive Care Med.* 2008;34:2248–55.
11. Fauroux B, Pigeot J, Polkey MI et al. Chronic stridor caused by laryngomalacia in children: Work of breathing and effects of noninvasive ventilatory assistance. *Am J Respir Crit Care Med.* 2001; 164:1874–8.
12. Essouri S, Nicot F, Clement A et al. Noninvasive positive pressure ventilation in infants with upper airway obstruction: Comparison of continuous and bilevel positive pressure. *Intensive Care Med.* 2005;31:574–80.
13. Pavone M, Verrillo E, Caldarelli V et al. Non-invasive positive pressure ventilation in children. *Early Hum Dev.* 2013;89:S25–31.
14. McDougall CM, Adderley RJ, Wensley DF, Seear MD. Long-term ventilation in children: Longitudinal trends and outcomes. *Arch Dis Child.* 2013;98:660–5.
15. Amaddeo A, Moreau J, Frapin A et al. Long term continuous positive airway pressure (CPAP) and non-invasive ventilation (NIV) in children: Initiation criteria in real life. *Pediatr Pulmonol.* 2016;51:968–74.
16. Fauroux B, Leroux K, Desmarais G et al. Performance of ventilators for noninvasive positive-pressure ventilation in children. *Eur Respir J.* 2008;31:1300–7.
17. Fauroux B, Pigeot J, Isabey D et al. In vivo physiological comparison of two ventilators used for domiciliary ventilation in children with cystic fibrosis. *Crit Care Med.* 2001;29:2097–105.
18. Fauroux B, Nicot F, Essouri S et al. Setting of pressure support in young patients with cystic fibrosis. *Eur Resp J.* 2004;24:624–30.
19. Gonzalez J, Sharshar T, Hart N et al. Air leaks during mechanical ventilation as a cause of persistent hypercapnia in neuromuscular disorders. *Intensive Care Med.* 2003;29:596–602.
20. Fauroux B, Lavis JF, Nicot F et al. Facial side effects during noninvasive positive pressure ventilation in children. *Intensive Care Med.* 2005;31:965–9.
21. Guilleminault C, Nino-Murcia G, Heldt G et al. Alternative treatment to tracheostomy in obstructive sleep apnea syndrome: Nasal continuous positive airway pressure in young children. *Pediatrics.* 1986;78:797–802.
22. Guilleminault C, Pelayo R, Clerk A et al. Home nasal continuous positive airway pressure in infants with sleep-disordered breathing. *J Pediatr.* 1995;127:905–12.

23. Waters WA, Everett FM, Bruderer JW, Sullivan CE. Obstructive sleep apnea: The use of nasal CPAP in 80 children. *Am J Respir Crit Care Med.* 1995; 152:780–5.
24. Giovannini-Chami L, Khirani S, Thouvenin G et al. Work of breathing to optimize noninvasive ventilation in bronchiolitis obliterans. *Intensive Care Med.* 2012;38:722–4.
25. Khirani S, Ramirez A, Aloui S et al. CPAP titration in infants with severe airway obstruction. *Crit Care.* 2013;17:R167.
26. Chihara Y, Tsuboi T, Hitomi T et al. Flexible positive airway pressure improves treatment adherence compared with auto-adjusting PAP. *Sleep.* 2013;36:229–36.
27. Marcus CL, Rosen G, Ward SL et al. Adherence to and effectiveness of positive airway pressure therapy in children with obstructive sleep apnea. *Pediatrics* 2006;117:e442–51.
28. Marcus CL, Beck SE, Traylor J et al. Randomized, double-blind clinical trial of two different modes of positive airway pressure therapy on adherence and efficacy in children. *J Clin Sleep Med.* 2012;8:37–42.
29. Fauroux B, Leroux K, Desmarais G et al. Performance of ventilators for noninvasive positive-pressure ventilation in children. *Eur Respir J.* 2008;31:1300–7.
30. Brochard L, Pluskwa F, Lemaire F. Improved efficacy of spontaneous breathing with inspiratory pressure support. *Am Rev Resp Dis.* 1987;136:411–5.
31. Rabec C, Emeriaud G, Amaddeo A et al. New modes in non-invasive ventilation. *Paediatr Respir Rev.* 2016;18:73–84.
32. Ramirez A, Delord V, Khirani S et al. Interfaces for long-term noninvasive positive pressure ventilation in children. *Intensive Care Med.* 2012;38:655–62.
33. Khirani S, Kadlub N, Delord V et al. Nocturnal mouthpiece ventilation and medical hypnosis to treat severe obstructive sleep apnea in a child with cherubism. *Pediatr Pulmonol.* 2013;48:927–9.
34. Lofaso F, Brochard L, Touchard D et al. Evaluation of carbon dioxide rebreathing during pressure support ventilation with airway management system (BiPAP) devices. *Chest.* 1995;108:772–8.
35. Gregoretti C, Navalesi P, Ghannadian S et al. Choosing a ventilator for home mechanical ventilation. *Breathe.* 2013;9:394–409.
36. Amaddeo A, Abadie V, Chalouhi C et al. Continuous positive airway pressure for upper airway obstruction in infants with Pierre Robin Sequence. *Plast Reconstr Surg.* 2016;137:609–12.
37. Piastra M, Antonelli M, Chiaretti A et al. Treatment of acute respiratory failure by helmet-delivered non-invasive pressure support ventilation in children with acute leukemia: A pilot study. *Intensive Care Med.* 2004;30:472–6.
38. Piastra M, Antonelli M, Caresta E et al. Noninvasive ventilation in childhood acute neuromuscular respiratory failure: A pilot study. *Respiration.* 2006;73:791–8.
39. Moerer O, Fischer S, Hartelt M et al. Influence of two different interfaces for noninvasive ventilation compared to invasive ventilation on the mechanical properties and performance of a respiratory system: A lung model study. *Chest.* 2006;129:1424–31.

57

Chronic non-invasive ventilation for children

ALESSANDRO AMADDEO, ANNICK FRAPIN AND BRIGITTE FAUROUX

INTRODUCTION

A growing population of children require non-invasive ventilation (NIV) due to neuromuscular disease, abnormalities of the airways, the chest wall and/or the lungs or disorders of ventilatory control.[1,2] These disorders are fundamentally hypoventilation disorders. As such, oxygen therapy *alone* is not only usually ineffective in relieving symptoms, but has also been shown to be dangerous and may lead to a marked acceleration of carbon dioxide (CO_2) retention.[3,4] NIV, by replacing or assisting the respiratory muscles in the case of neuromuscular or lung diseases, or by maintaining airway patency during the breathing cycle in the case of obstructive sleep apnoea (OSA), improves alveolar ventilation. There is some evidence of decreased mortality with NIV, but the main benefit is indisputably a benefit to the family experience and health-related quality of life.[2,5–8] However, the increase in NIV use contrasts with the lack of validated initiation criteria and the limited proven physiological benefits. The adequate choice of equipment and careful monitoring are important factors contributing to the success of NIV. The tremendous heterogeneity of the disorders, ages, prognosis and outcomes of the patients underlines the necessity of management by experienced paediatric multidisciplinary centres.

This chapter focuses on chronic NIV for children, with a special focus on indications and contraindications, before concluding on future developments.

PATHOPHYSIOLOGY

The ability to sustain spontaneous ventilation can be viewed as a balance between neurological mechanisms controlling ventilation together with respiratory muscle power on one hand and the respiratory load, determined by lung, thoracic and airway mechanics on the other (Figure 57.1). The significant dysfunction of any of these components of the respiratory system may impair the ability to spontaneously generate efficacious breaths. In healthy individuals, central respiratory drive and ventilatory muscle power exceed the respiratory load, enabling them to sustain adequate spontaneous ventilation. However, if the respiratory load is too high and/or respiratory muscle power or central respiratory drive is too low, ventilation may be inadequate, resulting in hypercapnia. Chronic ventilatory failure, then, is the result of an imbalance in the respiratory system, in which respiratory muscle power and central respiratory drive are inadequate to overcome the respiratory load. If this imbalance cannot be corrected with medical treatment, long-term NIV may be indicated. NIV will be preferentially delivered by means of a non-invasive interface, which is associated with a greater comfort and less morbidity than a tracheostomy.

Three categories of respiratory system dysfunction may thus benefit from NIV: an increase in respiratory load (due to intrinsic lung diseases, upper airway abnormalities or skeletal deformities), respiratory muscle weakness (due to neuromuscular diseases or spinal cord injury) or failure of the neurological control of ventilation (with central hypoventilation syndrome being the most common presentation) (Figure 57.1).

Increase in respiratory load

Upper or lower airway obstruction and chest wall deformity are disorders characterised by an increase in respiratory load.

OSA is less common in children than in adults. The pathophysiology is also different with the predominant role of enlarged tonsils and adenoids. If adenotonsillectomy is not able to relieve upper airway obstruction, then non-invasive continuous positive airway pressure (CPAP) is proposed as a first therapeutic option.[9–11] Indeed, the maintenance of airway patency by means of CPAP reduces the respiratory muscle output, which translates into an improvement in alveolar ventilation.

An increase in respiratory load is also observed in patients with advanced pulmonary cystic fibrosis (CF) disease. Indeed, as lung disease progresses, indices reflecting

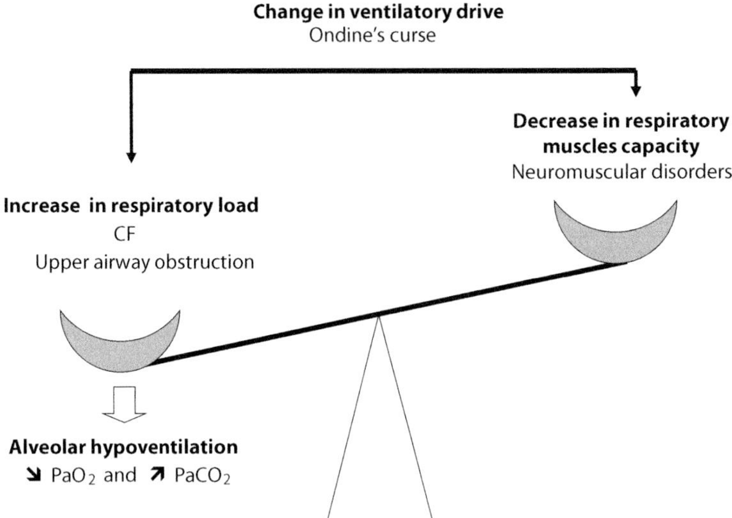

Figure 57.1 Spontaneous ventilation is the result of a balance between neurological mechanisms controlling ventilation together with ventilatory muscle power on one side and the respiratory load, determined by lung, thoracic and airway mechanics, on the other. If the respiratory load is too high and/or ventilatory muscle power or central respiratory drive is too low, ventilation may be inadequate, resulting in alveolar hypoventilation with hypercapnia and hypoxemia. CF, cystic fibrosis; $PaCO_2$, partial arterial carbon dioxide pressure; PaO_2, partial arterial oxygen pressure.

the respiratory muscle output, such as the oesophageal and diaphragmatic pressure time products and the elastic work of breathing, dramatically increase.[12] As a result, the patients develop a compensatory mechanism of rapid shallow breathing pattern in an attempt to reduce the increase in load, which translates into a rise in partial arterial carbon dioxide pressure ($PaCO_2$). Short-term physiological studies, during wakefulness and sleep, have demonstrated that NIV reduces respiratory muscle load and work of breathing,[13–15] which translates into an improvement in alveolar ventilation and gas exchange.

Respiratory muscle weakness

Respiratory muscles are rarely spared in neuromuscular diseases.[16] In general, inadequate gas exchange results from inspiratory muscle weakness, which limits inspiration thus leading to repeated atelectasis and hypoventilation, and from expiratory muscles involvement which causes cough inability and predisposes to lung infections. Respiratory muscle weakness, dysfunction or paralysis can occur because of neuromuscular disease, or as a result of spinal cord injury.

The most common neuromuscular diseases requiring NIV during childhood are Duchenne muscular dystrophy (DMD) and spinal muscular atrophy (SMA). DMD is a progressive disorder, and ventilatory failure is inevitable in the course of the disease, although the time course of progression to it varies between individuals. Home NIV counteracts the hypoventilation and has been shown to improve survival.[5,17,18] Respiratory failure is also common in children with SMA type I or II. Respiratory failure is less frequent in other muscular dystrophies, such as Becker, limb-girdle and facioscapulohumeral dystrophies. Congenital myopathies are often static.[16] However, some congenital myopathies such as collagen 6 myopathies are characterised by a predominant weakness of the diaphragm, exposing these children to sleep-disordered breathing, although their peripheral muscle strength remains relatively preserved.[19] Finally, the conditions of children with neuromuscular disease may functionally deteriorate with growth because weakened muscles are unable to cope with increasing body mass.

The importance of respiratory failure associated with spinal cord injury depends on the level of the injury. High spinal cord injury, above C3, causes diaphragm paralysis. In patients with lower cervical cord injury, expiratory muscle function is compromised, impairing cough and the clearance of bronchial secretions. As a result, the retention of secretions leading to atelectasis and bronchopneumonia frequently occurs. All these children with respiratory muscle weakness often do not have severe intrinsic or parenchymal lung disease; thus, they are good candidates for home NIV.

Failure of the neurological control of ventilation

Disorders of the neurological control of breathing that are severe enough to cause chronic respiratory failure are uncommon to rare. Congenital central hypoventilation syndrome (Ondine's curse) is the most common presentation in childhood and is characterised by failure of the autonomic control of breathing predominantly occurring during sleep.[20] A tracheostomy is nearly always mandatory in infants and young children, but older children may be switched to NIV when ventilatory assistance may be restricted to sleep.[21,22]

Table 57.1 Potential benefits of long-term NIV in children according to the underlying disease

	Neuromuscular disorders	Obstructive sleep apnoea	Cystic fibrosis
Improvement in nocturnal hypoventilation and gas exchange	Yes	Yes	Yes
Increase in survival	Yes (in patients with Duchenne muscular dystrophy)	Not applicable (tracheostomy is an alternative)	Not proven
Improvement in lung function	Not proven	Not applicable	Limited data
Improvement in respiratory muscle performance	Not proven	Not applicable	Limited data
Improvement in exercise tolerance	Not proven	Not applicable	Limited data
Preservation of normal pulmonary mechanics and lung growth	Not proven	Not applicable	Not applicable
Improvement of quality of life	Yes	Yes (as an alternative to tracheostomy)	Not proven

BENEFITS OF NIV

The benefits of NIV vary according to the underlying disease. Some beneficial effects, such as the correction of nocturnal alveolar hypoventilation, are common to the different diagnostic groups, whereas other effects, such as the increase in survival, may be specific to some disorders (Table 57.1). Evidence-based studies on the indications, benefits and weaning criteria of chronic NIV in children are scarce. This may be explained by the heterogeneity of underlying diseases and practical and ethical issues.

Correction of nocturnal hypoventilation and gas exchange

The correction of nocturnal hypoventilation by NIV has been documented for different causes of alveolar hypoventilation in children. Sleep is associated with changes in respiratory mechanics, such as an increase in ventilation–perfusion mismatch and in airflow resistance and a fall in functional residual capacity (Figure 57.2). Although the activity of the diaphragm is preserved, that of the intercostal and the upper airway muscles significantly decreases. Finally, central drive and chemoreceptor sensitivity are less efficient during sleep than during wakefulness. All these abnormalities explain a physiological degree of nocturnal hypoventilation causing a rise in $PaCO_2$ of up to 3 mmHg (0.4 kPa) in healthy adults.[23] This decrease in alveolar ventilation predominates during rapid eye movement sleep and explains why patients with chronic respiratory failure are more vulnerable during this sleep stage.

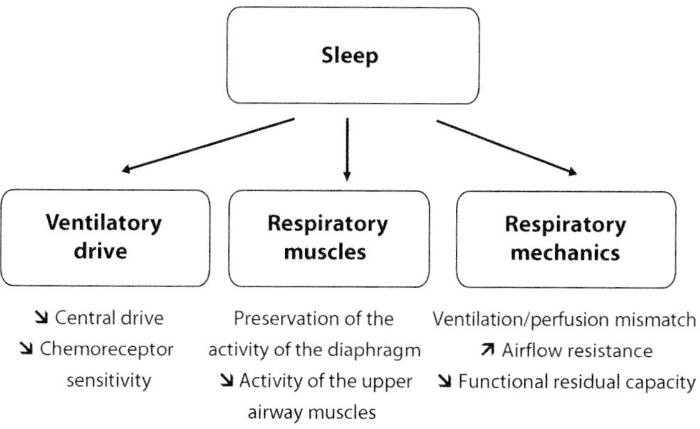

Figure 57.2 Physiological alterations during sleep explaining the worsening of respiratory failure during sleep.

NIV has been shown to correct nocturnal hypoventilation in children with OSA,[9–11,24] neuromuscular disease[25–28] and CF.[29–33]

Increase in survival

The improvement in survival represents a major expectation of NIV in patients with progressive neuromuscular or lung disease. This benefit has been observed only in patients with DMD in a case series[5] and in one nationwide study. Indeed, an analysis of the national DMD register in Denmark showed that mortality significantly fell between 1977 and 2001 due to the large increase in ventilator users.[18] NIV, associated with nutritional support and cough-assisted techniques, has also been shown to increase survival in infants with SMA type I.[34] An increase in survival has not been demonstrated in patients with CF.[33] In patients with OSA, survival is not an issue, because a tracheostomy may constitute an alternative to NIV.

Improvement in lung function, respiratory muscle performance and exercise tolerance

The stabilisation or the slowing of the decline in lung function by NIV in patients whose disease course is characterised by a decline in lung function, such as patients with neuromuscular disease or CF, represents a major expectation of long-term NIV. No data are presently available to support this hypothesis for patients with neuromuscular disease.[28,35] Data from the French Cystic Fibrosis Observatory have shown that NIV may be associated with a stabilisation of the decline in lung function in patients with advanced lung disease.[36] However, no change in lung function was observed after 6 weeks of NIV in eight adult patients with CF, but this study was limited by the use of too low NIV airway pressures.[15,32]

Few studies have analysed the effect of NIV on respiratory muscle function in patients with CF. An increase in maximal expiratory (PEmax) and inspiratory pressure (PImax) has been observed in four adults with CF after 1 month of NIV.[37] But because of the very small number of patients and the possibility of a learning effect or a better motivation, these results should be interpreted with caution. More interestingly, significant increases in PImax and PEmax have been observed in children and adults with CF after a physiotherapy session performed with NIV compared to standard physiotherapy session.[38,39]

Patients with chronic respiratory insufficiency are at risk of acute exacerbations, which are mainly triggered by respiratory tract infections. Although no prospective randomised trial is available (and would be ethically questionable), the use of NIV in patients with CF hospitalised for an acute respiratory exacerbation was associated with a more rapid recovery.[40–42] Within the same context, long-term NIV was associated with a decrease in hospitalisations for respiratory tract infection in children with neuromuscular disease.[27,43]

Preservation of normal pulmonary mechanics and lung growth

A major concern in children is the effect of chronic hypoventilation on lung and chest wall growth and, as a logical consequence, the effect of NIV in promoting or preserving physiologic lung growth in the developing child. An observational study in infants with neuromuscular disease showed that long-term NIV was associated with an improvement in chest wall shape.[44]

Improvement of quality of sleep and quality of life

In a small group of children with SMA, NIV was associated in an improvement in symptoms of nocturnal hypoventilation and the maintenance of the different modules of quality-of-life measures, with the exception of the physical module, which reflects the progression of the underlying neuromuscular disease.[45] NIV was also associated with an improvement in the quality of life in boys with DMD.[5] Such a benefit has not yet been demonstrated in patients with CF. However, NIV has been shown to reduce dyspnoea during physiotherapy[39] and in the long term.[32]

CLINICAL APPLICATIONS

Indications

There are no validated criteria for starting long-term NIV in children. A recent study analysing all the children who were started on long-term home NIV over a 1-year period showed that NIV was initiated during three different clinical scenarios: in the paediatric intensive care unit because of the inability to be weaned from ventilatory support after an acute respiratory failure requiring an acute initiation of NIV or an endotracheal intubation, in a subacute setting after a variable association of nocturnal gas exchange abnormalities alone and in a chronic setting after a scheduled polygraphy or a polysomnography in a child referred for sleep-disordered breathing symptoms or an underlying disease associated with a high risk of sleep-disordered breathing.[46] A major issue for the future will be to determine the efficacy of NIV according to these different clinical scenarios and the underlying disease.

In clinical practice, consensus conferences agree on the value of daytime hypercapnia and recurrent acute respiratory exacerbations to initiate NIV because these criteria are the signature of established ventilatory failure.[47–49] These criteria are valuable for patients with neuromuscular disease and lung disease such as CF.[50] But these classical criteria are preceded by a variable period of nocturnal hypoventilation during which treatable symptoms, such as frequent arousals, poor sleep quality, severe orthopnoea, daytime fatigue and alterations in cognitive function may deteriorate the daily life of the patient. A major issue is thus to determine the optimal timing of a sleep study to document nocturnal hypoventilation. Sleep-disordered breathing may be difficult to establish in children because of reliance on parents and second-hand caregivers, who have a different perception of the child's disease.[35] Patients with chronic disorders tend to underestimate symptoms such as fatigue before using NIV because onset is generally insidious. A study comparing symptoms associated with sleep-disordered breathing in children with neuromuscular disease did not observe a significant difference between children with or without objective alveolar hypoventilation.[51] Lung function parameters are poor indicators of nocturnal hypoventilation. In patients with neuromuscular disease, vital capacity (VC) and inspiratory VC have been shown to have some correlation with daytime and nocturnal gas exchange.[52,53] Daytime predictors of nocturnal hypoventilation have mainly been identified for patients with DMD who represent a more homogeneous group of patients. As such, the forced expiratory volume in 1 s (FEV1), daytime PaO_2 and $PaCO_2$, base excess and the rapid shallow breathing index are all significantly correlated to nocturnal hypoventilation in patients with DMD.[54–57] Another prospective study performed in a large group of children with various neuromuscular disorders did not observe a correlation between parameters evaluating lung or respiratory muscle function and nocturnal hypoxemia or hypercapnia.[58] In patients with CF, the correlation between objective and subjective parameters of sleep-disordered breathing was also weak.[59] A study showed that the initiation of NIV at the stage of nocturnal hypercapnia without daytime hypercapnia in children and adults with neuromuscular disorders and chest wall disease was associated with an improvement in nocturnal gas exchange.[60] Larger prospective studies, in a homogeneous group of patients, are warranted to confirm the benefit of the initiation of NIV at the stage of 'isolated' nocturnal hypoventilation.

Abundant recent data have underpinned the importance of neurocognitive dysfunction in children with even mild OSA.[61–63] This underlines the importance of a complete correction of OSA in children. Recent recommendations suggest that CPAP should be initiated in a child when the apnoea hypopnoea index (AHI) >5–10/hours after surgical (adenotonsillectomy), medical (anti-inflammatory treatment) and/or orthodontic treatment.[64]

Thus, future studies are mandatory to establish, for every diagnostic group, first the most pertinent criteria for a sleep study and, second, those which may require the initiation of NIV.

Contraindications, side effects and limits of NIV

NIV is preferred over invasive mechanical ventilation as the first therapy of severe sleep-disordered breathing. However, NIV is contraindicated in some circumstances which, however, continuously evolve (Table 57.2).[65] These contraindications also depend on the child's medical condition, the quality of the family training, the family structure and reliability and the experience of the medical team. Discharge at home care requires a motivated family, with adequate and appropriate training of the family and caregivers, a suitable home environment and adequate funding and healthcare resources.

Table 57.2 Contraindications for NIV

Relative Contraindications
- Severe swallowing impairment
- Inadequate family/caregiver support
- Need for full-time ventilatory assistance

Absolute Contraindications
- Complete persistent upper airway obstruction during NIV
- Uncontrollable secretion retention
- Inability to cooperate
- Inability to achieve adequate peak cough flow, even with assistance
- Inability to fit any non-invasive interface

Source: Hill NS, *Semin Respir Crit Care Med*, 23, 293–305, 2005.

NIV may be temporarily contraindicated in the case of recent pneumothorax, which may occur in patients with advanced CF lung disease. An upper airway examination is systematically recommended before the initiation of NIV. Indeed, in patients with CF, nasal polyps are common and should be treated before the initiation of NIV. In children with OSA, adenotonsillectomy is the first-line treatment; residual OSA should be checked by a control sleep study 2–4 months after the upper airway surgery.

Side effects of NIV are more often due to the interface than to NIV itself. Skin injury is the most common side effect of the interface.[66] In young children, there is also a potential risk of facial deformity, such as facial flattening and maxilla retrusion, caused by the pressure applied by the mask on growing facial structures. These potential side effects justify the first-line use of minimal contact interfaces such a nasal prongs (or canula) and systematic evaluation before the initiation and during the follow-up of children receiving NIV by a paediatric maxillofacial specialist. Abdominal distension caused by NIV may be observed and can be corrected by improving patient–ventilator interaction, decreasing the airway pressure or the tidal volume.[11]

NIV is not always successful in adequately relieving hypoventilation.[67] Air leaks have been shown to be an important cause of persistent hypercapnia in neuromuscular patients.[67] Simple practical measures, such as choosing an appropriate interface, increasing the ventilator settings, or changing the type of the ventilator, are able to reduce the volume of air leaks and improve the efficacy of NIV.[67,68]

In patients with neuromuscular disease, cough-assisted techniques should be associated to NIV. Several techniques are available such as manual physiotherapy, intermittent positive pressure breathing and mechanical insufflation–exsufflation.[69,70] These techniques, associated with daytime ventilation by means of a mouthpiece,[71,72] extends the use of NIV in patients having increasing ventilatory dependency.

However, despite these measures, in progressive diseases such as some neuromuscular diseases, a tracheotomy may become necessary. The close monitoring of the patient's physiological status and disease progression, together with clear information of the family, is essential for the decision of a tracheotomy. It is essential that the child, if the age permits it, and the parents have the opportunity to discuss the tracheotomy in advance. Discussion should start long enough before the anticipated need to allow the child and the family to thoroughly evaluate options and to discuss their feelings.

In conclusion, NIV is increasingly used in children and infants. Further studies should aim at validating the most pertinent criteria to initiate NIV according to the disease and the age of the patient, to evaluate the long-term benefits with regard to the increase in survival, stabilisation in the decline of lung function and respiratory muscle performance, promotion of lung growth and respiratory mechanics and, most importantly, the quality of life of the child and his family.

CHAPTER SUMMARY

Long-term NIV represents an efficient respiratory support, which has transformed the scope of chronic respiratory failure and severe sleep-disordered breathing in children. The tremendous heterogeneity of the disorders, ages, prognosis and outcomes of the patients underlines the necessity of management by experienced multidisciplinary centres, having technical competencies in paediatric NIV and an expertise in sleep studies and therapeutic education. The increased use of NIV contrasts with the limited proven benefits. Future studies should aim at defining disease- and age-appropriate initiations and weaning criteria, as well as the objective physiological and quality-of-life benefits.

REFERENCES

1. Pavone M, Verrillo E, Caldarelli V et al. Non-invasive positive pressure ventilation in children. *Early Hum Dev.* 2013;89:S25–31.
2. McDougall CM, Adderley RJ, Wensley DF, Seear MD. Long-term ventilation in children: Longitudinal trends and outcomes. *Arch Dis Child.* 2013;98:660–5.
3. Gay P, Edmonds L. Severe hypercapnia after low-flow oxygen therapy in patients with neuromuscular disease and diaphragmatic dysfunction. *Mayo Clin Proc.* 1995;70:327–30.
4. Masa J, Celli B, Riesco J et al. Noninvasive positive pressure ventilation and not oxygen may prevent overt ventilatory failure in patients with chest wall disease. *Chest.* 1997;112:207–13.
5. Simonds A, Muntoni F, Heather S, Fielding S. Impact of nasal ventilation on survival in hypercapnic Duchenne muscular dystrophy. *Thorax.* 1998;53:949–52.
6. Graham RJ, Fleegler EW, Robinson WM. Chronic ventilator need in the community: A 2005 pediatric census of Massachusetts. *Pediatrics.* 2007;119:e1280–7.
7. Marcus CL, Radcliffe J, Konstantinopoulou S et al. Effects of positive airway pressure therapy on neurobehavioral outcomes in children with obstructive sleep apnea. *Am J Respir Crit Care Med.* 2012;185:998–1003.
8. Nozoe KT, Polesel DN, Moreira GA et al. Sleep quality of mother-caregivers of Duchenne muscular dystrophy patients. *Sleep Breath.* 2016;20:129–34.
9. Waters WA, Everett FM, Bruderer JW, Sullivan CE. Obstructive sleep apnea: The use of nasal CPAP in 80 children. *Am J Respir Crit Care Med.* 1995;152:780–5.
10. Guilleminault C, Nino-Murcia G, Heldt G et al. Alternative treatment to tracheostomy in obstructive sleep apnea syndrome: Nasal continuous positive airway pressure in young children. *Pediatrics.* 1986;78:797–802.
11. Guilleminault C, Pelayo R, Clerk A et al. Home nasal continuous positive airway pressure in infants with sleep-disordered breathing. *J Pediatr.* 1995; 127:905–12.
12. Hart N, Polkey MI, Clément A et al. Changes in pulmonary mechanics with increasing disease severity in children and young adults with cystic fibrosis. *Am J Respir Crit Care Med.* 2002;166:61–6.
13. Fauroux B, Pigeot J, Isabey D et al. In vivo physiological comparison of two ventilators used for domiciliary ventilation in children with cystic fibrosis. *Crit Care Med.* 2001;29:2097–105.
14. Fauroux B, Louis B, Hart N et al. The effect of back-up rate during non-invasive ventilation in young patients with cystic fibrosis. *Intensive Care Med.* 2004;30:673–81.
15. Fauroux B, Nicot F, Essouri S et al. Setting of pressure support in young patients with cystic fibrosis. *Eur Resp J.* 2004;24:624–30.
16. Nicot F, Hart N, Forin V et al. Respiratory muscle testing: A valuable tool for children with neuromuscular disorders. *Am J Respir Crit Care Med.* 2006;174:67–74.
17. Vianello A, Bevilacqua M, Salvador V et al. Long-term nasal intermittent positive pressure ventilation in advanced Duchenne's muscular dystrophy. *Chest.* 1994;105:445–8.
18. Jeppesen J, Green A, Steffensen BF, Rahbek J. The Duchenne muscular dystrophy population in Denmark, 1977–2001: Prevalence, incidence and survival in relation to the introduction of ventilator use. *Neuromuscul Disord.* 2003;13:804–12.
19. Quijano-Roy S, Khirani S, Colella M et al. Diaphragmatic dysfunction in Collagen VI myopathies. *Neuromuscul Disord.* 2014;24:125–33.
20. Gozal D. Congenital central hypoventilation syndrome: An update. *Pediatr Pulmonol.* 1998; 26:273–82.
21. Nielson DW, Black PG. Mask ventilation in congenital central alveolar hypoventilation syndrome. *Pediatr Pulmonol.* 1990;9:44–5.
22. Zaccaria S, Braghiroli A, Sacco C, Donner CF. Central hypoventilation in a seven year old boy: Long-term treatment by nasal mask ventilation. *Monaldi Arch Chest Dis.* 1993;48:37–8.
23. Gothe B, Altose MD, Goldman MD, Cherniak NS. Effect of quiet sleep on resting and CO_2 stimulated breathing in humans. *J Appl Physiol.* 1981;50:724–30.
24. Fauroux B, Pigeot J, Polkey MI et al. Chronic stridor caused by laryngomalacia in children: Work of breathing and effects of noninvasive ventilatory assistance. *Am J Respir Crit Care Med.* 2001;164:1874–8.
25. Simonds AK, Ward S, Heather S et al. Outcome of paediatric domiciliary mask ventilation in neuromuscular and skeletal disease. *Eur Respir J.* 2000;16:476–81.

26. Mellies U, Ragette R, Dohna Schwake C et al. Long-term noninvasive ventilation in children and adolescents with neuromuscular disorders. *Eur Respir J.* 2003;22:631–6.
27. Katz S, Selvadurai H, Keilty K et al. Outcome of non-invasive positive pressure ventilation in paediatric neuromuscular disease. *Arch Dis Child.* 2004;89:121–4.
28. Annane D, Orlikowski D, Chevret S et al. Nocturnal mechanical ventilation for chronic hypoventilation in patients with neuromuscular and chest wall disorders. *Cochrane Database Syst Rev.* 2007;17:CD001941.
29. Regnis JA, Piper AJ, Henke KG et al. Benefits of nocturnal nasal CPAP in patients with cystic fibrosis. *Chest.* 1994;106:1717–24.
30. Gozal D. Nocturnal ventilatory support in patients with cystic fibrosis: Comparison with supplemental oxygen. *Eur Resp J.* 1997;10:1999–2003.
31. Milross MA, Piper AJ, Norman M et al. Low-flow oxygen and bilevel ventilatory support: Effects on ventilation during sleep in cystic fibrosis. *Am J Respir Crit Care Med.* 2001;163:129–34.
32. Young AC, Wilson JW, Kotsimbos TC, Naughton MT. Randomised placebo controlled trial of non-invasive ventilation for hypercapnia in cystic fibrosis. *Thorax.* 2008;63:72–7.
33. Moran F, Bradley JM, Piper AJ. Non-invasive ventilation for cystic fibrosis. *Cochrane Database Syst Rev.* 2013;30:CD002769.
34. Oskoui M, Levy G, Garland CJ et al. The changing natural history of spinal muscular atrophy type 1. *Neurology.* 2007;69:1931–6.
35. Young HK, Lowe A, Fitzgerald DA et al. Outcome of noninvasive ventilation in children with neuromuscular disease. *Neurology.* 2007;68:198–201.
36. Fauroux B, Le Roux E, Ravilly S et al. Long-term noninvasive ventilation in patients with cystic fibrosis. *Respiration.* 2008;76(2):168–74.
37. Piper AJ, Parker S, Torzillo PJ et al. Nocturnal nasal IPPV stabilizes patients with cystic fibrosis and hypercapnic respiratory failure. *Chest.* 1992;102:846–50.
38. Fauroux B, Boulé M, Lofaso F et al. Chest physiotherapy in cystic fibrosis: Improved tolerance with nasal pressure support ventilation. *Pediatrics.* 1999;103:e32–40.
39. Holland AE, Denehy L, Ntoumenopoulos G et al. Non-invasive ventilation assists chest physiotherapy in adults with acute exacerbations of cystic fibrosis. *Thorax.* 2003;58:880–4.
40. Sood N, Paradowski LJ, Yankaskas JR. Outcomes of intensive care unit care in adults with cystic fibrosis. *Am J Respir Crit Care Med.* 2001;163:335–8.
41. Ellafi M, Vinsonneau C, Coste J et al. One-year outcome after severe pulmonary exacerbation in adults with cystic fibrosis. *Am J Respir Crit Care Med.* 2005;171:158–64.
42. Texereau J, Jamal D, Choukroun G et al. Determinants of mortality for adults with cystic fibrosis admitted in intensive care unit: A multicenter study. *Respir Res.* 2006;7:14–24.
43. Dohna-Schwake C, Podlewski P, Voit T, Mellies U. Non-invasive ventilation reduces respiratory tract infections in children with neuromuscular disorders. *Pediatr Pulmonol.* 2008;43:67–71.
44. Chatwin M, Bush A, Simonds AK. Outcome of goal-directed non-invasive ventilation and mechanical insufflation/exsufflation in spinal muscular atrophy type I. *Arch Dis Child.* 2011;96:426–32.
45. Mellies U, Dohna-Schwake C, Stehling F, Voit T. Sleep disordered breathing in spinal muscular atrophy. *Neuromuscul Disord.* 2004;14:797–803.
46. Amaddeo A, Moreau J, Frapin A et al. Long term continuous positive airway pressure (CPAP) and noninvasive ventilation (NIV) in children: Initiation criteria in real life. *Pediatr Pulmonol.* 2016;51:968–7.
47. Robert D, Willig TN, Paulus J. Long-term nasal ventilation in neuromuscular disorders: Report of a consensus conference. *Eur Respir J.* 1993;6:599–606.
48. Rutgers M, Lucassen H, Kesteren RV, Leger P. Respiratory insufficiency and ventilatory support: 39th European Neuromuscular Centre International workshop. *Neuromuscul Disord.* 1996;6:431–5.
49. Clinical indications for noninvasive positive pressure ventilation in chronic respiratory failure due to restrictive lung disease, COPD, and nocturnal hypoventilation – A consensus conference report. *Chest.* 1999;116:521–34.
50. Hull J, Aniapravan R, Chan E et al. Respiratory management of children with neuromuscular weakness guideline group on behalf of the British Thoracic Society Standards of care committee. *Thorax.* 2012;67:i1–40.
51. Katz SL, Gaboury I, Keilty K et al. Nocturnal hypoventilation: Predictors and outcomes in childhood progressive neuromuscular disease. *Arch Dis Child.* 2010;95:998–1003.
52. Ragette R, Mellies U, Schwake C et al. Patterns and predictors of sleep disordered breathing in primary myopathies. *Thorax.* 2002;57:724–8.
53. Mellies U, Ragette R, Schwake C et al. Daytime predictors of sleep disordered breathing in children and adolescents with neuromuscular disorders. *Neuromuscul Disord.* 2003;13:123–8.
54. Barbé F, Quera-Salva MA, McCann C et al. Sleep-related respiratory disturbances in patients with Duchenne muscular dystrophy. *Eur Respir J.* 1994;7:1403–8.
55. Lyager S, Steffensen B, Juhl B. Indicators of need for mechanical ventilation in Duchenne muscular dystrophy and spinal muscular atrophy. *Chest.* 1995;108:779–85.
56. Hukins CA, Hillman DR. Daytime predictors of sleep hypoventilation in Duchenne muscular dystrophy. *Am J Respir Crit Care Med.* 2000;161:166–70.

57. Toussaint M, Steens M, Soudon P. Lung function accurately predicts hypercapnia in patients with Duchenne muscular dystrophy. *Chest*. 2007; 131:368–75.
58. Bersanini C, Khirani S, Ramirez A et al. Nocturnal hypoxemia and hypercapnia in children with neuromuscular disorders. *Eur Respir J*. 2012;39:1206–12.
59. Fauroux B, Pepin JL, Boelle PY et al. Sleep quality and nocturnal hypoxaemia and hypercapnia in children and young adults with cystic fibrosis. *Arch Dis Child*. 2012;97:960–6.
60. Ward S, Chatwin M, Heather S, Simonds AK. Randomised controlled trial of non-invasive ventilation (NIV) for nocturnal hypoventilation in neuromuscular and chest wall disease patients with daytime normocapnia. *Thorax*. 2005;60:1019–24.
61. Kheirandish L, Gozal D. Neurocognitive dysfunction in children with sleep disorders. *Dev Sci*. 2006;9:388–99.
62. Montgomery-Downs HE, Gozal D. Snore-associated sleep fragmentation in infancy: Mental development effects and contribution of secondhand cigarette smoke exposure. *Pediatrics*. 2006;117:e496–502.
63. Marcus CL, Moore RH, Rosen CL et al. A randomized trial of adenotonsillectomy for childhood sleep apnea. *N Engl J Med*. 2013;368:2366–76.
64. Kaditis AG, Alonso Alvarez ML et al. Obstructive sleep disordered breathing in 2- to 18-year-old children: Diagnosis and management. *Eur Respir J*. 2016;47:69–94.
65. Hill NS. Ventilator management for neuromuscular disease. *Semin Respir Crit Care Med*. 2002;23:293–305.
66. Fauroux B, Lavis JF, Nicot F et al. Facial side effects during noninvasive positive pressure ventilation in children. *Intensive Care Med*. 2005;31:965–9.
67. Paiva R, Krivec U, Aubertin G et al. Carbon dioxide monitoring during long-term noninvasive respiratory support in children. *Intensive Care Med*. 2009;35:1068–74.
68. Gonzalez J, Sharshar T, Hart N et al. Air leaks during mechanical ventilation as a cause of persistent hypercapnia in neuromuscular disorders. *Intensive Care Med*. 2003;29:596–602.
69. Chatwin M, Ross E, Hart N et al. Cough augmentation with mechanical insufflation/exsufflation in patients with neuromuscular weakness. *Eur Respir J*. 2003;21:502–8.
70. Fauroux B, Guillemot N, Aubertin G et al. Physiologic benefits of mechanical insufflation-exsufflation in children with neuromuscular diseases. *Chest*. 2008;133:161–8.
71. Toussaint M, Steens M, Wasteels G, Soudon P. Diurnal ventilation via mouthpiece: Survival in end-stage Duchenne patients. *Eur Resp J*. 2006;28:549–55.
72. Khirani S, Ramirez A, Delord V et al. Evaluation of ventilators for mouthpiece ventilation in neuromuscular disease. *Respir Care*. 2014;59:1329–37.
73. Kushida CA, Chediak A, Berry RB et al. Clinical guidelines for the manual titration of positive airway pressure in patients with obstructive sleep apnea. *J Clin Sleep Med*. 2008;4:157–71.
74. Khirani S, Ramirez A, Aloui S et al. CPAP titration in infants with severe airway obstruction. *Crit Care*. 2013;17:R167.

58

Non-invasive positive pressure ventilation in children with acute respiratory failure

GIORGIO CONTI, MARCO PIASTRA AND SILVIA PULITANÒ

INTRODUCTION

The term *non-invasive positive pressure ventilation* (NIV) refers to the application of inspiratory positive airway pressure to the airways, usually in combination with positive end-expiratory pressure (PEEP), in order to increase tidal volume, augment alveolar ventilation and decrease the work of breathing in patients with acute respiratory insufficiency.

In a large subset of patients, NIV avoids the need for an invasive interface (typically an endotracheal tube) and uses an external interface, a nasal, a facemask or a helmet usually in conjunction with a pressure targeted ventilator. The aim of this chapter is to briefly review the possible indications and advantages of NIV application in children with acute respiratory failure (ARF); we will not address other non-conventional forms of non-invasive ventilation (NIV), such as assistance with negative (subatmospheric) pressure devices or the use of NIV for children with chronic respiratory failure (see Chapter 57).

The major advantage of NIV over invasive mechanical ventilation is the capacity to treat disorders associated with hypoventilation and/or increased respiratory workload without an indwelling artificial airway. In adults, treatment with NIV has been associated with a dramatic reduction of the need for endotracheal intubation and ventilator-associated pneumonia (VAP),[1,2] and in acute exacerbations of chronic obstructive pulmonary disease or in hypoxaemic immunocompetent and immunocompromised patients, a significantly improved survival has been reported, compared with that observed in patients treated with conventional treatment and invasive mechanical ventilation.[3–5]

Conversely, the number of prospective and controlled clinical trials comparing NIV with standard treatments or conventional ventilation in paediatric patients is still extremely low, but several case series, including a large single-centre study[6] and a randomised controlled trial (RCT) in children with acute hypoxaemic respiratory failure, strongly support the use of NIV in children with ARF.[7]

EVIDENCE BASE

A large body of evidence, including several RCTs, support the early administration of NIV in adults with ARF of various aetiologies. In such patients, NIV has been shown to significantly decrease the need for endotracheal intubation, improve survival compared with standard care and decrease the incidence of VAP.[2] Conversely, there are relatively few published studies in support of NIV in paediatric patients with acute respiratory distress.[6–8] Despite the paucity of data from large prospective clinical trials in the paediatric population, which does not allow assuming that the benefits described earlier also occur in children, several case series and at least two large studies published in the past decade have suggested that NIV also has great potential as an alternative to standard treatment in infants and children with acute respiratory distress.

In the early case reports and small series, NIV was used in children with acute respiratory distress caused by pneumonia, advanced cystic fibrosis, non-cardiogenic pulmonary oedema and aspiration lung injury, generally showing its safety and effectiveness.[9–12] More recently, we reported the safe and successful use of NIV in patients with acute respiratory distress caused by pneumonia in neuromuscular disease infants,[13] in children with haematological malignancies complicated by ARF[14] and in children with myasthenia gravis[15] and with post-operative acute respiratory insufficiency after thoracic surgery for malignancy.[16]

The largest published experience on NIV application in the paediatric population was reported by Essouri et al.[6]; 114 consecutive unselected patients were treated with NIV during 5 consecutive years (including infants/children with pneumonia, bronchiolitis, acute lung injury/acute respiratory distress syndrome [ARDS], post-extubation ARF and acute chest syndrome complicating sickle cell disease). Of the 114 patients, 83 (77%) were successfully treated by NIV and avoided intubation (NIV success group). Interestingly, the success rate of NIV was significantly lower (22%) in the patients with ARDS than in the other patients. The Pediatric Risk of Mortality (PRISM) II and Pediatric Logistic Organ Dysfunction scores at admission were significantly higher in patients who were unsuccessfully treated with NIV (NIV failure group). Baseline values of PCO_2, pulse oximetry and respiratory rate did not differ between the two groups. Multivariate analysis showed that a diagnosis of ARDS and a high Pediatric Logistic Organ Dysfunction score were independent predictive factors for NIV failure. Only 11 patients (9.6%), all belonging to the NIV failure group, died during the study. The authors concluded that their study demonstrated the feasibility and efficacy of NIV in the daily practice of a paediatric ICU and that NIV could be proposed as a first-line treatment in children with acute respiratory distress, except in those with a diagnosis of ARDS.[6]

The first prospective randomised multicentre trial in the paediatric population was published by Yanez et al.,[7] comparing the benefits of NIV plus standard therapy with standard therapy alone in children with acute respiratory failure. Fifty patients with acute respiratory failure (mainly from respiratory syncityal virus [RSV] bronchiolitis) admitted to paediatric intensive care units (PICU) were recruited: 25 patients were randomly allocated to NIV plus standard therapy (study group); the remaining 25 were given standard therapy (control group). Both groups were comparable in demographic terms. The study group received NIV under inspiratory positive airway pressure ranging between 12 and 18 cm H_2O and PEEP between 6 and 12 cm H_2O. Heart rate and respiratory rate significantly improved with NIV. Detailed analysis revealed that both heart and respiratory rates were significantly lower after 1 hour of treatment compared with admission, and this trend continued over time. With NIV, PO_2/FIO_2 significantly improved from the first hour. The endotracheal intubation rate was significantly lower (28%) in the NIV group than in the control group (60%). The authors concluded that NIV reduces hypoxaemia and the signs and symptoms of acute respiratory failure, thus avoiding endotracheal intubation and related complications in these patients.

A useful tool for the clinical use of NIV in the paediatric population should be the identification of predictive factors for NIV failure and success: this aspect was evaluated in a prospective paper by Bernet et al.[17] Unfortunately the study included both NIV and CPAP given in a large age range (from newborns to children) making it difficult to interpret the results. More recently, Mayordomo-Colunga et al.[18] published a prospective observational study including 116 episodes of ARF. The clinical data collected were respiratory rate (RR), heart rate and FiO_2 before NIV. The same data and expiratory and support pressures were collected at 1, 6, 12, 24 and 48 hours. Conditions precipitating ARF were classified into two groups: type 1 hypoxaemic ARF (38 episodes) and type 2 hypercapnic ARF (78 episodes). Factors predicting NIV failure were determined by multivariate analysis. Most common admission diagnoses were pneumonia (81.6%) in type 1 and bronchiolitis (39.7%) and asthma (42.3%) in type 2. Complications secondary to NIV were detected in 23 episodes (20.2%). NIV success rate was 84.5% (68.4% in type 1 and 92.3% in type 2). Type 1 patients showed a higher risk of NIV failure compared with type 2 (odds ratio [OR], 11.108; 95% confidence interval [CI], 2.578–47.863). A higher PRISM score (OR, 1.138; 95% CI, 1.022–1.267) and a lower RR decrease at 1 hour and at 6 hours (OR, 0.926; 95% CI, 0.860–0.997 and OR, 0.911; 95% CI, 0.837–0.991, respectively) were also independently associated with NIV failure. The authors concluded that NIV is a useful respiratory support technique in paediatric patients. Type 1 group classification, higher PRISM score and lower RR decrease during NIV were independent risk factors for NIV failure. This is a very interesting study, including the large sample; however, unfortunately, the authors combined the data on children treated with NIV with those of children treated with CPAP alone, making the results more difficult to interpret: a large study on the prediction of NIV failure in the paediatric population is therefore still needed. Table 58.1 summarises the main clinical studies on NIV in paediatric patients, and Box 58.1 lists the advantages of using NIV in children.

More controversial is the use of NIV in children with severe hypoxaemia due to status asthmaticus.[22,23] Despite NIV being effective in improving oxygenation and the clinical picture in a subset of children admitted to a paediatric ICU with acute asthma, agitation that required treatment with intravenous sedatives was often reported.[23] Moreover, in the same study, NIV did not prevent endotracheal intubation in a subset of children with hypercarbia and acute asthma.

Recent paediatric experience seems to confirm the role of NIV in immunocompromised patients affected by early ARDS, as has been demonstrated in adults.[4,24–26] In our feasibility study, we reported that 13/23 (56%) of immunocompromised children with ARDS, deemed to require mechanical ventilation, were successfully managed with NIV, avoiding endotracheal intubation.[8] Children successfully ventilated with NIV also had a shorter PICU and hospital stay, a lower incidence of septic complications (including VAP and septic shock) and lower respiratory and heart rate at the end of treatment, suggesting better haemodynamic and respiratory stability. Notably, at PICU admission, severity scores and organ failure did not differ between the group successfully treated with NIV and that in which NIV failed. Our data suggest that an NIV trial could be considered in immunocompromised children with early ARDS. Moreover, the extensive application of NIV in a paediatric oncology setting has been reported, independent of the severity and grade of the respiratory condition.[21]

An increasing role for NIV in PICU has recently been reported in a cohort study[27] performed by the Italian PICU

Table 58.1 Main clinical studies on non-invasive positive pressure ventilation in paediatric patients

Authors	No. of patients	Diagnosis	No. intubated (%)	Comments
Akingbola et al.[19]	2	Down's, leukaemia, ARDS	0	Used post-extubation
Marino et al.[11]	1	Leukaemia	0	Avoided intubation
Piastra et al.[14]	4	Leukaemia, ARDS	2 (50)	Helmet-delivered NIV, prevented intubation
Fortenberry et al.[10]	28	Pneumonia, neurological disorders	3 (11)	Retrospective chart review. NIV improved oxygenation in hypoxaemic ARF
Padman et al.[20]	34	Neuromuscular disease, encephalopathy	3 (9)	Prospective clinical study. NIV avoided intubation
Bernet et al.[17]	42	Pneumonia, viral respiratory infection, post operative congenital heart disease, miscellaneous	18 (43)	Prospective clinical study. Level FiO_2 after 1 hour of NIV may be a predictive factor for the outcome of NIV
Essouri et al.[6]	114	Community-acquired pneumonia, acute lung injury/ ARDS, acute chest syndrome, post extubation ARF	31 (27)	Observational retrospective cohort study. NIV first-line treatment in children with ARF
Pancera et al.[21]	120	Haematological malignancy, solid tumours	31 (25,8)	Retrospective cohort study mechanical ventilation vs NIV: mortality rate lower in the NIV group
Yanez et al.[7]	50	Status asthmaticus, viral/ bacterial infection, respiratory syncytial virus, pneumoniae/ bronchiolitis, influenza A, pneumonia	7 NIV (28) 15 ST (60)	Prospective randomised study. NIV vs standard therapy: NIV reduced the need for intubation
Mayordomo-Colunga et al.[18]	116	Pneumonia, bronchiolitis, asthma	18 (16)	Prospective observational study; mixed children treated with NIV or continuous positive airway pressure
Piastra et al.[8]	23	ARDS in immunocompromised children	10 (44)	Observational clinical study; lower incidence of septic complications in non-invasive ventilation group

Note: ARDS, acute respiratory distress syndrome; ARF, acute respiratory failure.

BOX 58.1: Advantages of applying NIV in children

- Avoids local trauma due to endotracheal intubation
- No interference with swallowing and airway clearance mechanisms
- Offsets additional work of breathing due to the small endotracheal tube
- Possibility of intermittent use

network; 7111 children admitted over 1 year were compared with an historical cohort of children enrolled 3 years before. An overall NIV use of 8.8% ($n = 630$) was observed. Among children who were admitted in the PICU without mechanical ventilation ($n = 3819$), NIV was used in 585 patients (15.3%) with a significant increment among the study years (from 11.6% to 18.2%). In the group of children already intubated at admission, 17.2% received NIV at the end of the weaning process to prevent reintubation. This possible role for NIV in children who develop ARF after extubation has been recently evaluated in an RCT[28] comparing NPPV and standard oxygen therapy for preventing reintubation. One hundred eight children receiving invasive ventilation for at least 48 hours and developing respiratory failure after programmed extubation were prospectively enrolled and randomly assigned into NPPV or O_2 groups. There was no statistically significant difference in reintubation rate and length of stay in PICU or hospital, suggesting a reduced role for NPPV in children developing ARF after extubation.

The application of neurally adjusted ventilatory assist (NAVA), an innovative ventilation mode that utilises the electrical activity of the diaphragm to trigger and cycle-off breaths, avoiding or reducing the delays induced by

BOX 58.2: Timing of therapy in children

- *Early*: To prevent endotracheal intubation
- *Established*: As an alternative to intubation
- *Resolving*: As a bridge to wean from ventilation (rarely evaluated)
- *Post-extubation*: To prevent reintubation

pneumatic triggering to optimise child/ventilator synchrony during NIV, has been recently assessed during paediatric NIV. Ducharme-Crevier et al.[29] assessed the feasibility and tolerance of NIV–NAVA in children, evaluating its impact on synchrony and respiratory effort in a group of children in which conventional NIV was compared to NIV–NAVA and again to conventional NIV. NIV–NAVA was feasible and well tolerated, generating a significant reduction in inspiratory and expiratory asynchronies. Ineffective efforts were also decreased, suggesting that NIV–NAVA is feasible and well tolerated in PICU patients and improves patient–ventilator synchrony.

Box 58.2 lists the optimal timing of application of NIV in children.

CLINICAL MANAGEMENT OF NIV IN THE PAEDIATRIC POPULATION

An important technical aspect still unsolved is the selection of the optimal interface in children with acute respiratory distress treated with NIV. Whereas NIV for long-term use is typically well tolerated by paediatric patients using a nasal mask, this interface presents major problems with air leaks and inability to attain the set inspiratory pressure in the acute setting. Thus, facemasks are generally considered the first choice in critically ill children with acute respiratory failure. However, some disadvantages have also been reported for the facemasks, mainly due to the natural fear in children of any device that 'closes' their upper airways.

Although this problem can be partly relieved by an experienced team, it is quite common to use sedatives in the paediatric ICU setting. It is important to remember that (different from the adult setting) due to their immature gastro-oesophageal sphincter function, children with respiratory distress are relatively prone to the development of gastro-oesophageal reflux; moreover gastric distension with gas is very common during NIV and can induce the regurgitation of the gastric contents into the facemask. In order to increase tolerance, in older children, a new interface, the helmet,[13,14] has been proposed for NIV administration. This innovative interface is associated with better tolerance than the facemasks, but due to its large internal volume and dead space, it increases the risk for carbon dioxide rebreathing and patient–ventilator asynchronies. In our experience, the use of the helmet should therefore be reserved for children weighing more than 20–25 kg.

Minor complications are commonly reported in children treated with NIV and include dermal abrasion at the nasal bridge, eye irritation and gastric distension with air. Conversely, major complications have been rarely reported in the PICU setting where optimal monitoring, caregiver expertise and careful device choice are the norm. Children treated with NIV must be observed by expert staff using cardiovascular and respiratory monitors, pulse oximetry and frequent assessment of blood gases.

Important variables that need to be carefully analysed before starting NIV in paediatric patients are the age and the dimensions of the child, the kind of respiratory system dysfunction and the level of cardiovascular stability. Usually, NIV is considered difficult to apply in young infants with severe respiratory distress (Box 58.3). NIV is also absolutely contraindicated in children with significant cardiovascular/rhythm instability, in children with facial/cervical trauma and in patients with seizures or coma.

Conventional ICU ventilators can be used to administer NIV with inspiratory pressure support and PEEP in the PICU setting. Previous generation bi-level ventilators were not equipped for air leak compensation or limitation of the inspiratory time. In the presence of significant air leaks, as commonly observed in paediatric patients, the preset inspiratory cycling-off criteria are often not reached; thus, inspiratory flow is maintained and the device does not cycle to expiration (hang-up phenomenon). This problem is a frequent cause of ineffective NIV administration, gas exchange deterioration and agitation. The only solution is to minimise air leaks: this can be achieved either by using a better fitting mask or by reducing the pressure applied to the airways or, mainly in infants and smaller children, by obtaining a more correct position of neck and chin, eventually also with a cervical collar.

NIV is usually started with 8–10 cm H_2O of inspiratory pressure support and 5 cm H_2O of PEEP, with subsequent increase in increments of the pressure support to obtain an optimal reduction of respiratory rate and inspiratory efforts, with optimal gas exchange. The PEEP level should be set to achieve two objectives: increase functional residual capacity and maintain the patency of the upper airway at end-expiration. Usually, PEEP levels between 5 and 10 cm H_2O are sufficient in the paediatric clinical applications of NIV.

BOX 58.3: Indications for conversion to intubation and conventional ventilation

- Ca rdiovascular/rhythm instability
- SaO_2 below 90% with FiO_2 of 0.5 or higher
- pH stable below 7.30 after 2 hours of NIV
- Mental deterioration/seizures
- Absent cough or gag reflex
- Mask intolerance
- Need for heavy sedation

CONCLUSIONS

Despite the publication of a single multicentre prospective randomised study, a growing body of evidence, including several large studies, support the usefulness of NIV in the paediatric setting. Despite these encouraging results, there is still large scope for improvement on several aspects, including new interfaces specifically designed for paediatric use and new assisted modes for optimising child–ventilator interaction.

REFERENCES

1. Bencault N, Boulair T. Mortality rate attributed to ventilator-associated nosocomial pneumonia in an adult intensive care unit: A prospective case-control study. *Crit Care Med.* 2001;29:2303–9.
2. Girou E, Brun-Buisson C, Taille S et al. Secular trends in nosocomial infections and mortality associated with noninvasive ventilation in patients with exacerbation of COPD and pulmonary edema. *JAMA.* 2003;290:2985–91.
3. Brochard L, Isabey D, Piquet J et al. Reversal of acute exacerbations of chronic obstructive lung disease by inspiratory pressure assistance with a face mask. *N Engl J Med.* 1990;323:1523–30.
4. Hilbert G, Gruson D, Vargas F et al. Noninvasive ventilation in immunosuppressed patients with pulmonary infiltrates, fever, and acute respiratory failure. *N Engl J Med.* 2001;344:481–7.
5. Antonelli M, Conti G, Rocco M et al. A comparison of noninvasive positive-pressure ventilation and conventional mechanical ventilation in patients with acute respiratory failure. *N Engl J Med.* 1998;339:429–35.
6. Essouri S, Chevret L, Durand P et al. Noninvasive positive pressure ventilation: Five years of experience in a pediatric intensive care unit. *Pediatr Crit Care Med.* 2006;7:329–34.
7. Yanez L, Yunge M, Emilfork M et al. A prospective, randomized, controlled trial of noninvasive ventilation in pediatric acute respiratory failure. *Pediatr Crit Care Med.* 2008;9:484–9.
8. Piastra M, De Luca D, Pietrini D et al. Noninvasive pressure support ventilation in immuno-compromised children with ARDS: A feasibility study. *Intensive Care Med.* 2009;35:1420–7.
9. Padman R, Nadkarmi V, Von Nessen S et al. Noninvasive positive pressure ventilation in end-stage cystic fibrosis: A report of seven cases. *Respir Care.* 1994;39:736–9.
10. Fortenberry JD, Del Toro J, Jefferson LS et al. Management of pediatric acute hypoxemic respiratory insufficiency with bilevel positive pressure (B_iPAP) nasal mask ventilation. *Chest.* 1995;108:1059–64.
11. Marino P, Rosa G, Conti G et al. Treatment of acute respiratory failure by prolonged non-invasive ventilation in a child. *Can J Anaesth.* 1997;44:727–31.
12. Akingbola O, Palmisano J, Servant G et al. Bi-PAP mask ventilation in pediatric patients with acute respiratory failure. *Crit Care Med.* 1994;22:A144.
13. Piastra M, Antonelli M, Caresta E et al. Noninvasive ventilation in childhood acute neuromuscular respiratory failure: A pilot study. *Respiration.* 2006;73:791–8.
14. Piastra M, Antonelli M, Chiaretti A et al. Treatment of acute respiratory failure by helmet-delivered non-invasive pressure support ventilation in children with acute leukemia: A pilot study. *Intensive Care Med.* 2004;30:472–6.
15. Piastra M, Conti G, Caresta E et al. Noninvasive ventilation options in pediatric myasthenia gravis. *Pediatr Anaesth.* 2005;15:699–702.
16. Piastra M, De Luca D, Zorzi G et al. Noninvasive ventilation in large postoperative flail chest. *Pediatr Blood Cancer.* 2008;51:831–3.
17. Bernet V, Hug MI, Frey B. Predictive factors for the success of noninvasive mask ventilation in infants and children with acute respiratory failure. *Pediatr Crit Care Med.* 2005;6:660–4.
18. Mayordomo-Colunga J, Medina A, Rey C et al. Predictive factors of non invasive ventilation failure in critically ill children: A prospective epidemiological study. *Intensive Care Med.* 2009;35:527–36.
19. Akingbola OA, Servant GM, Custer JR et al. Noninvasive bi-level positive airway pressure in the management of pediatric lung disease. *Respir Care.* 1993;38:1092–8.
20. Padman R, Lawless ST, Kettrick RG. Noninvasive ventilation via bilevel positive airway pressure support in pediatric practice. *Crit Care Med.* 1998;26:169–73.
21. Pancera CF, Hayashi M, Fregnani JH et al. Noninvasive ventilation in immunocompromised pediatric patients: Eight years of experience in a pediatric oncology intensive care unit. *J Pediatr Hematol Oncol.* 2008;30:533–8.
22. Teague WG. Noninvasive ventilation in the pediatric intensive care unit for children with acute respiratory failure. *Pediatr Pulmonol.* 2003;35:418–26.
23. Teague WG, Lowe E, Dominick J et al. Non-invasive positive pressure ventilation (NPPV) in critically ill children with status asthmaticus. *Am J Respir Crit Care Med.* 1998;157:A542.
24. Antonelli M, Conti G, Bufi M et al. Noninvasive ventilation for the treatment of acute respiratory failure in patients undergoing solid organ transplantation: A randomized trial. *JAMA.* 2000;283:235–41.
25. Conti G, Marino P, Cogliati A et al. Noninvasive ventilation for the treatment of acute respiratory failure in patients with hematological malignancies: A pilot study. *Intensive Care Med.* 1998;24:1283–8.

26. Rocco M, Conti G, Antonelli M et al. Noninvasive pressure support ventilation in patients with acute respiratory failure after bilateral lung transplantation. *Intensive Care Med.* 2001; 27:1622–6.
27. Wolfler A, Calderini E, Iannella E et al. Network of pediatric intensive care unit study group: Evolution of noninvasive mechanical ventilation use: A cohort study among Italian PICUs. *PCCM.* 2015;16:418–27.
28. Fioretto JR, Ribeiro CF, Carpi MF et al. Comparison between noninvasive mechanical ventilation and standard oxygen therapy in children up to 3 years old with respiratory failure after extubation: A pilot prospective randomized clinical study. *Pediatr Crit Care Med.* 2015;16:124–30.
29. Ducharme-Crevier L, Beck J, Essouri S et al. Neurally adjusted ventilatory assist (NAVA) allows patient-ventilator synchrony during pediatric noninvasive ventilation: A crossover physiological study. *Crit Care.* 2015;19:44.

PART 13

Special situations

59 Bronchoscopy during non-invasive ventilation 540
Massimo Antonelli and Giuseppe Bello

60 Non-invasive positive pressure ventilation in the obstetric population 544
Daniel Zapata, David Wisa and Bushra Mina

61 Diaphragm pacing (by phrenic nerve stimulation) 547
Jésus Gonzalez-Bermejo

62 Tracheostomy 554
Piero Ceriana, Paolo Pelosi and Maria Vargas

63 Swallowing and phonation during ventilation 564
Hélène Prigent and Nicolas Terzi

59

Bronchoscopy during non-invasive ventilation

MASSIMO ANTONELLI AND GIUSEPPE BELLO

INTRODUCTION

Fibreoptic bronchoscopy (FB) with bronchoalveolar lavage (BAL) has a central role in the diagnosis of pneumonia in critically ill patients. A prompt identification of the responsible pathogens is crucial to start an appropriate antimicrobial therapy and avoid the empirical administration of unnecessary and often toxic antibiotics. Non-intubated spontaneously breathing patients with hypoxaemia should not undergo FB because of the high risk of worsening respiratory failure or developing serious cardiac arrhythmias.[1] Until a few years ago, the available options in hypoxaemic patients with the suspicion of pneumonia were (1) avoiding FB and to institute empirical treatment or (2) performing endotracheal intubation and administering mechanical ventilation to ensure adequate respiratory assistance during FB. Non-invasive ventilation (NIV) has been demonstrated to be a valuable tool to assist spontaneous breathing during diagnostic bronchoscopy, successfully avoiding the need for endotracheal intubation in high-risk patients.[2–6]

The areas covered here include the rationale for using NIV to assist patients undergoing FB, the available literature supporting this method and some procedural considerations.

In this chapter, continuous positive airway pressure delivered non-invasively is referred to as CPAP. The use of intermittent positive pressure ventilation with or without positive end-expiratory pressure (PEEP) is referred to as NIV.

RATIONALE

FB is associated with transient alterations in pulmonary mechanics and gas exchange.[7,8] PaO_2 may fall significantly below its baseline value during FB and remain decreased for a few minutes to several hours after removing the bronchoscope.[7,8] In a large group of critically ill mechanically ventilated patients undergoing FB, the mean drop in PaO_2 at the end of the procedure was of 26% compared with the control value.[9] Hypoxaemia may be more pronounced when BAL is performed because of ventilation and perfusion abnormalities created by the saline solution instillation.[10]

In a non-intubated adult male, a 5.7 mm outside diameter flexible bronchoscope has been calculated to occupy about 10% of the tracheal cross-sectional area and about 15% of the cross-sectional area at the cricoid ring.[7] Placing the bronchoscope into the major airways decreases the area available for airway flow and, consequently, increases airway resistance.[7] Transnasal insertion of a 5.2 mm bronchoscope into an 11 mm inside diameter trachea would increase airway resistance approximately twofold.[8] The high exhalation resistance very quickly results in an increase in functional residual capacity (FRC) and, therefore, in the development of an intrinsic PEEP.[8] This may exert deleterious effects, such as imposing additional work of breathing or risk of barotrauma, particularly during coughing.

Besides the physical presence of the bronchoscope in the airway, ongoing suction through the instrument working channel is another cause of the alterations in pulmonary mechanics and gas exchange during FB. Removing tracheobronchial gas by excessive use of suction evacuates respiratory gas from the lungs and decreases FRC, with consequent hypoxaemia.[7]

In the 1990s, the encouraging results obtained in the treatment of acute respiratory failure by using NIV[11–13] stimulated investigations on various applications of NIV in the acute care setting. In hypoxaemic patients needing FB with BAL, NIV was employed to prevent gas-exchange deterioration associated with FB and compensate for the increase in work of breathing occurring during the procedure, thus avoiding endotracheal intubation and its complications.

EVIDENCE BASE

Several investigators have evaluated the use of NIV in hypoxaemic patients needing diagnostic FB. Antonelli et al.[2] originally described the application of facemask NIV during FB in eight immunocompromised hypoxaemic (i.e. PaO_2 to inspired oxygen fraction [FiO_2] ratio, <100) patients with suspected pneumonia. NIV was associated with a significant improvement in PaO_2/FiO_2 during FB. The technique was well tolerated, and no patient required endotracheal intubation.

The successful application of NIV during FB was also reported in patients with chronic obstructive pulmonary disease (COPD). Da Conceiçao et al.[3] investigated 10 consecutive COPD patients with pneumonia who were admitted to the intensive care unit with hypercapnia (i.e. arterial carbon dioxide tension [$PaCO_2$], 67 ± 11 mmHg) and hypoxaemia (i.e. PaO_2, 53 ± 13 mmHg). During FB with NIV, the arterial oxygen saturation of haemoglobin measured by pulse oximetry (SpO_2) increased from 91 ± 4.7% at baseline up to 97 ± 1.7%. There were no changes in $PaCO_2$ and PaO_2 during the hour following the end of the procedure, and no patients were intubated within 24 hours.

Maitre et al.[4] conducted a randomised double-blind study of 30 patients with PaO_2/FiO_2 < 300 to compare a new CPAP treatment to oxygen administration in maintaining oxygenation during FB. The facemask CPAP device was based on four funnel-shaped microchannels connected to an oxygen source and generating high-velocity microjets and, thus, positive pressure. CPAP allowed minimal alterations in gas exchange and prevented subsequent respiratory failure. During FB and 30 min thereafter, SpO_2 was significantly higher in the CPAP group than in the oxygen group. Arterial blood gas measurements 15 min after the termination of FB showed that the PaO_2 had increased by 10.5 ± 16.9% in the CPAP group and decreased by 15 ± 16.6% in the oxygen group ($p = 0.01$).[4] Five patients in the oxygen group, but none in the CPAP group, developed respiratory failure and required intubation in the 6 hours following the FB procedure.

In a subsequent trial, Antonelli et al.[5] randomised 26 hypoxaemic (i.e. PaO_2/FiO_2, <200) patients needing diagnostic FB to receive an FiO_2 of 0.9 via facemask or NIV via oronasal mask with pressure support ventilation of 15–17 cm H_2O, expiratory pressure of 5 cm H_2O and FiO_2 of 0.9. PaO_2/FiO_2 was substantially higher both during FB (261 vs. 139 mmHg) and 1 hour after FB (176 vs. 140 mmHg), although both groups started at essentially the same PaO_2/FiO_2 at baseline (143 vs. 155 mmHg). After undergoing FB, three patients required non-emergent intubation, one patient in the NIV group (7 hours after the procedure) and two patients in the control group (9 and 5 hours after the procedure). In all three cases, the intubation was not apparently related to FB.

A more recent study showed that in patients with hypoxaemic acute respiratory failure receiving NIV through the helmet, FB with BAL is a safe and feasible technique, capable of avoiding endotracheal intubation and discontinuation of assisted ventilation.[6] Finally, a prospective study on 40 critically ill patients with hypoxaemic ARF suggested that bronchoscopy can be performed with an acceptable risk in patients who are already in need of NIV prior to the decision to perform bronchoscopy.[14]

CLINICAL APPLICATIONS

Performing FB during the delivery of NIV has been used either to assist spontaneous breathing in patients at risk for developing acute respiratory failure during FB or to avoid the discontinuation of NIV in patients scheduled to undergo FB.

The risks associated with either the NIV application or bronchoscopic examination should be weighed against the benefits in the patient who needs the procedure. The criteria for excluding patients from NIV treatment include severe central neurological disturbances, the inability to protect the airway, unstable haemodynamic conditions; vomiting; facial deformities; and recent oral, oesophageal or gastric surgery. However, even though the patient has no contraindications to NIV, the following circumstances are considered contraindications to FB: (1) absence of consent from the patient; (2) lack of trained personnel; (3) refractory hypoxaemia even during NIV; (4) inability to normalise platelet count and coagulation if biopsy or brushing are anticipated; (5) unstable cardiac disease (the risks of FB are thought to be reduced 4–6 weeks after myocardial infarction[15]); and (6) uncontrolled bronchospasm.[16]

The complication rate of FB has been shown to be increased in COPD patients.[17] In these patients, oxygen supplementation as well as intravenous sedation should be avoided or given with extreme caution to prevent dangerous increases in $PaCO_2$.

TECHNICAL CONSIDERATIONS

The bronchoscopic technique is slightly different depending on the type of interface which is used to deliver NIV. When NIV is delivered through a facial mask, a T-adapter is attached to the mask for the insertion of the bronchoscope through the nose or the mouth (Figure 59.1). Differently, if the helmet is adopted, the bronchoscope is passed through the specific seal connector placed in the plastic ring of the helmet. This connector can also be used to spray local anaesthetics into the nostrils and pharynx of the patient. The internal adjustable diaphragm of the seal connection can prevent loss of the respiratory gases, maintaining ventilation and PEEP throughout FB.[6]

Prior to performing FB, NIV is administered (if not yet started) for at least 5 min in order to obtain an adequate patient–ventilator interaction. NIV is maintained during FB and for at least 30 min after the termination of the procedure, after which it is discontinued if the patient is not showing respiratory difficulties or significant gas exchange deterioration. The FiO_2 is kept at 0.9–1 while the patient adjusts to the ventilator and during the examination. Over the first 30 min after the completion of FB, the applied FiO_2 is gradually reduced to the pre-FB requirements as long as the patient is able to maintain SpO_2 at >92%.

The topical anaesthesia of the nose and pharynx can be obtained by spraying a 10% lidocaine solution. The topical

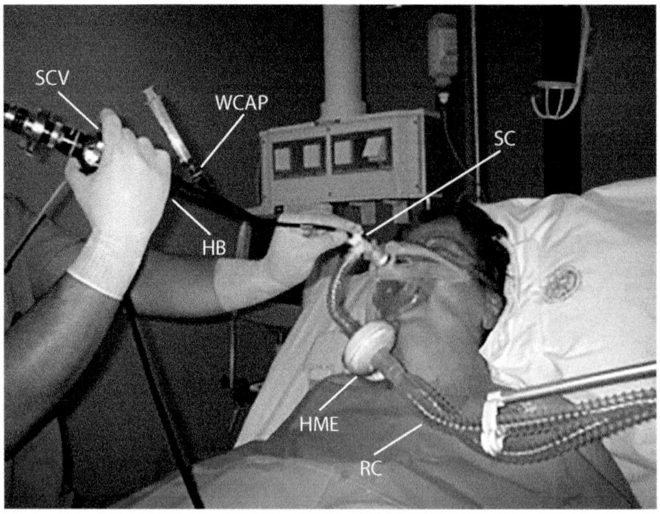

Figure 59.1 FB performed during NIV delivered through an oronasal mask. HB, handle of the bronchoscope; HME, heat and moisture exchanger; RC, respiratory circuit; SC, seal connection; SCV, suction control valve; WCAP, working channel access port. (Photograph printed with the permission of the patient.)

anaesthesia of the larynx and vocal cords can be performed by injecting 2% lidocaine through the working channel of the bronchoscope. When FB is used to obtain samples from the lower respiratory tract for the diagnosis of pneumonia, the sampling area is selected by localising new or progressive infiltrate on chest radiograph or the segment visualised during FB as having purulent secretions.[18] Information is unclear about the sampling site in patients with diffuse lung infiltrates. In the supine patient, the BAL fluid recovery is best from the right middle lobe or lingula. When BAL is performed, the tip of the bronchoscope is wedged as far as possible into a distal airway, generally fourth- to fifth-order bronchi, and sterile saline solution is instilled through the bronchoscope and then aspirated into a sterile trap. Additional aliquots of 20–60 mL are injected and aspirated back after each instillation. The total amount of fluid used to obtain BAL ranges from 140 to 240 mL.[17] Bacterial pneumonia is diagnosed when at least 10,000 colony-forming units per millilitre of bacteria are measured in the BAL fluid.[19]

It is necessary for the patient to have no oral feeding (or enteral nutrition) for 4 hours and no clear oral fluids for 2 hours before FB.[16] Subjects with a history of asthma should be premedicated with a bronchodilator before FB.

An accurate cardiorespiratory monitoring is necessary during the procedure, including continuous electrocardiogram and SpO_2, continuous intra-arterial blood pressure or intermittent cuff blood pressure measurement at least every 5 min, tidal volume, minute ventilation and airway pressure.

Finally, the type of NIV interface may affect the feasibility of the technique. When the helmet is used, performing FB could be difficult if there is a large distance between the plastic ring of the helmet and the patient's nose or mouth. This problem is easily solved by reducing this distance by gently pushing the plastic ring towards the face of the patient. Also, the specific seal connector placed in the plastic ring of the helmet, which is used to pass the cord of the bronchoscope, may be located too markedly out of line with the mouth or the nose of some patients, thus increasing the difficulty of the technique. In this case, the plastic ring of the helmet should be gently shifted in order to make the cord of the bronchoscope as straight as possible. Anyway, opening the patient access port of the helmet for just a few seconds could facilitate the procedure, by allowing holding of the insertion cord of the bronchoscope with one hand inside the helmet and rapidly introducing it into the patient's nose or mouth. Soon after, the patient access port is closed and NIV is resumed.

Transnasal FB in patients undergoing facemask NIV may involve some technical difficulties if the opening of the facemask, which is attached to the ventilator circuit, is not positioned above the patient's nose. When it occurs, it may be difficult either to introduce the bronchoscope into the nose or to manoeuvre the instrument through the airways. Replacing the facemask with another model can overcome this problem.

Conscious sedation using popofol target-controlled infusion (TCI) techniques seems to be a promising approach to assist bronchoscopy in hypoxaemic patients under NIV.[20] Similarly, sedation with remifentanil TCI has been safely and effectively used in critically ill patients with spontaneous ventilation undergoing bronchoscopy.[21] During the last years, dexemedetomidine use has been widely implemented in the clinical practice as a sedative agent, although few data are available in patients receiving NIV.[22] Due to its favourable pharmacological profile, its use might be suitable as an adjuvant agent during bronchoscopy in spontaneous breathing critically ill patients with respiratory failure.

FUTURE RESEARCH

Performing FB during NIV has been described either in at-risk patients who were initially breathing spontaneously and who started NIV to assist FB or in patients who were already receiving NIV and who were scheduled to undergo FB during NIV. In all cases, FB was needed to obtain BAL specimens for the diagnosis of pneumonia. It could be interesting to investigate the safety and usefulness of FB during NIV in at-risk patients who need a bronchoscopic examination for diagnostic purposes other than BAL, such as biopsies, or for therapeutic procedures, such as laser treatment and removal of retained secretions.

REFERENCES

1. Goldstein RA, Rohatgi PK, Bergofsky EH et al. Clinical role of bronchoalveolar lavage in adults with pulmonary disease. *Am Rev Respir Dis.* 1990;142:481–6.
2. Antonelli M, Conti G, Riccioni L et al. Noninvasive positive-pressure ventilation via face mask during bronchoscopy with BAL in high-risk hypoxemic patients. *Chest.* 1996;110:724–8.
3. Da Conceiçao M, Genco G, Favier JC et al. Fiberoptic bronchoscopy during noninvasive positive-pressure ventilation in patients with chronic obstructive lung disease with hypoxemia and hypercapnia. *Ann Fr Anesth Reanim.* 2000;19:231–6.
4. Maitre B, Jaber S, Maggiore SM et al. Continuous positive airway pressure during fiberoptic bronchoscopy in hypoxemic patients: A randomized double-blind study using a new device. *Am J Respir Crit Care Med.* 2000;162:1063–7.
5. Antonelli M, Conti G, Rocco M et al. Noninvasive positive-pressure ventilation vs. conventional oxygen supplementation in hypoxemic patients undergoing diagnostic bronchoscopy. *Chest.* 2002;121:1149–54.
6. Antonelli M, Pennisi MA, Conti G et al. Fiberoptic bronchoscopy during noninvasive positive pressure ventilation delivered by helmet. *Intensive Care Med.* 2003;29:126–9.
7. Lindholm CE, Ollman B, Snyder JV et al. Cardiorespiratory effects of flexible fiberoptic bronchoscopy in critically ill patients. *Chest.* 1978;74:362–8.
8. Matsushima Y, Jones RL, King EG et al. Alterations in pulmonary mechanics and gas exchange during routine fiberoptic bronchoscopy. *Chest.* 1984;86:184–8.
9. Trouillet JL, Guiguet M, Gibert C et al. Fiberoptic bronchoscopy in ventilated patients: Evaluation of cardiopulmonary risk under midazolam sedation. *Chest.* 1990;97:927–33.
10. Lin CC, Wu JL, Huang WC: Pulmonary function in normal subjects after bronchoalveolar lavage. *Chest.* 1988;93:1049–53.
11. Meduri GU, Conoscenti CC, Menashe P, Nair S. Noninvasive face mask ventilation in patients with acute respiratory failure. *Chest.* 1989;95:865–70.
12. Brochard L, Isabey D, Piquet J et al. Reversal of acute exacerbations of chronic obstructive lung disease by inspiratory assistance with a face mask. *N Engl J Med.* 1990;323:1523–30.
13. Elliott MW, Steven MH, Phillips GD, Branthwaite MA. Non-invasive mechanical ventilation for acute respiratory failure. *BMJ.* 1990;300:358–60.
14. Baumann HJ, Klose H, Simon M et al. Fiber optic bronchoscopy in patients with acute hypoxemic respiratory failure requiring noninvasive ventilation – A feasibility study. *Crit Care.* 2011;15:R179.
15. Eagle KA, Brundage BH, Chaitman BR et al. Guidelines for perioperative cardiovascular evaluation for noncardiac surgery: Report of the American College of Cardiology/American Heart Association Task Force on Practice Guidelines. Committee on Perioperative Cardiovascular Evaluation for Noncardiac Surgery. *Circulation.* 1996;93:1278–317.
16. British Thoracic Society Bronchoscopy Guidelines Committee. British Thoracic Society guidelines on diagnostic flexible bronchoscopy. *Thorax.* 2001;56:i1–21.
17. Peacock MD, Johnson JE, Blanton HM. Complications of flexible bronchoscopy in patients with severe obstructive pulmonary disease. *J Bronchol.* 1994;1:181–6.
18. Meduri GU, Chastre J. The standardization of bronchoscopic techniques for ventilator-associated pneumonia. *Chest.* 1992;102:557S-64S.
19. American Thoracic Society; Infectious Diseases Society of America. Guidelines for the management of adults with hospital-acquired, ventilator-associated, and healthcare-associated pneumonia. *Am J Respir Crit Care Med.* 2005;171:388–416.
20. Clouzeau B, Bui HN, Guilhon E et al. Fiberoptic bronchoscopy under noninvasive ventilation and propofol target-controlled infusion in hypoxemic patients. *Intensive Care Med.* 2011;37:1969–75.
21. Chalumeau-Lemoine L, Stoclin A et al. Flexible fiberoptic bronchoscopy and remifentanil target-controlled infusion in ICU: A preliminary study. *Intensive Care Med.* 2013;39:53–8.
22. Devlin JW, Al-Qadheeb NS, Chi A et al. Efficacy and safety of early dexmedetomidine during noninvasive ventilation forpatients with acute respiratory failure: A randomized, double-blind, placebo-controlled pilot study. *Chest.* 2014;145:1204–12.

60

Non-invasive positive pressure ventilation in the obstetric population

DANIEL ZAPATA, DAVID WISA AND BUSHRA MINA

RESPIRATORY FAILURE IN PREGNANCY

It is found that 9.1% of obstetric ICU admissions are due to pulmonary complications with the most common reasons being secondary to respiratory failure from asthma, pneumonia, cystic fibrosis, pulmonary oedema, pulmonary embolism, acute respiratory distress syndrome (ARDS) and amniotic fluid embolism (Table 60.1).[1] Acute respiratory failure (ARF) in pregnancy occurs in less than 0.1% of pregnant patients,[2] but is considered one of the most common indications for obstetric admissions into the intensive care units and cause for maternal and foetal mortality to be as high as 14% and 11%, respectively.[3,4] These are risks that are predisposed in these patients due to the anatomic and physiologic changes in the respiratory system that can affect overall management. Respiratory failure in pregnancy may be due to a pregnancy-specific disease or exacerbation of previously existing respiratory disease.

UTILISATION OF NIV IN PREGNANCY

In the pregnant patient, it is well described that intubation failure is eight times more common[5] with an incidence of fatal failed intubation to be 13 times higher when compared to the non-parturient.[6,7] As a result, NIV can be considered to avoid the potential complications of endotracheal intubation. However, the same goals and contraindications apply to the pregnant patient as they do to other populations.

The primary goal is to maintain adequate ventilation and oxygenation to provide haemodynamic support to assist in determining the best timing for delivery when the mother is in respiratory distress or impending respiratory failure. In the review of the literature, the use of NIV in pregnant patients with respiratory failure has been demonstrated only in multiple case reports and case series. These reports convey favourable use of NIV in a number of clinical scenarios ranging from obstructive lung diseases and neuromusculoskeletal disorders and in the perioperative setting. NIV has also been described to be beneficial for sleep disorders during pregnancy.[8–10]

Ventilatory failure associated with neuromuscular diseases and severe kyphoscoliosis[11–13] were the first cases described to utilise NIV in the pregnant patient. Kahler et al.[13] described the use of nasal NIV starting in the 20th week of gestation, which was adapted throughout the pregnancy which led to corrected exercise tolerance, fatigue and nocturnal oxygen desaturations, which led to a successful caesarean with intraoperative NIV. Bach[14] reported four cases of continuous NIV in three females with poliomyelitis developing chronic respiratory failure and another developing ventilator insufficiency due to severe kyphoscoliosis. In all these cases, NIV was utilised to successfully permit the natural completion of pregnancy. NIV has also been successfully reported in mitochondrial myopathies.[15,16]

The utilisation of NIV for hypoxemic respiratory failure has not been proven and at best is controversial. Nonetheless, its successful utilisation has been described in the parturient developing hypoxaemic respiratory failure, where causes can range from pneumonia to pulmonary oedema associated with tocolytic therapy and severe pre-eclampsia.[17–23] Asthma is a frequent chronic condition associated with complications during pregnancy. Its prevalence among pregnant females is increasing, which subsequently increases perinatal risks, which include pre-eclampsia, preterm birth, low birth weight, spontaneous abortion and perinatal mortality.[24] Severe attacks from asthma are usually seen at 21–24 weeks, but can occur at any stage of pregnancy. NIV and its use in asthma exacerbations is a provocative modality. However, it has been proven to be beneficial in chronic obstructive pulmonary disease where hypercarbic respiratory failure is the main pathophysiology.[25] An example of its successful use in asthma is demonstrated in the case of a 28-year-old female in her 16th week

Table 60.1 Most common causes of respiratory failure in pregnancy

- Asthma
- Pulmonary infections
- Pulmonary oedema
- Thromboembolic disease
- Amniotic fluid embolism
- ARDS
- Restrictive lung disease
- Aspiration

of pregnancy with community-acquired pneumonia, who presented during an asthma attack with NIV use, significantly decreasing her oxygen requirements.[26]

NIV application in ARDS has also been described to be efficacious as in the case depicted by Al-Ansari et al.,[27] which involved four pregnant patients with sickle cell disease, who presented with acute chest syndrome and ARDS, and successful treatment with NIV was achieved while avoiding endotracheal intubation. Cases of ARDS related to all-transretenoic acid syndrome,[28] community-acquired pneumonia, sepsis and influenza have also been found in the literature.[29]

In terms of H1N1-related ARDS, mortality rate can reach as high as 60% for those who require mechanical ventilation, which, as discussed in the pregnant population, may be possibly higher. In 2012, a prospective multicentred study found that the early application of NIV, with the aim to avoid invasive ventilation during the H1N1 pandemics, was associated with an overall success rate of 48% of patients with elevated Simplified Acute Physiology Score II score, ARF and pulmonary infiltrates and a 75% success rate in patients not needing immediate intubation for a life-threatening condition.[30] This success is further depicted in the case of a 28-year-old pregnant female with ARDS from the H1N1 virus; the patient was successfully treated without the means of mechanical ventilation.[31] This brings out the point of a possible role for NIV in reducing this morbidity by decreasing the number of required intubations in isolated respiratory failure and ARDS from influenza.

In addition to salvaging respiratory therapies, other descriptions of NIV in pregnancy have also been noted in the perioperative setting.[32–34] Sedation and NIV have also been a topic of interest for many years. Duan et al.[17] described a case of successfully applying NIV with dexmedetomidine in a pregnant patient.

NIV is a modality that should not be routinely applied in pregnancy as there are theoretical concerns for aspiration risk and obtaining a proper fit for oxygenation. Despite the lack of large-scale evidence, its use has been successfully described in many case reports and series. Using similar indications, contraindications and, lastly, an experienced team, the use of NIV may be successfully used in the pregnant patient population.

REFERENCES

1. Ananth CV, Smulian JC. Epidemiology of critical illness in pregnancy, In: Belfort M, Saade G, Foley M, Phelan J, Dildy III, G, eds. *Critical Care Obstetrics*, 5th ed. Hoboken, NJ: Blackwell Publishing; 2010.
2. Chen CY, Fau-Chen C-P, Chen CP et al. Factors implicated in the outcome of pregnancies complicated by acute respiratory failure. *J Reprod Med.* 2003;48:641–8.
3. Jenkins TM, Troiano NH, Graves CR et al. Mechanical ventilation in an obstetric population: Characteristics and delivery rates. *Am J Obstet Gynecol.* 2003;188:549–2.
4. Christiansen L, Collin K. Pregnancy associated deaths: A 15-year retrspective study and overall review of maternal pathophysiology. *Am J Foren Med Path.* 2006;27:11–9.
5. King TA, Adams AP. Failed tracheal intubation. *Br J Anaesth.* 1990;65:400–14.
6. Lyons G. Failed intubation: Six years' experience in a teaching maternity unit. *Anaesthesia.* 1985; 40:759–62.
7. Glassenberg R. General anesthesia and maternal mortality. *Semin Perinatol.* 1991;15:386–96.
8. Edwards N, Blyton DM, Kirjavainen T et al. Nasal continuous positive airway pressure reduces sleep-induced blood pressure increments in preeclampsia. *Am J Respir Crit Care Med.* 2000;162:252–7.
9. Blyton DM, Sullivan CE, Edwards N. Reduced nocturnal cardiac output associated with preeclampsia is minimized with the use of nocturnal nasal CPAP. *Sleep.* 2004;27:57, 79–84.
10. Guilleminault C, Kreutzer M, Chang JL. Pregnancy, sleep disordered breathing and treatment with nasal continuous positive airway pressure. *Sleep Med.* 2004;5:43–51.
11. Reddy R, Evans E, Khoo O, Allen MB. Pregnancy in kyphoscoliosis: Benefit of non-invasive ventilatory support. *J Obstet Gynaecol.* 2005;25:267–8.
12. Sawicka EH, Branthwaite MA. Respiration during sleep in kyphoscoliosis. *Thorax.* 1987;42:801–8.
13. Kähler CM, Högl B, Habeler R et al. Management of respiratory deterioration in a pregnant patient with severe kyphoscoliosis by non-invasive positive pressure ventilation. *Wien Klin Wochenschr.* 2002; 114:874–7.
14. Bach JR. Successful pregnancies for ventilator users. *Am J Phys Med Rehabil.* 2003;82:226–9.
15. Díaz-Lobato S, Gómez Mendieta MA, Moreno García MS et al. Two full-term pregnancies in a patient with mitochondrial myopathy and chronic ventilatory insufficiency. *Respiration.* 2005;72:654–6.
16. Yuan N, El-Sayed YY, Ruoss SJ et al. Successful pregnancy and cesarean delivery via noninvasive ventilation in mitochondrial myopathy. *J Perinatol.* 2009;29:166–7.

17. Duan M, Lee J, Bittner EA. Dexmedetomidine for sedation in the parturient with respiratory failure requiring noninvasive ventilation. *Respir Care.* 2012;57(11):1967–9.
18. Allred CC, Matías Esquinas A, Caronia J et al. Successful use of noninvasive ventilation in pregnancy. *Eur Respir Rev.* 2014;23:142–4.
19. Fujita N, Tachibana K, Takeuchi M, Kinouchi K. Successful perioperative use of NIPPV in a pregnant woman with acute pulmonary edema. *Masui.* 2014;63:557–60.
20. Perbet S, Constantin JM, Bolandard F, Bazin JE. Ventilation non-invasive pour œdème pulmonaire attribue aux tocolytiques lors du travail d'une grossesse gé mellaire (Non-invasive ventilation for pulmonary edema associated with tocolytic agents during labour for a twin pregnancy). *Can J Anaesth.* 2008;55:769–73.
21. Jalilian L, Delgado Upegui C, Ferreira R et al. Intraoperative treatment of fetal asystole after endovascular repair of aortic coarctation in a pregnant woman with mitral stenosis. *A A Case Rep.* 2015;6:150–3.
22. Terajima K, Suzuki R, Suganuma R, Sakamoto A. Non-invasive positive pressure ventilation and subarachnoidal blockade for caesarean section in a parturient with pulmonary oedema. *Acta Anaesthesiol Scand.* 2006;50:1307–8.
23. Rojas-Suarez J, Cogollo-González M, García-Rodríguez MC et al. Ventilación mecánica no invasiva como estrategia adyuvante en el manejo del fallo respiratorio agudo secundario a edema pulmonar periparto por preeclampsia severa (Non-invasive mechanical ventilation as adjuvant strategy in the management of acute respiratory failure secondary to peripartum pulmonary edema in severe preeclampsia). *Med Intensiva.* 2011;35:518–9.
24. Murphy VE, Clifton VL, Gibson PG. Asthma exacerbations during pregnancy: Incidence and association with adverse pregnancy outcomes. *Thorax.* 2006;61:169–76.
25. Ferrer M, Esquinas A, Leon M et al. Noninvasive ventilation in severe hypoxemic respiratory failure: A randomized clinical trial. *Am J Respir Crit Care Med.* 2003;168:1438–44.
26. Dalar L, Caner H, Eryuksel E, Kosar F. Application of non-invasive mechanical ventilation in an asthmatic pregnant woman in respiratory failure: A case report. *J Thorac Dis.* 2013;5:97–100.
27. Al-Ansari MA, Hameed AA, Al-jawder SE et al. Use of noninvasive positive pressure ventilation during pregnancy: Case series. *Ann Thorac Med.* 2007;2:23–5.
28. Bassani MA, de Oliveira AB, Oliveira Neto AF. Noninvasive ventilation in a pregnant patient with respiratory failure from all-trans-retinoic-acid (ATRA) syndrome. *Respir Care.* 2009;54:969–72.
29. Banga A, Khilnani GC. Use of non-invasive ventilation in a pregnant woman with acute respiratory distress syndrome due to pneumonia. *Indian J Chest Dis Allied Sci.* 2009;51:115–7.
30. Nicolini A, Tonveronachi E, Navalesi P et al. Effectiveness and predictors of success of noninvasive ventilation during H1N1 pandemics: A multicenter study. *Minerva Anestesiol.* 2012;78:1333–40.
31. Djibré M, Berkane N, Salengro A et al. Non-invasive management of acute respiratory distress syndrome related to *Influenza A* (H1N1) virus pneumonia in a pregnant woman. *Intensive Care Med.* 2010;36:373–4.
32. Polin CM, Hale B, Mauritz AA et al. Anesthetic management of super-morbidly obese parturients for cesarean delivery with a double neuraxial catheter technique: A case series. *Int J Obstet Anesth.* 2015;24:276–80.
33. Guterres AP, Newman MJ. Total spinal following labour epidural analgesia managed with non-invasive ventilation. *Anaesth Intensive Care.* 2010;38:373–5.
34. Erdogan G, Okyay DZ, Yurtlu S et al. Non-invasive mechanical ventilation with spinal anesthesia for cesarean delivery. *Int J Obstet Anesth.* 2010; 19:438–40.

61

Diaphragm pacing (by phrenic nerve stimulation)

JÉSUS GONZALEZ-BERMEJO

INTRODUCTION

Certain neurological diseases cause patients to become ventilator-dependent due to a defect of the production or transmission of respiratory control ('central respiratory paralysis') while the main effector of inspiration, the diaphragm, remains intact. Mechanical ventilator dependence is responsible for loss of autonomy, making it difficult for these patients to return home. Implanted phrenic nerve stimulation is a therapeutic approach that allows patients to be weaned from the constraints of mechanical ventilation. It must be stressed that diaphragm pacing by implanted phrenic nerve stimulation consists of nerve stimulation and not direct stimulation of the diaphragm muscle.

Ventilator dependence of quadriplegic patients following a high cervical spinal cord injury (SCI) is the most common indication for implanted phrenic nerve stimulation.[1,2] Other indications (congenital or acquired central hypoventilation) are much less common. Two phrenic nerve stimulation techniques are currently available: intrathoracic phrenic nerve stimulation and intramuscular diaphragm pacing. Unfortunately, the overall quality of the literature on phrenic nerve stimulation is fairly poor. A recent review simply suggested that phrenic nerve stimulation is a safe and effective option to decrease ventilator dependence in patients with high spinal cord injuries and central hypoventilation.[3]

PHRENIC NERVE STIMULATION TECHNIQUES

Two phrenic nerve stimulation techniques are currently available (Figure 61.1a and b).

Intrathoracic phrenic nerve stimulation (Figure 61.1a)

Intrathoracic phrenic nerve stimulation is the older technique,[4,5] based on radiofrequency transmission of energy and information generated and modulated by an external stimulator (Atrostim®, Atrotech, Tampere, Finland, or Avery®, Avery Medical System, United States) to a receptor implanted underneath the skin and connected to phrenic nerve electrodes, via antennae fixed onto the skin. Stimulation may be either bipolar (Avery) or quadripolar and sequential (Atrostim). Electrodes are implanted via a minimally invasive thoracotomy onto each phrenic nerve (over the superior vena cava for the right phrenic nerve and over the pulmonary artery for the left phrenic nerve). The correct functioning of the electrodes must be tested intraoperatively by determining the stimulation threshold of each electrode, which must be less than 1 mA.

Intramuscular diaphragm pacing (Figure 61.1b)

This implantation technique has been proposed more recently[6] (NeurRxDP4®, Synapse, Oberlin, Ohio, United States). Stimulation electrodes are laparoscopically implanted following intraoperative stimulation mapping designed to identify the phrenic nerve motor points in each hemidiaphragm; two stimulation electrodes are then implanted at these sites. The most distal portion of the phrenic nerve is therefore stimulated by two intramuscular diaphragm electrodes. The electrode leads are then subcutaneously tunnelled and connected to the phrenic nerve stimulator via a connector and a cable.

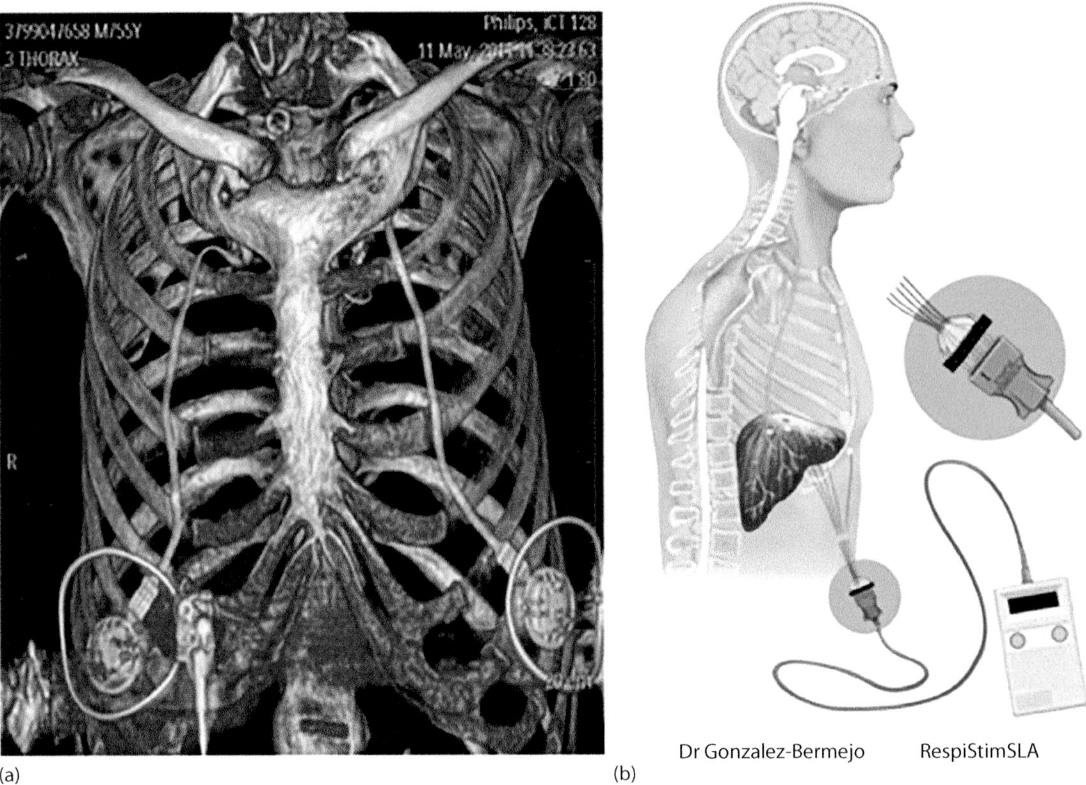

(a) (b)

Figure 61.1 Phrenic nerve stimulation techniques. **(a)** Intrathoracic phrenic nerve stimulator (Atrostim, Atrotech, Tampere, Finland). Four multipolar electrodes are implanted around the two phrenic nerves and subcutaneous receptors receive information from cutaneous antennae. **(b)** Intramuscular diaphragm pacing system (NeurRxDP4, Synapse, Oberlin, Ohio, United States). Four electrodes are implanted in the diaphragm by laparoscopy.

ADVANTAGES AND DISADVANTAGES

Intrathoracic phrenic nerve stimulation is the gold standard, and many patients have been implanted by this technique all over the world for nearly 40 years. Intrathoracic phrenic nerve stimulation ensures the stimulation of all phrenic nerve fibres with stimulation intensities ranging from 1 to 2 mA. However, this technique requires thoracotomy, a fairly invasive procedure, and is associated with a potential risk of intraoperative phrenic nerve injury and a possibly more complicated post-operative course than after laparoscopy.[7] It is an expensive technique, as the Atrostim stimulator from Atrotech (Tampere, Finland) costs about €50,000. The intramuscular diaphragm pacing system (Synapse-Biomedical®) requires minimally invasive surgery with no risk of phrenic nerve injury. This system costs less than €20,000. This system does not stimulate all phrenic nerve fibres and delivers high-intensity stimulation of up to 25 mA. The efficacy of intramuscular diaphragm pacing can be compromised in patients with intact sensory pathways (congenital or acquired central hypoventilation, certain incomplete spinal cord injuries, referred pain to the shoulder induced by the stimulation of phrenic nerve sensory afferents).[4] This pain can limit the efficacy of stimulation and may require the use of analgesics targeting neuropathic pain.

INDICATIONS AND CONTRAINDICATIONS

Indications

The validated indications for implanted phrenic nerve stimulation are ventilator dependence secondary to a respiratory control disorder in the context of the following:

1. Quadriplegia secondary to a high SCI (usually traumatic); the objective of phrenic nerve stimulation is to achieve weaning from mechanical ventilation, at least during the day. Implantation must be performed a considerable time after the injury, when the lesions have become stable. However, in order to avoid SCI-induced diaphragm atrophy, an interval of 6–18 months after the injury appears to be reasonable. Nevertheless, cases of successful implantation more than 5 years after the injury have been reported.[5]
2. Congenital or acquired (degenerative diseases, after surgical resection of a posterior fossa or brainstem tumour, stroke or encephalitis etc.) and permanent or sleep-related central hypoventilation; the objective of stimulation in this context, in the absence of motor deficit, is to improve the patient's quality of life by eliminating the need for mechanical ventilation. The indication for phrenic nerve stimulation is relatively simple in adults with acquired permanent central hypoventilation.

However, no consensus has been reached concerning the optimal timing of implantation in patients with congenital central hypoventilation syndrome (Ondine curse).[3,8] Phrenic nerve stimulation can be considered, especially when central hypoventilation persists when the patient is awake and particularly following failure of mechanical ventilation alone.[9]

Contraindications

It must be stressed that diaphragm pacing by implanted phrenic nerve stimulation consists of nerve stimulation and not the direct stimulation of the diaphragm muscle. Any lesion of the phrenic nerve therefore constitutes a contraindication to phrenic nerve stimulation. Phrenic nerve lesions can be due to SCIs involving phrenic motoneurons (C4 SCI), nerve root injury (for example by traumatic avulsion) or a phrenic nerve trunk injury. The frequency of these lesions is unknown, and the presence of such lesions must therefore be excluded prior to implantation. Phrenic nerve stimulation also requires an intact diaphragm; any intrinsic muscle lesion therefore constitutes a contraindication. The only exception is denervation diaphragm muscle atrophy due to SCI, which can be reversed by the muscle reconditioning obtained by diaphragm pacing. However, severe malnutrition can considerably interfere with this reconditioning. The patient's clinical context can also constitute a contraindication. For example, the patient's psychiatric or psychological state can predispose to the failure of diaphragm pacing. Implantation should also be avoided in patients with an active disease and a limited life expectancy. Finally, the social and family context and the patient's life project must also be taken into account in the decision to perform diaphragm pacing.

Preimplantation assessment

The preimplantation assessment must evaluate phrenic nerve and diaphragm function and assess central conduction pathways by delivering phrenic nerve stimulation[10] and recording the electromyographic and mechanical responses of the diaphragm[11] (Figure 61.2). The analysis of the diaphragm response to transcranial magnetic stimulation provides information about the status of central conduction pathways, particularly in patients with acquired central respiratory paralysis.[12] The absence of response to transcranial magnetic stimulation indicates the complete interruption of respiratory control transmission pathways, excluding any hope of recovery and consequently confirms the indication for phrenic nerve stimulation (when the phrenic nerve is intact, see the following). On the contrary, a persistent response to transcranial magnetic stimulation suggests the possibility of recovery, and the patient must be reviewed at a later date in order to determine the indication for implanted phrenic nerve stimulation.[13] Cervical magnetic stimulation confirms the integrity of the phrenic nerve and diaphragm.[14]

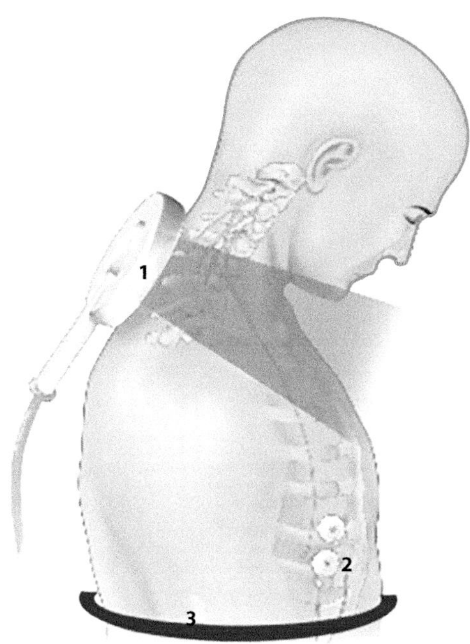

Figure 61.2 Electrophysiological examination of the diaphragm. **(1)** Magnetic stimulation; **(2)** electromyography electrodes; and **(3)** abdominal belt.

A psychological and social assessment is also necessary before confirming the indication for implanted phrenic nerve stimulation.

Alternative treatments

When the implantation of a phrenic nerve stimulator is contraindicated because of a phrenic nerve lesion, no other alternative treatment is currently available for the patient. Intermittent abdominal compression can help promote diaphragm function for several hours, when patients refuse to be connected to a ventilator at the neck. The functional electrical stimulation of abdominal muscles to induce 'reversed' ventilation (active expiration, passive inspiration by abdominal muscle relaxation) has been the subject of numerous physiological studies, but no clinical applications have yet been reported. A phrenic nerve transfer protocol, consisting of reinnervating the phrenic nerve by a superior laryngeal branch, is currently underway (NCT00213616).

PRACTICAL ASPECTS

Initiation of diaphragm pacing and reconditioning

Intrathoracic phrenic nerve stimulation is initiated about 2–8 weeks after implantation to allow the stabilisation of the electrodes by the formation of scar tissue. Intramuscular diaphragm pacing can be initiated after only 48 hours. Stimulation thresholds are checked for each electrode.

A period of diaphragm reconditioning is necessary for quadriplegic patients due to the presence of denervation atrophy.[15,16] One diaphragm reconditioning session is performed each day within the limits of fatigue (generally identified by a 50% reduction of the tidal volume initially induced by phrenic nerve stimulation or signs of clinical intolerance). The initial duration of stimulation cannot be predicted; it may be less than 5 min in patients with severe atrophy or up to 20–30 min. In the most severe forms of diaphragm atrophy, reconditioning may be possible only under mechanical ventilation, in which case, the initial duration of stimulation is 10 min and is gradually increased to reach 2 hours/day after 4 weeks according to the protocol currently used in our department. Reconditioning under conditions of stimulated ventilatory autonomy is then possible when the tidal volume reaches 400 mL, which generally takes 6 weeks to 3 months.[16]

Clinical surveillance and cycle-to-cycle monitoring of the tidal volume are necessary to ensure the patient's safety throughout the reconditioning period. The monitoring of tidal volume is performed by an electronic spirometer, usually connected to the tracheostomy cannula. Once a stable tidal volume has been achieved, the tidal volume needs to be measured only in case of problems.

It should be stressed that the transfer of quadriplegic patients from the supine position to the sitting position is associated with decreased mechanical efficacy of the diaphragm secondary to abdominal muscle weakness.[17] The stimulator must therefore always be adjusted in the sitting position and generally with abdominal compression, which must not cover the zones of costal insertion of the diaphragm to avoid impairing effective diaphragm contraction.

Surveillance and follow-up

After the completion of diaphragm reconditioning, the risk of short-term or long-term diaphragmatic muscle fatigue is low, or even non-existent. Phrenic nerve stimulation is unlikely to cause injury to the phrenic nerve or diaphragm, as illustrated by the efficacy of phrenic nerve stimulation in some patients with a follow-up of more than 20 years.[17–19] In practice, the duration of diaphragm pacing essentially depends on the patient's wishes and especially the possibility of nighttime respiratory surveillance, as, unlike mechanical ventilators, phrenic nerve stimulators are not equipped with devices designed to monitor their own efficacy and are fitted only with battery or electronic dysfunction alarms. Consequently, when nighttime respiratory surveillance is not possible, patients should be advised to spend the night on mechanical ventilation.

What becomes of the tracheostomy?

Tracheostomy closure is possible and is performed very regularly in the United States,[16,20] both in quadriplegic patients and in patients with central hypoventilation. However, tracheostomy closure raises two types of problems. It makes access to the upper airways more difficult, requiring intubation when surgery is required or in life-threatening situations (including those induced by stimulator dysfunction). Phrenic nerve stimulation does not induce physiological inspiration, as the diaphragmatic contraction induced by stimulation is not preceded by the opening of the upper airways and is not associated with the contraction of upper chest wall muscles to stabilise the upper airways, resulting in paradoxical movement of the upper chest wall during diaphragmatic contraction,[21] exerting pressure on the upper airways with a risk of upper airway obstruction during inspiration induced by phrenic nerve stimulation.[22]

Precautions and risks of dysfunction

Phrenic nerve stimulators do not induce any risk of implanted cardiac pacemaker dysfunction.[23] Magnetic resonance imaging (MRI) and lithotripsy are formally contraindicated in the presence of an intrathoracic phrenic nerve stimulator due to the risks of electromagnetic interference. MRI is also currently contraindicated in patients with an intramuscular diaphragm pacing system. However, plain X-rays and computed tomography and the use of electrical scalpels are not contraindicated.

Finally, covering the intrathoracic phrenic nerve stimulator transmission antennae by a space blank immediately blocks the transmission of information and stops diaphragm pacing.[24]

The life span of the intrathoracic phrenic nerve stimulator is unknown at the present time, but is estimated to be about 10 years, as the internal components often need to be changed after this time. The life span of intramuscular diaphragm pacing is unknown, as the longest follow-up for patients implanted in France is less than 10 years.

RESULTS

Implanted phrenic nerve stimulation has been performed in several thousands of patients since the 1970s. This technique has allowed many patients to be weaned from mechanical ventilation. However, most of the published studies are purely observational, sometimes comparative, but based on retrospective analysis, making it difficult to precisely determine the benefit provided by implanted phrenic nerve stimulation compared to mechanical ventilation, although this benefit is undeniable.[3]

Weaning from mechanical ventilation

Published studies have concerned the Atrotech intrathoracic implantation system. The largest international multicentre study was based on a cohort of 64 patients, composed of 35 children and 29 adults.[18] Implanted phrenic nerve stimulation was mostly indicated in the context of traumatic quadriplegia (71%) or congenital central hypoventilation syndrome (22%). Phrenic nerve stimulation was considered to be successful with no complications in 60%

of children and 52% of adults. The following complications were reported: infections in 6% of cases, iatrogenic phrenic nerve injury in 3.8% of cases, electrode dysfunction in 3.1% of cases and receptor dysfunction in 5.9% of cases. Following the resolution of these complications, phrenic nerve stimulation was considered to be effective in 94% of paediatric patients and 86% of adult patients. Another single-centre study reported weaning from mechanical ventilation in 81.8% of patients, mostly presenting traumatic quadriplegia (72%).[17] More recently, a North American centre reported its experience acquired since 2000 with the intramuscular diaphragm pacing system (Synapse®). Forty-nine high SCI patients were implanted, allowing complete weaning from mechanical ventilation in 96% of cases.[25]

Improvement of quality of life

Weaning from mechanical ventilation as a result of implanted phrenic nerve stimulation considerably improves the patient's autonomy, facilitating the nursing care of quadriplegic patients (toilet, transfer to the armchair) and their everyday life (allowing them to leave home).[26,27] Lighter nursing care also facilitates return home[28] or transfer to other accommodation facilities (for example discharge from the intensive care unit) for some patients. Phrenic nerve stimulation also eliminates the noisy environment of the ventilator for both the patient and the family.

In some quadriplegic patients, diaphragm pacing restores phonation that was impossible on mechanical ventilation because of poor tolerance of non-invasive ventilation. Finally, phrenic nerve stimulation restores airflow in the upper airways and consequently restores olfaction.[29] These positive effects are major determinants in the patient's self-reported improvement of quality of life.

Reduction of morbidity and mortality

Continuous positive airway pressure ventilation predisposes to the development of thromboembolic complications by reducing intrathoracic venous return, as observed in intensive care unit patients.[30] In contrast, implanted phrenic nerve stimulation creates negative intrathoracic pressure and consequently promotes venous return, which should theoretically reduce the risk of thromboembolic complications in quadriplegic patients, although this effect has not been formally demonstrated.

Tracheostomy-related complications, such as tracheal injury or tracheoesophageal fistula, are facilitated by conflict between the cannula and the trachea occurring, for example during patient mobilisation. It would therefore be intuitively possible for implanted phrenic nerve stimulation to reduce the incidence of mechanical ventilated-related tracheal injury.

However, the main expected medical benefit is the reduction of infectious complications, as implanted phrenic nerve stimulation allows more physiological inspiration and improves drainage of bronchial secretions, while reducing basal atelectasis. Phrenic nerve stimulation is often associated with a decreased frequency of bronchial aspiration and a lower incidence of bronchial and lung infections.[31]

Finally, implanted phrenic nerve stimulation ensures more effective ventilation of the lung bases with improved pulmonary perfusion. This phenomenon can probably be explained by reduction of the alveoloarterial oxygen gradient observed during diaphragm pacing compared to mechanical ventilation for a comparable level of ventilation.[32]

CONCLUSIONS AND PROSPECTS

Implanted phrenic nerve stimulation in carefully selected patients (appropriate indications, satisfactory electrophysiological investigations) can restore ventilatory autonomy associated with medical and probably economic benefits. However, the target population remains extremely limited on the basis of currently validated indications, but this population could be increased on the basis of the results recently obtained in patients with central sleep apnoea and Cheyne–Stokes respiration[33] showing that implanted phrenic nerve stimulation effectively correct these disorders and could therefore possibly decrease the associated morbidity and mortality. These results observed in central sleep apnoea, which are particularly promising for the future of this technique, were obtained following the development of fully implantable endovascular phrenic nerve stimulators (so-called transvenous pacing) not requiring open surgery (Remedē System®, Respicardia, Minneapolis, Minnesota, United States).

Other applications of implanted phrenic nerve stimulation are currently under investigation, no longer designed to provide ventilatory support, as in the case of respiratory control disorders, but to correct or prevent diaphragm atrophy, as it has been hypothesised that implanted phrenic nerve stimulation could slow diaphragm degeneration during amyotrophic lateral sclerosis (ALS).[34] However, two randomised controlled trials reported concordant negative results demonstrating excess mortality in the arm treated by phrenic nerve stimulation. Implanted phrenic nerve stimulation could also reduce respiratory complications related to particularly high-risk surgery (heart surgery and supramesocolic surgery), which would require temporary diaphragm pacing by means of electrodes that are easy to implant and easy to remove, such as the electrodes inserted into the subclavian vein to treat central sleep apnoea by transvenous pacing nerve (LungPacer®, Lungpacer medical, Burnaby, British Columbia, Canada). Transvenous phrenic nerve stimulation could have a wide range of applications in intensive care, as an adjuvant treatment to mechanical ventilation, as preliminary data suggest that this technique could prevent ventilator-induced diaphragm dysfunction[35] and could therefore limit the impact of diaphragm dysfunction on weaning from mechanical ventilation.

FINANCIAL DISCLOSURE

Jésus Gonzalez-Bermejo received honoraria from Synapse Biomedical in 2009 for conducting two training sessions in centres managing patients with implanted phrenic nerve stimulation.

SCIENTIFIC DISCLOSURE

Jésus Gonzalez-Bermejo has been a coinvestigator in several public-funded studies, essentially concerning intrathoracic phrenic nerve stimulation, and has contributed to the official recognition of implanted phrenic nerve stimulation in France and to the reimbursement of Atrostim (Atrotech) and NeurRxDPS® (Synapse) stimulators by French national health insurance.

He was also a coinvestigator in an open-label study of intramuscular diaphragm pacing for patients with amyotrophic lateral sclerosis (ALS) funded by Synapse Biomedical. This study has now been completed (NCT00420719), and French data have been published[36] and contributed to the Food and Drug Administration approval for Synapse Biomedical to use this technique in patients with ALS at the stage of alveolar hypoventilation.

He was principal investigator in a study funded by a Public Hospital Clinical Research Programme grant, an ALS research association, and the Thierry de Latran Foundation designed to determine whether early implantation can postpone the need for mechanical ventilation (NCT01583088). Synapse Biomedical provided stimulators at a reduced price for this study.

None of these studies has raised any financial conflicts of interests for the author.

REFERENCES

1. Creasey GH, Ho CH, Triolo RJ et al. Clinical applications of electrical stimulation after spinal cord injury. *J Spinal Cord Med.* 2004;27:365–75.
2. DiMarco AF. Restoration of respiratory muscle function following spinal cord injury: Review of electrical and magnetic stimulation techniques. *Respir Physiol Neurobiol.* 2005;147:273–87.
3. Sieg EP, Payne RA, Hazard S, Rizk E. Evaluating the evidence: Is phrenic nerve stimulation a safe and effective tool for decreasing ventilator dependence in patients with high cervical spinal cord injuries and central hypoventilation? *Childs Nerv Syst.* 2016;32:1033–8.
4. Morélot-Panzini C, Le Pimpec-Barthes F, Menegaux F et al. Referred shoulder pain (C4 dermatome) can adversely impact diaphragm pacing with intramuscular electrodes. *Eur Respir J.* 2015;45:1751–4.
5. DiMarco AF. Phrenic nerve stimulation in patients with spinal cord injury. *Respir Physiol Neurobiol.* 2009;169:200–9.
6. DiMarco AF, Onders RP, Ignagni A et al. Phrenic nerve pacing via intramuscular diaphragm electrodes in tetraplegic subjects. *Chest.* 2005;127:671–8.
7. Weese-Mayer DE, Silvestri JM, Kenny AS et al. Diaphragm pacing with a quadripolar phrenic nerve electrode: An international study. *Pacing Clin Electrophysiol.* 1996;19:1311–1319.
8. Ali A, Flageole H. Diaphragmatic pacing for the treatment of congenital central alveolar hypoventilation syndrome. *J Pediatr Surg.* 2008;43:792–6.
9. Morélot-Panzini C, Gonzalez-Bermejo J, Straus C, Similowski T. Reversal of pulmonary hypertension after diaphragm pacing in an adult patient with congenital central hypoventilation syndrome. *Int J Artif Organs.* 2013;36:434–8.
10. Shaw RK, Glenn WW, Hogan JF, Phelps ML. Electrophysiological evaluation of phrenic nerve function in candidates for diaphragm pacing. *J Neurosurg.* 1980;53:345–54.
11. Alshekhlee A, Onders RP, Syed TU et al. Phrenic nerve conduction studies in spinal cord injury: Applications for diaphragmatic pacing. *Muscle Nerve.* 2008;38:1546–52.
12. Estenne M, De Troyer A. Mechanism of the postural dependence of vital capacity in tetraplegic subjects. *Am Rev Respir Dis.* 1987;135:367–71.
13. Duguet A, Demoule A, Gonzalez J et al. Predicting the recovery of ventilatory activity in central respiratory paralysis. *Neurology.* 2006;67:288–92.
14. Similowski T, Straus C, Attali V et al. Assessment of the motor pathway to the diaphragm using cortical and cervical magnetic stimulation in the decision-making process of phrenic pacing. *Chest.* 1996;110:1551–7.
15. Nochomovitz ML, Hopkins M, Brodkey J et al. Conditioning of the diaphragm with phrenic nerve stimulation after prolonged disuse. *Am Rev Respir Dis.* 1984;130:685–8.
16. Perez IA, Kun S, Keens TG. Diaphragm pacing by phrenic nerve stimulation. *Am J Respir Crit Care Med.* 2016;193:P13–4.
17. Le Pimpec-Barthes F, Gonzalez-Bermejo J, Hubsch JP et al. Intrathoracic phrenic pacing: A 10-year experience in France. *J Thorac Cardiovasc Surg.* 2011;142:378–83.
18. Dobelle WH, D'Angelo MS, Goetz BF et al. 200 cases with a new breathing pacemaker dispel myths about diaphragm pacing. *Asaio J.* 1994;40:M244–52.
19. Elefteriades JA, Quin JA, Hogan JF et al. Long-term follow-up of pacing of the conditioned diaphragm in quadriplegia. *Pacing Clin Electrophysiol.* 2002;25:897–906.
20. Bolikal P, Bach JR, Goncalves M. Electrophrenic pacing and decannulation for high-level spinal cord injury: A case series. *J Spinal Cord Med.* 2012;35:170–4.

21. Danon J, Druz WS, Goldberg NB, Sharp JT. Function of the isolated paced diaphragm and the cervical accessory muscles in C1 quadriplegics. *Am Rev Respir Dis.* 1979;119:909–19.
22. Hyland RH, Hutcheon MA, Perl A et al. Upper airway occlusion induced by diaphragm pacing for primary alveolar hypoventilation: Implications for the pathogenesis of obstructive sleep apnea. *Am Rev Respir Dis.* 1981;124:180–5.
23. Onders RP, Khansarinia S, Weiser T et al. Multicenter analysis of diaphragm pacing in tetraplegics with cardiac pacemakers: Positive implications for ventilator weaning in intensive care units. *Surgery.* 2010;148:893–7; discussion 897–8.
24. Boissel N, Vaananen L, Michoux J et al. Dysfunction of phrenic pacemakers induced by metallic rescue blankets. *Pacing Clin Electrophysiol.* 2001;24:241–3.
25. Onders RP, Elmo M, Khansarinia S et al. Complete worldwide operative experience in laparoscopic diaphragm pacing: Results and differences in spinal cord injured patients and amyotrophic lateral sclerosis patients. *Surg Endosc.* 2009;23:1433–40.
26. Chervin RD, Guilleminault C. Diaphragm pacing for respiratory insufficiency. *J Clin Neurophysiol.* 1997;14:369–37.
27. Fodstad H. Phrenicodiaphragmatic pacing. In: Roussos C, ed. *The Thorax*, 2nd ed. New York: Marcel Dekker; 1995:2597–617.
28. Esclarin A, Bravo P, Arroyo O et al. Tracheostomy ventilation versus diaphragmatic pacemaker ventilation in high spinal cord injury. *Paraplegia.* 1994;32:687–93.
29. Adler D, Gonzalez-Bermejo J, Duguet A et al. Diaphragm pacing restores olfaction in tetraplegia. *Eur Respir J.* 2009;34:365–70.
30. Cook D, Crowther M, Meade M et al. Deep venous thrombosis in medical-surgical critically ill patients: Prevalence, incidence, and risk factors. *Crit Care Med.* 2005;33:1565–1571.
31. Hirschfeld S, Exner G, Luukkaala T, Baer GA. Mechanical ventilation or phrenic nerve stimulation for treatment of spinal cord injury-induced respiratory insufficiency. *Spinal Cord.* 2008;46:738–742.
32. Gonzalez-Bermejo J, Morélot-Panzini C, Georges M et al. Can diaphragm pacing improve gas exchange? Insights from quadriplegic patients. *Eur Respir J.* 2014;43:303–6.
33. Abraham WT, Jagielski D, Oldenburg O et al. Phrenic nerve stimulation for the treatment of central sleep apnea. *JACC Heart Fail.* 2015;3:360–9.
34. Gonzalez-Bermejo J, Morélot-Panzini C, Salachas F et al. Diaphragm pacing improves sleep in patients with amyotrophic lateral sclerosis. *Amyotroph Lateral Scler.* 2012;13:44–54.
35. Masmoudi H, Coirault C, Demoule A et al. Can phrenic stimulation protect the diaphragm from mechanical ventilation-induced damage? *Eur Respir J.* 2013;42:280–3.
36. Gonzalez-Bermejo J, Morélot-Panzini C, Tanguy ML et al. Early diaphragm pacing in patients with amyotrophic lateral sclerosis (RespiStimALS): A randomised controlled triple-blind trial. *Lancet Neurol.* 2016;15(12):1217–27. Oct 11. PubMed PMID: 27751553.

62

Tracheostomy

PIERO CERIANA, PAOLO PELOSI AND MARIA VARGAS

INTRODUCTION

Approximately 40% of patients admitted to the intensive care unit (ICU) for respiratory failure, regardless of origin, require mechanical ventilation.[1,2] With the exception of a percentage ranging between 5% and 15% of patients that can be managed with non-invasive mechanical ventilation (NIMV),[3,4] the vast majority receive translaryngeal intubation and invasive mechanical ventilation (IMV). While in about 70% of cases, respiratory failure resolves within a few days, thus allowing extubation, the remaining 30% of patients require maintenance of IMV and translaryngeal tube for a longer period,[5] because the advancements in the care of critically ill patients have increased the number of patients surviving the acute phase and undergoing prolonged IMV. Protracted translaryngeal intubation not only bypasses and impairs the upper airway protective mechanisms, thus increasing the risk of ventilator-associated pneumonia (VAP),[6] but can also cause severe laryngeal injury[7] and sinusitis,[8] when nasal intubation is performed instead of oral intubation. Based on these issues, it is common and accepted practice to convert the interface for IMV from a translaryngeal tube into a tracheostomy cannula in those patients who require prolonged mechanical ventilation. Besides the reduction in translaryngeal tube-related complications, tracheostomy carries other potential advantages such as less need for sedation, better airway hygiene, improved patient's comfort and decreased airway resistance.[9]

HISTORY

Tracheostomy is one of the most ancient surgical procedures, since the first reports of a technique very similar to it can be found in books older than 4000 years.[10] But it was only after the polio epidemics during the fifth decade of the twentieth century that tracheostomy became a technique for airway management during mechanical ventilation,[11] and not only a technique for relieving upper airway obstruction. From then on, its application became more and more popular due to the development of tracheostomy tubes designed to minimise tracheal injury and percutaneous dilational techniques that made this procedure simpler and feasible at the bedside. Despite their frequent interchangeable use, the terms *tracheostomy* and *tracheotomy* are distinct and indicate an opening in the trachea with or without a surgical attachment to the skin, respectively.[12]

EPIDEMIOLOGY

The practice of tracheostomy can be variable in different countries according to local attitudes, protocols and ethical issues. There has been, however, a general increase in the number of tracheotomies over the past decades mainly due to the advancement in technology and manufacture of percutaneous tracheostomy kits. Over a 9-year period in North Carolina, the incidence of tracheostomy increased from 8.3 per 100,000 to 24.2 per 100,000.[13] It is now calculated that approximately 100,000 tracheostomy procedures are performed each year in the United States,[14] and this accounts for about more than 12% of patients receiving mechanical ventilation.[15] A similar figure has been reported by other authors[16] in a multicenter study involving different countries, while in a study conducted in Norway, the incidence of tracheostomy was about 16% of all patients admitted to the ICU.[17] This last study also documented how, besides the total number of tracheostomies, a significant change has occurred in the type of technique used; in fact, surgical tracheostomies, which in 1996 accounted for almost 95% of all procedures, only 7 years later represented only 15% of all tracheostomies, since the majority were carried out with the percutaneous technique. The first global picture of current practices with regard to tracheostomy insertion demonstrated considerable international variation in practice, suggesting a need for greater standardisation of approaches to tracheostomy.[18] Besides all advantages of tracheotomy, it must be said that many health systems provide a significant reimbursement for tracheostomy, especially if the procedure is carried out within a few days from ICU admission.[19] This kind of payment could represent a theoretical driver and incentive to the performance of early procedures and even generate dissimilarities of treatment according to the different reimbursement system.[20]

PATHOPHYSIOLOGY

Tracheostomy, dead space and humidification

Breathing through a tracheal cannula partially diverts the flow of air from the upper native airways: this implies a reduction in the distance covered by air from the atmosphere to the alveolar spaces and of dead space by about 80–100 mL. Moreover, the anatomical site where inspired air is warmed and humidified is bypassed, and tracheostomised patients, in the absence of artificial humidification, can develop chronic inflammation and dehydration of the tracheobronchial tree, with subsequent reduced ciliary function and thickened secretions.

Effects on airflow resistance

The flow through artificial conduits obeys Poiseuille's law, according to which resistance is directly proportional to the tube length and inversely proportional to the fourth or fifth power of the tube radius for, respectively, laminar or turbulent flow. Therefore, in every case in which the airflow is increased (high inspiratory demand) or the tube radius is reduced (small and long cannula, apposition of secretions), the patient has to cope with a higher resistive load. Tube design and features, however, allow the clinician to minimise the increased resistive load imposed by the tracheostomy cannula: the presence of fenestrationl,[21] removal of the inner cannula[22] and deflation of the cuff[23] are all means of decreasing the airflow resistance and the inspiratory work of breathing.

Tracheostomy and swallowing

The presence of a tracheostomy tube, per se, can impair the process of swallowing through the following mechanisms: reduced laryngeal elevation, hindered glottic closure, decreased larynx sensitivity to the penetration of foreign material, reduced efficiency of protective cough[24] and impaired coordination between respiration and swallowing.[25] Then, the leak created by tracheostomy in the normally closed subglottic system causes the loss of subglottic pressure, a mechanism normally important for the protection of airways from aspiration.[26] The presence of an inflated tracheostomy cuff represents a worsening situation, since it favours anchoring of the larynx to the anterior neck, which limits the process of elevation, delays the onset of the swallowing reflex and increases the amount of bolus retention in the pharyngeal valleculae[27] (Figure 62.1).

Resumption of oral feeding after tracheostomy requires a preliminary clinical assessment for the evaluation of the following items:

- Tongue and oral muscle strength
- Dry swallowing

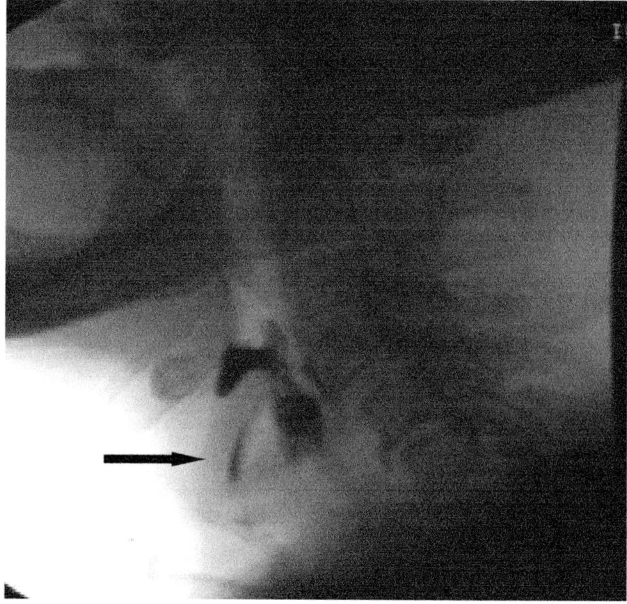

Figure 62.1 After oral administration of a small bolus of thickened barium, the patient is invited to swallow it while a slow-motion X-ray sequence is performed. Part of the bolus is retained in the vallecula and pharyngeal recesses, and part of it penetrates in the airway (see the arrow).

- Presence of gag reflex
- Presence and efficiency of volitional and reflex cough

The following step includes performance of a modified Evans blue test[28]: a positive result (aspiration of blue-dyed secretions) is indicative of aspiration, while in the presence of a negative test, dysphagia cannot be ruled out, so a supervised oral feeding can be resumed with the cuff deflated. Further instrumental evaluation with fibre-optic endoscopy and/or videophluoroscopy[29] must be carried out in patients with a positive dye test and in those that, despite a negative dye test, present witnessed or suspected episodes of inhalation. Besides cuff deflation, the placement of a speaking valve on the tracheotomy tube seems to improve swallowing efficiency,[30] probably through the resumption of subglottic pressure.[26]

Tracheostomy and phonation

The possibility to preserve speech and to communicate has a great relevance for a tracheotomised patient, mainly for the maintenance of social relationships and of an acceptable quality of life (QOL). From the physiological point of view, phonation requires a subglottic pressure of at least 2–3 cm H_2O and a flow through the vocal cords greater than 3 L/min.[31] A further basic requirement for proper phonation is the preserved glottic function, including vocal cord mobility and the absence of upper airway stenosis. In a spontaneously breathing patient, phonation can be simply obtained by deflating the cuff and occluding the proximal tube opening with a finger, with a cap or with a one-way speaking

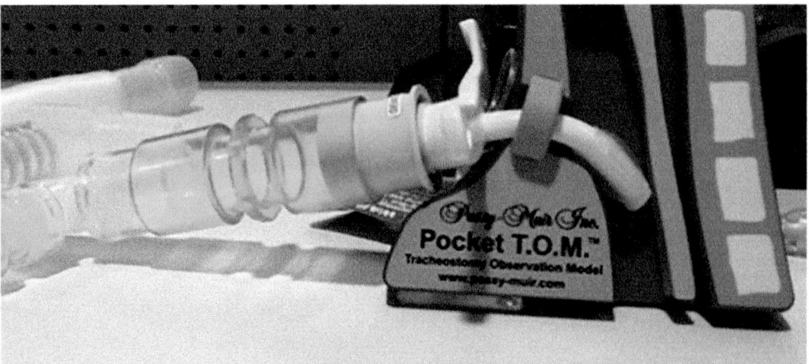

Figure 62.2 The speaking valve (Passy Muir®) is positioned at the distal end of the catheter mount before the tracheostomy tube.

valve. In a mechanically ventilated patient with a cuffed cannula, phonation can be facilitated only if the cannula is fenestrated. In alternative, 'open' ventilation, using cuffless tubes enables phonation provided that good glottis function is preserved. Furthermore, the quality of speech can be significantly ameliorated with proper adjustment of the ventilator mode and setting[32] or placing a one-way speaking valve between the ventilator circuit and the tracheotomy tube[33] (Figure 62.2).

Indications

The general and most common indications for tracheostomy are the following:

1. Weaning failure from mechanical ventilation in patients in which weaning success can be attempted at a later time after clinical stabilisation
2. Respiratory failure requiring long-term mechanical ventilation in patients not amenable to subsequent weaning (e.g. amyotrophic lateral sclerosis patients)
3. Failure to protect the lower airways as in cases of severe neurologic insult or copious secretions
4. Relief of upper airway obstruction[34]

In some cases, tracheostomy must be considered permanent as in category 2 patients, while in other groups, the placement of a tracheostomy cannula can be considered temporary provided that the underlying condition, as in groups 3 and 4, has come to resolution. For patients belonging to group 1, the increased use of NIMV allows many patients to be weaned from tracheostomy even when mechanical ventilation is still needed and the patient must be enrolled in a programme of domiciliary NIMV.

Timing

The procedure of tracheostomy should not follow strict rules regarding time, but should be tailored to the individual patient, taking into account the underlying cause of respiratory failure and the clinical course. The search for advantages of early (2–10 days after intubation) versus late tracheostomy (>10 days of intubation) failed to show clear advantages in term of reduced VAP incidence[35] mortality[36] or median ICU stay.[37] One large randomised controlled trial, in particular, showed that only 45% of patients assigned to the late tracheostomy group (>10 days) received it, since many of them were liberated from IMV before the 10th day without the need for tracheostomy.[37] This means that, in the absence of better criteria for predicting which patient will need prolonged IMV, it is reasonable, in the majority of cases, to wait at least 10 days before deciding to perform tracheostomy.

Tracheostomy and weaning from mechanical ventilation

Conversion of the translaryngeal tube into tracheostomy implies the potential advantage of a reduced resistive work of breathing. This has been also demonstrated in a group of difficult-to-wean patients[38] in which after tracheostomy, there was less ventilatory demand, respiratory drive, work of breathing and intrinsic positive end-expiratory pressure. Other advantages of tracheostomy include easier airway suctioning, better patient comfort and oral care, easier and more secure airway fastening, less need for sedation, enhanced ability to communicate, greater mobility and the possibility of transferring the patient from the ICU. The process of weaning from prolonged IMV is complex and multifactorial, so that the link between tracheostomy and weaning cannot be linear nor consequential. It is likely, however, that, for a subset of patients, tracheostomy could play a crucial role in the weaning process.[39]

PRACTICAL APPLICATIONS

Choice of cannula

Metal tubes, formerly used for permanent placement after laryngectomy, are seldom used nowadays due to their high cost and design limitations. Plastic tubes, on the other hand, are currently available in a huge variety of models, size and design and can fit almost any kind of patient and any

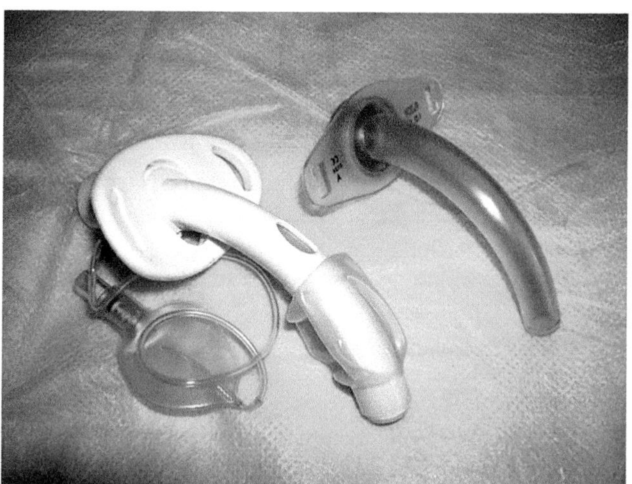

Figure 62.3 *Left side*: cuffed and fenestrated cannula. *Right side*: non-fenestrated cuffless cannula with speaking valve. Both have the inner cannula.

individual need and peculiarity (Figure 62.3). The choice of the cannula depends on several factors:

- Need for IMV
- Ability to protect the lower airways
- Temporary or permanent use
- Specific anatomical problems (neck size and length, deformities)
- Presence of tracheal or glottic stenosis

The ideal tracheostomy tube should meet all the preceding requirements, should facilitate proper speech and swallowing function and should minimise complications. One of the first features to consider is the size: this should be proportional to the size of the native airway, to achieve a proper airway seal without the need to overinflate the cuff. Tubes are identified by three measurements: inner diameter (ID), outer diameter and length, can be angled or curved and can be available in standard size as well as with the proximal or the distal segment longer, to adjust to different anatomical variants.[40] Some tubes have a suction port just above the cuff, to aspirate subglottic secretions; others are made of silicone and are reinforced by an inner spiral wire, so that they never kink or collapse: they are especially helpful for tracheal stenosis, tracheomalacia and thoracic deformities. In different types of cannula, the presence of an adjustable flange allows the clinician to easily advance or withdraw it up to the desired length.

Fenestration

Fenestrated tubes are similar to non-fenestrated ones, but have an opening in the posterior curved portion above the cuff, which can be single or multiple. These cannulas have a disposal inner cannula available with and without fenestration: only when the fenestrated inner cannula is in place, the opening is complete and effective. During expiration, air passes through the fenestration and crosses the glottis, thus facilitating phonation. This process can be enhanced by the deflation of the cuff and by capping the cannula and requires, of course, optimal adaptation to the patient's anatomy, so that the fenestration is properly positioned in the middle of the tracheal lumen. Our suggestion is to leave the fenestration open only temporarily. If the fenestration is left open permanently, the posterior tracheal wall can be drawn inwards by suction, leading to adherence and granulation inside the cannula with problems during airway suctioning and serious risks during cannula replacement.

Inner cannula

The presence of an inner cannula, in the so-called dual-cannula tubes, prevents the deposition of thickened secretions into the internal lumen, thus maintaining its full patency and postponing the time of replacement: the reusable inner cannula is removed and cleaned while the new one is positioned. The presence of an inner cannula, however, reduces the true ID, and this can have an influence on the inspiratory resistive load[22] and the imposed work of breathing. The advantages of the inner cannula are better appreciated in long-term domiciliary management, where delayed replacement and the possibility of relieving a sudden obstruction by simply pulling out the inner cannula are highly desirable.

Cuff management

Tracheostomy tubes may or may not have an inflatable cuff, which is designed to seal the residual natural airspace between the cannula and the tracheal wall. The maintenance of a closed system is desirable for those patients who cannot protect their lower airways from spillage of nose and mouth secretions, to prevent respiratory tract infections, but it is mainly indicated during IMV to avoid leaks and to achieve full control and easier manipulation of gas exchange. This is not mandatory, since open ventilation using cuffless tubes can be effectively performed[41] in patients with preserved glottic function and adequate pulmonary compliance. The cuff should be inflated with air up to a pressure not higher than the tracheal capillary perfusion pressure, to avoid mucosal ischaemia: for this purpose, it is generally agreed that a maximum intracuff pressure of 25 mmHg (or 35 cm H_2O) is acceptable. Monitoring cuff pressure with only manual appreciation of the pilot balloon tension can be misleading; therefore, the manoeuvre should be done with a manometer every time that the cuff is inflated or deflated, in case of leaks, or when the cannula is repositioned or replaced.

Cuffs are available in three different kinds:

- Tight-to-shaft cuffs, when deflated, perfectly adhere to the tube surface without forming wrinkles. They are silicone made and permeable to gas, so that they must be filled with sterile water instead of air. The advantage

of these tubes is the easier insertion through the stoma and the better air passage when the cuff is deflated.
- High-volume low-pressure cuffs are most commonly used for the specific design that reduces the risk of tracheal damage. Compared with tight-to-shaft tubes, the cuff, when deflated, forms protruding wrinkles and folds.
- Foam-cuffed tubes have a large cuff made of polyurethane foam lined on the outer surface by a sheath of silicone. Before insertion, the cuff is evacuated, then it is allowed to reexpand without manual syringe inflation: the pilot conduit remains open to the atmosphere, so that the intracuff pressure equals ambient pressure. This cannula is specifically designed to avoid mucosal ischaemia and to minimise tracheal injury, but, despite this sound rationale, it has not gained widespread use.

Weaning from tracheostomy

When the initial cause of respiratory failure that required tracheostomy has resolved, the patient can be evaluated for possible decannulation, taking into account age, past history and baseline disease. If upper airway obstruction was the cause, restoration of adequate upper airspace must be carefully evaluated by means of endoscopy. In patients still on IMV, tracheostomy should be maintained only for ventilator-dependent patients, while for the remaining ones, a possible conversion to non-invasive ventilation and subsequent decannulation can be considered. For these patients, it is advisable to start NIMV, leaving the capped tracheostomy cannula with the deflated cuff for some 'crucial' days of adaptation to NIMV, and to remove the cannula when this process is completely achieved (Figure 62.4).

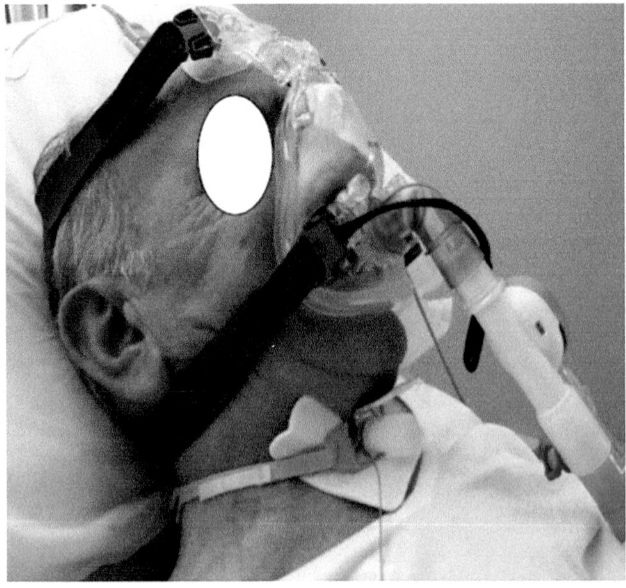

Figure 62.4 During the conversion from IMV to NIMV, the patient is kept with the capped cannula while the process of adaptation to NIMV is carried out.

In summary, the baseline checklist for screening candidates for tracheostomy removal should include the following items:

- Clinical stability
- Mental alertness and integrity, including the capacity to understand the benefits and risks of decannulation
- Consent of both patient and relatives
- Sufficient pulmonary reserve and stability of blood gas values
- Absence of tracheal or glottic stenosis
- Limited volume of airway secretions and proper cough efficiency
- Adequate airway protection and swallowing mechanisms

Cough efficiency can be evaluated by measuring the peak cough flow and maximal expiratory pressure that can be reliably measured by connecting the manometer directly to the cuffed tracheostomy tube.[42] Values as high as 160 L/min[43] and 40 cm H_2O[44] for, respectively, peak cough flow and maximal expiratory pressure, have been indicated as desirable during the process of decannulation. The following step is to cap the tube for gradually longer periods to assess the patency of native airways; if the patient can comfortably breathe around a capped 8 mm ID tube with deflated cuff, it is likely that his or her native airways are intact and they have sufficient pulmonary reserve. Even in this case, however, control of upper airway with fibre-optic endoscopy is highly desirable before decannulation. In presence of all favourable criteria, straight cannula removal can be carried out; if successful decannulation is uncertain, the channel can be kept open by applying caps or buttons to bridge the following days, applying a wait-and-see strategy, even taking into account a process of cannula downsizing.[45] After tube removal, the stoma of a percutaneous dilational tracheostomy (PDT) will usually shrink spontaneously within a short time; only in very rare cases is there circumferential skin growth and lining over the mucosal edge, which prevents stoma closure and requires surgical closure.

Quality of life after percutaneous tracheostomy

Literature about QOL after percutaneous tracheostomy is very scant, and only a few studies are available. Table 62.1 shows a summary of findings related to common tools for measurement of QOL in critically ill patients.

Furthermore, different scales can measure QOL, and no standardised methods are actually proposed. Antonelli et al.[46] evaluated the QOL after tracheostomy using the Short Form 12 Health Survey scores.[46] In this paper, the authors compared the QOL between critical patients with translaryngeal tracheostomy and surgical tracheostomy. The authors found no difference in QOL between the considered groups; however, half of the interviewed patients reported a physical status of moderate to severely compromised and

Table 62.1 Summary of findings related to common tools for measurement of QOL in critically ill patients

Instrument	Purpose	Description/ no. of domains	Physical status	Mental status	Emotional status	Pain
EuroQol-5D (EQ-5D)	State of health	Five domains classified with three levels	Yes	Yes	Yes	Yes
Short Form 36 Health Survey (SF-36)	General health	Eight domains evaluated with 36 items	Yes	Yes	Yes	Yes
Nottingham Health Profile	General health	Six domains evaluated with 38 + 7 items	Yes	Yes	Yes	Yes
Sickness impact profile	State of health	Twelve domains evaluated with 136 items	Yes	Yes	Yes	Yes

worst emotional status. Interestingly, in this paper, patients with closed stomas had a better QOL than patients with open stomas.[46] In the Stroke-Related Early Tracheostomy versus Prolonged Orotracheal Intubation in Neurocritical Care Trial (SETPOINT), the authors evaluated the QOL, as functional status with modified Rankin scale, in neurosurgical and neurological patients with early or late tracheostomy.[47] The modified Rankin scale is a method for assessing the degree of disability or dependence in daily activities in neurological patients. The scale runs from 0 to 6: 0 – no symptoms; 1 – no significant disability; 2 – slight disability; 3 – moderate disability; 4 – moderately severe disability; 5 – severe disability; and 6 – death.[48] In the SETPOINT trial, poor functional outcome, defined as modified Rankin scale of 5–6, was found 6 months after ICU admission.[47] However, this study is about a selected category of patients, the neurological one, in which the QOL and functional status largely depend on neurological damage. Engoren et al.[49] evaluated the functional outcome with SF-36 in a group of patients tracheostomised for respiratory failure. The patients were divided into three groups at discharge: patients with ventilator, patients without ventilator but with tracheostomy tube still present and patients without ventilator and decannulated. The authors found no difference in physical functioning, pain, general health, vitality, emotional status and mental health. However, decannulated patients had better social functioning compared with partially or totally dependent patients.[49]

Evaluation of QOL in tracheostomised patients is very difficult. First, the available questionnaires evaluated the status of patients related to the underlying disease rather than to tracheostomy per se. Actually, there are no scores or questionnaires that evaluate the impact of tracheostomy cannula and/or management on the social, mental and physical status of critically ill patients. Second, the QOL after tracheostomy is poorly investigated probably because follow-up is difficult to be performed in critically ill patients who suffer from high morbidity and mortality. Third, critical care researchers routinely evaluate short-term acute outcome than long-term outcome or chronic sequelae after ICU.

The Italian Society of Anesthesia and Intensive Care actually promotes a study with the aim to assess the QOL after tracheostomy. In this study, the QOL is evaluated with EQ-5D and with the performance status scale for head and neck surgery. This scale is used by eye, nose and throat specialists for tracheostomy after glottis cancer. In our opinion, this scale can be used also for percutaneous tracheostomy. This scale evaluates the normalcy of diet, public eating and the understandability of speech. In the evaluation of the normalcy of diet, patients are asked to declare which food they eat and if there are some difficulties in eating solid or liquid food. The scale for public eating asks which kind of food the patients eat in public and if there is limitation for solid of food, for example. The scale for the understandability of speech is based on the interviewer's ability to understand the patient during conversation. This scale may evaluate the QOL of patients due to tracheostomy limitation and not due to the underlying disease.

TECHNICAL CONSIDERATIONS

Percutaneous dilational tracheostomy

The percutaneous dilatational technique was proposed by Ciaglia et al.[50] in 1985. These authors carried out progressive dilatation with blunt-tipped dilators; since then, several other methods have been proposed for performing percutaneous tracheostomy at the bedside.[51–54] Some of them are characterised by the insertion of the tracheostomy cannula from outside the trachea: the modified original Ciaglia technique ('single-step' Blue Rhino)[51]; the guide wire dilating forceps technique proposed by Griggs et al.[52]; and the PercuTwist as proposed by Frova and Quintel.[53] Another one is characterised by the fact that the tracheostomy cannula is inserted from inside the trachea: the translaryngeal technique proposed by Fantoni and Ripamonti.[54]

The Blue Rhino is characterised by a modification of the original Ciaglia technique simplified with only one single dilator. An initial skin incision and blunt preparation of the pretracheal tissue may be helpful in identifying the tracheal rings, thus avoiding either too high or too low tracheal puncture. After dilatation with the maximal available dilator, a tracheal cannula (ID up to 9 mm) can be inserted while mounted on a corresponding dilator. The main problems related to this technique are difficult ventilation, bleeding and rupture or dislocation of the tracheal rings.

The Griggs technique is characterised by the use of forceps for blunt dilatation of the pretracheal and intercartilaginous tissue after insertion of the guide wire into the trachea and skin incision. Applying this method on patients with a short and or thick neck may be difficult, if not dangerous, particularly while attempting to perform intercartilaginous dilation. The main problems of this technique are that dilation with forceps is not easily calibrated with the cannula diameter, rupture or dislocation of tracheal rings and difficult ventilation. The PercuTwist technique is characterised by controlled rotating dilation performed by an external spiral, which should reduce tracheal wall collapse during the manoeuvre. One problem encountered with this technique is the rupture or dislocation of tracheal rings. All these percutaneous techniques are characterised by the dilation of the tissues, with the forces being applied from the outside to the inside of the tracheal wall.

The translaryngeal technique is different from the previous ones because the cannula is stripped from inside to outside. In contrast with other techniques, the initial puncture of the trachea is carried out with the needle directed cranially and the tracheal cannula inserted with a pull-through technique along the orotracheal route. This modification in the direction of the forces should favour much less injury of the tissues and tracheal wall itself, in both the anterior and posterior walls; reduced bleeding; the possibility to ventilate during the manoeuvre; and possible application of this technique in paediatric patients in which all other techniques are contraindicated. The major problems related to this technique are difficulty in intubating the patients with a rigid fibrescope; need for several intubations and extubations (thus, this technique is contraindicated in patients with difficult intubation and in those in whom the extension of the neck has to be avoided); difficulties in ventilation during the manoeuvre; and unsuitability in an emergency.

While performing percutaneous tracheostomy, independently from the technique, several tools have been suggested to improve the safety of the manoeuvre:

- Bronchoscopy with simple endoscopy or video-assisted endoscopy to facilitate and reduce possible complications[55]
- Previous evaluation by chest radiography, magnetic resonance imaging and ultrasound assessment prior to PDT in patients with altered neck and tracheal anatomy[56]
- Chest X-ray following dilatational percutaneous tracheostomy after procedures noted to be difficult by the physician[57]

In particular clinical situations, the usefulness of ultrasound-guided control and the use of a laryngeal mask have also been reported.[58,59]

Finally, the following must be standardised: correct ventilatory procedure in pressure control, inspired oxygen fraction of 1.0 and positive end-expiratory pressure of 0 cm H_2O, although some authors have demonstrated that the procedure is safe even with the use of high positive end-expiratory pressures in patients with severe respiratory failure.[60]

With the PDT procedure, only a narrow opening in the tracheal wall is generated and the stoma takes a few days (at least 1 week) to become more stable. Therefore, during the first week, dislocation or unintentional removal of the cannula must be avoided, since reinsertion may result in life-threatening misplacement; it is therefore recommended to postpone at least 7–8 days after PDT the first replacement of cannula.

Surgical tracheostomy

Surgical tracheostomy is usually carried out in the operating theatre, despite similar outcomes being achievable in the ICU, provided that proper equipment and adequate staff are available. After a horizontal incision, superficial vessels are ligated and the thyroid isthmus is transected or moved away from the incision. The second or third tracheal ring is identified and cut about 1.5–2 cm below the cricoid membrane; it is in fact important to create the stoma far from the cricoid cartilage to avoid damaging this structure, as it is the only complete cartilaginous ring in the upper airway. Subglottic stenosis is a likely occurrence after cricoid cartilage injury, due to the loss of laryngeal integrity. The stoma is made through the anterior tracheal wall by means of an incision that can be horizontal, vertical or cruciate, although most surgeons seem to prefer the horizontal incision.

Comparison of percutaneous dilatational technique with surgical tracheostomy

Percutaneous tracheostomy can be performed immediately once the decision has been made, whereas surgical tracheostomy requires more organisation and, if it is to be done in the operating theatre, scheduling. The time required for percutaneous tracheostomy is generally shorter than that for the surgical route and implies less stress to the patient and better use of resources. Although a cost comparison between percutaneous and surgical tracheostomies is not easy because of varying reimbursement systems and hospital structures, available studies show that percutaneous tracheostomy is considerably cheaper than the surgical route: it is in fact common sense that if fewer personnel and no operating theatre are required, the overall cost of percutaneous tracheostomy will be lower than that of surgical tracheostomy.[61] The majority of prospective randomised trials reported that the potential advantages of the percutaneous technique relative to surgical tracheostomy include ease of performance, lower incidence of peristomal bleeding and post-operative infection associated with lower costs, although the real clinical impact of these study results is limited by the heterogeneity of the samples and percutaneous techniques employed.[62–65]

FUTURE RESEARCH

In conclusion, tracheostomy can offer several advantages in the management of critically ill patients who need mechanical ventilation and/or control of airways. The right timing of tracheostomy remains controversial, but it appears that early tracheostomy in selected patients, such as in severe trauma and neurological patients, could be effective in reducing ICU stay and associated costs. For other patients, it could be reasonable to wait at least 10 days, but clinicians need to improve their capacity to predict which patients will need prolonged IMV. Percutaneous tracheostomy techniques are becoming the procedure of choice in the majority of cases, because these are safe, easy and quick to do and the complications and costs, compared with those of surgical tracheostomies, seem to be lower. The surgical technique should be considered when contraindications to percutaneous techniques are present, such as anatomical difficulties or previously failed percutaneous techniques. No one percutaneous technique seems superior in comparison with the rest, but the experience of the operator and clinical, individual, anatomical and physiopathological characteristics of the patient should always be considered.

REFERENCES

1. Goligher E, Ferguson ND. Mechanical ventilation: Epidemiological insight into current practices. *Curr Opin Crit Care*. 2009;15:44–51.
2. Smischney NJ, Velagapudi VM, Onigkeit JA et al. Derivation and validation of a search algorithm to retrospectively identify mechanical ventilation initiation in the intensive care unit. *BMC Med Inform Decis Mak*. 2014;14:55–60.
3. Esteban A, Anzueto A, Frutos F et al. Characteristics and outcomes in adult patients receiving mechanical ventilation. *JAMA*. 2002;287:345–55.
4. Demoule A, Chevret S, Carlucci A et al. Changing use of noninvasive ventilation in critically ill patients: Trends over 15 years in francophone countries. *Intensive Care Med*. 2016;42:82–92.
5. Nevins ML, Epstein SK. Weaning from prolonged mechanical ventilation. *Clinics Chest Med*. 2001;22:13–33.
6. Ranes JL, Gordon SM, Chen P et al. Predictors of long-term mortality in patients with ventilator-associated pneumonia. *Am J Med*. 2006;119:897.e13–9.
7. Schönhofer B, Kluge S. Consequences of endotracheal intubation and tracheostomy, In: Stevens RD, Hart N, Herridge MS, eds., *Textbook of Post-ICU Medicine: The Legacy of Critical Care*. Oxford: Oxford University Press; 2014:180–94.
8. Holzapfel L, Chevret S, Madinier G et al. Influence of long-term oro- or nasotracheal intubation on nosocomial maxillary sinusitis and pneumonia: Results of a prospective randomized clinical trial. *Crit Care Med*. 1993;21:1132–8.
9. Nieszkowska A, Combes A, Luyt CE et al. Impact of tracheotomy on sedative administration, sedation level, and comfort of mechanically ventilated intensive care unit patients. *Crit Care Med*. 2005;33:2527–33.
10. Lassen HC. A preliminary report on the 1952 epidemic of poliomyelitis in Copenhagen with special reference to the treatment of respiratory insufficiency. *Lancet*. 1953;1:37–41.
11. Szmuk P, Ezri T, Evron S et al. A brief history of tracheostomy and tracheal intubation from the Bronze Age to the Space Age. *Int Care Med*. 2008;34:222–8.
12. Reibel JF. Tracheotomy/tracheostomy. *Respir Care*. 1999;44:820–3.
13. Cox Ce, Carson SS, Holmes GM et al. Increase in tracheostomy for prolonged mechanical ventilation in North Carolina, 1993–2002. *Crit Care Med*. 2004;32:2219–26.
14. Yu M. Tracheostomy patients on the ward: Multiple benefits from a multidisciplinary team? *Crit Care*. 2010;14:109.
15. Wunsch H, Linde-Zwirble WT, Angus TC et al. The epidemiology of mechanical ventilation use in the United States. *Crit Care Med*. 2010;38:1947–53.
16. Penuelas O, Frutos-Vivar F, Fernandez C et al. Characteristics and outcome of ventilated patients according to time to liberation from mechanical ventilation. *Am J Respir Crit Care Med*. 2011;184:430–7.
17. Flaatten H, Gjerde S, Heimdal JH, Aardal S. The effect of tracheostomy on outcome in intensive care unit patients. *Acta Anesthesiol Scand*. 2006;50:92–8.
18. Vargas M, Sutherasan Y, Antonelli A et al. Tracheostomy procedures in the intensive care unit: An international survey. *Crit Care*. 2015;19:291.
19. Centers for Medicare & Medicaid Services. Acute impatient PPS: List of final MSDRGs, relative weighting factors and geometric and arithmetic mean length of stay. Available at http://cms.gov/medicare/medicare-fee-for-service-payment/acuteinpatientpps/fy-2013-ipps-final-rule-home-page-items/fy-2013-final-rule-tables.html.
20. Shaw JJ, Santry HP. Who gets early tracheostomy? Evidence of unequal treatment at 185 academic medical centers. *Chest*. 2015;148:242–50.
21. Hussey JD, Bishop MJ. Pressures required to move gas through the native airway in the presence of a fenestrated vs a nonfenestrated tracheostomy tube. *Chest*. 1996;110:494–7.
22. Cowan T, Op't Holt TB, Gegenheimer C et al. Effect of inner cannula removal on the work of breathing imposed by tracheotomy tubes: A bench study. *Respir Care*. 2001;46:460–5.

23. Ceriana P, Carlucci A, Navalesi P et al. Physiological responses during a T-piece weaning trial with a deflated tube. *Int Care Med.* 2006;32:1399–403.
24. Nash M. Swallowing problems in the tracheotomized patient. *Otolaryngol Clin North Am.* 1988;21:701–9.
25. Shaker R, Dodds WJ, Dantas RO et al. Coordination of deglutitive glottic closure with oropharyngeal swallowing. *Gastroenterology.* 1990;98:1478–84.
26. Eibling DE, Diez Gross R. Subglottic air pressure: A key component of swallowing efficiency. *Ann Otol Rhinol Laryngol.* 1996;105:253–8.
27. Ceriana P, Carlucci A, Schreiber A et al. Changes of swallowing function after tracheostomy: A videofluoroscopy study. *Minerva Anestesiol.* 2015;81:389–97.
28. Thompson-Henry S, Braddock B. The modified Evan's blue dye procedure fails to detect aspiration in tracheotomized patients: Five case reports. *Dysphagia.* 1995;10:172–4.
29. Logemann JA. *Manual for the Videophluorographic Study of Swallowing*, 2nd ed. San Diego, CA: College-Hill Press;1993.
30. Suiter DM, McCullough GH, Powell PW. Effects of cuff deflation and one-way tracheotomy speaking valve placement on swallow physiology. *Dysphagia.* 2003;18:284–92.
31. Hess D. Facilitating speech in the patient with a tracheostomy. *Respir Care.* 2005;50:519–25.
32. Hoit JD, Banzett RB, Lohmeier HL et al. Clinical ventilator adjustments that improve speech. *Chest.* 2003;124:1512–21.
33. Passy V, Baydur A, Prentice W, Darnell-Neal R. Passy–Muir tracheostomy speaking valve on ventilator-dependent patients. *Laryngoscope.* 1993;103:653–8.
34. De Leyn P, Bedert L, Delcroix M et al. Tracheotomy: Clinical review and guidelines. *Eur J Cardiothorac Surg.* 2007;32:412–21.
35. Terragni PP, Antonelli M, Fumagalli R et al. Early vs late tracheostomy for the prevention of pneumonia in mechanically ventilated adult ICU patients: A randomized controlled trial. *JAMA.* 2010;303:1483–9.
36. Gomes Silva BN, Andriolo RB, Saconato H et al. Early vs late tracheostomy for critically ill patients. *Cochrane Database Syst Rev.* 2012;3:CD007271.
37. Young D, Harrison DA, Cuthbertson TH et al. Effect of early vs late tracheostomy placement on survival in patients receiving mechanical ventilation: The TrachMan randomized trial. *JAMA.* 2013;309:2121–9.
38. Diehl JL, Atrous S, Touchard D et al. Changes in the work of breathing induced by tracheotomy in ventilator-dependent patients. *Am J Respir Crit Care Med.* 1999;159:383–8.
39. Heffner JE. The role of tracheotomy in weaning. *Chest.* 2001;120:477S–81S.
40. Hess DR. Tracheostomy tubes and related appliances. *Respir Care.* 2005;50:497–510.
41. Gregoretti C, Squadrone V, Fogliati C et al. Transtracheal open ventilation in acute respiratory failure secondary to severe chronic obstructive pulmonary disease exacerbation. *Am J Respir Crit Care Med.* 2006;173:877–81.
42. Vitacca M, Paneroni M, Bianchi L et al. Maximal inspiratory and expiratory pressures measurement in tracheotomised patients. *Eur Respir J.* 2006;27:343–9.
43. Bach JR, Saporito LR. Criteria for extubation and tracheotomy tube removal for patients with ventilatory failure. *Chest.* 1996;110:1566–71.
44. Ceriana P, Carlucci A, Navalesi P et al. Weaning from tracheotomy in long-term mechanically ventilated patients: Feasibility of a decisional flowchart and clinical outcome. *Int Care Med.* 2003;29:845–8.
45. Veelo DP, Schultz MJ, Phoa KY et al. Management of tracheostomy: A survey of Dutch intensive care units. *Respir Care.* 2008;53:1709–15.
46. Antonelli M, Michetti V, Di Palma A et al. Percutaneous translaryngeal versus surgical tracheostomy: A randomized trial with 1-yr double blind follow-up. *Crit Care Med.* 2005;33:1015–20.
47. Bosel J, Schiller P, Hook Y et al. Stroke-related early tracheostomy versus prolonged orotracheal intubation in neurocritical care trial (SETPOINT): A randomized pilot trial. *Stroke.* 2013;44:21–8.
48. Rankin J. Cerebral vascular accidents in patients over the age of 60: II. Prognosis. *Scott Med J.* 1957;2:200–15.
49. Engoren M, Engoren CA, Buderer NF. Hospital and long-term outcome after tracheostomy for respiratory failure. *Chest.* 2004;125:220–7.
50. Ciaglia P, Firshing R, Syniec C. Elective percutaneous dilatational tracheostomy: A new simple bedside procedure: Preliminary report. *Chest.* 1985;87:715–9.
51. Byhahn C, Wilke HJ, Halbig S et al. Percutaneous tracheostomy: Ciaglia Blue Rhino versus the basic Ciaglia technique of percutaneous dilatational tracheostomy. *Anesth Analg.* 2000;91:882–6.
52. Griggs WM, Worthley LIG, Gilligan JE et al. A simple percutaneous tracheostomy technique. *Surg Gynec Obstet.* 1990;170:543–5.
53. Frova G, Quintel M. A new simple method for percutaneous tracheostomy: Controlled rotating dilating – A preliminary report. *Int Care Med.* 2002;28:299–303.
54. Fantoni A, Ripamonti D. A non-derivative, non-surgical tracheostomy: The translaryngeal method. *Int Care Med.* 1997;23:386–92.
55. Oberwalser M, Weis H, Nehoda H et al. Videobronchoscopic guidance makes percutaneous dilational tracheostomy safer. *Surg Endosc.* 2004;18:839–42.
56. Muhammad JK, Major E, Patton DW. Evaluating the neck for percutaneous dilatational tracheostomy. *J Craniomaxillofac Surg.* 2000;28:336–42.

57. Datta D, Onyirimba F, McNamee MJ. The utility of chest radiographs following percutaneous dilatational tracheostomy. *Chest.* 2003;123:1603–6.
58. Rustic A, Zupan Z, Antoncic I. Ultrasound-guided percutaneous dilatational tracheostomy with laryngeal mask airway control in a morbidly obese patients. *J Clin Anesth.* 2004;16:121–3.
59. Dosemeci L, Yilmaz M, Gurpinar F et al. The use of the laryngeal mask airway as an alternative to the endotracheal tube during percutaneous dilatational tracheostomy. *Int Care Med.* 2002;28:63–7.
60. Beiderlinden M, Groeben H, Peters J. Safety of percutaneous dilatational tracheostomy in patients ventilated with high positive end expiratory pressure (PEEP). *Int Care Med.* 2003;29:944–8.
61. Kaylie DM, Andersen PE, Wax MK. An analysis of time and staff utilization for open versus percutaneous tracheostomies. *Otolaryngol Head Neck Surg.* 2003;128:109–14.
62. Freeman BD, Isabella K, Cobb JP et al. A prospective, randomized study comparing percutaneous with surgical tracheostomy in critically ill patients. *Crit Care Med.* 2001;29:926–30.
63. Massick DD, Yao S, Powell DM et al. Bedside tracheostomy in the intensive care unit: A prospective randomized trial comparing open surgical tracheostomy with endoscopically guided percutaneous dilatational tracheotomy. *Laryngoscope.* 2001;111:494–500.
64. Antonelli M, Michetti V, Di Palma A et al. Percutaneous translaryngeal versus surgical tracheostomy: A randomized trial with 1-yr double blind follow-up. *Crit Care Med.* 2005;33:1015–20.
65. Silvester W, Goldsmith D, Uchino S et al. Percutaneous versus surgical tracheostomy: A randomized controlled study with long-term follow-up. *Crit Care Med.* 2006;34:2145–52.

63

Swallowing and phonation during ventilation

HÉLÈNE PRIGENT AND NICOLAS TERZI

Over the past decades, non-invasive positive pressure ventilation (NIV) has become the first-line treatment and the standard of care in restrictive chronic respiratory failure.[1–4] With the improvement of the ventilation devices and ventilation modes, and the diversification of ventilation interfaces, NIV has been used increasingly, even in patients with severe respiratory failure.[5,6] While a few decades back, invasive ventilation with a tracheostomy was the only long-term option in ventilator-dependent patients; the development of NIV has offered a valuable alternative to invasive ventilation, allowing efficient ventilatory support even in patients with no respiratory autonomy. Long-term mechanical ventilation has been successfully used, prolonging survival in several neuromuscular or neurological diseases such as Duchenne muscular dystrophy,[7–9] amyotrophic lateral sclerosis,[10,11] spinal cord injury[12] and post-polio syndrome[13] as well as in thoracic disorders such as scoliosis.[14] More recently, the specific study of the impact of NIV has confirmed its efficiency on survival in long-term use in this population.[8,15,16]

While non-invasive ventilation has been used since the 1980s for both acute and chronic respiratory failures, its increasing use in ventilator-dependent patients raises new questions concerning its interaction with functions such as speaking and swallowing. Indeed, the extensive use of NIV is liable to interfere with these basic functions and has received little attention. Yet in ventilator-dependent patients, maintaining a correct speech is essential as it determines quality of communication and, consequently, quality of life.[17,18] Likewise, the impact of NIV on swallowing is also of interest as complications such as inhalation and respiratory infections can jeopardise patient's prognosis. Moreover, malnutrition is frequent in patients with severe respiratory failure[19–21]; the improvement of swallowing may lead to better nutritional status and prognosis.

SPEAKING WITH NIV

Speech and respiratory failure

Speech requires the involvement and the coordination of several muscle groups, including respiratory, postural, oropharyngeal and laryngeal muscles. It requires to produce and to sustain sufficient tracheal pressure during expiration through the vocal cords in order to produce sounds and ultimately speech.

Speech is an example of voluntary control of respiration as important modifications of the respiratory cycle occur during speech production.[22] Most notably, in order to speak, normal subjects modify the structure of their respiratory cycle, decreasing inspiratory time and increasing, sometimes considerably, expiratory time to allow speech production. It also involves a modification of respiratory muscle involvement as the inspiratory volume increases just before phonation while expiration is active with a delayed relaxation of the diaphragm and the external intercostal muscles followed by the activation of expiratory muscles.[22–26] These adaptations prolong expiration and allow maintaining a stable tracheal pressure under the vocal cords to obtain the desired speech output and prosody (the capacity to give various intonations to speech).

Patients with chronic restrictive respiratory failure exhibit modifications of their breathing pattern as they present a decreased spontaneous tidal volume to an increased respiratory frequency associated.[27,28] These modifications can interfere with the quality of speech and prosody by reducing the ability to generate longer expiration and to maintain sufficient subglottic pressure.

Patients with respiratory muscle weakness commonly report alteration of their speech.[17,29,30] Draper et al.[25] observed that spinal cord injury patients were unable to modulate loudness and that these impairments of speech modulation were more pronounced as the level of spinal cord injury was higher with a more severe dysfunction of the respiratory muscle. Likewise, neuromuscular patients with severe chronic respiratory failure describe an alteration of speech with decreased intensity and pitch variation, which alters the quality of their communication.[30,31]

Speech and mechanical ventilation

While in invasive ventilation with leak ventilation on tracheostomy, modifications of ventilation parameters have been used to support and improve speech in those patients, mainly by using positive expiratory pressure, which contributes to increase expiratory flow towards the upper airways and improves speech quality,[32–37] the same is not true for NIV.

In this situation, ventilation can contribute to significantly alter the quality of speech. The choice of the ventilation interface used in that situation is crucial in obtaining a good speech quality. Indeed, facemasks covering the mouth during ventilation prevent patients from speaking and are not appropriate to maintain a correct level of communication especially during daytime. Correct speech will require an interface which liberates the mouth, using either a nasal interface (nasal masks or pillows) or a mouthpiece for mouthpiece ventilation (MPV). However, nasal interfaces may interfere with the quality of speech during NIV. Indeed, during speech, the variations of flow and pressures in the upper airways are liable to interact with the ventilator and to induce modifications of frequency rate and autotriggering (Figure 63.1). This reduces the ability of the patients to control their respiratory cycle in order to promote correct speech and interferes with prosody.[17,31,38] Moreover, when patients are ventilated with a pressure-controlled mode, the increasing leaks during speech may result in a wide variation of the volume delivered by the ventilator impairing the quality of speech as air leaks from the nose to the buccal cavity interfering with speech production.

In this situation, the most appropriate interface is the use of a mouthpiece. With MPV, patients are able to discontinue ventilation when they wish to speak and can resume ventilator support whenever they want by taking sips with their interface. This requires, however, that the interface is appropriately fixated for the patient to be able to release it and to take it up again when he or she wishes to do so. It also requires sufficient mouth closure on the mouthpiece to receive adequate air volume, and mouth leaks may be a limit to this technique.[39,40] MPV offers several additional advantages for patients. It allows them to use NIV right before speaking, benefiting from an increased inspiratory volume provided by the ventilator liable to improve expiratory flow and duration and therefore speech production. Patients with severe respiratory failure and decreased spontaneous tidal volume can therefore achieve a situation close to that observed in normal subjects, i.e. increasing prephonatory inspiratory volume.

Moreover, if patients are ventilated in a volume-controlled mode, they can do breath stacking to improve speech quality. Breath stacking is usually used as a cough assistance technique to enhance airway clearance; it consists of the inhalation by the patient of several consecutive tidal

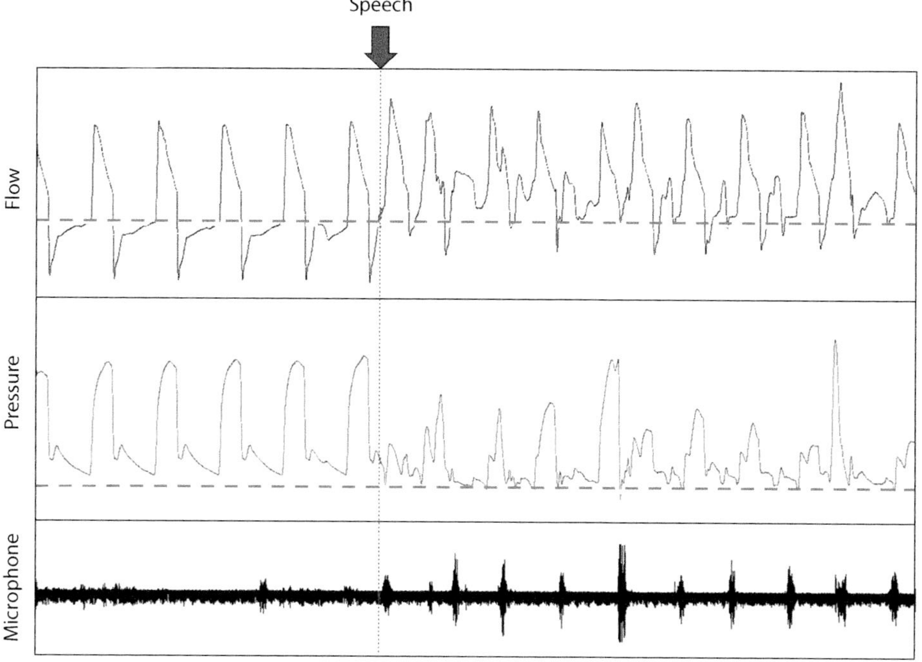

Figure 63.1 Speaking with NIV. The ventilation with a nasal mask of a neuromuscular patient under NIV is disrupted as soon as the patient starts to speak (reading a list of words). Respiratory rate increases with unintentional triggering, and flow delivery is impaired. The patient is unable to modify his or her respiratory cycle to adapt to speech production.

volumes delivered by the ventilator without exhaling in order to increase inspiratory volume. If used for speech, the additional tidal volumes increase the prephonatory inspiratory volume and allow patients to improve speech duration, loudness and prosody, once again putting them in a situation closer to that of a normal subject.

Unsurprisingly, when surveyed, patients mention speech quality as one of the main reasons for preferring MPV during daytime ventilation.[41]

SWALLOWING WITH NIV

Swallowing and respiratory failure

Swallowing is a fundamental function which ensures two main purposes: not only the propulsion of the food bolus from the oropharynx to the stomach via the pharynx and the oesophagus but also the protection of the respiratory tract with the swallowing reflex.[42,43] Indeed, the latter evacuates the oropharynx while closing the nasopharynx and the larynx, in order to prevent any aspiration of saliva or food remnants. It is a complex action not only involving the precise and sequenced activation of numerous muscles but also requiring a precise coordination with breathing in order to protect from the aspiration of the ingested boluses and to ensure adequate gas exchanges.[43,44]

Swallowing involves modifications of the respiratory cycle and interacts with the control of respiration. An interruption of the respiratory cycle occurs during the pharyngeal phase of swallowing in order to prevent aspiration in the respiratory tract.[42] In healthy adults, the occurrence of this apnoea is predominantly followed by an expiration, which constitutes an important protective mechanism as expiratory flow contributes to prevent the aspiration of any remnants of the bolus (Figure 63.2). In addition, when swallowing interrupts the expiratory phase, the elastic recoil of the lungs and the chest wall can generate a subglottic positive pressure which is considered as a key component of swallowing efficiency.[45–48]

While swallowing and its interaction have been extensively studied in normal subjects,[49–53] the impact of respiratory failure on these interactions has received much less attention. However, experimental hypercapnia is associated with perturbations of the breathing swallowing synchronisation and an increasing occurrence of aspiration.[54] Chronic obstructive pulmonary disease (COPD) patients, in stable state, present the disrupted coordination of the respiratory cycle with deglutition and increased swallowing occurrence during inspiration, which worsens during acute respiratory failure.[53,55–57] In 29 neuromuscular patients, Terzi et al.[58] observed the fragmentation of deglutition (interruption of the swallowing of a single bolus by respiratory cycles) and piecemeal deglutition; the swallowing disorders were directly correlated with inspiratory muscle strength, suggesting a close relationship between respiratory failure and swallowing disorders. Therefore, one might ponder on the potential effect of ventilatory support on the swallowing quality of patients with respiratory failure.

Ventilation impact on swallowing

Eating and drinking during NIV is usually not recommended by manufacturers as it may expose patients to inhalation if the air delivered by the ventilator pushes the

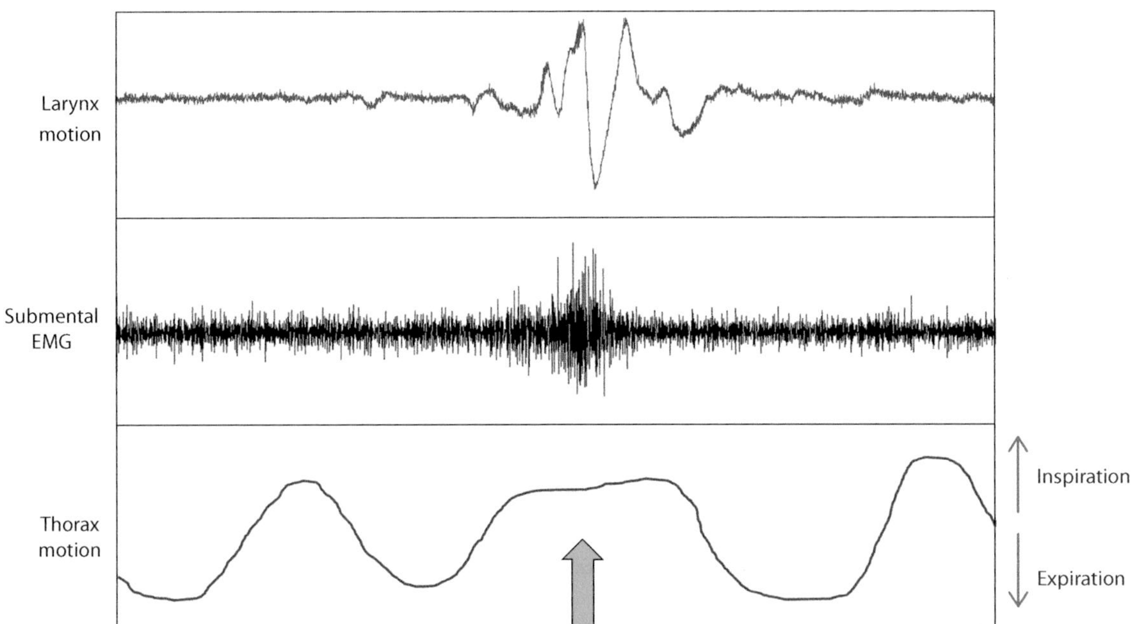

Figure 63.2 Deglutition apnoea. Swallowing is detected by the submental EMG and the laryngeal motion detector. Once swallowing is initiated, the subject ventilation withholds ventilation (*arrow*) at the end of the inspiratory cycle, as evidenced by the thoracic movements. When swallowing is completed, respiration is resumed with expiration.

bolus in the airways. However, some ventilator-dependent patients, regardless of those recommendations, report eating while using ventilation, which relieves the dyspnoea they experience during meals.[31,59] To support this clinical observation, Terzi et al.[58,60] observed that in tracheostomised neuromuscular patients, all swallowing parameters improved when patients swallowed while they were ventilated with a significant decrease of perceived dyspnoea during swallowing.

In keeping with these observations, NIV use in COPD patients, during acute respiratory failure, was associated with an improvement of breathing and swallowing synchronisation and of all swallowing parameters (swallowing duration, fragmentation, number of swallows per bolus and percentage of swallows followed by an expiration).[57] However, with regular ventilation devices, the negative pressure generated in the upper airways by swallowing could induce autotriggering, which is liable to jeopardise patients if the bolus swallowing is not complete. In order to ensure patients' security and reduce this type of side effects, Terzi et al.[57] used a modified home ventilation device which allowed patients to manually withhold ventilation while swallowing to prevent any risk of aspiration. Using the same device, Garguilo et al.[61] also observed significant improvement of swallowing and breathing interactions in neuromuscular patients with severe chronic respiratory failure requiring ventilation for more than 14 hours/day. Most notably, the number of swallows followed by expiration significantly increased regardless of the size and the texture of bolus. Therefore, although there is evidence that NIV use is liable to improve swallowing in severe patients, its extensive use is prevented by the lack of available devices providing the control of ventilation necessary to avoid potential deleterious side effects of unintentional triggering.

Again, the more adapted interface currently available seems to be MPV. Indeed, patients may use MPV to take a sip if they wish to rest during mealtime. However, it does not provide the same respiratory support as continuous ventilation, and the time required to properly chew and swallow solid food may interfere with the ventilatory requirements as patients cannot use MPV until swallowing is completed. The use of larger tidal volumes has been proposed for MPV.[16,39,40] If used before swallows, this may promote more efficient deglutition as swallowing at higher lung volumes is faster and more efficient[46,58]; moreover, the increased inspiratory volume may contribute to raise subglottic pressure, which protects the lower airways against aspiration after the reopening of the larynx at the end of the swallowing apnoea.[45,47]

Although formal evaluations of the impact of MPV on breathing–swallowing synchronisation are lacking, patients report the improvement of eating comfort with the use of MPV.[31,41] Further studies would be helpful to confirm these clinical observations.

CONCLUSION: SUMMARY

In an era of increasing use of NIV, the improvement of NIV efficiency has allowed its use in severe ventilator-dependent patients. Understanding the interactions of NIV with function such as speech and swallowing is therefore crucial as it pertains to not only the quality of care but also the quality of life of these patients.

As of now, the best speech quality is obtained with MPV, which greatly contributes to make it a preferred interface for daytime ventilation.

Breathing and swallowing interactions can be significantly improved by NIV support, but its extensive use would require an evolution of home ventilator devices in order to avoid aspiration risk in case of unintentional triggering. MPV may help relieve the dyspnoea perceived by patients during swallowing.

REFERENCES

1. Clinical indications for noninvasive positive pressure ventilation in chronic respiratory failure due to restrictive lung disease, COPD, and nocturnal hypoventilation – A consensus conference report. *Chest.* 1999;116:521–34.
2. Hull J, Aniapravan R, Chan E et al. British Thoracic Society guideline for respiratory management of children with neuromuscular weakness. *Thorax.* 2012;67:i1–40.
3. Make BJ, Hill NS, Goldberg AI et al. Mechanical ventilation beyond the intensive care unit: Report of a consensus conference of the American College of Chest Physicians. *Chest.* 1998;113:289S–344S.
4. Windisch W, Walterspacher S, Siemon K et al. Guidelines for non-invasive and invasive mechanical ventilation for treatment of chronic respiratory failure. *Pneumologie.* 2010;64:640–52.
5. Janssens JP, Derivaz S, Breitenstein E et al. Changing patterns in long-term noninvasive ventilation: A 7-year prospective study in the Geneva Lake area. *Chest.* 2003;123:67–79.
6. Leger P, Bedicam JM, Cornette A et al. Nasal intermittent positive pressure ventilation: Long-term follow-up in patients with severe chronic respiratory insufficiency. *Chest.* 1994;105:100–5.
7. Eagle M, Baudouin SV, Chandler C et al. Survival in Duchenne muscular dystrophy: Improvements in life expectancy since 1967 and the impact of home nocturnal ventilation. *Neuromusc Disord.* 2002;12:926–9.
8. Ishikawa Y, Miura T, Ishikawa Y et al. Duchenne muscular dystrophy: Survival by cardio-respiratory interventions *Neuromusc Disord.* 2011;21:47–51.
9. Kieny P, Chollet S, Delalande P et al. Evolution of life expectancy of patients with Duchenne muscular dystrophy at AFM Yolaine de Kepper centre between 1981 and 2011. *Ann Phys Rehab Med.* 2013;56:443–54.

10. Aboussouan LS, Khan SU, Meeker DP et al. Effect of noninvasive positive-pressure ventilation on survival in amyotrophic lateral sclerosis. *Ann Intern Med.* 1997 15;127:450–3.
11. Bourke SC, Tomlinson M, Williams TL et al. Effects of non-invasive ventilation on survival and quality of life in patients with amyotrophic lateral sclerosis: A randomised controlled trial. *Lancet Neurol.* 2006;5:140–7.
12. DeVivo MJ, Ivie CS, 3rd. Life expectancy of ventilator-dependent persons with spinal cord injuries. *Chest.* 1995;108:226–32.
13. Bach JR. Management of post-polio respiratory sequelae. *Ann New York Acad Sci.* 1995 25;753:96–102.
14. Gustafson T, Franklin KA, Midgren B et al. Survival of patients with kyphoscoliosis receiving mechanical ventilation or oxygen at home. *Chest.* 2006;130:1828–33.
15. Soudon P, Steens M, Toussaint M. A comparison of invasive versus noninvasive full-time mechanical ventilation in Duchenne muscular dystrophy. *Chron Respir Dis.* 2008;5:87–93.
16. Toussaint M, Steens M, Wasteels G, Soudon P. Diurnal ventilation via mouthpiece: Survival in end-stage Duchenne patients. *Eur Respir J.* 2006; 28:549–55.
17. Laakso K, Markström A, Hartelius L. Communication and quality of life in individuals receiving home mechanical ventilation. *Int J Ther Rehab.* 2009; 16:648–55.
18. Leder SB. Importance of verbal communication for the ventilator-dependent patient. *Chest.* 1990;98:792–3.
19. Finder JD, Birnkrant D, Carl J et al. Respiratory care of the patient with Duchenne muscular dystrophy: ATS consensus statement. *Am J Respir Crit Care Med.* 2004 15;170:456–65.
20. Willig TN, Bach JR, Venance V, Navarro J. Nutritional rehabilitation in neuromuscular disorders. *Semin Neurol.* 1995;15:18–23.
21. Vermeeren MA, Schols AM, Wouters EF. Effects of an acute exacerbation on nutritional and metabolic profile of patients with COPD. *Eur Respir J.* 1997;10:2264–9.
22. Hoit JD, Lohmeier HL. Influence of continuous speaking on ventilation. *J Speech Lang Hear Res.* 2000;43:1240–51.
23. Bunn JC, Mead J. Control of ventilation during speech. *J Appl Physiol.* 1971;31:870–2.
24. Draper MH, Ladefoged P, Whitteridge D. Respiratory muscles in speech. J *Speech Hear Res.* 1959;2:16–27.
25. Draper MH, Ladefoged P, Whitteridge D. Expiratory pressures and air flow during speech. *Br Med J.* 1960 18;1:1837–43.
26. Hoshiko MS. Sequence of action of breathing muscles during speech. *J Speech Hear Res.* 1960;3:291–7.
27. De Troyer A, Borenstein S, Cordier R. Analysis of lung volume restriction in patients with respiratory muscle weakness. *Thorax.* 1980;35:603–10.
28. Vitacca M, Clini E, Facchetti D et al. Breathing pattern and respiratory mechanics in patients with amyotrophic lateral sclerosis. *Eur Respir J.* 1997;10:1614–21.
29. Hoit JD, Banzett RB, Brown R, Loring SH. Speech breathing in individuals with cervical spinal cord injury. *J Speech Hear Res.* 1990;33:798–807.
30. Laakso K, Markstrom A, Idvall M et al. Communication experience of individuals treated with home mechanical ventilation. *Int J Lang Commun Disord/Royal College Speech Lang Ther.* 2011;46:686–99.
31. Britton D, Benditt JO, Hoit JD. Beyond tracheostomy: Noninvasive ventilation and potential positive implications for speaking and swallowing. *Semin Speech Lang.* 2016;37:173–84.
32. Garguilo M, Leroux K, Lejaille M et al. Patient-controlled positive end-expiratory pressure with neuromuscular disease: Effect on speech in patients with tracheostomy and mechanical ventilation support. *Chest.* 2013;143:1243–51.
33. Hoit JD, Banzett RB. Simple adjustments can improve ventilator-supported speech. *Am J Speech-Lang Pathol.* 1997;6:87–96.
34. Hoit JD, Banzett RB, Lohmeier HL et al. Clinical ventilator adjustments that improve speech. *Chest.* 2003;124:1512–21.
35. Prigent H, Garguilo M, Pascal S et al. Speech effects of a speaking valve versus external PEEP in tracheostomized ventilator-dependent neuromuscular patients. *Intensive Care Med.* 2010;36:1681–7.
36. Prigent H, Samuel C, Louis B et al. Comparative effects of two ventilatory modes on speech in tracheostomized patients with neuromuscular disease. *Am J Respir Crit Care Med.* 2003 15;167:114–9.
37. Hoit JD, Shea SA, Banzett RB. Speech production during mechanical ventilation in tracheostomized individuals. *J Speech Hear Res.* 1994;37:53–63.
38. Laakso K, Markstrom A, Havstam C et al. Communicating with individuals receiving home mechanical ventilation: The experiences of key communication partners. *Disabil Rehab.* 2014;36:875–83.
39. Benditt JO, Boitano LJ. Pulmonary issues in patients with chronic neuromuscular disease. *Am J Respir Crit Care Med.* 2013;187:1046–55.
40. Hess DR. The growing role of noninvasive ventilation in patients requiring prolonged mechanical ventilation. *Respir Care.* 2012;57:900–18; discussion 18–20.
41. Khirani S, Ramirez A, Delord V et al. Evaluation of ventilators for mouthpiece ventilation in neuromuscular disease. *Respir Care.* 2014;59:1329–37.

42. Ertekin C, Aydogdu I. Neurophysiology of swallowing. *Clin Neurophysiol.* 2003;114:2226–44.
43. Miller AJ. Deglutition. *Physiol Rev.* 1982;62:129–84.
44. Smith J, Wolkove N, Colacone A, Kreisman H. Coordination of eating, drinking and breathing in adults. *Chest.* 1989;96:578–82.
45. Eibling DE, Gross RD. Subglottic air pressure: A key component of swallowing efficiency. *Ann Otol Rhinol Laryngol.* 1996;105:253–8.
46. Gross RD, Atwood CW, Jr., Grayhack JP, Shaiman S. Lung volume effects on pharyngeal swallowing physiology. *J Appl Physiol.* 2003;95:2211–7.
47. Gross RD, Carrau RL, Slivka WA et al. Deglutitive subglottic air pressure and respiratory system recoil. *Dysphagia.* 2012;27:452–9.
48. Gross RD, Carrau RL, Slivka WA et al. Direct measurement of subglottic air pressure while swallowing. *Dysphagia.* 2006;116:753–61.
49. Hardemark Cedborg AI, Sundman E et al. Co-ordination of spontaneous swallowing with respiratory airflow and diaphragmatic and abdominal muscle activity in healthy adult humans. *Exp Physiol.* 2009;94:459–68.
50. Martin-Harris B, Brodsky MB, Michel Y et al. Breathing and swallowing dynamics across the adult lifespan. *Arch Otolaryngol Head Neck Surg.* 2005;131:762–70.
51. Nishino T, Hiraga K. Coordination of swallowing and respiration in unconscious subjects. *J Appl Physiol.* 1991;70:988–93.
52. Paydarfar D, Gilbert RJ, Poppel CS, Nassab PF. Respiratory phase resetting and airflow changes induced by swallowing in humans. *J Physiol.* 1995 15;483:273–88.
53. Shaker R, Li Q, Ren J, Townsend WF et al. Coordination of deglutition and phases of respiration: Effect of aging, tachypnea, bolus volume, and chronic obstructive pulmonary disease. *Am J Physiol.* 1992;263:G750–5.
54. Nishino T, Hasegawa R, Ide T, Isono S. Hypercapnia enhances the development of coughing during continuous infusion of water into the pharynx. *Am J Respir Crit Care Med.* 1998;157:815–21.
55. Gross RD, Atwood CW, Jr., Ross SB et al. The coordination of breathing and swallowing in chronic obstructive pulmonary disease. *Am J Respir Crit Care Med.* 2009 1;179:559–65.
56. Mokhlesi B, Logemann JA, Rademaker AW et al. Oropharyngeal deglutition in stable COPD. *Chest.* 2002;121:361–9.
57. Terzi N, Normand H, Dumanowski E et al. Noninvasive ventilation and breathing-swallowing interplay in chronic obstructive pulmonary disease. *Crit Care Med.* 2014;42:565–73.
58. Terzi N, Orlikowski D, Aegerter P et al. Breathing-swallowing interaction in neuromuscular patients: A physiological evaluation. *Am J Respir Crit Care Med.* 2007 1;175:269–76.
59. Toussaint M, Davidson Z, Bouvoie V et al. Dysphagia in Duchenne muscular dystrophy: Practical recommendations to guide management. *Disabil Respir.* 2016;38:2052–62.
60. Terzi N, Prigent H, Lejaille M et al. Impact of tracheostomy on swallowing performance in Duchenne muscular dystrophy. *Neuromuscul Disord.* 2011;20:493–8.
61. Garguilo M, Lejaille M, Vaugier I et al. Noninvasive mechanical ventilation improves breathing-swallowing interaction of ventilator dependent neuromuscular patients: A prospective crossover study. *PloS One.* 2016;11:e0148673.

PART 14

Prolonged weaning

64	End-of-life care and non-invasive ventilation *Christina Faull*	571
65	Pathophysiology of weaning failure *Theodoros I. Vassilakopoulos*	582
66	Non-invasive ventilation for weaning and extubation failure *Scott K. Epstein*	591
67	Weaning strategies and protocols *Michele Vitacca and Luca Barbano*	607
68	Specialised weaning units *Aditi Satti, James Brown, Gerard J. Criner and Bernd Schönhofer*	615
69	Psychological problems during weaning *Amal Jubran*	623

64

End-of-life care and non-invasive ventilation

CHRISTINA FAULL

INTRODUCTION

Non-invasive ventilation (NIV) is a medical treatment that is used in the care of several groups of patients for the purposes of improving the symptoms of respiratory failure and prolonging survival. Most patients who use NIV have a progressive disease. Some require NIV for support during a crisis from which they may or may not recover; others use NIV on an intermittent basis dictated by symptoms, at least initially; and some are or have become completely dependent on the ventilator to avoid overwhelming breathlessness and rapid oxygen desaturation. Although all patients using NIV have respiratory failure, they are diverse in other aspects of their illness. A patient with advanced heart failure who has acutely decompensated has needs different from those of a patient with motor neurone disease (MND) who has lost all independence and uses NIV for 16 hours or more a day. A young man who has lived with his muscular dystrophy for 30 years has needs, expectations and approaches to decision-making different from those of a frail elderly person with multiple comorbidities including chronic obstructive pulmonary disease (COPD). Thus, end-of-life care considerations must always be individualised.

NIV undoubtedly offers many patients with respiratory failure significant benefits. Without this medical intervention, life may end and mechanically assisting ventilation can often provide effective management of the symptoms of breathlessness, fatigue, anxiety and other effects of hypoventilation and hypercapnia. The use of NIV, however, does have significant burdens for the patient and for their family (see Table 64.1). Prolongation of life can be a double-edged sword as it may not always be associated with a satisfactory quality of life and may create complex and emotional future decisions about the withdrawal of treatment.

The quality of life for patients with advanced and progressive diseases, who are nearing the end of their lives, is first and foremost about weighing the benefits and burdens of treatments. The best outcomes for patients are achieved by clinicians sharing information about prognosis, discussing choices and helping patients to formulate their goals for life and for care and their preferences for treatments and place of care in the last months, weeks and days of their life.

NIV is an intervention that requires close monitoring and consideration of the patient's goals of care. The patient's underlying disease will progress despite NIV, and NIV has the potential to prolong a life with unacceptable quality. Evidence, in MND at least, suggests that too few patients know about their potential choices or are asked about their views of continuing assisted ventilation.[1] There is a clear need for more information sharing and improvement in facilitated decision-making. This information and discussion should be introduced when starting NIV and throughout the disease progression, so that decisions can be made with full involvement of the patient and those close to them.

END OF LIFE: DEFINITIONS, DUTIES AND AMBITIONS

Appropriate care for patients at the end of life is being increasingly focused on in many countries.[2] In the late 1960s, the hospice movement[3] shone a light on the experiences of patients who were dying and their families. Over the subsequent years, this has led to understanding of how dying patients are often ignored or overtreated by health services; how symptoms, especially pain, can be effectively managed[4]; and what may from the patient's perspective constitute a 'good' death.[5]

Table 64.1 Benefits and burdens of NIV as a palliative intervention

Benefits	Burdens
Buys time to treat potentially reversible cause of respiratory failure May postpone death to allow a desired goal to be achieved May improve dyspnoea May allow other treatments for dyspnoea time to work	Medicalises the dying process, making speaking, kissing, smiling, drinking and communication problematic May be uncomfortable and add to suffering May require a decision to withdraw treatment seeming like a decision to end life May make it difficult for people to die anywhere but in clinical institutions May provide false hope that death can be avoided May create discord in the family about conflicting direction of care and regret after death May increase anxiety because of alarms May shift the focus of the patient and family from preparing for dying and saying goodbye Patients may feel obliged to try

In the United Kingdom, the first national end-of-life care strategy was published in 2008.[6] End-of-life care is the care needed by everyone as they approach the end of their lives; Box 64.1 shows the British Medical Association definition for this.[7]

End-of-life care is often regarded as a focus on the last 6–12 months of life. Although this terminology can be ambiguous to both clinicians and patients and their families (*end of life* may commonly be used to communicate that someone is imminently dying), it is important that end-of-life care is seen as a longer period time or phase of illness, requiring a change in focus from primarily curative to one which balances burdens and benefits of treatments and interventions and facilitates shared decision-making. In the United Kingdom, the General Medical Council has recommended that death should be an explicit discussion point when patients are thought likely to die within 12 months or have an existing condition that puts them at risk of dying from a sudden acute crisis in their condition.[8] All patients who have respiratory failure and are offered NIV meet these criteria.

BOX 64.1: British Medical Association definition of 'end-of-life care'

The total care of a person with an advanced incurable illness and does not just equate with dying. The end-of-life care phase may last for days, weeks, months or even longer. It is defined as care that helps those with advanced, progressive, incurable illness to live as well as possible until they die. It includes the prevention and relief of suffering through the assessment and treatment of pain and other problems, whether physical, psychosocial or spiritual.

Source: BMA (British Medical Association), End-of-life care and physician assisted dying – Volume 1: Setting the scene, BMA, London, 2016.

The 2016 'Ambitions for end-of-life care'[9] seeks to ensure a personal experience of life that is as good as possible:

> I can make the last stage of my life as good as possible because everyone works together confidently, honestly and consistently to help me and the people who are important to me, including my carer(s).[10]

The end-of-life care strategy in England and Wales defined a pathway for optimising the quality of care in the last months of life (Figure 64.1),[6] and the Gold Standards Framework (GSF) provides a operational framework for end-of-life care in primary care.[11] All patients who use NIV should be on the practice GSF register and discussed at GSF/palliative care multidisciplinary practice meetings.

There are themes common to people's views about a good death and concerns and fears about dying. The factors that are seen generally to be important in end-of-life care are the following[12,13]:

- Pain and symptom relief
- Not being a burden
- Being with family and friends
- Being listened to and receiving respect
- Privacy and dignity
- Access to healthcare professionals and support

Lacking the capacity to make their end-of-life wishes known or end-of-life wishes not being met is the aspect of dying which most concerned people in a UK survey.[14]

There have been no studies specifically about patients who use NIV and their perspectives on what constitutes a good death. Studies in COPD identify the great fear of severe breathlessness or 'suffocating'.[15]

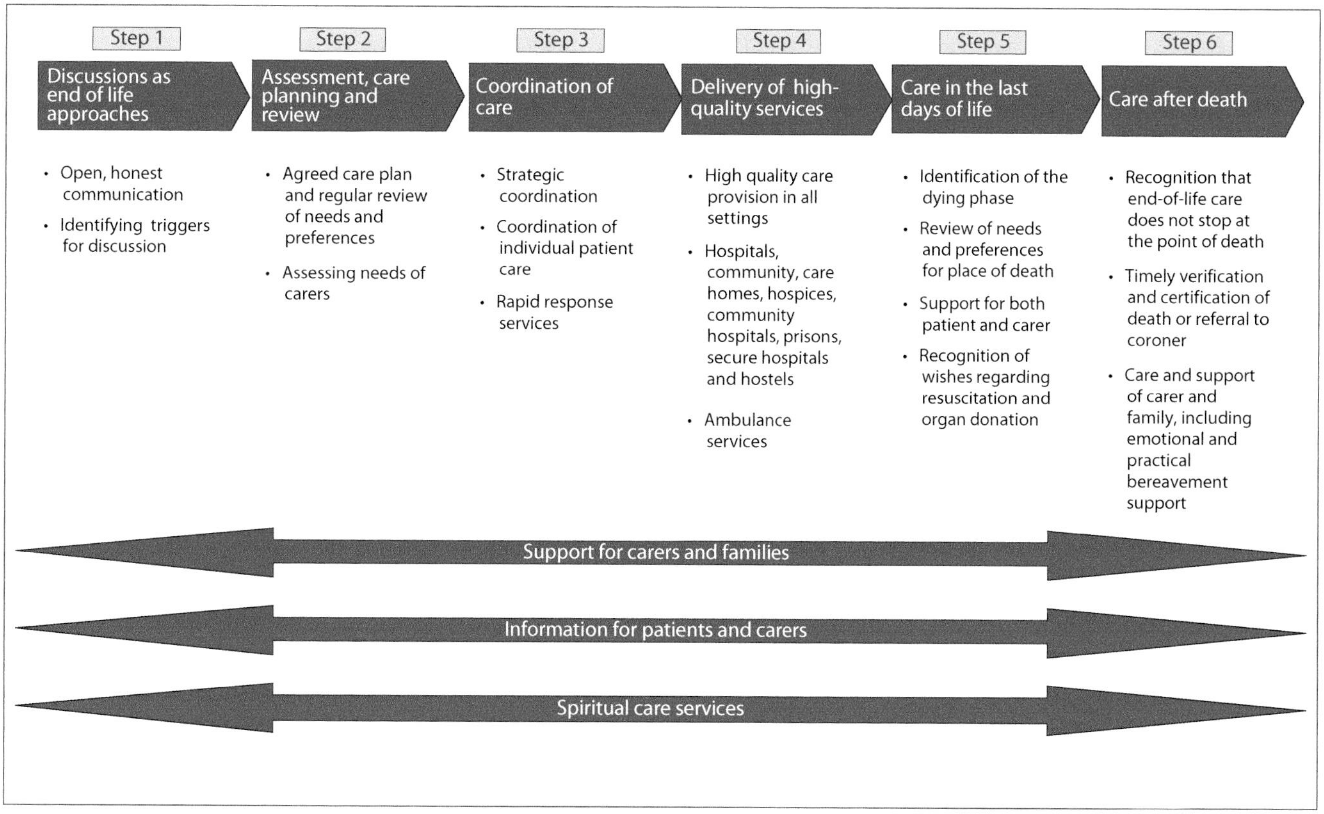

Step 1	Step 2	Step 3	Step 4	Step 5	Step 6
Discussions as end of life approaches	Assessment, care planning and review	Coordination of care	Delivery of high-quality services	Care in the last days of life	Care after death
• Open, honest communication • Identifying triggers for discussion	• Agreed care plan and regular review of needs and preferences • Assessing needs of carers	• Strategic coordination • Coordination of individual patient care • Rapid response services	• High quality care provision in all settings • Hospitals, community, care homes, hospices, community hospitals, prisons, secure hospitals and hostels • Ambulance services	• Identification of the dying phase • Review of needs and preferences for place of death • Support for both patient and carer • Recognition of wishes regarding resuscitation and organ donation	• Recognition that end-of-life care does not stop at the point of death • Timely verification and certification of death or referral to coroner • Care and support of carer and family, including emotional and practical bereavement support

Support for carers and families

Information for patients and carers

Spiritual care services

Figure 64.1 End-of-life care pathway. (Reproduced from Department of Health, *End of life Care strategy*, Department of Health, London, 2008.)

The last part of end-of-life care is care for the patient who is in the last days of life and for their family. Guidelines from the UK National Institute for Health and Care Excellence (NICE) use the terminology *care of the dying* and describe best practice in holistic care and symptom management.[16]

The lack of recognition of the fact that patients are nearing the ends of their lives and an open discussion of this with patients and their families are the major barriers to achieving best outcomes, including enabling people to die where they would most want to.[17–19] Just under half of patients with advanced non-malignant conditions report a preference for a home death.[20] This is notably lower than among cancer patients. The reasons for this difference are not fully understood, and it is undoubtedly multifactorial. One aspect will certainly be that for any episode of acute deterioration for a patient with advanced illness, there is substantial uncertainty about the outcome of treatment. Some such patients will recover, but others will die. Prognostication for patients is very inexact; thus, patients, families and clinicians must work within a context of considerable uncertainty.

Studies in the United States have found that patients were sceptical of the ability of expanded care in their home to treat acute illness, since they perceived home care as low intensity and low frequency of care. They associated hospital with the greatest chance of survival. If the sites proved equal in terms of survival, then they preferred home because of the freedom from constraints and the associated comfort of home. Those who did prefer hospital largely found home a lonely and frightening place to be sick.[21] Views were shaped by social support, self-reliance, religion and past illness experience. Preferences were also shaped by concerns about being a burden and the family's ability to provide care.[22]

TRANSITIONS TO AN END-OF-LIFE CARE APPROACH

It is not straightforward to identify prospectively when a patient is in the last 6–12 months of their life, especially for those patients with non-cancer long-term progressive conditions. In COPD for instance, studies have shown that the 1-year mortality after an exacerbation may be as high as 43%,[23] but even in severe disease, there is a high degree of uncertainty, so that it is difficult to predict which exacerbation may prove fatal. The 'chaos' illness narrative of living with COPD[24] and probably also for patients with progressive neurological conditions, such as muscular dystrophy, which have become 'a way of life' makes a distinct transition point to palliative care elusive. However, many if not most patients with advanced illness do want end-of-life issues to be discussed with them,[25,26] but the prognostic uncertainty often means that clinicians feel unable to take this forward.

Much thought has been given to how indicators may help identify people at risk of deterioration and dying; Box 64.2 outlines the clinical indicators for helping identify such

BOX 64.2: Clinical indicators for identifying patients who are at risk of deterioration and dying

GENERAL INDICATORS

- Unplanned hospital admissions
- Deteriorating performance status
- Weight loss or BMI < 20
- Dependent on others for care

SPECIFIC CLINICAL INDICATORS

Respiratory disease

- Severe chronic lung disease
- Breathless at rest or on minimal exertion
- Meets criteria for long-term oxygen therapy
- Has needed ventilation for respiratory failure

Heart disease

- New York Heart Association III/IV heart failure or untreatable coronary artery disease
- Breathlessness or chest pain at rest or on minimal exertion

Neurological disease

- Progressive deterioration in physical and/or cognitive function despite optimal therapy
- Increasing difficulty in communicating
- Progressive swallowing difficulties
- Recurrent aspiration

Source: Based on the Supportive and Palliative Care Indicators Tool; Highet G et al., *BMJ Support Palliat Care*, 4, 285–90, 2014.

people.[27] The initiation of NIV should always trigger consideration of a transition in the approach to care if this has not already been thought about.

Having identified people that may be in the last months of life, a key challenge is to communicate this to them and to discuss choices about the future and negotiate a change in the focus of care from purely curative to one where benefits and burdens are weighed and the patient's values and goals are elucidated and drive the plan of care.

This transition may be countercultural and difficult for clinicians, especially those in hospital settings. Gott et al.[28] found that structured transitions to a palliative care approach early in the patient's disease trajectory rarely happened in the hospital setting. Participants cited that a focus on acute (curative intent) medicine was one of the reasons for this, and discussion about prognosis with patients and their families was not routine. A phased transition between active and palliative care was rarely evident in the hospital setting. Instead, some participants identified there to be an 'either/or mentality', and a transition to palliative care mostly happened close to death.

The decision to make the transition to palliative care earlier in a disease trajectory was seen as 'challenging' and described as 'taking courage'. Primary care participants confirmed that there were barriers to the communication of information from secondary to primary care, with hospital clinicians failing to tell patients they now needed palliative care, giving them a false hope of cure. Disagreement exists over whether hospital doctors or primary care doctors (general practitioners) are best placed to communicate that a change in focus is now appropriate, and evidence suggests that most patients with long-term conditions are not having such discussions.[29,30]

Communication skills are a vital component of these transitional conversations and an area in which clinicians commonly lack confidence.[31,32] Specific concerns for professionals are about how and when to initiate such discussions and how to ascertain a patient's preferences. The patient's and relatives' reticence and ambivalence with regard to initiating discussions exacerbate the challenges. There is also evidence that some patients strongly prefer not to discuss such matters.[33] Parry et al.[34] found from a systematic review that the use of hypothetical questions about future scenarios is an effective way to open discussions and encourage talk about deterioration and preferences. They also found that since many clinicians find it uncomfortable to be alongside patients who become upset, a shifting of conversation towards more 'optimistic' aspects was frequently used to close further talk. A key recommendation was that clinicians learn how to delay this shift.

Comprehensive and very practical clinical practice guidelines for communicating prognosis and end-of-life issues with adults in the advanced stages of life-limiting illness and their caregivers have been published.[35] Not only do these detail structural guidance for such conversations but they also provide useful phrases for discussions in all areas, including appropriate strategies to facilitate hope and coping. Detailed exploration of how such conversations are conducted with patients by experienced doctors are also proving helpful in developing the evidence base on which to base training and self development.[36]

The transition to a palliative approach may usefully include integration of palliative care services with other services that the patient is receiving. These services may enhance the patient's and family members' quality of life, improve the management of physical and non-physical symptoms and support preparation for the end of life.[37] Palliative care services may be, however, very unfamiliar with NIV and may require education and practical support to allow confidence in supporting such patients and safe access to their services.[38]

ADVANCE CARE PLANNING

Advance care planning (ACP) is a process whereby individuals can discuss and prepare for their care in the event of future decisional incapacity, usually with input from healthcare or other professionals.[39] It has become associated predominantly with the refusal of specific medical technologies (for example not wishing to have assisted ventilation) in advance of a loss of capacity. To limit its remit to such narrow practice would be to underestimate the scope and potential of ACP and also to misunderstand the key principles of the process. A medical model of ACP, where medical information alone is given and medical decisions alone are made, lacks sufficient utility for individuals and their families. ACP should additionally include exploring an individual's general understanding of what end-of-life events may entail and what their hopes or fears may be for this time, giving them an opportunity to discover more information about their condition(s), reflect on their concerns and look at their life values in the context of all of this.[40]

The important principle is that patient involvement in any future decision-making process is maximised, be it when they lose capacity or when they still have it. Enabling patients to think ahead and refine and rehearse their decisions is a valuable underpinning to achieving good patient-related outcomes.

Whilst the legislation and guidance surrounding ACP differs between countries and jurisdictions within countries, in general there are three possible ways of formally stating an individual's position:

1. *Advance statements* indicate an individual's preferences for care; they are not legally binding. In the United States, this may be known as a values history.
2. *Refusals of treatment* may be legally binding. In England and Wales, an Advance Decision to Refuse Treatment (ADRT) is a legally binding record of informed consent for withholding or withdrawal of certain treatments, including life-sustaining measures, under particular health scenarios. For the withholding or withdrawal of life-sustaining measures, the records must be in writing and signed by both the individual and a witness and include the clause 'even if my life is at risk'.
3. *Proxies for healthcare decisions* may be appointed. Such surrogate decision makers are known in England and Wales as Lasting Powers of Attorney for Health and Welfare. Elsewhere these may be known as Welfare Powers of Attorney (Scotland), Durable Powers of Attorney for Health Care (Australia, Canada and United States) or Representatives (Canada). These appointments may pertain to decision-making for health and welfare and/or financial matters. Where appointments are made for health and welfare decisions, there will usually be a requirement to assign specific decision-making rights over life-sustaining measures.

Understanding of both the principles and legal aspects of ACP is vital in the support of patients who use NIV, especially those with MND, where it can be anticipated that the ability to communicate will deteriorate and may be lost completely. Both UK (NICE) and European (European Federation of Neurological Societies) guidelines in MND care recommend that discussions on end-of-life care and advance directives and or naming of a proxy should be introduced when NIV is started and discussed further when the patient is becoming increasingly dependent on NIV as well as at times when/if the patient asks for information. These discussions should include consideration of care plans and strategies for potential withdrawal of ventilation.

Planning for future deterioration is complex and a person's 'actual' decisions cannot be easily predicted. This is well illustrated by a case report of a patient with MND.[41] In this case, the patient never lost capacity to make decisions, being always able to communicate his wishes. Although stating that he would not wish, in this case invasive, ventilation, when the need for it arose because of pneumonia, he accepted it, thinking it would be required short term only. This proved not to be the case, and he later requested that it be withdrawn. This has resonance with the findings of the seminal research in ACP, the Study to Understand Prognoses and Preferences for Outcomes and Risks of Treatment (SUPPORT), which found that outcomes often did not match preferences stated in advance of the clinical need.[42]

Despite those caveats, in general, ACP does seem to help patients who maintain capacity to be able to engage better in decision-making when the time comes, and reduces the distress of relatives if best-interest decisions need to be made when the patient loses capacity.[43]

There is evidence of the lack of opportunity given to patients who are using assisted ventilation to make choices about their future. Interviews with patients with MND using assisted ventilation in the United States (mostly receiving ventilation via tracheostomy) found that whilst most patients wanted to issue a direction in advance about circumstances in which they would wish to stop assisted ventilation, few had had opportunity to do so.[44] Many patients with MND using NIV have been found to lack sufficient information on their disease, its likely progress and what happens in the very advanced and terminal phases.[1,45] Although some of the studies were undertaken many years ago, there is evidence of continued need for improvement. Whitehead et al.[46] explored end-of-life decision-making with patients and with bereaved carers, identifying a need for more information and shared decision-making; one participant challenged the lack of support for progression to tracheotomy.[46] The study also highlighted the challenges that people faced; healthcare professionals and systems sometimes failed to support the wishes that patients had expressed in advance of their loss of capacity and a deterioration in their health, findings that were supported by another work.[47]

The willingness to make end-of-life decisions with patients also varies geographically. Sprung et al.[48] found that south European physicians are more reluctant to make end-of-life decisions than their northern European colleagues and the percentage of patients with do-not-intubate (DNI) decisions varies accordingly.

NIV IN ADVANCED DISEASE: BURDENS AND BENEFITS

NIV is the gold standard in COPD-related respiratory failure,[49] and some patients may use it long term, intermittently or even continuously. Patients with COPD are now the most common users of home NIV.[50] Exploration of the experiences of patients and their family's personal views on the outcomes of using NIV is, however, very limited.

NIV has the potential to profoundly impact the outcome of end-stage COPD and lead to improved survival of COPD patients who may otherwise succumb to acute exacerbation.[51] COPD patients can now live longer with advanced or end-stage illness with fragile, minimal functional respiratory reserve and an unstable propensity to recurrent respiratory failure. It is important that clinicians evaluate with patients whether the NIV is enhancing living and not adding to their burden of living and delaying dying. The appropriateness of NIV may change in the same patient, both in different settings and as their disease progresses and the respiratory function becomes increasingly compromised.[52]

For patients with advanced diseases, NIV may be used as a bridge to support ventilatory failure whilst disease-directed therapies are given a chance to work. There is a growing literature on its use and value in patients with DNI decisions: when a patient has expressed a wish not to receive intubation or clinicians have decided that there should be no plan to escalate care further.[53–55] The DNI orders made by clinicians may be based on very low pulmonary capacity, very low physical ability, low quality of life, referral from a nursing home or extensive comorbidities with poor prognosis.[53] There are, however, no agreed or firm criteria for assessing the ineffectiveness of ventilation via intubation. Around 25% of patients for whom NIV is the ceiling of care are later discharged, and although maybe half of these survivors die within 6 months, one study found that the others lived for several years with only one to two admissions a year in that time.[53]

In an acute critical situation where a patient would otherwise die from respiratory failure and recovery is uncertain, it is vital that the burdens and benefits of treatment are acknowledged and weighed by the clinical team and discussed with the patient, including if the patient agrees with their family. Table 64.1 summarises these considerations.

Of utmost importance in these scenarios is that goals of care are defined at the start of treatment, that the use of NIV is regularly reviewed to weigh the burdens and benefits and the contribution of NIV to the stated goals is assessed. Declared time limitations to trials are also important.[56] In the United Kingdom, many hospitals are using the AMBER care bundle to support the delivery of care for patients where recovery is uncertain.[57] This provides a framework for teams to provide active treatments in parallel with discussion of potential deterioration with patients, enabling patient-centred decision-making.

It is always tempting to 'do something', especially when patients and families are in crisis. NIV must not be used without careful thought as it has the potential to turn a good death into a bad one by providing no benefits and only false hopes of recovery.[58] NIV may be used as a last-ditch effort for uncertain recovery when intensive care admission is not appropriate, but it must be clear whether the intent is to improve symptoms or to prolong survival. The latter may be very valuable to the patient if they need time to say goodbye, to put their affairs in orders or to be part of a key family event. For others it may painfully prolong the inevitable.

LAST DAYS OF LIFE

The care for patients and families in the last days of life is often excellent, but for a substantial number of people it can fall far short of what they need. Many complaints relate to poor end-of-life care, and a key feature of this is the inadequacy of communication between clinicians and their patients and families. In the United Kingdom, there have been multiple reports and enquiries exposing the suffering caused to many.[59] The five priorities for the care of dying people[60] are outlined in Figure 64.2. These priorities are generic. For patients using NIV the individualised plan of care has additional elements to other patients, specifically what happens to the NIV.

Some patients using NIV intermittently may at a certain point wish to have their symptoms managed in a different way and not put their mask back on. For some patients that have lost capacity (due to, for example, confusion or drowsiness), the doctor may make this best-interest decision or a legally delegated attorney may direct the care.

Many patients will die with their NIV in situ, usually requiring additional approaches to the management of their symptoms. It is important that all involved with these patients realise that the NIV may still cause the patient's chest to move after they have died. Relatives and some nurses may need to discuss in advance exactly how it can be certain that the patient has died if they are still 'breathing'. The process for the removal of the NIV after the patient has died also needs to be discussed. Care staff need to know who has the authority to remove the mask and stop the machine, including if it is permissible for the patient's family to do this for a patient that dies at home (it is!).

For some patients who are completely dependent on assisted ventilation, the support may be withdrawn and symptoms managed in an alternative way. This may be because the patient requests it or because the NIV is no longer of any clinical benefit and is not in line with the agreed goals of care.

NICE has published guidelines for the care of a dying adult.[16] These recommend a holistic approach to assessment and management of patient needs. Pharmacological strategies for management of breathlessness comprise opioid or benzodiazepine alone or in combination. Additionally, benzodiazepines are recommended for the management of anxiety. Thus, most patients with refractory breathlessness

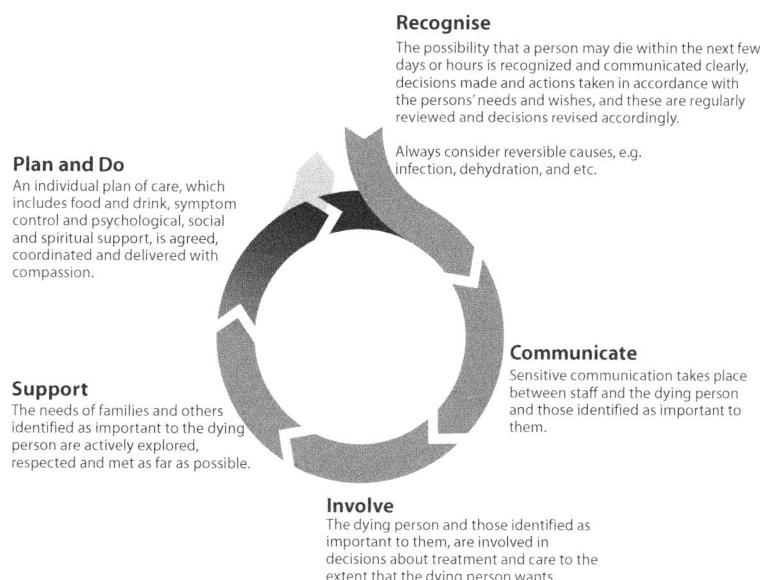

Figure 64.2 Five priorities for the care of dying people. (Reproduced from Leadership Alliance for the Care of Dying People, *One chance to get it right: Improving people's experience of care in the last few days and hours of life*, Department of Health and Social Care, London, 2014.)

typically benefit from a combination of morphine (or diamorphine) and midazolam delivered in a continuous infusion, often subcutaneously, and with intermittent additional 'as-required' doses.

WITHDRAWAL OF NIV AT THE REQUEST OF A PATIENT

A small minority of patients who are ventilator dependent request that their assisted ventilation is withdrawn, because for them, the burdens outweigh the benefits. These patients are likely to develop acute and severe breathlessness without the ventilator, so the process of withdrawal needs to be managed in a planned and proactive way to ensure that they receive appropriate symptom management and that unnecessary distress is avoided. There are degrees of ventilator dependence. Some patients will be unable to tolerate the lack of assisted ventilation for even a few minutes, whereas others will be able to tolerate it for several hours. This variability, which likely has both patient and disease factors, requires an individualised plan of care.

In the United Kingdom and many other but not all countries, it is the legal right of a patient to decide to refuse assisted ventilation, and the duty of care of professionals to manage the physical and emotional impact of this decision on the patient and family members. Phelps et al.[1] explored the experiences of professionals and families of patients with MND in the United Kingdom and found that whilst there were examples of good outcomes, there was considerable variation in outcomes for patients and care often fell short of what patients and families needed. Research concerning the withdrawal of NIV at the request of patients with diseases other than MND is scant. Exploration of the views of young men with Duchenne muscular dystrophy is in progress.[61]

A patient who is ventilator dependent and who decides that they no longer wish to have assisted ventilation has made a difficult decision. This life-ending decision may evolve over time, but often the patient's final decision around treatment withdrawal arises in the setting of a clinical deterioration, either secondary to an acute problem such as infection or in the setting of a decline in function that leads to a persistently unacceptable quality of life. A decreasing ability to communicate effectively (and thus ability to control care) may play a significant role in making the decision that the burdens of continued ventilation outweigh the benefits. Some patients may make a written statement or an ADRT with respect to the withdrawal of NIV at a time when communication is lost, and some may appoint an attorney for decisions about life-sustaining treatments in advance of their losing the ability to communicate or losing capacity for another reason.

Professionals have said that providing the care for a ventilator-dependent patient who has asked for assisted ventilation to be withdrawn is practically and emotionally challenging and that the lack of guidance on practical aspects of withdrawal, poor ACP, lack of experience and the need to support all involved in order to prevent conflict were significant factors in the impact of this care on themselves and others.[62] Additionally, although the ethics and legality are, in theory, very clear, in practice many voiced considerable uncertainty as to what constitutes ethical and legal defensibility in these scenarios.[1]

The Association for Palliative Medicine of Great Britain and Ireland (APM) has published guidance for professionals to support their practice in this very challenging area of care.[63,64] The guidance, developed by a multiprofessional

Table 64.2 Summary of the guidance for the withdrawal of assisted ventilation at the request of a patient with MND

Timing	Standard	Process for addressing the standard(s)
When commencing assisted ventilation and throughout care	**Standard 1** A patient should be made aware that assisted ventilation is a form of treatment and they can choose to stop it at any time. They should be in no doubt that this is legal and that healthcare teams will support them.	Inform patients that they can choose to stop the treatment at any time, that it is entirely their right and legal and that their healthcare team will manage their symptoms in a different way. Offer patients and, with due regard for confidentiality, families the opportunity to discuss future scenarios when assisted ventilation is being considered. Promote the concept of ACP and discussion of wishes and values with patients who use assisted ventilation, especially those who have lost one modality of communication. Assess and discuss capacity for the decision about treatment and its continuation.
Withdrawal of assisted ventilation	**Standard 2** Senior clinicians should validate the patient's decision and lead the withdrawal.	Affirm the decision by assessing the patient's capacity or validity and applicability of an ADRT and that this is a settled view, allowing time for discussion and reflection between the initial conversation and the patient's final decision. Planning, coordination and communication are vital tasks.
	Standard 3 Withdrawal should be undertaken within a reasonable timeframe after a validated request	Discuss with the patient and family when, where and how withdrawal will happen, including the potential for living for some hours without the ventilator and occasionally longer. Discuss with the professionals when, where and how withdrawal will happen; identify key people and their roles. Ensure that members of the team understand the ethical principles and the legal position.
	Standard 4 Symptoms of breathlessness and distress should be anticipated and effectively managed	Make a plan for symptom management. The key decisions are as follows: • Does the patient require sedation before assisted ventilation withdrawal: ventilator-dependent patients using >16 hours a day, very short periods of ventilator before distress? Or • Does the patient require *augmented symptom control*: patient can manage some hours off assisted ventilation? • What drugs, doses and route? • Who will prescribe and administer? • Who will manage the ventilator and how will settings be adjusted and mask/tubing removed? Administer anticipatory medication, titrating opioids and benzodiazepine to manage symptoms. For those who are ventilator dependent, assess the effectiveness of symptom management by reducing or stopping assisted ventilation for a few minutes <u>before</u> full removal. Continue to titrate opioids and benzodiazepine to manage symptoms.
After death	**Standard 5** After the patient's death, family members should have appropriate support and opportunities to discuss the events with the professionals involved.	Consider the needs of family and professionals after death: • Plan who will provide support to family members. • Debrief for professionals/significant event analysis. Submit data set and share key learning.

Source: Faull C, Oliver D, *BMJ Supp Palliat Care*, 6,144–6, 2016.

group, identifies five standards for care and the processes that will support achievement of these (Table 64.2). The guidance is underpinned by the following principles:

- Communication between the patient, the family and the professionals involved is of fundamental importance in achieving sensitive, safe and effective care.
- Teamwork is key to achieving best outcomes for the patient and requires senior clinical leadership.
- The need for psychological support for the patient, the family and the professional team should be anticipated and planned for.
- The principles for the management of symptoms are generalisable but the precise methodology requires individual tailoring to the patient.

The guidance also calls for continued gathering of data and outcomes seeking submission of a defined data set by those who undertake this care. The guidance is for the care of patients with MND, but it recognises that the ethical and clinical principles go beyond that population. An evidence base in all populations is greatly needed to make sure that outcomes are safe and satisfactory for patients, families and professionals. Because this area of care is rare, most practitioners have very limited experience to draw upon. The guidance signposts to the support available from experienced colleagues via a list held by the APM secretariat.

CONCLUSION

NIV is a valuable treatment but has significant implications for the optimum care of people when their disease is very advanced. Initiating NIV is a key trigger for integration of a palliative care approach alongside 'curative' disease management strategies. Patients require us to sensitively share information about prognosis and the burdens and benefits of treatment and to help them make decisions that fit with their values and wishes. This setting of the goals of care and ACP is an ongoing process that is helpful to patients and families.

Symptom management for patients with refractory breathlessness is well described for patients in the last days of life. For patients that request withdrawal of their ventilation, a guidance is available from the APM to ensure that care is safe and effective for patients, families and the professionals that support them, who may find this a challenging area of care.

REFERENCES

1. Phelps KP, Regen EL, Oliver D et al. Withdrawal of ventilation at the patient's request in MND: A retrospective exploration of the ethical and legal issues that have arisen for doctors in the UK. *BMJ Support Palliat Care.* 2015;bmjspcare-2014-000826.
2. Gawande A. Letting go: What should medicine do when it can't save your life? *The New Yorker* 2010 (2 August):36–49. Available at http://www.newyorker.com/magazine/2010/08/02/letting-go-2 (accessed 13 June 2016).
3. Clark D. *Cicely Saunders – Founder of the Hospice Movement 1959–1999.* Oxford: Oxford University Press; 2005.
4. Faull C, De Caestecker S, Nicholson A, Black F, eds. *Handbook of Palliative Care*, 3rd ed. Hoboken, NJ: Wiley-Blackwell; 2012.
5. Meier EA, Gallegos JV, Thomas LP et al. Defining a good death (successful dying): Literature review and a call for research and public dialogue. *Am J Geriatr Psychiatry.* 2016;24:261–71.
6. DH (Department of Health). *End of Life Care Strategy.* London: DH; 2008.
7. BMA (British Medical Association). *End-of-Life Care and Physician Assisted Dying – Volume 1: Setting the Scene.* London: BMA; 2016.
8. GMC (General Medical Council). *Treatment and care towards the End of Life: Good Practice in Decision Making.* London: GMC; 2010.
9. National Partnership for Palliative and End of Life Care. Ambitions for palliative and end of life care: A national framework for local action: 2015–2020. 2015. Available at http://endoflifecareambitions.org.uk/ (accessed 13 June 2016).
10. National Voices and the National Council for Palliative Care (NCPC) and NHS England. Every moment counts: A narrative for person centred coordinated care for people near the end of life. London: National Voices; 2015. Available at http://www.nationalvoices.org.uk/every-moment-counts-new-vision-coordinated-care-people-near-end-life-calls-brave-conversations (accessed 13 June 2016).
11. Shaw KL, Clifford C, Thomas K et al. Review: Improving end-of-life care: A critical review of the Gold Standards Framework in primary care. *Palliat Med.* 2010;24:317–29.
12. Seymour J, Kennedy S, Arthur A et al. Public attitudes to death, dying and bereavement: A systematic synthesis – Executive summary. 2009. Available at https://www.nottingham.ac.uk/research/groups/srcc/documents/projects/srcc-project-summary-public-attitudes.pdf (accessed 13 June 2016).
13. Ryder S, Demos. A time and a place: What people want at the end of life. 2013. Available at https://www.sueryder.org/~/media/files/about-us/a-time-and-a-place-sue-ryder.ashx (accessed 13 June 2016).
14. ComRes. National Council for Palliative Care – Public opinion on death and dying. 2015. Available at http://www.dyingmatters.org/sites/default/files/files/National%20Council%20for%20Palliative%20Care_Public%20opinion%20on%20death%20and%20dying_5th%20May.pdf (accessed 13 June 2016).

15. Hall S, Legault A, Cote J. Dying means suffocating: Perceptions of people living with severe COPD facing the end of life. *Int J Palliat Nurs.* 2010;16:451–7.
16. NICE (National Institute for Health and Care Excellence). *Clinical guidelines for care of dying adults in the last days of life (NG31).* London: NICE; 2015.
17. Lakhani M. Let's talk about dying. *BMJ.* 2011;342: d3018.
18. Boyd K, Murray SA. Recognizing and managing key transitions in end of life care. *BMJ.* 2010;341:c4863.
19. National Audit Office. *End of life care.* London: Stationary Office; 2008.
20. Murtagh FEM, Bausewein C, Petkova H et al. *Understanding place of death for patients with non-malignant conditions: A systematic review.* London: HMSO; 2012. Available at http://www.netscc.ac.uk/hsdr/files/project/SDO_FR_08-1813-257_V01.pdf (accessed 7 June 2016).
21. Fried TR, van DC, Tinetti ME et al. Older persons' preferences for site of treatment in acute illness. *J Gen Intern Med.* 1998;13:522–7.
22. Fried TR, van Doorn C, O'Leary JR et al. Older people preferences for home vs hospital care in treatment of acute illness. *Arch Int Med.* 2000;160:1501–6.
23. Almagro P, Calbo E, Ochoa de Echaguen A et al. Mortality after hospitalization for COPD. *Chest.* 2002;121:1441–8.
24. Pinnock H, Kendall M, Murray SA et al. Living and dying with severe chronic obstructive pulmonary disease: A multi-perspective longitudinal qualitative study. *BMJ.* 2011;342:d142.
25. Gaber KA, Barnett M, Planchant Y et al. Attitudes of 100 patients with COPD to artificial ventilation and CPR. *Palliat Med.* 2004;18:626–9.
26. Gardiner C, Gott M, Payne S et al. Exploring the care needs of patients with advanced COPD: An overview of the literature. *Respir Med.* 2010;104:159–65.
27. Highet G, Crawford D, Murray SA et al. Development and evaluation of the Supportive and Palliative Care Indicators Tool (SPICT): A mixed-methods study. *BMJ Support Palliat Care.* 2014;4:285–90.
28. Gott M, Ingleton C, Bennett MI et al. Transitions to palliative care in acute hospitals in England. *BMJ.* 2011;342:d1773.
29. Newbould J, Burt J, Bower P et al. Experiences of care planning in England: Interviews with patients with long term conditions. *BMC Fam Pract.* 2012;13:71.
30. Abarshi E, Echteld M, Donker G et al. Discussing end-of-life issues in the last months of life: A nationwide study among general practitioners. *J Palliat Med.* 2011;14:323–30.
31. Almack K, Cox K, Moghaddam N et al. After you: Conversations between patients and healthcare professionals in planning for end of life care. *BMC Palliat Care.* 2012;11:15.
32. Munday D, Petrova M, Dale J. Exploring preferences for place of death with terminally ill patients: Qualitative study of experiences of general practitioners and community nurses in England. *BMJ.* 2009;339:b2391.
33. Parker SM, Clayton JM, Hancock K et al. A systematic review of prognostic/end-of-life communication with adults in the advanced stages of a life-limiting illness: Patient/caregiver preferences for the content, style, and timing of information. *J Pain Symptom Manage.* 2007;34:81.
34. Parry R, Land V, Seymour S. How to communicate with patients about future illness progression and end of life: A systematic review. *BMJ Supp Pall Care.* 2014;4:331–4.
35. Clayton JM, Hancock KM, Butow PN et al. Clinical practice guidelines for communicating prognosis and end-of-life issues with adults in the advanced stages of a life-limiting illness, and their caregivers. *Med J Aust.* 2007;186:77.
36. Pino M, Parry R, Land V et al. Engaging terminally ill patients in end of life talk: How experienced palliative medicine doctors navigate the dilemma of promoting discussions about dying. *Plos ONE.* 2016;11:e0156174.
37. Boland J, Martin J, Wells AU et al. Palliative care for people with non-malignant lung disease: Summary of current evidence and future direction. *Palliat Med.* 2013;27:811–6.
38. Khan N, Monday D. Noninvasive ventilation in management of end-stage COPD: The implications for palliative care. *Eur J Palliat Care.* 2012;19:218–21.
39. Conroy S, Fade P, Fraser A et al. Advance care planning: Concise evidence-based guidelines. London: RCP; 2009.
40. NHS Improving Quality. Capacity, care planning and advance care planning in life limiting illness: A guide for health and social care staff. London: NHS Improving Quality; 2014. Available at http://www.nhsiq.nhs.uk/resource-search/publications/eolc-ccp-and-acp.aspx (accessed 14 June 2016).
41. Berger JT. Preemptive use of palliative sedation and amyotrophic lateral sclerosis. *J Pain Symptom Manage.* 2012;43:802–5.
42. Teno J, Lynn J, Wenger N et al. Advance directives for seriously ill hospitalized patients: Effectiveness with the patient self-determination act and the SUPPORT intervention. *J Am Geriatr Soc.* 1997;45:500–7.
43. Wong R. Advance care planning. In: Faull C, De Caestecker S, Nicholson A, Black F, eds. *Handbook of Palliative Care*, 3rd ed., pp. 93–108 Hoboken, NJ: Wiley-Blackwell; 2012.
44. Moss AH, Oppenheimer EA, Casey P et al. Patients with amyotrophic lateral sclerosis receiving long-term mechanical ventilation: Advance care planning and outcomes. *Chest.* 1996;110:249–55.

45. Kaub-Wittemer D, von Steinbuchel N, Wasner M et al. Quality of life and psychosocial issues in ventilated patients with amyotrophic lateral sclerosis and their caregivers. *J Pain Symp Manage*; 2003;24:890–6.
46. Whitehead B, O'Brien M, Jack B et al. Experiences of dying, death and bereavement in motor neurone disease: A qualitative study. *Palliat Med.* 2011;26:368–78.
47. Preston H, Cohen Fineberg I, Callagher P et al. The preferred priorities for care document in motor neurone disease: Views of bereaved relatives and carers. *Palliat Med.* 2011;25:1–7.
48. Sprung C, Maia P, Bülow HH et al. The importance of religious affiliation and culture on end-of-life decisions in European intensive care units. *Int Care Med.* 2007;33:1732–9.
49. NICE. Quality standard: Chronic obstructive pulmonary disease (QS10). London: NICE; 2011. Available at https://www.nice.org.uk/guidance/qs10/chapter/Quality-statement-7-Noninvasive-ventilation (last update February 2016) (accessed 14 June 2016).
50. Lloyd-Owen SJ, Donaldson GC, Ambrosino N et al. Patterns of home mechanical ventilation use in Europe: Results from the Eurovent survey. *Eur Resp J.* 2005;25:1025–31.
51. Nava S, Grassi M, Fanfulla F et al. Non-invasive ventilation in elderly patients with acute hypercapnic respiratory failure: A randomised controlled trial. *Age Ageing.* 2011;40:444–50.
52. Scala R, Nava S. NIV and palliative care. *Eur Resp Soc Monograph.* 2008;41:287–306.
53. Bülow HH, Thorsager B. Noninvasive ventilation in do-not-intubate patients: Five-year follow-up on a two-year prospective, consecutive cohort study. *Acta Anaesthesiol Scand.* 2009;53:1153–7.
54. Quill CM, Quill TE. Palliative use of noninvasive ventilation: Navigating murky waters. *J Palliat Med.* 2014;17:657–61.
55. Azoulay E, Kouatchet A, Jaber S et al. Noninvasive mechanical ventilation in patients having declined tracheal intubation. *Intensive Care Med.* 2013; 39:292–301.
56. Quill TE, Holloway R. Time-limited trials near the end of life. *JAMA.* 2011;306:1483–4.
57. The Amber Care Bundle. Available at http://www.ambercarebundle.org/homepage.aspx. (accessed 14 June 2016).
58. Short K, Whitnack J. Letter to the editor. *Crit Care Med*, 2006;34:1855.
59. PHSO (Parliamentary and Health Service Ombudsman). *Dying without dignity: Investigations by the Parliamentary and Health Service Ombudsman into complaints about end of life care.* London: PHSO; 2015.
60. Leadership Alliance for the Care of Dying People. *One chance to get it right: Improving people's experience of care in the last few days and hours of life.* London: Department of Health and Social Care; 2014.
61. Abbott D. Exploring the views of men with Duchenne muscular dystrophy on end-of life care decision making. Available at http://www.musculardystrophyuk.org/grants/exploring-the-views-of-men-with-duchenne-muscular-dystrophy-on-end-of-life-care-decision-making/ (accessed 26 June 2016).
62. Faull C, RoweHaynes C, Oliver D. The issues for palliative medicine doctors surrounding the withdrawal of NIV at the request of a patient with MND: A scoping study. *BMJ Support Palliat Care.* 2014;4:43–9.
63. Faull C, Oliver D. Withdrawal of ventilation at the request of a patient with motor neurone disease: Guidance for professionals. *BMJ Supp Palliat Care.* 2016;6:144–6.
64. Faull C. *Withdrawal of Ventilation at the Request of A Patient with Motor Neurone Disease: Guidance for Professionals.* Fareham, UK: Association for Palliative Medicine of Great Britain and Ireland; 2015.

65

Pathophysiology of weaning failure

THEODOROS I. VASSILAKOPOULOS

INTRODUCTION

Mechanical ventilation (MV) is a life-saving 'therapeutic' intervention for patients with respiratory failure. For most mechanically ventilated patients, the resumption of spontaneous ventilation can be a rapid and uneventful process. However, there is a substantial number of mechanically ventilated patients (20%–30%) in whom weaning is difficult and likely to fail, posing a great challenge for clinicians because the pathophysiology of weaning failure is complex.[1,2]

Failure to sustain spontaneous breathing is usually due to the incomplete resolution of the illness requiring ventilatory support or to a new pathological condition that has developed. In either case, weaning failure is usually caused by the inability of the respiratory muscle pump to tolerate the load imposed upon it. Consequently, weaning a patient from the ventilator will be successful whenever an appropriate relationship exists between ventilatory needs and neuromuscular capacity of the respiratory muscles and will ultimately fail whenever this relationship becomes imbalanced. Less often, failure to wean is due to cardiovascular dysfunction, hypoxaemia or dyspnoea/anxiety that develops on transition to spontaneous breathing.

VENTILATORY NEEDS AND NEUROMUSCULAR CAPACITY

To take a spontaneous breath, the inspiratory muscles must generate sufficient force to overcome the elastic loads of the lungs and chest wall as well as the resistive load of the airways and tissue (Figure 65.1). This requires an adequate central respiratory drive, functional nerve integrity, unimpaired neuromuscular transmission, an intact chest wall and adequate muscle strength. Under normal conditions, there are reserves that permit a considerable increase in load. However, a single breath is not enough to sustain life. Respiratory muscles must continuously contract throughout life lacking the ability to rest in order to sustain 'breathing' and be functionally flexible in order to sustain acid–base balance and minute ventilation. The ability of the respiratory muscles to sustain this load without the appearance of fatigue is called 'endurance' and is determined by the balance between energy supplies (Us) and energy demands (Ud)[3] (Figure 65.2).

On the one hand, energy supplies depend on the inspiratory muscle blood flow, the blood substrate concentration and arterial oxygen content, the ability to extract and utilise energy sources and the energy stores of the muscle. On the other hand, energy demands proportionally increase with the mean tidal pressure developed by the inspiratory muscles (P_I), expressed as a fraction of the maximum inspiratory pressure ($P_I/P_{I,max}$), the minute ventilation ($V'E$), the inspiratory duty cycle (T_I/T_{TOT}) and the mean inspiratory flow rate (V_t/T_I) and are inversely related to the efficiency of the muscles.[4,5]

Bellemare and Grassino[6] have suggested that the ratio of T_I/T_{TOT} and the mean transdiaphragmatic pressure expressed as a fraction of maximal ($P_{di}/P_{di,max}$) defines a useful index, the 'tension–time index' (TTIdi), that is related to the endurance time of the diaphragm:

$$\text{TTIdi} = (P_{di}/P_{di,max}) \times (T_I/T_{TOT})$$

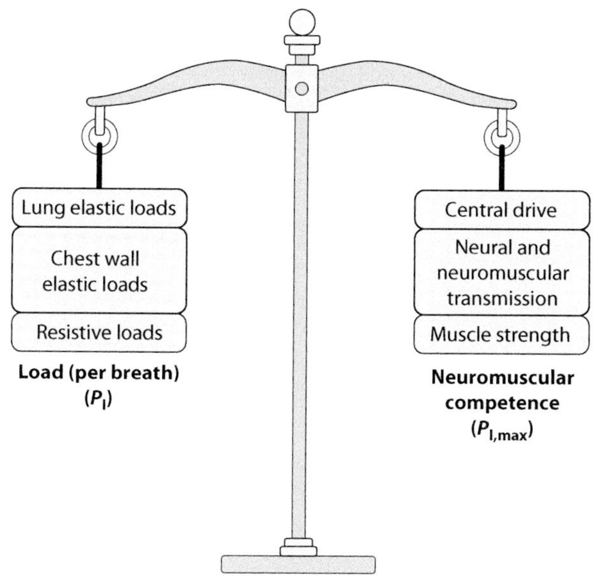

Figure 65.1 The ability to take a spontaneous breath is determined by the balance between the load imposed upon the respiratory system (P_I) and the neuromuscular competence of the ventilatory pump ($P_{I,max}$). Normally, this balance weighs in favour of competence permitting significant increases in load. However, if the competence is, for whatever reason, reduced below a critical point (e.g. drug overdose or myasthenia gravis), the balance may then weigh in favour of load, rendering the ventilatory pump insufficient to inflate the lungs and chest wall. (Adapted from Vassilakopoulos T et al., *Eur Respir J*, 9, 2383–400, 1996.)

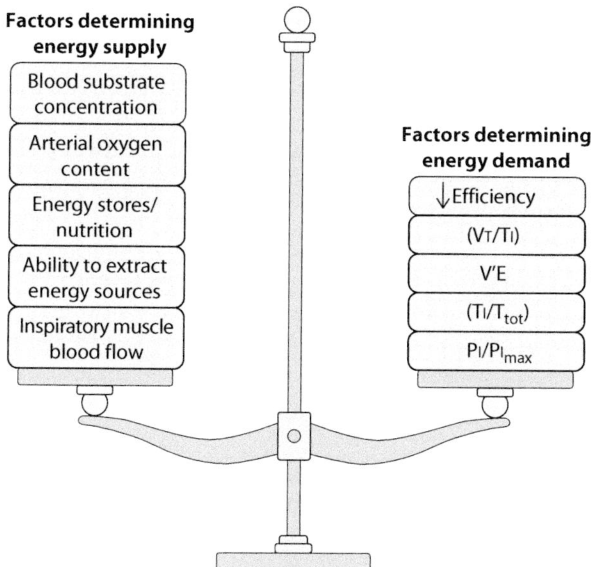

Figure 65.2 Respiratory muscle endurance is determined by the balance between energy supplies and demands. Normally, the supplies meet the demands, and a large reserve does exist. Whenever this balance weighs in favour of demands, the respiratory muscles ultimately become fatigued, leading to inability to sustain spontaneous breathing. (Adapted from Vassilakopoulos T et al., *Eur Respir J*, 9, 2383–400, 1996.)

Whenever TTIdi value is less than the critical value of 0.15, the load can be sustained indefinitely, but when it exceeds the critical zone of 0.15–0.18, the load can be sustained only for a limited time (endurance time). A TTIdi is assumed to exist not just for the diaphragm but also for the respiratory muscles as a whole.

$$\mathrm{TTI} = (P_I/P_{I,\max}) \times (T_I/T_{TOT})$$

Given that T_I/T_{TOT} and $P_I/P_{I,max}$ are among the determinants of energy demands, an increase in either will also increase the energy demands, which might not be met by the energy supplies.

Interestingly, Roussos et al.[7] have directly related $P_I/P_{I,max}$ with the endurance time. The critical value of $P_I/P_{I,max}$ that could be indefinitely generated at functional residual capacity (FRC) was around 0.60. Greater values of $P_I/P_{I,max}$ were inversely related to the endurance time in a curvilinear fashion. This means that in the case of hyperinflation, i.e. when FRC increases, endurance time decreases.

But what determines the ratio $P_I/P_{I,max}$? The numerator is determined by the elastic and resistive loads imposed on the inspiratory muscles. The denominator is determined by the neuromuscular competence. It follows that the value of $P_I/P_{I,max}$ is determined by the balance between load and competence (see Figure 65.1). But $P_I/P_{I,max}$ is also one of the determinants of energy demands (see Figure 65.2), so the two balances, i.e. between load and competence and energy supply and demand, are in essence linked, creating a system. This can be schematically represented by two linked balances (Figure 65.3), in which the $P_I/P_{I,max}$, one of the determinants of energy demands, is replaced by its equivalent, the balance between load and neuromuscular competence. When the central hinge of the system is at the horizontal level or moves upwards, the neurorespiratory capacity exceeds the ventilatory needs, and spontaneous ventilation can be sustained. When the central hinge of the system moves downwards, spontaneous breathing cannot be sustained and weaning will ultimately fail.[3]

Table 65.1 summarises all possible factors that can lead to an inappropriate relationship between ventilator needs and neurorespiratory capacity and thus to weaning failure. Diaphragmatic weakness is a major contributor to this inappropriate relationship. Accordingly, impaired diaphragmatic contractile function has been demonstrated in permeabilised single-diaphragm fibres isolated from human diaphragm biopsy specimens of mechanically ventilated intensive care unit (ICU) patients in both slow and fast twitch fibres[8,9] with evidence of impaired calcium sensitivity. In the following paragraphs, we will discuss some common disease entities affecting the respiratory muscles in the ICU specifically related to weaning failure.

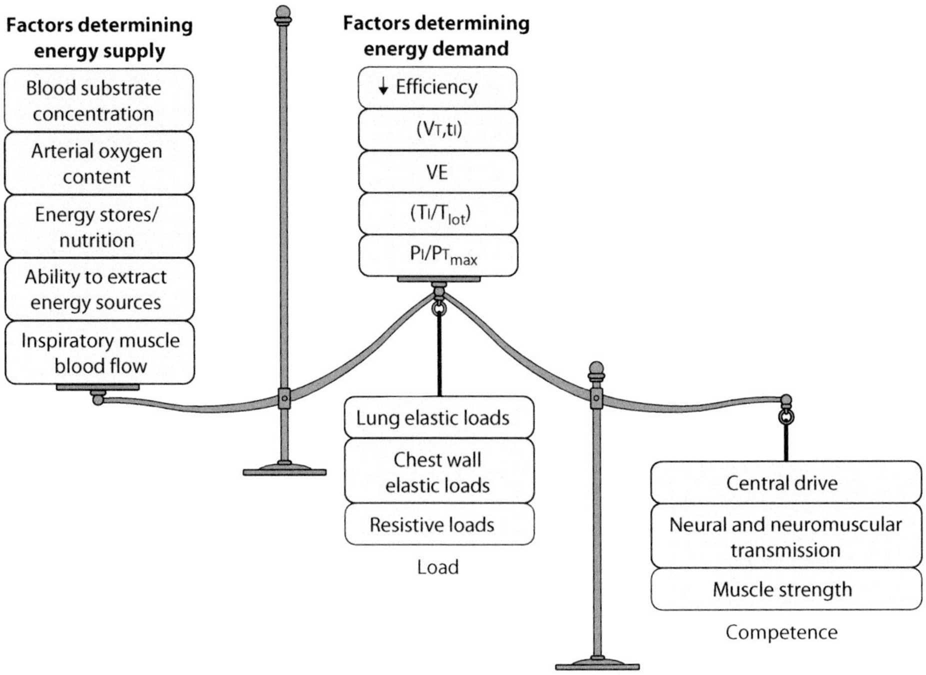

Figure 65.3 The system of two balances incorporating the various determinants of load, competence, energy supplies and demands is schematically represented. The $P_I/P_{I,max}$ that was one of the determinants of energy demands (see Figure 65.1) is replaced by its equivalent: the balance between load and neuromuscular competence (see Figure 65.2). In fact, this is the reason why the two balances are linked. When the central hinge of the system moves upwards or is at least at the horizontal level, an appropriate relationship between ventilatory needs and neurorespiratory capacity exists, and spontaneous ventilation can be sustained. In healthy persons, the hinge moves far upwards, creating a large reserve. (Adapted from Vassilakopoulos T et al., *Eur Respir J*, 9, 2383–400, 1996.)

VENTILATOR INDUCED DIAPHRAGMATIC DYSFUNCTION

Controlled MV (CMV) is a mode of ventilator support where the ventilator takes full responsibility for inflating the respiratory system using the minute ventilation set by the clinician (i.e. ventilator assumes all the work of breathing, and the respiratory muscles are theoretically inactive). Extensive animal research[10,11] and few human studies[12–15] have provided evidence that CMV can also cause dysfunction of the diaphragm, an entity named ventilator induced diaphragm dysfunction (VIDD).

VIDD is characterised by diaphragmatic weakness resulting from both atrophy and impairment of the force-generating capacity of the muscle (specific force production). Initial animal studies revealed that as few as 6–12 hours of CMV were adequate to induce contractile dysfunction of the diaphragm, followed by atrophy of all types of diaphragmatic fibres.[10,11] This is a progressive phenomenon, i.e. the longest the duration of CMV, the greater the degree of atrophy and contractile impairment. Diaphragmatic force production impairment precedes fibre atrophy.[16,17] Contractile dysfunction is due to impaired force-generating capacity of the muscle itself and not due to impaired neural and neuromuscular transmissions.[18] It is important to mention that (1) compared to peripheral skeletal muscles that are also inactive during CMV, the diaphragm develops atrophy earlier[19,20] and (2) some aspects of VIDD develop during partial support modes, when the support is excessive, but at a later time point.[21–23] Human studies confirmed animal data showing that the atrophy of both slow and fast twitch fibres and ultrastructural injury is evidenced at diaphragmatic specimens from organ donor patients after 24–48 hours of CMV.[8,9,13,14] Atrophy correlates with time spent on CMV.[13]

Atrophy can result from decreased protein synthesis, increased proteolysis or both. Studies in animal and humans support that both of these mechanisms play an important role in VIDD development.[10,11] All systems of proteases that mammalian cells have for intracellular proteolysis (lysosomal proteases, calpains, caspases and the proteasome system) are activated under CMV in humans.[9,12,14,24,25] Oxidative stress[12,14] that is evidenced very early in the course of CMV is important for the initiation of the cascade that leads to VIDD. Animal and human studies outline the importance of mitochondrial derived reactive oxygen species (ROS) on the pathogenesis of VIDD.[22,26,27] Picard et al.[27] showed mitochondrial dysfunction, impaired mitochondrial biogenesis and mitochondrial genome damage together with intramyocellular lipid accumulation in the human diaphragm of organ donor patients. Although the reason for the increased mitochondrial ROS production is not clear, lipid accumulation in the diaphragm

Table 65.1 Various factors that can lead to an inappropriate relationship between ventilatory needs and neurorespiratory capacity

	↑ Energy demands				↓ Neuromuscular competence		
	↓ Efficiency	↑ Load					
↓ Energy supplies	↑ V_i/Ti ↑ Ti/T_{TOT} ↑ Minute Ventilation loads	↑ Resistive loads	↑ Lung elastic loads	↑ Chest wall elastic loads	↓ Drive	Impaired nerve/ neuromuscular transmission	Muscle weakness
↓ Energy stores 1. Poor nutrition 2. Catabolic states 3. Prolonged submaximal breathing 4. Blood fuel Extreme inanition Inability to utilise Energy 1. Sepsis 2. CN^- poisoning ↓ Arterial O_2 content 1. Hypoxemia 2. Anemia ↓ Respiratory muscle blood flow 1. ↓ C.O. (shock LVF) 2. ↑ Force of contraction 3. ↑ Ti/T_{TOT}	A) ↑ V_{CO_2} 1. Fever 2. Sepsis 3. Shivering 4. Tetanus 5. Pain/agitation 6. Trauma/severe burns 7. Excess carbohydrates B) ↑ V_D/V_T 1. Pulmonary embolism 2. Emphysema 3. ARDS 4. Hypovolemia 5. Endotracheal tube connectors and filters 6. ↑ FRC (Hyperinflation)	1. Bronchospasm 2. Airway oedema, secretions 3. Upper airway obstruction 4. Obstructive sleep apnoea 5. Endotracheal tube kinking and secretion encrustation 6. Ventilatory circuit resistance	1. Hyperinflation [PEEPi] 2. Alveolar oedema 3. Infection 4. Atelectasis 5. Interstitial inflammation or oedema 6. Lung tumor	1. Pleural effusion 2. Pneumothorax 3. Flail chest 4. Tumor 5. Obesity 6. Ascites 7. Abdominal distention	1. Drug overdose 2. Brainstem lesion 3. Sleep deprivation 4. Hypothyroidism 5. Starvation/ malnutrition 6. Metabolic alkalosis 7. Toxic metabolic encephalopathy 8. Bulbar poliomyelitis 9. Acid maltase deficiency 10. Myotonic dystrophy 11. Sleep-induced hypoventilation	I. Phrenic nerve injury 2. Spinal cord lesion 3. Neuromuscular blockers 4. Myasthenia gravis 5. Aminoglycosides 6. Guillian barre 7. Botulism 8. Critical illness poly-neuropathy 9. Poliomyelitis	1. Electrolyte derangement 2. Malnutrition 3. Myopathy 4. Hyperinflation 5. Drugs—corticosteroids 6. Disuse atrophy (VIDD) 7. Sepsis

Source: Vassilakopoulos, T. et al., *Eur Respir J*, 9, 2383–400, 1996.

Note: CaO_2, arterial oxygen content; Q', perfusion; CO, cardiac output; CN, cyanide; LVF, left ventricular failure; $V'CO_2$, carbon dioxide elimination; V_D/V_T, physiologic dead space/tidal volume ratio; ARDS, adult respiratory distress syndrome; PEEPi, intrinsic positive end-expiratory pressure; ↑, increased; and ↓, reduced.

(toxic effect of fatty acids),[27] disruption of the normal mitochondrial fission/fusion balance and reduced blood flow to the diaphragm[28] may play some role. Autophagy that is induced in the diaphragm during VIDD in both humans[12] and animals[29] has been proposed to be an adaptive–protective event, as it is the mechanism responsible for the removal of damaged organelles (speculatively mitochondria) in the case of VIDD.[15,29]

The decline in diaphragmatic force production due to VIDD cannot be explained solely by disuse atrophy, but can be attributed to a reduction in the number of attached cross-bridges due to myofibrillar damage. Accordingly, Hussain et al.[24] studied an isolated myofibril preparation and showed that the brain dead organ donors on prolonged CMV exhibited reduced maximal active and passive specific force generation in myofibrils and reduced force redevelopment during activation and in response to imposed shortening. In this study, the impairment in contractility was associated with reduced protein levels of contractile proteins.

Ultrasound imaging studies of the diaphragm in mechanically ventilated humans showed that CMV results in the progressive loss of diaphragmatic thickness.[30–32] Within a week, nearly half of mechanically ventilated patients had evidence of more than 10% decline in diaphragmatic thickness, and this correlated well with increased ventilatory support.[31] The decline of diaphragmatic thickness is already evidenced after 24 hours of MV.[32] Although ultrasound is not the ideal monitoring tool for VIDD, it can be used as a surrogate marker of atrophy in the ICU.

A rational approach to the problem of VIDD would be to limit to the extent possible the use of controlled modes of MV and the amount of assist-pressure provided by the ventilator in ICU patients. However, the degree of diaphragm loading we should aim in mechanically ventilated patients to prevent or reverse VIDD is not known and has not even been adequately addressed even in animal studies.

INTENSIVE CARE ACQUIRED WEAKNESS

Intensive care unit-acquired weakness (ICUAW) is defined as the generalised muscle weakness that develops during critical illness and ICU admission that is attributed to the acute illness itself, i.e. no other identifiable causes can be found. It is what, in 1892, Sir William Osler reported as 'rapid loss of flesh' in patients with prolonged severe life-threatening infections.[33–35] Although clinicians suspect its existence when they face difficulty in the process of weaning patients from MV and/or mobilisation due to functional disability, it is a frequent event especially among the group of patients with prolonged ICU stay. At present, we know that it can present as critical illness polyneuropathy (CIP), critical illness myopathy (CIM) or both (different phenotypes of a probable similar clinical entity). CIP is an acute axonal sensorimotor polyneuropathy that affects limb and respiratory muscles. Electrophysiological studies shows abnormal motor and sensor responses. CIM is characterised by limb and respiratory muscle weakness with retained sensory function. Atrophy preferentially with loss of myosin filaments and/or muscle necrosis are the findings on muscle biopsies. Aetiology is multifactorial, and the severity of illness (shock, sepsis, multiorgan failure), ICU interventions (hyperglycaemia, drugs etc.) and age are among the risk factors. The presence of ICUAW results in prolonged ICU stay and ventilatory dependence, worst ICU outcome and prolonged functional impairment.[33–35]

RESPIRATORY MUSCLE FATIGUE

The consideration of the imbalance between energy supply and demand of the respiratory muscles (Figure 65.2) suggests that inspiratory muscle fatigue is frequently a final common pathway leading to weaning failure.

During weaning trials, patients who fail to wean show electromyographic evidence of excessive inspiratory muscle load, which is prevented by the application of pressure support.[36,37] The load that the respiratory muscles of patients who fail to wean are facing (assessed as the TTI) is increased to the range that would predictably produce fatigue in respiratory muscles,[38] if patients were allowed to continue spontaneous breathing without ventilator assistance. When these same patients successfully wean, the load is reduced below the fatiguing threshold.[38,39]

It is common in daily practice to use CMV in cases of weaning failure after a spontaneous breathing trial (SBT) or after extubation, based on the premise that respiratory muscle fatigue (requiring rest to recover) is the cause of weaning failure.[3,40] The results of the study by Laghi et al.[41] do not support the existence of low-frequency fatigue (the type of fatigue that is long lasting, taking more than 24 hours to recover) in patients who fail to wean despite the excessive respiratory muscle load. The twitch transdiaphragmatic pressure elicited by the magnetic stimulation of the phrenic nerve was not altered before and after the failing weaning trials.[41] The (TTIdi was 0.17–0.22 during failing weaning trials.[41] In fact, Bellemare and Grassino[6] had reported that the relationship between the TTIdi and time to task failure in healthy subjects follows an inverse power function: time to task failure = 0.1 $(\text{TTIdi})^{-3.6}$. Based on this formula, the expected times to task failure would be 28–59 min. The average value of the TTIdi during the last minute of the trial was 0.26, and the weaning failure patients would be predicted to sustain this effort for another 13 min before developing diaphragmatic fatigue.[41] Thus, the lack of the development of low-frequency respiratory muscle fatigue despite the excessive load is due to the fact that physicians have adopted criteria for the definition of SBT failure, which led them to put patients back on the ventilator before the development of low-frequency respiratory muscle fatigue. Thus, no reason exists to completely unload the respiratory muscles with CMV for low-frequency fatigue reversal if weaning is terminated based on widely accepted predefined criteria. This approach would also reduce the risk of VIDD.

During weaning, the diaphragm, the main respiratory muscle, becomes the major pathophysiologic determinant of weaning failure or success.[3] In the ICU, the interplay of excessive ventilator support (VIDD) with the other ICU insults (sepsis, critical illness myopathy, electrolyte disturbances, hyperinflation, to name a few out of a long list[3]) renders the diaphragm weak in a time-dependent manner[13,42] and thus weaning is difficult in a significant proportion of ICU patients.

CARDIOVASCULAR DYSFUNCTION

Approximately, 20%–30% of weaning failures resulted from congestive heart failure.[3,43] Patients with underlying ventricular dysfunction may increase their pulmonary artery occlusion pressure (PAOP) and sometimes ultimately decrease their cardiac output on removal from positive pressure MV.[44] Transition from positive pressure ventilation to spontaneous breathing induces changes that can lead to weaning-induced left ventricular (LV) dysfunction.[45] During spontaneous breathing, the increase in respiratory muscle work load as well as anxiety and sympathetic discharge result in an abrupt increase in oxygen and cardiac demands. The failing left ventricle is unable to normally respond, and left ventricular end-diastolic pressure (LVEDP) rises, causing interstitial, peribronchial and alveolar oedema, which reduces lung compliance, increases airway resistance and worsens ventilation–perfusion mismatching, leading to hypoxaemia. Energy demands of the respiratory muscles are increased, whereas energy supplies are either diminished or not sufficiently increased (inadequate cardiac output and hypoxaemia). This eventually leads to the inability to sustain spontaneous ventilation at a level adequate to achieve normocapnia, and PCO_2 rises. The abnormal blood gases depress cardiac contractility and, at the same time, respiratory muscle function. This worsens blood gases more and creates a vicious cycle that may culminate in failure to wean.[44]

Several factors may be responsible,[45] the most important being the changes in intrathoracic and intra-abdominal pressures on the initiation of spontaneous breathing. Normally, spontaneous inspiration increases abdominal pressure, and at the same time, it decreases pleural pressure due to diaphragmatic contraction and descent. The role of the decreased pleural pressure on venous return is already known. An increase in abdominal pressure would compress the abdominal venous system, through which two-thirds of the venous return passes,[46] and this would increase the amount of blood returning to the heart.[47] At the same time, the negative intrathoracic pressure increases the afterload of both ventricles, and this, combined with the increased venous return, may lead to right ventricular distention. Because the two ventricles are constrained by a common pericardial sac and share the interventricular septum, changes in the volume of one ventricle may affect the function of the other; thus, right ventricular distention impedes the filling of the left ventricle.[48] This occurs both through a generalised increase in pericardial pressure and because of a shift of the interventricular septum towards the left. Left ventricular filling impediment increases its diastolic stiffness at the same time that its afterload is elevated due to the decreased pleural pressure. These combined effects lead to the elevation of LVEDP, culminating in weaning failure.

The seminal study by Lemaire et al.[44] was the first to show evidence of pulmonary oedema as a major cause of weaning failure. This study as well as many others that followed measured PAOP as an index of LVEDP and showed that a value above 18 cm H_2O or a marked elevation from baseline characterised patients that were failing the weaning process.[49,50]

As pulmonary catheterisation is an invasive process, effort was made to establish less invasive methods to be used in everyday practice.

With transthoracic echocardiography, the estimation of LV filling pressures can be done by using the ratio of early (E) to late (A) peak diastolic velocities (E/A) of the transmittal inflow or the ratio of E to peak early diastolic mitral annular velocity (Ea) – E/Ea. The diastolic dysfunction of the heart detected as increases in E/Ea and E/A during the weaning process can predict weaning failure.[51,52] The evidence of diastolic dysfunction before the SBT in patients with preserved systolic function was a key factor associated with weaning outcome.[53]

B-type natriuretic peptide (BNP) and N-terminal–pro-BNP are markers of myocardial stretch that are elevated due to increases in left ventricular filling pressures. Baseline values of both BNP and pro-BNP (at the beginning of SBT) predict weaning failure due to cardiac dysfunction,[54,55] whereas their changes/increases during SBT can diagnose heart failure.[55] A BNP-driven strategy of fluid management can shorten ventilatory dependence especially in patients with systolic dysfunction.[56] Signs of haemoconcentration such as increase in haemoglobin or plasma protein concentration as well as increases in extravascular lung water during SBT can diagnose weaning-induced pulmonary oedema.[49,57]

Another cardiovascular cause of weaning failure is myocardial ischaemia due to the increased cardiac workload on the resumption of spontaneous breathing.[58–61] In the literature, many studies have found either electrocardiographic evidence of myocardial ischaemia[58,59] or evidence from myocardial scintigraphy with thallium 201 during the discontinuation of MV.[60] Ischaemia was detected more frequently (10%) in patients with a history of coronary artery disease (CAD) and was associated with weaning failure in 22% of these patients.[59] However, a small study in the medical ICU population detected the evidence of silent ischaemia in 70% of patients at some point, and this was associated with difficulty in weaning (35% of patients required more than one trial). Interestingly, only 21% of these patients had a diagnosis of CAD.[62]

The haemodynamic and ventilatory changes associated with the resumption of spontaneous breathing may increase myocardial oxygen demands to such an extent that they cannot be met by the available coronary oxygen supply, probably due to coronary atherosclerosis or spasm, thus leading to ischaemia. The incidence of myocardial ischaemia might be underestimated because the methods usually used (electrocardiographic criteria) to detect it are inherently faced with the weakness of false-negative findings. The available data suggest that myocardial ischaemia is relatively infrequent in the usual ICU population, although its incidence increases in susceptible patient populations, such as those with CAD, where it is more likely associated with weaning failure. Myocardial ischaemia should be suspected in the susceptible patient who fails to wean, even in the absence of electrocardiogram changes.[40]

DYSPNOEA/ANXIETY: COGNITIVE IMPAIRMENT

During weaning trials, patients display fearfulness and apprehension related to the anticipation of dyspnoea[63] rather than the stress of the activity per se. This sense is frequently underestimated by their physicians.[63]

Dyspnoea is closely associated with anxiety,[63] which has four physiological consequences:

1. Muscle tone is increased, and this leads to increased $V'O_2$ (oxygen consumption); at the same time, the respiratory muscles also increase their $V'O_2$. Increased muscle tone also elevates the chest wall elastic load via its effect on the intercostals,[64] which, in turn, makes inspiration more difficult, since they are expiratory muscles.
2. Anxiety causes muscle deconditioning, and this leads to uncoordinated breathing, again increasing the load.[64]
3. Anxiety increases the concentration of circulating catecholamines. This increases the afterload of the heart (by increasing systemic vascular resistance), its preload (by constricting the great veins and forcing blood towards the heart) and the myocardial oxygen demands.
4. Breathing frequency may increase, which, in turn, would increase the energy demands of the respiratory muscles and generate dynamic hyperinflation.

The development of cognitive impairment in the form of delirium is frequent in ICU patient during their course of illness. During the weaning process, the presence of delirium delays weaning, prolongs MV dependence and is associated with the development of complications (respiratory–neurological).[65,66] The fact that brain function affects the weaning process is appreciated especially in neurocritical patients, where a low Glascow coma scale (GCS 7-9) and the inability to follow commands result in the prolongation of ventilatory dependence.[67]

REFERENCES

1. Brochard L, Rauss A, Benito S et al. Comparison of three methods of gradual withdrawal from ventilatory support during weaning from mechanical ventilation. *Am J Respir Crit Care Med.* 1994;150:896–903.
2. Esteban A, Frutos F, Tobin MJ et al. A comparison of four methods of weaning patients from mechanical ventilation: Spanish Lung Failure Collaborative Group. *N Engl J Med.* 1995;332:345–50.
3. Vassilakopoulos T, Zakynthinos S, Roussos C. Respiratory muscles and weaning failure. *Eur Respir J.* 1996;9:2383–400.
4. Macklem PT. Respiratory muscle dysfunction. *Hosp Pract (Off Ed).* 1986;21:83–6.
5. Roussos C, Macklem PT. The respiratory muscles. *N Engl J Med.* 1982;307:786–97.
6. Bellemare F, Grassino A. Effect of pressure and timing of contraction on human diaphragm fatigue. *J Appl Physiol Respir Environ Exerc Physiol.* 1982;53:1190–5.
7. Roussos C, Fixley M, Gross D et al. Fatigue of inspiratory muscles and their synergic behavior. *J Appl Physiol Respir Environ Exerc Physiol.* 1979;46:897–904.
8. Hooijman PE, Beishuizen A, de Waard MC et al. Diaphragm fiber strength is reduced in critically ill patients and restored by a troponin activator. *Am J Respir Crit Care Med.* 2014;189:863–5.
9. Hooijman PE, Beishuizen A, Witt CC et al. Diaphragm muscle fiber weakness and ubiquitin-proteasome activation in critically ill patients. *Am J Respir Crit Care Med.* 2015;191:1126–38.
10. Powers SK, Wiggs MP, Sollanek KJ et al. Ventilator-induced diaphragm dysfunction: Cause and effect. *Am J Physiol Regul Integr Comp Physiol.* 2013;305:R464–77.
11. Vassilakopoulos T, Petrof BJ. Ventilator-induced diaphragmatic dysfunction. *Am J Respir Crit Care Med.* 2004;169:336–41.
12. Hussain SN, Mofarrahi M, Sigala I et al. Mechanical ventilation-induced diaphragm disuse in humans triggers autophagy. *Am J Respir Crit Care Med.* 2010;182:1377–86.
13. Jaber S, Petrof BJ, Jung B et al. Rapidly progressive diaphragmatic weakness and injury during mechanical ventilation in humans. *Am J Respir Crit Care Med.* 2011;183:364–71.
14. Levine S, Nguyen T, Taylor N et al. Rapid disuse atrophy of diaphragm fibers in mechanically ventilated humans. *N Engl J Med.* 2008;358:1327–35.
15. Petrof BJ, Hussain SN. Ventilator-induced diaphragmatic dysfunction: What have we learned? *Curr Opin Crit Care.* 2016;22:67–72.
16. Mrozek S, Jung B, Petrof BJ et al. Rapid onset of specific diaphragm weakness in a healthy murine model of ventilator-induced diaphragmatic dysfunction. *Anesthesiology.* 2012;117:560–7.
17. Corpeno R, Dworkin B, Cacciani N et al. Time course analysis of mechanical ventilation-induced diaphragm contractile muscle dysfunction in the rat. *J Physiol.* 2014;592:3859–80.
18. Radell PJ, Remahl S, Nichols DG et al. Effects of prolonged mechanical ventilation and inactivity on piglet diaphragm function. *Intensive Care Med.* 2002;28:358–64.

19. Ochala J, Gustafson AM, Diez ML et al. Preferential skeletal muscle myosin loss in response to mechanical silencing in a novel rat intensive care unit model: Underlying mechanisms. *J Physiol.* 2011;589:2007–26.
20. Shanely RA, Zergeroglu MA, Lennon SL et al. Mechanical ventilation-induced diaphragmatic atrophy is associated with oxidative injury and increased proteolytic activity. *Am J Respir Crit Care Med.* 2002;166:1369–74.
21. Ge H, Xu P, Zhu T et al. High-level pressure support ventilation attenuates ventilator-induced diaphragm dysfunction in rabbits. *Am J Med Sci.* 2015;350:471–8.
22. Hudson MB, Smuder AJ, Nelson WB et al. Both high level pressure support ventilation and controlled mechanical ventilation induce diaphragm dysfunction and atrophy. *Crit Care Med.* 2012;40:1254–60.
23. Jung B, Constantin JM, Rossel N et al. Adaptive support ventilation prevents ventilator-induced diaphragmatic dysfunction in piglet: An in vivo and in vitro study. *Anesthesiology.* 2010;112:1435–43.
24. Hussain SN, Cornachione AS, Guichon C et al. Prolonged controlled mechanical ventilation in humans triggers myofibrillar contractile dysfunction and myofilament protein loss in the diaphragm. *Thorax.* 2016;71:436–45.
25. Levine S, Biswas C, Dierov J et al. Increased proteolysis, myosin depletion, and atrophic AKT-FOXO signaling in human diaphragm disuse. *Am J Respir Crit Care Med.* 2011;183:483–90.
26. Hudson MB, Smuder AJ, Nelson WB et al. Partial support ventilation and mitochondrial-targeted antioxidants protect against ventilator-induced decreases in diaphragm muscle protein synthesis. *PLoS One.* 2015;10:e0137693.
27. Picard M, Jung B, Liang F et al. Mitochondrial dysfunction and lipid accumulation in the human diaphragm during mechanical ventilation. *Am J Respir Crit Care Med.* 2012;186:1140–9.
28. Davis RT, III, Bruells CS, Stabley JN et al. Mechanical ventilation reduces rat diaphragm blood flow and impairs oxygen delivery and uptake. *Crit Care Med.* 2012;40:2858–66.
29. Azuelos I, Jung B, Picard M et al. Relationship between autophagy and ventilator-induced diaphragmatic dysfunction. *Anesthesiology.* 2015;122:1349–61.
30. Grosu HB, Lee YI, Lee J et al. Diaphragm muscle thinning in patients who are mechanically ventilated. *Chest.* 2012;142:1455–60.
31. Goligher EC, Fan E, Herridge MS et al. Evolution of diaphragm thickness during mechanical ventilation: Impact of inspiratory effort. *Am J Respir Crit Care Med.* 2015;192:1080–8.
32. Schepens T, Verbrugghe W, Dams K et al. The course of diaphragm atrophy in ventilated patients assessed with ultrasound: A longitudinal cohort study. *Crit Care.* 2015;19:422.
33. Batt J, dos Santos CC, Cameron JI et al. Intensive care unit-acquired weakness: Clinical phenotypes and molecular mechanisms. *Am J Respir Crit Care Med.* 2013;187:238–46.
34. Hermans G, Van den Berghe G. Clinical review: Intensive care unit acquired weakness. *Crit Care.* 2015;19:274.
35. Jolley SE, Bunnell A, Hough CL. Intensive care unit acquired weakness. *Chest.* 2016.
36. Brochard L, Harf A, Lorino H et al. Inspiratory pressure support prevents diaphragmatic fatigue during weaning from mechanical ventilation. *Am Rev Respir Dis.* 1989;139:513–21.
37. Cohen CA, Zagelbaum G, Gross D et al. Clinical manifestations of inspiratory muscle fatigue. *Am J Med.* 1982;73:308–16.
38. Vassilakopoulos T, Zakynthinos S, Roussos C. The tension-time index and the frequency/tidal volume ratio are the major pathophysiologic determinants of weaning failure and success. *Am J Respir Crit Care Med.* 1998;158:378–85.
39. Carlucci A, Ceriana P, Prinianakis G et al. Determinants of weaning success in patients with prolonged mechanical ventilation. *Crit Care.* 2009;13:R97.
40. Vassilakopoulos T, Roussos C, Zakynthinos S. Weaning from mechanical ventilation. *J Crit Care.* 1999;14:39–62.
41. Laghi F, Cattapan SE, Jubran A et al. Is weaning failure caused by low-frequency fatigue of the diaphragm? *Am J Respir Crit Care Med.* 2003;167:120–7.
42. Hermans G, Agten A, Testelmans D et al. Increased duration of mechanical ventilation is associated with decreased diaphragmatic force: A prospective observational study. *Crit Care.* 2010;14:R127.
43. Epstein SK. Etiology of extubation failure and the predictive value of the rapid shallow breathing index. *Am J Respir Crit Care Med.* 1995;152:545–9.
44. Lemaire F, Teboul JL, Cinotti L et al. Acute left ventricular dysfunction during unsuccessful weaning from mechanical ventilation. *Anesthesiology.* 1988;69:171–9.
45. Teboul JL. Weaning-induced cardiac dysfunction: Where are we today? *Intensive Care Med.* 2014; 40:1069–79.
46. Robotham JL, Becker LC. The cardiovascular effects of weaning: Stratifying patient populations. *Intensive Care Med.* 1994;20:171–2.
47. Permutt S. Circulatory effects of weaning from mechanical ventilation: The importance of transdiaphragmatic pressure. *Anesthesiology.* 1988;69:157–60.

48. Biondi JW, Schulman DS, Matthay RA. Effects of mechanical ventilation on right and left ventricular function. *Clin Chest Med.* 1988;9:55–71.
49. Anguel N, Monnet X, Osman D et al. Increase in plasma protein concentration for diagnosing weaning-induced pulmonary oedema. *Intensive Care Med.* 2008;34:1231–8.
50. Jubran A, Mathru M, Dries D et al. Continuous recordings of mixed venous oxygen saturation during weaning from mechanical ventilation and the ramifications thereof. *Am J Respir Crit Care Med.* 1998;158:1763–9.
51. Lamia B, Maizel J, Ochagavia A et al. Echocardiographic diagnosis of pulmonary artery occlusion pressure elevation during weaning from mechanical ventilation. *Crit Care Med.* 2009;37:1696–701.
52. Moschietto S, Doyen D, Grech L et al. Transthoracic echocardiography with Doppler tissue imaging predicts weaning failure from mechanical ventilation: Evolution of the left ventricle relaxation rate during a spontaneous breathing trial is the key factor in weaning outcome. *Crit Care.* 2012;16:R81.
53. Papanikolaou J, Makris D, Saranteas T et al. New insights into weaning from mechanical ventilation: Left ventricular diastolic dysfunction is a key player. *Intensive Care Med.* 2011;37:1976–85.
54. Mekontso-Dessap A, de PN, Girou E et al. B-type natriuretic peptide and weaning from mechanical ventilation. *Intensive Care Med.* 2006;32:1529–36.
55. Zapata L, Vera P, Roglan A et al. B-type natriuretic peptides for prediction and diagnosis of weaning failure from cardiac origin. *Intensive Care Med.* 2011;37:477–85.
56. Mekontso DA, Roche-Campo F, Kouatchet A et al. Natriuretic peptide-driven fluid management during ventilator weaning: A randomized controlled trial. *Am J Respir Crit Care Med.* 2012;186:1256–63.
57. Dres M, Teboul JL, Anguel N et al. Extravascular lung water, B-type natriuretic peptide, and blood volume contraction enable diagnosis of weaning-induced pulmonary edema. *Crit Care Med.* 2014;42:1882–9.
58. Abalos A, Leibowitz AB, Distefano D et al. Myocardial ischemia during the weaning period. *Am J Crit Care.* 1992;1:32–6.
59. Chatila W, Ani S, Guaglianone D et al. Cardiac ischemia during weaning from mechanical ventilation. *Chest.* 1996;109:1577–83.
60. Hurford WE, Lynch KE, Strauss HW et al. Myocardial perfusion as assessed by thallium-201 scintigraphy during the discontinuation of mechanical ventilation in ventilator-dependent patients. *Anesthesiology.* 1991;74:1007–16.
61. Hurford WE, Favorito F. Association of myocardial ischemia with failure to wean from mechanical ventilation. *Crit Care Med.* 1995;23:1475–80.
62. Frazier SK, Brom H, Widener J et al. Prevalence of myocardial ischemia during mechanical ventilation and weaning and its effects on weaning success. *Heart Lung.* 2006;35:363–73.
63. Knebel AR, Janson-Bjerklie SL, Malley JD et al. Comparison of breathing comfort during weaning with two ventilatory modes. *Am J Respir Crit Care Med.* 1994;149:14–8.
64. Holliday JE, Hyers TM. The reduction of weaning time from mechanical ventilation using tidal volume and relaxation biofeedback. *Am Rev Respir Dis.* 1990;141:1214–20.
65. Mekontso DA, Roche-Campo F, Launay JM et al. Delirium and Circadian rhythm of melatonin during weaning from mechanical ventilation: An ancillary study of a weaning trial. *Chest.* 2015;148:1231–41.
66. Salluh JI, Wang H, Schneider EB et al. Outcome of delirium in critically ill patients: Systematic review and meta-analysis. *BMJ.* 2015;350:h2538.
67. Wang S, Zhang L, Huang K et al. Predictors of extubation failure in neurocritical patients identified by a systematic review and meta-analysis. *PLoS One.* 2014;9:e112198.

66

Non-invasive ventilation for weaning and extubation failure

SCOTT K. EPSTEIN

INTRODUCTION

Non-invasive ventilation (NIV) has become a standard therapeutic intervention for many forms of acute respiratory failure, with a goal of improving outcome by avoiding intubation and its attendant complications.[1] With increasing skill in application, clinicians have extended the use of NIV to shorten the duration of mechanical ventilation by facilitating weaning (earlier extubation),[2–4] preventing reintubation in surgical patients in the post-operative period,[5] and for patients after planned extubation.[6–9] In the latter instance, NIV is used as a preventive strategy with application immediately post-extubation in patients predicted to be at increased risk for extubation failure.[8,9] On the other hand, NIV has been used in patients who develop clear signs of respiratory failure after extubation.[6,7] The use of NIV for these various applications has significantly increased. An observational study found that 30% of applications of NIV for acute respiratory failure were for facilitating weaning or after extubation.[10] In another observational study, 21% of NIV applications were for post-extubation respiratory failure.[11] Finally, in a prospective observational study in 54 French and Belgian intensive care units (ICUs), 11% of intubated patients received post-extubation NIV, a significant increase from the author's analysis more than a decade earlier.[12] In this analysis, 64% of post-extubation NIV applications were to prevent the development of acute respiratory failure, while 36% were used after post-extubation respiratory failure occurred. In this chapter, the rationale for using NIV to facilitate weaning and to prevent extubation failure will be discussed first. Subsequently, a detailed review of randomised controlled trials (RCTs) will lead to recommendations for effective use.

RATIONALE: THE IMPORTANCE OF FACILITATING WEANING AND EXTUBATION

Mechanical ventilation, delivered via an endotracheal tube, provides essential and life-saving support for patients intubated with various forms of acute respiratory failure. The invasive delivery of ventilatory support is predictably associated with clinically significant complications including injury to the upper airway (vocal cord dysfunction, tracheal stenosis, tracheomalacia), increase risk for gastrointestinal bleeding and for thromboembolism (consequences of increased stress and immobility), injury to lung parenchyma (e.g. volutrauma, barotrauma) and infection (e.g. sepsis, sinusitis, ventilator-associated pneumonia).[13] In general, the risk for complications increases with the duration of mechanical ventilation. Approximately 20% of intubated patients for acute respiratory failure will require 7 or more days of mechanical ventilation.[14] Up to 40%–60% of mechanical ventilation time is spent weaning the patient, a procedure that is dependent on the process of care.[15] Weaning patients as soon as possible is crucial because mortality increases with duration of intubation.[14]

Once ventilatory support is no longer required, attention shifts to removing the endotracheal tube (i.e. extubation). Both delayed extubation and failed extubation (reintubation) are associated with poor outcomes. The importance of timely extubation was demonstrated in a study of 136 mechanically ventilated brain-injured patients.[16] These patients were screened daily to ascertain readiness for extubation. The 27% of patients with delayed extubation (failure to extubate within 48 hours of achieving readiness criteria) experienced more pneumonia, longer ICU and hospital stay and increased mortality when compared with the patients extubated without delay.

Extubation failure is a common event. It is usually defined as respiratory failure necessitating the reinstitution of mechanical ventilatory support (reintubation or NIV), within 48–72 hours of endotracheal tube removal.[17] In one multicentre study, 25% of 980 extubated patients developed, within 48 hours of extubation, signs of respiratory distress with at least two of the following: hypercapnia ($PaCO_2$ > 45 mmHg or >20% increase from pre-extubation), respiratory acidosis (pH < 7.35 with $PaCO_2$ > 45 mmHg), clinical signs of respiratory muscle fatigue or increased work of breathing, respiratory rate (RR) of >25 breaths/min for two consecutive hours and hypoxaemia (SpO_2 < 90% or PaO_2 < 80 mmHg on FiO_2 > 0.50).[6] Fifty per cent of these patients required reintubation. In another study, 29% of 1152 extubated patients met objective criteria for extubation failure with 54% of those patients requiring reintubation.[18] Rates of extubation failure depend on many factors (Box 66.1). Extubation failure is more common in paediatric, medical, multidisciplinary and neurological ICU patients with rates averaging 15%.[17,19]

Extubation failure markedly prolongs the duration of invasive mechanical ventilation. In medical ICU patients, extubation failure led to 12 additional days on mechanical ventilation, 3 additional weeks in the ICU and 30 additional days in the hospital.[20] Patients experiencing extubation failure are significantly more likely to require tracheostomy.[20–25]

Extubation failure is associated with increased mortality; univariate analyses show mortality rates 2–10 times that experienced by successfully extubated patients.[18,20–22,26,27] Mortality rates of 40%–50% were observed in general surgical, medical, multidisciplinary and paediatric patients with extubation failure. In contrast, trauma and cardiothoracic surgical patients experience mortality rates of approximately 10%. With multivariate analyses adjusted for severity of illness and comorbid conditions, most studies found extubation failure to be independently associated with mortality.[18,21,27] Mortality rates are lower when reintubation results from upper airway obstruction, aspiration or excess pulmonary secretions compared with reintubation from respiratory or cardiac failure.[23]

A number of explanations have been offered for the association of extubation failure and increased mortality. Extubation failure may be another marker for increased severity of illness. Reintubation results in direct complications (e.g. sustained hypotension, hypoxaemia, pneumonia) that may contribute to poor outcome.[28] Once reintubated, patients experience more prolonged intubation and are subject to the risks mentioned earlier. Lastly, clinical deterioration can occur between extubation and reintubation, especially when there are delays in re-establishing ventilatory support in the patient with post-extubation respiratory distress. This hypothesis is supported by the observation that mortality is lowest in patients who are relatively rapidly reintubated. As an example, patients reintubated after self-extubation do not have excess hospital mortality, perhaps because the vast majority are reintubated within 1 hour of extubation.[29] In a study that controlled for cause of extubation failure, increased time from planned extubation to reintubation was independently associated with mortality.[23] Four additional studies found more delayed reintubation associated with poor outcome.[24,30–32] A potential mechanism was suggested by a study that found a lower incidence of pneumonia in patients immediately reintubated compared to patients with more delayed reintubation.[32] Another study found that organ failure and complications (most frequently pneumonia) frequently developed after reintubation.[18] This concept is further supported by the observation that, in contrast to successfully extubated patients,

BOX 66.1: Factors associated with increased risk of extubation failure

Patient factors

- Type of patient (medical, paediatric, multidisciplinary, neurologic vs. surgical or trauma)
- Older age (>65 years)
- COPD
- Congestive heart failure (especially severe left ventricular systolic dysfunction)
- Pneumonia as a cause for mechanical ventilation
- Higher severity of illness at the time of extubation
- ICU-acquired paresis
- Longer duration of mechanical ventilation (>7 days prior to extubation)
- Longer duration of weaning
- Positive fluid balance prior to extubation (increased BNP prior to extubation)
- Ineffective cough (peak cough flow rate ≤ 60 L/min)
- Abundant respiratory secretions (required airway suctioning more often than every 2 hours)
- Abnormal mental status, delirium
- Low cuff leak volume (cuff leak test) suggesting increased risk for upper airway obstruction
- Rapid shallow breathing prior to or during a SBT
- Hypercapnia at the conclusion of a SBT or immediately after extubation ($PaCO_2$ > 45 mmHg)
- Post-extubation dysphagia
- Morbid obesity

Process of care factors

- Use of continuous intravenous sedation (vs. bolus dosing)
- Semirecumbent positioning
- Transport out of the ICU for procedures
- Reduced physician and nurse staffing the ICU

those who fail demonstrate progressive clinical deterioration after extubation as indicated by worsening sequential organ failure assessment or SOFA scores.[33] This relationship between time to reintubation and outcome suggests that the earlier re-establishment of ventilatory support, using NIV, may improve outcome.

PATHOPHYSIOLOGY OF WEANING AND EXTUBATION FAILURE

The pathophysiology of weaning failure has been extensively investigated by comparing patients who fail with those who pass a trial of spontaneous breathing (SBT). Alternatively, a cohort of patients serves as their own controls, studied at the time of weaning failure, then again at the time of weaning success. Patients intolerant of spontaneous breathing demonstrate rapid shallow breathing, increased elastic and resistive work of breathing, increased intrinsic PEEP, abnormal gas exchange, respiratory muscle weakness and increased tension–time index.[34] The latter finding suggests that weaning failure is characterised by a potentially fatiguing set of conditions. Fortunately, overt respiratory muscle fatigue may be avoided by careful monitoring during the SBT. Returning the patient to full ventilator support at the earliest sign of trouble during the trial avoids the development of respiratory muscle fatigue.[35] Weaning failure is also characterised by an abnormal cardiovascular response manifested as a failure to increase oxygen transport to the respiratory muscles.[36] Studies indicate a range of additional cardiovascular abnormalities during weaning failure (weaning-induced cardiac dysfunction) including an increased transmural pulmonary artery occlusion pressure, abnormal left ventricular ejection fraction (detected by echocardiogram), ischaemia (detected by electrocardiogram), failure to appropriately increase cardiac output (detected by right heart catheterisation, non-invasively by partial CO_2 rebreathing or by passive leg raising) and an elevated brain natriuretic peptide (BNP) or pro-BNP.[37–41]

The physiological effects of NIV can reverse many of the abnormalities seen with weaning failure (Box 66.2). Non-invasive ventilation is associated with decreased rapid shallow breathing, improved gas exchange, improved alveolar ventilation and decreased work of breathing.[42,43] Pressure–time product, an indicator of work of breathing, is consistently reduced by NIV in proportion to the level of non-invasive pressure support applied.[44] This effect results in a 17%–93% reduction in the diaphragmatic electromyography (EMG) signal.[44] NIV can deliver extrinsic positive end-expiratory pressure (PEEP) to counterbalance intrinsic PEEP, decreasing work of breathing and reducing the inspiratory threshold load that results from dynamic hyperinflation.[42,43] The positive intrathoracic pressure associated with NIV reduces both cardiac preload and afterload, improving cardiovascular function.

A number of additional potential benefits occur when NIV permits the removal of the endotracheal tube (Box 66.3). These benefits must be weighed against the fact that unlike mechanical ventilation delivered via an endotracheal tube, there is no guaranteed minute ventilation with NIV. NIV does not enhance airway clearance and does not provide the convenient access of an endotracheal tube to suction copious airway secretions. Sedating the agitated patient on mechanical ventilation can be challenging without the airway protection of an endotracheal tube. Fortunately, agitation usually decreases when the endotracheal tube is removed, and therefore, sedation requirements should diminish as a result.

BOX 66.2: Physiological effects of NIV that favourably counterbalance pathophysiologic causes of weaning failure

- Reduces work of breathing
- Counterbalances intrinsic PEEP
- Increases dynamic compliance
- Unloads diaphragm (reduces EMG signal of diaphragm)
- Decreases RR
- Increases tidal volume
- Reduces rapid shallow breathing
- Increases PaO_2
- Decreases $PaCO_2$
- Increases pH
- Decreases cardiac preload
- Decreases cardiac afterload

BOX 66.3: Advantages of removing an endotracheal tube

- Eliminates imposed work of breathing that can occur with a narrow endotracheal tube
- Decreases risk for nosocomial infection and pneumonia
- Improves verbal communication
- Improves patient comfort and reduces the need for sedation
- Allows for effective cough
- Improves mucociliary secretion clearance
- Improves sinus drainage

NON-INVASIVE VENTILATION TO FACILITATE WEANING

Evidence base

Uncontrolled studies published in the 1990s indicated that NIV could be used to wean patients from mechanical ventilation. The earliest reports used NIV in patients with prolonged mechanical ventilation with a tracheostomy.[45–47]

In this way, these studies substantially differ from the RCTs discussed subsequently. The initial three reports suggested a success rate approaching 90% with weaning by NIV.[45–47] The lack of controls makes it impossible to determine the actual effectiveness of the technique.

Subsequently, enthusiasm was tempered by a study where NIV was used in 22 intubated trauma patients.[48] After a T-piece trial to assess the patient's capacity for spontaneous breathing, all 22 patients were extubated to NIV. The authors found no difference in blood gases and respiratory parameters when comparing measurements made with equivalent settings of either invasive or non-invasive pressure support. Of concern, nine patients (36%) required reintubation, and six eventually died on mechanical ventilation.

One additional observational study used NIV in 15 patients intubated for acute respiratory failure.[49] Patients were extubated after satisfying the following criteria: $PaO_2 \geq$ 40 mmHg (on FiO_2 0.21), $PaCO_2 \leq 55$ mmHg, pH > 7.32, RR ≤ 40 breaths/min, tidal volume ≥ 3 mL/kg, frequency/tidal volume ratio ≤ 190 breaths/L/min and negative inspiratory force ≥ 20 cm H_2O. These criteria are substantially more liberal than usual and would not typically indicate readiness for weaning and extubation. NIV (continuous positive airway pressure [CPAP] of 5 cm H_2O and pressure support ventilation [PSV] of 15 cm H_2O) was applied after extubation and maintained for a median of 2 days. Both modes of NIV resulted in physiological benefits including improved oxygenation, increased tidal volume and decreased RR. Non-invasive PSV ventilation reduced $PaCO_2$, increased minute ventilation and increased pH. Thirteen of 15 patients were successfully extubated. Although this success rate appears impressive, we cannot be certain that all 15 patients were true weaning failure patients.

A number of RCTs using NIV to facilitate weaning (vs. weaning in those who remain intubated) in patients failing at least one SBT have been subsequently reported (Table 66.1).[50–59] Four additional trials, published in Chinese and summarised in a meta-analysis, studied chronic obstructive pulmonary disease (COPD) patients with pneumonia randomised to NIV versus continued invasive mechanical ventilation after pulmonary infection was thought to be under control.[60] These four studies fundamentally differ from the studies listed in Table 66.1 in that patients did not fail an SBT before randomisation.

The first randomised trial, by Nava et al.,[4] screened 68 COPD patients intubated with severe acute-on-chronic respiratory failure. Patients had an average $PaCO_2$ of 90 mmHg prior to intubation and approximately 40% failed NIV prior to intubation. Once intubated, patients were ventilated in volume-assist control mode facilitated by heavy sedation and neuromuscular blockade (Figure 66.1). Patients were then changed, after approximately 12 hours, to pressure support. A 2-hour SBT was then performed, approximately 48 hours after intubation. The 50 patients failing the T-piece trial were randomised. Twenty-five patients remained intubated and underwent weaning by gradual reduction in the level of pressure support with a goal RR of <25 breaths/min. They also received SBTs twice daily on either CPAP or T-tube. The remaining 25 patients were extubated to NIV via an oronasal mask using an ICU ventilator in pressure support mode. Patients extubated to NIV underwent a weaning protocol similar to that for the invasive group. When compared to patients who remained intubated, those randomised to NIV experienced significantly better outcomes including a reduction in the duration of mechanical ventilation, shorter length of ICU stay, increased weaning success and improved 60-day survival (Table 66.2). Complications associated with NIV were common, but not severe, with the most frequent being nasal bridge abrasions. No NIV patient developed pneumonia compared with 25% of those remaining intubated, suggesting a possible mechanism for improved outcome with NIV. This study is also notable for demonstrating that failure of NIV as the primary therapy did not preclude the successful use of NIV at a later time.

Girault et al.[3] published a randomised controlled trial with a design similar to that of Nava. Thirty-three patients with acute-on-chronic respiratory failure who failed a 2-hour T-tube trial were randomised to extubation to NIV or continued invasive weaning using pressure support mode.[3] In contrast to Nava, in the Girault study, NIV was delivered by either nasal or oronasal mask and with either pressure support or volume-assist control modes. Using this approach, weaning using NIV resulted in a 3-day reduction in the duration of intubation (4.6 vs. 7.7 days). Yet no significant differences were noted in rate of weaning success, ICU or hospital length of stay, rate of reintubation (23% vs. 25%) or mortality at 3 months. This study is notable as it shows that NIV may decrease the duration of intubation while increasing the total ventilation time (invasive plus non-invasive).

Ferrer et al.[2] studied 43 patients (77% with chronic lung disease) randomised after failing at least *three* trials of spontaneous breathing. NIV was applied for a minimum of 24 hours using a bi-level mode (initial settings: inspiratory positive airway pressure [IPAP] of 10–20 cm H_2O and expiratory positive airway pressure [EPAP] of 4–5 cm H_2O) delivered with a nasal or oronasal mask. The study was halted early after the first interim analysis. Compared to invasive weaning, weaning facilitated by extubation with NIV was associated with significant decreases in the duration of invasive mechanical ventilation, duration of ICU and hospital stay and incidence of septic shock and pneumonia (Table 66.3). Weaning using NIV was associated with decreased ICU and 90-day mortality. This investigation is notable for the dramatic benefits seen with NIV despite the relatively small cohort studied.

In a trial published in abstract form, 303 patients with acute respiratory failure were screened including 45 who failed a 30-min T-piece trial.[50] Sixteen patients met exclusion criteria because of either excessive secretions or the presence of abnormal mental status. Of the remaining patients, 21 of 29 were enrolled and randomised, with 9 remaining

Table 66.1 RCTs using NIV to facilitate weaning from mechanical ventilation

Authors (year) (enrolment criteria)	Percentage with chronic obstructive pulmonary disease	No. of patients	Effects of NIV versus control group weaning with endotracheal tube in place
Nava et al. (1998) (failed single 2-hour SBT)[4]	100	50	↓ Duration of intubation ↓ ICU length of stay ↓ Hospital length of stay ↓ Pneumonia ↑ 60-day survival
Girault et al. (1999) (failed single 2-hour SBT)[3]	76	33	↓ Duration of intubation ↑ Total duration of mechanical ventilation (invasive plus non-invasive)
Hill et al. (2000) (failed single 30 min SBT)[50]	33	21	↓ Duration of intubation
Chen et al. (2001)[51]	100	24	↓ Duration of intubation ↓ Hospital length of stay ↓ Pneumonia
Ferrer et al. (2003) (failed at least 3 SBTs)[2]	58	43	↓ Duration of intubation ↓ ICU length of stay ↓ Hospital length of stay ↓ Septic shock ↓ Pneumonia ↓ Need for tracheostomy ↑ ICU survival ↑ 90-day survival
Rabie et al. (2004) (failed single 2-hour SBT)[52]	100	37	↓ Duration of intubation ↓ ICU length of stay ↓ Hospital length of stay ↓ Pneumonia ↑ Weaning success
Trevisan and Vieira (2008) (failed single 30-min SBT)[53]	35[a]	65	↓ Complications ↓ Need for tracheostomy
Prasad et al. (2009) (failed a single 120 min SBT)[54]	100	30	None
Girault et al. (2009) (failed single 5–120 min SBT)[b][55]	100	208	↓ Weaning failure[c]
Vaschetto et al. (2012) (achieved PSV + PEEP of ≤25 cm H_2O, PEEP of <14 cm H_2O, PaO_2/FiO_2 of 200–300 on FiO_2 of ≤0.6)[56]	0	20	↑ Invasive ventilation-free days
Tawfeek and Ali-Elnabtity (2012) (failed single 30-min SBT)[57]	21	42	↑ Weaning success ↓ Pneumonia
Rabie Agmy and Metwally (2012) (failed single 120 min SBT)[58]	100	264	↑ Weaning success ↓ Pneumonia ↓ Mortality
Carron et al. (2014) (failed single 30-min SBT)[59]	63	64	↓ Duration of intubation ↓ Complications ↓ Pneumonia

Note: ICU, intensive care unit; SBT, spontaneous breathing trial.

[a] Includes patients with COPD and asthma.

[b] Includes third randomisation group that was extubated to oxygen alone.

[c] Weaning failure defined as either post-extubation acute respiratory failure, reintubation within 7 days or death within 7 days of extubation.

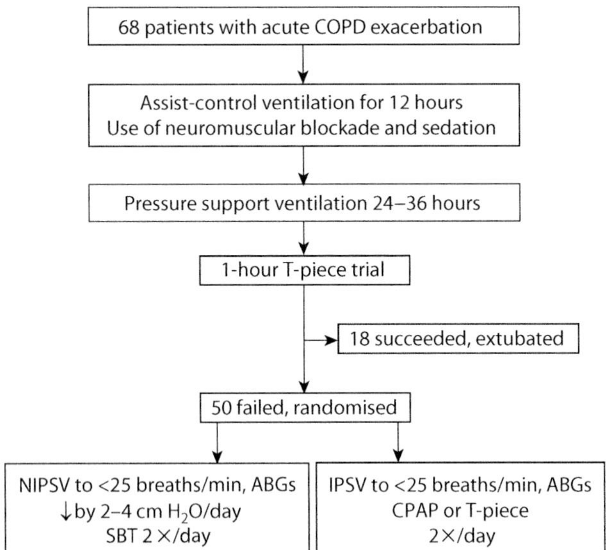

Figure 66.1 Design of a randomised controlled trial using NIV to wean patients with acute-on-chronic respiratory failure secondary to COPD. Patients failing a T-piece trial were randomised to continued intubation with pressure support weaning (IPSV) or weaning with NIV (NIPSV). ABG, arterial blood gas; ACV, volume assist control ventilation; CPAP, continuous positive airway pressure; PSV, pressure support ventilation; SBT, spontaneous breathing trial. (From Nava S *Ann Intern Med*, 128, 721–8, 1998.)

Table 66.2 Results from the RCT by Nava et al.[4] comparing weaning with NIV and continued intubation

	NIV	Intubation	*p* value
Duration of mechanical ventilation (days)	10	17	<0.05
ICU length of stay (days)	15	25	<0.05
Weaning success at 60 days (%)	88	68	<0.05
Survival at 60 days (%)	92	72	<0.05
Pneumonia after randomisation (%)	0	25	<0.05

Table 66.3 Results from the RCT by Ferrer et al.[2] comparing weaning with NIV and continued intubation

	NIV	Intubation
Duration of intubation (days)	9.5	20.1
ICU length of stay (days)	14	25
Hospital length of stay (days)	28	49
Tracheostomy (%)	5	59
ICU mortality (%)	10	41
90-day mortality (%)	29	59
Nosocomial pneumonia (%)	24	59
Septic shock (%)	10	41
Reintubation (%)	14	27

Note: All comparisons were statistically significant except for reintubation.

intubated and 12 extubated to NIV. Four of 12 NIV patients failed and required reintubation, while 8 of 9 controls successfully weaned. No difference was observed in hospital survival. NIV was associated with the decreased duration of intubation. Full appraisal of this study is difficult as only limited details have been reported. The study is nevertheless important in demonstrating that among patients intubated for acute respiratory failure, NIV for weaning is applicable for fewer than 10%. In addition, this study is one of the few that also employed a sedation protocol.

Another study used a quasi-randomised design (allocation to groups based on order rather than blind randomisation) in 24 COPD patients intubated for 3 days or more for an acute exacerbation.[51] NIV was associated with a significant decrease in the incidence of pneumonia, reduced duration of invasive ventilation and length of hospitalisation after randomisation. No difference was found in mortality, but the study was underpowered to adequately examine this outcome.

Rabie Agmy et al.[52] enrolled 37 COPD patients, intubated for acute-on-chronic respiratory failure, who failed a 2-hour SBT. When compared with patients who remained intubated, those weaned using NIV (using proportional assist ventilation, or PAV, delivered by face or nasal mask) were more likely to experience successful weaning and extubation and had a shorter duration of intubation, decreased ICU and hospital length of stay and fewer pneumonias. As with the study of Hill et al., this study, published only in abstract form, is difficult to fully appraise. In a subsequent study, these authors randomised 264 patients with acute-on-chronic respiratory failure secondary to COPD who failed a 120 min SBT. Weaning with NIV was associated with a decrease in pneumonia, increase in weaning success and decreased mortality.[58]

Trevisan and Vieira[53] randomised 65 patients, ventilated for at least 48 hours, who failed a 30 min SBT. The patients substantially differed from those discussed earlier where 58%–100% had COPD. In contrast, this study population was heterogeneous and consisted of patients with obstructive lung disease (35%, COPD or asthma), post-surgery/thoracic trauma (28%), pneumonia/tuberculosis/other respiratory disease (18%) and heart disease (16%). Thirty-seven patients remained intubated and underwent weaning with daily SBTs. The remaining 28 patients were extubated to NIV (bi-level positive airway pressure) using an IPAP from 10–30 cm H_2O delivered via a facemask. NIV weaning was carried out by systematically decreasing the level of pressure support. Weaning with NIV produced similar results to that performed in intubated patients with regard to ICU length of stay, hospital length of stay, hospital survival and duration of time on mechanical ventilation. NIV weaning was associated with a reduction in complications (pneumonia, sepsis, congestive heart failure), and fewer patients required tracheostomy. Six of 28 (21%) extubated to NIV required reintubation.

Girault et al.[55] conducted a 17-centre RCT of 208 patients (69% with COPD). Patients with acute-on-chronic respiratory failure were eligible if they were intubated for at least 48 hours and had failed an SBT lasting from 5 to 120 min. Using an innovative study design, patients were randomised to three groups: continued intubation with conventional weaning by pressure support, immediate extubation to NIV or immediate extubation to oxygen but without NIV. It is this third randomised group that makes this study unique. No differences were found in reintubation, complications, ICU and hospital length of stay and hospital survival. NIV was associated with a decrease in weaning failure, an outcome that combined post-extubation acute respiratory failure, reintubation within 7 days or death within 7 days (Table 66.4). It is important to note that NIV was used as salvage therapy in 45% of patients invasively weaned (successfully in 45%) and 57% patients extubated to oxygen alone (successfully in 58%).

Vaschetto et al.[56] randomised 20 patients with hypoxaemic respiratory failure for at least 48 hours to invasive weaning or non-invasive weaning using the helmet interface. This study also differs from those discussed earlier because eligibility was determined by ventilator settings (inspiratory pressure support of <25 cm H2O, PEEP of 8-13 cm H2O, PaO_2/FiO_2 of 200–300 on FiO_2 of ≤0.6) rather than failing an SBT. With this approach, NIV was associated with an increase in invasive ventilation-free days without other benefits.[56]

Prasad et al.[54] studied 30 patients with COPD and acute hypercapnic respiratory failure. Patients were randomised to invasive weaning or weaning via NIV once they had failed a 120-min SBT. In this study, the investigators found no difference between invasive and non-invasive weaning when comparing ventilator-associated pneumonia, weaning duration, duration of mechanical ventilation, length of stay and mortality.[54]

Table 66.4 Comparison of patients randomised to weaning via continued intubation, extubation to oxygen alone or extubation to NIV

	NIV	Oxygen	Intubation
Patients (number)	69	70	69
Reintubation within 7days (%)	30	37	32
Weaning failure (%)[a,b]	54	71	33
Complications (%)	51	61	52
ICU length of stay (days)	7.5	7.5	7.5
Hospital length of stay (days)	18.5	19.5	17.5
Hospital survival (%)	87	87	77

Source: Girault C et al., *Am J Respir Crit Care Med*, 184, 672–9, 2011.

[a] Includes post-extubation acute respiratory failure, reintubation (≤7 days) and death (≤7 days).

[b] $p < 0.001$.

Tawfeek and Ali-Elnabtity[57] randomised 42 patients with various causes for acute respiratory failure after they had failed a 120-min SBT. NIV was delivered using PAV, and invasive weaning was carried out using synchronised intermittent mandatory ventilation (SIMV). NIV was associated with improved weaning success and less pneumonia, but this did not translate into a mortality benefit.

Burns et al.[60] conducted a meta-analysis of 16 studies with a total of 994 patients (mostly COPD) who had been invasively ventilated for a minimum of 24 hours. Of these studies, nine exclusively enrolled patients with COPD while seven studies enrolled a mixed patient population. The meta-analysis included the 12 studies discussed earlier and 4 Chinese studies that significantly differed in study design. These latter investigations randomised a total of 227 COPD patients with pneumonia. Unlike the previously discussed trials where randomisation occurred only after a patient failed a SBT (with the exception of the Prasad study), these studies randomised when control of pulmonary infection was indicated by a separate set of criteria. Therefore, many of these patients might have, if given the chance, tolerated an SBT and been successfully extubated. An uneven allocation of such patients would bias the results. These studies are also questionable because three of four used different weaning strategies for NIV (pressure support) versus the intubated controls (SIMV plus pressure support). Hence, differences in outcome might have resulted from the ventilator modes. With these limitations in mind, the meta-analysis found that NIV weaning significantly reduced mortality (RR of 0.53), weaning failures (RR of 0.63), ventilator-associated pneumonia (RR of 0.25), ICU length of stay (−5.6 of days), hospital length of stay (−6.0 days), total duration of ventilation (−5.6 days) and duration of invasive ventilation (−7.4 days). NIV was associated with fewer tracheostomies (RR of 0.19) and decreased reintubation (RR of 0.65). The mortality benefit was greatest in those studies that exclusively enrolled COPD patients. The meta-analysis showed no benefit with regard to the duration of ventilation related to weaning.

One additional study, published after the meta-analysis, examined the use of a helmet for weaning patients from mechanical ventilation. Sixty-four patients, intubated for at least 48 hours for either hypoxaemic or hypercapnic respiratory failure (63% with exacerbation of COPD), were randomised if they failed to tolerate 30 min of spontaneous breathing on 7 cm H_2O of pressure support. When compared to invasive weaning, NIV via the helmet was associated with decreased duration of intubation, reduced complication and less ventilator-associated pneumonia.[59]

Taken together, these RCTs and the meta-analysis indicate that using NIV to facilitate weaning is associated with better outcomes than weaning performed in the intubated patient with COPD. Yet, one must be cautious in considering the evidence base given the significant heterogeneity between the various randomised control trials (see Table 66.5).

Why is weaning by NIV superior to invasive weaning? One explanation is that NIV is associated with fewer complications. When used as primary therapy for acute

Table 66.5 Factors contributing to the heterogeneity of studies of NIV to facilitate weaning from mechanical ventilation

Factor	Differences between studies and within studies
Patient population	COPD versus mixed; acute-on-chronic respiratory failure due to COPD exacerbation vs. COPD complicated by pneumonia; hypercapnic respiratory failure versus hypoxaemic respiratory failure
Enrolment criteria	Randomisation after failing one or more 120 min SBT versus randomisation after achieving control of respiratory infection or satisfying defined ventilator thresholds without undergoing an SBT; 30 min SBT versus 120 min SBT; failing a single SBT versus failing multiple SBTs; SBT conducted on T-piece of PSV
Experience of the centre in performing NIV	Highly experienced centres versus less experienced centres
Method of weaning when comparing invasive to non-invasive groups	PSV or PAV versus PSV or SIMV-PSV
Interface used to deliver NIV	Facemask versus nasal mask versus helmet
Ventilator used to deliver NIV	Standard ICU ventilator versus NIV-dedicated device
Use of weaning protocols	Use of strict protocol driven by objective data versus weaning driven by clinician preference
Use of sedation protocols	Sedation driven by objective scoring system with 'mandated' adjustments to medications versus sedation driven by clinician preference
Criteria for success	Timing of reintubation (48 hours vs. 7 days); diagnosis of pneumonia (patients who remain intubated are more likely to have airway secretions sampled)

respiratory failure, NIV, when compared to intubation, is associated with a lower risk of pneumonia and other infections. Similar findings have been noted in some of the studies (and the meta-analyses) where NIV was used to facilitate weaning (Table 66.1). NIV is more comfortable than intubation and therefore probably reduces the need for sedation, especially continuous intravenous sedation, a factor associated with increased duration of mechanical ventilation.[61] NIV may allow the clinician to identify the patient who, although seemingly intolerant of weaning, is ready to be weaned and extubated. Two circumstances where this can occur are weaning intolerance resulting from psychological reasons (e.g. anxiety) and that caused by the imposed work of breathing from a narrow endotracheal tube. The latter was demonstrated in a study that determined the imposed work of breathing from the endotracheal tube in a cohort of surgical patients intolerant of a CPAP trial.[62] More than 90% of patients failed the trial with significant tachypnoea, but with a normal physiological work of breathing (e.g. elevated work of breathing attributable to the endotracheal tube), were successfully extubated. If NIV were used in these settings, patients would appear to respond with improved outcome, although it would be the removal of the endotracheal tube, rather than a direct beneficial effect of NIV, that disclosed the patient's readiness for extubation. In this regard, the study by Girault is instructive.[55] By randomising patients to a third option, supplemental oxygen alone, these investigators demonstrated that some patients intubated with chronic hypercapnic respiratory failure who are intolerant of SBTs are nevertheless ready for extubation. Indeed, 20 of 70 (29%) patients in this arm of the study were successfully extubated (e.g. did not require NIV or reintubation and did not die).

Clinical application

When individually assessed, the majority of the investigations discussed earlier found NIV to be superior to invasive weaning: *none* found NIV to be the inferior strategy. The latter consideration is of considerable importance as mechanical ventilation delivered by NIV is more comfortable than via an endotracheal tube. This is relevant as total ventilation time (measured as total time intubated plus total time on NIV) may not be reduced by NIV, even though the time with an endotracheal tube does decrease. The RCTs and the meta-analysis indicate that NIV is an effective tool for facilitating weaning but only *in a very select group of patients*, those with acute exacerbation of COPD (e.g. acute-on-chronic respiratory failure). The efficacy of NIV in this population mimics that seen when NIV is used as primary therapy in COPD.[63] The study of Girault et al.[55] suggests that NIV may not need to be applied immediately, as some patients with apparent weaning intolerance are actually ready to be extubated (they will do well without NIV),

BOX 66.4: Caveats to consider prior to using NIV to facilitate weaning

- NIV to facilitate weaning should be used only in patients with acute-on-chronic respiratory failure (COPD).
- Primary failure of NIV (e.g. prior to intubation) does not preclude effective use of NIV after extubation.
- Patients must satisfy SBT readiness criteria:
  - P/F ≥ 120 – 150 on FiO_2 or ≤0.4–0.5 on PEEP ≤5–8 cm H_2O
  - Haemodynamically stable
  - Spontaneous breathing noted while on mechanical ventilation
- Patients should have failed between one and three SBTs before consideration is given to using NIV to facilitate weaning.
- Patients must satisfy extubation readiness criteria:
  - Adequate cough (spontaneously or in response to airway suctioning)
  - Absence of increased airway secretions (requiring suctioning less than every 2 hours)
  - Adequate mental status
  - No evidence of upper airway obstruction (assessed by cuff leak test)
- Patient must be a good candidate for NIV
  - An adequate interface can be established
  - Adequate mental status
  - Not a difficult reintubation from technical standpoint
  - Must be able to tolerate 5–10 min of spontaneous breathing to allow for adjustment of the interface and NIV settings
- Initial settings should be the following:
  - IPAP of 10–20 cm H_2O titrated to achieve the desired level of ventilation and $PaCO_2$
  - EPAP of 5 cm H_2O titrate to achieve the desired oxygen saturation of PaO_2
- An expert in airway management must be immediately available.

and in others, NIV can be successfully used at the first signs of respiratory distress. Indeed, as will be seen in the following, NIV appears to be effective in COPD patients at high risk for extubation failure[8,9] and those who develop respiratory distress after extubation.[64] That said, as will be shown in the following, the application of NIV to non-COPD patients who experience post-extubation respiratory failure has not been shown to be effective.

Prior to using NIV, it is important to assess whether the patient is a good candidate for this technique. Airway assessment should ensure that the patient will not have a difficult reintubation. Patients should be able to sustain spontaneous breathing for at least 5–10 min as it may take that long to adequately adjust the interface and arrive at optimal settings (Box 66.4). Specifically, IPAP should be adjusted in response to ventilatory needs, and EPAP should be adjusted based on oxygenation. There must be a capacity to closely monitor the patient over the ensuing hours to ensure that NIV is being tolerated and the patient is not deteriorating.

NON-INVASIVE VENTILATION TO TREAT POST-EXTUBATION RESPIRATORY FAILURE

Evidence Base

Uncontrolled studies suggest that NIV effectively reverses post-extubation respiratory failure preventing the need for reintubation in 65%–70% of patients. In an observational study, NIV was applied in 158 patients with acute hypoxaemic or hypercapnic respiratory failure. In 39 (17 with COPD) patients, NIV was used for post-extubation respiratory distress manifested by a RR of 30 breaths/min, a pH of 7.31 and $PaCO_2$ of 63 mmHg.[65] Eight-six per cent showed improvement or correction in blood gases with NIV, and reintubation was averted in 65%. In another observational study of 19 patients (five unplanned extubations), NIV was successful in 11; NIV failures were associated with mask leaks, secretions and hypoxaemia.[66]

Hilbert et al.[64] performed a case control study of NIV in 30 COPD patients who developed respiratory distress, within 72 hours of extubation, defined as either an RR of >25 breaths/min or $PaCO_2$ increase of >25% with pH of <7.35. Pressure support mode, applied using a full face mask, was used to administer NIV. The application of NIV was for a minimum of 30 min every 4 hours with patients receiving NIV for a mean of 5 days. A mean inspiratory pressure of 16 cm H_2O was needed to achieve predefined targets of RR ≤ 25 breaths/min and tidal volume ≥ 7 mL/kg. When compared with 30 matched controls, NIV was associated with significant reductions in reintubation (20% vs. 67%), ICU length of stay (8 vs. 14 days) and duration of ventilatory assistance in survivors (6 vs. 11 days).

Two RCTs examined whether NIV can improve outcome for patients with established post-extubation respiratory failure.[6,7] Keenan et al.[7] enrolled 358 patients, ventilated for at least 48 hours with cardiac or pulmonary disease, who underwent extubation after successful weaning. Post-extubation respiratory distress was defined as a RR of >30 breaths/min (or >50% increase from baseline) or signs of increased work of breathing including the use of accessory respiratory muscles or thoracoabdominal paradox.[7] The 81 (23%) patients developing respiratory distress within 48 hours of extubation were randomised to standard post-extubation care (controls) or NIV (bi-level mode) continuously administered for at least the first 12 hours. In this negative study, NIV did not improve outcome in terms of the need for reintubation, the development of pneumonia and ICU or hospital survival. This relatively small study may have been underpowered to detect differences between the groups. Another important limitation is that after the first year, COPD patients were excluded from enrolment. Presumably, physicians were reluctant to have these patients, in whom NIV is effective as primary therapy, 'risk' randomisation to the control group. As a result, only 11% of study patients had COPD. The 70% reintubation rate further suggests that NIV may not have been used early enough in these patients. Indeed, the study raises the question of whether the earlier application of NIV, immediately after extubation or at the first sign of respiratory distress, might be a better strategy. Another possible explanation of reduced effect of NIV may be the chosen setting; i.e. low inspiratory pressures may not sufficiently reduce the work of breathing.

The second RCT tried to overcome the limitations of the Keenan study by enrolling more patients and applying NIV earlier, at the very first signs of post-extubation respiratory distress. Therefore, Esteban et al.,[6] using 37 ICUs in eight countries, enrolled nearly 1000 patients, ventilated for at least 48 hours, who had passed a SBT. Patients were randomised if they satisfied two or more of the following criteria within 48 hours of extubation:

- RR of >25 breaths/min for two consecutive hours
- Clinical signs of respiratory muscle fatigue or increased work of breathing
- Hypercapnia ($PaCO_2$ of >45 mmHg or >20% increase from pre-extubation)
- Respiratory acidosis (pH of <7.33 with $PaCO_2$ of >45 mmHg)
- Hypoxaemia (SpO_2 of <90% or PaO_2 of <80 mmHg on FiO_2 of ≤0.50)

Two hundred and forty-four patients (25%) developed post-extubation respiratory distress and 221 were randomised (NIV 114, control 107). Twenty-three patients were not randomised as they required emergent reintubation. The groups were similar in age, gender, severity of illness (Simplified Acute Physiology Score or SAPS II), duration of mechanical ventilation prior to extubation, pre-extubation respiratory variables and the method used to carry out the SBT. No differences were noted in time from extubation to satisfying criteria for post-extubation respiratory distress (mean: 9 hours). In comparing the NIV group with the controls, no difference was noted in the need for reintubation and length of stay in the ICU (Figure 66.2). NIV was associated with significantly increased ICU mortality (25% vs. 14%) with mortality higher in reintubated NIV patients when compared to control patients who needed reintubation. One possible explanation for the increased ICU mortality was the longer time between the onset of post-extubation respiratory distress and reintubation in those randomised to NIV (12.7 vs. 2.4 hours). As with the Keenan study, this investigation suffers from the relatively small number (10%) of randomised patients with COPD. For reasons that remain unclear, when NIV was used in control

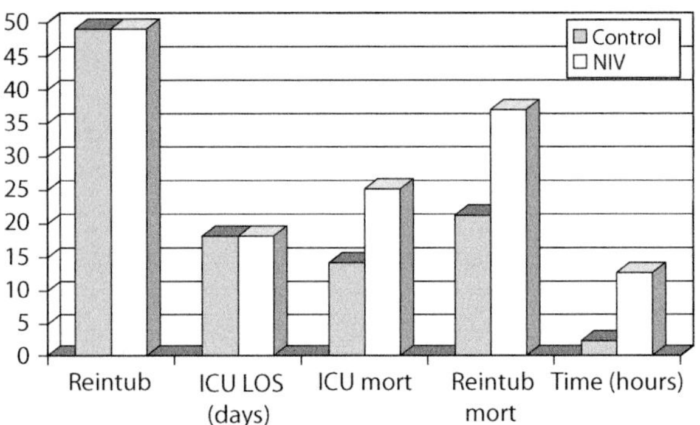

Figure 66.2 Results of a randomised controlled trial of NIV in post-extubation respiratory failure.[7] Two hundred and twenty-one patients were assigned to either NIV or standard care after extubation. The *y*-axis represents the percentage of patients, days (as indicated) or hours (as indicated). LOS, length of stay; Mort, mortality; Reintub, reintubation; Time, time between extubation and reintubation. (Redrawn from Epstein SK, *Respir Care*, 54, 198–208, discussion 11, 2009. With permission.)

patients as salvage therapy, the success rate was higher (75%) than in patients randomised to NIV (50%).

Clinical application

Uncontrolled studies found NIV to be the effective therapy for post-extubation respiratory failure. In contrast, RCTs indicate that NIV is not effective in this setting (Table 66.6).[67–73] This may not be true for COPD patients because RCTs contained few COPD patients. In addition, the case control study of Hilbert found NIV to be effective in COPD patients developing extubation failure.[64] Whether NIV may be harmful in non-COPD patients is unclear. Rather, the adverse results (increased ICU mortality) seen with NIV may be explained by delayed reintubation rather than a direct negative effect of NIV. More careful monitoring of patients with NIV and timely reintubation, when indicated, may avoid potential harm (see the following).[74]

NON-INVASIVE VENTILATION TO PREVENT POST-EXTUBATION RESPIRATORY FAILURE

Evidence base

As is the case with studies using NIV to facilitate weaning, studies of NIV to prevent or treat extubation failure are characterised by heterogeneity (Table 66.7). In an RCT of 93 patients, Jiang et al.[67] compared standard care (oxygen alone) to the application of NIV after extubation. The patient cohort was notable for containing both planned (60%) and unplanned (40%) extubations. NIV was applied via an oronasal mask using a bi-level device.[67] No significant difference was found in the need for reintubation. A much larger study randomised 406 mixed respiratory

Table 66.6 Summary of case control and RCTs of NIV to treat or prevent extubation failure

Authors (year), study design	Study type (patient population)	Number of patients	Effects of NIV versus control group
Hilbert et al. (1998), case control[64]	Treatment (COPD)	60	↓ Reintubation ↓ ICU length of stay ↓ Duration of ventilatory assistance in survivors
Jiang et al. (2000), RCT[67]	Prevention (all extubated patients)	93	None
Keenan et al. (2002), RCT[7]	Treatment (mixed)	81	None
Esteban et al. (2004), RCT[6]	Treatment (mixed)	221	↑ ICU mortality
El-Solh et al. (2006), case control[68]	Prevention (morbidly obese)	124	↓ Post-extubation respiratory failure ↓ Reintubation
Nava et al. (2006), RCT[8]	Prevention (high risk for extubation failure)	97	↓ Reintubation ↓ ICU mortality
Ferrer et al. (2006), RCT[9]	Prevention (high risk for extubation failure)	162	↓ Post-extubation respiratory distress ↓ ICU mortality ↑ 90-day survival in patients with hypercapnia
Ferrer et al. (2009), RCT[69]	Prevention (chronic respiratory disorders with hypercapnia during SBT, 70% COPD)	106	↓ Post-extubation respiratory failure ↑ 90-day survival
Khilnani et al. (2011), RCT[70]	Prevention (extubated patients with COPD)	40	None
Su et al. (2012), RCT[71]	Prevention (all extubated patients, 10% COPD)	406	None
Ornico et al. (2013), RCT[72]	Prevention (all extubated patients, 25% COPD)	40	↓ Reintubation ↑ Hospital survival
Mohamed et al. (2013), RCT[73]	Prevention (all extubated patients, 30% COPD)	120	↓ Reintubation ↓ ICU length of stay ↑ Hospital survival

failure patients (~10% COPD) who passed a 2-hour SBT and underwent planned extubation. No differences were noted in post-extubation respiratory failure, reintubation or ICU mortality when comparing NIV to conventional therapy.[71]

By studying all extubated patients, these studies were essentially underpowered to find a difference between standard care and NIV (e.g. the reintubation rate was too low in the conventional therapy groups). Extubation success rates range between 80% and 95%, so only 5%–20% will require reintubation, making it difficult to show the superiority of NIV. A better approach is to select patients deemed to be at high risk for extubation failure.[74]

Two studies conducted in patients with mixed aetiologies for acute respiratory failure showed NIV to be superior to conventional management after planned extubation. These positive effects could relate to the higher proportion of COPD patients randomised. As an example, Ornico et al.[72] randomised 40 patients intubated for a minimum of 72 hours (mean: 9 days) with hypoxaemic or hypercapnic acute respiratory failure of different aetiologies (~25% with COPD) to either oxygen or NIV immediately after planned extubation. Among the 38 patients completing the study, those in the NIV group were less likely to be reintubated within 48 hours (5% vs. 39%, RR: 0.13) and more likely to survive the hospitalisation (100% vs. 78%).[72] In another study, Mohamed and Abdalla[73] randomised 120 patients who had been intubated for at least 48 hours and who had passed a 120 min trial of pressure support ventilation at 7 cm H_2O. Patients randomised to NIV were less likely to need reintubation, had shorter ICU length of stay and increased hospital survival. These differences were greatest among the ~30% of patients in the study with COPD.[73]

What is the role of preventive NIV in patients deemed to be at high risk for extubation failure? In a case control study, El-Solh et al.[68] applied NIV immediately post-extubation in morbidly obese patients (body mass index of >35) mechanically ventilated for a minimum of 48 hours. Bi-level NIV was delivered, on average for 16 hours/day, using initial settings of an IPAP of 12 cm H_2O and EPAP of 4 cm H_2O. A nasal mask was used with NIV titrated to keep the RR of <25 breaths/min. Control subjects were matched for age, body mass index, Acute Physiology and Chronic Health Evaluation (APACHE) II score and weaning protocol. Compared with controls, NIV was associated with

Table 66.7 Factors contributing to the heterogeneity of studies of NIV to prevent or treat extubation failure

Factor	Differences between studies and within studies
Patient population	COPD versus mixed; hypoxaemic or hypercapnic acute respiratory failure
Study design	RCT versus case control study
Enrolment criteria	Prevention of extubation failure versus treatment of extubation failure; for prevention – high risk for extubation failure versus all extubated patients; variable definitions of 'high risk' for extubation failure; randomisation after passing SBTs of variable duration and SBT conducted on different modes
Experience of the centre in performing NIV	Highly experienced centres versus less experienced centres
Interface used to deliver NIV	Face mask versus nasal mask
Application of NIV	NIV administered for variable lengths of time after extubation and using variable settings
Ventilator used to deliver NIV	Standard ICU ventilator versus NIV-dedicated device
Criteria for success	Post-extubation respiratory failure vs. reintubation. timing of reintubation (48 hours vs. 7 days)

decreased post-extubation respiratory failure (10% vs. 26%) and fewer reintubations (10% vs. 21%). Mortality was similar between the two groups. The prevalence of obstructive sleep apnoea, a condition expected to benefit from NIV, was similar between the groups (NIV: 22% vs. controls: 27%).

RCTs have examined the effect of NIV, applied soon after extubation as preventive therapy, in patients predicted to be at high risk for extubation failure. The first, by Nava et al.,[8] randomised 97 patients who tolerated an SBT but were assessed to be at risk for extubation failure based on the presence of at least one of the following criteria:

- More than one consecutive failed weaning trial
- Chronic heart failure
- $PaCO_2$ of >45 mmHg (measured 1 hour post-extubation)
- Greater than one comorbidity
- Weak cough

One-third of patients had COPD and 10% had heart failure. NIV was administered using either a bi-level device or a standard ICU ventilator and was required for a minimum of 6 out of 24 hours. Immediate post-extubation NIV decreased the need for reintubation (4.8% vs. 12.2%) and was associated with lower ICU mortality. No significant differences were found in other outcomes including hospital mortality and length of stay.

A second study by Ferrer et al.[9] identified patients at high risk for extubation failure using different criteria. Randomised patients had to have one or more of the following:

- Age of >65 years
- Cardiac failure
- APACHE II score of >12 at the time of extubation[9]

The investigators randomised 162 patients to NIV or standard care. Half of the patients had chronic respiratory disease, and 50% of the time, acute exacerbations of these conditions were the precipitant for acute respiratory failure and intubation. A bi-level device was used with inspiratory pressure of 12–20 cm H_2O and expiratory pressure range of 4–6 cm H_2O. When compared to controls, NIV resulted in important improvements in outcome including a reduction in post-extubation respiratory distress (13% vs. 27%), a trend towards reduced need for reintubation (2% vs. 12%) and reduced ICU mortality. Differences were not found in either length of stay or mortality (hospital or 90 days). Subgroup analysis demonstrated that NIV in patients with hypercapnia was associated with improved 90-day survival. In a subsequent study, using a similar design, these authors randomised patients with chronic respiratory disease who manifested hypercapnia during a trial of spontaneous breathing. When compared to post-extubation oxygen alone, NIV was associated with decreased respiratory failure and improved 90-day survival.[69]

Khilnani et al.[70] randomised 40 patients with COPD and acute exacerbation to NIV or conventional therapy after planned extubation and found no statistically significant differences in reintubation or length of stay. This study was likely underpowered to detect a difference between the groups. In addition, the NIV group may have been disadvantaged because the ventilator used did not have real-time assessment of mask pressure or effective leak compensation. Also, the initial pressure settings (IPAP of 8 cm H_2O and EPAP of 4 cm H_2O) may have been inadequate to effectively support ventilation and counterbalance dynamic hyperinflation.[70]

A meta-analysis was conducted on the preceding RCTs and included two additional studies of patients with acute-on-chronic respiratory failure (one published in Chinese, the other in abstract form). The meta-analysis showed that NIV decreased the need for reintubation in COPD patients (RR of 0.33) and those at high risk for extubation failure (RR of 0.47). The analysis also suggested decreased ICU and hospital mortality rates with NIV. In contrast, no difference in outcomes was noted in studies examining mixed medical ICU patients.[75]

What about oxygen delivered by high-flow nasal cannula (HFNC)? Although this modality differs from NIV, the very high flow rates (up to 60 L/min) are capable of creating a PEEP effect and washing out the pharyngeal dead space. In addition, to deliver a constant FiO_2, secretion clearance is enhanced by the heated humidification system. Like NIV, the use of HFNC reduces dyspnoea and breathing frequency when compared to conventional methods of oxygen delivery. Hernandez et al.[76] randomised 527 patients at low risk for extubation failure to either HFNC or conventional oxygen after planned extubation. Post-extubation respiratory failure was less common in patients receiving HFNC, and those patients were less likely to be reintubated.[76]

Clinical application

The routine use of NIV, applied very soon after extubation, cannot be recommended except for patients assessed to be at significantly increased risk for extubation failure (Table 66.6, Box 66.1). The case control study of El-Solh et al.[76] indicates that NIV is an effective preventive therapy in morbidly obese patients. The RCTs reviewed earlier and a meta-analysis indicate that the immediate application of NIV in high-risk patients reduces the need for reintubation and may improve survival.

Prior to using NIV, it is important to assess whether the patient in question is a good candidate for this technique. Whenever NIV is used in the post-extubation setting, the patient must be closely monitored. Frequent assessment should document that the patient is responding to NIV based on reduced dyspnoea, decreased use of accessory respiratory muscles, decreased RR and decreasing $PaCO_2$. If unequivocal evidence of improvement cannot be demonstrated after the initial 2–4 hours of NIV, the patient should (if appropriate) be reintubated (Box 66.5).

> **BOX 66.5: Summary of NIV use in extubation failure**
>
> - Only use NIV as a preventive strategy in high-risk patients (see Box 66.1).
> - Patients must satisfy extubation readiness criteria:
>   - Adequate cough (spontaneously or in response to airway suctioning)
>   - Absence of increased airway secretions (requiring suctioning less than every 2 hours)
>   - Adequate mental status
>   - No evidence of upper airway obstruction (assessed by cuff leak test)
> - Patient must be a good candidate for NIV.
>   - An adequate interface can be established
>   - Adequate mental status
>   - Not a difficult reintubation from technical standpoint
> - Apply NIV immediately after extubation.
> - Initial settings should be the following:
>   - IPAP of 10–20 cm H_2O titrated to achieve the desired level of ventilation and $PaCO_2$
>   - EPAP of 5 cm H_2O titrate to achieve the desired oxygen saturation of PaO_2
> - An expert in airway management must be immediately available.
> - With established post-extubation respiratory failure
>   - Only use NIV in patients with COPD
>   - If NIV is used, monitor closely
>   - Reintubate the patient within 2–4 hours if no signs of improvement of NIV

FUTURE RESEARCH

Although RCTs provide a strong evidence base for providing recommendations, many important questions remain unanswered:

- The studies cited earlier used either ICU ventilators or smaller portable devices to deliver NIV. Whether one or the other is superior in using NIV to facilitate weaning or prevent extubation failure is unknown. That said, the increased risk for reintubation would argue for a ventilator that can used with either a facemask (with necessary leak compensation) or an endotracheal tube.
- Most studies of NIV use a pressure-targeted flow-cycled mode. This mode can lead to difficulties in patient–ventilator interaction, especially during the transition from inspiration to expiration in COPD patients. Ventilators that allow for the adjustment of the expiratory cycle criteria may improve the interaction. It remains to be seen whether these devices or pressure-targeted ventilation using a time-cycled mode will be more effective.
- RCTs used either a nasal mask, an oronasal mask or a helmet, but a direct comparison of interfaces for this application has not been performed.
- Care for the patient with NIV can be time consuming for ICU nurses and respiratory therapists especially during the initial hours of application. It is not yet known whether nursing or respiratory therapy needs change in going from invasive weaning to weaning with NIV.
- As noted earlier, NIV is an effective mode of weaning in patients with COPD. Further work is needed in patients who have been intubated with other forms of acute respiratory failure.
- The studies of NIV as prevention against extubation failure used (with the exception of cardiac failure) two different sets of criteria to identify patients at increased risk. Further work is needed to refine these criteria. In addition,

larger studies may be required to convincingly demonstrate that each individual criterion (e.g. age of >65 years) is truly predictive of high risk for extubation failure.
- Further work is needed to define the optimal settings (inspiratory positive airway pressure) that effectively reduce work of breathing to optimise outcomes.
- Further work is needed to better define how much experience an NIV team must possess to optimise outcomes.

CHAPTER SUMMARY

Non-invasive ventilation is increasingly used after extubation from mechanical ventilation. The analysis of more than a dozen RCTs indicates that NIV can facilitate weaning in patients with acute-on-chronic respiratory failure and COPD who are failing SBTs. In so doing, NIV shortens the duration of intubation, reduces length of stay, lessens the risk for acquiring pneumonia, decreases the need for tracheostomy and improves survival. NIV is also used after extubation in patients who tolerate SBTs and undergo planned extubation. Among patients predicted to be at increased risk for extubation failure (especially with COPD), this preventive application of NIV, used immediately after extubation, improves outcome in the form of decreased post-extubation respiratory distress, reduced need for reintubation and improved survival. In contrast, the use of NIV in patients with established post-extubation respiratory failure does not appear to be effective and may be harmful. The exception is in patients with COPD, where case control data indicate that NIV is effective in patients who develop respiratory distress after extubation.

REFERENCES

1. Demoule A, Girou E, Richard JC et al. Increased use of noninvasive ventilation in French intensive care units. *Intensive Care Med.* 2006;32:1747–55.
2. Ferrer M, Esquinas A, Arancibia F et al. Noninvasive ventilation during persistent weaning failure: A randomized controlled trial. *Am J Respir Crit Care Med.* 2003;168:70–6.
3. Girault C, Daudenthun I, Chevron V et al. Noninvasive ventilation as a systematic extubation and weaning technique in acute-on-chronic respiratory failure: A prospective, randomized controlled study. *Am J Respir Crit Care Med.* 1999;160:86–92.
4. Nava S, Ambrosino N, Clini E et al. Noninvasive mechanical ventilation in the weaning of patients with respiratory failure due to chronic obstructive pulmonary disease: A randomized, controlled trial. *Ann Intern Med.* 1998;128:721–8.
5. Jaber S, Lescot T, Futier E et al. Effect of noninvasive ventilation on tracheal reintubation among patients with hypoxemic respiratory failure following abdominal surgery: A randomized clinical trial. *JAMA.* 2016;315:1345–53.
6. Esteban A, Frutos-Vivar F, Ferguson ND et al. Noninvasive positive-pressure ventilation for respiratory failure after extubation. *N Engl J Med.* 2004;350:2452–60.
7. Keenan SP, Powers C, McCormack DG et al. Noninvasive positive-pressure ventilation for postextubation respiratory distress: A randomized controlled trial. *JAMA.* 2002;287:3238–44.
8. Nava S, Gregoretti C, Fanfulla F et al. Noninvasive ventilation to prevent respiratory failure after extubation in high-risk patients. *Crit Care Med.* 2005; 33:2465–70.
9. Ferrer M, Valencia M, Nicolas JM et al. Early noninvasive ventilation averts extubation failure in patients at risk: A randomized trial. *Am J Respir Crit Care Med.* 2006;173:164–70.
10. Girault C, Briel A, Hellot MF et al. Noninvasive mechanical ventilation in clinical practice: A 2-year experience in a medical intensive care unit. *Crit Care Med.* 2003;31:552–9.
11. Schettino G, Altobelli N, Kacmarek RM. Noninvasive positive-pressure ventilation in acute respiratory failure outside clinical trials: Experience at the Massachusetts General Hospital. *Crit Care Med.* 2008;36:441–7.
12. Demoule A, Chevret S, Carlucci A et al. Changing use of noninvasive ventilation in critically ill patients: Trends over 15 years in francophone countries. *Intensive Care Med.* 2016;42:82–92.
13. Epstein S. Complications in ventilator supported patients. In: Tobin M, ed. *Principles and Practice of Mechanical Ventilation.* New York: McGraw Hill; 2006;877–902.
14. Sellares J, Ferrer J, Cano E et al. Predictors of prolonged weaning and survival during ventilator weaning in a respiratory ICU. *Intensive Care Med.* 2011;37:775–84.
15. Esteban A, Alia I, Ibanez J et al. Modes of mechanical ventilation and weaning: A national survey of Spanish hospitals: The Spanish Lung Failure Collaborative Group. *Chest.* 1994; 106:1188–93.
16. Coplin WM, Pierson DJ, Cooley KD et al. Implications of extubation delay in brain-injured patients meeting standard weaning criteria. *Am J Respir Crit Care Med.* 2000;161:1530–6.
17. Epstein SK. Decision to extubate. *Intensive Care Med.* 2002;28:535–46.
18. Frutos-Vivar F, Esteban A, Apezteguia C et al. Outcome of reintubated patients after scheduled extubation. *J Crit Care.* 2011;26:502–9.
19. Thille AW, Richard JM, Brochard L. The decision to extubate in the intensive care unit. *Am J Respir Crit Care Med.* 2013;187:1294–1302.
20. Epstein SK, Ciubotaru RL, Wong JB. Effect of failed extubation on the outcome of mechanical ventilation. *Chest.* 1997;112:186–92.

21. Gowardman JR, Huntington D, Whiting J. The effect of extubation failure on outcome in a multidisciplinary Australian intensive care unit. *Crit Care Resusc.* 2006;8:328–33.
22. de Lassence A, Alberti C, Azoulay E et al. Impact of unplanned extubation and reintubation after weaning on nosocomial pneumonia risk in the intensive care unit: A prospective multicenter study. *Anesthesiology.* 2002;97:148–56.
23. Epstein SK, Ciubotaru RL. Independent effects of etiology of failure and time to reintubation on outcome for patients failing extubation. *Am J Respir Crit Care Med.* 1998;158:489–93.
24. Esteban A, Alia I, Tobin MJ et al. Effect of spontaneous breathing trial duration on outcome of attempts to discontinue mechanical ventilation: Spanish Lung Failure Collaborative Group. *Am J Respir Crit Care Med.* 1999;159:512–18.
25. Frutos-Vivar F, Esteban A, Apezteguia C et al. Outcome of mechanically ventilated patients who require a tracheostomy. *Crit Care Med.* 2005;33:290–8.
26. Penuelas O, Frutos-Vivar F, Fernandez C et al. Characteristics and outcomes of ventilated patients according to time to liberation from mechanical ventilation. *Am J Respir Crit Care Med.* 2011;184:430–37.
27. Esteban A, Alia I, Gordo F et al. Extubation outcome after spontaneous breathing trials with T-tube or pressure support ventilation: The Spanish Lung Failure Collaborative Group. *Am J Respir Crit Care Med.* 1997;156:459–65.
28. Elmer J, Lee S, Rittenberger JC et al. Reintubation in critically ill patients: Procedural complications and implications for care. *Crit Care.* 2015;19:12.
29. Epstein SK, Nevins ML, Chung J. Effect of unplanned extubation on outcome of mechanical ventilation. *Am J Respir Crit Care Med.* 2000;161:1912–16.
30. Tahvanainen J, Salmenpera M, Nikki P. Extubation criteria after weaning from intermittent mandatory ventilation and continuous positive airway pressure. *Crit Care Med.* 1983;11:702–7.
31. Demling RH, Read T, Lind LJ et al. Incidence and morbidity of extubation failure in surgical intensive care patients. *Crit Care Med.* 1988;16:573–7.
32. Torres A, Gatell JM, Aznar E et al. Re-intubation increases the risk of nosocomial pneumonia in patients needing mechanical ventilation. *Am J Respir Crit Care Med.* 1995;152:137–41.
33. Thille AW, Harrois A, Shortgen F et al. Outcome of extubation failure In medical intensive care unit patients. *Crit Care Med.* 2011;39:2612–18.
34. Vassilakopoulos T, Zakynthinos S, Roussos C. The tension-time index and the frequency/tidal volume ratio are the major pathophysiologic determinants of weaning failure and success. *Am J Respir Crit Care Med.* 1998;158:378–85.
35. Laghi F, Cattapan SE, Jubran A et al. Is weaning failure caused by low-frequency fatigue of the diaphragm? *Am J Respir Crit Care Med.* 2003;167:120–7.
36. Jubran A, Mathru M, Dries D et al. Continuous recordings of mixed venous oxygen saturation during weaning from mechanical ventilation and the ramifications thereof. *Am J Respir Crit Care Med.* 1998;158:1763–9.
37. Dres M, Teboul JL, Monnet X. Weaning the cardiac patient from mechanical ventilation. *Curr Opin Crit Care.* 2014;20:493–8.
38. Lemaire F, Teboul JL, Cinotti L et al. Acute left ventricular dysfunction during unsuccessful weaning from mechanical ventilation. *Anesthesiology.* 1988;69:171–9.
39. Grasso S, Leone A, De Michele M et al. Use of N-terminal pro-brain natriuretic peptide to detect acute cardiac dysfunction during weaning failure in difficult-to-wean patients with chronic obstructive pulmonary disease. *Crit Care Med.* 2007;35:96–105.
40. Mekontso-Dessap A, de Prost N, Girou E et al. B-type natriuretic peptide and weaning from mechanical ventilation. *Intensive Care Med.* 2006;32:1529–36.
41. Tanios M, Epstein S, Sauser S, Chi A. Noninvasive Monitoring of cardiac output during weaning from mechanical ventilation: A pilot study. Am *J Crit Care.* 2016;25:257–65.
42. Appendini L, Patessio A, Zanaboni S et al. Physiologic effects of positive end-expiratory pressure and mask pressure support during exacerbations of chronic obstructive pulmonary disease. *Am J Respir Crit Care Med.* 1994;149:1069–76.
43. Vitacca M, Ambrosino N, Clini E et al. Physiological response to pressure support ventilation delivered before and after extubation in patients not capable of totally spontaneous autonomous breathing. *Am J Respir Crit Care Med.* 2001;164:638–41.
44. Kallet RH, Diaz JV. The physiologic effects of noninvasive ventilation. *Respir Care.* 2009;54:102–15.
45. Goodenberger DM, Couser JI Jr, May JJ. Successful discontinuation of ventilation via tracheostomy by substitution of nasal positive pressure ventilation. *Chest.* 1992;102:1277–9.
46. Restrick LJ, Scott AD, Ward EM et al. Nasal intermittent positive-pressure ventilation in weaning intubated patients with chronic respiratory disease from assisted intermittent, positive-pressure ventilation. *Respir Med.* 1993;87:199–204.
47. Udwadia ZF, Santis GK, Steven MH et al. Nasal ventilation to facilitate weaning in patients with chronic respiratory insufficiency. *Thorax.* 1992;47:715–18.
48. Gregoretti C, Beltrame F, Lucangelo U et al. Physiologic evaluation of non-invasive pressure support ventilation in trauma patients with acute respiratory failure. *Intensive Care Med.* 1998;24:785–90.

49. Kilger E, Briegel J, Haller M et al. Effects of noninvasive positive pressure ventilatory support in non-COPD patients with acute respiratory insufficiency after early extubation. *Intensive Care Med.* 1999;25:1374–80.
50. Hill N, Lin D, Levy M et al. Noninvasive positive pressure ventilation (NPPV) to facilitate extubation after acute respiratory failure: A feasibility study. *Am J Respir Crit Care Med.* 2000;161:A263.
51. Chen J, Qiu D, Tao D. Time for extubation and sequential noninvasive mechanical ventilation in COPD patients with exacerbated respiratory failure who received invasive ventilation. *Zhonghua Jie He He Hu Xi Za Zhi.* 2001;24:99–100.
52. Rabie Agmy GM, Mohamed A, Mohamed R. Noninvasive ventilation in the weaning of patients with acute-on-chronic respiratory failure due to COPD. *Chest.* 2004;126:755S.
53. Trevisan CE, Vieira SR. Noninvasive mechanical ventilation may be useful in treating patients who fail weaning from invasive mechanical ventilation: A randomized clinical trial. *Crit Care.* 2008;12:R51.
54. Prasad SB, Chaudhry D, Khanna R. Role of noninvasive ventilation in weaning from mechanical ventilation in patients with chronic obstructive pulmonary disease: An Indian experience. Indian *J Crit Care. Med.* 2009;13:207–12.
55. Girault C, Bubenheim M, Abroug F et al. Non invasive ventilation and weaning in patients with chronic hypercapnic respiratory failure. *Am J Respir Crit Care Med.* 2011;184:672–9.
56. Vaschetto R, Turucz E, Dellapiazza F et al. Noninvasive ventilation after early extubatoin in patients recovering from hypoxemic respiratory failure: A single center feasibility study. *Intensive Care Med.* 2012;38:1599–606.
57. Tawfeek MM, Ali-Elnabtity AM. Noninvasive proportional assist ventilation may be useful in weaning patients who failed a spontaneous breathing trial. *Egyptian J Anaesthes.* 2012;28:89–94.
58. Rabie Agmy GM, Metwally MM. Noninvasive ventilation in the weaning of patients with acute-on-chronic respiratory failure due to COPD. *Egyptian J Chest Dis Tuberculosis.* 2012;28:84–91.
59. Carron M, Rossi S, Carollo C et al. Comparison of invasive and noninvasive positive pressure ventilation delivered by means of a helmet for weaning of patients from mechanical ventilation. *J Crit Care.* 2014;29:580–5.
60. Burns KEA, Meade MO, Premji A et al. Noninvasive ventilation as a weaning strategy for mechanical ventilation in adults with respiratory failure: A Cochrane systematic review. *CMAJ.* 2014;186:E112–22.
61. Kress JP, Pohlman AS, O'Connor MF et al. Daily interruption of sedative infusions in critically ill patients undergoing mechanical ventilation. *N Engl J Med.* 2000;342:1471–7.
62. Kirton OC, DeHaven CB, Morgan JP et al. Elevated imposed work of breathing masquerading as ventilator weaning intolerance. *Chest.* 1995;108:1021–5.
63. Keenan SP, Sinuff T, Cook DJ et al. Which patients with acute exacerbation of chronic obstructive pulmonary disease benefit from noninvasive positive-pressure ventilation? A systematic review of the literature. *Ann Intern Med.* 2003;138:861–70.
64. Hilbert G, Gruson D, Portel L et al. Noninvasive pressure support ventilation in COPD patients with postextubation hypercapnic respiratory insufficiency. *Eur Respir J.* 1998;11:1349–53.
65. Meduri GU, Turner RE, Abou-Shala N et al. Noninvasive positive pressure ventilation via face mask. First-line intervention in patients with acute hypercapnic and hypoxemic respiratory failure. *Chest.* 1996;109:179–93.
66. Chiang AA, Lee KC. Use of noninvasive positive pressure ventilation via nasal mask in patients with respiratory distress after extubation. Zhonghua Yi Xue Za Zhi (Taipei) 1995;56:94–101.
67. Jiang JS, Kao SJ, Wang SN. Effect of early application of biphasic positive airway pressure on the outcome of extubation in ventilator weaning. *Respirology.* 1999;4:161–5.
68. El-Solh AA, Aquilina A, Pineda L et al. Noninvasive ventilation for prevention of post-extubation respiratory failure in obese patients. *Eur Respir J.* 2006;28:588–95.
69. Ferrer M, Sellares J, Valencia M et al. Non-invasive ventilation after extubation in hypercapnic patients with chronic respiratory disorders: A randomized controlled trial. *Lancet.* 2009;374:1082–8.
70. Khilnani GC, Galle AD, Hadda V et al. Non-invasive ventilation after extubation in patients with chronic obstructive airways disease: A randomised controlled trial. *Anaesth Intensive Care.* 2011;39:217–23.
71. Su CL, Chiang LL, Yang SH et al. Preventive use of noninvasive ventilation after extubation: A prospective, multicenter randomized controlled trial. *Respir Care.* 2012;57:204–10.
72. Ornico SR, Lobo SM, Sanches HS et al. Noninvasive ventilation immediately after extubation improves weaning outcome after acute respiratory failure: A randomized controlled trial. *Crit Care.* 2013;17:R39.
73. Mohamed KAE, Abdalla MH. Role of non invasive ventilation in limiting re-intubation after planned extubation. *Egyptian J Chest Dis Tuberculosis.* 2013;62:669–74.
74. Epstein SK. Noninvasive ventilation to shorten the duration of mechanical ventilation. *Respir Care.* 2009;54:198–208;discussion 11.
75. Bajaj A, Rathor P, Shegal V et al. Efficacy of non-invasive ventilation after planned extubation: A systematic review and meta-analysis of randomized controlled trials. *Heart Lung.* 2015;44:150–7.
76. Hernandez G, Vaquero C, Gonzalez P et al. Effect of postextubation high-flow nasal cannula vs conventional oxygen therapy on reintubation in low-risk patients. *JAMA.* 2016;315:1354–61.

67

Weaning strategies and protocols

MICHELE VITACCA AND LUCA BARBANO

INTRODUCTION

In the past 15 years, the availability of beds intensive care units (ICUs), new technologies and improved levels of care have increased the population of patients defined as 'survivors of catastrophic illness', often requiring prolonged weaning procedures.[1] About 80% of patients admitted to an ICU and mechanically ventilated because of acute respiratory failure (ARF) resume spontaneous breathing quite easily after a few days of ventilation.[2] The weaning success rate differs among studies depending on the case mix and referrals to an individual ICU. The 20% unsuccessful cases are mainly concentrated in specific populations, in which age, residual or premorbidity impairment of the cardiorespiratory or neuromuscular systems renders the discontinuation from mechanical ventilation particularly difficult.[2] These patients represent <10% of ICU admissions but account for a huge demand on financial resources.[1] In addition, from a financial point of view, prolonged mechanical ventilation (>30 days) in the ICU results in high costs for the healthcare system.[3] To this end, new strategies and protocols for weaning from mechanical ventilation are clearly needed in the daily practice of healthcare.

Weaning from mechanical ventilation: Rarely early, often too late

While unnecessary delays in withdrawing mechanical ventilation can increase the risk of complications, prolong ICU stay and significantly amplify healthcare costs, premature attempts at withdrawal of mechanical ventilation might lead to the development of severe distress, hamper the recovery process and further delay weaning.[4] Physicians often fail to recognise patients who may already be ready for extubation. Studies among patients who are accidentally or self-extubated demonstrate that 23% of patients receiving full mechanical ventilation and 69% of patients who have begun weaning do not require reintubation.[5,6] On the other hand, 5%–20% of patients who are successfully weaned and possibly extubated need subsequent tracheal reintubation within the next 48–72 hours.[7] In one study, 35% of tracheostomised patients who were considered ineligible for weaning, once referred from one facility to another, underwent spontaneous breathing without any additional weaning attempt.[8] For all these reasons, in current clinical practice, the variability regarding weaning decisions is evident in terms of correct time of extubation, types of ventilation needed, how to use these techniques, criteria for poor tolerance on the spontaneous breathing test (SBT) and personnel involved in the weaning process. That is, there are different approaches depending on the underlying disease and definition of definitive weaning failure. Tobin[9] proposed a series of stages in the process of care, from intubation and initiation of mechanical ventilation through initiation of the weaning effort to the ultimate liberation from mechanical ventilation and successful extubation. These six stages are described as follows[9]: (1) treatment of ARF; (2) suspicion that weaning may be possible; (3) assessment of readiness to wean; (4) SBT; (5) extubation; and possibly (6) reintubation. It is important to recognise that delay in reaching stage 2, the suspicion that weaning may be possible, and beginning stage 3, assessing readiness to wean, is a common cause of delayed weaning. Stage 2 begins when the clinician first thinks there is a reasonable probability of weaning success. Stage 3 begins when the clinician actually initiates a process of daily tests of readiness to wean in order to confirm this suspicion. Stage 3 ends when the results of the daily test cause a reassessment of the probability to a high enough level to justify an SBT. The weaning process begins with the first SBT, defined as a T-tube trial or a low-level pressure support (PS).[4]

Definition of successful weaning

Brochard during the International Consensus Conference of Budapest, in 2007, proposed a classification of patients according to difficulty and length of the weaning process[4] (Figure 67.1): Group 1 includes patients who successfully

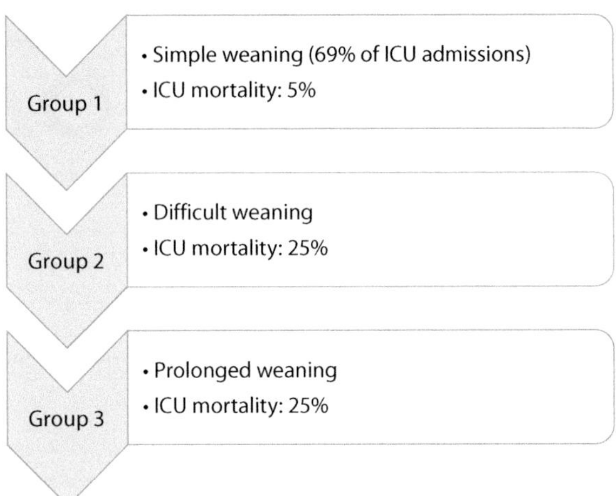

Figure 67.1 Group 1: patients who successfully pass the initial SBT and are successfully extubated on the first attempt; group 2: patients who require up to three SBT or as long as 7 days from the first SBT to achieve successful weaning; group 3: patients who require more than three SBTs or 7 days of weaning after the first SBT.

pass the initial SBT and are successfully extubated on the first attempt; group 2 includes patients with difficult weaning and patients who require up to three SBT or as long as 7 days from the first SBT to achieve successful weaning. Group 3, prolonged weaning, includes patients who require more than three SBT or 7 days of weaning after the first SBT. As has been recently, and correctly, stated, 'the physician should distinguish between liberation (no need for the ventilator) and extubation (no need for endotracheal tube)', so that after a patient has successfully undergone a trial of unassisted breathing, one must re-evaluate the continuing need for an artificial airway. The other crucial point, never systematically addressed, is to define the minimum time patients must remain disconnected from a ventilator to consider them as 'weaned'. Most of the published studies specify that a time interval of 48 hours is enough to believe that any reintubation would be for reasons other than premature extubation. A national survey performed in Spain addressed weaning problems.[10] It was reported that 41% of the total time of mechanical ventilation was devoted to weaning, with large differences among patients with different diseases.[10] For example, the process of discontinuation from mechanical ventilation was ≥50% only in patients with chronic obstructive pulmonary disease (COPD), chronic heart failure or neurological problems.

How the weaning process should be conducted

Strategies shown to be effective in promoting timely weaning include weaning attempts and weaning protocols. There are various strategies that may also promote timely and successful weaning including bundling of SBTs with sedation and delirium monitoring/management as well as early mobility, the use of automated weaning systems and modes that improve patient–ventilator interaction, mechanical insufflation–exsufflation as a weaning adjunct, early extubation to non-invasive ventilation and high-flow humidified oxygen.[11] A variety of mechanical ventilation strategies have been proposed to facilitate the separation or release of the patient from mechanical ventilation. Among different modalities, the most used and studied have been pressure support ventilation (PSV) and SBT.[12–14] In a recent meta-analysis published in 2014, Blackwood et al.[15] consider 17 studies (period of 1993–2014) and, in a subgroup analysis, show a reduction of days of ventilation with a method of stepwise reduction (either intermittent mandatory ventilation or PSV, six trials included studies with automatic system) compared to SBT protocol (eight trials) in total duration of mechanical ventilation.[15] In another recent meta-analysis, Ladeira et al.[16] have found evidence of generally low quality from studies comparing PSV and a T-tube. The effects on weaning success, ICU mortality, reintubation, ICU and Longterm Weaning Unit (LWU) length of stay and pneumonia were imprecise. However, PSV was more effective than a T-tube for successful SBTs among patients with simple weaning. Based on the findings of single trials, three studies presented a shorter weaning duration in the group undergoing PS SBT; however, a fourth study found a shorter weaning duration with a T-tube.[16] More recently, Bosma et al.[17] enrolled 54 intubated patients with various pathologies, excluded neuromuscular diseases and compared weaning process on PS to proportional assist ventilation (PAV) and showed feasibility safety and utility about the utilisation of this modality of ventilation. The duration of ventilator support is shorter if weaning is contemplated at the earliest possible time during the period of mechanical ventilation, and repeated assessments of patients expedite the process.[18] The development of ventilators that enable computerized weaning draw attention to a major problem in ventilator management: clinicians are slow to initiate weaning.[19] The risk that protocols hinder rather than expedite weaning seems reasonable. Difficulties in ventilator weaning can result from respiratory muscle weakness, abnormal respiratory mechanics, impaired gas exchange, cardiac dysfunction, psychological distress and other factors.[18] Determining the reason for difficulty in weaning in a particular patient requires an astute clinician rather than a sophisticated protocol.[20] Few aspects of critical care medicine are more dependent on diagnostic acumen and individualised care.[19] Individualised care is the antithesis of protocolised care, which has been proposed in literature.[20]

Automated systems

Given that protocolised weaning is a complex intervention with multiple interrelated and interdependent components, interpretation of literature should take into account the contextual and intervention factors that are likely to have impact on protocolised weaning. Box 67.1 summarises the most frequent automated closed-loop systems available for weaning.[11] The most frequent automated systems are

BOX 67.1: Automated closed-loop systems available for weaning

PAV: Adjusts airway pressure based on measurement of compliance and resistance throughout the inspiratory cycle to maintain a clinician selected % degree of support.
Mandatory minute ventilation: closed-loop control of the mandatory breath rate while considering the patient's spontaneous breath rate based on a clinician predetermined MV.
SmartCare: closed-loop control of PS based on monitoring of respiratory rate, tidal volume and end-tidal carbon dioxide.
ASV: closed-loop control of inspiratory pressure and mandatory breath rate on a breath-by-breath basis to maintain pre-set minimum MV; automatically switches to PSV and adapts PS based on respiratory rate and tidal volume.
Automode: Switches from a controlled mode (for example pressure control ventilation) to a support mode (for example PSV) based on the detection of patient triggering of two consecutive breaths.
Proportional pressure support (PPS): PS is proportionately provided to changes in airway resistance and lung compliance. PPS is based on the PAV algorithm.
NAVA: Partial ventilatory support proportional to inspiratory diaphragmatic electrical activity measured via an oesophageal catheter.
INTELLIVENT-ASV®: Extension of ASV that uses closed-loop control to adjust MV using end-tidal carbon dioxide and oxygenation by adjusting PEEP and the fraction of inspired oxygen.
Mandatory rate ventilation: closed-loop control to adjust PS based on a respiratory rate target.

Adapted from Rose L, *Intensive Crit Care Nurs*, 31, 89–95, 2015.

SmartCare/PS™ and Adaptive Support Ventilation (ASV). SmartCare is a closed-loop control of PS based on the monitoring of respiratory rate, tidal volume and end-tidal carbon dioxide with tests for extubation readiness using a one hour spontaneous breath trial. The ASV is a closed-loop control of inspiratory pressure and mandatory breath rate on a breath-by-breath basis to maintain preset minimum minute ventilation (MV), automatically switches to PSV and adapts PS based on respiratory rate and tidal volume. Neurally adjusted ventilatory assist (NAVA) is a partial ventilatory support proportional to inspiratory diaphragmatic electrical activity measured via an oesophageal catheter extension of ASV that uses closed-loop control to adjust MV using end-tidal carbon dioxide and oxygenation by adjusting positive end-expiratory pressure (PEEP) and the fraction of inspired oxygen. There are controversial results about the use of this systems. Recently, various studies compare weaning duration by type of approach: professional led versus computed driven. The subgroup analysis of a previous meta-analisis by Blackwood et al.[15] shows a significant reduction of time of weaning (hours) with professional led compared to computed led. In this meta-analysis only 2 studies analysed computed led versus 12 studies that analysed professional led weaning. Otherwise, a meta-analysis performed by Burns et al.,[21] who collected 10 trials with 654 patients (two of these with high risks of bias), compared non automated weaning strategies with weaning with SmartCare. Smart Care weaning significantly decreased mechanical ventilation time, time to successful extubation, ICU stay and percentage of patients receiving ventilation for longer than 7 and 21 days. It also showed a favourable trend towards fewer patients receiving ventilation for longer than 14 days; however, the estimated effect was imprecise. Summary estimates from review suggest that these benefits may be achieved without increasing the risk of adverse events, especially reintubation; however, the quality of the evidence ranged from low to moderate, and evidence was derived from 10 small randomised controlled trials. A more recent meta-analysis[22] collected data from 21 trials (1676 participants) until year 2013 and showed that automated systems (SmartCare and ASV) may reduce weaning and ventilation duration and ICU stay. No conclusion is possible to be drawn with other systems of computed driven weaning. No difference was found in surgical population due to substantial trials heterogeneity. Hence an adequately powered, high quality, multicentre randomized controlled trial is needed.

Weaning protocols

Respiratory care protocols (i.e. nurse- or therapist-driven) have been extensively investigated for the discontinuation of mechanical ventilation.[23–26] These protocols are drawn from a medical critical care population where the duration of mechanical ventilation greatly exceeds that seen in mixed surgical populations.[27] Weaning protocols are a consensus of medical knowledge and opinions: they are synthesised into a care plan or algorithm to guide the weaning on changes in measurable patients variables.[28] The weaning protocol team usually consists of a physician, a patient, a family, a nurse and a respiratory therapist.[28] The daily tasks in a weaning protocol consist of recording functional activities early in the morning, followed by a rest period before initiating the weaning process in the best position, e.g. sitting upright in bed or in a chair.[29] The plan for a weaning protocol also addresses the prevention and amelioration of the deleterious effects of lying in bed, communication, emotional support and psychological well-being.[29] Initial evaluation includes the assessment of the patient and ventilator status and patient–ventilator synchrony. This evaluation is usually performed routinely within a range of 2–4 hours and together with change in each ventilator setting.

Box 67.2 summarises the criteria proposed in the literature to start and conduct a weaning protocol. In a survey of 460 ICUs in 17 European countries, the respiratory therapist was reported to be active in the adjustment of mechanical ventilation in 12%, in weaning from mechanical ventilation in 22%, in extubation in 25% and in the implementation of non-invasive mechanical ventilation (NIV) in 46% of ICUs.[30] The implementation of weaning protocols decreased the duration of mechanical ventilation[31,32] and ICU stay[24–27] by increasing the number of safe extubations[26] and reducing by 50% the complications related to the ventilator.[24,27,33] The use of weaning protocols has also been found to be cost-effective.[24,25] The importance of a motivated weaning team has been stressed by Henneman et al.[34] and Chan et al.[35] as well as the importance of improving the technology behind the use of weaning protocols.[36] In neurosurgical patients,[37] in infants or children when the majority of patients are rapidly extubated,[38] in traumatic patients[39] or in ICU with doctors with a particular interest in weaning and already providing high-quality critical care,[40] weaning protocols have been shown to give similar results to those observed in typical daily care. To this end, Krishan et al.[40] study deserves a special comment: the doctor hours dedicated to each patient were very high (9.5 hours/bed/day) when compared to other studies, and this may be the real explanation for the lack of superiority of a strict protocol in comparison with the doctor's job. A recent previously cited meta-analysis[15] confirms our review on main results. Blackwood collected 17 studies (2434 pts) and showed that standardised weaning protocols reduced the duration of mechanical ventilation, weaning duration and ICU length of stay. Reductions are most likely to occur in medical, surgical and mixed ICUs, but not in neurosurgical ICUs. However, significant heterogeneity among studies indicates caution in generalising results. Few patients with primarily ventilatory impairment due to neuromuscular weakness are weaned from mechanical ventilation. The same patients are considered at high risk of post-extubation failure.

BOX 67.2: Criteria used in the literature to start weaning or to test weaning steps failure

Objective measurements

- PaO_2: >60–65 mmHg; SaO_2: >88%–90%, FiO_2: 40%–60%, PaO_2/FiO_2: ≥200; PEEP: <5–10 cm H_2O
- Haemodynamic stability: no vasopressors or inotropic substances, dopamine <5 g/kg/min, no arrhythmia; systolic pressure: >90 and <180 mmHg; HR: >50 and <140 beats per minute
- Temperature: <37°C–38°C
- No respiratory acidosis under MV: pH: >7.35, $PaCO_2$: <50 mmHg
- Haemoglobin: >8/10 g/dL
- Glasgow Coma Scale score: ≥10–13
- No infusion of sedatives
- Peak expiratory flow measured after cough under endotracheal tube or tracheostomy >160 L/min
- Normal electrolytes
- MIP: ≥20–22 cm H_2O
- Static compliance: >25 mL/cm H_2O

Subjective measurements

- No use of accessory muscles
- Good neurological level
- Able to open the mouth
- No signs of distress
- Possibility of cough
- No distress during an SBT

Ventilator parameters

- Respiratory rate: ≤35/min
- MV: ≤10–15 L/min
- Tobin index (*f*/*Vt*): ≤105
- Vital capacity: >10 mL/kg or double of VTe
- Vte: >5 mL/kg or >0.3 L

Weaning in neuromuscular patients

Conventional weaning protocols for advanced neuromuscular patients have a significant risk of extubation failure: neuromuscular patients unable to pass the SBT should undergo tracheostomy.[4,41] A dedicated protocol for extubation in non-bulbar neuromuscular patients has been developed by Bach et al.[41] using continuous NIV and mechanically assisted cough. Briefly, a nasogastric tube was removed and a non-invasive interface was placed for immediate post-extubation. NIV was set with PSV or assist-control volumes. No supplemental oxygen was added and, for episodes of SpO_2 < 95%, NIV and mechanically assisted coughing were used at pressures of 40–60 cm H_2O to −40 to −60 cm H_2O as needed until SpO_2 returned to ≥95% via the airway tube and subsequently via the oronasal interface.[41] This protocol has demonstrated that neuromuscular patients who are unable to pass ventilator weaning trials, with very low vital capacity and peak cough flow, can be successfully extubated, suggesting that early tracheostomy somehow facilitates ventilator weaning. The implementation of a validated weaning protocol is feasible as is a respiratory therapist-driven protocol without daily supervision by a weaning physician or a specific team.[42] Scheinhorn et al.[43] reported an expected variability in the daily application of a well-designed weaning protocol, leading to the conclusion that both doctors and respiratory therapists may be confident in using this approach, which, over the years, has resulted in improvement in several aspects. More recently, Zhu et al.,[44] in a very large study which involved 1428 patients, demonstrated that a quality improvement programme defined as systematic data-guided activities designed to bring about immediate improvements in healthcare delivery in particular settings and characterised by strict observation of patients by residents of ICU involving protocol-directed weaning is associated with beneficial clinical outcomes in mechanically ventilated patients. A protocol to start weaning or whether to decide the extubation time is mandatory. However, less evidence is available about the need of a strict protocol on performing weaning in terms of modality and time to dedicate to each step of weaning.[45] Weaning processes are necessary as feedback for young doctors, for ICUs with a high turnover and in operative units with a rapid turnover in expertise to better integrate different sanitary professionals creating a weaning team and to better document the clinical activity.[45] Whatever the explanation, it is important for us to highlight that in the weaning process, the method employed is probably less important than the confidence and familiarity with the technique adopted and that the same ventilatory approach may result in different outcomes depending on the underlying diseases. The way to conduct weaning and patient's underlying conditions – rather than ventilator modality per se – may influence weaning outcome as days of MV and percentage of success but will have no effect on survival.[46]

Factors influencing weaning outcome

REHABILITATION

The prevention of ICU-acquired weakness, which has been found to prolong the period of weaning from mechanical ventilation, combined with daily sedation interruption (DSI) and SBT, could result in a shorter duration of mechanical ventilation. A strategy for whole-body rehabilitation – consisting of the interruption of sedation and physical and occupational therapy in the earliest days of critical illness – was safe and well tolerated and resulted in better functional outcomes at hospital discharge, a shorter duration of delirium and more ventilator-free days compared with standard care.[47] For the first time, Martin et al.[48] showed a relationship between upper limb motor strength and weaning time, demonstrating that higher was the arm strength obtained during rehabilitation and shorter were the days spent under mechanical ventilation. The sonographic diaphragmatic parameters can provide valuable information in the assessment and follow-up of patients with diaphragmatic weakness, in terms of patient–ventilator interactions during controlled or assisted modalities of mechanical ventilation and can potentially help understand post-operative pulmonary dysfunction or weaning failure from mechanical ventilation.[49]

FLUID MANAGEMENT

Dessap et al.[50] shows that fluid management guided by daily B-type natriuretic peptide (BNP) plasma concentrations improves weaning outcomes compared with empirical therapy dictated by clinical acumen. They enrolled in a controlled multicentre study 304 patients to either a BNP-driven or a physician-driven strategy of fluid management during ventilator weaning. To standardise the weaning process, patients in both groups were ventilated with an automatic computer-driven weaning system. Time to successful extubation was significantly shorter with the BNP-driven strategy. The BNP-driven strategy increased the number of ventilator-free days but did not change the length of stay or mortality. The effect on weaning time was strongest in patients with left ventricular systolic dysfunction.

SEDATION

Continuous infusions of sedative drugs in the ICU may postpone the weaning process from mechanical ventilation. The necessity to follow protocols to correctly use sedative drugs has been recently studied. The use of protocol-directed sedation with daily withdrawal of sedative drug infusions can reduce, in critically ill patients with ARF, the duration of mechanical ventilation[51–54]; ICU and hospital length of stay[51–54]; need for tracheostomy[51]; or other complications such as ventilator-associated pneumonia, upper gastrointestinal haemorrhage, barotraumas and venous thromboembolic disease[53]; during the year after enrolment, patients in the group of protocol sedation were less likely to die than were patients in the control group.[54] Otherwise, Burry et al.[55] in a meta-analysis published in 2014 did not find strong evidence that DSI alters the duration of mechanical ventilation, mortality, length of ICU or hospital stay, adverse event rates, drug consumption or quality of life for critically ill adults receiving mechanical ventilation compared to sedation strategies that do not include DSI. These results should be considered unstable rather than negative for DSI given the statistical and clinical heterogeneity identified in the included trials.[55]

CARE FACILITY AVAILABILITY

Long-term acute care hospitals play an increasingly important role in patients with chronic critical illness. Yet few data exist to guide decision-making about transfer or to inform policy decisions about whether to support or restrict this rapidly growing cost centre. The main benefits of chronic ventilator facilities seems to be (1) the possibility of relieving congestion of ICU beds, (2) maintaining a high level of nursing assistance, (3) responding to sudden changes in a patient's clinical condition, (4) allowing enough time for a multidisciplinary rehabilitation approach and (5) acting as a bridge to home care programs or other forms of continuous chronic assistance (e.g. telemedicine or dedicated long-term units).[45]

Specific populations

TRACHEOSTOMISED

Our data[8] show that SBTs and decreasing levels of inspiratory PSV are equally effective in weaning COPD tracheostomised patients undergoing mechanical ventilation for >15 days. Whatever the explanation, it is important to highlight that in the weaning process, the method employed is probably less important than the confidence in and familiarity with the technique adopted and that the same ventilatory approach may produce different outcomes depending on the underlying pathologies. Otherwise, Jubran et al.[56]

in a 2013 paper say that among patients requiring prolonged mechanical ventilation and treated at a single long-term care facility, unassisted breathing through a tracheostomy, compared with PS, resulted in shorter median weaning time, although weaning mode had no effect on survival at 6 and 12 months. Hernandez et al.[57] performed a single-centre randomised trial conducted in a general ICU and compared the effects of deflating the tracheal cuff during disconnections from mechanical ventilation in tracheostomised patients and found that deflating the tracheal cuff in those patients shortens weaning, reduces respiratory infections and probably improves swallowing.[57]

NEUROLOGICAL PATIENTS

In neurosurgical patients, when physicians do not extubate patients following a successful SBT,[30] weaning protocols have been shown to give similar results to those observed in typical daily care. Roquilly et al.[58] enrolled 499 brain-injured patients and assessed the effectiveness of an evidence-based extubation readiness bundle associating protective ventilation, early enteral nutrition, local protocol for the probabilistic treatment of hospital-acquired pneumonia and systematic approach to extubation. They showed that was associated with a reduction in the duration of mechanical ventilation and in the rates of hospital-acquired pneumonia and of unplanned extubation.[58]

Future research

As most critically ill patients requiring mechanical ventilation will tolerate extubation with minimal weaning, the identification of strategies to improve the management of those patients experiencing difficult and prolonged weaning should be a priority for clinical practice, quality improvement initiatives and weaning research. Future studies should define the minimal criteria required for assessing the correct weaning time in view of the different underlying diseases; the need for a screening test prior to the SBT; the identification of patients who are successful on an SBT but who fail extubation; the role of constant positive airway pressure/PEEP in the COPD patient undergoing an SBT; required duration of the SBT in patients who failed the initial trial; and which specific aspects improve the weaning outcome. In the last few years, there have been significant advances that have allowed an improvement in the duration and the withdrawal of mechanical ventilation in critically ill patients. However, more clinical research is needed to identify patients at high risk for extubation failure, disconnection strategies of prolonged mechanical ventilation and application of new techniques of weaning that may contribute to the decrease in the mortality in critically ill patients. Future research will be focused on how the clinical context influences outcome as well as provide insights into aid implementation in other settings and an ability to separate effectiveness of the intervention from effectiveness of implementation. In addition, an economic evaluation taking into consideration the cost-effectiveness of protocolised weaning versus individualised care, not only from the payer's perspective, but also from that of service users and society as a whole, would be useful for decision makers.

CONCLUSIONS

Weaning should be considered in the early stages in patients receiving mechanical ventilation. The majority of patients can be successfully weaned at the first attempt. The duration of ventilator support is shorter if weaning is contemplated at the earliest possible time during the period of mechanical ventilation, and repeated assessments of patients expedite the process. For the majority of patients, the SBT is the major diagnostic test to determine if they can be successfully extubated. The initial SBT should last for 30 min and consist of either T-tube breathing or low levels of PSV with or without 5 cm H_2O PEEP. Synchronised intermittent mechanical ventilation should be avoided as a weaning modality. The major limitation of weaning protocols is the lack of generalisability in different diseases and conditions: different diseases require different physiopathological approaches and thus require different weaning approach. A protocol to start weaning or to decide the extubation time is mandatory. Conversely, less evidence is available about the need for a rigid protocol to perform weaning in terms of the modality chosen or the time dedicated for each step of weaning. The risk that protocols hinder rather than expedite weaning seems reasonable. The art of weaning is often dependent on diagnostic acumen and individualized care that is the antithesis of protocolized care. Anyway, weaning protocols seems useful as feedback for young doctors, for ICUs with a high turnover, for units with a rapid change in expertise, for better cooperation between the different members of a weaning team and to better document the clinical activity, for COPD patients and for prolonged or difficult to wean patients.

How the weaning is conducted and the patient's underlying condition may be more influential than the ventilator modality per se when considering weaning outcomes (days of mechanical ventilation and rate of success but not survival).

REFERENCES

1. Nava S, Vitacca M. Chronic ventilator facilities. In: Tobin M, ed. *Principles and practice of mechanical ventilation*. New York: McGraw-Hill; 2006:691–704.
2. Carlet J, Artigas A, Bihari D et al. The first European Consensus Conference in intensive care medicine: Introductory remarks. *Intensive Care Med.* 1992; 18:180–1.
3. Halpern NA, Bettes L, Greenstein R. Federal and nationwide intensive care units and healthcare costs: 1986–1992. *Crit Care Med.* 1994;22:2001–7.

4. Boles JM, Bion J, Connors A et al. Task force weaning from mechanical ventilation statement of the Sixth International Consensus Conference on intensive care medicine. *Eur Respir J.* 2007;29:1033–56.
5. Epstein SK, Nevins ML, Chung J. Effect of unplanned extubation on outcome of mechanical ventilation. *Am J Respir Crit Care Med.* 2000;161:1912–16.
6. Betbese AJ, Perez M, Bak E et al. A prospective study of unplanned endotracheal extubation in intensive care unit patients. *Crit Care Med.* 1998;26:1180–6.
7. Nevins ML, Chung J. Effect of unplanned extubation on outcome of mechanical ventilation. *Am J Respir Crit Care Med.* 2000;161:1912–16.
8. Vitacca M, Vianello A, Colombo D et al. Comparison of two methods for weaning patients with chronic obstructive pulmonary disease requiring mechanical ventilation for more than 15 days. *Am J Respir Crit Care Med.* 2001;164:225–30.
9. Tobin MJ. Role and interpretation of weaning predictors. As presented at the 5th International Consensus Conference in Intensive Care Medicine: Weaning from Mechanical Ventilation. Hosted by ERS, ATS, ESICM, SCCM and SRLF, Budapest, April 28–29, 2005. Available at: http://www.ersnet.org/ers/lr/browse/default.aspx?id52814.
10. Esteban A, Alia I, Ibanez J et al. Modes of mechanical ventilation and weaning: A national survey of Spanish hospitals: The Spanish Lung Failure Collaborative Group. *Chest.* 1994;106:1188–93.
11. Rose L. Strategies for weaning from mechanical ventilation: A state of the art review. *Intensive Crit Care Nurs.* 2015;31:189–95.
12. Brochard L, Rauss A, Benito S et al. Comparison of three methods of gradual withdrawal from ventilatory support during weaning from mechanical ventilation. *Am J Respir Crit Care Med.* 1994;150:896–903.
13. Esteban A, Frutos F, Tobin MJ et al. A comparison of four methods of weaning patients from mechanical ventilation. *N Engl J Med.* 1995;332:345–50.
14. Esteban A, Alia I, Tobin MJ et al. Effect of spontaneous breathing trial duration on outcome of attempts to discontinue mechanical ventilation. *Am J Respir Crit Care Med.* 1999;159:512–18.
15. Blackwood B, Burns KEA, Cardwell CR et al. Protocolized versus non-protocolized weaning for reducing the duration of mechanical ventilation in critically ill adult patients (Review) *Cochrane Database Syst Rev.* 2014;11.
16. Ladeira MT, Vital FMR, Andriolo RB et al. Pressure support versus T-tube for weaning from mechanical ventilation in adults (Review). *Cochrane Database Syst Rev.* 2014;5.
17. Bosma KJ, Read BA, Bahrgard Nikoo MJ et al. A Pilot randomized trial comparing weaning from mechanical ventilation on pressure support versus proportional assist ventilation. *Crit Care Med.* 2016.
18. Tobin MJ, Jubran A. Weaning from mechanical ventilation. In: Tobin MJ, ed. *Principles and practice of mechanical ventilation*, 2nd ed. New York, NY: McGraw-Hill; 2006:1185–220.
19. Tobin MJ. Remembrance of weaning past: The seminal papers. *Intensive Care Med.* 2006;32:1485–93.
20. Adlgüzel N, Güngör G, Tobin MJ. Hippocrates is alive and weaning in Brazil. *Crit Care.* 2009;13:142.
21. Burns KEA, Lellouche F, Nisenbaum R et al. Automated weaning and SBT systems versus non-automated weaning strategies for weaning time in invasively ventilated critically ill adults (Review). *Cochrane Database Syst Rev.* 2014:CD008638.
22. Rose L, Schultz MJ, Cardwell CR et al. Automated versus non-automated weaning for reducing the duration of mechanical ventilation. *Crit Care.* 2015;19:48.
23. Ely EW, Meade MO, Haponik EF et al. Mechanical ventilator weaning protocols driven by non physician health-care professionals: Evidence-based clinical practice guidelines. *Chest.* 2001;120:454S–63S.
24. Ely EW, Baker AM, Dunagan DP et al. Effect of the duration of mechanical ventilation of identifying patients capable of breathing spontaneously. *N Engl J Med.* 1996;335:1864–9.
25. Kollef MH, Shapiro SD, Silver P et al. A randomized, controlled trial of protocol-directed versus physician-directed weaning from mechanical ventilation. *Crit Care Med.* 1997;25:567–74.
26. Saura P, Blanch L, Mestre J et al. Clinical consequences of the implementation of a weaning protocol. *Intensive Care Med.* 1996;22:1052–6.
27. Marelich GP, Murin S, Battistella F et al. Protocol weaning of mechanical ventilation in medical and surgical patients by respiratory care practitioners and nurses: Effect on weaning time and incidence of VAP. *Chest.* 2000;118:459–67.
28. Durbin C. Therapist driven protocols in adult intensive care unit patients. In: Stoller JK, Kester L, eds. *Therapist driven protocols*. Philadelphia, PA: Saunders Company; 1996.
29. ACCP, AARC, ACCCM task force. Evidence based guidelines for weaning and discontinuing ventilatory support. *Chest.* 2001;120:375s–95s.
30. Norrenberg M, Vincent JL. A profile of European intensive care unit physiotherapists: European Society of Intensive Care Medicine. *Intensive Care Med.* 2000;26:988–94.
31. Horst HM, Mouro D, Hall-Jenssens RA et al. Decrease in ventilation time with a standardized weaning process. *Arch Surg.* 1998;133:483–9.
32. Kollef MH, Levy NT, Ahrens TS et al. The use of continuous IV sedation is associated with prolongation of mechanical ventilation. *Chest.* 1998;114:541–8.
33. Dries DJ, McGonigal MD, Malian MS et al. Protocol-driven ventilator weaning reduces use of mechanical ventilation, rate of early reintubation, and ventilator-associated pneumonia. *J Trauma.* 2004;56:943–51.

34. Henneman E, Dracup K, Ganz T et al. Effect of a collaborative weaning plan on patient outcome in the critical care setting. *Crit Care Med.* 2001;29:297–303.
35. Chan PK, Fischer S, Stewart TE et al. Practising evidence-based medicine: The design and implementation of multidisciplinary team-driven extubation protocol. *Crit Care.* 2001;5:349–54.
36. Iregui M, Ward S, Clinikscale D et al. Use of handheld computer by respiratory care practitioners to improve the efficacy of weaning patients from MV. *Crit Care Med.* 2002;30:2038–204.
37. Namen AM, Ely W, Tatter SB et al. Predictors of successful extubation in neurological patients. *Am J Respir Crit Care Med.* 2001;163:658–64.
38. Randolph AG, Wypij D, Venkataraman ST et al. Effect of mechanical ventilator weaning protocols on respiratory outcomes in infants and children. A randomised controlled trial. *JAMA.* 2002;288:2561–8.
39. Duane TM, Riblet JL, Golay D et al. Protocol driven ventilator management in a trauma Intensive care unit population. *Arch Surg.* 2002;137:1223–7.
40. Krishan JA, Moore D, Robeson C et al. A prospective controlled trial of a protocol-based strategy to discontinue mechanical ventilation. *Am J Respir Crit Care Med.* 2004;169:673–8.
41. Bach JR, Gonçalves MR, Hamdani I et al. Extubation of patients with neuromuscular weakness: A new management paradigm. *Chest.* 2009.
42. Ely EW, Bennett PA, Bowton DL et al. Large scale implementation of a respiratory therapist-driven protocol for ventilator weaning. *Am J Respir Crit Care Med.* 1999;159:439–46.
43. Scheinhorn D, Chao DC, Stearn-Hassenpflug M et al. Outcome in post-ICU mechanical ventilation: A therapist implemented weaning protocol. *Chest.* 2001;119:236–42.
44. Zhu B, Li Z, Jiang L et al. Effect of a quality improvement program on weaning from mechanical ventilation: A cluster randomized trial *Intensive Care Med.* 2015;41:1781–90.
45. Nava S, Vitacca M. Chronic ventilator facilities. In: Martin T, ed. *Principles and practice of mechanical ventilation.* New York: McGraw-Hill; 2006:691–704.
46. Vitacca M. The magic formula of weaning: The doctors' holy grail. *Rev Port Pneumol.* 2011.
47. Schweickert WD, Pohlman MC, Pohlman AS et al. Early physical and occupational therapy in mechanically ventilated, critically ill patients: A randomised controlled trial. *Lancet.* 2009;373:1874–82.
48. Martin UJ, Hincapie L, Nimchuk M et al. Impact of whole-body rehabilitation in patients receiving chronic MV. *Crit Care Med.* 2005;33:2259–65.
49. DiNino E, Gartman EJ, Sethi JM et al. Diaphragm ultrasound as a predictor of successful extubation from mechanical ventilation. *Thorax.* 2014;69:423–7.
50. Dessap AM, Roche-Campo F, Kouatchet A et al. Natriuretic peptide-driven fluid management during ventilator weaning: A randomized controlled trial. *Am J Respir Crit Care Med.* 2012;186:1256–63.
51. Brook AD, Ahrens TS, Stiff R et al. Effect of a nursing-implemented sedation protocol on the duration of mechanical ventilation. *Crit Care Med.* 1999;27:2609–15.
52. Kress JP, Pohlman AS, O'Connor MF et al. Daily interruption of sedative infusions in critically ill patients undergoing mechanical ventilation. *N Engl J Med.* 2000;342:1471–7.
53. Schweickert WD, Gehlbach BK, Pohlman AS et al. Daily interruption of sedative infusions and complications of critical illness in mechanically ventilated patients. *Crit Care Med.* 2004;32:1272–6.
54. Girard TD, Kress JP, Fuchs BD et al. Efficacy and safety of a paired sedation and ventilator weaning protocol for mechanically ventilated patients in intensive care (Awakening and Breathing Controlled trial): A randomised controlled trial. *Lancet.* 2008; 371:126–34.
55. Burry L, Rose L, McCullagh IJ et al. Daily sedation interruption versus no daily sedation interruption for critically ill adult patients requiring invasive mechanical ventilation. *Cochrane Database Syst Rev.* 2014:CD009176.
56. Jubran A, Grant BJB, Duffner LA et al. Effect of pressure support vs. unassisted breathing through a tracheostomy collar on weaning duration in patients requiring prolonged mechanical ventilation: A randomized trial. *JAMA.* 2013;309:671–7.
57. Hernandez G, Pedrosa A, Ortiz R et al. The effects of increasing effective airway diameter on weaning from mechanical ventilation in tracheostomized patients: A randomized controlled trial. *Intensive Care Med.* 2013;39:1063–70.
58. Roquilly A, Cinotti R, Jaber S et al. Implementation of an evidence-based extubation readiness bundle in 499 brain-injured patients. *Am J Respir Crit Care Med.* 2013;188:958–66.

68

Specialised weaning units

ADITI SATTI, JAMES BROWN, GERARD J. CRINER AND BERND SCHÖNHOFER

INTRODUCTION

The advancement of care on the intensive care unit (ICU) has improved survival in the catastrophically ill patient. The improvement in medical technology and a greater understanding of many disease states have led to an increased demand for intensive care beds and have created an increased strain on our current healthcare system. It is projected that by 2017, healthcare spending will reach over US$4.3 trillion. Forty percent of healthcare resources are consumed by critical care medicine; critical care costs account for 1% of the US gross domestic product. It is generally accepted that the cost of a critical care bed is three times the cost of a non-critical care bed.[1] Critical care costs have increased by 190% from 1985 to 2000.[2] Chronic ventilated patients require expensive care that is inadequately reimbursed. In addition, the number of chronically ventilated patients is projected to double between years 2012 and 2020.[3] Mechanical ventilation (MV) has also been found to substantially drive costs in the ICU. In a study of approximately 51,000 adult patients in 253 US hospitals in 2002, MV was associated with both higher mean costs, $31,574 versus $12,931, and longer mean ICU length of stay, 14.4 days versus 8.5 days, when compared to non-ventilated patients.[4] Moreover, the increased demands for ICU care have led to competing demands for the use of a relatively small number of ICU beds. Efforts to decrease ICU length of stay for chronic ventilated patients are desperately needed to contain the costs associated with critical care medicine and to free up ICU beds for other types of critically ill patients who do not require chronic ventilation.

On this background, the goal of specialised weaning units is to improve weaning potential of the chronic ventilated patient.

WEANING: CLASSIFICATION

The International Task Force defines three weaning categories (Table 68.1).[5] Categories 1–3 are distributed in a ratio of about 60:25:15%.[6] Compared to categories 1 and 2, patients with prolonged weaning have the highest mortality rate. Category 3 comprises a heterogeneous population with different diagnoses, severity of illnesses and comorbidities.

MUSCULAR WEAKNESS IN THE INTENSIVE CARE UNIT

A prolonged ICU stay and the presence of a chronic critical illness are associated with muscle weakness, deconditioning, decreased mental and physical functioning and an impaired quality of life. Acute respiratory distress syndrome (ARDS), a common condition encountered in the ICU, is an example of an illness that requires prolonged ventilation and is associated with long-term psychological and functional dysfunctions. In a study reviewing 109 survivors of ARDS, muscle fatigue, weakness and weight loss were the major reasons given for the patient's persistent functional limitations. These functional limitations were evident in the lower than predicted distance walked in 6 min at 1 year after ICU discharge.[7] We found that survivors of prolonged ventilation also experienced a marked impairment in their physical quality of life, even though their mental health was preserved.[8]

There is an increased need for mobility in the ICU because of the harmful consequences of prolonged bed rest. A prolonged ICU stay and chronic critical illness not only are associated with weakness, deconditioning, decreased whole-body function and quality of life, but also increase the risk for hospital-acquired pneumonia, venous thromboembolism and the development of decubitus ulcers.

The effects of limb muscle deconditioning are primarily known from studies done in healthy people placed on bed rest in space programmes constructed to evaluate the effects of low-gravity environments on skeletal muscle structure and function in normal healthy volunteers.[9] Muscle atrophy, loss of force generation and changes in muscle fibre types rapidly occur with bed rest alone and even more so in hypercatabolic ICU patients who have increased oxidant stress. It has been found that even short periods of bed rest adversely affect skeletal muscle performance. After 14 and 35 days,

Table 68.1 Weaning categories defined by the International Task Force

Group	Category	Definition
1	Simple weaning	Successful weaning and extubation with the first SBT
2	Difficult weaning	Successful weaning and extubation after initial failure but at the latest with the third SBT or within 7 days of MV after initiation of the weaning process
3[a]	Prolonged weaning	Successful weaning after at least three failed SBTs or MV longer than 7 days after the first failed SBT

Source: Boles JM, *Eur Respir J*, 29, 1033–56, 2007.
Note: SBT, spontaneous breathing trial; NIV, non-invasive ventilation.
[a] Subgroup 3b consists of (1) of patients with intermittent NIV, which is finished during the stay in hospital, and (2) of patients who continue to depend on NIV after discharge from hospital.

muscle force decreases by 15% and 25%, respectively, and thigh and calf muscle volumes significantly decrease.[9] Limb skeletal muscle atrophy that occurs with disuse also occurs in the diaphragm; diaphragm atrophy occurs even in normal subjects more rapidly than previously believed.

The so-called ventilator-induced diaphragm dysfunction (VIDD) is caused by the inactivity of the diaphragm during MV, which leads to loss of contractile force and muscle mass.[10]

Diaphragm biopsy specimens from previously normal brain-dead thoracic organ donors who were placed on MV for only 18–69 hours showed significant atrophy of both the slow- and fast-twitch diaphragm muscle fibres.[11] This indicates that diaphragm muscle weakness can very rapidly occur in patients receiving controlled ventilation even in previously normal hosts and indicates the profound effects that rest and catabolic illness (e.g. oxidant injury) may have on skeletal muscle in the ICU patients.

Obviously, these changes could markedly impair weaning from MV and worsen the patients' overall functional status.

In the recent years, the generalised muscle weakness, which develops during the course of an ICU admission and for which no other cause can be identified is called 'ICU-acquired weakness' (ICUAW).[12] ICUAW can be evoked either by critical illness polyneuropathy, by critical illness myopathy, or by both during the course of critical illness.

WEANING UNIT

In general, the goal of specialised weaning units is to improve the weaning potential of the chronic ventilated patient, as well as their overall physical, psychological and social functions to avoid the complications associated with immobility through whole-body and respiratory rehabilitation, aggressive nutritional support and speech and swallowing therapy.

In a weaning unit, the weaning success in difficult and prolonged weaning can be improved by comprehensive weaning strategies with a multidisciplinary approach to weaning that involves the physician, nurses, physical therapists, respiratory therapists and nutritionists.

In the following, some important strategies in the complex weaning process are elaborated.

EARLY MOBILITY

ICU patients are a special population who benefit from early mobility. The ability to sit, stand and ambulate not only improves their quality of life and functional status, but also mitigates the complications of immobility, such as deep venous thrombosis, pulmonary embolism and decubitus ulcers.

The benefits of rehabilitation in respiratory failure have been demonstrated in different studies.

We previously evaluated and reported the efficacy of aggressive whole-body rehabilitation in 49 chronically ventilated patients.[13] All patients had been ventilated for at least 14 days, and none had underlying neuromuscular disorders. Physical therapy was started on admission to our ventilator rehabilitation unit after transfer from the ICU. The rehab programme consisted of trunk control, active and passive upper and lower extremity resistance trainings and ambulation and inspiratory muscle training. Deconditioning was assessed daily using a five-point motor score looking at strength and range of motion of all muscle groups. Improvements in patient strength were seen after a whole-body rehabilitation programme. All patients, initially bed bound, were able to sit and stand, and the majority (81%) were able to ambulate prior to discharge. Increased upper motor strength decreased the amount of time spent on the ventilator. This may have been due to strengthening of the pectoralis muscles and an improvement in inspiratory and expiratory functions.

Past studies in different patient populations have shown an improvement in ventilatory mechanics (increased mean inspiratory pressure and expiratory reserve volume) with pectoralis muscle training.[14] Table 68.2 summarises the results of upper extremity training and the effect on ventilatory muscle strength and endurance.[14–16] It can be concluded from our study that whole-body rehabilitation should be an integral part of the care of a chronically ventilated patient and, if started earlier, may have additional benefit.

An early mobility programme, consisting of sitting, standing and ambulation, can be safely done in the majority of ICU patients. A study that examined the safety of early activity showed that the majority of respiratory patients were able to participate in a physical therapy programme in the ICU, even while orally intubated, without adverse events (1%).[17] Comprehensive guidelines that can be used to assess the safety of mobilising critically ill patients are available.[18] The main safety factors that should be addressed include intrinsic factors related to the patient (e.g. medical background, cardiovascular and respiratory reserve and haematological considerations) and factors extrinsic to the patient (e.g. patient attachments, environment and staffing).[18]

Table 68.2 Summary of studies of upper extremity training on ventilatory muscle strength and endurance

Author, year	Subject	Results
Keens et al., 1977[14]	Cystic fibrosis	57% increase in ventilatory muscle endurance
Clanton et al., 1987[15]	Female swimmers	25% increase in maximum inspiratory pressure (MIP), 100% in ventilatory endurance
Estenne et al., 1989[16]	C8-C8 quads	Six weeks of isometric pectoralis major training increased expiratory reserve volume (ERV) by 47%

Note: MIP, maximum inspiratory pressure; ERV, expiratory reserve volume.

Schweickert et al.[19] demonstrated that a strategy for whole-body rehabilitation consisting of the interruption of sedation and physical and occupational therapy in the earliest days of critical illness is safe and well tolerated and resulted in better functional outcomes at hospital discharge, a shorter duration of delirium and more ventilator-free days compared with standard care.

The European Respiratory Society and European Society of Intensive Care Medicine Task Force suggest that rehabilitation can begin when certain stability criteria have been met (Figure 68.1).[20]

Portable ventilators now allow patients to be mobilised earlier in their hospital course despite higher needs for oxygenation or even continuous MV. Invasive ventilation can be provided by 'laptop'-sized ventilators that are suspended from wheelchairs or walkers to allow standing and ambulation despite the requirements for full ventilation.

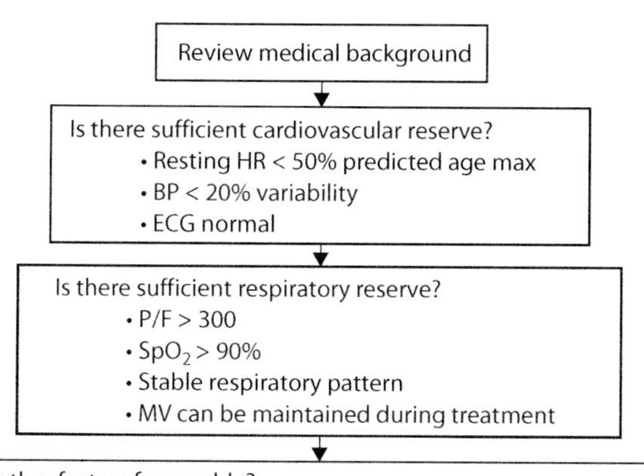

Figure 68.1 ERS/ESICM guidelines for mobilisation of the critically ill patient. ERS, European Respiratory Society; ESICM, European Society of Intensive Care Medicine. (Adapted from Gosselink R et al., *Intensive Care Med*, 34, 1188–99, 2008.)

Additionally, other new respiratory therapy techniques provide methods to unload the respiratory work in the non-intubated ICU patient and include continuous positive airway pressure, bi-level positive airway pressure, helium–oxygen administration and high-flow oxygen. All these methods can also be organised to be made portable and provided non-invasively to unload the patient's work of breathing during periods of ambulation or higher levels of whole-body rehabilitation.

RESPIRATORY MUSCLE TRAINING

Spontaneous breathing provides ventilatory muscle endurance training, but inspiratory muscle strength training may also be beneficial to increase respiratory muscle strength and improve weaning outcome. A substantial body of literature demonstrates the ability of loaded inspiratory breathing training on increasing respiratory muscle strength in quadriplegics, normal controls and patients with chronic obstructive pulmonary disease (COPD). Martin et al.[21] demonstrated that daily inspiratory muscle training in 10 chronically ventilated patients resulted in an increase in inspiratory muscle strength and success in weaning 9 out of 10 patients from MV after its implementation. In order to provide inspiratory muscle strength training, at our facilities, we routinely institute inspiratory muscle training at one-third the maximum inspiratory pressure for 10 min daily, or twice daily in patients able to spontaneously breathe by tracheal collar.

A recently published systematic review underlined that inspiratory muscle training for selected patients in the ICU facilitates weaning, with potential reductions in length of stay and the duration of non-invasive ventilatory support after extubation.[22]

Strategies of mechanical ventilation in difficult and prolonged weaning

Recently, there has been a great expansion in our knowledge of VIDD. In general, the strategy how MV is performed in difficult and prolonged weaning aims at reconditioning the weak diaphragm. This may be achieved by avoiding continuous controlled MV and encourage sufficient diaphragmatic use. This may be reached by the gradual continuous reduction of ventilator support or intermittent spontaneous breathing trials where the patient is disconnected from the ventilator.

In a study of more than 300 tracheostomised patients cared for in long-term acute care hospitals, investigators compared the effect of unassisted breathing through a tracheostomy collar and pressure support on weaning duration.[23] In that study, weaning by unassisted breathing through a tracheostomy resulted in shorter median weaning time (15 days with tracheostomy collar vs. 19 days with pressure support). Weaning mode had no effect on survival at 6 months (51% with tracheostomy collar vs. 56% with pressure support) and 12 months (60% with tracheostomy collar vs. 66% with pressure support).

SPEECH AND SWALLOWING

The ability to speak and eat also has a benefit on overall psychological well-being. These issues are extremely important, and therapy should be instituted as early as feasible when caring for chronically ventilated patients. Most patients report that their inability to communicate is the most important factor contributing to the sense of fear and isolation. Speech therapists are an integral part of the multidisciplinary rehabilitation team. The use of an electrolarynx, one-way speaking valve or even periods of cuff deflation with finger occlusion of the tracheostomy tube can be individualised to assist in their speech.

The reinstitution of eating is also a primary concern for chronically ventilated patients and their families. Although the conversion of an endotracheal to tracheostomy tube may allow the resumption of oral intake, patients receiving chronic ventilation may have a significant incidence of swallowing abnormalities.

When we evaluated the effects of chronic MV on swallowing function, we found that 43% of patients who received prolonged MV had evidence of aspiration on a modified barium swallow study with videoflouroscopy.[24] A modified barium swallow study is particularly important because it helps to point out the mechanism(s) responsible for the high incidence of aspiration detected on bedside examination in the patient with tracheostomy and MV. Furthermore, fibreoptic endoscopic examination of swallowing is an established method to evaluate the swallowing procedure.[25] Finally, scintigraphy is another method to evaluate early aspiration after oral feeding in patients receiving prolonged ventilation via tracheostomy.[26]

Neuromuscular disorders, medications, underlying medical illness, weakness of the oropharyngeal muscles and laryngeal oedema are all factors that may contribute to swallowing dysfunction. Speech therapists should evaluate swallowing, oral motor strength and adequate cough and gag reflexes. The initial goal in a patient with swallowing dysfunction is to prevent aspiration. Proper patient positioning, alternative routes of nutrition and assessment for other neurological conditions contributing to swallowing dysfunction should be included in the management of these patients. The ability to eat, speak and socially interact reengages the patient in normal human behaviour, which is vital to their overall well-being. After appropriate swallowing evaluation and training, most patients receiving chronic ventilation without obvious severe neuromuscular diseases can successfully resume normal oral intake.

Nutritional status and metabolism

Being over- or underweight can prolong the weaning period. In the presence of pulmonary cachexia, which is often present due to underlying pulmonary disease, inadequate nutrition is especially deleterious[27] and should be avoided. Nutrition should be preferably provided by the enteral route. If a MV time of more than 4–6 weeks is expected, a percutaneous gastrotomy should be considered early. With respect to recommendations for nutrition, the guideline refers to national and international guidelines on nutritional therapy.[28]

SLEEP

Other issues that contribute to psychological dysfunction in the ventilated patient are sleep deprivation.[29] Patients admitted to the ICU are susceptible to sleep deprivation due to underlying illnesses, medications and the ICU environment itself; the ICU is a noisy environment that provides the patient with continuous, meaningless sensory input. Normal sleep architecture is disturbed in the ICU and can lead to ICU-related delirium. Sleep has a role in healing, and deprivation may impair immunity and tissue repair. Steps to improve sleep such as creating a diurnal environment and minimising interruptions should be taken.[30] Some steps that may be beneficial are placing patients in individual rooms with a window, regular orientation with a clock and calendar, early mobilisation and uninterrupted sleep.

PSYCHOLOGICAL DYSFUNCTION

Psychological disorders such as delirium and anxiety are commonly seen in the ICU. The incidence of delirium in the ICU is 30%–40% with an increased incidence in the elderly population.[31] Delirium is associated with poor outcomes such as prolonged hospitalisation, functional decline, increased use of chemical and physical restraints and an increased mortality (>30%). Risk factors for delirium include older age, prior cognitive impairment, the presence of infection, multiple comorbidities, dehydration and psychotropic medication use. Individuals at high risk for delirium should be assessed daily using a standardised tool to facilitate prompt identification and management. The Confusion Assessment Method (CAM) is a simple validated tool used for the detection of delirium in both the clinical and research settings. The CAM-ICU uses four key delirium criteria to rapidly assess the patient's cognition: acute change in mental status, inattention, disordered thinking and an altered level of consciousness, to determine the presence of delirium. The CAM-ICU uses picture recognition and non-verbal responses to assess delirium. The CAM assessment has been shown to be useful and reproducible in ventilated and non-ventilated patients.[31] Non-pharmacologic interventions to improve delirium include the use of assistive devices to facilitate speech, the ability to eat, improved mobility and the promotion of good sleep. Creating a diurnal environment and normalising a patient's daily routine by getting a patient out of bed and ambulating may minimise confusion and delirium. Haloperidol and atypical antipsychotics are also used in the treatment of delirium.

A recently published guideline provides a roadmap for developing integrated, evidence-based and patient-centred protocols for preventing and treating pain, agitation and delirium in critically ill patients.[32]

WEANING FAILURE AND LIFE ON LONG-TERM MV

Patients with prolonged weaning (category 3 of the international consensus conference) comprises a heterogeneous

Table 68.3 Three subgroups (groups 1–3) of prolonged weaning (category 3)

Group	Category	Definition
3a	Prolonged weaning without NIV	Successful weaning after at least three failed SBTs or MV longer than 7 days after the first failed SBT without NIV
3b	Prolonged weaning with NIV	Successful weaning after at least three failed SBTs or MV longer than 7 days after the first failed SBT in combination with NIV; if necessary, continued into out-of-hospital (home) MV[a]
3c	Weaning failure	Death or discharge with invasive MV via tracheostomy

Source: Barr J et al., *Crit Care Med*, 41, 263–306, 2013.
Note: SBT, spontaneous breathing trial; NIV, non-invasive ventilation.
[a] Subgroup 3b consists of both patients with intermittent NIV, which is finished during the stay in hospital, and patients who continue to depend on NIV after discharge from hospital.

population with different diagnoses, severity of illnesses and comorbidities. Therefore, in the German guideline of prolonged weaning,[33] category 3 was further divided into three subgroups (groups 1–3) according to their weaning course (Table 68.3).

Patients with persistent ventilatory insufficiency after prolonged weaning (group 3b) may benefit from non-invasive ventilation (NIV). The discharge process in this situation is usually focused on the provision of technical equipment such as ventilators and accessory parts, and future caregivers are being instructed how to handle them correctly.

In weaning failure category 3c, patients with NIV failure and continuous invasive MV, discharge to an out-of-hospital facility or to the patient's home is feasible.

Observational studies report that up to 30% of patients with prolonged weaning are treated with home MV after being weaned, most commonly due to COPD, obesity–hypoventilation syndrome, kyphoscoliosis and neuromuscular diseases with hypercapnic respiratory failure.[34,35]

In patients with indication for long-term MV, a structured discharge and planning the care of patients at home or in out-of-hospital facilities should be organised in a specialised weaning unit. In general, different models of care exist for patients still dependent on MV[33]:

- Self-care in the patient's home (predominantly when treated with NIV)
- Home care with support from outpatient nursing services or personalised assistance (1:1 care – in particular, in high-dependency invasive MV)
- Outpatient care in an assisted care facility/living group for patients with long-term MV
- Specialised long-term ventilation care facility
- Palliative care facility with special expertise in MV

EXPERIENCE WORLDWIDE

The process of weaning from MV support may be long and frustrating and time consuming for patients, their families and the healthcare team. The financial and medical implications of caring for these patients have led to the development of intermediate and specialised weaning facilities. These facilities often utilise a multidisciplinary team approach and emphasise the rehabilitation, medical and psychosocial issues of the patient and their family. Caring for an increased population of patients on prolonged MV in an optimal and cost-effective manner has become a global challenge.

North American perspective

Unlike in Europe, intensive care medicine in the United States has always been closely linked to respiratory medicine. Specialised weaning facilities are much more common in the United States and play an important role in patients on prolonged MV. The number of facilities has increased due to the improved reimbursement and diagnosis-related group exemption. These long-term facilities often have differing admission and discharge criteria, patient care staffing ratios and weaning approaches. One of the first specialised units was a 24-bed prolonged respiratory care unit started at Bethesda Lutheran Medical Center in 1979.[36] Their 18-month trial showed cost savings when compared to an acute care centre. Elpern et al.[37] showed a decrease in the daily cost of care of US$2000 per patient in those transferred to the weaning facility.

Temple University Hospital was one of the four original sites selected to participate in a study funded by the Health Care Financing Administration Chronic Ventilator Dependent Unit Demonstration Project.[38] The ventilator rehabilitation unit (VRU) at Temple is an 18-bed non-invasive respiratory care unit in a tertiary care hospital and has provided care to over 2500 patients with prolonged respiratory failure. One of the goals in the VRU is to achieve maximum functional status despite the ongoing need of the patient for MV. The VRU is composed of a multidisciplinary team, each with a unique role. The team is composed of a pulmonary attending, pulmonary fellow, nurse coordinator, speech therapist, pharmacist, respiratory therapists, physical and occupational therapists and a nutritionist. Appropriate consultations are made to otolaryngologists and psychiatrists on an as-needed basis. The purpose of the study was to examine the effect of a multidisciplinary rehabilitation programme, costs, survival and quality of life in patients requiring prolonged MV. The study showed that patients in a specialised ventilator-dependent unit (VDU) were more likely to be weaned from the ventilator and be discharged to home. These patients were also found to be more functionally independent at the time of discharge. Patients treated in the VDU generated lower costs per day compared with matched patients who received conventional care in the ICU. The success of the Temple VRU was dependent on the organisation of the treatment team and quality of the rehabilitation programme. Similar experiences have been documented in other institutions.

The experience of the respiratory special care unit (ReSCU) at the Cleveland Clinic showed that of 212 patients, 60% were successfully weaned from the ventilator.[39] There was a mortality rate of 18%. A cost analysis was done comparing the charges for patients in the special weaning unit versus those in the ICU. To make the comparison, it was assumed that those patients who were transferred to the weaning unit would have stayed in the ICU for the entire length of stay. The difference in daily cost per bed between the ICU and ReSCU is US$585. This is a cost saving of US$13,339 per patient for those transferred to ReSCU. Although lacking prospective supportive data, specialised weaning units may provide a clinically and cost-effective alternative to ICU care.

European perspective

There has been a growing interest in specialised weaning facilities in Europe over the past decade.[40] Respiratory ICUs (RICUs) specialise in non-invasive and prolonged MV and provide a step-down unit from the ICU to the general ward. There is a nurse–patient ratio of 1:4 or 1:5, accounting for some of the cost savings. Germany and Italy have the largest number of RICUs of all European countries. The management of the RICU by a respiratory specialist is a new and emerging trend.

Driven by chest physicians, the contemporary status of weaning centres was evaluated in 2006 with a nationwide German survey.[41] In the year 2009, the network of weaning units of the German Respiratory Society has been founded. Figure 68.2 illustrates the three components of the certified weaning centres in the *WeanNet*.

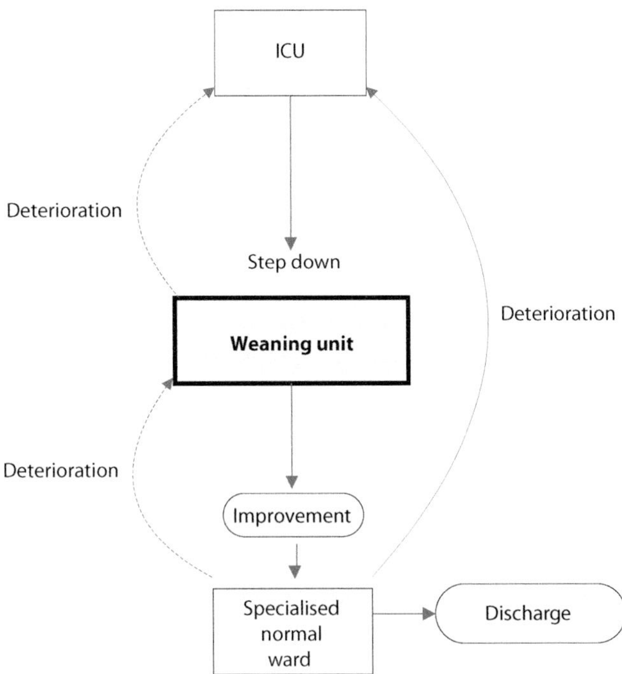

Figure 68.2 Three components of the certified weaning centres in the WeanNet: ICU, weaning unit, specialised ward on home MV. (From Schönhofer B et al., *Dtsch Med Wochenschr*, 133, 700–4, 2008.)

A 3-month prospective cohort study done in 26 Italian RICUs provides insight into the prevalence and description of these units.[42] The study showed that the presence of RICUs contributed to increased ICU bed availability. Of the 756 patients, 61% had tracheostomies and were considered ventilator dependent. The predicted mortality according to the Acute Physiology and Chronic Health Evaluation (APACHE) 2 score was 22% with an actual mortality of 16%. The study showed that patients admitted to the Italian RICU achieved ventilator independence rates similar to the studies done in the United States and were able to successfully manage patients with acute-on-chronic respiratory failure.

OUTCOMES

Multiple studies have evaluated the outcomes and survival of patients transferred to a weaning facility. The evidence is mainly limited to observational, retrospective, single-centre non-randomised studies. The patient population, outcome reporting and weaning methods often differ between studies. Despite these confounding variables, there has been documented success in weaning and a proven financial benefit in these specialised units. Scheinhorn et al.[43] studied 1123 ventilator-dependent patients transferred to a regional weaning facility over an 8-year period.[43] Patients were transferred earlier to a weaning facility; 55% of patients were successfully weaned and 29% died in the unit. During the time period, the survival rate 1 year after discharge had improved from 29% to 37%. Differences in patient population can be clearly seen when comparing the prior study with that of Gracey et al.[44] in 2000. In this study, 60% of patients were successfully weaned and 6% died. The patient population was predominately post-surgical and younger and had fewer comorbidities.

Recently, data from WeanNet on epidemiology and outcomes of 6899 patients with prolonged weaning from the WeanNet register were published.[45] The majority of patients (62.2%) were successfully weaned from the ventilator and discharged from the weaning unit without invasive ventilator after a median of 33 days. NIV was initiated in 19.4% of patients with chronic ventilatory insufficiency after prolonged weaning. Patients who were discharged with NIV were significantly younger than the average (68 vs. 71 years). In 22.9% of the patients, weaning definitively failed, and continuous invasive ventilation was needed. Compared to other main reasons for MV, patients with COPD were rarely completely weaned from the respirator and more often needed NIV for home MV. In total, 14.9% of the 6899 patients died during the treatment in the weaning unit.

Despite the substantial differences in patient make-up between the studies, these studies do demonstrate the safety and success of weaning patients in a less costly environment than the ICU with the use of specialised weaning units. The major studies and their findings are given in Table 68.4.[46–49]

Table 68.4 Studies of weaning outcomes

First author and reference	Pilcher et al.[35]	Schönhofer et al.[46]	Gracey et al.[47]	Scheinhorn et al.[48]	Bagley and Cooney[49]
Patients (*n*)	153	232	132	421	278
Mean age (years)	62	65	67	70	67
Diagnosis					
COPD (%)	27	54	13	24	30
Surgery (%)	24	7	63	24	11
Amyotrophic lateral sclerosis (%)	–	5	1	32	28
Neuromuscular (%)	31[a]	16	–	8	19
Miscellaneous (%)	18	18	23	12	12
Weaning					
Ventilation days	26	44	14	49	–
Days to wean	19	7.5	16	39	–
Weaning success (%)	38	65	70	53	38
Survival					
At discharge (%)	73	72	90	71	53
Long-term (%)	58 (1 year)	64 (3 months)	–	28 (1 year)	–

SUMMARY

Multiple retrospective and observational studies have shown that specialised weaning units can provide effective care to the patient on prolonged MV, both financially and medically. The multidisciplinary approach to care, with an emphasis on rehabilitation, strategies of MV, sleep, nutrition, speech and swallowing has improved patients' overall psychological well-being and facilitated weaning from the ventilator. Prospective randomised controlled trials are still needed to improve the care and utility of these specialised units.

REFERENCES

1. Hopkins RO, Spuhler VJ, Thomsen GE. Transforming ICU culture to facilitate early mobility. *Crit Care Clin.* 2007;23:81–96.
2. Halpern NA, Pastores SM, Greenstein RJ. Critical care medicine in the United States: 1985–2000: An analysis of bed numbers, use and cost. *Crit Care Med.* 2004;32:1254–9.
3. Donahoe MP, Current venues of care and related costs for the chronically critically ill. *Respir Care.* 2012;57:867–86.
4. Dasta JF, Pilon D, Mody SH et al. Daily costs of hospitalization in non-valvular atrial fibrillation patients treated with anticoagulant therapy. *J Med Econ.* 2015;18:1041–9.
5. Boles JM, Bion J, Connors A et al. Weaning from mechanical ventilation. *Eur Respir J.* 2007;29:1033–56.
6. Funk GC, Anders S, Breyer MK et al. Incidence and outcome of weaning from mechanical ventilation according to new categories. *Eur Respir J.* 2010;35:88–94.
7. Herridge MS, Cheung AM, Tansey CM et al. One-year outcomes in survivors of the acute respiratory distress syndrome. *N Engl J Med.* 2003;348:683–93.
8. Euteneuer S, Windisch W, Suchi S et al. Health-related quality of life in patients with chronic respiratory failure after long-term mechanical ventilation. *Respir Med.* 2006;100:477–86.
9. Adams GR, Caiozzo VJ, Baldwin KM. Skeletal muscle unweighting: Space flight and ground based models. *J Appl Physiol.* 2003;95:2185–201.
10. Jaber S, Jung B, Matecki S, Petrof BJ. Clinical review: Ventilator-induced diaphragmatic dysfunction – Human studies confirm animal model findings. *Crit Care.* 2011;15:206.
11. Levine S, Nguyen T, Taylor N et al. Rapid disuse atrophy of diaphragm fibers in mechanically ventilated humans. *N Engl J Med.* 2008;358:1327–35.
12. Hermans G, Van den Berghe G. Clinical review: Intensive care unit acquired weakness. *Crit Care.* 2015;19:274.
13. Martin U, Hincapie L, Nimchuk M et al. Impact of whole-body rehabilitation in patients receiving chronic mechanical ventilation. *Crit Care Med.* 2005;33:2259–65.
14. Keens TG, Krastins IR, Wannamaker EM et al. Ventilatory muscle endurance training in normal subjects and patients with cystic fibrosis. *Am Rev Respir Dis.* 1977;116:853–60.
15. Clanton TL, Dixon GF, Drake J et al. Effects of swim training on lung volumes and inspiratory muscle conditioning. *J Appl Physiol.* 1987;62:39–46.
16. Estenne M, Knoop C, Vanvaerenbergh J et al. The effect of pectoralis muscle training in training tetraplegic subjects. *Am Rev Respir Dis.* 1989;139:1218–22.

17. Bailey P, Thomsen GE, Spuhler VJ et al. Early activity is feasible and safe in respiratory failure patients. *Crit Care Med.* 2007;35:139–45.
18. Stiller K. Safety issues that should be considered when mobilizing critically ill patients. *Crit Care Clin.* 2007;23:35–53.
19. Schweickert WD, Pohlman MC, Pohlman AS et al. Early physical and occupational therapy in mechanically ventilated, critically ill patients: A randomised controlled trial. *Lancet.* 2009;373(9678):1874–82.
20. Gosselink R, Bott J, Johnson M et al. Physiotherapy for adult patients with critical illness: Recommendations of the European Respiratory Society and European Society of Intensive Care Medicine Task Force on Physiotherapy for Critically Ill Patients. *Intensive Care Med.* 2008;34:1188–99.
21. Martin DA, Davenport PD, Franceschi AC et al. Use of inspiratory muscle strength training to facilitate ventilator weaning. *Chest.* 2002;122:192–6.
22. Elkins M, Dentice R. Inspiratory muscle training facilitates weaning from mechanical ventilation among patients in the intensive care unit: A systematic review. *J Physiother.* 2015;61:125–34.
23. Jubran A, Grant BJ, Duffner LA et al. Effect of pressure support vs unassisted breathing through a tracheostomy collar on weaning duration in patients requiring prolonged mechanical ventilation: A randomized trial. *JAMA.* 2013;309:671–7.
24. Tolep K, Getch CL, Criner GJ et al. Swallowing dysfunction in patients receiving prolonged mechanical ventilation. *Chest.* 1996;109:167–72.
25. Hiss SG, Postma GN. Fiberoptic endoscopic evaluation of swallowing. *Laryngoscope.* 2003;113:1386–93.
26. Schönhofer B, Barchfeld T, Haidl P et al. Scintigraphy for evaluation of early aspiration after oral feeding in patients receiving prolonged ventilation via tracheotomy. *Intensive Care Med.* 1999;25:311–14.
27. Cahill NE, Dhaliwal R, Day AG et al. Nutrition therapy in the critical care setting: What is 'best achievable' practice? An international multicenter observational study. *Crit Care Med.* 2010;38:395–401.
28. McClave SA, Martindale RG, Vanek VW et al. Guidelines for the provision and assessment of nutrition support therapy in the adult critically Ill patient: Society of Critical Care Medicine (SCCM) and American Society for Parenteral and Enteral Nutrition (A.S.P.E.N.). *J Parenter Enter Nutr.* 2009;33:277–316.
29. Kamdar BB, Needham DM, Collop NA. Sleep deprivation in critical illness: Its role in physical and psychological recovery. *J Intensive Care Med.* 2012;27:97–111.
30. Krachman SL, D'Alonzo GE, Criner CJ et al. Sleep in the intensive care unit. *Chest.* 1995;107:1713–20.
31. Criner G. Psychological disturbances in the ICU. In: *Critical Care Study Guide.* New York: Springer;2002.
32. Barr J, Fraser GL, Puntillo K et al. Clinical practice guidelines for the management of pain, agitation, and delirium in adult patients in the intensive care unit. *Crit Care Med.* 2013;41:263–306.
33. Schönhofer B, Dellweg D, Geiseler J et al. S2k-Guideline on prolonged weaning. *Pneumologie.* 2014;68;19–75.
34. Schönhofer B, Euteneuer S, Nava S et al. Survival of mechanically ventilated patients admitted to a specialised weaning centre. *Intensive Care Med.* 2002;28:908–16.
35. Pilcher DV, Bailey MJ, Treacher DF et al. Outcomes, cost and long term survival of patients referred to a regional weaning centre. *Thorax.* 2005;60:187–92.
36. Indihar FJ, Forsberg DP. Experience with a prolonged respiratory care unit. *Chest.* 1982;81:189–92.
37. Elpern EH, Silver MR, Rosen RL et al. The noninvasive respiratory care unit. *Chest.* 1999;1:205–8.
38. Criner G. Long term ventilation: Introduction and perspectives. *Respir Care Clin.* 2002;8:345–53.
39. Dasgupta A, Rice R, Mascha E et al. Four year experience with a unit for long-term ventilation at the Cleveland Clinic Foundation. *Chest.* 1999; 116:447–55.
40. Corrado A, Roussos C, Ambrosino N et al. Respiratory intermediate care units: A European survey. *Eur Respir J.* 2002;20:1343–50.
41. Schönhofer B, Berndt C, Achtzehn U et al. Weaning from mechanical ventilation: A survey of the situation in pneumologic respiratory facilities in Germany. *Dtsch Med Wochenschr.* 2008;133:700–4.
42. Confalonieri M, Cuvelier A, Elliott M et al. Respiratory intensive care units in Italy: A national census and prospective cohort study. *Thorax.* 2001;56:373–8.
43. Scheinhorn DJ, Chao DC, Stearn-Hassenpflug MA et al. Post ICU mechanical ventilation: Treatment of 1123 patients at a regional weaning center. *Chest.* 1997;11:1654–9.
44. Gracey DR, Hardy DC, Koenig GE. The chronic ventilator-dependent unit: A lower cost alternative to intensive care. *Mayo Clin Proc.* 2000;75:445–9.
45. WeanNet-Study-Group: Register of German Weaning units. *Dtsch Med Wochenschr.* 2016, in press.
46. Schönhofer B, Haidl P, Kemper P et al. Withdrawal from the respirator (weaning) in long-term ventilation: The results in patients in a weaning centre. *Dtsch Med Wochenschr.* 1999;124:1022–8.
47. Gracey DR, Naessens JM, Viggiano RW et al. Outcomes of patients cared for in a ventilator-dependent unit in a general hospital. *Chest.* 1995;107:494–9.
48. Scheinhorn DJ, Artinian BM, Catlin JL. Weaning from prolonged mechanical ventilation. *Chest.* 1994;105:534–9.
49. Bagley PH, Cooney E. A community-based regional ventilator weaning unit: Development and outcomes. *Chest.* 1997;111:1024–9.

69

Psychological problems during weaning

AMAL JUBRAN

Critically ill patients who require mechanical ventilation are at risk for mental stress because they know that their ability to breathe depends on assistance from a machine. The presence of an endotracheal (or tracheostomy) tube makes it extremely difficult for most ventilated patients to communicate their physical and emotional needs.[1] The inability to talk decreases a patient's sense of control, leading to feelings of helplessness, anger and despair.[2] Weaning from the ventilator can be particularly stressful; patients commonly experience increased respiratory work, gas exchange abnormalities and cardiovascular derangements.[3–6] Some patients panic as soon as they perceive the active withdrawal of a life-preserving therapy,[7] fearing that they will be unable to sustain ventilation on their own. As the duration of mechanical ventilation increases, adverse emotional reactions are likely to increase, which may negatively impact a patient's ability to wean from the ventilator.[8,9] Research on ventilator weaning has primarily focused on physiological variables that predict weaning outcomes[10–12] and the use of different techniques to facilitate weaning.[13–15] In contrast, studies that explore the impact of mental well-being on weaning outcome are limited.

In a study focused on the pathophysiology of weaning failure, investigators found that 18% of patients who failed a T-tube trial of weaning from mechanical ventilation did not demonstrate any greater pathophysiologic abnormalities than those seen in weaning success patients.[4] As such, it is reasonable to suspect that weaning failure in those patients may have been caused by psychological factors.[16] The most commonly described psychiatric disturbances in patients requiring mechanical ventilation include depression, delirium, anxiety and post-traumatic stress disorder (PTSD).

DEPRESSION

To assess the occurrence of depression and its impact on outcome, Jubran et al.[9] conducted a prospective study in 478 patients transferred to a specialised facility (known as a long-term acute hospital [LTACH]) for weaning from prolonged ventilation. A clinical psychologist conducted a psychiatric interview and classified patients as having *depressive disorders* if they met the *Diagnostic and Statistical Manual of Mental Disorders, 4th edition* (DSM-IV) criteria for depressive disorders.[17] Of the 478 patients, 142 had persistent coma or delirium and were unable to be evaluated for depressive disorders. Of the remaining 336 patients, 142 (42%) were diagnosed with depressive disorders; specifically, 17 (12%) were diagnosed with major depression, 6 (4%) with dysthymic disorder and 119 (84%) were diagnosed with depressive disorder not otherwise specified. Independent predictors for the presence of depressive disorders included functional dependence before the acute illness (odds ratio [OR], 1.70), comorbidity score (OR, 1.23) and history of psychiatric disorders (OR, 3.04). Importantly, patients with depressive disorders had a higher rate of weaning failure than those without depressive disorders (61% vs. 33%) (Figure 69.1).

The presence of depressive disorders may contribute to weaning failure by interfering with the pragmatics of weaning.[9] Weakened or deconditioned respiratory muscles are believed to be a major reason that patients repeatedly fail weaning attempts.[18] One approach to reconditioning the respiratory muscles is the use of daily trials of spontaneous breathing.[15,19] Apathy, loss of energy and diminished motivation are commonly seen with depression.[20,21] As such, depressed patients may not have the energy and motivation necessary to tolerate the challenge of daily spontaneous breathing trials. If so, depressive disorders would contribute to weaning failure.

In the Jubran et al.[9] study, hospital mortality was higher among patients with depressive disorders than among those without such disorders (23.9% vs. 10.3%). The presence of depressive disorders was independently associated with mortality (OR, 4.3); age (OR, 1.06) and comorbidity score (OR, 1.24) also predicted mortality. Treatment with antidepressants was associated with a decreased risk for dying (OR, 0.95). The fact that treatment for depressive disorders was associated with a decrease in mortality suggests a link between depressive disorders and mortality. Conceivably, the presence of depressive disorders may add to the distress that patients experience while receiving mechanical

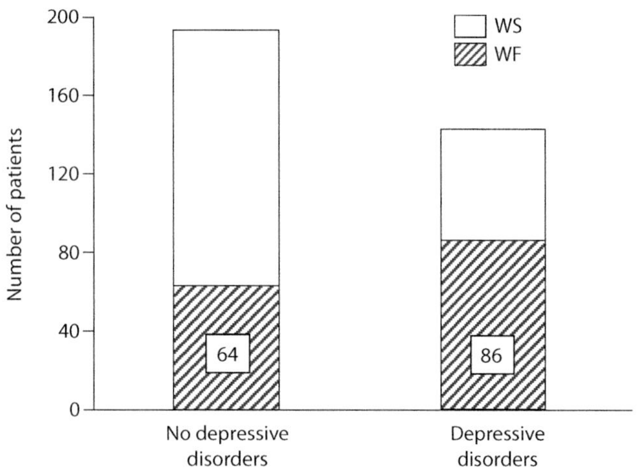

Number of patients
200
160
120
80
40
0
WS
WF
64
86
No depressive disorders
Depressive disorders

Figure 69.1 Number of patients with and without a depressive disorder. Hatched area of each column represents the number of patients who failed weaning (WF); clear area represents the number of patients who were successfully weaned (WS). Ventilator weaning was less frequent among patients with depressive disorders than among those without such disorders ($p < 0.0001$).

ventilation. Under such circumstances, coping mechanisms may become overwhelmed, and thus, a feeling of giving up may have occurred.[22]

DELIRIUM

Patients with depressive symptoms are at an increased risk for developing delirium.[23,24] Delirium is a serious disturbance in mental abilities that commonly occurs during a critical illness. According to the DSM-IV,[17] the diagnostic criteria for delirium include disturbance of consciousness, change in cognition and disturbance that develops over a short period and tends to fluctuate during the course of the day.

To identify delirium in intensive care unit (ICU) patients, most studies have employed screening tools, such as the Confusion Assessment Method for the intensive care unit or Intensive Care Delirium Screening Checklist. Using such screening questionnaires, investigators have reported that the incidence of delirium in ICU patients requiring short-term ventilation ranges between 16% and 82%.[25–29] The wide range in delirium rates most likely reflects different population being studied and the different diagnostic criteria employed[30]. Delirium has been associated with increased mortality up to 1 year after ICU admission[26,31] and decreased long-term cognitive function.[32]

In patients transferred to a LTACH for weaning from prolonged ventilation, the incidence of delirium was investigated using semi-structured interviews conducted by a psychologist within 3 days of admission to the facility.[9] Patients were categorised as delirious using the DSM-IV criteria for delirium.[17] Of the 478 patients evaluated, 246 (51.5%) were categorised as having delirium on arrival to the weaning facility, and of those delirious patients, 61.5% improved during the stay at the facility. Mortality rate was equivalent in the delirium and normal mentation group: 18% versus 16%.[9]

The observation that delirium was not associated with increased mortality in difficult-to-wean patients is in sharp contrast with studies of ICU ventilated patients, where delirium was associated with increased mortality.[27,29,31,33] Several factors may account for the differences. Patients managed at the weaning facility were in the recovery stage, whereas ICU patients were in the acute phase of a critical illness. Conceivably, it is the acute illness, not delirium per se, which explains the association between delirium and increased mortality in ICU patients. In ventilated patients, delirium paralleled shock and Acute Physiology and Chronic Health Evaluation (APACHE) score as a predictor of ICU mortality.[33] Second, the daily dose of sedation that patients received at a weaning facility was substantially less than the dose reported in ICU ventilated patients[9]; sedation has been associated with delirium, longer ventilator duration and longer hospital stay.[32,34]

POST-TRAUMATIC STRESS DISORDER

PTSD is a complex, chronic and severe psychiatric disorder that is triggered by events that pose a serious threat to a person's well-being, such as critical illness.[35,36] The patient's reaction is one of intense fear, horror or helplessness. Survivors of a life-threatening illness who develop PTSD have persistent symptoms that fall into three groups: reliving (or intrusion) symptoms, avoidance and numbing symptoms and increased arousal symptoms. To satisfy the diagnosis of PTSD, the symptoms must be present for 1 month or longer.[17]

In ICU survivors who required short-term mechanical ventilation (average duration of 6 days), the prevalence of PTSD or PTSD-related symptoms ranged from 8% to 51%.[37–41] These prevalence studies, however, have mostly relied on screening questionnaires to detect PTSD. When using the DSM-IV criteria for PTSD, the rate of PTSD among ICU survivors ranges from 8% to 13%.[42–44]

The prevalence of PTSD among survivors of prolonged ventilation (average duration of ventilation is 42 days) managed at weaning facility was investigated.[8] The diagnosis of PTSD was established by an experienced psychologist who conducted a structured clinical interview[45,46]; this interview is considered the reference standard for diagnosing PTSD.[17] To ensure that symptoms were related to PTSD rather than to an acute stress disorder, the interview was conducted at 3 months after weaning.[47] To assess for the presence of PTSD-related symptoms, the Post Traumatic Stress Syndrome 10-questions inventory was also administered 1 week after weaning and 3 months later.[44,48,49]

The psychologist diagnosed PTSD in 12% of patients 3 months after ventilator weaning.[8] Of the 10 PTSD symptoms, sleep disturbance, nightmares, jumpiness, wishing to withdraw from others, frequent changes in mood, guilt, fear of places and situations that reminded the patient of the time of weaning and increased muscle tension were

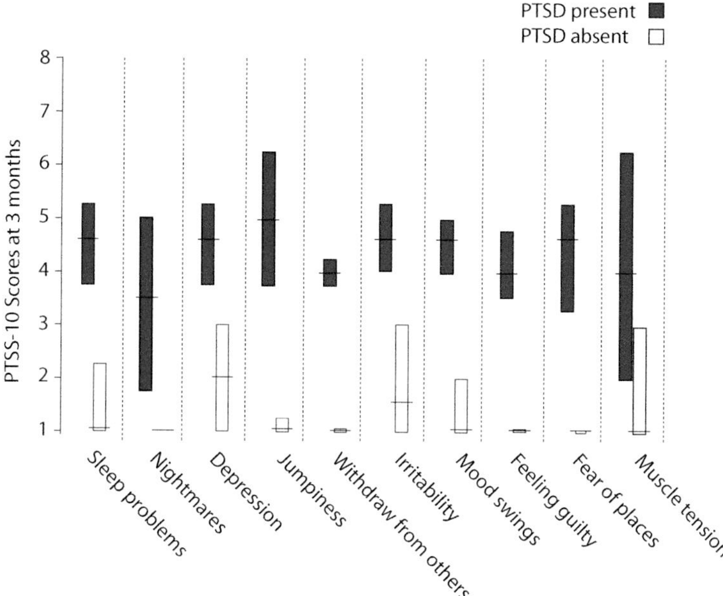

Figure 69.2 Box plots showing median and interquartile ranges of the scores for each of the 10 symptoms on the PTSS-10 questionnaire obtained 3 months after ventilator weaning in patients diagnosed with PTSD (*blue columns*) and in patients not diagnosed with PTSD (*white columns*). Each symptom in the PTSS-10 questionnaire is rated from 1 (never) to 7 (always); the total score ranges from 10 to 70 points. The severity of each symptom on the PTSS-10 questionnaire was greater in patients with PTSD than that in patients without PTSD ($p < 0.01$ for each instance).

reported more in patients with PTSD than in patients without PTSD ($p < 0.02$); depression and generalised irritability were reported equally by both groups (Figure 69.2).

All patients diagnosed with PTSD 3 months after ventilator weaning had a previous history of a psychiatric disorder compared to 31% of patients not diagnosed with PTSD.[8] The development of PTSD was not associated with ventilator duration nor severity of illness[8]; the lack of such an association has also been reported in ICU survivors.[36,38,43]

Patients with PTSD are more likely to develop mood, anxiety and substance abuse disorders than patients without PTSD.[50] In addition, patients with PTSD are six times more likely than matched controls to attempt suicide.[50] Accordingly, the earliest possible identification of patients at increased risk for PTSD might permit the implementation of preventive measures.[51] To determine whether a screening questionnaire is reliable as an early screen for PTSD, the PTSS-10 questionnaire was administered 1 week after weaning from prolonged ventilation and then compared with the psychologist's diagnosis of PTSD obtained 3 months later.[8] A PTSS-10 score greater than 20, 1 week after weaning, reliably identified patients who were diagnosed with PTSD 3 months later: sensitivity, 1.0; specificity, 0.76; area under receiver operating characteristic curve, 0.91. This finding suggests that a simple questionnaire administered before hospital discharge can identify patients at risk for developing PTSD.

ANXIETY

Anxiety is one of the most stressful psychological experiences in patients requiring mechanical ventilation. Clinical features include agitation, excessive fears or worries, hypervigilance, diaphoresis, palpitations and restlessness.[52] When 43 patients were questioned 48–96 hours after extubation (mean duration of mechanical ventilation was 14 days), half reported diffuse anxiety and 37% reported an intense fear of dying at least once during the ventilation period.[53] When 158 patients were interviewed as long as 4 years after receiving mechanical ventilation, almost 50% of patients said they had experienced anxiety and/or fear, and the same proportion said that they had found it very frustrating not to be able to talk.[7] Severe psychological distress in the form of agony and/or panic had at one time or another been experienced by 30% of the patients. Inability to talk and communicate was found to be the dominant reason for evoking anxiety/fear and agony/panic emotions. It also made it more difficult for patients to sleep.

To quantify the level of anxiety during mechanical ventilation, a State-Trait Anxiety Inventory was administered to 200 patients receiving mechanical ventilation.[54] While the level of anxiety considerably varied among patients, the average level of anxiety was 48.5 – a level consistent with moderate levels of anxiety. Patients receiving mechanical ventilation for more than 22 days report the highest level of anxiety.

FACTORS CONTRIBUTING TO MENTAL DISCOMFORT DURING MECHANICAL VENTILATION

Dyspnoea

Dyspnoea is the most common symptom of anxiety and panic disorder.[55] On the other hand, anxiety can cause dyspnoea in the absence of cardiopulmonary pathology. Because of this two-way interaction, the conditions for a vicious circle are present in ventilated patients: dyspnoea causing anxiety and anxiety exacerbating dyspnoea. In mechanically ventilated patients reporting dyspnoea, respiratory discomfort was associated with anxiety (OR, 8.84).[56] In a subgroup of patients in which dyspnoea was lessened by altering ventilator settings, anxiety was also reduced, suggesting that the dyspnoea caused the anxiety.[56] An association between anxiety and dyspnoea may have also been reported in patients as they are weaned from mechanical ventilation.[57]

The prevalence of dyspnoea in ventilated patients widely varies with as much as 19% of patients reporting moderate to severe discomfort.[58] In one study, patients were asked to characterise the quality of their discomfort – 42% reported experiencing air hunger, 20% reported excessive work/effort and 17% reported both air hunger and work/effort.[56]

Several mechanisms can cause dyspnoea during mechanical ventilation. Excessive work of breathing secondary to increased resistance or elastance is an important cause of dyspnoea in ventilated patients.[58] In difficult-to-wean patients, Leung et al.[59] showed that the patients' rating of dyspnoea proportionally increased as the percentage of work done by the ventilator decreased.

Unpleasant dyspnoea, such as air hunger, can also be present in the absence of any respiratory work.[60] Air hunger arises from chemoreceptor stimulation; a rise in partial pressure of carbon dioxide (PCO_2) will induce air hunger.[58] In a study of 16 healthy, ventilated subjects in which the PCO_2 was acutely raised, subjects reported air hunger when the PCO_2 increased by as little as 4 mmHg. An increase in PCO_2 of 10 mmHg produced a level of respiratory discomfort that subjects could not tolerate even for a few minutes.[61] Average PCO_2 increase in weaning failure patients is greater than 10 mmHg[4]; such an increase in PCO_2 may lead to severe dyspnoea and distress.

Using functional brain images, investigators have shown that in humans, air hunger caused the activation of the paralimbic cortex, a region of the brain associated with emotional responses and learning.[58,62] Air hunger has been shown to activate the insula, which has been found to be essential for the perception of other primal sensations (hunger and thirst). Air hunger also activates the amygdala, which is implicated in the perception of fear and anxiety.[62] Thus, it is conceivable that air hunger that occurs in ventilated patients may lead to severe psychological trauma.

Inability to communicate

Patients being weaned from the ventilator are unable to speak and are totally dependent on others for their physical needs. When interviewed about the experience of mechanical ventilation, survivors were emphatic that trouble speaking was the most bothersome experience.[63] In addition, when patients attempted to speak after deflating the cuff, the abnormal quality of their speech, especially unwanted pauses and inadequate loudness, was very frustrating to them.[1]

Sleep disruption

Subjectively, one-third of patients who received mechanical ventilation reported difficulty resting and sleeping in the ICU, and one-fourth had nightmares.[7,63] Indeed, several sleep studies have shown that ICU patients suffer from sleep deprivation, sleep fragmentation and frequent arousals.[64,65] When ICU patients were interviewed about the quality of sleep, all perceived sleep quality to be much poorer than sleep at home. Neither the perceived quality of sleep nor daytime sleepiness improved over the course of the ICU stay.[66]

In the past, the aetiology of sleep disruption was thought to be related to noise in the ICU. When audio and video signals in synchrony with polysomnography were obtained in ventilated patients, Gabor et al.[67] found that loud noise and frequent patient care activities accounted for less than 30% of the observed sleep disruption. Other sources of sleep disruption may be related to the ventilatory mode. In 11 critically ill patients, higher frequency of arousals and awakenings were observed during pressure support than during assist control ventilation.[68] In 13 patients weaned from mechanical ventilation, the lower number of arousals and improved sleep architecture were observed with proportional assist ventilation than with pressure support.[69] In 14 non-sedated patients during weaning from mechanical ventilation, a lower duration of rapid eye movement sleep and higher sleep fragmentation were observed with pressure support than with neurally adjusted ventilatory assist.[70]

ASSESSMENT OF PSYCHOLOGICAL PROBLEMS

The diagnosis of psychological disturbances in a ventilated patient is a difficult task, complicated by the variety of pathophysiological and psychological processes that play a role in the origin of disturbances. The patient has to be alert enough to be able to participate in a psychiatric evaluation. In addition, the presence of an endotracheal tube makes it extremely difficult for most ventilated patients to communicate their physical and emotional needs. Moreover, capturing descriptors that bests fit the patient's discomfort is challenging.

Mental stress is not a uniform concept: patients report different experiences depending on the questions asked and on the condition causing discomfort. When interviewed after being weaned from the ventilator, some patients were uneasy when first removed from the ventilator.[71] Other patients complained of the readjustment in breathing pattern after being put back on the ventilator. Self-rated questionnaires, such as Beck's depression inventory, State-Trait Anxiety Inventory, or Hospital anxiety–depression scale,[38,54,72–75] are commonly used to detect psychiatric disturbances in hospitalised patients; preliminary data, however, suggest that they may not be reliable in ventilated patients.[76] Because of the challenges in measuring mental stress, it is not surprising why psychological assessments are rarely included in research studies.[77]

In assessing the emotional state of a ventilated patient, a comprehensive medical history and physical examination should be first undertaken to determine if there are organic causes contributing to the psychological distress. Observing for specific symptoms (depressed mood, loss of interest in participating in physical therapy, daily grooming and sleep disturbance) and physical signs (flat or constricted affect, tears, agitation and irritability) of mental distress should be undertaken.[52] Observing the manner in which a patient interacts with family and treatment staff may be helpful. Questions about patient's previous psychiatric problems and his or her coping strategies when faced with life stresses or illnesses should also be included in the psychological assessment.[52]

STRATEGIES TO MINIMISE PSYCHOLOGICAL PROBLEMS DURING MECHANICAL VENTILATION

Alleviate dyspnoea

Altering the level of ventilator support can relieve dyspnoea.[58] Increasing the level of ventilatory support in critically ill patients was associated with a proportional decrease in the rating of 'difficulty breathing'.[59] In ventilated patients who reported dyspnoea, the increasing level of support reduced (defined as 1 cm decrease in dyspnoea rating on a visual analogue scale) dyspnoea in 35% of cases.[56] Non-respiratory interventions, such as cool air directed over the face and phasic vibration of intercostals spaces, have also been shown to decrease dyspnoea[78,79]; these interventions, however, have not been studied in the context of mechanical ventilation.

Improve speech

Simple adjustments to the ventilator, such as increasing inspiratory time and positive end-expiratory pressure, or ventilating with bi-level pressure support ventilation, can safely improve ventilator-supported speech.[80,81] Some patients can also benefit from a talking tracheostomy tube, which provides a separate air source to produce speech while the tracheostomy tube cuff is inflated.[1]

Improve sleep

Minimising noise, excessive light and nursing interventions may improve sleep in the ICU.[82] White noise has been shown to decrease arousals during exposure to recorded ICU noise in the sleep laboratory.[83] Avoiding excessive sleep during the day and re-establishing a regular sleep schedule may also be helpful. Finally, tailoring ventilator settings and mode to meet patient's efforts may improve sleep in the ICU.[65,82]

Relaxation techniques (biofeedback and music therapy)

Biofeedback technique has been shown to reduce anxiety.[84] To determine if biofeedback can reduce weaning time, 40 difficult-to-wean patients were randomly assigned to a biofeedback group or to a control group.[85] The biofeedback group received 30–50 min training sessions 5 days a week until extubation. The biofeedback group weaned 12 days earlier than the control group. The reduction in weaning time in biofeedback group was associated with a decrease in anxiety and an increase in respiratory drive and respiratory muscle efficiency.

Music therapy has been shown to decrease anxiety, respiratory rate and heart rate.[86,87] In a clinical trial assessing the effect of music therapy on anxiety, ventilated patients were randomly assigned to self-initiated music therapy group, self-initiated noise-cancelling headphones group or usual care group.[75] On average, patients in the music therapy group listened to music for 78.8 ± 126 min/day; patients in the headphones group wore the headphones for 34.0 ± 89.6 min/day. At any point, anxiety score (quantified using a 100 mm visual analogue scale) was 19.5 points lower in the music therapy group than that in the usual care group; the score was comparable in music therapy group and headphone group.

SUMMARY

Psychological problems are common in patients weaning from mechanical ventilation. Depression occurs in 40% of patients who are weaning from mechanical ventilation and is associated with weaning failure and mortality. PTSD is not uncommon, and full-blown PTSD has been reported in 12% of patients 3 months after weaning from prolonged mechanical ventilation. Dyspnoea, inability to communicate and lack of sleep are the three major stressors contributing to psychological disturbances in ventilated patients. Measurements of mental stress are largely ignored in research studies; this stems, in part, from researcher's underappreciation of the importance of the emotional state in weaning a patient from the ventilator. Treatment plans in ventilated patients should focus on identifying and reversing factors contributing to psychological distress.

REFERENCES

1. Hoit JD, Banzett RB, Brown R. Ventilator-supported speech. In: Tobin MJ, ed. *Principles and Practice of Mechanical Ventilation*, 3rd ed. New York: McGraw-Hill; 2013:1281–92.
2. Riggio RE, Singer RD, Hartman K, Sneider R. Psychological issues in the care of critically ill respirator patients: Differential perceptions of patients, relatives, and staff. *Psychol Rep.* 1982;51:363–9.
3. Jubran A, Mathru M, Dries D, Tobin MJ. Continuous recordings of mixed venous oxygen saturation during weaning from mechanical ventilation and the ramifications thereof. *Am J Respir Crit Care Med.* 1998;158:1763–9.
4. Jubran A, Tobin MJ. Pathophysiologic basis of acute respiratory distress in patients who fail a trial of weaning from mechanical ventilation. *Am J Respir Crit Care Med.* 1997;155:906–15.
5. Jubran A, Tobin MJ. Passive mechanics of lung and chest wall in patients who failed or succeeded in trials of weaning. *Am J Respir Crit Care Med.* 1997;155:916–21.
6. Tobin MJ, Laghi F, Jubran A. Ventilatory failure, ventilator support, and ventilator weaning. *Compr Physiol.* 2012;2:2871–21.
7. Bergbom-Engberg I, Haljamae H. Assessment of patients' experience of discomforts during respirator therapy. *Crit Care Med.* 1989;17:1068–72.
8. Jubran A, Lawm G, Duffner LA et al. Post-traumatic stress disorder after weaning from prolonged mechanical ventilation. *Intensive Care Med.* 2010;36:2030–7.
9. Jubran A, Lawm G, Kelly J et al. Depressive disorders during weaning from prolonged mechanical ventilation. *Intensive Care Med.* 2010;36:828–35.
10. Yang K, Tobin MJ. A prospective study of indexes predicting outcome of trials of weaning from mechanical ventilation. *N Engl J Med.* 1991;324:1445–50.
11. Jubran A, Grant BJ, Laghi F et al. Weaning prediction: Esophageal pressure monitoring complements readiness testing. *Am J Respir Crit Care Med.* 2005;171:1252–9.
12. Tobin MJ, Jubran A. Variable performance of weaning-predictor tests: Role of Bayes' theorem and spectrum and test-referral bias. *Intensive Care Med.* 2006;32:2002–12.
13. Brochard L, Rauss A, Benito S et al. Comparison of three methods of gradual withdrawal from ventilatory support during weaning from mechanical ventilation. *Am J Respir Crit Care Med.* 1994;150:896–903.
14. Esteban A, Frutos F, Tobin MJ et al. A comparison of four methods of weaning patients from mechanical ventilation: Spanish Lung Failure Collaborative Group. *N Engl J Med.* 1995;332:345–50.
15. Jubran A, Grant BJ, Duffner LA et al. Effect of pressure support vs unassisted breathing through a tracheostomy collar on weaning duration in patients requiring prolonged mechanical ventilation: A randomized trial. *JAMA.* 2013;309:671–7.
16. Tobin MJ, Jurban A. Weaning from mechanical ventilation. In: Tobin MJ, ed. *Principles and Practice of Mechanical Ventilation*, 3rd ed. New York: McGraw-Hill; 2013:1307–51.
17. American Psychiatric Association. *Diagnostic and Statistical Manual of Mental Disorders.* Washington, DC: American Psychiatric Association; 1994.
18. Cattapan SE, Laghi F, Tobin MJ. Can diaphragmatic contractility be assessed by airway twitch pressure in mechanically ventilated patients? *Thorax.* 2003;58:58–62.
19. Laghi F, Tobin MJ. Disorders of the respiratory muscles. *Am J Respir Crit Care Med.* 2003;168:10–48.
20. Koenig HG, Blazer DG. Epidemiology of geriatric affective disorders. *Clin Geriatr Med.* 1992;8:235–51.
21. Stoudemire A, Thompson TL, 2nd. Medication noncompliance: Systematic approaches to evaluation and intervention. *Gen Hosp Psychiatry.* 1983;5:233–9.
22. Engel GL. A life setting conducive to illness. The giving-up–give-up comples. *Ann Intern Med.* 1968; 69:293–300.
23. Givens JL, Jones RN, Inouye SK. The overlap syndrome of depression and delirium in older hospitalized patients. *J Am Geriatr Soc.* 2009;57:1347–53.
24. McAvay GJ, Van Ness PH, Bogardus ST, Jr et al. Depressive symptoms and the risk of incident delirium in older hospitalized adults. *J Am Geriatr Soc.* 2007;55:684–91.
25. Bergeron N, Dubois MJ, Dumont M et al. Intensive Care Delirium Screening Checklist: Evaluation of a new screening tool. *Intensive Care Med.* 2001;27:859–64.
26. Ely EW, Shintani A, Truman B et al. Delirium as a predictor of mortality in mechanically ventilated patients in the intensive care unit. *JAMA.* 2004;291:1753–62.
27. Ouimet S, Kavanagh BP, Gottfried SB, Skrobik Y. Incidence, risk factors and consequences of ICU delirium. *Intensive Care Med.* 2007;33:66–73.
28. Plaschke K, von Haken R, Scholz M et al. Comparison of the confusion assessment method for the intensive care unit (CAM-ICU) with the Intensive Care Delirium Screening Checklist (ICDSC) for delirium in critical care patients gives high agreement rate(s). *Intensive Care Med.* 2008; 34:431–6.
29. Reade MC, Finfer S. Sedation and delirium in the intensive care unit. *N Engl J Med.* 2014;370:444–54.
30. Skrobik Y. Psychological problems in the ventilated patient. In: Tobin MJ, ed. *Principles and Practice of Mechanical Ventilation*, 3rd ed. New York: McGraw-Hill; 2013:1259–66.

31. Pisani MA, Kong SY, Kasl SV et al. Days of delirium are associated with 1-year mortality in an older intensive care unit population. *Am J Respir Crit Care Med.* 2009;180:1092–7.
32. van den Boogaard M, Schoonhoven L, Evers AW et al. Delirium in critically ill patients: Impact on long-term health-related quality of life and cognitive functioning. *Crit Care Med.* 2012;40:112–8.
33. Lin SM, Liu CY, Wang CH et al. The impact of delirium on the survival of mechanically ventilated patients. *Crit Care Med.* 2004;32:2254–9.
34. Kress JP, Pohlman AS, O'Connor MF, Hall JB. Daily interruption of sedative infusions in critically ill patients undergoing mechanical ventilation. *N Engl J Med.* 2000;342:1471–7.
35. Schelling G, Stoll C, Vogelmeier C et al. Pulmonary function and health-related quality of life in a sample of long-term survivors of the acute respiratory distress syndrome. *Intensive Care Med.* 2000;26:1304–11.
36. Davydow DS, Gifford JM, Desai SV et al. Posttraumatic stress disorder in general intensive care unit survivors: A systematic review. *Gen Hosp Psychiatry.* 2008;30:421–34.
37. Weinert CR, Sprenkle M. Post-ICU consequences of patient wakefulness and sedative exposure during mechanical ventilation. *Intensive Care Med.* 2008;34:82–90.
38. Samuelson KA, Lundberg D, Fridlund B. Stressful memories and psychological distress in adult mechanically ventilated intensive care patients – A 2-month follow-up study. *Acta Anaesthesiol Scand.* 2007;51:671–8.
39. Kress JP, Gehlbach B, Lacy M et al. The long-term psychological effects of daily sedative interruption on critically ill patients. *Am J Respir Crit Care Med.* 2003;168:1457–61.
40. Jones C, Griffiths RD, Humphris G, Skirrow PM. Memory, delusions, and the development of acute posttraumatic stress disorder-related symptoms after intensive care. *Crit Care Med.* 2001;29:573–80.
41. Cuthbertson BH, Hull A, Strachan M, Scott J. Post-traumatic stress disorder after critical illness requiring general intensive care. *Intensive Care Med.* 2004;30:450–5.
42. Jones C, Backman C, Capuzzo M et al. Intensive care diaries reduce new onset post traumatic stress disorder following critical illness: A randomised, controlled trial. *Crit Care.* 2010;14:R168.
43. Patel MB, Jackson JC, Morandi A et al. Incidence and risk factors for intensive care unit-related post-traumatic stress disorder in veterans and civilians. *Am J Respir Crit Care Med.* 2016;193:1373–81.
44. Nickel M, Leiberich P, Nickel C et al. The occurrence of posttraumatic stress disorder in patients following intensive care treatment: A cross-sectional study in a random sample. *J Intensive Care Med.* 2004;19:285–90.
45. Spitzer R, Williams J, Gibbon M, First M. *Structured Clinical Interview for DSM-III-R.* Washington, DC: American Psychiatric Association; 1990.
46. Watson CG, Juba MP, Manifold V et al. The PTSD interview: Rationale, description, reliability, and concurrent validity of a DSM-III-based technique. *J Clin Psychol.* 1991;47:179–88.
47. Koren D, Arnon I, Klein E. Acute stress response and posttraumatic stress disorder in traffic accident victims: A one-year prospective, follow-up study. *Am J Psychiatry.* 1999;156:367–73.
48. Deja M, Denke C, Weber-Carstens S et al. Social support during intensive care unit stay might improve mental impairment and consequently health-related quality of life in survivors of severe acute respiratory distress syndrome. *Crit Care.* 2006;10:R147.
49. Stoll C, Kapfhammer HP, Rothenhausler HB et al. Sensitivity and specificity of a screening test to document traumatic experiences and to diagnose post-traumatic stress disorder in ARDS patients after intensive care treatment. *Intensive Care Med.* 1999;25:697–704.
50. Kessler RC. Posttraumatic stress disorder: The burden to the individual and to society. *J Clin Psychiatry.* 2000;61:4–12; discussion 13–14.
51. Ballenger JC, Davidson JR, Lecrubier Y et al. Consensus statement update on posttraumatic stress disorder from the international consensus group on depression and anxiety. *J Clin Psychiatry.* 2004;65:55–62.
52. Misra S, Ganzini L. Delirium, depression, and anxiety. *Crit Care Clin.* 2003;19:771–87.
53. Pochard F, Lanore JJ, Bellivier F et al. Subjective psychological status of severely ill patients discharged from mechanical ventilation. *Clin Intensive Care.* 1995;6:57–61.
54. Chlan LL. Description of anxiety levels by individual differences and clinical factors in patients receiving mechanical ventilatory support. *Heart Lung.* 2003;32:275–82.
55. Smoller JW, Pollack MH, Otto MW et al. Panic anxiety, dyspnea, and respiratory disease: Theoretical and clinical considerations. *Am J Respir Crit Care Med.* 1996;154:6–17.
56. Schmidt M, Demoule A, Polito A et al. Dyspnea in mechanically ventilated critically ill patients. *Crit Care Med.* 2011;39:2059–65.
57. Knebel AR, Janson-Bjerklie SL, Malley JD et al. Comparison of breathing comfort during weaning with two ventilatory modes. *Am J Respir Crit Care Med.* 1994;149:14–8.
58. Banzett RB, Similowski T, Brown R. Addressing respiratory discomfort in the ventilated patient. In: Tobin MJ, ed. *Principles and Practice of Mechanical Ventilation*, 3rd ed. New York: McGraw-Hill; 2013:1267–92.

59. Leung P, Jubran A, Tobin MJ. Comparison of assisted ventilator modes on triggering, patient effort, and dyspnea. *Am J Respir Crit Care Med.* 1997;155:1940–8.
60. Schmidt M, Banzett RB, Raux M et al. Unrecognized suffering in the ICU: Addressing dyspnea in mechanically ventilated patients. *Intensive Care Med.* 2014;40:1–10.
61. Banzett RB, Lansing RW, Reid MB et al. 'Air hunger' arising from increased PCO2 in mechanically ventilated quadriplegics. *Respir Physiol.* 1989;76:53–67.
62. Evans KC, Banzett RB, Adams L et al. BOLD fMRI identifies limbic, paralimbic, and cerebellar activation during air hunger. *J Neurophysiol.* 2002;88:1500–11.
63. Rotondi AJ, Chelluri L, Sirio C et al. Patients' recollections of stressful experiences while receiving prolonged mechanical ventilation in an intensive care unit. *Crit Care Med.* 2002;30:746–52.
64. Cooper AB, Thornley KS, Young GB et al. Sleep in critically ill patients requiring mechanical ventilation. *Chest.* 2000;117:809–18.
65. Parthasarathy S, Tobin MJ. Sleep in the intensive care unit. *Intensive Care Med.* 2004;30:197–206.
66. Freedman NS, Kotzer N, Schwab RJ. Patient perception of sleep quality and etiology of sleep disruption in the intensive care unit. *Am J Respir Crit Care Med.* 1999;159:1155–62.
67. Gabor JY, Cooper AB, Crombach SA et al. Contribution of the intensive care unit environment to sleep disruption in mechanically ventilated patients and healthy subjects. *Am J Respir Crit Care Med.* 2003;167:708–15.
68. Parthasarathy S, Tobin MJ. Effect of ventilator mode on sleep quality in critically ill patients. *Am J Respir Crit Care Med.* 2002;166:1423–9.
69. Bosma K, Ferreyra G, Ambrogio C et al. Patient-ventilator interaction and sleep in mechanically ventilated patients: Pressure support versus proportional assist ventilation. *Crit Care Med.* 2007;35:1048–54.
70. Delisle S, Ouellet P, Bellemare P et al. Sleep quality in mechanically ventilated patients: Comparison between NAVA and PSV modes. *Ann Intensive Care.* 2011;1:42.
71. Jablonski RS. The experience of being mechanically ventilated. *Qual Health Res.* 1994;4:186–207.
72. Rincon HG, Granados M, Unutzer J et al. Prevalence, detection and treatment of anxiety, depression, and delirium in the adult critical care unit. *Psychosomatics.* 2001;42:391–6.
73. Spielberger C. *State-Trait Anxiety Inventory Manual.* Redwood City, CA: Mind Garden; 1983.
74. Beck AT, Steer RA, Brown GK. *Beck Depression Inventory: Second Edition Manual.* San Antonio, TX: Psychological Corporation, Harcourt, Brace; 1980.
75. Chlan LL, Weinert CR, Heiderscheit A et al. Effects of patient-directed music intervention on anxiety and sedative exposure in critically ill patients receiving mechanical ventilatory support: A randomized clinical trial. *JAMA.* 2013;309:2335–44.
76. Baugh MJ, Lawm G, Kelly J et al. Screening for depressive disorders during weaning from prolonged mechanical ventilation. *Am J Respir Crit Care Med.* 2010;181:A3043.
77. Girard TD, Kress JP, Fuchs BD et al. Efficacy and safety of a paired sedation and ventilator weaning protocol for mechanically ventilated patients in intensive care (Awakening and Breathing Controlled trial): A randomised controlled trial. *Lancet.* 2008; 371:126–34.
78. Schwartzstein RM, Lahive K, Pope A et al. Cold facial stimulation reduces breathlessness induced in normal subjects. *Am Rev Respir Dis.* 1987;136:58–61.
79. Manning HL, Basner R, Ringler J et al. Effect of chest wall vibration on breathlessness in normal subjects. *J Appl Physiol (1985).* 1991;71:175–81.
80. Hoit JD, Banzett RB, Lohmeier HL et al. Clinical ventilator adjustments that improve speech. *Chest.* 2003;124:1512–21.
81. Prigent H, Samuel C, Louis B et al. Comparative effects of two ventilatory modes on speech in tracheostomized patients with neuromuscular disease. *Am J Respir Crit Care Med.* 2003;167:114–9.
82. Hanly PJ. Sleep in the ventilator-supported patient. In: Tobin MJ, ed. *Principles and Practice of Mechanical Ventilation*, 3rd ed. New York: McGraw-Hill; 2013:1293–306.
83. Stanchina ML, Abu-Hijleh M, Chaudhry BK et al. The influence of white noise on sleep in subjects exposed to ICU noise. *Sleep Med.* 2005;6:423–8.
84. Hannich HJ, Hartmann U, Lehmann C et al. Biofeedback as a supportive method in weaning long-term ventilated critically ill patients. *Med Hypotheses.* 2004;63:21–5.
85. Holliday JE, Hyers TM. The reduction of weaning time from mechanical ventilation using tidal volume and relaxation biofeedback. *Am Rev Respir Dis.* 1990;141:1214–20.
86. Chlan L. Effectiveness of a music therapy intervention on relaxation and anxiety for patients receiving ventilatory assistance. *Heart Lung.* 1998;27:169–76.
87. Wong HL, Lopez-Nahas V, Molassiotis A. Effects of music therapy on anxiety in ventilator-dependent patients. *Heart Lung.* 2001;30:376–87.

PART 15

The physiotherapist and assisted ventilation

70 Respiratory physiotherapy (including cough assistance techniques and glossopharyngeal breathing) 632
Miguel R. Gonçalves and João Carlos Winck

71 Rehabilitation 645
Rik Gosselink, Bruno Clerckx, T. Troosters, J. Segers and D. Langer

70

Respiratory physiotherapy (including cough assistance techniques and glossopharyngeal breathing)

MIGUEL R. GONÇALVES AND JOÃO CARLOS WINCK

INTRODUCTION

The effective elimination of airway mucus and other debris is one of the most important factors that allows the successful use of chronic and acute ventilation support (non-invasive and invasive) for patients with either ventilatory or oxygenation impairment. In ventilatory-dependent patients, the goals of intervention are to maintain lung compliance and normal alveolar ventilation at all times and to maximise cough flows for adequate bronchopulmonary secretion clearance.

Techniques for augmenting the normal mucociliary clearance and cough efficacy have been used for many years to treat patients with respiratory disorders from different aetiologies. In recent years, new technologies and more advanced techniques have been developed to be more comfortable and effective for the majority of patients. Postural drainage with manual chest percussion and shaking has, in most parts of the world, been replaced by more independent and effective techniques.

Inspiratory and expiratory muscle aids are devices and techniques that involve the manual or mechanical application of forces to the body or intermittent pressure changes to the airway to assist inspiratory or expiratory muscle function. In recent years, new technologies and more advanced techniques have been developed to be more comfortable and effective for airway clearance and lung expansion. The evidence in support of these techniques is variable, and the literature is confusing and sometimes conflicting regarding the clinical indication for each technique.[1] Moreover, it can be confusing for healthcare professionals, patients and their caregivers when it comes to choosing and utilising the most appropriate airway clearance techniques and products.

Although the use of respiratory muscle aids is an important intervention for eliminating airway secretions for patients with muscle weakness, as for normal coughing, these aids may not adequately eliminate secretions that are obstructing the smaller airways.[2] In these situations, it is important to consider secretion mobilisation techniques to gradually loosen and mobilise secretions to assist mucociliary clearance from the lower airway into the upper airway to avoid the risk of atelectasis and pneumonia, which can often lead to numerous hospitalisations and even premature death.

In patients with primarily ventilatory impairment, such as neuromuscular disease, 90% of episodes of respiratory failure are a result of the inability to effectively clear airway mucus during intercurrent chest colds. Although the use of respiratory muscle aids is the single most important intervention for eliminating airway secretions for these patients, as for normal coughing, these aids may not adequately remove secretions from the very small peripheral airways more than six divisions from the trachea; the flows they create may not be sufficient to eliminate secretions that are obstructing the smaller airways. In these situations, it is important to consider secretion mobilisation techniques to gradually loosen and mobilise secretions to assist mucociliary clearance from the lower airway into the upper airway where they then need to be cleared by either assisted coughing techniques or the patient's natural cough.

One of the techniques that may be very helpful for patients with ventilatory impairment is glossopharyngeal breathing (GPB). This technique was commonly used in the 1950s with poliomyelitis patients to enhance their breathing capabilities.[3] This same technique can be used in both patients with neuromuscular disease[4] and individuals with high spinal cord injury (SCI)[5] to improve their forced vital capacity (FVC) and peak cough flow (PCF). It has been shown that in SCI patients, ventilatory-free breathing increases on more than 3 hours with GPB,[6] and the GPB maximum single breath capacity can be increased with training.[4]

A great majority of episodes of secretion encumbrance develop in acute respiratory failure, and it has been demonstrated that morbidity and mortality can be avoided without hospitalisations with a correct and effective secretion management protocol.[7] Moreover, it has been reported that conventional chest physical therapy for secretion management does not increase the chances of weaning and extubation success in critically ill patients.[8] However, some of these patients may have normal mucociliary clearance but ineffective PCFs, which itself has been associated with extubation failure.[9,10] A protocol that includes assisting coughing techniques as adjunct to an efficient non-invasive ventilation (NIV) application may increase the success rates of extubation in difficult to wean patients.

IMPAIRMENT OF MUCUS ELIMINATION AND CLINICAL INDICATIONS FOR AIRWAY CLEARANCE PHYSIOTHERAPY TECHNIQUES

For patients with chronic airways disease, mucus stasis can contribute to bronchial obstruction, and chronic expectoration can be a physically and socially disabling problem. Mucus retention can also cause pathological changes in the lungs and is thought to contribute to the progression of airway disease. It is, therefore, not surprising that for patients with chronic airways disease, mucus hypersecretion has been associated with increased mortality,[11] and it is thought to contribute to the development of respiratory tract infections.

Mucus clearance and bronchial hygiene is often decreased in patients with airway disease, as well as in both paediatric and adult patients with neuromuscular disorders (NMDs) and consequent dysfunctional cough or glottis control.

Patients with airway diseases

Hypersecretion is usually present in the acute episodes of asthma, and normally, mucus transport is impaired due to the reduction of ciliary activity.[12] In these patients, mucus transport can be recovered or remain reduced, despite favourable changes in mucus viscoelasticity after an exacerbation.

In patients with chronic obstructive pulmonary disease (COPD), there is a persistent and permanent dyspnoea and airway obstruction, with incomplete reversibility with therapy. Normally, in these patients, the mucociliary transport is not so impaired, until an acute exacerbation occurs. Secretion encumbrance has been associated with failure of NIV in COPD, where endotracheal intubation and mechanical ventilation may become necessary during acute exacerbations.

Cystic fibrosis (CF) is a relatively common, inherited life-limiting disorder. The genetic defect causes abnormal mucus secretion in the airways, potentially leading to airway obstruction and mucus plugging.

Treatment methods, which improve mucus clearance, are considered essential in optimising respiratory status and reducing the progression of lung disease in these patient populations. The goal is to reduce disease progression by augmenting the normal mucociliary clearance mechanism of the lungs and facilitating expectoration.[13]

Patients with neuromuscular disorders

The effectiveness in eliminating secretions is determined by the amount of flow generated in the expulsive phase. These factors depend on the linear velocity of gas flow, the diameter of the segment and dynamic compression, and they are basically manifested in the value of PCF.[14]

In NMD, there is a progressive decrease in vital capacity (VC), which is mainly related to the combination of muscle weakness and alterations of the mechanical properties of the lungs and chest wall.[15]

Changes in the ability to cough, understood as the inability to expel secretions effectively or finding it difficult to do so, may precede alterations in alveolar ventilation and place patients at risk for atelectasis, mucus plugging and pneumonia. Such alterations are the main cause of morbidity and mortality in patients with NMD.[7]

Along with hypoventilation, these alterations represent the most important problem from the patient's point of view.[16]

Severe bulbar dysfunction and glottic dysfunction most commonly occur in patients with amyotrophic lateral sclerosis (ALS), spinal muscle atrophy (SMA) type 1 and the pseudobulbar palsy of central nervous system aetiology.[17] The inability to close the glottis and vocal cords results in complete loss of the ability to cough and swallow.

CONTROL OF MUCUS AND AIRWAY CLEARANCE TECHNIQUES

Airway clearance refers to two separate, but connected, mechanisms: mucociliary clearance and cough clearance.

Approaches to preventing airway secretion retention include pharmacotherapy to reduce mucus hypersecretion or to liquefy secretions and the application of chest physiotherapy (CPT) techniques. These techniques do not appear to benefit patients during recovery from acute exacerbations of COPD or pneumonia. These conditions are characterised by interstitial pathology, which cannot be influenced by physical interventions in the airways.[18–20] Further studies are needed to identify the patients and more circumstances, which are at risk from complications or adverse effects of manual CPT.

An effective cough is based on expiratory muscle force, capable of producing effective PCFs. The PCF is a routine measure in the evaluation of neuromuscular patients, and clinical investigations suggest that it should be used in SCI patients as well. The patient with partial or complete abdominal muscle paralysis is unable to produce an effective cough.[21,22]

Positioning, breathing control techniques and CPT

Positioning the patient to enable gravity to assist the flow of bronchial secretions from the airways has been a standard treatment for some time in patients with retained secretions.[23] The combination of positioning with breathing techniques and manual CPT increases the effectiveness of airway clearance in patients with different aetiologies (Figure 70.1).

Positioning can also place the patient at risk for skin and cardiac complications, cerebral blood flow or intracranial pressure changes and gastro-oesophageal reflux.[24]

Breathing control techniques include autonomous breathing exercises such as forced and deep expirations, and diaphragmatic breathing to optimise airway mucus clearance. One of the techniques described as the most efficient in mucus clearance is the active cycle of breathing technique (ACBT)[23] that consists of repeated cycles of three ventilatory phases: breathing control, thoracic expansion exercises and the forced expiration technique. Huffing to low lung volumes will assist in mobilising and clearing the more peripherally situated secretions, and when secretions have reached the larger and proximal upper airways, a huff or cough from a high lung volume can be used to clear them. The concept of the equal pressure point explains the mechanism of the effectiveness of huffing in airway clearance. The period of breathing control is essential between the huffing phases to prevent bronchospasm. In patients with asthma, CF and chronic airflow limitation, there is no evidence of any increase in airflow obstruction. The ACBT technique may be performed by a patient independent of a caregiver, but it has also been shown to be equally effective with assistance.

Another breathing control technique that is widely used is autogenic drainage.[23,25] This technique is based on breathing at different lung volumes (low volume, tidal volume and high volume), and expiration is used to move the mucus. The aim is to maximise expiratory flow. When sufficient mucus has reached the upper airways, it may be cleared by a cough.

Both ACBT and autogenic drainage are not indicated in severe ventilatory-dependent patients; however, it may be used during weaning protocols.

Approaches to preventing the retention of airway secretions include the use of medication to reduce mucus hypersecretion or to liquefy secretions and the facilitation of mucus mobilisation. To complement this objective, CPT techniques can be very effective in preventing pulmonary complications in infant and adult patients with secretion accumulation.

Manual chest percussion (*clapping*) and *chest vibration* have been associated with an increase in airflow obstruction[26] and have been shown to cause an increase in hypoxaemia.[23] On the basis of three randomised controlled trials, CPT is ineffective and perhaps even detrimental in the treatment of patients with acute exacerbations of COPD.[27]

Guidebooks of manual thoracic techniques may have been published that demonstrate the hand placements and thrusting techniques in children and adults.[28]

Instrumental techniques for mucus mobilisation

Methods of promoting airway clearance using specific devices have been included in most respiratory therapy programmes.

Positive expiratory pressure (PEP) breathing is usually applied by breathing through a facemask or mouthpiece with an inspiratory tube containing a one-way valve and an expiratory tube containing a variable expiratory resistance. It results in PEP throughout expiration.[23,24,29,30]

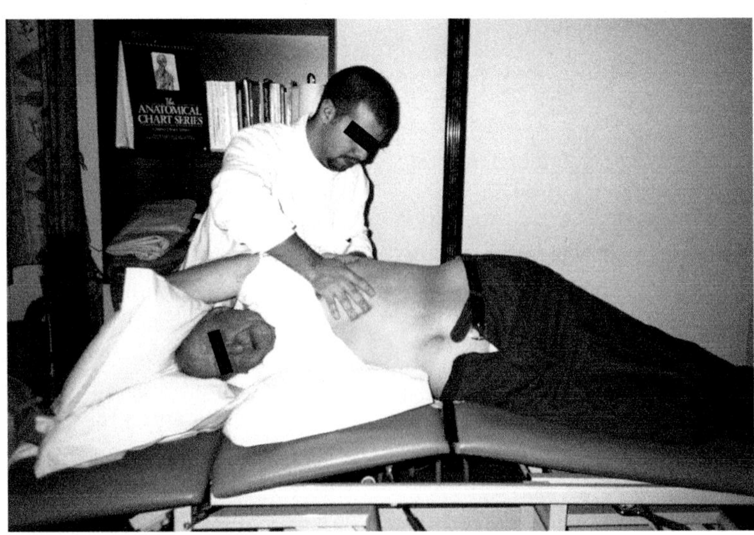

Figure 70.1 Manual CPT applied in an airway disease patient.

A combination of PEP and air column oscillation applied at the mouth can be obtained when the patient expires through a shaped device called oscillatory positive expiratory pressure (OPEP) device. The mucus mobilising effect is thought to be due to both a widening of the airways due to the increased expiratory pressure and the occurrence of airflow oscillations,[31] as secretions mobilised to the central airways are cleared by coughing or huffing. A list of available PEP and OPEP devices, as well as their main characteristics, is shown in Tables 70.1 and 70.2.

Manually assisted coughing and lung insufflation techniques

Manually assisted cough is the external application of pressure to the thoracic cage or epigastric area, coordinated with a forced exhalation. This action serves to simulate the normal cough mechanism by generating an increase in the velocity of the expired air and may be helpful in moving secretions towards the trachea. The abdominal thrust is an assisted coughing technique, which consists of the

Table 70.1 Characteristics of PEP breathing devices

PEP devices		Nebuliser	Flow-dependent resistance
EzPAP®		Yes	Yes
Resistex®		Yes	Yes
ThetaPEP®		No	Yes
ThresholdPEP®		No	No

Table 70.2 Characteristics of OPEP breathing devices

OPEP devices		Allows multiple positions	Nebuliser	Adjustable resistance	Boiling safe
Acapella®	DM DH Choice Duet	Yes	Due	Sim	Duet choice
Aerobika®		No	Yes	Yes	Yes
Flutter®		No	No	No	No
Lung Flute®		No	No	No	No
Quake®		Yes	No	Yes	Yes
RC-Cornet®		Yes	Yes	Yes	Yes
Shaker®	Classic Deluxe Plus	No	No	No	Plus

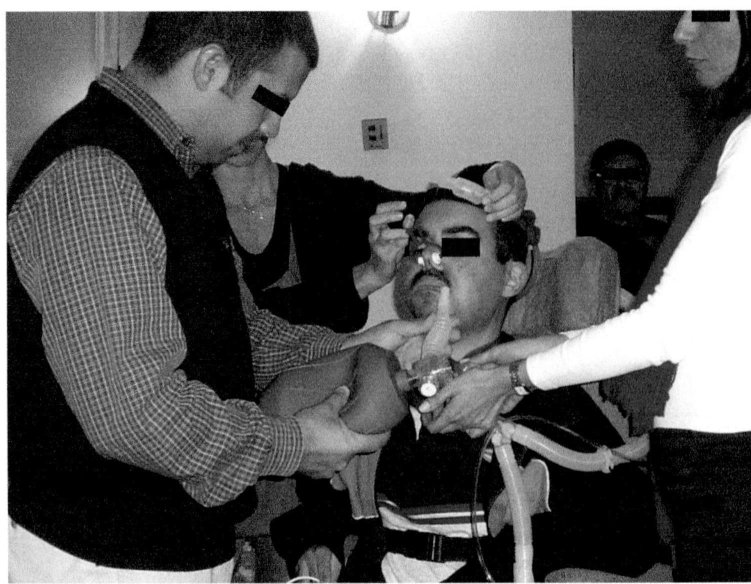

Figure 70.2 Air stacking with manual resuscitator via a mouthpiece in a Duchenne muscular dystrophy patient with low VC and suboptimal PCF.

association of two techniques: the costophrenic compression and the Heimlich manoeuvre.

The combination of deep lung insufflations to the maximal insufflation capacity (MIC)[32] (Figure 70.2) followed by manually assisted cough with abdominal thrust (Figure 70.3) has been shown to significantly increase PCFs values in NMD patients.[33,34] The MIC is the maximum, tolerable externally assisted insufflation capacity that is dependent on the glottic control of exhalation.[32] The 'lower end' of an MIC is the residual volume, as the 'upper end' of an MIC is assisted on top of the VC. This assistance may be provided by GPB, a bagging circuit, assisted inspiration by a volume-cycled ventilator. With respect to MIC generation, the hallmark of this measure is that the device delivered volume is typically pressure limited, and the expiratory control remains with the participant and her/his glottis.[22] The lung insufflation capacity is the maximum, tolerable externally assisted insufflation capacity that is independent of glottic control of exhalation.[35] This assistance may be provided by a bagging circuit with a one-way value, assisted inspiration by a volume cycled ventilator or the inflation component of a mechanical insufflation–exsufflation (MI-E) device.

Although an optimal insufflation followed by an abdominal thrust provides the greatest increase in PCF, it can also be significantly increased by providing only a maximal insufflation or providing only an abdominal thrust. Interestingly, PCFs are significantly increased more by the maximal insufflation than by the abdominal thrust.[36,37] Manually assisted coughing and MIC manoeuvre require a cooperative patient and a good coordination between the patient and caregiver (Figures 70.4 and 70.5).

Abdominal compressions should not be used for 1–1.5 hours following a meal; however, chest compressions can be used to augment PCF. Chest thrusting techniques must be performed with caution in the presence of an osteoporotic rib cage. Unfortunately, since it is not widely taught to healthcare professionals, manually assisted coughing is underutilised.[38]

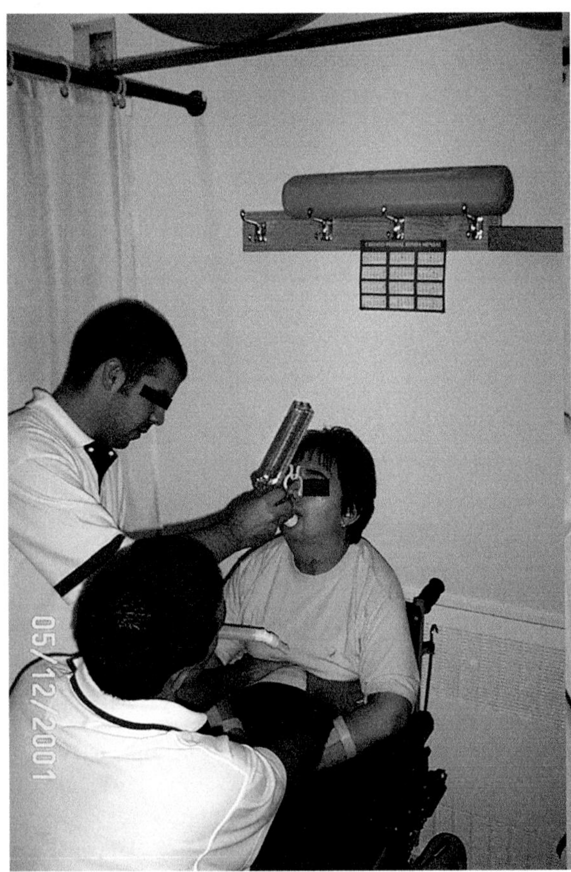

Figure 70.3 Manually assisted cough with abdominal thrust to measure PCF in sitting position in an NMD patient.

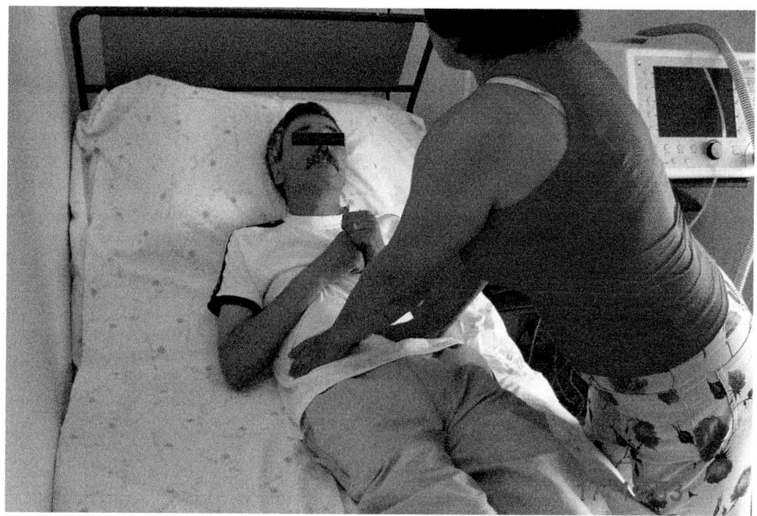

Figure 70.4 Air stacking in a patient with NMD, performed by the family caregiver.

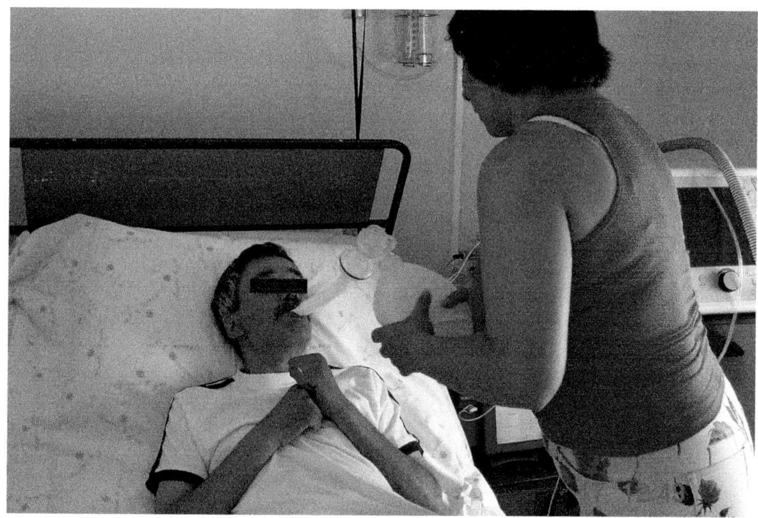

Figure 70.5 Manually assisted cough in a patient with NMD, performed by the family caregiver.

GLOSSOPHARYNGEAL BREATHING

Both inspiratory and, indirectly, expiratory muscle function can be assisted by GPB. The technique involves the use of the glottis to add to an inspiratory effort by projecting (gulping) boluses of air into the lungs. The glottis closes with each 'gulp'. One breath usually consists of six to nine gulps of 40–200 mL each.[4] During the training period, the efficiency of GPB can be monitored by spirometrically measuring the millilitres of air per gulp, gulps per breath and breaths per minute.

GPB (or 'frog' breathing) uses the muscles of the tongue (the glossa) and the throat (pharyngeal muscles) to force air into the trachea and lungs through a repetitious process.

Neuromuscular and SCI patients are perfect candidates because of their intact bulbar function, but most of them need considerable instruction and encouragement to learn this technique, as well as hours of practice to master it. Approximately 60% of ventilator users with no autonomous ability to breathe and good bulbar muscle function can use GPB for autonomous breathing from minutes to up to all day.[39,40]

Many daily activities can interfere with an individual's ability to perform GPB. The reason is because these daily activities involve the mouth and throat muscles, thus causing interference. With a great deal of practice and confidence, patients can learn to master these daily requirements and still be able to effectively perform GPB.[41]

Although extremely useful, GPB is rarely taught since there are few healthcare professionals familiar with the technique. This technique is also rarely useful in the presence of an indwelling tracheostomy tube. It cannot be used when the tube is uncapped as it is during tracheostomy intermittent positive pressure ventilation (IPPV), and even when capped, the gulped air tends to leak around the outer walls of the tube and out the stoma. The safety and versatility afforded by GPB are key reasons to eliminate tracheostomy in favour of non-invasive aids.

MECHANICAL RESPIRATORY MUSCLE AIDS FOR SECRETION MANAGEMENT

Respiratory muscle aids for secretion management are devices and techniques that involve the mechanical application of forces to the body or intermittent pressure changes to the airway to assist expiratory muscle function and airway mucus clearance.

Intrapulmonary percussive ventilation

The intrapulmonary percussive ventilator (IPV) is an airway clearance positive-pressure breathing pneumatic device that simultaneously delivers aerosolised solution and intrathoracic percussion. This modified method of intermittent positive-pressure breathing imposes high-frequency minibursts of gas (at 100–300 cycles/min) on the patient's own respiration. This creates a global effect of the internal percussion of the lungs, which could promote clearance of the peripheral bronchial tree.

The high-frequency gas pulses expand the lungs, vibrate and enlarge the airways and deliver gas into distal lung units, beyond accumulated mucus.[25,42,43] The physiological effects of IPV have been studied in vitro.[44] Increasing frequency increases positive end-expiratory pressure (PEEP) and percussion (i.e. the peak of pressure), but decreases ventilation. Increasing inspiratory/expiratory (I/E) time increases PEEP and decreases percussion. Increasing pressure increases PEEP and ventilation. Interestingly, higher expiratory than inspiratory flows are always produced by IPV.

Parameters of IPV devices can be set as follows: in order to obtain the highest peaks of pressure, high-frequency and short inspiration are recommended.[45] However, lower frequencies and higher pressures are required when patients need assisted ventilation. Lower pressures and higher frequencies will be set in infants and children. Again, pressures will be increased to obtain normal SpO_2 and $PaCO_2$ in those ventilator-dependent patients such as type 1 SMA. The length of IPV session is related to the comfort of patients.

This technique has been shown to be as effective as a standard CPT and to assist mucus clearance in patients with secretion encumbrance from different aetiologies, such as CF,[46] acute exacerbations of COPD[47] and Duchenne muscle dystrophy.[42] In CF, IPV was shown to be as effective as the other methods of airway clearance in sputum mobilisation, when the amount of sputum produced was assessed by dry weight.[48]

IPV can be delivered through a mouthpiece and a facial mask and through a endotracheal and tracheostomy tube. The primary aims of this technique are to reduce secretion viscosity, promote deep lung recruitment, improve gas exchange, deliver a vascular 'massage' and protect the airway against barotrauma. The main contraindication is the presence of diffuse alveolar haemorrhage with haemodynamic instability. Relative contraindications include active or recent gross haemoptysis, pulmonary embolism, subcutaneous emphysema, bronchopleural fistula, oesophageal surgery, recent spinal infusion, spinal anaesthesia or acute spinal injury, presence of a transvenous or subcutaneous pacemaker, increased intracranial pressures, uncontrolled hypertension, suspected or confirmed pulmonary tuberculosis, bronchospasm, emphysema or large pleural effusion and acute cardiogenic pulmonary oedema.[49]

The BTS guidelines on airway clearance techniques in the spontaneously breathing adult[50] highlight that 'the ATS consensus statement on the management of patients with DMD[51] concludes there is insufficient evidence to make any firm recommendations on the use of IPV with self-ventilating patients, but that the use of airway clearance devices dependent on a normal cough is likely to be ineffective without the concurrent use of other assisted cough techniques. Therefore, other techniques, alone or in combination, may be required to clear secretions once mobilised centrally following intrapulmonary percussive ventilation. Further research is required to evaluate the safety and efficacy of IPV in the care of patients with neuromuscular disease.'

High-frequency chest wall oscillation

During high-frequency chest wall oscillation (HFCWO), positive pressure air pulses are applied to the chest wall. The compressive force is usually via an inflatable jacket adjusted to snugly fit over the thorax. The air pulse generator then delivers intermittent positive airflow into the jacket. As the jacket expands, compressing the chest wall, it produces a transient/oscillatory increase in airflow in the airways, vibrating the secretions from the peripheral airways towards the mouth. Recommended starting settings for this device are a frequency of 5 Hz building up to 10–15 Hz, and the jacket pressure should be inflated to comfort, but the oscillations should be felt by the patient within the lungs and not just superficially. HFCWO can also be delivered via a cuirass with negative pressure ventilation devices.

Mechanical vibration is applied during the entire breathing cycle or during expiration only. The adjustable I/E ratio permits asymmetric inspiratory and expiratory pressure changes (for example +3 to −6 cm H_2O), which favour higher exsufflation flow velocities to mobilise secretions. The average length of time spent in each treatment session will vary according to patient tolerance, amount and consistency of secretions and the phase of the patient's illness (acute or chronic).[43] The simultaneous use of an aerosolised medication or saline is recommended throughout the treatment. This humidifies the air to counteract the drying effect of the increased airflow.[47]

HFCWO may act like a physical mucolytic, reducing the viscoelasticity of mucus and enhancing clearance by coughing.[24,25,52] HFCWO has demonstrated efficacy in assisting mucus clearance in patients with CF.[52–55]

These beneficial effects upon both mucus clearance and clinical parameters are not so evident in other groups of patients such as COPD. Moreover, side effects of percussion and vibration include increasing obstruction to airflow for patients with COPD.[20,56,57] The proven value of HFCWO in patients with relatively normal mucus composition and characteristics but neuromuscular weakness is still under investigation, especially as a long-term treatment modality. In one study, the addition of HFCWO to randomly selected patients with ALS failed to achieve any significant clinical benefits in relation to the time of death (survival days). In addition, HFCWO failed to modify the rate of decline in FVC, given the progressive nature of this chronic neurodegenerative disease process.[58] On another hand, Lange et al.[59] also compared lung function parameters in ALS patients who were randomised to 12 weeks of HFCWO or no treatment. Results showed the maintenance of FVC and decreased fatigue and dyspnoea in the HFCWO group compared to the untreated group.

Contraindications for HFCWO are mostly the same as those for IPV, plus head or neck injury not yet stabilised, burns, open wounds, infection or recent thoracic skin grafts, osteoporosis, osteomyelitis, coagulopathy, rib fracture, lung contusion, distended abdomen and chest wall pain.[24,54] The major limitation of this technique in patients with neuromuscular disease is that there is still the ongoing need to use cough augmentation devices to clear secretions from the central airways. There is also the potential to mobilise a vast amount of secretions into the central airways. This has the potential to cause a respiratory arrest. Therefore, it is essential to have equipment readily available to clear secretions from the airway.

Mechanical insufflation–exsufflation

In 1951, Barach et al.[60] described an exsufflator attachment for iron lungs. The device used a vacuum cleaner motor with a 5 in. solenoid valve attached to an iron lung portal. These techniques were sufficiently effective for the investigators to report that the exsufflation produced by this device 'completely replaced bronchoscopy as a means of keeping the airway clear of thick tenacious secretions'. These investigations led to the construction and implementation of an exsufflation-with-negative pressure device called a Cofflator that initiated the concept of MI-E for secretion clearance.[61]

MI-E devices deliver deep insufflations (at positive pressures of 30–70 cm H_2O) immediately followed by deep exsufflations (at negative pressures of −30 to −70 cm H_2O). The insufflation and exsufflation pressures and delivery times are independently adjustable.[62] With a correct inspiratory and expiratory time, there is a very good correlation between the pressures used and the flows obtained.[63,64]

Except after a meal, an abdominal thrust is applied in conjunction with the exsufflation (mechanically assisted coughing [MAC]).[37] MI-E can be provided via an oral–nasal mask, a simple mouthpiece or a translaryngeal or tracheostomy tube. When delivered via the latter, the cuff, when present, should be inflated.[65]

MI-E applied with an oronasal mask (Figure 70.6) can generate PCFs greater than 2.7 L/s in motor neuron disease patients, with the exception of those with very acute bulbar dysfunction,[66] in whom there exists great instability of the upper airways.[67]

The CoughAssist™ can be manually or automatically cycled. Manual cycling facilitates caregiver–patient coordination of inspiration and expiration with insufflation and exsufflation, but it requires hands to deliver an abdominal thrust, to hold the mask on the patient and to cycle the machine. One treatment consists of about five cycles followed by a short period of normal breathing or ventilator use to avoid hyperventilation.[68] Insufflation and exsufflation pressures are almost always from +35 to +60 cm H_2O to −35 to −60 cm H_2O. Most patients use 35–45 cm H_2O pressures for insufflations and exsufflations. In experimental models, +40 to −40 cm H_2O pressures have been shown to provide maximum forced deflation VCs and flows.[36,64,69] Multiple treatments are given until no further secretions are expulsed and any secretion or mucus-induced dessaturations are reversed.[70]

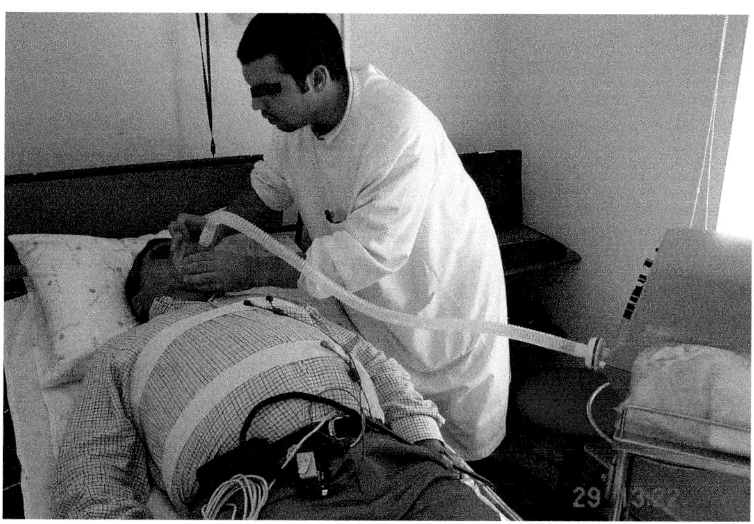

Figure 70.6 MI-E provided via an oral–nasal mask in a monitorised patient with neuromuscular disease.

A PCF lower than 2.7 L/s has been proposed as indicating an ineffective cough on the basis of flows below this level resulting in extubation failure.[42] Baseline PCF values lower than 4.5 L/s have also been reported to be associated with a high risk for pulmonary complications during respiratory tract infections because during chest infections, the pressure generated by expiratory muscles is reduced, and consequently, PCF decreases further. In this way, PCF generated by MI-E is the most common outcome measure in order to value MI-E effectiveness. A recently designed device allows PCF monitoring during MI-E sessions to improve pressure adjustments.

The use of MI-E via the upper airway can be effective for children as long as they permit its effective use by not crying or closing their glottises. Between 2 and 5 years of age, most children become able to cooperate and cough with MI-E.[71]

The abduction of the glottis is fundamental for the free flow of air in and out of the lungs during respiration with the least possible resistance. One study investigated the laryngeal response to MI-E via laryngoscopy. Interestingly, an abduction of the vocal folds was observed in all healthy subjects, during both the insufflation and exsufflation phases.[72] Various constricting laryngeal movements were observed in some subjects, such as narrowing of the vocal folds, retroflexion of the epiglottis, hypopharyngeal constriction and backwards movement of the base of the tongue. This technique may help in assessing MI-E in patients with bulbar muscle weakness.[72]

Whether via the upper airway or via indwelling airway tubes, routine airway suctioning misses the left main stem bronchus about 90% of the time. MI-E, on the other hand, provides the same exsufflation flows in both left and right airways without the discomfort or airway trauma of tracheal suctioning, and it can be effective when suctioning is not. Patients almost invariably prefer MI-E over suctioning for comfort and effectiveness, and they find it less tiring.[73,74]

Contraindications of the technique include previous barotrauma, the existence of bullae, emphysema or bronchial hyperreactivity.[75] Even when used following abdominal surgery and following extensive chest wall surgery, no disruption of recently sutured wounds was noted.[76,77] As patients with spinal shock can present bradycardias, MI-E should be carried out with caution, with gradual increase in pressures or premedication with anticholinergics.[78] In patients with very low VC who have not previously received maximum insufflations, the use of high pressures may cause thoracic muscle discomfort; thus, progressive increase is also indicated.

Patients in the intensive care setting often have impaired airway clearance. There are studies showing the importance of cough strength and the amount of secretions for a successful extubation.[9] Therefore, following extubation, all patients should be closely monitored, and an early airway secretion clearance must be performed in order to prevent re-intubation. Gonçalves et al. found that secretion management with MI-E may work as a useful complementary technique to prevent re-intubation in patients in whom acute respiratory failure develops in the first 48 hours after extubation, suggesting that MI-E is safe and efficient in ICU respiratory patients with indications for mechanical ventilation. In this study, the re-intubation rates related to NIV failure were significantly lower in the group using MI-E when compared with controls not using MI-E.[79]

The use of MI-E has been demonstrated to be very important in extubating NMD patients following general anaesthesia despite their lack of any breathing tolerance and to manage them successfully with NIV with reduced complications related to secretion encumbrance.[2,7,80,81] It has also been proved to be effective in avoiding intubation or, together with NIV, as a strategy to quickly extubate NMD and high SCI patients (Figure 70.7) in acute ventilatory failure with no breathing tolerance and profuse airway

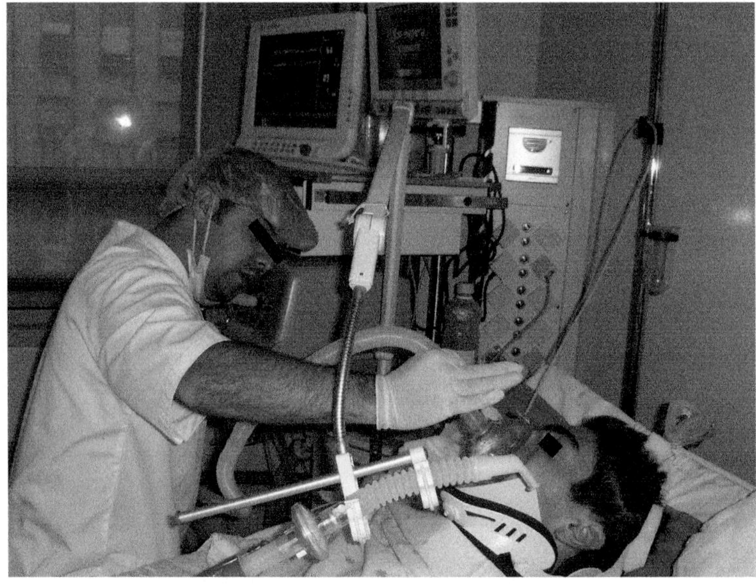

Figure 70.7 Twenty-one-year-old man with a high-level SCI (C2), extubated with a VC of 120 mL and a PCF of 125 L/min, using MAC with the CoughAssist (Phillips Respironics International) via an oronasal interface at pressures of 40 to −40 cm H_2O, after extubation to continuous NIV. MAC was performed by a trained respiratory therapist.

secretions due to intercurrent chest infections.[81–84] MI-E in a protocol with manually assisted coughing, oximetry feedback and home use of non-invasive IPPV was shown to effectively decrease hospitalisations and respiratory complications and mortality for patients with NMD.[85,86]

A survey of 37 NMD patients using MI-E at home showed that 46% used MI-E daily and 27% weekly. One-third of patients had used MI-E to resolve a choking episode and 88% agreed that home MI-E had improved their/their child's overall respiratory health. One-third reported negative features using MI-E, which were related to the size and weight of the device and the time required to manage and administer the setting of the device.[87]

MI-E is very effective in the resolution of acute respiratory failure in NMD patients, but rarely ever needed for stable patients with intact bulbar function who can air stack to maximum lung volumes and close the glottis against high pressures with an abdominal thrust. However, even in stable patients, it may be advisable to use it in a routine basis, just to stay in practice so that they can apply it in an effective way during upper respiratory tract infections (that is when they really need it).

CONCLUSION

There continues to be widespread debate as to which airway clearance regimen should be used and when. In most comparisons, bronchial hygiene physical therapy produced no significant effects on pulmonary function, apart from clearing sputum in COPD and in bronchiectasis.[20] However, there is strong evidence that supports the use of respiratory physical therapy techniques for secretion clearance in neuromuscular disease to improve quality of life and survival.[7,80]

So, in conclusion, in patients with ventilatory impairment, NIV is a very efficient technique in respiratory management; however, in the majority of the cases, secretions are excessive, and NIV alone is likely to fail. The role of respiratory physiotherapy is important and should be based on the actual evidence and directed to the goals of intervention described in this chapter to permit an efficient treatment while the patient is hospitalised and prevent hospitalisations when the patient is at home, where family members must be trained to provide the treatments and maintain the achievement of the goals and therefore maximise the potential of airway clearance to avoid respiratory problems.

REFERENCES

1. van der Schans CP, Postma DS, Koeter GH, Rubin BK. Physiotherapy and bronchial mucus transport. *Eur Respir J.* 1999;13:1477–86.
2. Gomez-Merino E, Bach JR. Duchenne muscular dystrophy: Prolongation of life by noninvasive respiratory muscle aids. *Am J Phys Med Rehabil.* 2002;81:411–5.
3. Dail CW. Glossopharyngeal breathing by paralyzed patients: A preliminary report. *California Med.* 1951;75:217–8.
4. Bach J, Bianchi C, Vidigal-Lopes M et al. Lung inflation by glossopharyngeal breathing and 'air stacking' in Duchenne muscular dystrophy. *Am J Phys Med Rehabil.* 2007;86:295–300.
5. Nygren-Bonnier M, Wahman K, Lindholm P et al. Glossopharyngeal pistoning for lung insufflation in patients with cervical spinal cord injury. *Spinal Cord.* 2009;47:418–22.
6. Bach JR. Alternative methods of ventilatory support for the patient with ventilatory failure due to spinal cord injury. *J Am Paraplegia Soc.* 1991;14:158–74.
7. Tzeng AC, Bach JR. Prevention of pulmonary morbidity for patients with neurosmucular disease. *Chest.* 2000;118:1390–96.
8. Templeton M, Palazzo MG. Chest physiotherapy prolongs duration of ventilation in the critically ill ventilated for more than 48 hours. *Intensive Care Med.* 2007;33:1938–45.
9. Smina M, Salam A, Khamiees M et al. Cough peak flows and extubation outcomes. *Chest.* 2003; 124:262–8.
10. Bach JR, Saporito LR. Criteria for extubation and tracheostomy tube removal for patients with ventilatory failure: A different approach to weaning. *Chest.* 1996;110:1566–71.
11. American Thoracic Society. Standards for the diagnosis and care of patients with chronic obstructive pulmonary disease. *Am J Respir Crit Care Med.* 1995;152:S77–120.
12. Hondras MA, Linde K, Jones AP. Manual therapy for asthma. *Cochrane Database Syst Rev.* 2000: CD001002.
13. Bradley JM, Moran FM, Elborn JS. Evidence for physical therapies (airway clearance and physical training) in cystic fibrosis: An overview of five Cochrane systematic reviews. *Respir Med.* 2006; 100:191–201.
14. Sancho J, Servera E, Diaz J, Marin J. Comparison of peak cough flows measured by pneumotachograph and a portable peak flow meter. *Am J Phys Med Rehabil.* 2004;83:608–12.
15. Schneerson JM, Simonds AK. Noninvasive ventilation for chest wall and neuromuscular disorders. *Eur Respir J.* 2002;20:480–7.
16. Bach JR, Campagnolo DI, Hoeman S. Life satisfaction of individuals with Duchenne muscular dystrophy using long-term mechanical ventilatory support. *Am J Phys Med Rehabil.* 1991;70:129–35.
17. Chaudri MB, Liu C, Hubbard R et al. Relationship between supramaximal flow during cough and mortality in motor neurone disease. *Eur Respir J.* 2002;19:434–8.
18. Plant PK, Owen JL, Elliot MW. Non-invasive ventilation in acute exacerbations of chronic obstructive pulmonary disease: Long term survival and predictors of in-hospital outcome. *Thorax.* 2001;56:708–12.

19. van der Schans CP, Piers DA, Beekhuis H et al. Effect of forced expirations on mucus clearance in patients with chronic airflow obstruction: Effect of lung recoil pressure. *Thorax.* 1990;45:623–7.
20. Jones AP, Rowe BH. Bronchopulmonary hygiene physical therapy for chronic obstructive pulmonary disease and bronchiectasis. *Cochrane Database Syst Rev.* 2000:CD000045.
21. Gonçalves MR. Noninvasive ventilation and mechanical assisted cough: Efficacy from acute to chronic care. PhD thesis in BioMedicine, Faculty of Medicine University of Porto, Porto, 2010.
22. Kang SW, Bach JR. Maximum insufflation capacity: Vital capacity and cough flows in neuromuscular disease. *Am J Phys Med Rehabil.* 2000;79:222–7.
23. Pryor JA. Physiotherapy for airway clearance in adults. *Eur Respir J.* 1999;14:1418–24.
24. van der Schans C, Bach J, Rubin BK. Chest Physical Therapy: Mucus-mobilization Techniques. In: Bach JR, ed. *Noninvasive Mechanical Ventilation*, 1st ed. Philadelphia, PA: Hanley & Belfus; 2002: 259–84.
25. Hess DR. The evidence for secretion clearance techniques. *Respir Care.* 2001;46:1276–93.
26. Wolmer P, Ursing K, Midgren B, Eriksson L. Ineficiency of chest percussion in the physical therapy of chronic bronchitis. *Eur J Respir Dis.* 1985:233–9.
27. Bach PB, Brown C, Gelfand SE, McCrory DC. Management of acute exacerbations of chronic obstructive pulmonary disease: A summary and appraisal of published evidence. *Ann Intern Med.* 2001;134:600–20.
28. Hubert J. Mobilisations du Thorax. *Les edicions Medicales et Paramedicales de Charleroi*, Montignies-sur-Sambre; 1989.
29. Lannefors L, Wollmer P. Mucus clearance with three chest physiotherapy regimes in cystic fibrosis: A comparison between postural drainage, PEP and physical exercise. *Eur Respir J.* 1992;5:748–53.
30. Bellone A, Spagnolatti L, Massobrio M et al. Short-term effects of expiration under positive pressure in patients with acute exacerbation of chronic obstructive pulmonary disease and mild acidosis requiring non-invasive positive pressure ventilation. *Intensive Care Med.* 2002;28:581–5.
31. Konstan MW, Stern RC, Doershuk CF. Efficacy of the Flutter device for airway mucus clearance in patients with cystic fibrosis. *J Pediatr.* 1994;124:689–93.
32. Kang SW, Bach JR. Maximum insufflation capacity. *Chest.* 2000;118:61–5.
33. Sivasothy P, Brown L, Smith IE, Shneerson JM. Effects of manually assisted cough and mechanical insufflation on cough flow of normal subjects, patients with chronic obstructive pulmonary disease (COPD), and patients with respiratory muscle weakness. *Thorax.* 2001;56:438–44.
34. Bach JR, Gonçalves MR, Paez S et al. Expiratory flow maneuvers in patients with neuromuscular diseases. *Am J Phys Med Rehabil.* 2006;85:105–11.
35. Bach JR, Mahajan K, Lipa B et al. Lung insufflation capacity in neuromuscular disease. *Am J Phys Med Rehabil.* 2008;87:720–5.
36. Bach JR. Mechanical insufflation–exsufflation: Comparison of peak expiratory flows with manually assisted and unassisted coughing techniques. *Chest.* 1993;104:1553–62.
37. Bach JR. Don't forget the abdominal thrust. *Chest.* 2004;126:1388–89; author reply, 1389–90.
38. Bach JR, Chaudhry SS. Standards of care in MDA clinics: Muscular Dystrophy Association. *Am J Phys Med Rehabil.* 2000;79:193–6.
39. Bach JR, Alba AS. Noninvasive options for ventilatory support of the traumatic high level quadriplegic patient. *Chest.* 1990;98:613–9.
40. Bianchi C, Grandi M, Felisari G. Efficacy of glossopharyngeal breathing for a ventilator-dependent, high-level tetraplegic patient after cervical cord tumor resection and tracheotomy. *Am J Phys Med Rehabil.* 2004;83:216–9.
41. Nygren-Bonnier M, Markstrom A, Lindholm P et al. Glossopharyngeal pistoning for lung insufflation in children with spinal muscular atrophy type II. *Acta Paediatr.* 2009;98:1324–8.
42. Toussaint M, De Win H, Steens M, Soudon P. Effect of intrapulmonary percussive ventilation on mucus clearance in duchenne muscular dystrophy patients: A preliminary report. *Respir Care.* 2003;48:940–7.
43. Langenderfer B. Alternatives to percussion and postural drainage: A review of mucus clearance therapies: Percussion and postural drainage, autogenic drainage, positive expiratory pressure, flutter valve, intrapulmonary percussive ventilation, and high-frequency chest compression with the ThAIRapy Vest. *J Cardiopulm Rehabil.* 1998;18:283–9.
44. Toussaint M, Guillet MC, Paternotte S et al. Intrapulmonary effects of setting parameters in portable intrapulmonary percussive ventilation devices. *Respir Care.* 2012;57:735–42.
45. Riffard G, Toussaint M. Intrapulmonary percussion ventilation: Operation and settings. *Rev Mal Respir.* 2012;29:347–54.
46. Varekojis SM, Douce FH, Flucke RL et al. A comparison of the therapeutic effectiveness of and preference for postural drainage and percussion, intrapulmonary percussive ventilation, and high-frequency chest wall compression in hospitalized cystic fibrosis patients. *Respir Care.* 2003;48:24–8.
47. Vargas F, Bui HN, Boyer A et al. Intrapulmonary percussive ventilation in acute exacerbations of COPD patients with mild respiratory acidosis: A randomized controlled trial [ISRCTN17802078]. *Crit Care.* 2005;9:R382–9.

48. Newhouse PA, White F, Marks JH, Homnick DN. The intrapulmonary percussive ventilator and flutter device compared to standard chest physiotherapy in patients with cystic fibrosis. *Clin Pediatr (Phila).* 1998;37:427–32.
49. Nava S, Barbarito N, Piaggi G et al. Physiological response to intrapulmonary percussive ventilation in stable COPD patients. *Respir Med.* 2006;100:1526–33.
50. Bott J, Blumenthal S, Buxton M et al. Guidelines for the physiotherapy management of the adult, medical, spontaneously breathing patient. *Thorax.* 2009;64:i1–51.
51. American Thoracic Society. Respiratory care of the patient with Duchenne muscular dystrophy: ATS consensus statement. *Am J Respir Crit Care Med* 2004;170:456–65
52. Hansen LG, Warwick WJ, Hansen KL. Mucus transport mechanisms in relation to the effect of high frequency chest compression (HFCC) on mucus clearance. *Pediatr Pulmonol.* 1994;17:113–8.
53. van der Schans C, Prasad A, Main E. Chest physiotherapy compared to no chest physiotherapy for cystic fibrosis. *Cochrane Database Syst Rev.* 2000:CD001401.
54. Scherer TA, Barandun J, Martinez E et al. Effect of high-frequency oral airway and chest wall oscillation and conventional chest physical therapy on expectoration in patients with stable cystic fibrosis. *Chest.* 1998;113:1019–27.
55. Darbee JC, Kanga JF, Ohtake PJ. Physiologic evidence for high-frequency chest wall oscillation and positive expiratory pressure breathing in hospitalized subjects with cystic fibrosis. *Phys Ther.* 2005;85:1278–89.
56. Hansen LG, Warwick WJ. High-frequency chest compression system to aid in clearance of mucus from the lung. *Biomed Instrum Technol.* 1990;24:289–94.
57. Jones A, Rowe BH. Bronchopulmonary hygiene physical therapy in bronchiectasis and chronic obstructive pulmonary disease: A systematic review. *Heart Lung.* 2000;29:125–35.
58. Chaisson KM, Walsh S, Simmons Z, Vender RL. A clinical pilot study: High frequency chest wall oscillation airway clearance in patients with amyotrophic lateral sclerosis. *Amyotroph Lateral Scler.* 2006;7:107–11.
59. Lange DJ, Lechtzin N, Davey C et al. High-frequency chest wall oscillation in ALS: An exploratory randomized, controlled trial. *Neurology.* 2006;67:991–7.
60. Barach AL, Beck GJ. Mechanical production of expiratory flow rates surpassing the capacity of human coughing. *Am J Med Sci.* 1953;226(3):241–49
61. Bach JR, Barrow SE, Gonçalves M. A historical perspective on expiratory muscle AIDS and their impact on home care. *Am J Phys Med Rehabil.* 2013;92:930–41.
62. Chatwin M. How to use a mechanical insufflator-exsufflator 'cough assist machine'. *Breathe.* 2008; 4:321–5.
63. Chatwin M, Ross E, Hart N et al. Cough augmentation with mechanical insufflation/exsufflation in patients with neuromuscular weakness. *Eur Respir J.* 2003;21:502–8.
64. Gomez-Merino E, Sancho J, Marin J et al. Mechanical insufflation–exsufflation: Pressure, volume, and flow relationships and the adequacy of the manufacturer's guidelines. *Am J Phys Med Rehabil.* 2002;81:579–83.
65. Bach JR, Smith WH, Michaels J et al. Airway secretion clearance by mechanical exsufflation for post-poliomyelitis ventilator-assisted individuals. *Arch Phys Med Rehab.* 1993;74:170–7.
66. Farrero E, Prats E, Povedano M et al. Survival in amyotrophic lateral sclerosis with home mechanical ventilation: The impact of systematic respiratory assessment and bulbar involvement. *Chest.* 2005;127:2132–8.
67. Sancho J, Servera E, Diaz J, Marin J. Efficacy of mechanical insufflation–exsufflation in medically stable patients with amyotrophic lateral sclerosis. *Chest.* 2004;125:1400–5.
68. Winck JC, Gonçalves MR, Lourenco C et al. Effects of mechanical insufflation–exsufflation on respiratory parameters for patients with chronic airway secretion encumbrance. *Chest.* 2004;126:774–80.
69. Sancho J, Servera E, Marin J et al. Effect of lung mechanics on mechanically assisted flows and volumes. *Am J Phys Med Rehabil.* 2004;83:698–703.
70. Gonçalves M, Winck J. Exploring the potential of mechanical insufflation–exsufflation. *Breathe.* 2008; 4:326–9.
71. Bach JR, Niranjan V, Weaver B. Spinal muscular atrophy type 1: A noninvasive respiratory management approach. *Chest.* 2000;117:1100–5.
72. Andersen T, Sandnes A, Brekka AK et al. Laryngeal response patterns influence the efficacy of mechanical assisted cough in amyotrophic lateral sclerosis. *Thorax.* 2016:1–9.
73. Garstang SV, Kirshblum SC, Wood KE. Patient preference for in-exsufflation for secretion management with spinal cord injury. *J Spinal Cord Med.* 2000;23:80–5.
74. Sancho J, Servera E, Vergara P, Marin J. Mechanical insufflation–exsufflation vs. tracheal suctioning via tracheostomy tubes for patients with amyotrophic lateral sclerosis: A pilot study. *Am J Phys Med Rehabil.* 2003;82:750–3.
75. Whitney J, Harden B, Keilty S. Assisted Cough: A new technique. *Physiotherapy.* 2002;88:201–7.
76. Williams EK, Holaday DA. The use of exsufflation with negative pressure in postoperative patients. *Am J Surg.* 1955;90:637–40.

77. Marchant WA, Fox R. Postoperative use of a cough assist device in avoiding prolonged intubation. *Br J Anaesth.* 2002;89:644–7.
78. Bach JR. Cough in SCI patients. *Arch Phys Med Rehabil.* 1994;75:610.
79. Gonçalves MR, Honrado T, Winck JC, Paiva JA. Effects of mechanical insufflation–exsufflation in preventing respiratory failure after extubation: A randomized controlled trial. *Crit Care.* 2012;16:R48.
80. Bach JR, Ishikawa Y, Kim H. Prevention of the pulmonary morbidity for patients with Duchenne muscular dystrophy. *Chest.* 1997;112:1024–8.
81. Bach JR, Gonçalves MR, Hamdani I, Winck JC. Extubation of patients with neuromuscular weakness: A new management paradigm. *Chest.* 2010;137:1033–9.
82. Vianello A, Corrado A, Arcaro G, Gallan F, Ori C, Minuzzo M, Bevilacqua M: Mechanical insufflation–exsufflation improves outcomes for neuromuscular disease patients with respiratory tract infections. *Am J Phys Med Rehabil.* 2005;84:83–88.
83. Servera E, Sancho J, Zafra MJ et al. Alternatives to endotracheal intubation for patients with neuromuscular diseases. *Am J Phys Med Rehabil.* 2005;84:851–7.
84. Bach JR, Saporito LR. Criteria for successful extubation and tracheostomy tube removal for patients with respiratory failure. *Chest.* 1996;110:1566–71.
85. Bach J, Gonçalves M. Ventilatory weaning by lung expansion and decanulation. *Am J Phys Med Rehabil.* 2004;83:560–8.
86. Bach JR. Prevention of morbidity and mortality with the use of physical medicine aids: The obstructive and paralytic conditions. In: Bach JR, ed. *Pulmonary Rehabilitation.* Philadelphia, PA: Hanley & Belfus; 1996:303–29.
87. Mahede T, Davis G, Rutkay A et al. Use of mechanical airway clearance devices in the home by people with neuromuscular disorders: Effects on health service use and lifestyle benefits. *Orphanet J Rare Diseases.* 2015;10:54.

71

Rehabilitation

RIK GOSSELINK, BRUNO CLERCKX, T. TROOSTERS, J. SEGERS AND D. LANGER

WHY REHABILITATION IN THE CRITICALLY ILL PATIENT?

The progress of intensive care medicine has dramatically improved the survival of critically ill patients, especially in patients with acute respiratory distress syndrome and sepsis.[1,2] This improved survival is, however, often associated with general deconditioning, muscle weakness, prolonged mechanical ventilation, dyspnoea, depression and anxiety and reduced health-related quality of life after intensive care unit (ICU) discharge.[3,4] Deconditioning and specifically muscle weakness have a key role in impaired functional status after ICU stay.[5,6]

Optimal physiological functioning depends on the upright position,[7–9] so bed rest and limited mobility during critical illness result in profound physical deconditioning and dysfunction of the respiratory, cardiovascular, musculoskeletal, neurological, renal and endocrine systems.[10] These effects can be exacerbated by inflammation and pharmacological agents, such as corticosteroids, neuromuscular blockers and antibiotics. The prevalence of skeletal muscle weakness in the ICU (ICU-acquired weakness [ICUAW]) varies up to 50%. Skeletal muscle wasting appears to be the highest during the first 2–3 weeks of ICU stay.[11–14] In addition, muscle weakness may already be present before ICU admission in patients with underlying chronic disease. The development of neuropathy or myopathy also contributes to weaning failure.[15] Although most patients under mechanical ventilation are extubated in less than 3 days, still approximately 20% require prolonged ventilatory support. Chronic ventilator dependence is a major medical problem, but it is also an extremely uncomfortable state for a patient, carrying important psychosocial implications. Finally, muscle weakness has been linked with ICU and hospital length of stay and increased 1-year mortality.[5,16]

The aforementioned changes in functional performance and limb muscle and respiratory muscle function not only indicate the need for rehabilitation *after* ICU stay,[17] but also underscore the need for assessment and measures to prevent deconditioning and loss of physical function *during* ICU stay. The amount of rehabilitation performed in ICUs is often inadequate,[18] and as a rule, rehabilitation is better organised in weaning centres or respiratory ICUs (RICUs).[19–21] The major reason is that the approach in rehabilitation is less driven by medical diagnosis; instead, rehabilitation is focusing on deficiencies in the broader scope of health problems as defined in the International Classification of Functioning, Disability and Health. This leads to the identification of problems and the prescription of one or more interventions at a level of *body structure and function* as well as *activities* and *participation*. Members of the rehabilitation team in the ICU (doctors, physiotherapists, nurses and occupational therapists) should be able to prioritise and identify aims and parameters of treatments, ensuring that these are both therapeutic and safe by appropriate monitoring of vital functions.[22] This team approach has been shown to be effective.[19,23–26]

Indeed, exercise and muscle training can improve muscle force and functionality in stable critically ill patients admitted to a RICU because of weaning failure.[21,27] However, it is important to prevent or attenuate muscle deconditioning as early as possible in patients with expected prolonged bed rest. To quote the 1944 paper 'The evil sequelae of complete bed rest'[28]: 'The physician must always consider complete bed rest as a highly *unphysiologic* and definitely *hazardous* form of therapy, to be ordered only for *specific indications* and *discontinued as early as possible*'. Mobilisation has been part of the physiotherapy management of acutely ill patients for several decades,[29] and the recommendation document of European Respiratory Society (ERS)/European Society of Intensive Care Medicine advises to start early with active and passive exercises in critically ill patients.[30] Over the last decade, increasing scientific and clinical interests and evidence have given support for a safe and early physical activity and mobilisation approach towards the critically ill patient by ICU team members.[31]

Assessment

The detrimental physiological effects of recumbency and restricted mobility on all systems, and the benefits of being upright and moving, have been widely reported. However, issues related to early physical activity and mobilisation of patients in the ICU as a therapeutic option including *safety*, *dose* and *implementation* have only recently been a shared focus of interest to interdisciplinary teams practising in the ICU.[19,23,25,32] The accurate assessment of cardiorespiratory reserve and rigorous screening for other factors that could preclude early mobilisation is of paramount importance.[22]

In addition to the assessment of the safety and readiness of the patient for exercise and physical activity, specific measures of function (e.g. muscle strength, joint mobility) and functional status (e.g. outcomes for functional performance such as the Functional Independence Measure, Berg Balance scale, Functional Ambulation Categories, Physical Function ICU Test [PFIT], Chelsea Critical Care Physical Assessment [CPAx] and quality of life [e.g. Medical Outcome Survey Short Form 36 {SF-36} and disease-specific questionnaires) must be considered (Box 71.1). See overview.[33]

Joint mobility

Knowledge on the epidemiology of major joint contractures is limited. A systematic review reported a high prevalence in patient population frequently admitted to ICU (spinal cord injuries, burns, brain injuries and stroke).[34] Functional significant contracture of major joints occurred in more than 30% of patients with prolonged ICU stay.[35] The elbow and ankle were the mostly affected joints at both ICU discharge and hospital discharge. This underlines the need for both the assessment and treatment of (passive) the range of motion (ROM) in ICU patients. The frequent assessment of joint mobility and causes of limitation of range of motion (muscle tone, muscle length, capsule, skin and oedema) is requested. The detailed assessment of joint mobility by physiotherapists can reveal undetected injuries.

Limb muscle strength testing

Muscle strength, or, more precisely, the maximum muscle force or tension generated by a muscle or (more commonly) a group of muscles, can be measured in several ways and with a range of different equipment. Manual muscle testing with the 0–5 Medical Research Council (MRC) scale is often used in clinical practice. The good reliability of the MRC sum score has been shown in critically ill patients.[36] This MRC sum score comprehends both upper limb muscles (arm abductors, forearm flexors and wrist extensors) and lower limb muscles (leg flexors, knee extensors and dorsal flexors of the foot). De Jonghe et al.[37] have proposed that a sum score less than 48 reflects significant ICUAW. Recently, the American Thoracic Society (ATS) has published a statement on the diagnosis of ICUAW and concluded that there is a lack of a gold standard. All available tests have their limitations, but until more data emerge, manual muscle testing is the preferred evaluation method.[38] However, manual muscle testing seems to be less sensitive to assess differences in muscle strength of values above grade 3 (active movement against gravity over the full ROM).[39] Therefore, several tools have been developed to more accurately measure muscle strength.

Dynamometry with mechanical or electrical equipment is used to measure isometric muscle force. Handgrip dynamometry has been shown to be reliable, and reference values are available.[36,40] For other upper and lower extremity muscle groups, handheld electrical devices have been developed. Two methods of isometric testing have been described: the make-test and the break-test. In the make-test, the maximal force the subject can exert is equal to the force of the assessor. In the break-test, the force of the assessor slightly exceeds the force of the patient. The test is reproducible in critically ill patients.[41] Handheld dynamometry is a viable alternative to costlier modes of isometric strength measurements,

BOX 71.1: Assessment of critically ill patient

Cooperation – level of confusion, agitation, sedation and consciousness

- Glasgow Coma Scale
- Confusion Assessment for the ICU
- Richmond Agitation and Sedation Scale
- Standardised 5 Questions

Joint mobility

- Active and Passive ROM

Muscle function

- MRC 0–5 scale/MRC sum score
- Handgrip dynamometry
- Muscle twitch stimulation force
- Muscle thickness with ultrasonography

Mobility – functional status

- Barthel Index
- Functional Independence Measure
- Katz Activities of Daily Living (ADL) Scale
- Berg Balance Scale
- Functional Ambulation Categories
- 4 m gait speed test
- PFIT
- CPAx

Well-being and quality of life

- Short-Form Health Survey
- Nottingham Health Profile
- Chronic Respiratory Disease Questionnaire

provided the assessor's strength is greater than that of the specific muscle group being measured. Reference values are available, also for elderly healthy subjects.[42] The limitation of the use of maximal voluntary contractions is the potential to observe submaximal contractions due to submaximal effort and cortical drive.[43] The use of superimposed electric or magnetic twitch contractions anticipates this potential variation in voluntary activation.[43] It is less painful than electrical stimulation, and the 'twitch' stimulations are relatively reproducible, but only clinically tested on the adductor pollicis. The ultrasound measurement of muscle thickness of the quadriceps was introduced and validated against magnetic resonance imaging, the gold standard for muscle cross-sectional area, and has recently been validated in ICU patients.[12,13] This allows the non-invasive and accurate assessment of muscle size in uncooperative critically ill patients.

Respiratory muscle testing

In clinical practice, respiratory muscle strength is measured as maximal inspiratory and expiratory mouth pressures (P_{Imax} and P_{Emax}, respectively). These pressure measurements are made via a small cylinder attached to the mouth with a circular mouthpiece. The ATS/European Respiratory Society statement describes respiratory muscle testing in more detail.[44] In ventilated patients, inspiratory muscle strength is estimated from temporary occlusion of the airway. The procedure involves a unidirectional expiratory valve to allow the patient to expire while inspiration is occluded. The optimal length of occlusion time is considered 25–30 s in adults.[45] Several groups have developed normal values; however, regardless of which set of normal values is used, the standard deviation is large. The presence of inspiratory weakness is accepted when P_{Imax} is lower than 50% of the predicted value. Goligher et al.[46] assessed diaphragm thickness and documented that a lower contractile activity of the diaphragm during mechanical ventilation was associated with further reduction of diaphragm thickness. More invasive techniques such as electric or magnetic diaphragm stimulation provide more accurate information on diaphragm function and are useful in the diagnosis of diaphragmatic paresis and weakness.[14]

FUNCTIONAL STATUS

The assessment of functional status may seem to be inapplicable for acutely ill ICU patients, but can be implemented in long-term weaning facilities and after ICU discharge. Functional assessment tools are also successfully used to monitor the progress of patients in several studies.[20,24,26,33,47] Furthermore, several of these tools are helpful in reconstructing the patient's functionality before ICU admission. The Barthel Index, Functional Independence Measure, Katz ADL Scale and Timed Up and Go test are commonly used and valid tools to score the patient's ability to independently perform a range of activities, mostly related to mobility (e.g. transfers from bed to chair, walking and stair climbing) and self-care (e.g. bathing, grooming, toileting, dressing and feeding). The Berg Balance Scale quantifies impairment in balance function by scoring the performance of simple functional tasks (e.g. sitting, standing, transfers, reaching forward and turning). Walking ability can also be simply assessed using the Functional Ambulation Categories. In patients who are able to walk, the Shuttle walk test, 6 min walking test or the 4 m gait speed test can be used to evaluate functional exercise capacity.[48,49]

Quality of life

As health-related quality of life is often reduced after prolonged ICU stay,[6,50] the appropriate evaluation of physical and mental health components is necessary. SF-36 is a widely used generic quality of life questionnaire, which includes eight multiple-item scales that assess physical functioning, social functioning, physical role, emotional role, mental health, pain, vitality and general health. An alternative tool is the Nottingham Health Profile, which covers six different quality of life areas: pain, energy, physical mobility, sleep, social isolation and emotional interaction. Both questionnaires have been frequently used in post-ICU quality of life studies. In patients with underlying chronic respiratory diseases, disease-specific questionnaires such as the Chronic Respiratory Disease Questionnaire or the St George's Respiratory Questionnaire can provide more specific information on the impact of the ICU stay on the disease perception.

TREATMENT: WHAT, WHEN AND HOW?

Exercise training is considered a cornerstone component of each rehabilitation programme, in addition to psychosocial interventions. Avoiding or minimising physical deconditioning and other complications and shortening of the duration of mechanical ventilation with early extubation are prime goals of the critical care team. Early mobilisation was shown to reduce the time to wean from mechanical ventilation 30 years ago and has been more recently proven in a randomised controlled trial.[24] It is the basis for long-term functional recovery. Evidence for the benefits of body positioning, mobilisation, exercise and muscle training, on the prevention and treatment of deconditioning in other patient groups as well as in healthy subjects, was confirmed in the management of critically ill patients.[31] In addition to safety issues, exercise should also be targeted at the appropriate intensity and exercise modality. These will be dependent on the stability and cooperation of the patient.

Acutely ill uncooperative patients are treated with modalities that will not need the cooperation of the patient and will not put stress on the cardiorespiratory system, such as passive ROM, muscle stretching, splinting, body positioning, passive cycling with a bed cycle or electrical muscle stimulation. On the other hand, the stable cooperative patient, beyond the acute illness phase but still on mechanical ventilation, will be able to be mobilised on the edge of the bed, transfer to a chair, perform resistance muscle training or active cycling with a bed cycle or chair cycle and walk with or without assistance. The flow diagram was developed by Gosselink et al.[51] and, based upon the scheme of Morris et al.[25] (Figure 71.1), has face validity and is an example of such step-up approach. A similar approach was followed in the study by Schweickert et al.[24]

The following paragraphs will deal with modalities of exercise training with progressive intensity and increasing need of cooperation of the patient. The risk of moving a critically ill patient is weighed against the risk of immobility and recumbency and, when employed, requires stringent monitoring to ensure that the mobilisation is instituted appropriately and safely.[22]

Uncooperative critically ill patient

The importance of body positioning ('stirring up' patients) was reported as early as the 1940s.[29] Since that time, positioning has been prescriptively used to remediate oxygen transport deficits such as impaired gas exchange by altering the distribution of ventilation (V) and perfusion (Q), V/Q matching, airway closure, work of breathing and work of the heart, as well as mucociliary transport (postural drainage). Recumbency during bed rest in patients who are critically ill exposes them to risk because the vertical gravitational gradient is eliminated, and exercise stress is restricted. To simulate the normal perturbations that the human body experiences in health, the patient who is critically ill needs to be positioned upright (well-supported) and rotated when recumbent. These perturbations need to be frequently scheduled to avoid the adverse effects of prolonged static positioning on respiratory, cardiac and circulatory functions. The potent and direct physiological effects of changing body position on oxygen transport and oxygenation are exploited when mobilisation is contraindicated. This evidence primarily comes from the space science literature in which bed rest has been used as a model of weightlessness. The prone position has been of particular interest in the management of the critically ill patient, but is underused. Knowledge of the physiologic effects of body position enables the physiotherapist to prescribe a positioning regimen to exploit its beneficial effects as well as minimise the effects of deleterious body positions. Other indications for active and passive positionings include the management of soft tissue contracture, protection of flaccid limbs and lax joints, nerve impingement and skin breakdown.

Although a specific body position may be indicated for a patient, varied positions and frequent body position changes, particularly extreme body positions, are based on the assessment findings. The efficacy of 2-hourly patient rotation, which is common in clinical practice, has not been scientifically verified. A rotation schedule that is more frequent and promotes turning from one extreme position to another approximates more normal heart–lung function than a standardised 2-hourly turning regimen. Medically unstable patients, who require a rotating or kinetic bed, benefit from continuous side-to-side perturbation, which supports the hypothesis that patients may benefit from frequent and extreme position changes rather than fixed, prolonged periods in given positions.

Bed design features in critical care should include hip and knee breaks so the patient can approximate upright sitting as much as can be tolerated. Heavy care patients such as those who are sedated, heavy or overweight may need chairs with greater support such as stretcher chairs. Lifts may be needed to safely change a patient's position.

Passive stretching or ROM exercise may have a particularly important role in the management of patients who are unable to spontaneously move. Studies in healthy subjects have shown that passive stretching decreases stiffness and increases the extensibility of the muscle. Evidence for using continuous dynamic stretching (and counterbalancing the 'silencing' of the muscle in critically ill patients) is based on the observation in patients with critical illness subjected to prolonged inactivity. Nine hours of continuous passive motion per day reduced the loss of muscle strength, muscle atrophy and protein loss, compared with passive stretching for 5 min, twice daily.[52,53]

For patients who cannot be actively mobilised and have high risk on soft tissue contracture, such as following severe burns, trauma and some neurological conditions, splinting may be indicated. Splinting of the periarticular structures in the stretched position for more than half an hour per day was shown to have a beneficial effect on the ROM in an animal model. In burn patients, fixing the position of joints reduced muscle and skin contraction.[54] In patients with neurological dysfunction, splinting may reduce muscle tone.[55]

The application of exercise training in the early phase of ICU admission is often more complicated due to the lack of cooperation and the clinical status of the patient. Technological development resulted in a bedside cycle ergometer for (active or passive) leg cycling during bed rest (Figure 71.2). The application of this training modality has been shown to be a safe and feasible exercise tool in (neuro) ICU patients.[26,56] The bedside cycle ergometer can perform a prolonged continuous mobilisation allowing rigorous control of exercise intensity and duration. A randomised controlled trial of early application of daily bedside leg cycling in critically ill patients showed improved functional status, muscle function and exercise performance at hospital discharge compared with patients receiving standard physiotherapy without leg cycling.[26]

In patients unable to perform voluntary muscle contractions, neuromuscular electrical stimulation (NMES) has been used to prevent disuse muscle atrophy. Daily NMES for at least 1 hour during an immobilisation period reduced in patients with lower limb fractures and cast immobilisation the decrease in cross-sectional area of the quadriceps and enhanced normal muscle protein synthesis.[57] In patients in the ICU not able to actively move, NMES was also introduced to preserve muscle strength and muscle

LEVEL 0	LEVEL 1	LEVEL 2	LEVEL 3	LEVEL 4	LEVEL 5
NO COOPERATION **S5Q[1] = 0**	**NO-LOW COOPERATION** **S5Q[1] < 3**	**MODERATE COOPERATION** **S5Q[1] ≥ 3**	**CLOSE TO FULL COOPERATION** **S5Q[1] ≥ 4/5**	**FULL COOPERATION** **S5Q[1] = 5**	**FULL COOPERATION** **S5Q[1] = 5**
FAILS BASIC ASSESSMENT[2]	**PASSES BASIC ASSESSMENT[3] +**	**PASSES BASIC ASSESSMENT[3] +**	**PASSES BASIC ASSESSMENT[3] +**	**PASSES BASIC ASSESSMENT[3] +**	**PASSES BASIC ASSESSMENT[3] +**
BASIC ASSESSMENT = -Cardiorespiratory unstable: MAP < 60 mmHg **or** $FiO_2 > 60\%$ **or** $PaO_2/FiO_2 < 200$ **or** RR > 30 bpm -Neurologically unstable -Acute surgery -Temp > 40°C	Neurological or surgical or trauma condition does not allow transfer to chair	Obesity or neurological or surgical or trauma condition does not allow <u>active</u> transfer to chair (even if MRCsum ≥ 36)	MRCsum ≥ 36 + BBS Sitto stand = 0 + BBS Standing = 0 + BBS Sitting ≥ 1	MRCsum ≥ 48 + BBS Sitto stand ≥ 0 + BBS Standing ≥ 0 + BBS Sitting ≥ 2	MRCsum ≥ 48 + BBS Sitto stand ≥ 1 + BBS Standing ≥ 2 + BBS Sitting ≥ 3
BODY POSITIONING[4] 2 hr turning	**BODY POSITIONING[4]** 2 hr turning Fowler's position Splinting	**BODY POSITIONING[4]** 2 hr turning Splinting Upright sitting position in bed Passive transfer bed to chair	**BODY POSITIONING[4]** 2hr turning Passive transfer bed to chair Sitting out of bed Standing with assist (2 ≥ pers)	**BODY POSITIONING[4]** Active transfer bed to chair Sitting out of bed Standing with assist (≥1 pers)	**BODY POSITIONING[4]** Active transfer bed to chair Sitting out of bed Standing
PHYSIOTHERAPY: No treatment	**PHYSIOTHERAPY[4]** Passive range of motion Passive bed cycling NMES	**PHYSIOTHERAPY[4]** Passive/Active range of motion Resistance training arms and legs Passive/Active leg and/or cycling in bed or chair NMES	**PHYSIOTHERAPY[4]** Passive/Active range of motion Resistance training arms and legs Active leg and/or arm cycling in bed or chair NMES ADL	**PHYSIOTHERAPY[4]** Passive/Active range of motion Resistance training arms and legs Active leg and/or arm cycling in chair or bed Walking (with assistance/frame) NMES ADL	**PHYSIOTHERAPY[4]** Passive/Active range of motion Resistance training arms and legs Active leg and arm cycling in chair Walking (with assistance) NMES ADL

[1] S5Q: response to 5 standardised questions for cooperation:

- Open and close your eyes
- Look at me
- Open your mouth and stick out your tongue
- Shake yes and no (nod your head)
- I will count to 5, frown your eyebrows afterwards

[2] *Fails* when at least one risk factor is present
[3] If basic assessment failed, decrease to level 0
[4] Safety: each activity should be deferred if severe adverse events (cv., resp. and subject. intolerance) occur during the intervention

Notes:
MRC (Medical Research Council) muscle strength sum scale (0–60)

BBS: Berg Balance Score

Sitting to standing
4: able to stand without using hands and stabilise independently
3: able to stand independently using hands
2: able to stand using hands after several tries
1: needs minimal aid to stand or stabilise
0: needs moderate or maximal assist to stand

Standing unsupported
4: able to stand safely for 2 minutes
3: able to stand 2 min with supervision
2: able to stand 30 s unsupported
1: needs several tries to stand 30 s unsupported
0: unable to stand 30 s unsupported

Sitting with back unsupported but feet supported on floor or on a stool
4: able to sit safely and securely for 2 min
3: able to sit 2 min under supervision
2: able to able to sit 30 s
1: able to sit 10 s
0: unable to sit without support 10 s

Figure 71.1 'Start to move' - Protocol Leuven: Step-up approach of progressive mobilisation and physical activity program. (Adapted from Gosselink R et al., *Neth J Int Care*, 15, 9, 2011.)

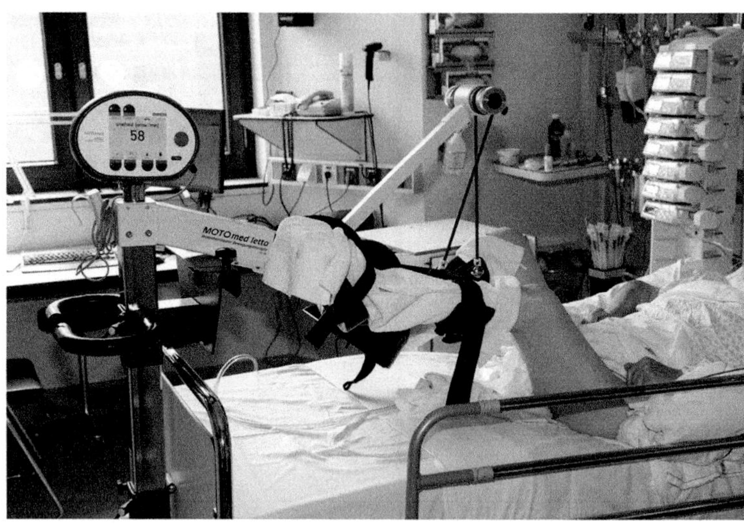

Figure 71.2 Device for active and passive cyclings in a bedridden patient in the intensive care.

mass in critically ill patients. Although the trend of the effectiveness is positive, results of the studies are conflicting.[58] Several reasons may account for these findings, such as patient characteristics (sepsis, oedema, use of vasopressives[59]), timing of NMES related to ICU admission and protocol for stimulation (devices, stimulation duration and frequency), and the methodology for the assessment of muscle function (muscle mass, strength) substantially varied. The NMES of the quadriceps, in addition to active limb mobilisation, enhanced muscle strength and hastened independent transfer from bed to chair in patients with prolonged critical illness.[60]

Cooperative patient

Mobilisation and ambulation have been part of the physiotherapy management of acutely ill patients for several decades.[29] Mobilisation refers to physical activity sufficient to elicit acute physiological effects that enhance ventilation, central and peripheral perfusion, circulation, muscle metabolism and alertness. Strategies – in order of intensity – include sitting over the edge of the bed, standing, stepping in place, transferring in bed and from bed to chair and walking with or without support. Although the approach of early mobilisation has face validity, its effectiveness was evaluated in two (randomised) controlled trials.[24,25] Morris et al.[25] demonstrated that patients receiving early mobility therapy had reduced ICU stay and hospital stay with no differences in weaning time. No differences were observed in discharge location or in hospital costs of the usual care and early mobility patients. Schweickert et al.[24] observed that early physical and occupational therapy improved functional status at hospital discharge, shortened duration of delirium and increased ventilator-free days. These findings did not result in differences in length of ICU or hospital stay.[24] The team approach (doctor, nurse, physiotherapist and occupational therapist) is an important and strong point in establishing an early ambulation programme. The early intervention approach is, although not easy, specifically in patients still in need of supportive devices (mechanical ventilation, cardiac assists) or unable to stand without support of personnel or standing aids, a worthwhile experience for the patient.[25,61] This difference in the mentality of the team was elegantly demonstrated in the study by Thomsen et al.[19] They studied 104 respiratory failure patients who required mechanical ventilation for more than 4 days. After correction for confounders, transferring a patient from the acute intensive care to the RICU substantially increased the number of patients ambulating threefold compared with pretransfer rates. Improvements in ambulation with transfer to the RICU were allocated to the differences in the team approach towards ambulating the patients.[19]

Standing and walking frames enable the patient to safely mobilise with attachments for bags, lines and leads that cannot be disconnected. The arm support on a frame or rollator has been shown to increase ventilatory capacity in patients with severe chronic obstructive pulmonary disease.[62] The frame needs to be able to accommodate either a portable oxygen tank or a portable mechanical ventilator and seat, or a suitable trolley for equipment can be used. Walking and standing aids, and tilt tables, enhance physiological responses[63] and enable early mobilisation of critically ill patients. The tilt table may be used when the patient is unable to move the legs to counter dependent fluid displacement and may be at risk of orthostatic intolerance. Abdominal belts need to be carefully positioned to support, not restrict, respiration during mobilisation. In patients with spinal cord injury, this improves vital capacity.[64] Transfer belts facilitate heavy lifts and protect both the patient and the physiotherapist or nurse. Non-invasive ventilation (NIV) during mobilisation may improve exercise tolerance for non-intubated patients, similar to that demonstrated in patients with stable chronic obstructive pulmonary disease.[65] However, no randomised trials have been performed in this setting. In ventilated patients, the ventilator settings may require adjustment to the patient's needs (i.e. increased minute ventilation).

Aerobic training and muscle strengthening, in addition to routine mobilisation, improved walking distance more than mobilisation alone in patients on long-term mechanical ventilation and chronic critical illness.[21,27] A randomised controlled trial showed that a 6-week upper and lower limb training programme improved limb muscle strength, ventilator-free time and functional outcomes in patients requiring long-term mechanical ventilation compared to a control group.[27] These results are in line with a retrospective analysis of patients on long-term mechanical ventilation who participated in whole-body training and respiratory muscle training.[20] In patients recently weaned from mechanical ventilation, the addition of upper limb exercise enhanced the effects of general mobilisation on exercise endurance performance and dyspnoea.[66] Low-resistance multiple repetitions of resistive muscle training can augment muscle mass, force generation and oxidative enzymes. Sets of repetitions (three sets of 8–10 repetitions at 50%–70% of one repetition maximum [1 RM]) within the patient's tolerance can be scheduled daily and commensurate with their goals. Resistive muscle training can include the use of pulleys, elastic bands and weight belts.

The chair cycle and the earlier mentioned bed cycle allow patients to perform an individualised exercise training programme. The intensity of cycling can be adjusted to the individual patient's capacity, ranging from passive cycling via assisted cycling to cycling against increasing resistance. The prescription of exercise intensity, duration and frequency is response dependent rather than time-dependent and is based on clinical challenge tests, such as the response to a nursing or investigative procedure, or to a specific mobilisation challenge. Exercise should be safely tolerated in any treatment session, and if the patient responds positively, greater intensity and duration can be applied. For acutely ill patients, frequent short sessions (analogous to interval training) allow for greater recovery than the less frequent longer sessions prescribed for patients with chronic stable conditions. Patients with haemodynamic instability, or with little to no oxygen transport reserve capacity (e.g. those on high concentrations of oxygen and high levels of ventilatory support or those with anaemia or cardiovascular instability), are not candidates for aggressive mobilisation. The risk of moving a critically ill patient is weighed against the risk of immobility and recumbency and, when employed, requires stringent monitoring to ensure that the mobilisation is instituted appropriately and safely.[22]

Weaning and respiratory muscle training

Fifteen to twenty per cent of patients fail liberation from mechanical ventilation, but they require a disproportionate amount of resources. Weaning failure has been extensively studied in the clinical literature, and several factors are likely to contribute to weaning failure. These factors include inadequate ventilatory drive, respiratory muscle weakness, respiratory muscle fatigue, increased work of breathing and cardiac failure.[67] The inability to spontaneously breathe relates to an imbalance between *load on* the respiratory muscles and the *capacity of* the respiratory muscles.[68] Respiratory muscle dysfunction in mechanically ventilated patients is observed in 80% of patients with ICUAW.[69] The decline in transdiaphragmatic pressure is approximately 2%–4% per day in the first weeks of ICU stay.[14] A rapid decline in diaphragm muscle strength is associated with sepsis.[15] There is accumulating evidence that weaning problems are associated with failure of the respiratory muscles to resume ventilation.[70] Indeed, high rates of respiratory muscle effort (ratio of workload and muscle capacity [P_I/P_{Imax}]) are a major cause of ventilator dependency and predict the outcome of successful weaning.[70] Since inactivity considerably contributes to muscle atrophy, 'mechanical silencing' has been identified as an important contributor to the loss of contractile properties.[52] A lower contractile activity of the diaphragm during mechanical ventilation was associated with further reduction of diaphragm thickness.[46] This observation supports the idea that the well-balanced intermittent loading of the respiratory muscles during the process of mechanical ventilation might be beneficial to prevent or ameliorate muscle atrophy. Indeed, modalities inducing (intermittent) loading of the respiratory muscles such as spontaneous breathing trials and early mobilisation have been shown to increase muscle strength and to shorten the duration of mechanical ventilation,[24] respectively. In patients at risk of failing the weaning process, *unloading* of the respiratory muscles with NIV has been shown to be successful.[71] Surprisingly, little attention has been given to specific interventions to enhance the strength and endurance of the respiratory muscles. Indeed, daily intermittent inspiratory loading with six to eight contractions repeated in three to four series at moderate to high intensity was safe, improved inspiratory muscle strength and weaning success in patients with difficult weaning.[72] One of the challenges of these studies is that patients who might benefit from the intervention are oftentimes not sufficiently capable of collaborating during the training sessions.

Alternatively, in patients unable to cooperate with respiratory muscle training, the intermittent electrical stimulation of the diaphragm through phrenic nerve pacing might be applied.[73] So far only studies in patients with spinal cord injury have been reported to support this concept.[74]

REFERENCES

1. Eisner MD, Thompson T, Hudson LD et al. Efficacy of low tidal volume ventilation in patients with different clinical risk factors for acute lung injury and the acute respiratory distress syndrome. *Am J Respir Crit Care Med.* 2001;164:231–6.
2. Kaukonen KM, Bailey M, Suzuki S et al. Mortality related to severe sepsis and septic shock among critically ill patients in Australia and New Zealand, 2000–2012. *JAMA.* 2014;311:1308–16.
3. Herridge MS. Recovery and long-term outcome in acute respiratory distress syndrome. *Crit Care Clin.* 2011;27:685–704.
4. Borges RC, Carvalho CR, Colombo AS et al. Soriano FG. Physical activity, muscle strength, and exercise capacity 3 months after severe sepsis and septic shock. *Intensive Care Med.* 2015;41:1433–44.
5. Hermans G, Van Mechelen H, Clerckx B et al. Acute outcomes and 1-year mortality of intensive care unit-acquired weakness. A cohort study and propensity-matched analysis. *Am J Respir Crit Care Med.* 2014; 190:410–20.
6. Wieske L, Dettling-Ihnenfeldt DS, Verhamme C et al. Impact of ICU-acquired weakness on post-ICU physical functioning: A follow-up study. *Crit Care.* 2015;19:196.
7. Convertino VA. Value of orthostatic stress in maintaining functional status soon after myocardial infarction or cardiac artery bypass grafting. *J Cardiovasc Nurs.* 2003;18:124–30.
8. Dittmer DK, Teasell R. Complications of immobilization and bed rest: Part 1: Musculoskeletal and cardiovascular complications. *Can Fam Phys.* 1993;39:1428–32, 35–7.
9. Teasell R, Dittmer DK. Complications of immobilization and bed rest: Part 2: Other complications. *Can Fam Phys.* 1993;39:1440–2, 5–6.
10. Parry SM, Puthucheary ZA. The impact of extended bed rest on the musculoskeletal system in the critical care environment. *Extrem Physiol Med.* 2015;4:16.
11. Gruther W, Benesch T, Zorn C et al. Muscle wasting in intensive care patients: Ultrasound observation of the M. quadriceps femoris muscle layer. *J Rehabil Med.* 2008;40:185–9.
12. Puthucheary ZA, Rawal J, McPhail M et al. Acute skeletal muscle wasting in critical illness. *JAMA.* 2013;310:1591–600.
13. Segers J, Hermans G, Charususin N et al. Assessment of quadriceps muscle mass with ultrasound in critically ill patients: Intra- and inter-observer agreement and sensitivity. *Intensive Care Med.* 2015;41:562–3.
14. Hermans G, Agten A, Testelmans D et al. Increased duration of mechanical ventilation is associated with decreased diaphragmatic force: A prospective observational study. *Crit Care.* 2010;14:R127.
15. De Jonghe B, Bastuji-Garin S, Durand MC et al. Respiratory weakness is associated with limb weakness and delayed weaning in critical illness. *Crit Care Med.* 2007;35:2007–15.
16. Ali NA, O'Brien JM, Jr., Hoffmann SP et al. Acquired weakness, handgrip strength, and mortality in critically ill patients. *Am J Respir Crit Care Med.* 2008;178:261–8.
17. Gosselink R. *Rehabilitation after Critical Illness: National Institute for Health and Clinical Excellence guidance.* London; 2009. https://www.nice.org.uk/guidance/cg83.
18. Corrado A, Roussos C, Ambrosino N et al. Respiratory intermediate care units: A European survey. *Eur Respir J.* 2002;20:1343–50.
19. Thomsen GE, Snow GL, Rodriguez L, Hopkins RO. Patients with respiratory failure increase ambulation after transfer to an intensive care unit where early activity is a priority. *Crit Care Med.* 2008;36:1119–24.
20. Martin UJ, Hincapie L, Nimchuk M et al. Impact of whole-body rehabilitation in patients receiving chronic mechanical ventilation. *Crit Care Med.* 2005; 33:2259–65.
21. Nava S. Rehabilitation of patients admitted to a respiratory intensive care unit. *Arch Phys Med Rehabil.* 1998;79:849–54.
22. Hodgson CL, Stiller K, Needham DM et al. Expert consensus and recommendations on safety criteria for active mobilization of mechanically ventilated critically ill adults. *Crit Care.* 2014;18:658.
23. Bailey P, Thomsen GE, Spuhler VJ et al. Early activity is feasible and safe in respiratory failure patients. *Crit Care Med.* 2007;35:139–45.
24. Schweickert WD, Pohlman MC, Pohlman AS et al. Early physical and occupational therapy in mechanically ventilated, critically ill patients: A randomised controlled trial. *Lancet.* 2009;373(9678):1874–82.
25. Morris PE, Goad A, Thompson C et al. Early intensive care unit mobility therapy in the treatment of acute respiratory failure. *Crit Care Med.* 2008;36:2238–43.
26. Burtin C, Clerckx B, Robbeets C et al. Early exercise in critically ill patients enhances short-term functional recovery. *Crit Care Med.* 2009;37:2499–505.
27. Chiang LL, Wang LY, Wu CP et al. Effects of physical training on functional status in patients with prolonged mechanical ventilation. *Phys Ther.* 2006;86:1271–81.
28. Dock W. The evil sequelae of complete bed rest. *JAMA.* 1944;125:5.
29. Dripps RD, Waters RM. Nursing care of surgical patients. *Am J Nursing.* 1941;41:4.
30. Gosselink R, Bott J, Johnson M et al. Physiotherapy for adult patients with critical illness: Recommendations of the European Respiratory Society and European Society of Intensive Care Medicine Task Force on Physiotherapy for Critically Ill Patients. *Intensive Care Med.* 2008;34:1188–99.

31. Castro-Avila AC, Seron P, Fan E et al. Effect of early rehabilitation during intensive care unit stay on functional status: Systematic review and meta-analysis. *PLoS One*. 2015;10:e0130722.
32. Stiller K. Safety issues that should be considered when mobilizing critically ill patients. *Crit Care Clin*. 2007;23:35–53.
33. Parry SM, Granger CL, Berney S et al. Assessment of impairment and activity limitations in the critically ill: A systematic review of measurement instruments and their clinimetric properties. *Intensive Care Med*. 2015;41:744–62.
34. Fergusson D, Hutton B, Drodge A. The epidemiology of major joint contractures: A systematic review of the literature. *Clin Orthop Relat Res*. 2007;456:22–9.
35. Clavet H, Hebert PC, Fergusson D et al. Joint contracture following prolonged stay in the intensive care unit. *CMAJ*. 2008;178:691–7.
36. Hermans G, Clerckx B, Vanhullebusch T et al. Interobserver agreement of Medical Research Council sum-score and handgrip strength in the intensive care unit. *Muscle Nerve*. 2012;45:18–25.
37. De Jonghe B, Sharshar T, Lefaucheur JP et al. Paresis acquired in the intensive care unit: A prospective multicenter study. *JAMA*. 2002;288:2859–67.
38. Fan E, Cheek F, Chlan L et al. An official American Thoracic Society Clinical Practice guideline: The diagnosis of intensive care unit-acquired weakness in adults. *Am J Respir Crit Care Med*. 2014;190:1437–46.
39. Bohannon RW. Norm references are essential if therapists are to correctly identify individuals who have physical limitations. *J Orthop Sports Phys Ther*. 2005;35:388.
40. Mathiowetz V, Kashman N, Volland G et al. Grip and pinch strength: Normative data for adults. *Arch Phys Med Rehabil*. 1985;66:69–74.
41. Vanpee G, Segers J, Van Mechelen H et al. The interobserver agreement of handheld dynamometry for muscle strength assessment in critically ill patients. *Crit Care Med*. 2011;39:1929–34.
42. Bohannon RW. Reference values for extremity muscle strength obtained by hand-held dynamometry from adults aged 20 to 79 years. *Arch Phys Med Rehabil*. 1997;78:26–32.
43. Allen GM, Gandevia SC, McKenzie DK. Reliability of measurements of muscle strength and voluntary activation using twitch interpolation. *Muscle Nerve*. 1995;18:593–600.
44. American Thoracic Society/European Respiratory Society. ATS/ERS Statement on respiratory muscle testing. *Am J Respir Crit Care Med*. 2002;166:518–624.
45. Marini JJ, Smith TC, Lamb V. Estimation of inspiratory muscle strength in mechanically ventilated patients: The measurement of maximal inspiratory pressure. *J Crit Care*. 1986;1:6.
46. Goligher EC, Fan E, Herridge MS et al. Evolution of diaphragm thickness during mechanical ventilation: Impact of inspiratory effort. *Am J Respir Crit Care Med*. 2015;192:1080–8.
47. Parry SM, Denehy L, Beach LJ et al. Functional outcomes in ICU – What should we be using? – An observational study. *Crit Care*. 2015;19:127.
48. Chan KS, Aronson Friedman L, Dinglas VD et al. Evaluating physical outcomes in acute respiratory distress syndrome survivors: Validity, responsiveness, and minimal important difference of 4–meter gait speed test. *Crit Care Med*. 2016;44:859–68.
49. Singh SJ, Puhan MA, Andrianopoulos V et al. An official systematic review of the European Respiratory Society/American Thoracic Society: Measurement properties of field walking tests in chronic respiratory disease. *Eur Respir J*. 2014;44:1447–78.
50. Herridge MS, Tansey CM, Matte A et al. Functional disability 5 years after acute respiratory distress syndrome. *N Engl J Med*. 2011;364:1293–304.
51. Gosselink R, Clerckx B, Robbeets C et al. Physiotherapy in the intensive care unit. *Neth J Int Care*. 2011;15:9.
52. Llano-Diez M, Renaud G, Andersson M et al. Mechanisms underlying ICU muscle wasting and effects of passive mechanical loading. *Crit Care*. 2012;16:R209.
53. Griffiths RD, Palmer TE, Helliwell T et al. Effect of passive stretching on the wasting of muscle in the critically ill. *Nutrition*. 1995;11:428–32.
54. Kwan MW, Ha KW. Splinting programme for patients with burnt hand. *Hand Surg*. 2002;7:231–41.
55. Hinderer SR, Dixon K. Physiologic and clinical monitoring of spastic hypertonia. *Phys Med Rehabil Clin N Am*. 2001;12:733–46.
56. Thelandersson A, Nellgard B, Ricksten SE, Cider A. Effects of early bedside cycle exercise on intracranial pressure and systemic hemodynamics in critically ill patients in a neurointensive care unit. *Neurocrit Care*. 2016.
57. Gibson JN, Smith K, Rennie MJ. Prevention of disuse muscle atrophy by means of electrical stimulation: Maintenance of protein synthesis. *Lancet*. 1988; 2(8614):767–70.
58. Maffiuletti NA, Roig M, Karatzanos E, Nanas S. Neuromuscular electrical stimulation for preventing skeletal-muscle weakness and wasting in critically ill patients: A systematic review. *BMC Med*. 2013;11:137.
59. Segers J, Hermans G, Bruyninckx F et al. Feasibility of neuromuscular electrical stimulation in critically ill patients. *J Crit Care*. 2014;29:1082–8.
60. Zanotti E, Felicetti G, Maini M, Fracchia C. Peripheral muscle strength training in bed-bound patients with COPD receiving mechanical ventilation: Effect of electrical stimulation. *Chest*. 2003;124:292–6.

61. Needham DM. Mobilizing patients in the intensive care unit: Improving neuromuscular weakness and physical function. *JAMA*. 2008;300:1685–90.
62. Probst VS, Troosters T, Coosemans I et al. Mechanisms of improvement in exercise capacity using a rollator in patients with COPD. *Chest*. 2004;126: 1102–7.
63. Chang AT, Boots R, Hodges PW, Paratz J. Standing with assistance of a tilt table in intensive care: A survey of Australian physiotherapy practice. *Aust J Physiother*. 2004;50:51–4.
64. Goldman JM, Rose LS, Williams SJ et al. Effect of abdominal binders on breathing in tetraplegic patients. *Thorax*. 1986;41:940–5.
65. van't Hul A, Gosselink R, Hollander P et al. Acute effects of inspiratory pressure support during exercise in patients with COPD. *Eur Respir J*. 2004;23:34–40.
66. Porta R, Vitacca M, Gile LS et al. Supported arm training in patients recently weaned from mechanical ventilation. *Chest*. 2005;128:2511–20.
67. Penuelas O, Frutos-Vivar F, Fernandez C et al. Characteristics and outcomes of ventilated patients according to time to liberation from mechanical ventilation. *Am J Respir Crit Care Med*. 2011;184:430–7.
68. Goldstone J, Moxham J. Assisted ventilation: 4. Weaning from mechanical ventilation. *Thorax*. 1991;46:56–62.
69. Jung B, Moury PH, Mahul M et al. Diaphragmatic dysfunction in patients with ICU-acquired weakness and its impact on extubation failure. *Intensive Care Med*. 2016;42:853–61.
70. Vassilakopoulos T, Zakynthinos S, Roussos C. The tension-time index and the frequency/tidal volume ratio are the major pathophysiologic determinants of weaning failure and success. *Am J Respir Crit Care Med*. 1998;158:378–85.
71. Nava S, Gregoretti C, Fanfulla F et al. Noninvasive ventilation to prevent respiratory failure after extubation in high-risk patients. *Crit Care Med*. 2005;33:2465–70.
72. Elkins M, Dentice R. Inspiratory muscle training facilitates weaning from mechanical ventilation among patients in the intensive care unit: A systematic review. *J Physiother*. 2015;61:125–34.
73. Pavlovic D, Wendt M. Diaphragm pacing during prolonged mechanical ventilation of the lungs could prevent from respiratory muscle fatigue. *Med Hypotheses*. 2003;60:398–403.
74. DiMarco AF, Onders RP, Ignagni A, Kowalski KE. Inspiratory muscle pacing in spinal cord injury: Case report and clinical commentary. *J Spinal Cord Med*. 2006;29:95–108.

PART 16

Outcome measures

72 Health status and quality of life 656
Wolfram Windisch

72

Health status and quality of life

WOLFRAM WINDISCH

INTRODUCTION

During the last century, enormous progress has been made in improving health standards, bringing with it an increase in life expectancy. Between 1900 and 2000, the average life expectancy at birth in the United States increased by nearly 30 years.[1] While the largest gains were made in the first two-thirds of the century, life expectancy still significantly increased by 6 years between 1970 and 2000. However, many of the patients who benefit from modern medicine in terms of increased life expectancy also have chronic, incurable diseases; thus, survival is increased in these patients without the amelioration of the underlying condition. In this scenario, information about the health status of each patient is needed to better understand the impact of chronic disease on subjective disease perception. For this reason, health-related quality of life (HRQL) evaluation is becoming increasingly important in healthcare practice and research. HRQL provides an important means of evaluating the human and financial costs and benefits of modern medical treatment modalities, which is particularly pertinent to patients with chronic and non-curable disorders.[2–4] The definition of HRQL is based on different components of subjectively reported health including physical state, psychological well-being, social relations and functional capacities that are influenced by a person's experience, beliefs, expectations and perceptions.[2–4]

There is particular interest to learn more about the limitations of HRQL in the most severely ill and obviously most severely disabled patients, such as those with chronic respiratory failure (CRF). Moreover, it is essential to know if treatment strategies such as home mechanical ventilation (HMV), delivered either non-invasively by a facial mask or invasively by the use of a tracheostoma, are capable of enhancing HRQL. Patients with CRF usually have severe dyspnoea and a medical history of several years or even decades and suffer from end-stage disease with objectively severe limitations of daily living. In addition, HMV is a time-consuming and cost-intensive therapy and can produce significant side effects. Therefore, it needs to be addressed if prolongation of life achieved by long-term HMV is associated with a subjectively acceptable health status and HRQL. Importantly, if HMV does increase the burden without producing an acceptable HRQL, this would raise ethical concerns. On the other hand, the prolongation of life is now well recognised to not necessarily be the primary goal of HMV, since improvements in HRQL after the commencement of HMV could still occur without actually improving survival.

Methodology for assessment of HRQL

Questionnaires are the most frequently used tool for HRQL assessment. There are, however, important psychometric properties which need to be established before these instruments can serve as tools for HRQL assessment in clinical trials.[2] First and foremost, the questionnaire must be objective, i.e. independent from the investigator. This refers to data assessment, data calculation and interpretation of the findings. Next, reliability needs to be established. This term describes the random error for data assessment, where the questionnaire must yield scale scores that are consistent or remain similar under constant conditions. Most importantly, validity needs to be established. In this regard, the question should be addressed as to whether a questionnaire postulating to measure HRQL actually *does* measure HRQL. For this reason, it must be guaranteed that the targets and measurements of the questionnaire are in accordance with its claims. In addition, changes in HRQL, such as those observed following treatment intervention, should be sufficiently assessed (responsiveness), and finally, changes in HRQL should be assessed as sensitively and accurately as possible (sensitivity).

Basically, there are two different types of questionnaires[2]: generic questionnaires, which are unspecific to any particular disease and, therefore, can be favourably applied to different diseases in a feasible manner. Another advantage is that these questionnaires are often standardised if reference values for a normal population are available.

However, the unspecific nature of such a generic instrument can lead to failing – or at least insufficient – responsiveness and sensitivity, particularly in the evaluation of specific treatment strategies. In contrast, disease- or condition-specific questionnaires are postulated to be most sensitive to HRQL changes, for example following treatment interventions; however, as a consequence, only limited application according to the specific disease or condition is reasonable.

HRQL QUESTIONNAIRES USED FOR PATIENTS WITH HMV

Several well-validated questionnaires have been repeatedly used for the assessment of HRQL in patients receiving HMV (Table 72.1).[5–16]

MOS 36-ITEM SHORT-FORM HEALTH STATUS SURVEY

The most commonly used instrument is the Medical Outcomes Study's (MOS) 36-Item Short-Form Health Status Survey (SF-36), a well-validated and widely used multipurpose survey of general health status in which the results from both the healthy reference population and different disease groups are available.[9–11] In addition, the SF-36 has been shown to be eligible for HRQL assessment in intensive care unit populations.[17–21] It consists of eight subscales measuring different aspects of health status. Each subscale produces a standardised score between 0 and 100, with lower scores indicating poorer health or higher disability. The scales can be aggregated into two summary measures (PCS, physical component summary; MCS, mental component summary). Recently, benchmark values were assessed specifically for patients receiving HMV, thus allowing comparisons to other disease categories.[22] In addition, patients with different underlying conditions causing CRF have been included in this study, whereby the SF-36 has been shown capable of discriminating between different underlying conditions of CRF.[22] Although the SF-36 has also been shown to assess changes in HRQL following treatment interventions in patients with CRF, i.e. the institution of HMV, the generic nature of the SF-36 might not provide a complete picture of HRQL impairments in CRF patients receiving HMV.

COPD-SPECIFIC QUESTIONNAIRES

There are two well-validated questionnaires which specifically focus on HRQL impairments in patients with chronic obstructive pulmonary disease (COPD), namely, the Chronic Respiratory Disease Questionnaire (CRQ)[12] and the St George's Respiratory Questionnaire (SGRQ).[13] Both questionnaires have been successfully used in COPD patients with different levels of disease severity and have become standard in the HRQL assessment of COPD patients. The CRQ and the SGRQ have also been used in the most severe COPD and CRF patients who require HMV.[23–26] However, it has been argued that both questionnaires were developed based on patients who, on average, had a more moderate form of the disease, when they should have otherwise been based on those with the most severe level of COPD.[14] In addition, it was pointed out that the most severe COPD patients lie at the extremes of the usable scoring range of these questionnaires, which means that in long-term follow-up studies, the questionnaires may not be able to detect deterioration over time in these patients.[14] Moreover, although the CRQ and SGRQ have been validated only for COPD patients, these questionnaires have also been used in patients with CRF secondary to diseases other than COPD.[27] However, specific determinants of HRQL in patients who require HMV because of CRF caused by restrictive thoracic deformities or neuromuscular diseases (NMDs) are not primarily targeted by the CRQ and the SGRQ. Therefore, despite the specific nature of the CRQ and the SGRQ, their suitability for patients with CRF is limited. This clearly calls for new instruments which specifically target the sphere of CRF patients who need HMV. Accordingly, two specific questionnaires have recently been developed for assessing HRQL in patients with CRF, the Maugeri Foundation Respiratory Failure item set (MRF-28) and the Severe Respiratory Insufficiency (SRI) questionnaire (Table 72.1).

MAUGERI FOUNDATION RESPIRATORY FAILURE ITEM SET

The MRF-28 is the first questionnaire developed for patients with CRF. It covers 28 items, some of which were drawn from previously developed and validated questionnaires including the Sickness Impact Profile (SIP)[5,6] and the

Table 72.1 Instruments used for HRQL assessment in patients receiving home mechanical ventilation

Instrument		First author	Scales (*n*)	Items (*n*)	Target
Sickness Impact Profile[5,6]	SIP	Bergner, M.	12	136	Generic
Nottingham Health Profile[7]	NHP	Hunt, S. M.	6	38	Generic
Hospital Anxiety and Depression scale[8]	HAD	Zigmond, A. S.	2	14	Generic
MOS 36-Item Short-Form Health Survey[9–11]	SF-36	Ware, J. E.	8	36	Generic
Chronic Respiratory Disease Questionnaire[12]	CRQ	Guyatt, G. H.	4	20	COPD
St George's Respiratory Questionnaire[13]	SGRQ	Jones, P. W.	3	76	COPD
Maugeri Foundation Respiratory Failure item set[14]	MRF-28	Carone, M.	3	28	CRF
Severe Respiratory Insufficiency Questionnaire[15,16]	SRI	Windisch, W.	7	49	CRF/HMV

Note: COPD, chronic obstructive pulmonary disease; CRF, chronic respiratory failure; and HMV, home mechanical ventilation.

SGRQ.[13] Three different subscales could be identified following validation: daily activity, cognitive function and invalidity. Two of the subscales (cognitive function and invalidity) had not been identified by previously developed questionnaires. This clearly indicates the significance of condition-specific questionnaires when assessing HRQL in patients with CRF. In addition, in the initial validation study on patients with CRF, only 39% of the possible scaling range was covered by the generic questionnaire (SIP). While the COPD-specific instrument (SGRQ) already produced a broader range of 76%, nearly the entire scaling range was covered by the MRF-28 alone.[14] This indicates the potential of best discriminating between different levels of subjectively impaired health in patients with CRF when using the condition-specific questionnaire. Moreover, improvements in HRQL following the initiation of HMV were not evident in COPD patients when the SGRQ was used, but were evident when the MRF-28 was used, again reflecting the superiority of condition-specific questionnaires when condition-related treatment interventions are being evaluated.[26] However, MRF-28 has been developed and validated only for patients with COPD and kyphoscoliosis, but its suitability in patients with different restrictive thoracic disorders (RTD), obesity hypoventilation syndrome (OHS) or NMDs still needs to be established. In addition, CRF in patients from the initial validation study was treated either by long-term oxygen therapy (LTOT) alone or invasive (tracheostomy) or non-invasive HMV (nasal mask).[14] Therefore, the MRF-28 is somewhat unspecific with regard to the treatment modality of CRF.

During the validation process, items were initially generated in English, translated into Italian and then back translated into English to ensure that the original meaning of the items had been correctly conveyed in Italian.[14] A French translation of the MRF-28 has also recently been published.[28]

SEVERE RESPIRATORY INSUFFICIENCY QUESTIONNAIRE[15,16]

In contrast to the MRF-28, the second questionnaire, the SRI, has been specifically developed for a broad spectrum of patients with CRF (including those with COPD, RTD, OHS and NMD) who exclusively receive non-invasive HMV.[15] Therefore, this questionnaire is postulated to be the most condition-specific instrument for patients with CRF receiving HMV.

The SRI consists of seven subscales covering 49 items (Figure 72.1): respiratory complaints, physical functioning, attendant symptoms and sleep, social relationships, anxiety, psychological well-being and social functioning. These seven subscales can be summarised to one summary scale (SRI-SS). All items are related to the patients' circumstances of the last week. A five-point Likert scale is provided, thereby attaining either positive or negative responses to a given statement with five possible grading steps ranging

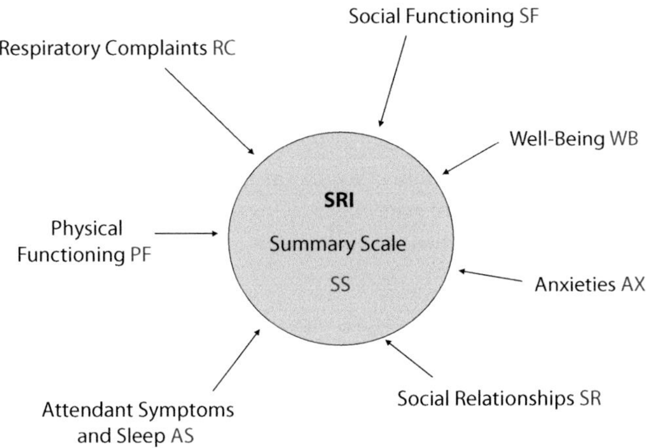

Figure 72.1 Structure of the SRI questionnaire with seven subscales and one summary scale.

from 'strongly agree' to 'strongly disagree'. Scores for all scales range between 0 and 100, with higher scores being attributed to better HRQL following transformation of raw values.

The initial multicentric validation study was performed in 226 CRF patients with various underlying diseases, including those with COPD, kyphoscoliosis, post-tuberculosis sequelae, Duchenne muscular dystrophy, polyneuropathy, myopathy, amyotrophic lateral sclerosis (ALS), OHS, poliomyelitis sequelae, phrenic nerve lesion and central hypoventilation syndrome.[15] High psychometric properties were established in this study. A high internal consistency reliability was shown by a Cronbach's α of >0.7 in all subscales and >0.8 in four subscales. High item discriminant validity was demonstrated by item–scale correlations. Construct validity was confirmed by factor analysis that indicated one summary scale accounting for 60% of the variance. Concurrent validity was confirmed by correlating subscales of the SRI and SF-36. Finally, different diagnostic groups could be discriminated by the SRI with best HRQL being measured in patients with kyphoscoliosis.

A subsequent validation study of 162 patients primarily focused on psychometric properties of the SRI when exclusively used for COPD.[16] Cross-validation was performed in two COPD groups each receiving HMV in addition to LTOT. Cronbach's α ranged from 0.73 to 0.88, indicating a high internal consistency reliability. Again, one factor could be established by explorative factor analysis, which explained 59% of the total variance confirming one summary scale (SRI-SS). For each of the seven subscales, confirmatory factor analysis revealed two factors, which were substantially correlated (r = 0.43–0.80). All scale scores covered a broad range of the scaling range (0–100) of the questionnaire, with the mean summary scale score of 52, indicating a homogenous scaling distribution. Therefore, this study extended the information on psychometric properties of the SRI by demonstrating that the SRI is a well-validated, multidimensional, highly specific tool for HRQL assessment in COPD patients with severe CRF receiving HMV.

The responsiveness of the SRI has also been established by several trials that applied the SRI to detect improvement in HRQL following commencement of HMV. Thereby, SRI scores for HRQL significantly increased in CRF patients with different underlying disorders including those with COPD, RTD, NMD and OHS.[29–32] Importantly, in one large study, the SRI – which specifically targets the sphere of CRF patients being dependent on HMV – was superior in detecting changes in HRQL when compared to SF-36, which is a generic instrument.[31] This once again highlights the inalienability of disease- or condition-specific instruments to reliably assess changes in HRQL in patients receiving HMV. The original language of the SRI is German. However, the author of the SRI is aiming to prepare and validate professional translations of the original German version. For this purpose, the original version needs to be professionally translated and then back-translated by two independent translators in order to warrant congruency. The final version needs then to be tested in a new validation study in the corresponding country. This indicates that the process of providing professionally translated versions is complex. The first completed translation is the recently published Spanish SRI.[33,34]

Finally, further information about the SRI, updates and new publications are provided via the homepage of the German Society of Pneumology and Mechanical Ventilation (http://www.pneumologie.de/808.0.html). Thereby, both the original German SRI and all professional translations can be downloaded free of charge for scientific purposes. Here, several international versions are in progress or have also recently been finished. The following SRI versions can be downloaded from the indicated homepage:

- Danish
- Dutch
- English
- French
- German
- Japanese
- Norwegian
- Polish
- Portuguese
- Spanish
- Swedish

There was one previous study comparing MRF-28 and the SRI in patients with CRF due to COPD, also including different questionnaires such as the CRQ.[35] Both questionnaires have been shown to be reliable and valid for COPD patients. In addition, while the emphasis in the MRF-28 was reportedly on activities of daily living, the SRI, like the CRQ, was more applicable to anxiety and depression. Recently, however, another study has concluded that the SRI performed slightly better than the other questionnaires including the CRQ and the MRF-28, which renders it the preferred questionnaire for scoring HRQL in patients with very severe COPD.[36]

Finally, the SRI has also recently been validated for COPD patients receiving LTOT without the addition of HMV.[37] Therefore, there is increasing evidence to suggest that the SRI is a very useful instrument to assess HRQL in advanced COPD patients receiving LTOT, long-term non-invasive ventilation (NIV) or both.

Evidence base and clinical applications

SIDE EFFECTS

The subjective benefit of a treatment modality should always counterbalance its burdens and side effects. Significant and frequent side effects of NIV in the chronic setting are already well recognised; thus, side effects can clearly deteriorate HRQL or might at least counteract the HRQL benefits gained from HMV. For this reason, side effects likely have the potential to negatively impact on adherence to treatment, and this should always be taken into consideration for patients who either stop HMV treatment or do not subjectively improve following HMV commencement. Most of the side effects are mask related, with a certain amount of pressure needed to fix the mask at the face, or airflow-related, with the latter significantly deteriorating in the event of leakage. The frequency and severity of side effects depend on the patient cohort, ventilator modes and settings, duration of HMV and materials used for HMV,[31,38,39] whereas technical refinements and new developments by manufacturers have clearly been aimed at reducing side effects and improving patient comfort. An estimation of side effect frequency in the chronic setting is given in Table 72.2.

CLINICAL STUDIES

Several clinical studies have addressed HRQL issues in patients with HMV. Thereby, cross-sectional studies have been performed, in which HMV patients were compared not only to normal populations and other chronic disorders,

Table 72.2 Frequency of the most important side effects when using NIV in the chronic setting according to the literature

Side effect	Frequency (%)
Facial soreness/skin lesions	20–40
Nasal congestion	20–40
Dryness of nose/mouth/throat	10–30
Sleep disruption	10–30
Not falling asleep	10–20
Abdominal distension/flatulence/pain	10–20
Eye irritation	10–20
Nasal bleeding	<10

Source: Windisch W, *Eur Respir J*, 32, 1328–36, 2008; Mehta S, Hill NS, *Am J Respir Crit Care Med*, 163, 540–77, 2001.

but also to different underlying conditions of CRF that required HMV, thus observing the impact of the underlying disease on HRQL in HMV patients. As a methodological consequence, most of the studies used generic instruments, particularly those including normal populations and different chronic disorders.

HRQL has, however, also been prospectively studied in longitudinal trials. In most of these studies, the impact of HMV on HRQL was addressed, since HRQL has previously been assessed prior to and following HMV commencement. The most recent studies used the two condition-specific questionnaires, the MRF-28 and the SRI, which have been specifically designed for the purpose of these studies (see preceding section).

CROSS-SECTIONAL TRIALS

The first study to extensively investigate HRQL issues in HMV patients was the Swedish study by Pehrsson et al.[40] in 1994. In this study, several instruments including the SIP[5,6] and the Hospital Anxiety and Depression scale (HAD scale)[8] were used to assess 39 patients with RTD and long-term HMV (mean of 50 months). Overall, HRQL was acceptable, given the severe objective limitations, and HRQL was no worse than that of patients with other chronic disorders such as chronic back pain or rheumatoid arthritis. However, only selected patients with long-term compliance and mild disease progression (mean daily duration of 7.7 hours per day after on average of 50 months of HMV) were included in the study, while patients with COPD and rapidly progressive NMDs such as ALS were excluded. In a similar, seminal study, Simonds et al.[41] investigated 136 patients with various disorders including COPD. In this study, SF-36 was filled in by 105 out of 116 patients, not only confirming the hypothesis that HRQL was impaired compared to the normal population, but also showing that HRQL was no worse than that of patients with other chronic medical conditions, such as diabetes, hypertension, recent myocardial infarction or cardiac failure. There were, however, some differences amongst the different underlying disorders, with COPD reportedly having the most HRQL impairments compared to patients with restrictive disorders.

The largest multicentric cross-sectional trial to date included 226 patients with HMV.[22] Patients with COPD (n = 78) and kyphoscoliosis (n = 57) formed the largest homogeneous subgroups that allowed comparative statistical analysis. The remaining patients suffered from post-tuberculosis sequelae, OHS and both rapidly and slowly progressing neuromuscular disorders. The analysis of SF-36 revealed that the overall HRQL was worse compared to a normal reference population, especially for the physical health parameter, but less so for mental health. In addition, when compared to a historical cohort of chronic lung diseases without CRF, physical health was still significantly impaired, whereas mental health was no worse in HMV patients compared to patients with less severe chronic lung disease. The comparison of COPD and kyphoscoliosis patients revealed no difference in physical health; however, mental health was more impaired in COPD patients, while kyphoscoliosis patients had no mental impairments at all compared to the normal reference population, according to the results of SF-36. Patients with Duchenne muscular dystrophy appeared to have even better mental health compared to the normal reference population, although the number of cases was too low to allow further statistical analysis. Another study also indicated that more severe limitations were only evident in physical functioning compared to other diseases, while other domains of HRQL related to mental health (SF-36) did not significantly differ even from age-matched male controls.[42] Therefore, robust data are now available to support the notion that even severe physical handicaps do not necessarily lead to mental limitation, at least in restrictive patients with CRF, once HMV has been successfully instituted. Finally, neither lung function parameters nor blood gases were reported predictors for HRQL.[22]

Specific instruments have also been used in cross-sectional trials. In a large Spanish trial, the SRI was employed to describe predictors of HRQL in a cohort of 115 patients who used HMV to treat CRF due to various underlying disorders including RTD, OHS, NMD and COPD.[43] In this study, the main predictors of HRQL domains were dyspnoea, the number of hospitalisations and the number of emergency room admissions in the preceding year. An obstructive pattern revealed by pulmonary function testing also predicted impairments in HRQL. In another large study that used the SRI, domains of HRQL in 231 CRF patients were reportedly predictive for long-term survival, in addition to established risk factors such as low body mass index, impairments in pulmonary function testing and elevated numbers of leukocytes.[44] This was particularly true for non-COPD patients (RTD, OHS and NMD), but not COPD patients. In contrast, according to another trial, HRQL was strongly and independently related to respiratory muscle function in patients with ALS.[45,46] These findings emphasise the impact of the underlying disease on HRQL.

LONGITUDINAL TRIALS

Early trials prospectively studied HRQL in small groups of COPD patients.[23–25,47] Thereby, the impact of HMV on HRQL changes has been addressed. The methodology of HRQL assessment considerably varied amongst these studies. In two studies using the CRQ[23] and SF-36,[47] respectively, HRQL did not improve following HMV commencement, but when using the SGRQ, HRQL was shown to improve following HMV.[24,25] However, none of these COPD studies used condition-specific questionnaires that specifically targeted the sphere of patients with CRF, as these instruments were not available at the time the studies were performed.

In the Italian multicentre randomised controlled trial (RCT) on NIV in COPD patients, the addition of HMV to LTOT, but not LTOT alone, resulted in improvements in HRQL, although survival benefits could not be achieved by the addition of HMV to LTOT.[26] However, improvements in

HRQL were detected only when using the condition-specific questionnaire MRF-28, whereas even the COPD-specific instrument, the SGRQ, failed to show any significant benefit. This clearly points out the impact of HRQL measurement methodology on the results and underlines the inevitability of using even the most specific HRQL measurement tools available when specific treatment interventions are being evaluated. Thus, in CRF patients requiring HMV, the instruments specific to CRF appear superior even to the disease-specific instruments developed in patients with milder forms of their disease, i.e. no presence of CRF (see also preceding text). In the most recent RCT, non-invasive positive pressure ventilation (NIV) produced mild survival benefits in stable hypercapnic COPD patients, but this appeared to be at the cost of worsening HRQL. However, worsening HRQL was only detectable by generic instruments, but not by the SGRQ.[48] This again emphasises that HRQL results depend on the instruments being used for assessment.

In a very recent RCT, the addition of NIV to pulmonary rehabilitation reportedly augmented the benefits of pulmonary rehabilitation in COPD patients, with greater improvements in HRQL.[32] In this study, both COPD-specific (CRQ) and condition-specific questionnaires (MRF-28 and SRI) were used. Therefore, this study again demonstrates that when specific instruments for HRQL assessment are used, NIV is shown to positively impact on HRQL, even in COPD patients.

HRQL benefits have also been established in non-COPD patients. Early studies again used unspecific questionnaires, with the SF-36 being the most frequently used. Thereby, HRQL improvements in both RTD and NMD patients were established.[49,50] However, in patients with more rapid NMD, particularly those with ALS, the evaluation of HRQL is by far more difficult. Early studies lacked consistency as they reported both non-significant[51] and significant[46,52] improvements following HMV commencement. For example, the application of the SF-36 showed that HMV improved the vitality domain score by as much as 25% for periods of up to 15 months, despite disease progression.[52] Although the other scores did not improve, a decline in HRQL was not observed despite disease progression.[52] However, more significant changes in either direction could have been missed as the SF-36 is suggested to be too unspecific for the problems unique to ALS patients.[53] Recently, in the largest study of 92 ALS patients, 22 patients were randomised to HMV and 19 patients were randomised to standard care without HMV, while 51 patients did not meet the criteria for randomisation during the surveillance period.[54] In this study, patients with no or moderate bulbar involvement had large HMV-associated benefits in survival and HRQL, as measured by a battery of instruments including the sleep apnoea quality-of-life index,[55] the SF-36 and the CRQ. In particular, the duration that HRQL was maintained above 75% of baseline was substantially longer in patients treated with HMV, compared to those with best supportive care alone. In contrast, there were no benefits in survival and only sparse HRQL benefits in patients with severe bulbar impairment.

There have also been several prospective trials in which the SRI served as the primary instrument of HRQL assessment. In the initial study, HRQL measured by the SRI significantly improved following HMV commencement, in both COPD and restrictive patients, and these improvements were correlated to the decline of $PaCO_2$ that resulted from HMV.[28] In another trial, the SRI-SS substantially improved following HMV in patients with OHS.[30] In this randomised crossover trial, these improvements were comparable in patients receiving bi-level pressure ventilation with or without the addition of target volume setting.

The largest prospective study using the SRI included 135 patients with different aetiologies of CRF from nine German HMV centres.[31] In this study, both short- and long-term effects of HMV were investigated. Interestingly, the overall HRQL improved after 1 month of HMV treatment, and these improvements could be maintained over the subsequent year during which HMV was continued, despite disease deterioration. Importantly, overall HRQL as measured by the SRI-SS revealed comparable improvements in patients with COPD, RTD and NMD. This is remarkable, since COPD patients are believed to have less HRQL benefits when HMV is instituted, with previous cross-sectional trials having indicated worse HRQL in COPD patients compared to restrictive patients.[15,22,35] In addition, the positive results on COPD patients obviously contrasts with the more pessimistic view derived from previous trials that used less specific tools for HRQL assessment. In particular, in the most recent Australian RCT, NPPV produced worsening of HRQL, but this was only detectable by generic instruments (see also preceding text).[48] Since the methodology of HRQL assessment is crucial, findings of studies, in which instruments specifically designed for severe respiratory failure have not been used, should be interpreted with caution. In the German multicentre trial,[35] however, a possible selection bias cannot be excluded with certainty, although patients in this trial were consecutively enrolled, as this was an uncontrolled prospective study. Nevertheless, this study clearly demonstrates that HRQL in COPD patients can substantially improve when HRQL is most specifically assessed.

Furthermore, it is also conceivable that HRQL improvement is dependent on the effectiveness of ventilatory support and, therefore, on the ability of HMV to improve alveolar ventilation as estimated from $PaCO_2$ levels. In the indicated study, $PaCO_2$ could be significantly reduced, and this could also explain improvements in HRQL. This could also explain that HRQL was not improved in the Australian study.[48] However, the impact of ventilatory strategies needs further investigation. Finally, subscale scores identified clear differences between patients with differing underlying aetiologies of CRF, indicating that HRQL benefits in particular domains of HRQL are disease related. For example, improvements in the subscale respiratory complaints were evident in all groups of patients, but this led to improvements in the subscale physical functioning only in patients with COPD, RTD and OHS, but not in those with NMD; this is conceivable as the latter group of patients is also substantially impaired by the weakness of the limbs. On the contrary, patients with NMD as well as those with OHS had the most remarkable improvements in the subscale attendant symptoms and sleep, although patients with COPD and RTD also improved. In addition, improvements in the subscale anxiety were most evident in OHS patients, although all other groups of patients significantly improved as well.

FUTURE RESEARCH

There is now a rich body of data to suggest that HMV positively impacts HRQL in CRF patients, in particular, if NIV is used for HMV. The application of new HRQL measurement tools specifically addressing the sphere of patients with CRF has recently shown that the HRQL benefit gained from HMV is even greater than that estimated by more unspecific or generic instruments. These highly specific instruments, namely, the MRF-28 and the SRI, are also postulated to be capable of discriminating between different treatment strategies. As an example, high-intensity NPPV aimed at maximally reducing $PaCO_2$ by using controlled modes of ventilation and inspiratory pressures around 30 cm H_2O has recently been introduced, with favourable results in COPD patients.[56–58] This type of treatment forgoes the more conventional approach of using assisted forms of ventilation and, on average, half the amount of inspiratory pressures.[56–58] More positive physiological results gained by high-intensity NPPV – particularly regarding the control of nocturnal hypoventilation, improved breathing pattern and lung function – must be balanced against the potential of more frequent side effects related to the increased airflow and mask pressures. A very recent short-term randomised crossover trial has clearly demonstrated the superiority of high-intensity over the more conventional low-intensity NIV, with particular reference to the capability of controlling nocturnal hypoventilation.[59] In this study, there is also a clear trend of more improved HRQL as assessed by the SRI in patients who received high-intensity NIV. Recently, the RCT by Köhnlein et al.[60] showed for the first time an impressive survival benefit gained by long-term NIV used for HMV in COPD patients when compared to controls, but this was only true when more aggressive NIV was aimed at improving $PaCO_2$, and importantly, HRQL as measured by the SRI significantly improved, also suggesting the importance of the ventilatory strategy.

Ultimately, these therapeutic refinements should always be guided towards improving patient comfort and HRQL.

Another important issue of future research targets invasively ventilated patients and their HRQL. This is particularly true for patients with weaning failure following prolonged ventilation. Initial research has shown that HRQL in these patients is severely heterogeneous, ranging from extremely good to unacceptably bad, with neuromuscular patients tending to have better SRI scores than those with COPD.[61] However, it is suggested that the questionnaires when used alone are not sufficient to address the complex issue of HRQL in patients with invasive HMV. This issue is important also in view of the steadily increasing numbers of patients with invasive HMV following weaning failure.[62]

Nevertheless, the international availability of specific instruments and multilanguage questionnaires is highly warranted.

REFERENCES

1. Lefant C. Clinical research to clinical practice – Lost in translation? *N Engl J Med.* 2003;349:868–74.
2. Testa MA, Simonson DC. Assessment of quality-of-life outcomes. *N Engl J Med.* 1996;334:835–40.
3. Wood-Dauphinee S. Assessing quality of life in clinical research: From where have we come and where are we going? *J Clin Epidemiol.* 1999; 52:355–63.
4. Higginson IJ, Carr AJ. Measuring quality of life: Using quality of life measures in the clinical setting. *BMJ.* 2001;322:1297–300.
5. Bergner M, Bobbitt RA, Pollard WE et al. The sickness impact profile: Validation of a health status measure. *Med Care.* 1976;14:57–67.
6. Bergner M, Bobbitt RA, Carter WB, Gilson BS. The sickness impact profile: Development and final revision of a health status measure. *Med Care.* 1981;19:787–805.
7. Hunt SM, McKenna SP, McEwen J et al. The Nottingham Health Profile: Subjective health status and medical consultations. *Soc Sci Med – Part A, Med Sociol.* 1981;15:221–9.
8. Zigmond AS, Snaith RP. The hospital anxiety and depression scale. *Acta Psychiatr Scand.* 1983;67: 361–70.
9. Ware JE, Jr., Sherbourne CD. The MOS 36-item short-form health survey (SF-36): I. Conceptual framework and item selection. *Med Care.* 1992;30:473–83.
10. Ware JE, Jr., Kosinski M, Bayliss MS et al. Comparison of methods for the scoring and statistical analysis of SF-36 health profile and summary measures: Summary of results from the Medical Outcomes Study. *Med Care.* 1995;33:AS264–79.
11. Ware JE, Jr. The SF-36 Health Survey. In: Spilker B (Hrsg), ed. *Quality of Life and Pharmacoeconomics in Clinical Trials.* Philadelphia, PA: Lippincott-Raven; 1996:337–45.
12. Guyatt GH, Berman LB, Townsend M et al. A measure of quality of life for clinical trials in chronic lung disease. *Thorax.* 1987;42:773–8.
13. Jones PW, Quirk FH, Baveystock CM. The St George's Respiratory Questionnaire. *Respir Med.* 1991;85:25–31.
14. Carone M, Bertolotti G, Anchisi F et al. Analysis of factors that characterize health impairment in

patients with chronic respiratory failure: Quality of Life in Chronic Respiratory Failure Group. *Eur Respir J.* 1999;13:1293–300.
15. Windisch W, Freidel K, Schucher B et al. The Severe Respiratory Insufficiency (SRI) Questionnaire: A specific measure of health-related quality of life in patients receiving home mechanical ventilation. *J Clin Epidemiol.* 2003;56:752–9.
16. Windisch W, Budweiser S, Heinemann F et al. The Severe Respiratory Insufficiency (SRI) Questionnaire was valid for patients with COPD. *J Clin Epidemiol.* 2008;61:848–853.
17. Chrispin PS, Scotton H, Rogers J et al. Short Form 36 in the intensive care unit: Assessment of acceptability, reliability and validity of the questionnaire. *Anaesthesia.* 1997;52:15–23.
18. Ridley SA, Chrispin PS, Scotton H et al. Changes in quality of life after intensive care: Comparison with normal data. *Anaesthesia.* 1997;52:195–202.
19. Welsh CH, Thompson K, Long-Krug S. Evaluation of patient-perceived health status using the Medical Outcomes Survey Short-Form 36 in an intensive care unit population. *Crit Care Med.* 1999;27:1466–1471.
20. Eddleston JM, White P, Guthrie E. Survival, morbidity, and quality of life after discharge from intensive care. *Crit Care Med.* 2000;28:2293–9.
21. Flaatten H, Kvale R. Survival and quality of life 12 years after ICU: A comparison with the general Norwegian population. *Intensive Care Med.* 2001;27:1005–11.
22. Windisch W, Freidel K, Schucher B et al. Evaluation of health-related quality of life using the MOS 36-Item Short-Form Health Status Survey in patients receiving noninvasive positive pressure ventilation. *Intensive Care Med.* 2003;29:615–21.
23. Elliott MW, Simonds AK, Carroll MP et al. Domiciliary nocturnal nasal intermittent positive pressure ventilation in hypercapnic respiratory failure due to chronic obstructive lung disease: Effects on sleep and quality of life. *Thorax.* 1992;47:342–8.
24. Meecham Jones DJ, Paul EA, Jones PW, Wedzicha JA. Nasal pressure support ventilation plus oxygen compared with oxygen therapy alone in hypercapnic COPD. *Am J Respir Crit Care Med.* 1995;152:538–44.
25. Perrin C, El Far Y, Vandenbos F et al. Domiciliary nasal intermittent positive pressure ventilation in severe COPD: Effects on lung function and quality of life. *Eur Respir J.* 1997;10:2835–9.
26. Clini E, Sturani C, Rossi A et al. The Italian multicentre study on noninvasive ventilation in chronic obstructive pulmonary disease patients. *Eur Respir J.* 2002;20:529–38.
27. Euteneuer S, Windisch W, Suchi S et al. Health-related quality of life in patients with chronic respiratory failure after long-term mechanical ventilation. *Respir Med.* 2006;100:477–86.
28. Janssens JP, Héritier-Praz A, Carone M et al. Validity and reliability of a French version of the MRF-28 health-related quality of life questionnaire. *Respiration.* 2004;71:567–74.
29. Windisch W, Dreher M, Storre JH, Sorichter S. Nocturnal non-invasive positive pressure ventilation: Physiological effects on spontaneous breathing. *Respir Physiol Neurobiol.* 2006;150:251–60.
30. Storre JH, Seuthe B, Fiechter R et al. Average volume assured pressure support in obesity hypoventilation: A randomized cross-over trial. *Chest.* 2006;130:815–21.
31. Windisch W. Impact of home mechanical ventilation on health-related quality of life. *Eur Respir J.* 2008;32:1328–36.
32. Duiverman ML, Wempe JB, Bladder G et al. Nocturnal non-invasive ventilation in addition to rehabilitation in hypercapnic patients with COPD. *Thorax.* 2008;63:1052–7.
33. Lopez-Campos JL, Failde I, Jimenez AL et al. Health-related quality of life of patients receiving home mechanical ventilation: The Spanish version of the severe respiratory insufficiency questionnaire. *Arch Bronconeumol.* 2006;42:588–93.
34. López-Campos JL, Failde I, Masa JF et al. Transculturally adapted Spanish SRI questionnaire for home mechanically ventilated patients was viable, valid, and reliable. *J Clin Epidemiol.* 2008;61:1061–6.
35. Duiverman ML, Wempe JB, Bladder G et al. Health-related quality of life in COPD patients with chronic respiratory failure. *Eur Respir J.* 2008;32:379–86.
36. Struik FM, Kerstjens HA, Bladder G et al. The Severe Respiratory Insufficiency Questionnaire scored best in the assessment of health-related quality of life in chronic obstructive pulmonary disease. *J Clin Epidemiol.* 2013;66:1166–74.
37. Walterspacher S, July J, Kohlhäufl M et al. The Severe Respiratory Insufficiency Questionnaire for subjects with copd with long-term oxygen therapy. *Respir Care.* 2016;61:1186–9.
38. Mehta S, Hill NS. Noninvasive ventilation. *Am J Respir Crit Care Med.* 2001;163:540–77.
39. Windisch W, Storre JH, Sorichter S, Virchow JC Jr. Comparison of volume- and pressure-limited NPPV at night: A prospective randomized cross-over trial. *Respir Med.* 2005;99:52–9.
40. Pehrsson K, Olofson J, Larsson S et al. Quality of life of patients treated by home mechanical ventilation due to restrictive ventilatory disorders. *Respir Med.* 1994;88:21–6.
41. Simonds AK, Elliott MW. Outcome of domiciliary nasal intermittent positive pressure ventilation in restrictive and obstructive disorders. *Thorax.* 1995;50:604–9.
42. Simonds AK, Muntoni F, Heather S, Fielding S. Impact of nasal ventilation on survival in

hypercapnic Duchenne muscular dystrophy. *Thorax*. 1998;53:949–52.
43. López-Campos JL, Failde I, Masa JF et al. Factors related to quality of life in patients receiving home mechanical ventilation. *Respir Med*. 2008; 102:605–12.
44. Budweiser S, Hitzl AP, Jörres RA et al. Health-related quality of life and long-term prognosis in chronic hypercapnic respiratory failure: A prospective survival analysis. *Respir Res*. 2007;17;8:92.
45. Bourke SC, Shaw PJ, Gibson GJ. Respiratory function vs sleep-disordered breathing as predictors of QOL in ALS. *Neurology*. 2001;57:2040–4.
46. Mustfa N, Walsh E, Bryant V et al. The effect of noninvasive ventilation on ALS patients and their caregivers. *Neurology*. 2006;66:1211–7.
47. Sivasothy P, Smith IE, Shneerson JM. Mask intermittent positive pressure ventilation in chronic hypercapnic respiratory failure due to chronic obstructive pulmonary disease. *Eur Respir J*. 1998;11:34–40.
48. McEvoy RD, Pierce RJ, Hillman D et al. Australian trial of non-invasive Ventilation in Chronic Airflow Limitation (AVCAL) Study Group: Nocturnal non-invasive nasal ventilation in stable hypercapnic COPD: A randomised controlled trial. *Thorax*. 2009;64:561–6.
49. Nauffal D, Doménech R, Martínez García MA et al. Noninvasive positive pressure home ventilation in restrictive disorders: Outcome and impact on health-related quality of life. *Respir Med*. 2002;96:777–83.
50. Doménech-Clar R, Nauffal-Manzur D, Perpiñá-Tordera M et al. Home mechanical ventilation for restrictive thoracic diseases: Effects on patient quality-of-life and hospitalizations. *Respir Med*. 2003;97:1320–7.
51. Pinto AC, Evangelista T, Carvalho M et al. Respiratory assistance with a non-invasive ventilator (Bipap) in MND/ALS patients: Survival rates in a controlled trial. *J Neurol Sci*. 1995;129:19–26.
52. Lyall RA, Donaldson N, Fleming T et al. A prospective study of quality of life in ALS patients treated with noninvasive ventilation. *Neurology*. 2001;57:153–6.
53. Bourke SC, Bullock RE, Williams RE et al. Non-invasive ventilation in ALS: Indications and effect on quality of life. *Neurology*. 2003;61:171–7.
54. Bourke SC, Tomlinson M, Williams TL et al. Effects of non-invasive ventilation on survival and quality of life in patients with amyotrophic lateral sclerosis: A randomised controlled trial. *Lancet Neurol*. 2006;5:140–7.
55. Flemons WW, Reimer MA. Development of a disease-specific healthrelated quality of life questionnaire for sleep apnoea. *Am J Respir Crit Care Med*. 1998;158:494–503.
56. Windisch W, Storre JH, Köhnlein T. Nocturnal non-invasive positive pressure ventilation for COPD. *Expert Rev Respir Med*. 2015;9:295–308.
57. Windisch W, Kostić S, Dreher M et al. Outcome of patients with stable COPD receiving controlled NPPV aimed at maximal reduction of $PaCO_2$. *Chest*. 2005;128:657–63.
58. Windisch W, Haenel M, Storre JH, Dreher M. High-intensity non-invasive positive pressure ventilation for stable hypercapnic COPD. *Int J Med Sci*. 2009;6:72–76.
59. Dreher M, Storre JH, C. Schmoor, Windisch W. High-intensity versus low-intensity non-invasive ventilation in stable hypercapnic COPD patients: A randomized cross-over trial. *Thorax*. 2010;65:303–8.
60. Köhnlein T, Windisch W, Köhler D et al. Non-invasive positive pressure ventilation for the treatment of severe stable chronic obstructive pulmonary disease: A prospective, multicentre, randomised, controlled clinical trial. *Lancet Respir Med*. 2014; 2:698–705.
61. Huttmann SE, Windisch W, Storre JH. Invasive home mechanical ventilation: Living conditions and health-related quality of life. *Respiration*. 2015;89:312–21.
62. Polverino E, Nava S, Ferrer M et al. Patients' characterization, hospital course and clinical outcomes in five Italian respiratory intensive care units. *Intensive Care Med*. 2010;36:137–42.

PART 17

The patient experience of NIV

73 Psychological issues for the mechanically ventilated patient 666
Linda L. Bieniek, Daniel F. Dilling and Bernd Schönhofer

74 The patient's journey 690
Stefano Nava

75 A patient's journey: NIV 691
Jeanette Erdmann and Andrea L. Klein

76 A carer's journey 697
Gail Beacock and Patrick Beacock

73

Psychological issues for the mechanically ventilated patient

LINDA L. BIENIEK, DANIEL F. DILLING AND BERND SCHÖNHOFER

INTRODUCTION

This chapter describes many of the psychological and emotional burdens that non-invasive ventilation (NIV) users experience. It illustrates how to improve ventilator users' lives by acting on an understanding of psychological health and its value to well-being. Home NIV has been consistently shown to be effective in improving health-related quality of life and emotional function in patients with chronic respiratory failure.[1–3]

Co-author Linda Bieniek has a wealth of experience using both NIV and invasive mechanical ventilation, and her psychological insights have enhanced the value of this chapter. She is a 65-year-old woman who contracted polio after childhood polio vaccination. She survived the disease, but it weakened her respiratory muscles. Severe kyphoscoliosis and post-polio syndrome compounded her respiratory problems, resulting in the initiation of NIV later in life. For more than 20 years, she successfully used various forms of NIV and appreciates its attendant complications and frustrations. Unfortunately, emergency surgery prompted the need for invasive mechanical ventilation, and in recovering from that operation, she was unable to wean from the ventilator, prompting placement of a tracheostomy. She remains on volume ventilation at night and during parts of each day. Her professional background includes more than 25 years of psychological training often with leading experts. During her 20-year career in a major corporation, she managed its employee assistance programme, assessing and referring individuals with psychological issues to appropriate resources. Since retiring, she has written and lectured at international conferences on psychological issues. Since the publication of the first edition of this book, she has become more consistently dependent on the ventilator and, with that, has developed an even deeper understanding of the emotional and psychological challenges of ventilator dependence.

In addition to Ms Bieniek's first-hand experiences, we include findings and examples from the literature and insights of Joan Headley, executive director of International Ventilator Users Network.

The more aware providers are of the psychological challenges that ventilator users face, the more they can employ the strategies identified in this chapter. Professionals will learn how to screen patients to identify symptoms and patterns that can adversely affect ventilator users' psychological and, potentially, physical health. When patients' symptoms indicate the need for professional assistance, providers should urge patients to pursue psychotherapy or other available behavioural health resources.

EMPOWER PATIENTS

The more patients depend on a ventilator to breathe, the greater the psychological challenges they may face. Loss of autonomy is among the most serious. It is extremely important that providers grasp the potential impact of this loss on patients' lives. Emotional vitality – a sense of enthusiasm, of hopefulness, of engagement in life and an ability to face life's stresses with emotional balance – has been associated with better health in later life.[4] With this understanding, providers can empower ventilator users in a number of ways. The key to empowerment is whenever choices exist, give the individuals information and control over decisions affecting their lives.

Empowerment requires presenting patients with clear information about treatment options, with attendant benefits and risks. Taking time to answer patients' questions and communicating honestly, directly, calmly and compassionately further equips patients to make informed decisions.

> What appears especially important to individuals is that providers show they believe their lives are worthwhile.
>
> *Headley JL*
> Interview, June 2009

Acknowledging the complexities that patients face, encouraging them to be resourceful in assessing options and then honouring their choices demonstrates respect for ventilator users' capabilities and rights.

RECOGNISE AND EDUCATE PATIENTS ABOUT THE IMPORTANCE OF PSYCHOLOGICAL HEALTH

Psychological health encompasses how one thinks, expresses thoughts and feelings, makes decisions and chooses to act. A psychologically healthy person is rational and open-minded, solves problems proactively, seeks to gain positive results and expresses feelings constructively. Spirituality – including both spiritual values and religious beliefs – is extremely important to the psychological health of many individuals.[5] Spirituality can provide a sense of meaning and purpose to life and support individuals in adapting to health changes. Any or all these factors may influence an individual's choices and responses to pain, suffering, loss and distress.

Ventilator users' responses to distress can affect emotional state, physical symptoms and quality of life. Providers empower patients first by educating them about the interrelationship of their minds, emotions, behaviours, spirituality and bodies and then about factors affecting psychological health, as described earlier. This education includes helping patients understand the value of reducing distress and of fulfilling emotional needs for support and assistance.

Several studies illustrate potential benefits of good psychological health. One demonstrated that individuals' beliefs, emotions, relationships and problem-solving skills can affect their physical health.[6] It concluded that individuals who use effective approaches to manage anxiety and depressive symptoms can reduce the frequency and intensity of somatic symptoms.[6] This is important for ventilator users to understand, as anxiety can increase shortness of breath, depression can exacerbate fatigue and distress may weaken physical resilience, increasing susceptibility to respiratory illness.

> For much of my life, I resented my body's limitations. In my 30s, work distress and relationship problems prompted me to seek psychotherapy. In the process, I discovered that significant past experiences were affecting my psychological and physical health. When my health forced me to leave my career, I entered a programme for depression. I learned how unresolved traumas triggered anxiety, depression, irritable bowel attacks and other somatic reactions. Most importantly, I learned how to transform negative beliefs and feelings and face myself with compassion. These skills continue to support me in adapting to the progression of post-polio syndrome and my respiratory condition.
>
> *Bieniek LL*
> Personal quote, 2009

A study of patients with motor neurone disease (MND) indicated that individuals who were proactive in confronting problems experienced lower levels of anxiety and depression while adjusting to physical and lifestyle changes.[5] This research revealed that levels of depression and loss of autonomy were determining factors affecting survival times of individuals with MND even when age, disease severity and time since diagnosis were controlled for.[5]

Generally, psychologically healthy people are better equipped to cultivate supportive relationships. Their connections can increase their emotional resilience, providing a buffer against psychological pain and reducing the risks of depression.[6]

RESPOND TO THE PSYCHOLOGICAL CHALLENGES VENTILATOR USERS FACE

Ventilator users contend with diverse psychological challenges from their medical conditions, external factors and unrelated life issues. External impediments and psychological effects of living with a neuromuscular condition appear more distressing to some individuals than their actual physical limitations.[5,7] The following publications contain valuable information about the psychological risks and obstacles they face:

- What psychotherapists should know about disability[8]
- University of Toronto's research on ventilator users' perspectives on the important elements of health-related quality of life[7]
- Post-Polio Health International's articles on resolving the effects of traumatic experiences related to childhood medical conditions and disabilities.[9–11]

The following sections describe potential causes of distress that may affect ventilator users' psychological health and well-being.

Difficulties adjusting to non-invasive ventilation

When introducing patients to NIV, communication is paramount. Providers need to explain potential problems, what to do and who to contact. The most effective approach requires the collaboration of patient, home health provider and the pulmonologist experimenting with different interfaces and settings until the patient can breathe comfortably on the ventilator.

Difficulties with equipment include, but are not limited to, leaking masks, finding suitable interfaces and synchronising settings.

> I cried the first few nights I used a ventilator. I recognized that I was entering a new stage of life. My tears also stemmed from my struggle to get in and out of the chest cuirass alone since I have weak hand muscles. Yet, after a few days, I was grateful for being able to breathe better on the ventilator. Once an orthotist made me a

custom-fitted polypropylene cuirass, my ventilator became my best friend.

Bieniek LL
Personal quote, 2009

Anxiety or claustrophobia related to a past trauma can resurface when using a facemask or mouthpiece. Individuals with history of trauma involving pressure on the face or in the mouth may develop post-traumatic symptoms while starting NIV. Examples of such traumas include near-drowning, domestic violence, war, assault, a medical experience and physical or sexual abuse.

Lack of self-acceptance may cause psychological struggles when individuals face the reality of how their medical conditions will impact the rest of their lives.

STRATEGIES FOR HEALTHCARE PROFESSIONALS

- Suggest that patients communicate with other ventilator users through disability and disease-related organisations (http://www.ventusers.org) and listservs (access at http://www.ventusers.org/net/VentDIR.pdf).
- Encourage patients to pursue resources to manage their anxieties. Refer them to 'Treatment Approach Options' at http://www.post-polio.org/edu/pphnews/pph19-1p9.pdf.
- Urge patients to seek professional assistance for ongoing distress.

Refusal to use non-invasive ventilation

Patients with conditions such as MND may decline ventilatory support because they cannot bear living with such a debilitating disease.[5] When they develop intense hopelessness about their future, dying may seem more acceptable than feeling like a 'burden' to their families, 'out of control', 'trapped' or dependent on others.[5]

STRATEGIES FOR HEALTHCARE PROFESSIONALS

- Acknowledge the complexities of patients' decisions; express compassion. Ask them to examine decisions with a behavioural health professional or spiritual director to ensure that they are grounded in the reality of their circumstances rather than despair from feelings of fear, grief, anger or shame – often resolvable through psychotherapy.
- Encourage patients to consider spiritual values and religious beliefs in making final decisions.
- Ask patients to talk with another person who navigates life with a ventilator successfully.
- Respect patients' rights to decline mechanical ventilation and life-sustaining therapies. Discuss options for comfortable end-of-life transitions.

Progression of neuromuscular conditions

As neuromuscular conditions progress, individuals often need to increase the time spent using NIV and mobility devices. Inaccessibility to external places impedes mobility, independence and travelling[7] – with significant loss of autonomy and development of dependencies. Losing basic abilities such as talking, seeing and eating may result from using a mouthpiece or mask with NIV during the day. Losing the ability to speak is especially traumatising. Consequently, it is imperative to find a means for the person to communicate needs and feelings, perhaps even through the use of a communication assist device.

Adjusting to loss may include loss of employment and income; relationships; living arrangements; professional and occupational identities and the ability to participate in social, recreational and spiritual activities.

It took me five years to accept my need to go on full-time disability. I valued my career and feared losing income and the ability to live independently. When I left work, I became depressed. I realized that I had lost part of my identity.

Bieniek LL
Personal quote, 2009

Accepting dependencies is one of the greatest challenges of living with physical limitations. Asking for and accepting help is difficult regardless of whether one has a disability and is especially challenging for people from families that believe in stoic self-reliance (Headley J. L., interview, June 2009).

As patients lose the ability to function independently, they may encounter episodes of anxiety, depression and loss of control. Additionally, their dependencies may trigger fears of abandonment, resentment or avoidance by friends and loved ones. Likewise, when individuals think of themselves as 'a burden' or are treated that way, they feel 'trapped' by their illnesses and can become hopeless and develop despair.[5]

A friend played chess with her neighbour who had MND and used NIV. She witnessed his wife's demeaning remarks to him, which would understandably cause him to feel like a 'burden'.

Bieniek LL
Personal quote, 2009

Even the hiring of care attendants can be a source of anxiety, especially when government programmes or individuals themselves cannot afford to pay them very well. This often hinders the hiring of reliable, trustworthy competent attendants who will not neglect ventilator users' needs, abuse them, or steal from them (Headley JL, interview, June 2009).

Experiencing chronic pain or fatigue can lead to sadness, anger, isolation or hopelessness, resulting in clinical depression. Emotional distress and spiritual emptiness can exacerbate physical pain.[7] Participating in sexual experiences creates anxiety for individuals when it causes dyspnoea. A pioneering study showed that the initiation of NIV markedly reduced patients' sexual activity; however, having a spouse or partner contributed to increases in ventilator use during sexual activities.[12] Another study cited positioning, fatigue and weakness as reasons for reducing sexual activities.[13]

STRATEGIES FOR HEALTHCARE PROFESSIONALS

- Urge patients to explore resources for strengthening emotional support. Refer them to the 'Treatment Approach Options' chart at http://www.post-polio.org/edu/pphnews/pph19-1p9.pdf.
- Emphasise the interrelationship of body, mind, emotions, spirituality and behaviours.
- Refer to specialists to help patients understand causes of pain and fatigue, exacerbating factors and strategies to reduce their impact.[8]
- Offer to discuss sexual activities with patients, including alternatives for expressing intimacy. Refer them to physical or occupational therapists for options on positioning and movement.

Medical emergencies

Providers should establish that patients understand their options in case of emergency. They should encourage patients to make autonomous decisions, and to inform surrogate decision makers of their wishes should they become incapacitated. Providers should avoid paternalistic attitudes, such as suggesting that chronic ventilator assistance is an undesirable way to live or that such individuals are a burden to society (Headley, J. L., interview, June 2009). If one becomes incapacitated, the patient's written instructions or designated surrogate should determine whether to employ or decline medical interventions during an emergency.

Ideally, providers should discuss patients' wishes before an emergency occurs and ask that patients document them in writing. Would they want to be tracheostomised to be kept alive? Are they willing and able to live with a tracheostomy? Do they have adequate verbal and written information about this option in order to make an informed decision?

Patients may become emotionally traumatised by a medical crisis. One study reported that 84% of patients with myasthenia gravis were diagnosed with an anxiety disorder and 69% developed a depressive disorder after unexpected respiratory failure and intubation.[14]

> My experience provides an example of the psychological impact of a medical crisis. While out of town without family, I needed emergency surgery. After recovering, I was shocked to learn I was conscious and in ICU, because I had no memory of this. Knowing my high risk for not surviving surgery, I must have been terrified and blocked out these memories. Trauma experts identify this phenomenon as 'dissociation', a coping strategy for managing overwhelming feelings.
>
> *Bieniek LL*
> Personal quote, 2009

Sometimes ventilator users panic if they sense that emergency personnel or providers do not understand their neuromuscular respiratory needs or other pre-existing conditions. It is imperative that providers become informed about a patient's particular conditions and special needs, consulting an expert to determine the most effective treatment options, if needed.

STRATEGIES FOR HEALTHCARE PROFESSIONALS

- Ensure that patients have emergency medical information in place to provide health professionals with key information. Ask them to complete the 'Take Charge, Not Chances' forms and carry them (stating their ventilator settings and special needs) when travelling and going to hospital. Access the forms at http://www.ventusers.org/vume/index.html.
- Ask patients to document emergency wishes and to designate surrogate decision makers.
- Provide patients with a copy of Appendix 73A: Exploring the Option of a Trach, available in the Vitalsource ebook edition.
- Insert pertinent documents into the medical record.
- Encourage patients to consider personal values, spiritual and religious beliefs and available support and resources when deciding about emergency interventions and future options.
- Implement stress reduction techniques such as patient education, music therapy, relaxation exercises and supportive touch while patients are in the intensive care unit (ICU) and transitioning to NIV.[15,16]
- Provide patients with psychological assistance to resolve psychological effects of a medical crisis.[15]
- Consult experts for advice on emergency interventions and treatment options. International Ventilator Users Network at +1-314-534-0475 provides referrals.

Lack of access to services and equipment

A lack of access to ventilator services causes significant distress for individuals who desire life-sustaining treatment and may lead to premature deaths. Patients in developing countries and remote areas often lack access to specialists who are knowledgeable about treating neuromuscular respiratory problems. Questions about the ethics of using home ventilation have been raised and remain important in some health systems, revolving around who should be offered home ventilation and around the impacts on the patient, the family and the healthcare system.[17] Vent users report that government programmes and insurance companies limit their choices of equipment, excluding more effective options (Headley JL, interview, June 2009).

STRATEGIES FOR HEALTHCARE PROFESSIONALS

- Encourage government programmes and insurance companies to ensure ventilator services are available in areas lacking them.

- Submit professional service information to International Ventilator Users Network for inclusion in the directory, a source of referrals for patients and professionals internationally. Contact info@ventusers.org. Access the directory at http://www.ventusers.org/net/vdirhm.html.

Emotional reactions

Until the actor Christopher Reeve used a ventilator in public, society did not understand mechanical ventilation as a part of some people's lives, and ventilator users were often avoided. Fortunately, Reeve reduced the stigma of using a ventilator by demonstrating that a ventilator-assisted person could live an active life (Headley JL, interview, June 2009). However, individuals still experience demeaning attitudes – and in some cultures and families, having a disability is still considered shameful.

Emotional reactions to living with progressive conditions include grief, fear, loneliness, hopelessness and anger. Individuals experiencing such reactions are especially susceptible to depression, substance abuse and self-destructive behaviours.[8] Shame and anxiety manifest as avoidance of public places and social events and descriptions of feeling 'embarrassed' about being seen with a ventilator.[7] These reactions increase isolation and, in turn, worsen anxiety symptoms.

> I tried to hide the fact that I used the machine, I put a tablecloth over it and then eventually I named it to make it more acceptable to my kids.[7]

Loneliness is a significant challenge for ventilator users who lack adequate support or cannot travel or communicate easily. Loneliness can lead to hopelessness, irrational beliefs and feelings of loss of control – precursors to anxiety and depression.[5] Unresolved anger can impair a person's ability to gain support and assistance when anger is suppressed or expressed destructively (directly or passive aggressively).

STRATEGIES FOR HEALTHCARE PROFESSIONALS

- Encourage patients to learn constructive strategies for expressing feelings and for seeking support. Refer them to 'Treatment Approach Options' chart at http://www.post-polio.org/edu/pphnews/pph19-1p9.pdf.
- Screen for dependency on alcohol and other substances and self-destructive patterns as advised in the following.

GENERAL STRATEGIES FOR HEALTH PROFESSIONALS

Use psychological screening tools

Individuals with disabilities are at high risk for substance abuse, addictions and physical and sexual abuse.[8] Screen for self-destructive behaviours and for anxiety, depressive and somatic symptoms. These can interfere with patients' health and functioning and exacerbate pain and fatigue. The use of substances to numb emotions (e.g. anxiety, grief, anger and loneliness) or physical pain may also increase breathing problems.

Studies report high rates of suicidal ideation in males with MND and in patients with multiple sclerosis.[15,18] If concern for self-harm or harm to another person exists, obtain immediate psychiatric assistance for the patient.

Ask open-ended questions to identify needs for psychological assistance:

- 'How is your mood or spirits?'
- 'What is your attitude towards life these days?'
- 'What do you spend most of your time doing?'
- 'How well do you sleep? Are you eating enough or too much?'
- 'What kind of support do you have? Do you feel safe?'
- 'How are you dealing with your health changes and loss of independence and control?'
- 'Do you have adequate assistance? How well do you communicate your needs?'
- 'If spirituality is important to you, how do you nurture your spiritual needs?'
- 'What do you do to relax when you get frustrated or you're stressed out?'
- 'What are any concerns or behaviours that family or friends see as problems?'
- 'How do you manage pain? What do you take?'
- 'What do you do when you get angry, sad or lonely?'
- 'What do you wish you would do differently to take better care of your health?'
- 'Have you thought about wanting to die or to harm yourself? Do you have a plan? When? How?'

Recommend proactive strategies

Encourage patients to pursue resources to reduce distress and fulfil their emotional needs. Refer them to 'Treatment Approach Options' chart at http://www.post-polio.org/edu/pph news/pph19-1p9.pdf and give them a copy of Appendix 73B: Ventilator User Guidelines for Emotional Health, available in the Vitalsource ebook edition. Patients can explore many of these options independently.

Prescribe psychotherapy or behavioural health resources when you identify the following:

- Ongoing or severe symptoms of anxiety, depression or other psychological conditions
- Distress that impairs cognitive or physical functioning
- Somatic symptoms, frequent illnesses
- Abuse or dependency on alcohol, other substances
- Addictions or other self-destructive behaviours
- Neglect of healthcare needs
- Inability to seek adequate personal care assistance

Refer patients to resources or therapists you know of; also offer them the choice of finding their own therapist. Finally, respect individuals' rights to decline psychological treatment unless they are at risk of harming themselves or others or of being harmed.

SUMMARY

This chapter has illustrated how professionals can raise their patient care to another level by acting on an understanding of psychological health to empower patients. Awareness of the psychological challenges that may interfere with patients' well-being provides opportunities to employ the strategies identified within this chapter. Providers can make significant differences to patients' lives by discussing treatment options, emphasising the importance of psychological health and honouring their choices. These perspectives indicate a need for further discussion and research of these critical issues.

Providers are encouraged to consult Appendices 73 A and B in the Vitalsource ebook edition and to give copies to patients. They are written by a ventilator user with psychological training and expertise for other ventilator users. One offers a wealth of strategies for deciding on the question of tracheostomy and another for pursuing resources, including psychotherapy, to manage anxieties and other psychological challenges related to using mechanical ventilation.

ACKNOWLEDGEMENTS

We are indebted to Veronica Cook, Laura Dowdle, Joan Headley, Audrey King, Nicole Lighthouse, Brigid Rafferty, Sarah Perz and Julie Truong for their assistance.

See Appendix 73A: Exploring the Option of a Trach and Appendix 73B: Ventilator Guidelines for Emotional Health in the Vitalsource ebook edition.

REFERENCES

1. Tsolaki V, Pastaka C, Kostikas K et al. Noninvasive ventilation in chronic respiratory failure: Effects on quality of life. *Respiration*. 2011;81:402–10.
2. Ali S, Kabir Z. Domiciliary non-invasive ventilation and the quality of life outcome of patients suffering from chronic respiratory failure. *Ir Med J*. 2007;100:336–8.
3. Hannan LM, Dominelli GS, Chen YW et al. Systematic review of non-invasive positive pressure ventilation for chronic respiratory failure. *Resp Med*. 2014;108:229–243.
4. Kubzansky LD, Thurston RC. Emotional vitality and incident coronary heart disease: Benefits of healthy psychological functioning. *Arch Gen Psychiatr*. 2007;64:1393–401.
5. McLeod JE, Clarke DM. A review of psychosocial aspects of motor neurone disease. *J Neurol Sci*. 2007;258:4–10.
6. Salovey P, Rothman AJ. Emotional states and physical health. *Am Psychol*. 2000;55:110–21.
7. Brooks D, Tonack M, King A. *Ventilator users' perspectives on important elements of health-related quality of life: A Canadian quality study*. Toronto, ON: University of Toronto; 2002:1–124.
8. Olkin R. *What Psychotherapists Should Know About Disability*. New York: Guilford Press; 1999.
9. Bieniek L, Kennedy K. Improving quality of life: Healing polio memories. *Polio Network News Winter* 2002;18:1–7.
10. Bieniek L, Kennedy K. A guide for exploring polio memories. *Polio Network News Summer* 2002; 18:3–7.
11. Bieniek L, Kennedy K. Pursuing therapeutic resources to improve your health. *Polio Network News Fall* 2002;18:3–8.
12. Schönhofer B, Von Sydow K, Bucher T et al. Sexuality in patients with noninvasive mechanical ventilation due to chronic respiratory failure. *Am J Respir Crit Care Med*. 2001;164:1612–17.
13. Lott D. IVUN joins those studying sexual activity and chronic illness. *Ventilator-Assisted Living* 2006; 20:4–9.
14. Kulaksizoglu IB. Mood and anxiety disorders in patients with myasthenia gravis: Aetiology, diagnosis and treatment. *CNS Drugs*. 2007; 21:473–81.
15. Thomas LA. Clinical management of stressors perceived by patients on mechanical ventilation. *AACN Clin Issues*. 2003;14:73–81.
16. Chlan LL. Music therapy as a nursing intervention for patients supported by mechanical ventilation. *AACN Clin Issues*. 2000;11:128–38.
17. Dybwik K, Nielsen EW, Brinchmann BS. Ethical challenges in home mechanical ventilation: A secondary analysis. *Nurs Ethics*. 2011;19:233–244.
18. Ziemssen T. Multiple sclerosis beyond EDSS: Depression and fatigue. *J Neurol Sci*. 2009; 277:S37–41.

APPENDIX 73A: EXPLORING THE OPTION OF A TRACH

LINDA L. BIENIEK

Planning for changes in your breathing condition takes courage. It is natural to avoid thinking about a possible breathing crisis. Yet, making informed decisions about your treatment options before a health crisis occurs has several benefits. First, it gives you the chance to consider factors that are important to you, such as spiritual and/or religious beliefs, personal values and practical needs. As a result, you can make a decision that brings you peace of mind. Then, it also helps to reduce the problems and distress that loved ones may experience, especially if your wishes are unknown. Finally, it helps to ensure that your wishes are respected. Otherwise, if you are unable to communicate your wishes and do not have written instructions, your health advocate, surrogate or closest family member will decide whether to employ or decline emergency interventions. This can make a difference between life and death!

Non-invasive ventilation (NIV) is the most appropriate form of ventilation for most people with neuromuscular respiratory conditions. However, when some vent users have needed stronger ventilation to breathe effectively, they have obtained a tracheostomy (trach). The main benefit of a trach is that it forces air directly into the lungs, providing greater respiratory assistance. This article offers a process for deciding whether you want, or do not want – and can afford – to use a trach in either of two scenarios: for the short-term, in order to save your life during an emergency and until you later recover; or for the long-term, if non-invasive ventilation no longer meets your needs.

In addition to helping you make a decision about using a trach, this article can help you talk with your pulmonologist about your options and decisions when:

- You encounter a life-or-death crisis and are unconscious.
- You cannot breathe and function adequately using non-invasive ventilation (NIV).
- You need to use NIV all day or for the majority of the day, and are interested in whether a trach's airway hole would enable you to function without a ventilator for extended periods.
- You are prone to pneumonia and respiratory infections **and** continue to have difficulty clearing mucous secretions even with techniques such as a Cough Assist machine or an Ambu bag.
- You need to be intubated periodically.
- You have irresolvable problems with your sinuses, digestive system, skin or teeth from using a nasal or full face mask, mouthpiece or nasal pillows.

If you decide you want to be trached in any of these situations, it is essential that you tell your physicians and write down that you are aware of the challenges of living with a trach, but consider it vital to your desire to stay alive.

> I would definitely prefer to use NIV if it enabled me to breathe and function adequately. After using NIV for more than 22 years, I experienced frequent breathing problems and spent increasing amounts of time during the day on my volume ventilator. Then, after an emergency surgery and respiratory failure, I could no longer breathe on my own when I was off the ventilator. Receiving a trach saved my life!
>
> With the trach, I am able to function off my ventilator during the day for extended periods. The airway hole allows me to inhale and exhale room air, enabling me to breathe easily. Since I still am unable to breathe through only my nose, I would need to be connected to NIV all day if I didn't have a trach. Even when I used NIV with custom-made masks, I had difficulties with air leaks. I also had bloating problems from air that traveled to my stomach. I value the mobility and freedom that my trach affords me. I am grateful that it keeps me alive and able to experience what gives meaning, satisfaction, and serenity to my life.
>
> *Linda Bieniek*
> Polio Survivor and Vent User: NIV 22 yrs, Trach 3 yrs

Learning about the pros and cons of a trach

Obtaining a trach requires a surgical procedure in which a physician creates an airway hole into a person's neck and places a tracheostomy tube into the trachea. When the trach tube is connected to a ventilator via tubing, the ventilator delivers air directly into the lungs, providing strong support to the breathing muscles. A trach also makes it easier to suction mucous secretions directly from the lungs.

Practical problems of living with a trach depend on where you live; the services and resources available to you from government programmes, social service agencies and health insurance benefits and your financial assets. At this time, many countries do not have health policies that pay for the ongoing expenses related to living with a trach. Unless you are physically able to do your own trach care and suctioning, having a trach normally requires a great deal of personal assistance that can be costly. Some areas provide in-home personal assistance, but often, it is limited and may be inadequate. Most individuals do not have enough family members and friends who can volunteer to provide the amount of assistance needed. If you face this dilemma, the costs for assistance may prevent you from affording to live with a trach. This is especially true unless you have access to significant financial resources or enough reliable volunteers to assist you. Most vent users want to live in the community, yet most areas lack accessible, affordable housing options. A few countries provide long-term living facilities; other areas have only a few government-funded facilities that accept only a limited number of trach users. Often, facilities may be located a distance from your family and friends. Questions in this article can help you identify your options and the additional resources you would need to afford to live safely with a trach.

> The cost of care and caregiver legislation and conditions become 'monumentally' more difficult if you have a trach (especially 24/7) and are trying to live in the community...the 'RN only'

restrictions in many areas create a huge liability, unless you can take care of your trach yourself – especially the suctioning.

Audrey King
Polio Survivor and Non-Invasive Ventilator User – Used a Trach for 2 years

When I got home from the hospital I did my own trach care. . . . I had help when doing a complete trach change, once a month at first and now once every other month. . . . I need to be suctioned, on average, about once a day. Sometimes I go a week between suctioning and sometimes I'll be suctioned two or three times in one day.

Richard Daggett
Polio Survivor and Ventilator User with a Trach since 1984

Emotional, psychological and spiritual issues are critical to consider when deciding whether to use a trach. These issues often affect your reactions to change, loss, pain, suffering and distress. For example, if spirituality (spiritual values or religious beliefs) is important to you, it may help you decide whether living with a trach matches your values and beliefs about life. On the other hand, if you have a short temper when you feel out of control, your negative reactions to difficulties related to a trach may result in your friends wanting to spend less time with you. For this reason, taking time to reflect on the emotional difficulties that you may encounter will help you identify the support and problem-solving strategies you would need to adapt to living with a trach. Potential emotional challenges include:

- **Feelings of loss:** of control, autonomy, independence, mobility, identity, quality of life, communication and participation in external events and activities.
- **Fears of:** dependencies, physical vulnerability, feeling trapped, abandonment by loved ones and friends, feeling like a burden, isolation, institutionalisation and being alone.
- **Emotional reactions:** grief, anger, spiritual emptiness, shame, disappointment, loneliness.
- **Physical, cognitive and emotional symptoms** of anxiety, depression and/or distress.

Such losses, reactions and experiences may affect many parts of your life including your relationships, employment, income, identity, living situation, spirituality, intimate experiences, roles in the family and sexual activities. You can ease the adjustments of living with a trach by learning about factors that affect your emotional health and how you can strengthen your skills to resolve potential difficulties.

If you decide to use a trach, changes in your life will most likely also impact loved ones and supportive friends. For this reason, it is important to discuss your needs openly and honestly with these individuals before getting a trach. Likewise, find out what others think they will need from you to keep your relationships mutually supportive of each other. This discussion will enable you to agree to how to support and respect each other's needs. Individuals who assist you must find ways to protect their personal needs. Otherwise, they can wear down physically and become distressed.

Lists at the end of the article identify sources of support for adjusting to and living with a trach. To learn how to strengthen your emotional health and reduce distress, ask your health provider or contact International Ventilator Users Network at info@ventusers.org or 001-314-574-0475 for a copy of 'Ventilator User Guidelines for Emotional Health.' Obtain a copy of the 'Treatment Approach Options Chart' from http://www.post-polio.org/edu/pphnews/pph19-1p9.pdf.

When I first came home with a trach, I was distressed about difficulties: infections; greater needs for assistance; costs of home care; and loneliness when I was unable to talk until an ENT gave me the right-sized trach. Yet, I have NO REGRETS about getting a trach.

Linda Bieniek
Trach User since 2006

BENEFITS AND DISADVANTAGES OF USING NIV OR A TRACH

Review the information below and note issues that will challenge you and/or potentially distress you.

By planning ahead, you can explore resources for potential assistance and support. If you are able to live in the community, family members, friends, volunteers and personal care assistants whom you hire can be trained to perform your trach care needs. If you hire assistants from a home health agency, legal restrictions may allow only nurses and respiratory therapists to provide trach care and ventilator assistance. Since hourly fees for these professionals are costly, most vent users hire non-agency assistants who charge more reasonable fees. However, if you only can afford to pay only low wages, you may find it difficult to hire competent, trustworthy, reliable assistants. In addition, if a non-agency assistant cannot work, you will need back-ups who are available and willing to help you on a short notice.

You also can seek volunteers from local non-profit and disability organisations, religious or spiritual communities and educational programmes for healthcare providers (such as those for pre-medical students, respiratory therapists, nurses) even if these groups do not have formal volunteer programmes. Before contacting the directors of these programs, find out their names (such as of the

Benefits of NIV with an interface	Disadvantages of NIV & interface	Benefits of a trach	Disadvantages of a trach
• Can save and extend your life by providing breathing assistance at night and/or during day • Presents less intense emotional, psychological and spiritual challenges • Enables you to obtain breathing assistance without creating a hole in your throat	• You may face emotional, psychological and spiritual challenges affecting your self-esteem, identity, work, income, relationships, activities, sexuality • May require continuous use of NIV for 24 hours or for extended periods during the day, limiting your abilities to see, eat and communicate easily	• Can save your life if you cannot breathe using NIV; experience respiratory failure; have dangerous blood gas levels and minimal lung vital capacity • May enable you to breathe through your airway hole while off the vent for periods during the day, reducing your need to be on your vent continuously	• You will face emotional adjustments and challenges that may distress you. See section on 'Emotional, Psychological, Spiritual Issues' above • Requires an invasive procedure to create an airway hole in your trachea

• Is increasingly a subject of interest in medical schools and healthcare programmes
• Has gained recognition as a cost-effective option for individuals needing breathing assistance
	• You may lack access to:
	  • Knowledgeable healthcare providers
	  • Home health services
	  • Effective ventilators, machines
	  • Mask and mouthpiece options
		• Is generally understood by emergency medical professionals	• You may lack access to:
			  • Knowledgeable healthcare providers
			  • Home health services needed for living with a trach

	• May leak air and limit the air that reaches your lungs via a mask, mouthpiece or nasal pillows	• Provides most direct delivery of air into your lungs	

• Reduces risk of infections by providing ventilation without an airway hole exposed to external bacteria
• You may use secretion management techniques to help release mucous
	• Increases difficulties removing secretions if you lack the ability to cough
	• May cause sinus congestion from using a mask or dryness from using nasal pillows
		Helps remove secretions:
		  • Can suction mucous through airway hole
		  • Provides direct access to lungs via Cough Assist machine or Ambu bag technique
			• Increases risks of infections from airway hole's exposure to bacteria and the external environment

	• May reduce your ability to see, talk and/or eat easily if you use a nasal or full face mask during the day • May interfere with speaking and/or eating if you use a mouthpiece continuously during the day • You may experience difficulty finding an interface (mask, mouthpiece, nasal pillows) that fits comfortably and securely	• Allows you to see and eat – essential functions of daily living	• May require use of a speaking valve to talk • May need a different sized trach – usually smaller – that will allow you to talk • May prevent your ability to talk. Need to consult specialists for different options. • You may need to find the brand and size of a trach that best suits your needs

(*Continued*)

Benefits of NIV with an interface	Disadvantages of NIV & interface	Benefits of a trach	Disadvantages of a trach

• Involves no risk of internal bleeding
• Results in less secretions
	• May cause problems:
	  • Bloating from air traveling into the stomach
	  • Distortion of teeth from long-term use of mask or mouthpiece
	  • Skin irritation from masks and/or straps
	  • Sinus dryness from nasal pillows
			• You may experience bleeding:
			  • From irritation of frequent suctioning
			  • From granulation tissue at trach opening and tracheal mucosa
			• Increases need to:
			  • Manage secretions
			  • Provide humidity
			  • Clean equipment

• Requires less need for assistance because there is less equipment to clean and fewer tasks to perform
• Increases your freedom and control if you are able to use your arms and hands
• Provides greater mobility if you need NIV during the night and for limited daytime hours or can easily attach the machine to your wheelchair or scooter, if needed
• Increases ability to travel because it requires less equipment and supplies
	• Requires assistance if you are unable to use your arms and hands to set up and clean humidifier
	• May require additional equipment for humidity
		• You may perform your own suctioning and trach care if you are physically able
		• May train family, friends, volunteers and non-agency personal assistants to suction and perform trach care
		• May mount ventilator equipment to wheelchair or scooter to increase mobility
			• Requires daily care for:
			  • Suctioning
			  • Cleaning trach site
			  • Maintaining equipment
			• May require a great amount of assistance if you cannot perform tasks independently
			• Reduces ease of mobility and traveling because of all the equipment and supplies needed

• Increases options to live:
  • Independently
  • In the community
  • In a long-term facility
			• May reduce options to live:
			  • Independently
			  • In the community
			  • In a long-term facility based on its availability in your country/area

• Reduces costs for assistance due to fewer tasks	• Requires out-of-pocket expenses depending on:
	  • Level of assistance needed
	  • Where you live and whether the area provides in-home care
		• Some countries cover costs for in-home assistance and/or care in a long-term facility	• May require significant out-of-pocket expenses based on:
			  • Your area's provisions for in-home services
			  • Your physical abilities
			  • Amount of assistance from volunteers
			  • Cost of non-agency assistants
			  • Legal requirements for hiring agency assistance

programme director or volunteer manager). You may need to make several calls and send emails or letters until you gain a positive response to your request. When an organisation provides or refers volunteers, you most likely will be asked to sign a legal waiver releasing the organisation and its volunteers of any legal responsibility for problems with your care. You are responsible for ensuring that volunteers are properly trained and managed to meet your needs when they assist you.

Healthcare providers, family and friends may vary in their views of living with a trach. For example, Dr John Bach believes that '*Nobody . . . should have a tracheostomy tube for respiratory management – ever.*' Dr Bach is extremely knowledgeable about human physiology and prescribes using NIV 24 hours each day for vent users with very low vital capacities. While using NIV throughout the day works for some individuals, it may not suit the lifestyles and preferences of others. Richard Daggett, a Post-Polio Support Group leader, wrote to Dr Bach about this viewpoint:

> Polio survivors differ and need medical care based on each individual's needs and not on a preconceived idea of what is best for 'everyone.' . . . I have had a trach since 1984. It was my decision. I breathe easier and manage colds much better. I asked for the trach. Certainly a trach is not for everyone. Non-invasive respiratory assistance should be tried first. I firmly believe, however, a trach is a viable option for some.

Some people believe that living with a trach results in poor quality of life. However, a Toronto study of vent users found that participants reported satisfaction with their overall quality of life. Also, the medical journal ***Chest*** published an article on the 'Quality-of-Life Evaluation of Patients with Neuromuscular and Skeletal Diseases Treated with Noninvasive and Invasive Home Mechanical Ventilation.' The article states that trach users with the following conditions reported better health than users of NIV:

> Patients receiving home mechanical ventilation reported a good perceived health, despite severe physical limitations. The patients with post-polio dysfunction and the patients with scoliosis treated with tracheostomy perceived the best health, compared with NIV for this diagnosis (Markström et al., 2002, p. 1695).

Other individuals view the amount of assistance that trach users need as a burden to families and society. What is important is that **you decide** whether you want to live and can adjust to a trach. Then you will need to find out if you have a suitable, affordable place to live and can obtain and afford the amount of assistance, supplies and equipment you will need to live safely and comfortably with a trach.

Deciding whether to use a trach

Since some of the following issues are complex and may trigger anxiety, you may want to work through this process with the support of a wise friend, mentor, counselor, therapist or spiritual director. Make sure that the person understands and values disability issues in the context of 'independent living.' For information about this philosophy, check out http://www.post-polio.org/adv/index.html.

> It is essential that every individual have a knowledgeable **health advocate** (surrogate) who understands their condition, past and recent experiences, personal preferences, and wishes. This advocate must be a person educated in the clinical need. . . . They should be kept abreast of new developments and usually should accompany the person in person when they access the health system, health facilities, use any health resources.
>
> *Allen Goldberg, MD*
> Honorary Board Member of International Ventilator Users Network

GATHER INFORMATION AND INSIGHTS

The process below can help you decide if you can adapt to living with a trach and if you can afford a place to live and the level of assistance and resources you will need to live safely and comfortably with it.

1. *Learn more using a tracheostomy from:*
   a. *International Ventilators Users Network (IVUN).* www.ventusers.org for information, articles and referrals to other vent users. See *Home Ventilator Guide and Resource Directory for Ventilator-Assisted Living.* Call 001-314.534.0476 or access at http://www.ventusers.org/net/VentDIR.pdf.
   b. West Park Health Centre's e-learning modules: www.westpark.org; www.ltvcoe.com/training_oelib_home.html.
   c. Ottawa Rehabilitation Institute's e-learning modules: www.irrd.ca/education.
   d. University of Toronto study on 'Ventilator Users' Perspectives on the Important Elements of Health-Related Quality of Life.' http://www.post-polio.org/res/QofLFINALREPORT-Sept2002.pdf.
   e. Feedback from other trach users. Join vent users' ListServs in the *Resource Directory for Ventilator Assisted Living* at http://www.ventusers.org/net/VentDIR.pd. Consider opinions of others objectively since personal attitudes differ for a variety of reasons.

   f. A *Chest* video of Audrey King describing her challenges of living with a trach for two years while recovering from an illness. Contact mlederer@chestnet.org for a copy.
2. *Obtain information and opinions to determine your options and available resources from:*
   a. Your pulmonologist: the pros and cons of a trach given your condition and circumstances.
   b. Other pulmonologists specialising in home mechanical ventilation. Obtain referrals from IVUN info@ventusers.org or 001-314-534-0475 or from the *Resource Directory for Ventilator-Assisted Living* that you can access at http://www.ventusers.org/net/vdirhm.html.
   c. Home health providers that service ventilator equipment and individuals with trachs in your area.
   d. Government programmes and/or your health insurance provider to determine the services and benefits for which you qualify and the procedures for obtaining them.
   e. Social service agencies for available services and how to apply for and obtain them.
   f. Family, relatives, friends and others to learn how much time and assistance they can provide.
3. *Think about what you have learned.* Do you want to explore the possibilities of using a trach further? If you do, the questions in the grid below can help you determine your needs.

Assess your resources and needs

As you ask yourself these questions, write down your responses. They will help you identify your ability to adapt to a trach, available resources and additional resources you would need. These include healthcare resources, personal assistance, emotional support and the ability to afford what you need.

Healthcare Resources:

- Do you have access to knowledgeable, responsive healthcare professionals: pulmonologist, home health providers and an accessible hospital equipped to handle ventilators and individuals with tracheostomies?

Emotional Resilience:

- Do you consider your life worth living? What makes life worthwhile for you?
- Do you have a purpose in life? How do you imagine you will fulfil your purpose while living with a trach?
- How creative and resourceful will you be in fulfilling your personal needs?
- What are healthy ways you will use to express your needs and feelings?
- How will you respond to distress? How will you support yourself emotionally?
- What access do you have to behavioural health professional(s) and resources for emotional assistance?
- Are your spiritual values and/or religious beliefs important to you? If yes, how will they affect your decision?
- What spiritual and religious resources are available to support you? What connections would you need?

Coordination of Care:

- Do you have a dedicated 'Health Advocate/Surrogate' who understands your medical conditions, special needs, preferences, and would speak on your behalf with health professionals? Who could you ask?
- Is this person willing and able to oversee the coordination of your care?
- Who would be your reliable 'Communication Coordinator' to inform your support network of your condition and needs and also relay their suggestions and messages back to you?

Daily Assistance:

- Are you capable of doing your own trach care and suctioning?
- How much additional assistance, from what you already have, will you need if you have a trach?
- Will you need help for 24 hours of each day? If yes, do you know who will provide that assistance?
- Do you have enough of reliable, trustworthy assistants to provide daily trach care, coordinate services and appointments, transport you to them, respond to emergency needs and enable you to function effectively?
- Can you hire and manage personal assistants or do you have reliable, skilled people who will do that for you?

Financial Costs:

- What costs will health insurance, government programmes and/or social services pay for?
- What do you estimate your out-of-pocket costs will total after coverage from these sources?
- Can you afford to pay for the unreimbursed costs for personal assistance, supplies and equipment?
- Do you have potential sources of income that you can use to cover these expenses?
- Will you be able to afford to continue living in your current residence or will you need to move to more affordable housing or a long-term residence that accepts and assists vent users with trachs?

(Continued)

Assess your resources and needs

Living Arrangement:

- Do you have a suitable place to live that will accommodate your additional needs with a trach?
- Are you physically strong enough to live alone with a medical alarm system that you wear and can operate?
- Do you have room for the additional equipment, supplies and personal assistants you will need?
- Do you have access to government housing or long-term care facilities that will accept vent users with trachs? Are there openings? Do you qualify? Are you willing to live in this kind of residence? What are the costs?
- Do you have other options of living with family, relatives or friends?

Support Network:

- Do you have reliable individuals to visit and assist you regularly? How many? How often?
- Do you have meaningful relationships you can depend on for emotional support and enjoyment?
- How could you stay connected with individuals and organisations? Through phone, computer, other means?
- Are you involved with organisations and/or spiritual or religious communities that could provide support or assistance or will help fulfil your spiritual or advocacy interests? Are you willing to pursue such options?

4. *Decide:*
   a. Does living with a trach match your beliefs about life and your values and goals?
   b. Do you think you can emotionally adjust to living with a trach?
   c. Will you have the resources and assistance you will need to live with a trach:
      i. For the short-term, during a medical emergency and your recovery?
      ii. For the long-term, if your breathing worsens and you need a trach to function?
5. *Inform appropriate individuals in writing of your decisions:*
   a. Persons with Power of Attorney for your health care. Include instructions in legal documents.
   b. Designated 'health advocate(s) or surrogate(s).'
   c. Your health care providers. Ask them to include your decisions in your medical records.
   d. Family and friends who may accompany you to a hospital during an emergency.
6. *Complete a copy of the 'Take Charge, No Chances' forms if you do not subscribe to a medical alert service which health providers can access.* Give copies of the TCNC forms to your assistants and designated individuals; instruct them to bring the forms along when you travel or go to a hospital. These forms will provide health providers with your ventilator settings and special needs. Access them at www.ventusers.org/vume/index or info@ventusers.org or by calling 001-314-574-0475.

Living with a trach

Once you decide you are willing to use a trach, these resources can support you in both your initial adjustment period and long-term use of a trach:

SOURCES OF SUPPORT FOR ADJUSTING TO A TRACH

Professional Assistance

- Highly-skilled, compassionate and communicative healthcare professionals
- A psychotherapist/behavioural health professional to assist in managing distress
- Physical, respiratory, occupational and speech therapists with expertise in your condition
- Case Manager or Coordinator who oversees authorisation for healthcare services in a hospital or facility
- Patient Relations Representative or Ombudsperson to assist in resolving problems in the healthcare facility

Personal Resources

- Your desire and determination to live and your inner strength
- An ability to communicate your needs, wishes and feelings – even if you cannot talk
- A designated 'Health Advocate(s) or Surrogate(s)' to represent you with health professionals
- Daily scheduled visitors to assist and intercede on your behalf in a hospital or other healthcare facility
- A 'Communication Coordinator' to update friends and convey messages to you. These websites may be used to facilitate communication: http://www.caringbridge.org/ or http://www.carepages.com/

Healing Resources

- Spirituality, prayers, kindred souls who share your values, beliefs and/or cultural traditions
- Supportive Touch: hand and foot massages, healing touch, gentle acupressure, back rubs
- Music Therapy: relaxing, uplifting music; your favourite songs and instrumental pieces
- Nutritional food and treats including fresh fruits and vegetables and good protein

ADDITIONAL SOURCES OF SUPPORT FOR LIVING WITH A TRACH

Physical Assistance

- Efficient, responsive and knowledgeable home health providers of ventilators and supplies
- Emergency plans: '***Take Charge, Not Chances***' forms or other medical information system; in-home

medical alert system; emergency evacuation plans; notifications to fire personnel and energy companies

- Reliable, efficient, competent and trustworthy personal care assistants and volunteers

Personal Support

- Loving, meaningful relationships that provide affirmation, comfort, serenity and joy
- Communication with other trach users who understand your challenges and encourage you
- Frequent visitors who provide assistance, share mutual interests and contribute good humour
- Membership and involvement in disability and/or disease-related organisations

Healing Resources

- Options for strengthening emotional health: see http://www.post-polio.org/edu/pphnews/pph19-1p9.pdf
- Meditation, mindfulness, visualisation, relaxation techniques, sitting yoga, tai chi, chi kung
- Bodywork: massages, cranial sacral therapy, gentle osteopathic manipulation therapy, if appropriate
- Opportunities for pleasure, comfort and laughter: children, pets, the arts, books, games
- Opportunities to fulfil your interests: spiritual, intellectual, artistic, recreational, professional/occupational
- Living in a healthy, uplifting, accessible environment; access to outdoors and Nature; uplifting views

Join International Ventilator Users Network (IVUN) to learn about living well with ventilator-assistance and to stay informed about ventilator issues, the latest equipment, research findings and opportunities to learn from other vent users and healthcare providers who generously share their expertise with IVUN.

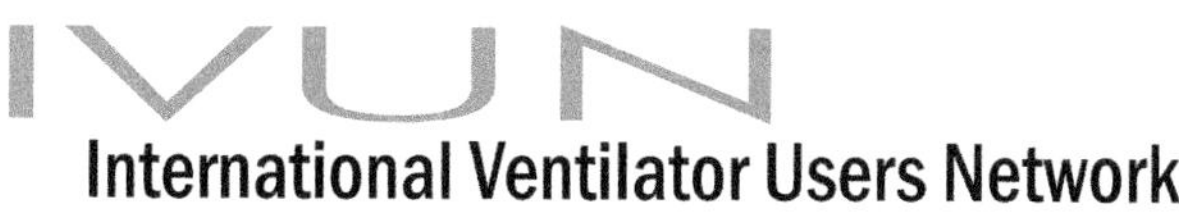

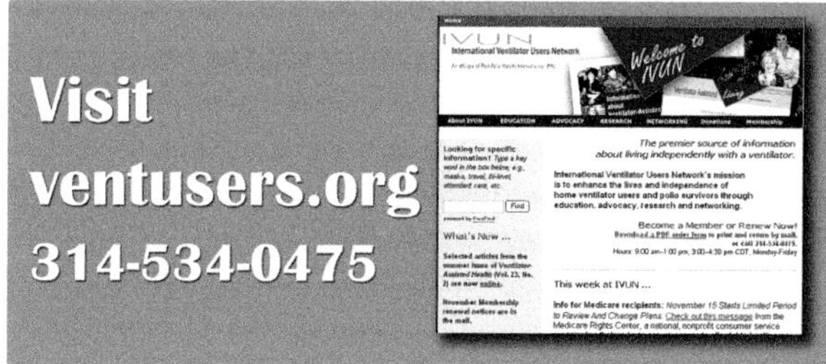

As a ventilator user for more than 25 years, Linda Bieniek advocates for the health and quality of life for vent users. From her personal experience, and her professional knowledge as a Certified Employee Assistance Professional, she shares strategies for deciding about using a trach and for strengthening emotional health. The opinions in this article are hers alone.

She is indebted to Veronica Cook for her insightful editing, to Julie Truong for her superb technical skills and to Norma Braun, MD, Virginia Brickley, Brenda Butka, MD, Richard Daggett, Laura Dowdle, Joan Headley, Marcy Kaplan, Audrey King and Brigid Rafferty for their astute suggestions.

APPENDIX 73B: VENTILATOR USER GUIDELINES FOR EMOTIONAL HEALTH

LINDA L. BIENIEK

Introduction

As ventilator users, we face challenges with our breathing, other physical limitations and unrelated difficulties we encounter while navigating through life. By using a ventilator, we protect our health and enhance our abilities to participate in life. Yet, we may have days when our spirits sag and our energy is in short supply. At times, we also are likely to encounter symptoms of distress, anxiety or depression – conditions common in the general public as well. This article hopes to shine light on the power of attending to our emotional health to restore our spirits and dramatically improve the quality of our lives.

To begin with, it is of foremost importance to understand that our minds, emotions, behaviours and spirits can affect our body and physical health – positively and negatively. While there are no magic cures as some self-help authors imply, we can pursue effective resources to learn how to improve aspects of our lives. Just as using our ventilators improves our breathing, using educational resources can ease our paths and enrich our ability to experience life's goodness.

Distress

As you may know, how we respond to ourselves, to others, and to stressful situations can affect us physically. Distress – negative effects of stress – can increase fatigue, shortness of breath or pain. It also can cause headaches, digestive problems or insomnia and interfere with our concentration, moods and relationships. As a result, we can benefit significantly from resolving causes of distress that are within our control and from managing the negative effects of situations that are out of our control. Our challenge is to learn how to do this and then to be able to do it!

EMOTIONAL HEALTH

Emotional health, or the absence of it, affects every aspect of our personalities. To start, it includes how we think, express our thoughts and feelings, make decisions, interact with others and choose what to do. An emotionally healthy person is rational and open-minded, takes initiative to solve problems, pursues positive goals and expresses thoughts and feelings respectfully and constructively. As our functioning declines, making positive changes that are within our control and accepting circumstances we cannot change are important for our emotional health. Quality relationships and a strong support network are also of extreme importance. Studies show that good relationships are the main source of happiness for many people and play a major role in enhancing our emotional well-being, and in some cases, physical health as well. For many of us, our spiritual values and/or religious beliefs also contribute significantly to our emotional health. They may offer a sense of purpose and meaning to our lives and support us in accepting parts of our lives that we cannot control.

Although we cannot wish away our progressive medical conditions, we can choose to improve the quality of our relationships and our lives in general. As our breathing and physical abilities change, emotional health can enable us to respond compassionately to ourselves and to others. It also can equip us to respond proactively to our needs and problems. **Research reinforces this point:**

- In one study, individuals who confronted their problems directly as their physical health declined, reduced their levels of anxiety and depression. (McLeod)
- Studies concluded that individuals who took action to resolve problems reduced the frequency and intensity of physical symptoms resulting from stress, slowed the progression of their neuromuscular condition and extended their longevity. (McLeod, p. 4–10) (Salovey, p. 110)
- Research has found that supportive relationships can strengthen a person's physical and emotional resilience, reducing suffering and increasing one's ability to cope with pain. (McLeod p. 6) (Salovey, p. 111)

Read: Rosen, E. and D'Elgin, T. (2001) *Think Like a Shrink: 100 Principles for Seeing Deeply into Yourself and Others* to learn about healthy ways of thinking, responding to others and making choices.

Guidelines

This article presents guidelines for strengthening our emotional health. Part I identifies resources for developing a supportive living situation to accommodate our physical and emotional needs. It also offers a step-by-step framework for achieving our goals and identifies resources and strategies that we can pursue independently or with an insightful, trustworthy friend, mentor or life coach.

Yet, when distress interferes with our ability to function or to make changes to protect our health, it's time to consider professional assistance, if that option is available. Part II of this article describes psychotherapy (therapy) as an invaluable resource. It also offers steps for selecting and working effectively with a psychotherapist (therapist) when that is an option, and for utilising other community resources that may be available.

PART I: DEVELOPING A LIVING SITUATION TO SUPPORT OUR PHYSICAL AND EMOTIONAL HEALTH

Personal characteristics

Investing in our overall health – our minds, bodies, emotions and spirits – requires time, energy, determination and resourcefulness. In some situations, we also may need assistance from others and money to pay for services. In addition, the process of improving our satisfaction with aspects of our lives calls for all our best qualities, including:

Acceptance: Of our physical limitations, needs for assistance and need for emotional support.
Courage: To face our thoughts, feelings and behaviours honestly. To learn how to make changes.
Awareness: Of what we do to manage distress, comfort ourselves, fulfil our needs for love and support.
Commitment: To resolve causes of distress and to manage negative effects of issues out of our control.
Humility: To reach out for support, assistance, comfort and enjoyment from good people.
Compassion: For ourselves and others affected by our losses and changes in life.
Open-mindedness: To explore options for achieving our goals and making our lives more gratifying.
Focus and Practice: To become aware of our choices and to choose healthy options to fulfil our needs

Resources contribute to building our emotional health

While on our journeys to build emotional health, we can tap a great number of resources, from specialised to simple. Here are some categories of resources that can protect our physical health, contribute to our well-being and enhance our abilities to live with greater ease and confidence.

Professional assistance

- Highly-skilled, compassionate and communicative healthcare professionals
- Physical, respiratory, occupational and speech therapists knowledgeable about treating our conditions
- Efficient, responsive and knowledgeable home health providers of equipment and supplies
- Behavioural health professionals (therapist, psychologist) to assist us in responding proactively to distress.

Supportive relationships

- Designated 'Health Advocate(s) or Surrogate(s)' to represent us with health professionals
- Loving, meaningful relationships; and frequent visitors who share our interests and values and provide humour
- A 'Communication Coordinator' to update others and convey messages if we are ill or hospitalised. Helpful websites: http://www.caringbridge.org/ or http://www.carepages.com/

Physical support

- Reliable, efficient, competent and trustworthy personal care assistants and/or volunteers
- Emergency plans: '*Take Charge, Not Chances*' forms www.ventusers.org/vume/index or another medical information system; in-home medical alert system; evacuation plans; notification to fire personnel, energy company
- Stretching, breathing and/or strengthening exercises tailored to our abilities; sitting yoga, tai chi, chi kung
- Supportive Touch: hand and foot massages, healing touch, gentle acupressure, back rubs
- Bodywork: massages, warm water therapy, cranial sacral therapy, gentle osteopathic manipulation therapy
- Nutritional food and treats including fresh fruits and vegetables and good protein

Self-expression

- Spirituality and/or religious values and visitors, prayers, participation in traditions and rituals
- Meditation, mindfulness, visualisation; relaxation techniques
- Music Therapy: relaxing or uplifting music; favourite songs; music performances or playing an instrument
- Opportunities for pleasure, comfort, humour, joy: children, pets, the arts, books, nature, games, sports
- Opportunities to fulfil our intellectual, artistic, recreational, professional and/or occupational interests
- Resources from the 'Treatment Approach Options Chart' at http://www.post-polio.org/edu/pphnews/pph19-1p9.pdf

Starting point: Deciding on our goals

In order to make changes, we need to identify what we need and want. Our goals must apply to ourselves and what we can realistically do. (Remember, we can't change someone else!) One way to identify our goals is to list issues in our lives that distress us. Then ask ourselves: '***What do I want instead?***' It is essential that you state your goal as a positive intention, not as what you do NOT want. Also, realise that 'doing' includes behaviours that do not require physical strength. Examples include how we think, solve problems or express ourselves. We also can discover our needs by asking ourselves: ***'What do I need to feel better about myself?' 'What do I wish I would do to take better care of my health?' 'What do I want to do that would bring me satisfaction?'*** Take time to develop two or three goals. The following are some examples.

Developing Self-Acceptance

- To learn how to accept my limitations and support myself in making necessary changes
- To learn how to face myself with understanding, compassion and patience instead of criticism

Learning Skills and Strategies

- To learn how to let go of anger and resentments that affect my relationships and health.
- To learn how to live in the present and appreciate the goodness that is available to me.
- To be able to ask for and accept help; and to be resourceful in obtaining assistance I need.
- To become creative in making and adapting to necessary lifestyles changes.
- To learn how to express my feelings honestly and directly, yet respectfully.
- To develop mutually loving, supportive relationships with individuals who share my values and interests.
- To negotiate options for sexual activities and for expressing affection with my spouse or partner.
- To make decisions and set priorities which reflect my values and beliefs.

Changing Coping Patterns

- To discover the causes and ways to change my self-destructive behaviors such as drinking alcohol excessively, overeating, being verbally abusive, spending hours on cybersex or overspending.
- To identify unmet emotional needs that result in self-defeating behaviours (procrastinating or isolating).
- To learn healthy ways of fulfilling my emotional needs.

Resources: Francis, L. & Zukav, G. (2001). *The heart of the soul: emotional awareness.* Simon & Schuster. O'Malley, M. (2004). *The gift of our compulsions: a revolutionary approach to self-acceptance and healing.*

Next step: Create a plan to achieve each goal

A goal without a plan may get us somewhere, but a plan gives wings to a goal. Here are effective steps for creating a plan. (Note: You may benefit from asking an insightful, trustworthy individual to assist with this process. Another option is to recruit a skilled, objective volunteer from a college or university programme. Or, if you can afford the fees, you may want to gain assistance from a Life Coach. These professionals are trained to assist individuals with achieving their goals; many are certified and work over the phone. In addition, you may contact the director of a certification training programme and request *pro bono* assistance from an individual in training who can assist you over the phone.)

> **Our mind, body, emotions, behaviours and spirit/spirituality are connected and affect each other.** Some vent users report they became less short of breath and more alert and energetic after they spoke up to settle a relationship conflict. Others say that having a good cry or receiving a neck massage can reduce muscle tension resulting from distress about a situation that was out of their control.

Before you begin, prepare how you will note your responses to the questions below. Notebook, pen, markers, post-em notes, laptop, computer dictation system?

1. **Now, state your goal.** Frame it in positive words. Make sure it applies to you and is realistic. Use the steps below for each goal that you set. Focus on one goal at a time!
2. **After you read each question, jot down any ideas that come to your mind.** Let your imagination go to work! Think logically, creatively and intuitively.
3. **Imagine when you reach your goal!** Be very specific in responding to these questions. Your answers will provide evidence of your achievements.
   a. What will you look like?
   b. How will you feel?
   c. How will you sound?
   d. What will you do or be doing?
   e. What will be different in your life?
4. **When do you want to reach your goal?**
5. **How will you benefit from achieving this goal?**
6. **Is there anyone who won't be in favour of your goal?** (Even if the person won't admit it.)
   a. Who?
   b. Why?
7. **Is there any part of YOU that is not totally convinced that this is a good goal for you to pursue?** For example, the part of you that is reluctant to ask for assistance?
8. **What are any possible negative consequences of your goal that may affect your life or others?**
   a. Your life?
   b. Others?
9. **Take time to list your own 'special personal qualities' that will help you achieve your goal.**
   For example: desire to learn, open-mindedness, sense of humour.
10. **Then, brainstorm: 'Who and what' can support you in reaching this goal?** For example: friends who will deliver library books or provide transportation, Internet access.
    a. Who?
    b. What?
11. **Next, try to identify any issues or obstacles that may limit or interfere with your ability to achieve your goal.** This list is very important because it may reveal the 'additional resources' you will need to reach your goal successfully. Include any objections or potentially negative consequences you identified in questions #6, #7, #8 above. For example: financial limitations; inadequate assistance
    a. Limitations
    b. Objections
    c. Possible negative consequences
12. **Now, try to identify the 'additional resources' you will need to reach your goal successfully.** List as many as you can think of. Consult the 'Treatment Approach Options Chart' at http://www.post-polio.org/edu/pphnews/pph19-1p9.pdf and creative friends for ideas.
    a. Who else could provide valuable support or skills to enable you to reach your goal?
    b. What additional resources? These can be skills, strategies, items, personal qualities.
13. **Logically and creatively, outline each step you will take: 1) to obtain the additional resources you need, and 2) to achieve your goal.** Create a way to map out your plans and then to track your progress. Some people use charts, lists, posters, journals or an excel spreadsheet. Include:
    a. What you will do to obtain additional resources?
    b. When you will do this?
    c. With whom?
    d. Where?
    e. What will you do to achieve your goals? When? With whom? Where?
14. **Finally, decide what you will do if you get stuck or encounter an unforeseen problem.**
    a. What will you do?
    b. Who will you consult for assistance?

Resources: ***This year I will...how to finally change a habit, keep a resolution, or make a dream come true*** by M. J. Ryan (2006). ***Embracing your inner critic*** by H. and S. Stone (1993). See the **'Treatment Approach Options Chart'** mentioned above and below for additional resources.

Pursue resources and develop strategies

Find other reputable resources that you can learn from on your own. The Self-Help industry offers numerous books, tapes, DVDs, Internet sites and television programs on personal development and behavioural health (mental health) topics. Some include sound information, useful and applicable to our lives. Others present unfounded claims that are misleading, and at times, unethical because of the unrealistic results they promise. Beware of approaches that seem too simple to be true or make almost magical promises. For example, '*If you change your thoughts, you can cure your physical condition.*' While thinking positively has benefits and may motivate you to improve aspects of your health, the reality is that very positive people have died from incurable conditions. Thus, look for authoritative information from well-respected professionals; search authoritative national or international mental health organisations for the additional suggestions.

> If I could leave you with only one tip for changing anything in your life, it would be this: recognizing you've blown it is progress! That is why I love the quote about the lighthouse... 'it is always darkest before dawn.' There is always a phase in creating forward motion when all you notice is how hard it is and how little you've moved....We can move through the stages of learning something new. But only if we're willing to treat ourselves encouragingly in the early parts so that we keep our spirits up, remind our brains that we are making progress, and mine our experiences for tomorrow.
>
> *M. J. Ryan*
> *This Year I Will . . . How to Finally Change a Habit, Keep a Resolution, or Make a Dream Come True*, pp. 132–133

Learn to manage distress and improve aspects of your life from resources and strategies identified on the 'Treatment Approach Options Chart.' Access at http://www.post-polio.org/edu/pphnews/pph19-1p9.pdf or request from info@ventusers.org or 001-314-574-0475. These approaches are used by reputable professionals and you can pursue many on your own.

Connect with people who share mutual interests and/or experiences

Learn ways to live well with your health condition and disabilities from others in similar situations. Join local, national, and international disability and disease-related organisations. Ask to be placed on email and/or mailing lists and to have membership dues waived, if you cannot afford them. Read reputable publications and websites for ideas about responding creatively to your challenges.

1. Join **International Ventilator Users Network (IVUN)** at www.ventusers.org for information about equipment, resources, advocacy and vent users' experiences. Contact info@ventusers.org or 001-314-534-0475 for referrals to other vent users and to knowledgeable health professionals.
2. Learn about the 'Independent Living' philosophy. http://www.post-polio.org/adv/index.html.
3. Read University of Toronto's study about 'Ventilator User's Perspectives on Important Elements of Health-Related Quality of Life' at http://www.post-polio.org/res/QofLFINALREPORT-Sept2002.pdf. You may find pages 50–64; 91–94; 97 most useful.

Join support groups if you are able to attend meetings and/or Internet groups. While initially a bit intimidating for some, support groups can develop into joyous lifelines over time. Sign up to receive ListServs emails for vent users at http://www.ventusers.org/net/VentDIR.pdf. Join groups that also relate to your personal interests such as book clubs, political discussion groups, arts and crafts gatherings or meeting with neighborhood sports enthusiasts. These are important for fulfilling your artistic, recreational and intellectual interests as well as building friendships with like-minded individuals. In any group, be cautious of people who try to impose their opinions on others. Also, share your personal information discreetly and maintain confidentiality to protect privacy and prevent others from using information inappropriately.

Connect with your Spiritual and/or Religious Values: For many, the challenge to grow emotionally into our best selves involves our faith and spiritual values and/or religious beliefs. If this is true for you, seek supportive connections with others who share them. Spirituality contributes to your emotional health when it supports you in making positive changes, pursuing life's goodness and facing life's difficulties with courage and creativity. If you do not belong to a spiritual or religious community, you may want to learn about those in your area to determine if any appeal to you.

- Contact religious or spiritual communities to find out if they would provide you with any assistance. Will they send visitors to your home? Volunteers to assist with tasks? Provide religious or spiritual services?
- Ask to receive information, if you are interested; even if you cannot afford to donate money.
- Consider counseling from a clergy member, spiritual director, pastoral counselor or parish representative, **if that counselor has the appropriate training, experience, integrity and professionalism** identified on pages 13–16. The person should never impose beliefs, try to convince you to join an organisation or religion or use the relationship for sexual purposes. See www.goodtherapy.org/blog/warning-signs-of-bad-therapy to learn about signs of unethical counseling.
- Join a committee or contribute your skills to a project as a way to meet like-minded individuals.

Experiences that signal a need for emotional health resources

Some among us may be all ready to set goals, create plans and take action, but find our spirits sagging and energy low, leaving us unable to do what we want. In these cases, the cause may be an unresolved experience or condition that cries out for our attention and for healing. Listed below are three major examples for you to review, along with specific suggestions for seeking relief and support.

Risk of Suicide or of Being Harmed or of Harming Another: If you are thinking about hurting yourself or someone else, or fear that someone may hurt you, or are experiencing a life-threatening crisis, get immediate help! Call your local law enforcement; go to the nearest hospital emergency room or call a Suicide Prevention or Domestic Violence Hotline listed in your local telephone book. Website resources include: http://suicidehotlines.com/ and http://www.evawintl.org/.

- Notify a physician of your impulses, risks and fears. Seek immediate assistance to protect yourself, including hospitalisation, if necessary. Work with a qualified professional (for example, psychologist, psychiatrist or psychotherapist) for ongoing assistance to resolve problems, reducing future risks.

Overuse or Dependency on Alcohol, Medications, Drugs, Food or Other Addictions and Self-Destructive Behaviors: Chemical dependency and substance abuse rates are higher in the disability community than in the general population (Olkin, p. 258). This is because these substances can temporarily help to numb physical pain and/or emotional distress resulting from issues such as loneliness, relationship conflicts, anger or traumatic experiences. If you overuse or depend on any substances or engage in other self-destructive behaviours (such as overspending, being verbally abuse, gambling, cybersex), seek assistance. Learn healthy, useful ways to respond to distress, boredom and your emotions (anger, fear, shame, sadness, anxiousness) and especially to fulfil your emotional needs.

- Approach yourself non-judgmentally – with compassion and curiosity. Pay attention to how you manage physical or emotional pain. Write down what happens just before you engage in a compulsive behavior.
- Learn about your addiction and behaviors from reputable resources: books, DVD, etc. Gain awareness of what you do and how it affects you and others. The more aware you become of your feelings and how you respond to them, the more power you will gain to consciously make healthy choices in your life.
- Attend self-help groups if you are able. Participate in reputable Internet groups. Seek support from skilled, knowledgeable and trustworthy individuals and support group members. Obtain a sponsor.
- Inform health providers of your unhealthy behavior patterns and their negative effects on your health, life and others. Seek their suggestions, support and referrals for professional assistance.
- Work with a therapist trained to treat your condition; participate in a self-help group, and in a treatment programme, if necessary. (Finney, p. 161–166) (Roberts, p. 27–28; 94–95; 248–256)

Experience of Emotional or Physical Abuse or Neglect, Sexual Abuse or a Life-Threatening Incident or a Life-Changing Loss: If you grew up in a household where a person had an addiction or another chronic problem such as mental illness, you were at greater risk for experiencing or witnessing neglect or abuse (Olkin, p. 232). Or, did you experience a life-threatening medical crisis? Or, did a parent die when you were a young child? If you struggle with anxiety, depression, negative attitudes, erratic or self-destructive behaviors or flashbacks or nightmares of bad memories, these problems may relate to unresolved traumatic experiences from your past.

- Obtain reputable information to learn about the possible effects of traumatic experiences. Read articles on healing early memories (Bieniek and Kennedy, Winter and Summer 2002). Access at www.post-polio.org or from 001-314-574-0475 or director@post-polio.org.
- Report your struggles, symptoms and physical problems to your physicians.
- Seek professional assistance, if you continue to experience difficulties after using self-help resources or if you become more anxious or depressed when you try to face these issues alone. It is important to work with professionals who have specialised training and expertise resolving the effects of a trauma safely and effectively. (Bieniek & Kennedy, Summer 2002) (Finney, p. 167–186) (Napier)

PART II: ALL ABOUT THERAPY

If you have used reputable self-help resources, but distress continues to interfere with your health, functioning, work, relationships or ability to make needed changes, it is time to take the next step. Likewise, if symptoms of anxiety or depression, an addiction or other self-destructive behaviour have prevented you from pursuing self-help resources, find the courage and support to seek available professional assistance.

In some parts of the world, psychotherapy (therapy) is the main type of professional assistance available to help a person in the situations described above. However, some areas may only offer treatment groups facilitated by professionals as a cost-effective option. Regardless of whether you participate in individual or group therapy, you may find it useful to think about seeking professional assistance like this: If you injure your back, your physician may prescribe physical therapy to reduce your pain and increase your functioning. Likewise, if distress impairs your health or functioning, your physician may recommend therapy, if it is available.

If your health provider has referred you to a therapist or programme for professional assistance, the following guidelines can help you make optimal use of that opportunity in the time allotted. They also can help you determine if a therapist is a good match for your needs, if you have a choice. Or, if you can afford to work with a therapist, the steps in this section can guide you in searching for and finding a good match. Understanding these guidelines also can empower you to understand the principles of ethical and effective counseling if you seek counseling services from a university, treatment center, religious or community organisation or a non-profit agency.

Therapy is a learning process. In therapy, you can learn how to resolve a problem that keeps you from falling asleep at night because you think about it over and over. Or if the problem is a situation that you can't change or influence, then you can learn how to manage your anxieties. If you find yourself unable to ask for needed assistance, therapy offers an opportunity to discover and change negative beliefs that may hold you back from taking care of your health. Therapy is especially useful when you want to change a self-destructive behaviour, such as using alcohol to cover up pain and loneliness; especially when it is combined with a 12-step program like Alcoholics Anonymous (AA). And, therapy can help you resolve problems that leave you depressed and unable to concentrate and meet deadlines at work.

Gaining positive results in therapy requires your determination and a therapist's dedication and expertise. It is important to work with a highly skilled psychotherapist (therapist) who understands how your physical disabilities may affect different aspects of your life and is creative in helping you achieve your goals. Your results also depend on you – your commitment, honesty and openness to work through difficulties. See 'Personal Characteristics' section on pages 2–3.

Your ability to obtain effective therapy may depend on various issues such as whether therapists are available in your area; whether you have coverage for the fees from a government programme or insurance benefits; what, if anything, you can afford to pay and your transportation options. You can ask if a therapist will accept an affordable, reduced rate or will provide any *pro bono* sessions, if you have little or no money. While in-person sessions are most useful, if you are unable to travel, ask if phone sessions are an option. Some therapists will assist periodically via email. However, always make sure you understand, what if any, services will be paid by your insurance benefits or a government programme, and which you are responsible to pay. If you need to appeal to an insurance provider or health programme for an accommodation to obtain coverage of such costs, ask your physician if he or she is willing to assist by documenting your physical limitations. Then, you can attach that to your request.

How long it takes to resolve the difficulties you face also depends on various factors. Individuals often can learn how to resolve a specific problem or to cope with a difficult situation in short-term focused therapy of 4–10 sessions. However, when a person needs to change ongoing self-defeating behaviors that stem from abusive childhood experiences, additional sessions may be needed to understand and learn healthy ways of responding to difficulties. Likewise, when a person faces complex issues such as an addiction, severe depression or anxiety or a long history of abuse and neglect, the person may need more than one type of assistance.

In some situations, appropriate medication may improve a person's condition, enabling that person, you, to work effectively in therapy, and possibly, reduce the amount of time in therapy. Non-addictive antidepressants may reduce distressing symptoms and increase a person's energy and ability to concentrate and to function more effectively. Studies report that the combination of psychotherapy and medication are most effective for treating conditions such as anxiety and depression. (Bruckner-Gordon, p. 34) (Roberts, p. 203–218) http://archpsyc.ama-assn.org/cgi/content/abstract/61/7/714

If available and costs are covered by a person's insurance benefits or a health programme, health professionals may refer individuals with ongoing complex conditions to an outpatient programme or to extended levels of treatment to facilitate their recovery. Outpatient programmes usually include educational sessions, individual and group therapy, medication assessments and development of prevention plans to support the recovery of the person returning home. Participating in self-help groups normally is part of all the above-mentioned treatment options, when they are available. Unfortunately, extended or intensive treatment programmes do not exist in many areas.

How therapy works

Therapy is a form of teamwork. Most often, you and a therapist will engage in a dialogue that includes, but is not limited to, sharing information, asking and responding to questions, gaining insights, discovering what holds you back from what you want, learning skills and strategies for making changes, changing negative beliefs and feelings and analysing benefits and consequences of future options. A therapist also may use other approaches, such as the expressive therapies, to teach you healthy ways to release intense feelings. Some therapists assign homework to discuss in a follow-up session.

> Psychotherapy helps individuals explore and resolve more enduring and deeply felt sources of conflict and dissatisfaction in their lives, so that they will gain confidence and inner wholeness. Psychotherapy is a specialized technique which is effective in helping you cope with a wide range of difficulties. It can produce lasting change in your life. Building an alliance of trust with the therapist leads to a reshaping of significant emotional experiences, and builds confidence and wholeness in new and enduring relationships.
>
> – *Gary Hellman*
> http://www.metanoia.org/choose/gethelp03.htm

Good therapy is a blend of art and science. The science includes the therapist's knowledge of psychological issues, therapeutic approaches and an understanding of your background, needs and learning style. The art relates to how the therapist applies that knowledge along his or her intuition, insights, skills and creativity to help you work through obstacles and enable you to achieve your goals.

The foundation of good therapy is the relationship you develop with your therapist. For this reason, it is important that you work with a therapist whom you feel safe revealing your deepest thoughts and feelings. A therapist's job is to show you how your therapy relationship is a practice ground for other relationships. The therapist can help you heal from negative experiences in your past by responding to you in ways that show understanding and build trust.

Finding an effective therapist

Finding a therapist who matches your personality and meets your needs enhances the success of your therapy experiences. If you have been in therapy or counseling before, and did not find it helpful, there are reasons why you may have been dissatisfied. These include but are not limited to: 1) the therapist and you did not set clear goals and agree on how you would determine that you reached them; 2) you may not have expressed your dissatisfaction to the therapist; 3) the therapist may not have had complete information about your situation either because you may not have relayed some important details, or the therapist did not ask enough of probing questions to identify the obstacles that you faced; 4) you may not have been emotionally ready to work through difficult issues you needed to make changes, often for a subconscious reason or 5) the therapist may not have had the expertise to help you resolve your problem.

For these reasons, when you have options, it is important to search for a therapist who is the '*most suitable match*' for your personality, goals, requirements and preferences. To search in this way, list your requirements which are ***'must haves'*** and preferences which are ***'would like to have'*** but are not necessary. Issues may range from the therapist's gender, location, personal qualities such as a sense of humour and fees, to religious background or use of a therapy approach that appeals to you.

Learn about Types of Professionals Who Work as Therapists: Professionals include, but are not limited to, social workers, psychologists and marriage and family therapists. Therapists' titles will differ based on their education and credentials. Titles, however, do not guarantee a professional's expertise and effectiveness. For more information, read the references and web links: (Finney, p. 44–49) (Striano, p. 5–19)

- www.planetpsych.com/zTreatment/psychotherapy.htm#How%20do%20I%20select%20a%20psychotherapist
- www.suicideandmentalhealthassociationinternational.org/psychother.html
- www.metanoia.org/choose/gethelp11.htm

Learn about Various Therapy Approaches: Any of the professionals who work as therapists as referred to above, may use a variety of approaches in working with clients. The website http://www.goodtherapy.org/types-of-therapy.html describes many types. What is important is that the therapist uses approaches that empower you to make changes that are within your control. Some approaches will help you gain awareness of the causes and effects of a problem – an important first step in making changes. However, other approaches often are needed for you to learn how to apply new behaviors into everyday life and minimise distress and subsequent problems. Also, it is important that your therapist train you to pay attention to your feelings and intuition – valuable sources of wisdom that can help you navigate life's challenges successfully.

Obtain Names of Therapists: Check out the following web link and references for sources from which you can obtain names of therapists: www.post-polio.org/edu/pphnews/pph18-4c.html (Bruekner-Gordon et al., p. 57–58) (Finney, p. 39–43; 210–217). Depending on your location, the web links below may provide additional names. Since none of these sources can determine a therapist's effectiveness and integrity, it is important for you to interview each therapist and decide if the person has the qualities identified in this section. Licensing and certifying boards can tell you if the therapist has a good record and has resolved any charges or complaints. If your choice of therapists is limited by an insurance provider or government programme, work through the steps of the system to obtain the best possible match for your needs.

- http://www.goodtherapy.org/find-therapist.html
- http://www.selfleadership.org/node/9002
- http://www.therapistlocator.net/ US, Canada, Overseas
- http://www.find-a-therapist.com/PublicHome/OutsideLearnAndExplore.aspx?&articleid=122&ind=Y
- http://therapists.psychologytoday.com/
- http://www.networktherapy.com/directory/find_therapist.asp?gclid=CPbu9eL7upwCFRINDQodX2Vzmw

Explore Community Mental Health Services and/or University Programmes if you can't afford therapists in private practice. These services often are based on your ability to pay. The counselors' expertise will vary; some still may be in training. Usually you are assigned to a counselor and are not given a choice. Yet, you can make requests, ask about the counselor's background, ask the counselor to read disability resources identified in this article and even check out the programme and counselor's reputation with other agencies. (Bieniek and Kennedy, Fall 2002) (Finney)

Qualities to seek in a therapist

Effective therapists will provide compassion, empathy, skillfulness, knowledge, understanding, intuitiveness and integrity, as demonstrated in the following ways:

An Interest in Learning about Your Health Condition and Disability Issues: If you are interested in working with a therapist who is not experienced with these issues, ask this professional if he or she is willing to learn about the risks, challenges, and social issues you may face by reading:

- Olkin's book, *What Psychotherapists Should Know about Disabilities*
- The 'Independent Living' philosophy at http://www.post-polio.org/adv/index.html.
- Information about your health conditions/disease from reputable websites or publications.
- University of Toronto's study about 'Ventilator User's Perspectives on Important Elements of Health-Related Quality of Life.' http://www.post-polio.org/res/QofLFINALREPORT-Sept2002.pdf (p. 50–64;91–94;97)
- Articles on healing early memories related to growing up with disabilities and chronic medical conditions. (Bieniek and Kennedy, Winter and Summer 2002)

Professionalism demonstrated when the therapist…

- Views the client/therapist relationship as a collaborative, team effort.
- Respects your spiritual values and/or religious beliefs and cultural or ethnic traditions.
- Encourages you to seek medical advice to rule out any medical causes of your symptoms.
- Consults more experienced professionals for advice in addressing your issues effectively.
- Provides you with a back-up therapist to contact for an emergency when he or she is away.

Therapeutic Approach demonstrated when the therapist…

- Provides a nurturing, judgment-free relationship that enables you to feel safe expressing your deepest thoughts and feelings, sharing reactions about the therapist and therapy and, asking any questions.
- Believes that you can develop, heal and improve your emotional health.
- Approaches you compassionately and patiently, understanding and accepting your limitations.
- Teaches you to pay attention to your feelings and helps you learn safe, productive ways to express them.
- Is an empathic, attentive listener who remembers key information you previously shared.
- Challenges you to work through difficulties and resistance you may encounter during therapy.
- Encourages you to take responsibility for your health, physically and emotionally.

Integrity demonstrated when the therapist…

- Maintains confidentiality and obtains informed consent except as required by law.
- Communicates consistently and clearly about policies and explains any exceptions or changes.
- Focuses completely on you during sessions. If an emergency interruption occurs, makes up your time.

Skills and Knowledge demonstrated when the therapist…

- Intervenes immediately if you are at risk of being harmed, harming yourself or another person.
- Understands your needs and uses effective approaches that help you achieve your goals.
- Affirms your strengths and uses empowering language to teach you positive ways to think about yourself.
- Provides insights about the effects of past experience on how you think, feel and behave.
- Recommends and introduces you to resources that you can pursue on your own.

Ethical Boundaries demonstrated when the therapist…

- Maintains clear, healthy boundaries. Does not exchange (barter) services, engage you in a personal or dual relationship or initiate any sexual contact with you. (Napier)
- Shares personal information about herself or himself in sessions only if it applies to your circumstances. (You are not there to listen to a report of the therapist's life.)

> In the past, universities and degree programmes for psychotherapists required students to work on their own issues in therapy as part of their education. Unfortunately, most programmes no longer require this. Thus, when you have choices, consider a therapist's own investment in therapy as an important factor in deciding whether to work with that therapist. (Bieniek & Kennedy, Fall 2002) (Bruckner-Gordon, et al. p.26) www.goodtherapy.org/blog/warning-signs-of-bad-therapy.

Interview therapists to find a good match for your needs

Before making an appointment, it is wise to first interview therapists over the phone for about 15 minutes. Take notes about: 1) the information the therapist provides; and 2) how you felt talking with that therapist. Ask each therapist some of the same questions. Here are some to consider:

Training and background

- What kind of education and license or certification do you have?
- What have you learned from your years in practice? How long have you worked as a therapist?
- What is your experience working with persons with disabilities and chronic health conditions?
- What training and experience do you have identifying and treating clients a) with addictions? b) who had a traumatic experience that is affecting their quality of life?
- Do you work with a supervisor or have a consultant with whom you discuss therapeutic problems?
- Have you worked on your own issues in therapy?

Therapy approaches

- Do you set treatment goals? If yes, how? How do you monitor them?
- How do you help clients reach their therapy goals?
- Do you specialise in any areas or in treating certain conditions?
- What types of therapy approaches do you use most often in working with clients?

Logistics

- Where is your office located?
- Are there any stairs or ramps to get into it? An accessible bathroom? Will I need to use an elevator?
- When do you have available appointments?

Policies and practices

- What are your fees? Will my insurance provider or a government-funded programme pay for them?
- Do you offer sliding scale fees?
- What are your policies regarding emergency phone consultations? Cancellations of appointments?
- Do you offer telephone sessions if I am unable to get to your office? Are these reimbursable?
- Do you provide a back-up therapist when you are away?
- Do you refer clients to a psychiatrist or physician if you think that medication would help the person?

(Bieniek and Kennedy, Fall 2002) (Bruckner-Gordon, et al. p. 61–65) (Finney, p. 64–65; 223) (Striano, p. 1–55) http://mentalhealth.samhsa.gov/publications/allpubs/KEN98-0046/default.asp

Making a final decision

In selecting a therapist consider asking yourself the following questions to gain insights about each therapist:

Trust Level: Is this therapist someone whom I can trust and would want to work with?

- How did I feel while talking with the therapist?
- What did I like about the therapist? What, if any, concerns do I have?
- What, if anything, did I learn about myself from talking with this therapist?
- How did the therapist communicate? Was I satisfied with the responses I received?

Background

- What about the therapist's experience, training and background appeals to me?
- Does the person fulfil my requirements? Preferences?
- Can I afford to work with this therapist?

If you have a choice of therapists, compare the information you've gathered and also consider your intuitive (gut) reactions in deciding which therapist is the best match for your needs. If you are unsure, continue searching to find a therapist you can talk with easily, if others are available to you. If you don't have other options, work with the available therapist keeping an open-mind, positive attitude and determination to learn how to resolve your difficulties in the time allotted, trusting this therapist can help you.

> *'Do not hire a therapist you do not like.' (Finney, p. 56)*

Understanding effective therapy

As you work with a therapist, you will gain insights about the therapist's qualities, integrity, skills and effectiveness. Each interaction with a therapist is an opportunity for learning and building trust. Even when you tell your therapist about a self-destructive behaviour that is affecting your health and creating problems in relationships, the therapist should approach you as a compassionate, wise teacher and not as a shaming critic. If you experience discomfort or resistance in therapy, learn about boundaries and warning signs of questionable therapy (Striano, p. 27–53) www.goodtherapy.org/blog/warning-signs-of-bad-therapy. This information will enable you to determine if your discomfort is because you feel reluctant (even subconsciously) to deal with an issue in your life or because of your dissatisfaction or a problem with your therapy or therapist. It is normal to want to avoid issues that are uncomfortable to face.

Yet, remember, when you solve a problem satisfactorily, you can gain not only peace of mind, but also mental energy, and confidence. Ultimately, effective therapy will strengthen your ability to reach out for support, make wise choices, adapt to your health's changes with greater ease, and develop satisfaction and fulfilment from life's goodness that is available to you. (Finney, p. 66–68) (Striano, p. 27–53)

REFERENCES: OBTAIN OUT-OF-PRINT BOOKS FROM LIBRARIES, WEBSITES AND BOOKSTORES OF USED BOOKS

Bieniek, L. Treatment Approach Options Chart. *Polio Network News.* http://www.post-polio.org/edu/pphnews/pph19-1p9.pdf

Bieniek L, Kennedy K. Improving quality of life: Healing polio memories. *Polio Network News.* Winter 2002;18(1).

Bieniek L, Kennedy K. A guide for exploring polio memories. *Polio Network News*. Summer 2002;18(3).

Bieniek L, Kennedy K. Pursuing therapeutic resources to improve your health. *Polio Network News*. Fall 2002;18(4).

Bruckner-Gordon, F. et al. (1988). *Making Therapy Work*. NY: Harper & Rowe. *(One of the best)*

Finney, L. (1995). *Reach for Joy: How to Find the Right Therapist and Therapy for You*. Freedom, CA: The Crossing Press.

Francis, L. and Zukav, G. (2001). *The Heart of the Soul: Emotional Awareness*. New York: NY: Simon & Schuster.

Hamstra, B. (1994). *How Therapists Diagnose: Professional Secrets You Deserve to Know*. New York, NY: St Martins Griffin.

Markstrom A. et al. *Chest* 2002;122(5): 1695–1700.

McLeod J.E. (2007). 'Review of psychosocial aspects of motor neuron disease.' *Journal of the Neurological Sciences* 258, 4–10. http://www.jns-journal.com/article/S0022-510X(07)00202-X/abstract.

Morella, J. (2008) *A Guide for Effective Psychotherapy*. Rockford, IL: Helm Publishing.

Napier, N. (1993) *Getting Through the Day: Strategies for Adults Hurt as Children*. New York, NY: W.W. Norton & Co.

Olkin, R. (1999) *What Psychotherapists Should Know About Disability*. New York, NY: Guilford Press.

O'Malley, M. (2004). *The Gift of Our Compulsions: A Revolutionary Approach to Self-Acceptance and Healing*. Novato, CA: New World Library.

Roberts, F. (2001) *The Therapy Sourcebook*. Los Angeles, CA: NTC/Contemporary Publishing Group.

Rosen, E. and D'Elgin, T. (2001) *Think Like a Shrink: 100 Principles for Seeing Deeply into Yourself and Others*. New York, NY: Simon and Schuster.

Ryan, M.J. (2006). *This Year I Will...How to Finally Change a Habit, Keep a Resolution, or Make a Dream Come True*, New York, NY: Broadway Books.

Salovey, P. et al. Emotional state and physical health. *American Psychologist*. 2000;55(1): 110–121.

http://heblab.research.yale.edu//pub_pdf/pub26_Saloveyetal.2000Emotionalstatesandphysicalhealth.pdf

Stone, H. and Stone, S. (1993). *Embracing Your Inner Critic: Turning Self-Criticism into an Asset*. New York, NY: HarperCollins.

Striano, J. (1987). *How to Find a Good Psychotherapist: A Consumer Guide*. Santa Barbara, CA: Professional Press.

ABOUT THE AUTHOR

Author Linda Bieniek urges other vent users to recognise the importance of proactively investing in our health and quality of life. She writes articles, presents at conferences and contributes to projects sponsored by International Ventilator Users Network (IVUN) for this purpose. Having used different types of ventilation for more than 25 years, she understands the various frustrations related to both non-invasive and invasive (with a tracheostomy) ventilation. As a former member of IVUN's Board of Directors, she also has witnessed other vent users besides herself recognise the many benefits of ventilators. She, as many, are grateful that our machines keep us alive, enabling us to experience and contribute to life's goodness.

In this article, she shares her research and insights for strengthening our emotional health and the quality of aspects of our lives. From her personal experience and her professional expertise, she understands the importance of working with a highly-skilled and dedicated therapist who matches our needs and personality when we seek professional assistance – if options are available. When choices are not available, she advocates that we gain knowledge to empower us to make the best use of the time we have to work with a designated counselor or therapist. The information and opinions in this article are solely hers unless referenced.

Linda has more than 20 years of behavioural health training, often with leading experts in the field. During her career at a major corporation, she managed its Employee Assistance Program, counseling individuals with personal and work problems. In that role, she often referred clients to appropriate resources they could pursue independently, and also to therapists and/or treatment programmes, as needed. Later, as the Mental Health Program Manager, she developed human resource strategies and successfully negotiated an expansion of behavioural health benefit coverage for employees and their families who needed treatment.

Linda was a Certified Employee Assistance Professional (CEAP) from 1986–2006; she is still certified as a Neuro-Linguistic Programming (NLP) Practitioner. The NLP training enhanced her skills needed to work effectively as a Life and Career Coach. Her career coaching expertise stems from attending Career Development Programmes of Loyola University in Chicago, Illinois, USA, and other professional development training programmes since the 1980s. Participating in those programmes combined with her gift of recognising 'possibilities' and her human resource experiences have equipped her to assist individuals in identifying and finding suitable careers and jobs in certain sectors of the economy.

As a Life and Career Coach, Linda is especially creative in enlightening individuals to discover and resolve obstacles that interfere with achieving their goals. In her phone-based consulting practice, she also assists persons seeking therapy by searching for therapists who appear to be a 'good match' based on the issues agreed upon with each individual.

The author is indebted to Virginia Brickley and Veronica Cook for their insightful editing and to Nicole Lighthouse, M.F.T., Sarah Perz and Julie Truong for their research and assistance. She also is grateful to Laura Dowdle, Joan Headley, Marcy Kaplan and Brigid Rafferty for their editing suggestions and to Audrey King and Alan Fiala for their feedback.

74

The patient's journey

STEFANO NAVA

In this video (https://youtu.be/EjiwtmdRWQs), we report the experience of a patient, facing more than one severe acute exacerbation of chronic obstructive pulmonary disease, until he was finally successfully treated with non-invasive ventilation.

75

A patient's journey: NIV

JEANETTE ERDMANN AND ANDREA L. KLEIN

KEY MESSAGES

For doctors

- Correct diagnosis is of utmost importance, especially for those with rare disorders.
- Be aware of weakened breathing muscles in congenital muscle disorders.
- Monitoring lung function in congenital myopathy disease patients is life saving.
- Every effort to keep a patient on NIV mobile is worth it.

For patients

- Never give up on getting a diagnosis or the appropriate care.
- Stay informed.
- Use social media to get connected.
- Do not restrain yourself from being mobile; travelling with a vent is always possible.

In an age of the Internet and Facebook, two women, almost the same age, diagnosed with the same very rare congenital muscle disorder, after more than decades long journey of unknown diagnosis, both on non-invasive ventilation (NIV), were living more than 5000 mi apart (Tennessee, United States and Germany). They met online, got connected and wrote this chapter about their lives with NIV. They share their background, diagnosis, experiences and their interactions with healthcare systems and professionals.

MORE THAN 45 YEARS UNTIL DIAGNOSIS

JEANETTE ERDMANN

My parents realised I was different shortly after my birth – I was delayed in starting to crawl, sit and walk. Despite suffering from a hip dislocation that was fixed by a plaster bed, the doctors could not do anything for me other than reassuring my parents that my health condition would stabilise over the years and everything would be fine in the end. However, my parents appeared to be concerned about my health, because they took me to see many doctors. At age 10, we finally learned that I had a benign muscle disease without any specific diagnosis.

My high school years, as well as my university years, were rather uneventful. I finished my diploma in biology in 1991 at the University of Cologne, Germany. Shortly after, I started to work on my PhD thesis at the Institute of Human Genetics in Bonn, Germany. At that time, I realised my scientific interest was to understand the genetic causes of diseases. However, it was more by chance that I ended up in the field of complex diseases and not monogenic disorders such as muscular dystrophies.

While working on my PhD thesis, my health deteriorated, and my lung function in particular started to cause major problems. I had great difficulties breathing at night, leading to severe headaches, fatigue, shortness of sleep in the night and microsleep during my laboratory work. However, it took me several years to finally realise and accept that my respiratory muscles had dramatically deteriorated.

The 'point of no return' was in New Orleans, United States, while I was attending the meeting of the American Society of Human Genetics in the fall of 1993. This week was extremely exhausting, and I was almost unable to attend the talks and stay awake. This extremely shattering week prompted me to make an appointment with a pulmonologist immediately after my homecoming. The diagnosis was devastating: I was told my blood had become hypoxic.

As a 28 year-old, I feared I was going to slowly suffocate. A turnaround was made in March 1994 by a courageous and very empathic physician (Bernd Schönhofer) who put me on NIV at night for the rest of my life.

I remember well that at first I was shocked after realising I had to live/sleep with a ventilator for the rest of my life. However, my condition, especially my headaches, improved almost immediately after the first night with only a few hours on NIV. I am fairly sure this is why I easily adapted to using a ventilator every night. In hindsight, I am extremely thankful for this decision, because this treatment allowed my respiratory muscles to rest so that I could return to my daily activities, and the beneficial effect has continued to this day.

Over the following years, I finished my PhD thesis and worked as a postdoctoral fellow in Berlin and Regensburg, Germany. During this time, NIV was part of my life with almost no problems, despite the fact that the nasal masks sometimes leaked and caused skin irritations. Living in Berlin and Regensburg, I lost contact with the clinic in Schmallenberg, because it was hundreds of kilometres away. However, the initial NIV settings helped me so much that I had no specific reason to have my settings checked for nearly 10 years. I now know this might not have been very smart, but I was so busy following my career during the late 1990s/early 2000s that I did not think about my NIV settings.

In 2004, I moved to Lübeck, working as an assistant professor, associate professor and full professor in cardiovascular genetics and, since 2013, as the director of a newly founded institute for cardiovascular genetics at the university with 25 staff members. I was fortunate to uncover genetic variants and mutations that increase the risk of myocardial infarction and other disorders. However, it had bothered me for a while that my own diagnosis remained elusive. Despite being on NIV, I experienced a slow progression of my muscular phenotype. Although my daily work was almost unaffected by my disorder, I started to think that it might be beneficial to finally have a diagnosis. This was particularly because of the tremendous advances that have been made over the last couple of years regarding treatment options for muscular dystrophies. I was scared that I might miss very important information by not knowing my diagnosis.

I again consulted an expert in congenital muscular disorders and underwent a complete check up with muscle biopsy, physical examination and blood work. In addition, we went through all the symptoms my mother and I could remember. However, the clinicians could not make any sense out of it, and I went home still undiagnosed. I remember very well lying in bed a few days after my return. I felt frustrated and sleepless. I do not know why exactly, but all of a sudden, I started to search on the Internet for some of my symptoms. I entered 'hip dislocation' and 'keloid' together with 'muscular dystrophy' in Google. Amazingly, all the hits on the front page referred to Bethlem myopathy or Ullrich muscular dystrophy, which is characterised by these and other coincidental symptoms. Another very common symptom of Bethlem/Ullrich is that the respiratory muscles are weakened, requiring people to use a ventilator to help them breathe, particularly during sleep. While reading this, I suddenly realised that my diagnosis was Bethlem/Ullrich or an intermediate form of it.

The next day, after my revealing Internet session, I decided to have my exome, the protein-coding part of my DNA, sequenced. I must admit that I could do this relatively easily because I had been working in the field of molecular genetics for more than 20 years. Therefore, my situation was special in this regard. I precisely remember the minute I got the confirmation by phone. It was on a Saturday afternoon while shopping in Lübeck. A colleague of mine who actually analysed my DNA called my mobile phone and told me that the sequencing was done and the results were ready. I just asked him to check if I am a carrier of a mutation in one of the Col6 genes, which have been repeatedly reported to cause Bethlem/Ullrich. It took him only seconds to check, and his answer was clear: yes. So, 2 months after my Internet session, I learned that I have a mutation located in the highly conserved codon 283 of the Collagen 6A2 gene that had been previously described to be mutated in patients with Bethlem/Ullrich muscular dystrophy. A very long journey, almost 45 years, was over.[1]

I have been often asked how the experts I have been seeing over the years could not diagnose Bethlem/Ullrich, one of the five most common myopathies; I do not have an answer. I was told that Bethlem/Ullrich is very rare, but is probably often underdiagnosed in adults. Moreover, the symptoms are heterogeneous and not well characterised in adults. I have met only two clinical neurologists in Germany who are seeing Bethlem/Ullrich patients. In Schleswig-Holstein (Germany), where I live, there is no neurologist with experience caring for patients with Ullrich/Bethlem myopathy. However, there must be something wrong with our healthcare system if a patient, just by using a search engine, can shed light on a disease and its cause, while doctors cannot. In this respect, I can only recommend and support Eric Topol and his famous book *The Patient Will See You Now*.[2]

Having a diagnosis, I immediately started to contact specialists in the United Kingdom and United States in order to learn more about my disorder. From the literature, I learned about the very low prevalence of my disease (less than 10 per million people), the prognosis, treatment options and specific preventive measures to avoid complications. While this knowledge was very helpful overall, it was sobering at the same time to understand my own disease and its implications. For almost my whole life, I managed to live with an unclear diagnosis. Somehow this made my life easier; because there was nothing to compare myself with, and the prognosis was absolutely open. However, after all, it is better to know rather than to guess about what to expect from my weakened muscles.

CHALLENGES ACCESSING NIV

ANDREA L. KLEIN

My journey with NIV had unexpected 'bumps in the road'. In the summer of 2007, my sister Cheryl developed a head cold that lasted 2 months. After it ended, she developed hand tremors. Her primary care physician advised it could be neurologic and was able to get her an appointment at a nearby Muscular Dystrophy Association (MDA) Clinic moved up by 2 weeks.

The tremors became more frequent, and during a phone call in November, Cheryl spoke nonsensical words. She admitted, 'I heard myself, but I don't know what I meant'.

I worried she might be developing a brain tumour that was affecting her speech. Later in November, she would fall asleep for brief periods during the day. During Thanksgiving dinner, she could barely stay awake. Next, she developed ankle swelling. By the end of November, Cheryl was blacking out and regaining consciousness a couple of times an hour. On December 1, it occurred every 15 min, and she felt a need for air. That night, she went to the emergency room (ER) where they administered supplemental oxygen for her very low oxygen saturation. After a few hours, she improved, and the staff mentioned discharge.

Instead, she was admitted to the hospital and had what seemed like a psychotic outburst. A nurse asked to do an arterial blood gas, and Cheryl had an uncharacteristic protest and lost consciousness. The staff maintained her breathing with an 'ambu bag' and intubated her with a paediatric tube after failed attempts with an adult one. On a ventilator in intensive care, she worsened. Her failure to achieve normal oxygen saturation caused the staff to recommend a tracheotomy. They implied she would improve, but more problems arose: pneumonia, blood clots in the lung and sepsis. She suffered lung collapse, multiple organ system failure and death at age 38, on my 33rd birthday.

Cheryl's death terrified me; naturally, I thought I would be next to die. On a quest to better understand what happened to my sister, I went to Amazon.com and found and ordered *Management of Patients with Neuromuscular Disease* and *Noninvasive Mechanical Ventilation* by Dr John R. Bach.[3,4] These books were enlightening. I became angry and saddened that ER staff failed to check her carbon dioxide (CO_2) level before administering supplemental oxygen (O_2). I understood that it was supplemental O_2 that led to her crash, because it disturbed the delicate balance of O_2 and CO_2 in her blood when she had symptoms of CO_2 retention.

Before her death, I had been seeing a pulmonary and critical care specialist who diagnosed me with severe asthma and mild diaphragmatic weakness. After Cheryl's death, he increased the frequency of my pulmonary function tests (PFTs) and ordered yearly arterial blood gas sampling and sleep studies.

In spring 2013, I began having morning headaches and worsening fatigue. A sleep study that fall confirmed my oxygen saturation was dropping into the low 70s. I was asked to use 2 L of O_2 during sleep and told to repeat the sleep study to check for improvement.

I was shocked and upset, since I had read supplemental O_2 was the wrong way to treat this. I told the nurse that my decision to not use supplemental oxygen was 'non-negotiable'. Days later, I dropped off articles about sleep disordered breathing in neuromuscular disease. An article in the MDA USA magazine *Quest* and peer-reviewed articles supported my opposition to supplemental O_2.

My pulmonologist agreed to delay prescribing supplemental O_2 and prescribed continuous positive airway pressure (CPAP). Some of the articles I had shared mentioned why CPAP was not advised, so I refused to try it. Months passed with no response from my doctor, and I worsened. I purchased a recording pulse oximeter to determine if my oxygen saturation was consistently dropping during sleep. Each morning, data downloads confirmed that it was.

During a check-up, my pulmonologist said the articles I shared did not apply to me, and his diagnosis from the sleep study was good news. He said it meant that I did not have breathing issues related to muscular dystrophy (MD) but that I had severe obstructive sleep apnoea. He explained that if I did not treat it, I could die in months or a year. I left the appointment confused and scared. Days later, I requested a second opinion referral to a pulmonologist that specialises in breathing issues in neuromuscular disease. Weeks later, the new pulmonologist who was 3 hours away prescribed bi-level positive airway pressure (BiPAP) spontaneous/timed (S/T) mode. She felt that I should have started NIV 6–7 years prior, based on my PFT results. This left me feeling I had been deprived of appropriate care.

The morning after my first night on NIV, I felt better than I had in years. I continued to see improvement in energy level, alertness and the ability to concentrate at my job as a business analyst in healthcare information technology.

Feeling better furthered my drive to determine if my sister and I truly had limb–girdle MD, our diagnosis from a 1980 muscle biopsy. After a free test for LGMD2i from a non-profit showed a negative result, I applied to participate in a free diagnostic study at the National Institutes of Health in Bethesda, Maryland, United States. I received my COL6A2 genetic diagnosis and clinical diagnosis of 'intermediate on the Bethlem/Ullrich spectrum' shortly after my 40th birthday.

Fourteen months later, I could sleep 10–12 hours a night and feel as if I had slept half that amount. My inspiratory and expiratory positive airway pressure settings were increased twice, but their effectiveness was limited. To alleviate fatigue, I began using NIV during an extended lunch break.

Later I started using average volume assured pressure support auto expiratory positive airway pressure on a multimode ventilator. It took many 'tweaks' to reduce the pulsating breaths delivered to reach my targeted volume. I struggled to get adequate sleep, but eventually a 'sweet spot' setting was implemented, and I felt well rested.

I also began mouthpiece ventilation (MPV). It was clear that the pulmonologist and respiratory therapist were still learning MPV, so I posted on patient support groups on Facebook to learn what settings others with my disease were using. When those were enabled, it was life changing. If I had not begun to use MPV, I could not have continued full-time employment.

My experiences have proven that NIV has more benefits than negatives, but I often awaken with a stomach full of swallowed air. I have increased nasal sensitivities with alternating congestion and runniness. Saline and allergy nasal sprays have helped. Weekly cleaning of tubing, masks and a water chamber and replacing supplies are added responsibilities.

GET CONNECTED: SOCIAL MEDIA, INTERNET AND BREATHE WITH MD

JEANETTE ERDMANN AND ANDREA L. KLEIN

Each day, Andrea felt a growing desire to help others understand NIV and prevent others from experiencing the loss her family endured. In memory of her sister, in 2014, she created *Breathe with MD*, an organisation to educate other MD patients about pulmonary function decline and its appropriate care and treatment.

On the public Facebook page, https://www.facebook.com/BreatheWithMD/, she shares articles and information on symptoms, mechanically assisted cough, NIV and related topics. The content encourages patients to be proactive and self-advocate. Andrea later created a website, http://www.breathewithmd.org/, and a close support group on Facebook that allows members to share experiences, ask questions and feel supported by others with similar challenges. The group is composed of members from all over the world with different forms of MD. Most use NIV; a few use invasive ventilation; but some are using only mechanically assisted cough or no interventions. It was through this Facebook group that Jeanette and Andrea met.

Jeanette posted in the group about her increasing need for NIV throughout the day. Several encouraged her to talk to her physician about increasing BiPAP settings and starting MPV. During her next check-up at the sleep lab, her physician made changes to her night settings and prescribed daytime MPV. Another member had symptoms of underventilation, and she was encouraged to get an evaluation before the symptoms became critical. Another member's wife battled repeated pneumonias. From others in the group, one learned about CoughAssist and advocated for his wife to get this device to prevent future hospitalisations. Others in the group have helped to troubleshoot settings and determine what settings the user might ask their physician about as their weakness progresses. Members have posted 'mask selfies', describing what they like and do not like about masks. This interactive communication between people around the world struggling with the same problems is extremely helpful. Being able to talk to each other via Skype and privately share is tremendously supportive. Although, sometimes it is also depressing to hear that many have been prescribed O_2 instead of ventilation, despite the fact that O_2 is the worst thing one can use, if they are already retaining CO_2.

Overall, it is amazing how informed self-educated patients can be and that they freely share information with each other.

STAY MOBILE

JEANETTE ERDMANN AND ANDREA L. KLEIN

After getting used to NIV, whether used during sleep or 24/7, the most important aspect is to stay mobile. Andrea and I are good examples of individuals on NIV with a positive work/life balance, and we travel, meeting friends and family, even hundreds of miles away from home. From the very beginning, I took my vent with me for traveling, to ensure that it did not get lost during a flight; I always declare it as hand baggage. After a while, you get used to the fact that it takes longer at the security counter to get your luggage checked, but I have never experienced any problems. I have visited many national and international conferences and meetings over the last 20 years, and my vent was always my companion. I must admit that I do not like traveling a lot, so I do not often travel for vacation; all the traveling for work is tiring enough. However, Andrea, being on NIV and MPV, travels for vacation. She road trips with her husband in their mobility van, and this requires advanced planning to ensure that accommodations and travel destinations are accessible. All the extra effort is worth the result: seeing new places and visiting family and friends.

REFERENCES

1. Erdmann J, Schunkert H. Forty-five years to diagnosis. *Neuromuscul Disord.* 2013;23:503–5.
2. Topol E. *The Patient Will See You Now: The Future of Medicine Is in Your Hands.* New York: Basic Books; 2015.
3. Bach JR. *Management of Patients with Neuromuscular Disease.* Philadelphia, PA: Hanley & Belfus; 2003.
4. Bach JR. *Noninvasive Mechanical Ventilation.* Philadelphia, PA: Hanley & Belfus; 2002.

ABOUT THE AUTHORS

Jeanette Erdmann, PhD, was born in 1965 and self-diagnosed with Bethlem/Ullrich myopathy at age 45. Her NIV started at age 30. She is still ambulatory, using a walker, with increasing problems to walk long distance. Since 2004, she lives in Lübeck, Germany, close to the Baltic Sea. Here she is working full time as the director of the Institute for Cardiogenetics at the University.

Andrea L. Klein, born in 1974, was diagnosed with Bethlem/Ullrich myopathy at the age of 40. She started NIV at the age of 39 and MPV at the age of 40. Andrea is using a power chair since 2014, but she is still able to walk short distances indoors. She lives in Cleveland, Tennessee, and works full time as a business analyst in healthcare information technology on a team developing , maintaining and supporting software applications for physical and occupational therapists and speech language pathologists. She served as Ms. Wheelchair Tennessee 2017 and competed in the National Ms. Wheelchair America 2018 disability advocacy pageant.

Pictures

Jeanette at the age of 33, shortly after she was put on NIV, just after her PhD defence at the University of Cologne, Germany.

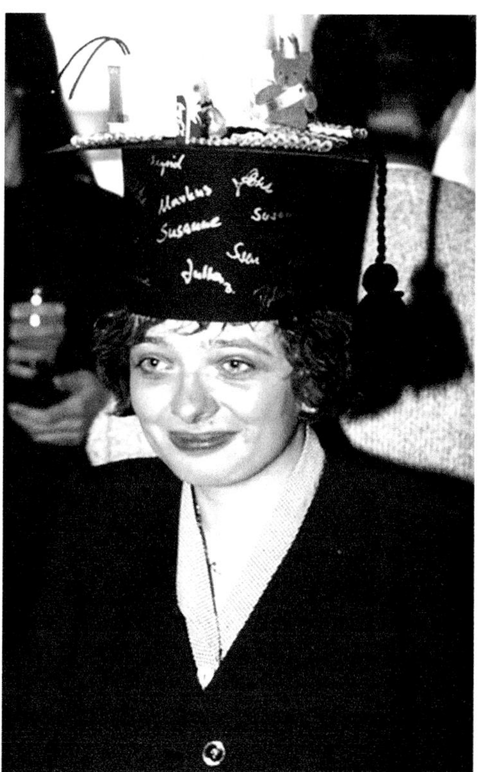

Jeanette, at the age of 45, receiving her appointment as professor at the University of Lübeck. Professor Heribert Schunkert (left) and Professor Peter Dominiak (right), former president of the University of Lübeck.

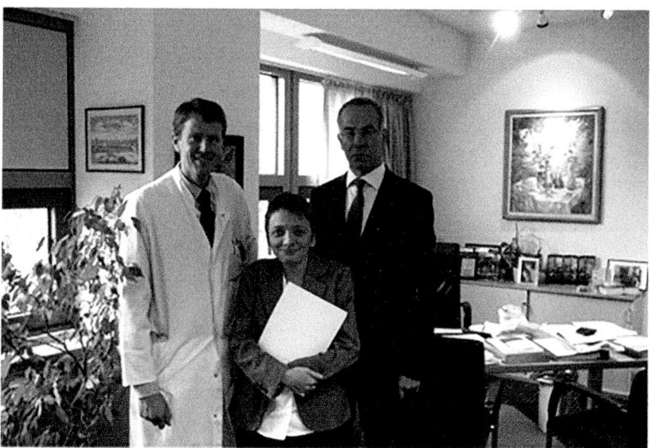

Jeanette, 2015, joining a panel discussion about 'genetics and public understanding' at the St Petri Church in Lübeck.

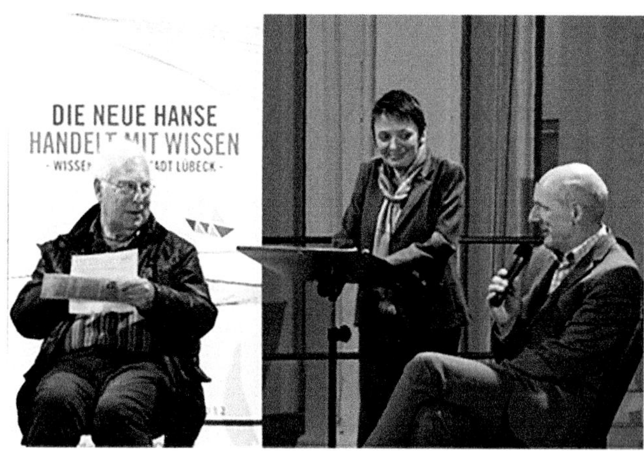

Andrea holding her award from the Speak Foundation 2015 Conference for Individuals with Neuromuscular Disease in Atlanta, Georgia, United States, where she was given an award of achievement for creating Breathe with MD and getting Dr. John R. Bach to come speak at the conference.

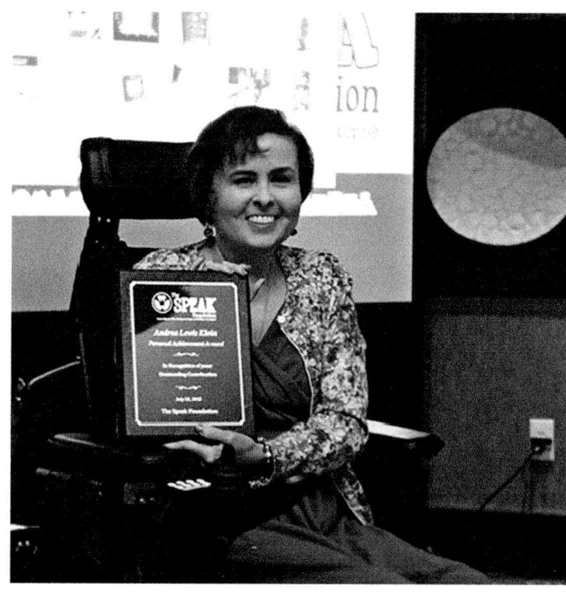

Andrea during a 2014 trip to the Epcot Center at Walt Disney World in Orlando, Florida, United States.

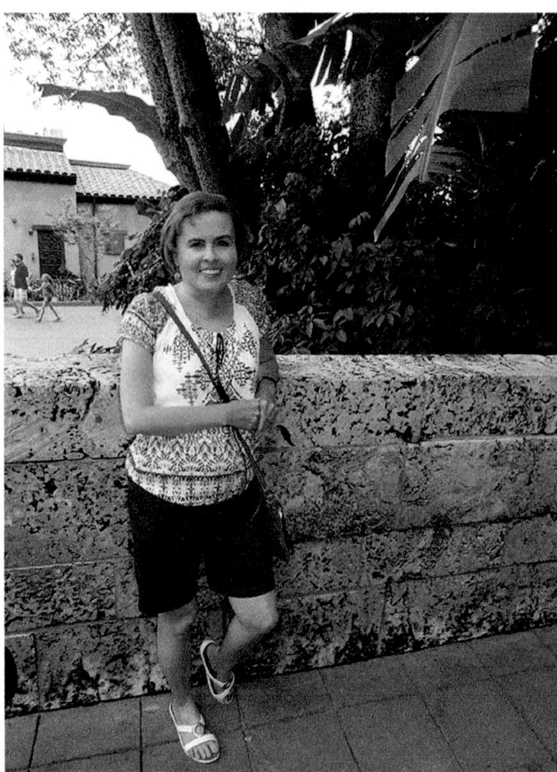

Andrea, at the age of 42 in her wheelchair with Trilogy Ventilator visible during a visit to see her husband's family in Lake Mills, Wisconsin, United States.

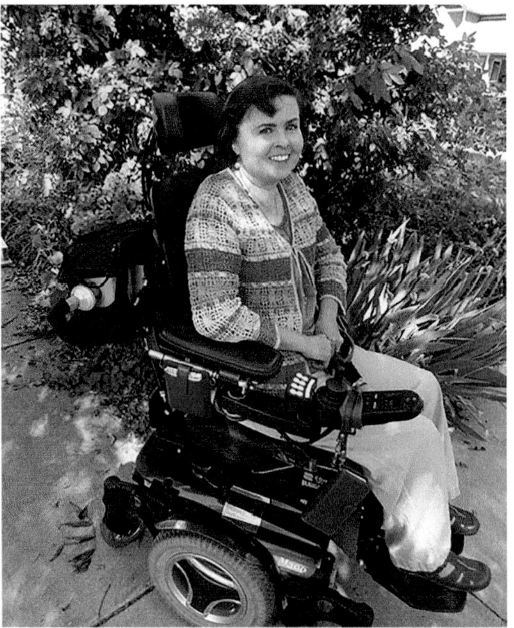

Andrea at the National Ms. Wheelchair America competition in August, 2017, in Erie, Pennsylvania, United States, delivering her platform speech as she represented her state of Tennessee.

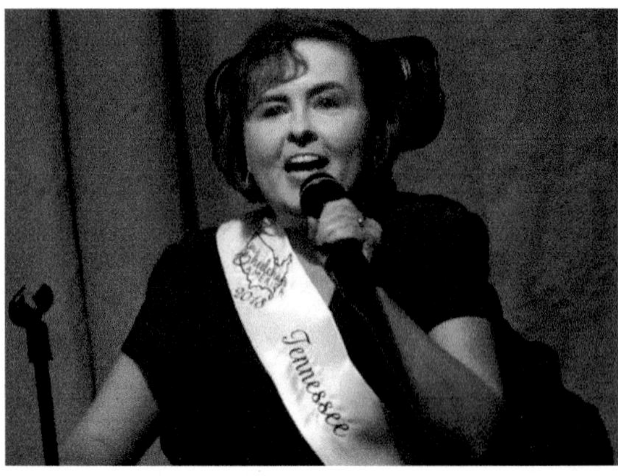

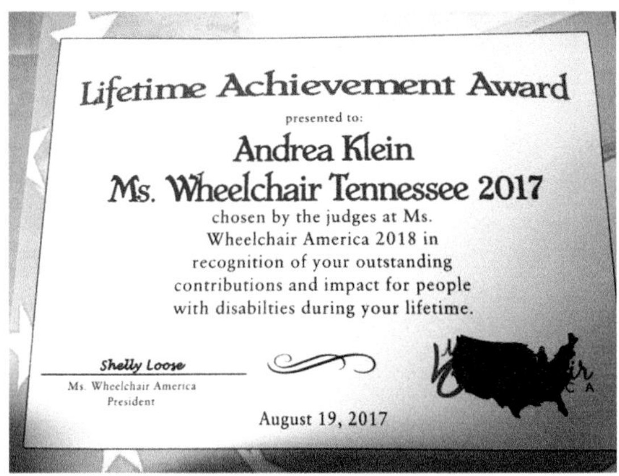

Lifetime Achievement Award

presented to:

Andrea Klein

Ms. Wheelchair Tennessee 2017

chosen by the judges at Ms. Wheelchair America 2018 in recognition of your outstanding contributions and impact for people with disabilties during your lifetime.

Shelly Loose

Ms. Wheelchair America President

August 19, 2017

76

A carer's journey

GAIL BEACOCK AND PATRICK BEACOCK

MY JOURNEY

GAIL BEACOCK

Gail is unable to speak – she communicates using a letter chart, spelling out words by blinking when the letter she wants is indicated.

I was an extrovert who had a lot to say and did everything at 100 miles per hour. The symptoms of motor neurone disease (MND) (amyotrophic lateral sclerosis [ALS]) came on rapidly, and soon, I was like a prisoner trapped in a prison, the prison being my own body.

Many men would have left, but not my Patrick. He stuck to our marriage vows, but he has only had the 'in sickness' part and is still waiting for the 'in health' part.

Six months after our wedding in 1995, I had a back operation to remove a slipped disc. After recovering, I was desperate to start a family, but MND put a stop to my dreams. I had heard that there was a 2–3-year life expectancy after MND diagnosis, and I feared I would only have 2 years to live. I was 35 years old.

In 2008, after my tracheotomy, a nurse said I would be lucky if I got to go into our back garden. I saw this as a gauntlet she had thrown down. My stubborn side saw this as a challenge. I was determined to prove that nurse wrong. I decided I would not be like most people and lay in bed and wait to die.

My husband, Patrick, describes our 'journey' in more detail. I would like to stress the following:

- Having the ventilator opened up my life. It enabled me to go anywhere.
- Many years ago, our flight was diverted, making an emergency landing, as I encountered respiratory problems with no access to a ventilator.
- My respiratory consultant Dr Mark Elliott gave me a new lease of life, and without Patrick, I would have no quality of life.

A CARER'S JOURNEY

PATRICK BEACOCK

It was in 1997 that Gail, then aged 34, first began experiencing walking/coordination difficulties, which led to the devastating diagnosis of MND (ALS) in 1998. We had been married for 3 years.

Around May 2002, Gail started experiencing occasional bouts of 'phlegm on her chest', as she described it, which would lead to bouts of coughing, which would invariably end up with her coughing and often end up with a spate of vomiting too. The subject would get raised on her periodic outpatient visits to the consultant neurologist, and I think the 'phenomenon' was put down to impaired respiratory muscles leading to an inability to clear her chest by coughing along with an element of inactivity (Gail had been wheelchair bound since 1999). Gail was prescribed carbocisteine to help manage the symptoms, but it was not very helpful. She was also provided with a suction machine, which would occasionally be used, but never taken out of the house with us.

At no time in this era did Gail ever feel her breathing was impaired, even when the nasty 'phlegm' problem was lurking. By 2006, occasional breathing difficulties seemed to surface, but if anything, the volume of phlegm seemed to be reduced, and the added-on vomiting had vanished.

At the same time, Gail was referred to Dr Mark Elliott, and I recall that initial consultations gave no concern by either party. Gail was provided with an ambu-bag, which we would occasionally use just to give a quick boost to her lungs and nothing more. A cough-assist machine was tried, but Gail found the experience extremely unpleasant, and this avenue was duly left behind. Overnight oximetry tests around this time yielded nothing worrying.

It was Christmas Day 2006 that Gail had a particularly unpleasant day – by this time, eating required more effort and would make her hot and slightly exhausted, and combined with a heated house full of family members and the notorious phlegm, which tried to rear its ugly head, it was a challenging Christmas Day for us both. A couple of weeks into the new year (2007), all seemed relatively calm, and the discomforts of the festive period seemed a distant memory.

So far the journey (for carer and patient) had been tricky, but this was soon to be followed by much rockier terrain, (to be followed later in this chapter by the present road, which we perceive, in comparison, to be relatively smooth. It may not be all that smooth, but at least, it is a consistent path now, with no totally unexpected twists and turns or pot-holes or abysses.)

It was in April 2007, after a very enjoyable holiday in Tenerife in March (with no dreaded phlegm attacks and nothing more dramatic than the very occasional use of the ambu-bag for a couple of big breaths here and there) that Gail felt less well than she had been. It was of no great concern, as there had always been up-and-down periods, on top of the underlying MND/ALS of the last 10 years. In the preceding months, we had perhaps not noticed that Gail was eating less and losing weight – eating/swallowing had gradually become more difficult and tiring, and the notorious phlegm episodes often led to an entire meal being missed.

In early May 2007, Gail was having her weekly visit by her physiotherapist Ann, who used to do passive exercises of her limbs, when Gail started to get one of her 'infamous' 'phlegm attacks'. As frequently happened, Ann had arrived considerably later than her scheduled appointment time, and what a good job she was late on this day. (At the time, Gail had care at certain times of the day, but there were spells when she was alone when I was at work. This was deemed acceptable to everyone including us for Gail's condition at the time). Gail's breathing rapidly became impaired. Ann quickly called the emergency services, and by the time they arrived a few minutes later, Gail had stopped breathing, and Ann, a slightly built lady nearing (or past) retirement age, immediately lifted her from her wheelchair, laid her on the floor and gave her life-saving mouth-to-mouth resuscitation. Simultaneously, Ann was ringing me to tell me what was happening, and I duly left work to head for the hospital that Gail was en route to by ambulance.

When I arrived at the hospital, Gail had been treated in the accident and emergency (A&E) department, was attached to a ventilator and mask and was in good spirits and relatively calm. She thought she had just fainted. She was duly transferred to the high dependency section of the respiratory ward, where it was confirmed that she had suffered a respiratory arrest. Gail felt fine and was reluctant to continue wearing the mask, but complied with the staff's instructions to do so. Due to the fact that she felt comparatively OK despite the abnormal readings, one has to wonder whether they had been less than satisfactory throughout the previous few weeks when she had felt less well than previously.

The following morning, Dr Elliott confirmed the severity of the episode, stating that she had been 'within an inch of being intubated'. Clearly, after years of struggles and challenges, we were in new uncharted territory now, and our thoughts turned to how things would pan out in the immediate future. Two or three days into the hospital admission, Gail had made remarkable progress and discharge from hospital appeared to be only days away. The ventilator and mask was not needed throughout the day, and ward staff were happy to provide minimal supervision. Dr Elliott's recommendation was that it be used overnight every night.

After 5 days in the hospital, Gail was being visited by her MND specialist nurse, when she experienced one of her legendary phlegm attacks. Despite years of these episodes, which had been mentioned on numerous occasions, nobody in the medical profession had actually witnessed one, until now. The cough-assist machine (which Gail had previously found unpleasant) was tried, to alleviate the symptoms, but to no avail, and Gail spent the afternoon on NIV. A couple of hours later, the situation had passed, and we continued thinking about the imminent discharge. The ward sister was keen that Gail should have 24-hour care at home on discharge, and we recognised that Gail could not have long spells alone at home as she had done previously. The waters were a bit muddied here as Gail had been in the process of working out a scheme with social services where she would have the services of a personal assistant for several hours a week for non-clinical duties (household duties etc), which Gail was reluctant to abort. Eventually, Gail relented on this idea and recognised that much more clinically led care at home was needed. The wheels in social services were turning at a moderate pace, which appeared to be in danger of delaying Gail's 'return to civvy street', but Gail was still determined to return to normal as soon as possible. Whilst in hospital, 2 days after the previous phlegm attack on the ward, Gail endured another one of these worrying episodes, just 24 hours before the mooted discharge date. Again the use of the NIV for a 'few hours' seemed to calm the problem. Social services officials visited Gail and I in the hospital on the morning of the planned discharge. What they had in mind for Gail was miles apart from what we felt was needed, and even further away from the ward's desires for Gail's care package at home. Social services indicated they could provide up to six pop-in visits per day at home – this was a long way short of our perception that Gail should have minimal or preferably no time alone. Not wishing to delay discharge from hospital for an indeterminate period, Gail arranged for her mother to spend the week at home with her, whilst social services worked on something more substantial than '6 pop-in visits per day', and 8 days after the initial emergency admission, Gail was home.

The next phase of the journey was about to begin. Gail was provided with a mains-powered portable ventilator. After we initially perceived that Gail would not leave the house due to the possible need to use the ventilator at any time, predominantly to manage any oncoming phlegm attack, we very soon took to venturing out and making short trips from the home. With previously booked summer holidays a few weeks away, I think we were establishing whether these were still viable propositions.

Week 1 at home was a mixed experience. Any hints of phlegm on the chest would cause Gail to panic that it might lead to another respiratory arrest, so she would immediately apply the mask/ventilator until the matter passed. This happened on two occasions in that first week at home, the second occasion going on for several hours, in fact for so long that her mum insisted that we return to the hospital. However we declined, and eventually that evening, everything was OK again. By the following week, social services had put (emergency) measures in place, and Gail was attended to by agency carers for most of the day, who were trained in applying the mask if it was needed. Gail was making progress in remarkable leaps and bounds, and by the end of the month of May 2007, we were able to take our previously booked long-weekend break in Jersey, accompanied (unlikely previously) by a ventilator and suction machine. Gail's insistence on having a bacon sandwich at the airport before the short flight was perhaps not so sensible – it caused rumblings of phlegm on her chest that she had to endure throughout the flight and the short car journey from the airport in Jersey to the hotel in St Helier, before a spell using the ventilator in the hotel room to restore matters. Thereafter, the three-night holiday and journey home passed without incident.

A month later, we ventured off on another previously booked holiday, a week in Bulgaria, in the middle of a heatwave, where temperatures soared as high as 47°C! Again, there was very little in the way of respiratory/phlegm-related concerns, even after the much longer flight, and Gail seemed to be doing well, with ostensibly the only change to the status quo of previous years being the overnight use of the ventilator, and possibly less of the dreaded phlegm attacks. A couple of days into the holiday, the evening meal gave rise to a chesty episode, with the rest of the evening being spent in the room on NIV. This was not to be repeated in the rest of the week, and I do not think either of us gave much thought to what to do in the event of such an occurrence at a less convenient time, such as when out sightseeing, or heaven forbid, at the airport or midflight. So despite the heat, the holiday was enjoyable, although I (Patrick) picked up a nasty cold on the last couple of days.

After we returned home, Gail picked up my streaming cold, which meant increased use of the mask, and at the same time, her skin, particularly on her nose, was becoming marked from the use of the tightly fitting mask. Over the next few weeks, this caused a very painful break in the skin on the bridge of her nose, which became badly infected and was treated (professionally in the community) with a series of unsightly padded dressings on her nose. This seemed to be the limit of knowledge in this field in the community, and we bizarrely never thought to seek specialist advice from the respiratory people at the hospital. Gail needed the mask to assist her breathing, but the mask pressed painfully on the already painful skin break on her nose.

In August 2007, we took a bank holiday weekend break in Majorca, something we had talked about doing for the previous 12 months or so. In the circumstances, this turned out not to be the best decision we had ever made. Aside from the exorbitant peak season flight and hotel costs, Gail's skin on her nose was very sore and painful, and she had just started a course of antibiotics (for a possible chest infection), which were making her feel a little unwell. The heat in Majorca was humid and stifling, and Gail was not comfortable in it and preferred to spend long spells in the cooler room on NIV. By the end of the last full day of the break, Gail had not managed to fulfil her wish to take a dip in the sea in a special wheelchair buggy that this resort (and several others) provided on the beach. Not wishing to return to the United Kingdom without doing this, and with a relatively late flight home, we duly did this in the afternoon (without incident), before departing for the airport in the early evening. The heat was still humid and uncomfortable, but Palma airport was cool. Unfortunately, the flight was delayed by 2 or 3 hours. Gail declined my suggestion to find somewhere to use her (mains-powered) ventilator, as she felt fine. Just before we were due to board the plane, after a quick visit to the airport toilets, Gail started to experience some worrying 'phlegm on the chest'. With boarding imminent, there was nothing to do except hope that things could be kept at bay until we landed in the United Kingdom. After take-off, the situation became more uncomfortable. Cabin crew provided some smelling salts, which were of minimal benefit. Gail was struggling to breathe and was offered oxygen, but this had no effect, despite the cabin steward saying Gail was OK. As the cabin steward assured me again that Gail was OK, I looked across at her and sensed that she was not breathing. Her eyes appeared glazed over. What happened next is a bit of a blur, but I think I dragged Gail from her seat and laid her down in the area at the front of the cabin and gave her mouth-to-mouth resuscitation. Her ambu-bag was duly located in the hand luggage, and the cabin crew put out an announcement for any medical professionals amongst the passengers; a midwife and a student nurse came forward. One of them used the ambu-bag and claimed to be able to feel a faint pulse. The ventilator was duly located, but need a US-style adaptor to plug into the power supply of the aircraft. Cabin crew asked me if we needed to make an emergency landing, and I said 'yes'. As we descended, a passenger came forward with a US-style mains adaptor, and the ventilator was brought into use. Gail immediately responded, and by the time we landed, she was breathing quite normally on the ventilator. The plane had landed in France, and we were taken to the local hospital, arriving in the early hours of the morning. I never worked out what department of the hospital this was, but it appeared to be a small high-dependency unit with three or four beds in separate rooms. I was also unsure what the roles of the various medical staff were, as the colours of their uniforms were different to the colours used in England; I did not know if I was being spoken to by a doctor, nurse or healthcare assistant! Gail was monitored/observed etc., over 24+ hours, whilst various different members of staff told me at various times that it was/was not possible, that she could fly home unaided/fly home with in-flight medical assistance, etc. Their English was excellent, but something was getting lost in translation, with the word *not* being used or omitted at random! On Wednesday morning, we were told we could fly home, and fortunately, that evening, there was a flight to Manchester. Booking a flight at 8 hours notice was not inexpensive. We duly left the hospital, with the staff waving us off with their best wishes as we boarded a taxi for the airport. I was somewhat relieved not to be presented with a bill at the time by the hospital (but that would follow in the post some weeks later!) The heat the previous day in France had been unbearable, but fortunately, it was now cool and breezy. After the trauma 2 days earlier, this flight was going to be a very nervous experience. (I had purchased a US-style mains adaptor earlier that day, in case midair ventilator use was required). The 2-hour flight passed without incident. One could sense the sheer relief in Gail when the plane commenced its descent into Manchester. Arriving at the airport, we were met by Gail's parents, who waited with her while I went to find our car, and we then went to their home. We spent some time talking to them and trying to come to terms with our ordeal, before getting home in the early hours of Thursday morning. I went to work on Thursday afternoon, where an uncompassionate boss presented me with a holiday form for the extra 2 and a half days I had taken off work!

Taking stock in the aftermath of this significant event, it appeared obvious to most that our travelling days were pretty much over. As we had always immensely enjoyed our holidays, somewhat selfishly, I was devastated if we would not be able to continue these. I also made the specialist team aware of our predicament (infected skin break on nose from mask use and major risks to Gail's health of not having rapid access to NIV). Our visit to the 'sleep service' was productive on both counts – Gail was supplied with a new type of mask (called nasal pillows), which avoided the damaged bridge of the nose, and a ventilator with an external battery source as well as mains supply. The bridge of Gail's nose healed up very quickly, leaving only minimal scarring. And with the new ventilator with the scope to use away from mains electricity, I set about exploring the possibility of continuing our beloved pursuit of holidays in the sun, with an aim of taking our usual November break in Tenerife, 3 months down the line, although neither Gail nor Dr Elliott shared my enthusiasm or optimism at the time.

Gail had no setbacks in the ensuing period, and the Canarian holiday duly went ahead (with the battery-powered Nippy in the aeroplane cabin with us, although it was not needed on either leg of the flight). There was the odd anxious moment, however, during the holiday – one day, we set off from the hotel, just as we had done in years gone by. We had not given a thought to taking the Nippy with us, and a mile or so away from the hotel, that awful feeling of phlegm on Gail's chest reared its ugly head, and I was faced with a mad uphill dash, with Gail in her wheelchair, back to the hotel, to connect the mask and Nippy. Thereafter, we wisely did not venture too far from the hotel, and one or two afternoons or evenings had to be curtailed early for mask/Nippy use in the room.

As the year turned 2008, we continued to manage the respiratory matters fairly adequately, and our main focus was now on trying to maintain/increase Gail's weight, as the previously mentioned eating difficulties had led to a fairly sizeable weight loss, and we were reluctant to not postpone the advent of enteral feeding. With the benefit of hindsight, we ought to have been more receptive to the idea. In the early months of 2008, Gail felt continually unwell, but a succession of visits from the general practitioner surgery and a variety of different medications did not really pinpoint the problem. By the springtime, Gail was feeling much better, until one day in May 2008, she felt mildly unwell and thought that she could sleep the ailments off – something she had done before on a number of occasions. When I arrived home, Gail's carer had just checked on her minutes earlier and felt she was fine. When I went to see Gail, she appeared to be semiconscious.

Without thinking, I immediately moved her from her lying position in bed and sat her in her wheelchair. I gave her mouth-to-mouth resuscitation, which seemed to instantly revive her. I and the carer felt that Gail needed to be seen by a doctor. Gail thought an ambulance was needed. I decided to let a doctor take a look first. The on-call doctor came fairly quickly, but could not identify what the problem was, if any, and recommended she be checked over in the hospital and arranged for an ambulance to take us. On arrival at the A&E department, Gail was immediately seen and, despite being attached to the Nippy, stopped breathing whilst being examined by the A&E consultant. Gail has no memory of this episode, and I was ushered out of the way so that the medical professionals could do their work. A few minutes later, I was informed that Gail had stopped breathing again and that now her heart had stopped. I pleaded with them to do all they could for Gail. The A&E consultant told me that Gail had a major infection (pneumonia) and that there was a risk that my 45-year old wife may not survive. It was suggested that I contact relatives. Gail was transferred to intensive care and placed on life support for several days. I doubt I can accurately quote all the details now, but I do recall hearing the intensive care unit consultant express his concern after a couple of days that Gail was not improving. Four days later Gail regained consciousness.

Progress from here was very slow, with numerous setbacks along the way, including emergency surgery on a near-fatal stomach perforation. It would not be distorting the facts too much to say that the surgeon himself was pushing the bed rather quickly along the hospital corridors to the operating theatre one Sunday morning to operate on Gail as soon as possible.

One month on from the initial hospitalisation, Gail was still not managing to breathe unaided; indeed for much of the time, she appeared to be fighting for every breath provided by the ventilator/mask. The overwhelming expert advice from all quarters at this stage was that Gail needed a tracheotomy if she was to make progress. (This had previously been discussed with Dr Elliott shortly after Gail regained consciousness near the start of the hospitalisation and faced with the hypothetical stark choice of trache/live or no trache/die, we both instantly proffered the former to Dr Elliott.) So with little further consideration, Gail had the tracheostomy operation in early June 2008, and the long, long hospital recovery process continued. The main advantage of the trachy, we found out very quickly, is that secretions (the 'dreaded phlegm' as we had called it for years) could be cleared from the chest very easily through the trachy tube via a thin catheter tube attached to a suction machine.

Part of the recovery process involved 'weaning', or spending spells off the ventilator. Initially, it was 5 minutes, then a few minutes more, until Gail was delighted to hit the milestone of 1 hour. Dr Elliott's Senior House Officer said this was good. Two hours would be better, but he did not think Gail could do it. Gail duly went 3 and three-quarter hours the next day.

Nearly 6 months after being admitted, and one or two more hurdles/setbacks later (including a very painful bout of pancreatitis), Gail was ready for discharge, with a comprehensive near 24-hour care package of specially trained agency carers in place. (I was at home full time at this point, as the same uncompassionate boss from the drama 12 months earlier had terminated my employment midway through Gail's hospitalisation by way of redundancy). Also in place was a comprehensive stock of trache-related consumables/supplies and now not one but two portable ventilators, both the upgraded Nippy 3+, which has an internal battery with around a 5-hour life, and a 5-hour external battery too, which is much smaller than the battery pack that accompanied the Nippy 3 some 12 months earlier. In October 2008, Gail was home. Mostly, thereafter, the main problems tended not to be with Gail's health, but with the complexities of the operation of such a complex care package, involving numerous areas of the National Health Service and a number of external bodies, all of whom were and still are striving to function on extremely stretched resources.

In the early months of Gail's 'new life' as a trachy patient, she would frequently spend several hours not using the Nippy (although it was sensibly never out of range); although within 2 or 3 years, and after two or three setbacks to Gail's health, this gradually declined to almost continuous use of the Nippy (connected to the trachy with the tubing invariably neatly hidden under a neck scarf) for the past 8 years. The aforementioned setbacks included a repeat of pneumonia in December 2009 (both lungs, this time), from which Gail recovered despite an initial less than optimistic prognosis, successive mystery illness/viral infection/small bowel ileus in December 2010 and mystery rib pain in October 2011 onwards (which eventually led to a cholecystectomy over 2 years later). The increased reliance on the ventilator was, to me, disappointing in some respects, but on the other hand, it was reassuring that Gail was accordingly 'safe' at all times, without constantly having to look every second to make sure Gail's breathing was OK.

Also, since the 2008 hospitalisation, which effectively prevented us both from doing anything at all for nearly 6 months, we both seem to have adopted a mind set to 'do things'. Clearly, in the post-2008 circumstances, there would be challenges to overcome, not least related to the additional equipment that needs to be on hand at all times. Our activities initially started out as trips to the shops (accompanied by a carer) and, in the ensuing 12 months, extended to trips to the theatre, cinema, horse racing and greyhound racing. May 2009 represented something of a milestone, as we took our first overnight trip away from home and without a carer. It was just a couple of nights on the coast in caravan, but a big step forward; the biggest challenge appeared to be fitting all the equipment in the car – as well as two Nippys, suction machine etc.; there was bed raising equipment (Gail is deemed to be safer sleeping in a slightly elevated position, enteral feed pump [no longer used as Gail has had bolus feeds enterally since mid-2009]) and a commode (no longer needed due to a catheter since September 2009, predominantly for the purpose of avoiding inconvenient calls of nature and the associated moving and handling, sometimes in barely accessible or inaccessible places).

The greatest step forward in the ongoing patient-and-carer journey was in September 2009, when we resumed our beloved pursuit of overseas holidays in warmer climes. The trip to Mallorca took a fair bit of logistical planning, particularly in terms of transporting all the equipment, consumables, medication and feeds required within airlines permitted baggage allowances! This we have indeed managed now on countless occasions (see the selection of photographs from some of our trips), and indeed, each overseas trip seems easier than the last one, in that we learn a little bit more each time. I am pleased to say there have been no respiratory-related problems on any of these vacations – although there have been a couple of trips where the suction machine charger has become faulty; this is now countered by taking two spare chargers and a manual suction device. Table 76.1 shows my checklist for any trip away from home.

This is our journey so far.

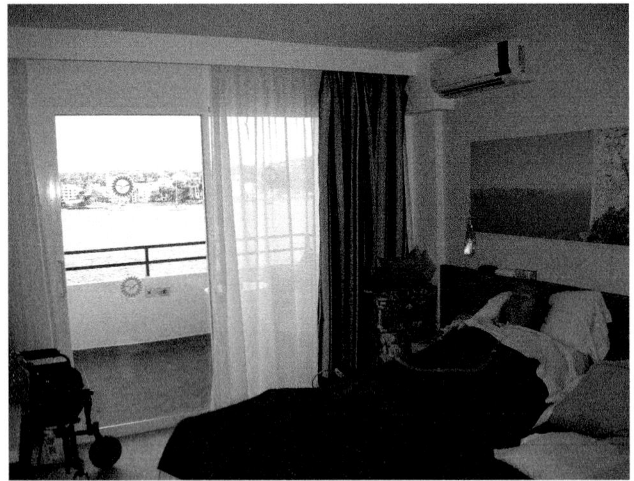

2013 (May) Mallorca.

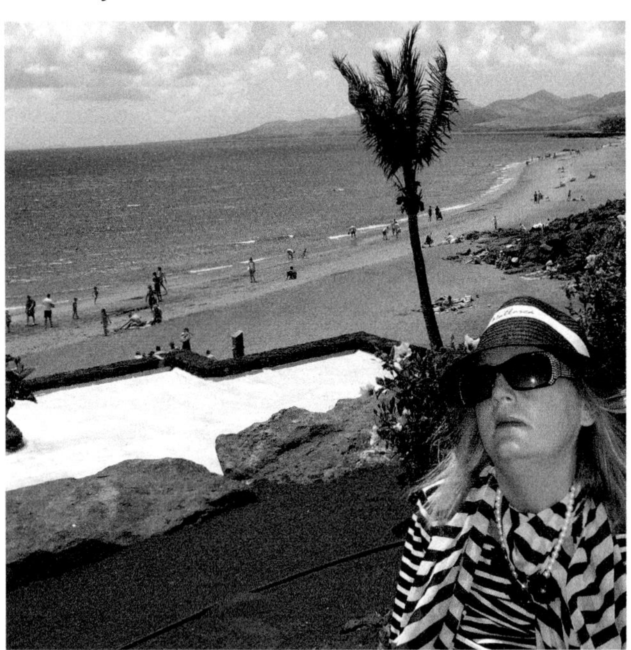

2014 Lanzarote.

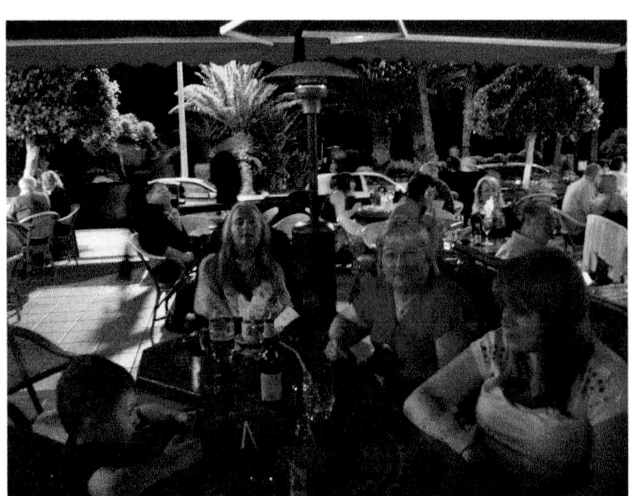

2015 Lanzarote.

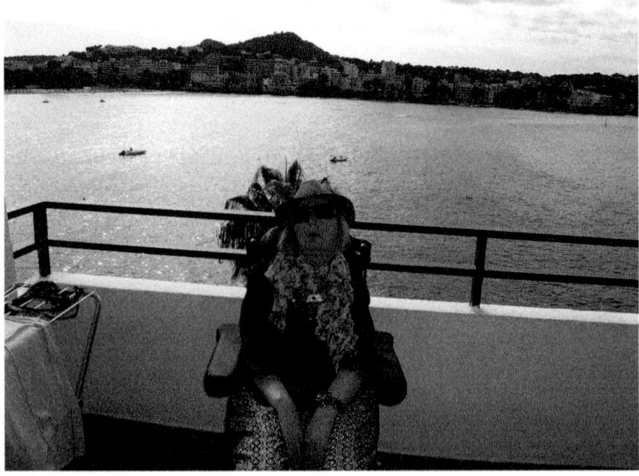

2015 Lanzarote.

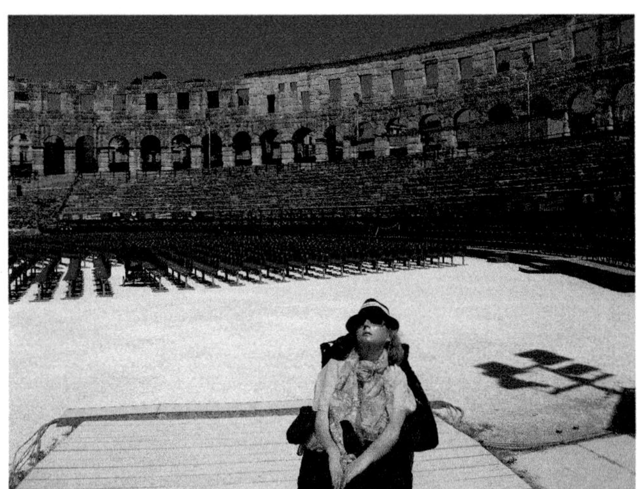

2015 Pula Amphitheatre.

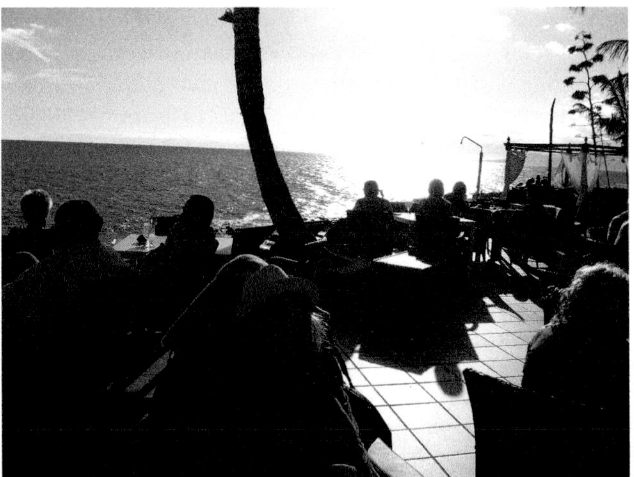

2016 (January) Lanzarote Cafe La Ola.

Table 76.1 Travel checklist

Must be taken as cabin luggage to be accessible during the flight
• Nippy 1 ventilator
• Power Lead
• Spare enteral feeding peg kit
• Travel adaptors
• Extension lead – 5 m
• Four-way socket[a]
• Inner tubes for trachy
• Suction catheters
• Trachy size 7
• Trachy size 6
• Trachy tapes
• Trachy dressings
• Sterile gloves
• Exhale valves (whisper)
• Nippy 2 ventilator
• Power lead
• Suction machine
Hold Baggage
• Medication
• Charger for suction machine
• Car charger for suction machine
• European charger for suction machine
• Second spare enteral feeding peg kit[b]
• Catheter mounts
• Water for inhalation
• Syringes: 2.5, 10 and 50 mL
• Swedish noses
• Dry air humidifiers
• Tracheal suction catheters
• Yankeur suction
• Trachy tapes
• Trachy dressings
• Gloves
• Cleaning granules
• Bed raiser
• Inflatable mattress (to go on top of hotel bed)
• Ambu-bag
• Bolus feeds
• Jugs and measuring pots
• Incontinence sheets
• Pads
• Conti wipes
• Baby wipes
• Face wipes
• Buzzer
• Spare button for buzzer in case of malfunction
• Heated humidifier
• Humidifier chamber and circuit
• Circuit wires for humidifier
• Manual suction device
• Hand warmers
• Wheelchair

[a] Hotel bedrooms may have very limited numbers of sockets and may be inconveniently situated.

[b] In the unlikely event that a change is needed, it is a safety net if the first spare kit is ruined when changing (specialist knowledge potentially limited by local doctors/nurses).

Index

Note: Page numbers followed by 'f' and 't' represent figures and tables respectively.

A

A′-profile, 193, 194f
A_1-adenosine receptor antagonists, 336
α2-adrenergic receptors, 125
Abdominal surgery, post-surgery non-invasive ventilation, 501–502
Absolute humidity (AH), inadequate, 63, 64t
Acceptance
 CPAP, 26
 telemonitoring processes, 229
ACE inhibitors, 336, 403
Acetazolamide, 411, 412
Acetylcysteine, 116
Acid maltase deficiency, lysosomal (Pompe's disease), 355, 360–361, 381
Acid–base balance, 177, 240–241
Acidaemia, severity and timing of, 151
ACP, *see* Advance care planning (ACP)
Acute cardiac failure, 143
Acute cardiogenic pulmonary oedema (APO), 341, 344
Acute Decompensated Heart Failure National Registry (ADHERE), 328, 333, 334, 335
Acute exacerbation COPD (AECOPD)
 ARF, 139–141
 ECCO2R in, 39, 40
Acute Heart Failure Global Survey of Standard Treatment (ALARM-HF), 328, 333
Acute heart failure syndrome (AHFS), 326–336
 assessment, diagnosis and prognostication, 327–328
 clinical management, 328–332
  association with myocardial infarction, 330
  discrepancies in evidence, 331–332
  evidence base, 329
  health economics, 330
  in-hospital trials, 329–330
  mechanism of action, 328–329
  non-invasive ventilation, 328–332
  overview, 328
  place in, 332
  pooled data, 330–331
  practical considerations, 332
  pre-hospital NIV, 330
  summary of evidence, 332
 definition and classification, 326–327
 pharmacological treatment, 333–336
  diuretics, 333–334
  opiates, 334–335
  other agents, 335–336
  vasodilators, nesiritide, 334–335
  vasodilators, nitrates and sodium nitroprusside, 334
 prognostic variables, 333
 risk variables, 333t
Acute hypercapnic respiratory failure (AHFR), 462
 base mortality rate, 150–152
  COPD, 150
  investigations, 151
  observations, 151–152
  post initiation, 152
  predictive tools, 152
  severity and timing of respiratory acidaemia, 151
  steady-state variables, 150–151
 during exacerbation, 38
 predicting outcome in patients, 149–154
  asthma, 153
  clinicians, 150
  current practice, 149–150
  IPF, 153
  NMD, 153
  OHS, 153
  other conditions, 152–153
  overview, 149
  pneumonia, 153
  pulmonary oedema, 153–154
Acute hypoxaemic respiratory failure, 144, 298–301, 315
Acute NIV
 ARF, *see* Acute respiratory failure (ARF)
 care settings, 3–5
 education programmes/assessment of staff competencies, *see* Education programmes/assessment
 in obesity related respiratory failure, 452
 monitoring during, *see* Monitoring, during acute NIV
 set-up, *see* Setup, acute NIV
Acute oxygen therapy, 287–293
 clinical assessment of potentially hypoxic patient, 287, 288
 future research, 292–293
 investigations, 288–289
 overview, 287, 288t
 oxygen therapy, 289–290
 supplementary oxygen, 290–292
  overview, 290–291
  prescription, administration and monitoring, 291–292
  vulnerable to oxygen, patients, 291
Acute respiratory distress syndrome (ARDS), 23, 30, 475
 ECCO2R in patients with, 36, 37–38, 40
 HFOT for, 298
 LUCI in ventilated patient with, 194–195
Acute Respiratory Distress Syndrome Network (ARDSNet), 37–38
Acute respiratory failure (ARF), 139–146, 481
 acute cardiac failure, 143
 acute hypoxaemic respiratory failure, 144
 COPD exacerbation, 139–141

COPD patients in, 24
effects of PAV in, 31
gold standard in, 122
HFNCO, 145–146
hypoxaemic, 298–301, 315
IMV, discontinuation of, 141–143
effects of NIV during unsuccessful weaning, 142–143
pathophysiology of weaning failure, 141–142
in amyotrophic lateral sclerosis, 394–395
in bronchiectasis, evidence-based use of NIV in, 471
in CF evidence-based use of NIV in, 471
in obesity and obesity–hypoventilation syndrome, 462
NIV and CPAP, 460–462
interfaces for, 43
NIV in children with, 533–536
clinical management, 536
evidence base, 533–536
overview, 533
nosocomial pneumonia, risk of, 57
oronasal masks for, 47
overview, 2, 3, 5, 47, 147
pressure support and volume control, 14
prevention
COPD and hypercapnic respiratory failure, exacerbation, 131
CPO, 131
de novo hypoxic respiratory failure, 132, 133–134
starting NIV, 73–77
equipment, 76, 77
location, 74–75
personnel, 73, 74f
practical issues, 77
selection of patients, 75–76, 77t
Acute setting
CPAP in, 25
guidelines for NIV in, 113
Acute-on-chronic respiratory failure
amyotrophic lateral sclerosis, 394
intubation in, 249–252
benefit of NIV, 249–250
Acute/acute-on-chronic respiratory failure, development of, 243–244
Adaptive pressure support, 16
Adaptive servo ventilation (ASV), 414
Adaptive Servo Ventilation on Survival and Hospital Admissions in Heart Failure (ADVENT-HF), 348
Adaptive servo-ventilation (ASV), 341, 347, 348–349
heart failure and central sleep apnoea, 415
Adenosine triphosphate and ventilatory control, 448
Adherence, reduced, in NIV, 64
Administering NIV, out of ICU, 251–252
Administration, supplementary oxygen therapy, 291–292
Adrenaline, 328
Advance care planning (ACP), 574–575
Advanced physiological measurements, pulmonary mechanics, 178, 179
ADVENT-HF trial, 349
Adverse effects, of ECCO2R, 39
Aerosol therapy, in NIV, 67–70
characteristic factors of technique, 67–69
airway flow, 69
BiPAP mode, 68–69
CPAP mode, 68
interface, leaks, generator position, 67, 68f
type of device, level of positive pressure and drug dose, 69
ventilatory mode, 68
factors depending on patient, 67
two factors derived from, 69–70
aerosolised bronchodilators during NIV, 69–70
ASTHMA-NIV, 70
COPD-NIV, 69
position of generator, 69
type of drug and dose, 69
type of generator, nebuliser *vs.* MDI, 69
Aerosolised bronchodilators, during NIV, 69–70
COPD-NIV, 69
Agitation, for NIV intolerance and failure, 115
Air leaks
for successful NIV, 30, 31
minimisation and comfort, 43
physiological aspects, interfaces, 45
technical factors contributing NIV failure, 118–119
Airway clearance, 377
Airway flow, aerosol therapy, 69
Airway pressurization, patient–ventilator interaction, 182
Airways
upper
in heart failure and central sleep apnoea with Cheynes-Stokes respiration, obstruction, 415
washout of dead space in, 296
Alarms, positive pressure ventilators, 17
Alternatives, to home in HMV, 210–211
Alveolar capillary diffusion, impaired, 239
Alveolar hypoventilation, 364, 365, 366
decreased respiratory muscle performance during sleep, 366–367
decreased respiratory muscle performance during wakefulness, 366
decreased respiratory muscle performance in ICU, 367
impaired cardiovascular performance, 367
impaired chest wall, 365
lung mechanics, 365
type 2 respiratory failure, 240
upper airway obstruction, 365
Alveolar overdistension, 23
Alveolar PCO_2 ($PaCO_2$), 411
Alveolar ventilation, 177, 411
Alveolar-to-arterial oxygen gradient (A-aDO_2), 364
Alveolar–capillary membrane, thickness, 289
Amantadine, 379
Ambulatory oxygen therapy
assessment for, 283–284
indications for, 282–283
overview, 279–280
American Academy of Neurology, 382
American Academy of Sleep Medicine (AASM) guidelines, 218, 219
American Society of Anesthesiologist (ASA), 161
American Thoracic Society, 181, 250
AMP-activated protein kinase (AMPK), 448
Amyotrophic lateral sclerosis (ALS), 5, 151, 365, 388–395
advanced malignant condition, 201
airway clearance, 390
arterial $PaCO_2$, 390
clinical features and investigations, 393–395
early respiratory evaluation, 211
EFNS guideline, 394
epidemiology, 388
gastrostomy tube placement, 395
interface, 395
lung volume recruitment, 390
NIV, 390–393
clinical application, 393–395
current guidelines and practice, 390–391
future research, 394–395

prognosis, 390
survival, 390–391
survival and, 390–391
technical aspects, 395
tracheostomy vs, 392
use of, 390
respiratory involvement, 388
respiratory muscle function, 388
signs, 388–389
symptoms, 388–389
tests of, 389–390
saliva, 395
strain, anxiety, depression and QoL, 391
technical aspects of NIV, 395
using MPV, 421
Anaemia, 287, 289
Analgesic agents, 123–125
morphine, 124
remifentanil, 124–125
Analgosedation, 123, 124, 128t
Anatomy, of nasal mucosa, 63, 65f
Angina, oxygen therapy, 290, 291
Angiotensin-converting enzyme (ACE) inhibitor drugs, 400
ANTADIR series, 432
Anti-asphyxia and vent systems, 44f, 45
Anti-tuberculous chemotherapy, 428
Anticipatory respiratory, 382
Apnoea, central, 15
Apnoea–hypopnoea index (AHI), 218–219, 393, 408, 443
Apnoea–hypopnoea score, 371
Apnoeic threshold in non-hypercapnic central sleep apnoea, 408–409
Appleton Consensus, 200
ARDS, *see* Acute respiratory distress syndrome (ARDS)
Arterial blood gases (ABG), 434
measurements, 412
NIV on, 249
Arterial carbon dioxide, 432
Arterial carbon dioxide tension ($PaCO_2$), 235–236, 240, 249, 259, 260–261, 262
Arterial oxygen tension (PaO_2), 235–236, 237, 259
Assessment of patients for HMV, diagnostic tests in, 175–187
clinical assessment, 176
gas exchange
acid–base balance, 177
carbon dioxide, 177
overview, 176
oxygen, 176, 177
overnight physiological monitoring, 184–187
advanced sleep studies, 185, 187f
overview, 184
oximetry, 184, 186f
transcutaneous capnography, 185
overview, 175, 176f
patient–ventilator interaction, 182, 184, 185f
pulmonary mechanics, 177–180
advanced physiological measurements, 178, 179
compliance, 179
lung volumes, 177, 178
overview, 177, 178f, 178t
PEEP, 179–180
WOB, 180
respiratory muscle testing, 180–182
invasive tests, 181–182, 183f
non-invasive tests, 181
overview, 180
Assisted/controlled mode (ACV), 421
Association Nationale pour les Traitements à Domicile, l'Innovation et la Recherche (ANTADIR), 170
Asthma
CAOS, 150
exacerbations, NIV for, 160–161
predicting outcome in patients with AHFR, 153
ASTHMA-NIV, 70
Asynchrony
defined, 105
patient–ventilator, *see* Patient–ventilator asynchrony
Atelectasis, 22, 23, 25, 38, 133, 144, 161
obstructive, 195
occurrence of, 133
ATP and ventilatory control, 448
Atrial fibrillation (AF), 409
Auto-CPAP in obesity-hypoventilation syndrome, 464
Auto-positive end-expiratory pressure (auto-PEEP), 12, 13, 118, 247
Auto-titrating CPAP, 25
Auto-Trak, 12
Auto-triggering, 105, 106f
Autonomic effects, mechanism of NIV in HF, 347
Autonomic nervous system, hypercapnic central sleep apnoea and, 411
Average volume assured pressure support (AVAPS) ventilation, 401, 464
obesity-hypoventilation syndrome, 464
Average volume-assured pressure support (AVAPS), 16, 33
Avicenne sign, 193

B

B-lines, 193
Bach's centre, 434
Balloon pressure monitoring catheter, 179
Barometric pressure, low, 236
Base mortality rate, AHFR, 150–152
COPD, 150
investigations, 151
observations, 151–152
post initiation, 152
predictive tools, 152
severity and timing of respiratory acidaemia, 151
steady-state variables, 150–151
Battery power, positive pressure ventilators, 17, 18f
Becker muscular dystrophy (BMD), 356, 357–358, 399
Belgian survey, hypoxaemic ARF, 316
Bench test study, 218
Benzodiazepines, 122, 126–127, 319
Berlin definition, of ARDS, 298
Beta-blockers, 400
Bi-level positive airway pressure (BiPAP)
AHFS, NIV in, 328–329, 330, 331
mode, aerosol therapy, 68–69
NIV mechanical ventilators, 17f, 65, 66
non-COPD-related ARF, treatment, 316, 318
post-surgery non-invasive ventilation, 497
Bi-level ventilation (pressure support ventilation and PEEP/BiPAP)
Duchenne muscular dystrophy, 402
failure, 378
myasthenia gravis, 378
obesity-hypoventilation syndrome, 464–465
scoliosis, 433
Bi-level ventilators, 10, 11, 12–13, 14, 15, 16
Bias, cognitive, 150
Bicarbonate in chronic hypercapnic respiratory failure, accumulation, 432
Bicarbonate–carbonic acid system, 241
BLUE points, 190, 191f
BLUE-protocol, 193
Body mass index (BMI), 441
arterial oxygen concentration and, 442
cardiovascular risk factors, 442
daytime hypercapnia, 457
longitudinal changes of, 442
low, AHFR and, 151

Bradyarrhythmias, 360
myotonic dystrophy, 360
Bradycardia, incidence of, 125
Brain (and neurological function)
Duchenne muscular dystrophy, 399, 403
myotonic dystrophy, 360
Brain natriuretic peptide (BNP), 327–328, 403
Breathlessness
clinical effects of HFOT, 297
oxygen reduced, 282–283
British Thoracic Society (BTS) working group, 284
Bronchiectasis; *see also* Cystic fibrosis (CF)
defined, 470
evidence-based use of NIV
chronic respiratory failure, 471
in acute respiratory failure, 471
future research ideas, 472
incidences, 470
initiation and weaning of NIV, 472
non-CF bronchiectasis, 470
pathophysiology, 470–471
technical considerations, 472
therapeutic strategies, 472
Bronchodilatation
mechanism of NIV in HF, 345
Bronchodilator drugs, for aerosol therapy, 69
Bronchoscopy
during NIV, 319, 540–543
clinical applications, 541
evidence base, 540–541
future research, 543
overview, 540
rationale, 540
technical considerations, 541–542, 542f
fibreoptic, 303, 304
Bulbar (muscle) function/dysfunction
neuromuscular diseases, amyotrophic lateral sclerosis, 392, 393, 395
Bulbar impairment, 395
Bulbar muscles, dysfunction of, 367

C

Calf hypertrophy, 357
Canadian Continuous Positive Airway Pressure for Patients with Central Sleep Apnea and Heart Failure Trial (CANPAP), 348, 349
Cancer
background, 481
clinical use of NIV in, 482
in patients with limitations of care, 483–484, 484*f*
patients without limitations of care, 482–483, 483f
pathophysiology of NIV in, 481–482
Candidates, selection of, chronic COPD, 260–261
Cannula selection, tracheostomy, 556–557, 557f
Cannulae, nasal, 310
CANPAP trial, 348, 349
Capillary diffusion, impaired alveolar, 239
Captopril, 336
Carbohydrate metabolism, 236
Carbon dioxide (CO_2)
ECCO2R, *see* Extracorporeal CO_2 removal (ECCO2R)
gas exchange, 177
in central sleep apnoea (non-hypercapnic), reserve, 409
in obesity, chronic retention, 444
rebreathing, dead space and, 45–46
removal technology, principles and circuitry
catheters, 37
membrane 'lung,' 37
pump, 37
removal, exacerbation of COPD, 253
Carboxyhaemoglobin levels, 289
Cardiac afterload, mechanism of NIV in HF, 346
Cardiac arrest, targeted whole-body ultrasound in, 195
Cardiac arrhythmias, 361
Cardiac disease, in muscular dystrophy
Becker muscular dystrophy, 357–358
Duchenne muscular dystrophy, 356–357
Cardiac dystrophin expression, 357
Cardiac failure
AHFS, *see* Acute heart failure syndrome (AHFS)
central sleep apnoea and, 408–410, 412–415
chronic congestive, *see* Chronic congestive cardiac failure
Cardiac performance, NIV on, 249
Cardiac surgery, post-surgery non-invasive ventilation, 498
Cardiogenic pulmonary oedema (CPE), 157, 316, 318, 319, 329, 331–332, 334, 335
ARF, prevention, 131
endotracheal intubation and reintubation, 132–133
invasive ventilation, alternative to, 134
treatment, 23
Cardiovascular dysfunction, weaning failure and, 587–588
Cardiovascular effects, effectiveness of NIV, 259
Care in HMV, organisation, 209–212
alternatives to home, 210–211
coordinator, 209, 210
networks, strong and weak relationships, 211–212
team working and coordination of care, 209, 210
Care team, characteristics of, 209, 210
Care, continuity of, *see* Continuity of care
Caregiver team factors, in NIV failure, 112
Caregivers
education, 204; *see also* Education
health of, in amyotrophic lateral sclerosis, 393
Carer, progressive and debilitating condition, 391
Carer's journey, 697–703
Cares, standards, Duchenne muscular dystrophy, 403–404
Case studies, chronic ventilatory failure, 80–81
Cataracts, 360
Catheter(s)
CO_2 removal technology, principles and circuitry, 37
nasal, 309–310
transtracheal, 311–312
Catheter-linked occult thrombosis (CLOT-protocol), 196
Central apnoea index (CAI), 408
Central sleep apnoea (CSA), 342–343, 345, 348–349, 408, 409
associated with central nervous system and spinal cord injury, 414
treatment, 414
atrial fibrillation (AF), 409
CPAP-emergent, management of, 415
epoch of periodic breathing, 410
hypercapnic, 412
idiopathic, 410–411
treatment of, 411
in asymptomatic cardio-/cerebrovascular pathology, 414
in chronic spinal cord injury, 414
in endocrine disorders, 415
in pacemaker recipients, 410
opioids, 412–414

periodic breathing, 410
treatment-emergent, 415
Centronuclear (myotubular) myopathy, 382–383
Cephalic mask, 46, 48, 49
Cervical spinal deformities, 426
CF, *see* Cystic fibrosis (CF)
Challenges for NIV, in COPD exacerbation, 250–252
as alternative to intubation, 251
continue NIV after acute phase, 251
delivering NIV outside ICU, 251–252
proportion of patients, receiving NIV, 250
safety reasons, 251–252
success rate, improving, 250–251
Chest infections, 358
Chest wall deformity, 429
Chest wall diseases, 457
Chest wall, mechanical disadvantage due to, 242, 243f
Cheyne-Stokes breathing (CSB), 366, 408
Cheyne–Stokes respiration, 185, 343
Children, *see* Paediatric ventilatory failure
Chronic central hypoventilation, 510
Chronic congestive cardiac failure, 341–350
limitations of studies
CPAP titration in CSA, 349
supplemental oxygen, 349
technical aspects, 349
overview, 341
pathophysiology, 341–343
heart failure, 341–342
sleep-disordered breathing, 342–343
pulmonary effects, 343, 344–349
evidence base, 347–349
mechanisms of NIV, 345–347
overview, 343, 344–345
Chronic COPD, 258–263
clinical application and selection of candidates, 260–261
clinical evidence, 259–260
economic considerations, 260
future research, 262
overview, 258
pathophysiology and effect of NIV, 258–259
practical recommendations, 262–263
technical considerations, 262
Chronic hypercapnic respiratory failure, 460–461
bicarbonate accumulates in patients, 432
Chronic hypercapnic respiratory failure, development of, 243
Chronic hypoxaemia, 280–281
Chronic NIV
CVS, *see* Chronic ventilator service (CVS)
monitoring during sleep, *see* Monitoring during sleep during chronic NIV
ultrasound, *see* Ultrasound
Chronic NIV, in children, 525–529
benefits of NIV, 527–528, 528t
correction of nocturnal hypoventilation and gas exchange, 527
increase in survival, 527
lung function improvement, 527–528
clinical applications, 528–529
contraindications, side effects and limits of NIV, 529, 530t
indications, 528–529
overview, 525
pathophysiology, 525–526, 526f
increase in respiratory load, 525–526, 526f
neurological control failure, 526
respiratory muscle weakness, 526
Chronic obesity-related respiratory failure, management of acute/acute, 453–454
Chronic obstructive pulmonary disease (COPD), 429, 453, 457
acute hypercapnic exacerbations of, 452
advanced malignant condition, 201
alveolar hypoventilation, 235
ASTHMA-NIV, 70
base mortality rate, AHFR, 150
chronic, *see* Chronic COPD
COPD and asthma outcomes study (CAOS), 150
COPD-NIV, 69
cost, 223
CPAP in, 25
diagnosis, 92
ECCO2R devices, 36
ECCO2R in patients with, 38–39
Exacerbations, *see* Exacerbations, COPD
hyper-inflation, 13
in ARF, 24
individualised prognosis for, 213
management, 167
mechanically ventilated, 24
triggering systems, 12
ventilatory failure in patients with, 241–242
hyperinflation and intrinsic PEEP, 242
increased expiratory resistance and expiratory flow limitation, 242
increased inspiratory resistance, 241–242
increased static compliance and reduced elastic recoil, 242
mechanical disadvantage due to chest wall and diaphragm position, 242, 243f
overview, 241
Chronic obstructive pulmonary disease (COPD), NIV in, 266–270
overview, 266
subtypes
comorbidities, on mortality and hospitalisation outcomes, 268, 268f, 269
comorbidities, on NIV compliance, tolerance and settings, 269–270
relevance for management and, 267, 267f
Chronic respiratory failure (CRF)
effects of PAV in, 31
home oxygen therapy in, *see* Home oxygen therapy, in CRF
hypercapnic, 258
in bronchiectasis, evidence-based use of NIV in, 471
in CF, evidence-based use of NIV in, 471
maintaining and worsening, 259
organisational complexity, 224, 225f
signs and symptoms, 78
starting NIV, 77–80
education, 77–78
equipment, 79–80
location, 78, 79
practical issues, 80
timing, 78
Chronic respiratory insufficiency, telemonitoring for, 226
Chronic ventilation service (CVS), 165–173
in community, 169–171
definition and goals, 169
HMV in Netherlands, 171–173
monitoring patient treated by HMV, 171, 172t
RHCSs, obligations, organisation and costs, 170–171
transition to home, 169–170
in hospital, 166–169
dedicated staff, 167–168
equipment, 168

monitoring, 169
organisation, 166–167
overview, 165
Chronic ventilatory failure, case study, 80–81
Cigarette smoking, secondary polycythaemia, 281
Circuitry, CO_2 removal technology
catheters, 37
membrane 'lung,' 37
pump, 37
Circuits, positive pressure ventilators, 10, 11f
Circulatory failure, causes, 341–342
Circulatory system, physiology of CPAP, 24
Classes, of NIV interfaces, 44
Claustrophobia, 115
CNBP gene, 358
CO_2 chemosensitivity, 409
CO_2 monitoring, end-tidal and transcutaneous, 377
Cobb angle, 427
Cochrane systematic review, 282, 283
CPAP, 25
Code of Federal Regulations Title 21 (CFR 21), 55–56
Coenzyme Q, 379
Cognitive bias, in medical practice, 150
Coma, 288
hypercapnic, 102
Comet-tail artifacts, 193
Comfort, patient, 101, 102
Community acquired pneumonia (CAP), 133, 134
Community, CVS in, 169–171
definition and goals, 169
HMV
in Netherlands, 171–173
monitoring patient treated by, 171, 172t
RHCSs, obligations, organisation and costs, 170–171
transition to home, 169–170
continuum of in-hospital education program, 169
home care setting, 170
social considerations, 170
Community-acquired pneumonia (CAP), 318
Comorbidities, COPD subtypes
NIV compliance, tolerance and settings, 269–270
on mortality and hospitalisation outcomes, 268, 268f, 269
Competence based learning process, 201
Competencies
assessing, 97
staff, education programmes/assessment, *see* Education programmes/assessment
Complex assessments, nocturnal ventilatory PG or PSG, 219–220
Compliance
data provided by software of home ventilators, 218
low, in NIV, 64
NIV, COPD subtypes and comorbidities, 269–270
pulmonary mechanics, 179
static, increased, 242
Computational fluid dynamics (CFD) software, numerical simulations with, 46
Concentrators, oxygen
static, 308
transportable and portable, 308–309
Confusion Assessment Method for ICU (CAM-ICU), 102, 127
Congenital kyphoscoliosis, 172
Congenital myopathies, 240, 382
Congenital myotonic dystrophy, 359
Continuity of care, 224–230
future research, 229–230
overview, 223
technical and clinical considerations, 224–226
telemonitoring, 226–229
cost, 226
design and acceptance, 229
for chronic respiratory insufficiency, 226
rationale for, 226
standard management, 226, 229
summary, 227t–228t
to gold standard, 229
Continuous non-invasive ventilatory support (CNVS), 419
Continuous positive airway pressure (CPAP), 22–27, 412, 443, 457
36 OHS patients, 459
acceptance and tolerance, 26
AHFS, NIV in, 328–329, 330, 331
application, 23, 24
auto-CPAP titration, 464
auto-titrating, 25
bench tests in, 218
equipment, 26
history, 22
in acute hypercapnic respiratory failure, 462
in acute setting, 25
in chronic hypercapnic respiratory failure, 460–461
in COPD, 25
in oncologic patients with ARF, 318
indications and contraindications, 25–26
mechanism of NIV in HF, 345–348
mode, aerosol therapy, 68
mode, positive pressure ventilators, 14
n-CPAP, 133
NIV and, 315
NIV titration in OHS, 464
NIV-CPAP, 1
outside hospital setting, 26–27
overview, 22
PAV, 31
physiology, 23–24
circulatory system, 24
overview, 23
respiratory system, 23–24
post-surgery non-invasive ventilation, 497
potential mechanisms to achieve improvement, 458
recommended treatment election, 463
sleep apnoea (OSA), 458
titration in CSA, 349
treatment, 459
types, 24–25
Continuous positive airway pressure (CPAP) therapy, 454
Continuum, of in-hospital education program, 169
Controlled mechanical ventilation (CMV), 57–58
Conventional vital signs, 102
Coordination of care, 209, 210
Coordinator, care, 209, 210
COPD-specific questionnaires, 657
Core team, 209
Costs
BIPAP equipment, 26
chronic COPD, 260
COPD, 223
CPAP equipment, 26
for ECCO2R, 40
HMV, 200
NIV, 91–92
RHCSs, 170–171
telemonitoring, 226
Cough effectiveness, 151
CPAP, *see* Continuous positive airway pressure (CPAP)
Criteria, for NIV discontinuation and ETI, 319t
Critical care ventilators, 11, 12
Critically ill, lung sliding in, 191
CRQ dyspnoea, 391

Cuff management, tracheostomy, 557–558
Curriculum for learning, designing, 96–97
Cycle, positive pressure ventilators, 13
Cycling-off phase, patient–ventilator asynchrony during, 107–108
  exhalation valve
    delayed opening of, 107–108
    premature opening of, 107
Cylinders, oxygen, 307–308
Cystic fibrosis (CF)
  characteristics, 470
  evidence-based use of NIV
    chronic respiratory failure, 471
    in acute respiratory failure, 471
  future research ideas, 472
  incidences, 470
  initiation and weaning of NIV, 472
  pathophysiology, 470–471
  technical considerations, 472
  therapeutic strategies, 472
Cystic fibrosis transmembrane conductance regulator (CFTR) gene, 470

D

D-Day, 208
Data Monitoring and Ethics Committee, 392
Data, pooled, AHFS, 330–331
Data, provided by software of home ventilators, 217–219
  AHI, 218–219
  compliance, 218
  estimated tidal volume and minute ventilation, 218
  flow and pressure tracings, 219
  leaks, 218
  overview, 217–218
  respiratory rate, 218
Databases, observations using, 159–160
Daytime hypercapnoea, 380
Daytime ventilatory support, mouthpiece ventilation for, 419
De novo hypoxic respiratory failure
  ARF, prevention, 132
  ETI and reintubation, 133–134
  invasive ventilation, alternative to, 134–135
Dead space
  and humidification, tracheostomy and, 555
  CO_2 rebreathing and, 45–46
Dedicated staff, CVS, 167–168
Deep-vein thrombosis (DVT), 196
Delayed opening, of exhalation valve, 107–108
Delirium, 102, 115, 127, 128t; *see also* Sedation
Delivered gas, warming and humidification of, 295–296
Delivery systems, oxygen, 309–312
  enclosures
    oxygen hat/hood, 312
    oxygen tent, 312
  mask systems, 310–311
    face masks with reservoir bag, 310
    simple face masks, 310
    tracheostomy mask, 311
    use of, 311
    Venturi mask, 311
  nasal systems
    cannulae, 310
    catheter, 309–310
    reservoir, 310
    use, 310
  overview, 309
  OxyArm, 312
  tracheal systems
    transtracheal catheter, 311–312
Depression, among caregivers, 204
Designing curriculum for learning, 96–97
Detecting, nocturnal hypoventilation, 216, 217
Developing outcomes for learning, 96
Dexmedetomidine, 123, 125–126, 127, 319
Diagnostic tests, in assessment of patients for HMV, 175–187
  clinical assessment, 176
  gas exchange, 176, 177
  overnight physiological monitoring, 184–187
    advanced sleep studies, 185, 187f
    overview, 184
    oximetry, 184, 186f
    transcutaneous capnography, 185
  overview, 175, 176f
  patient–ventilator interaction, 182, 184, 185f
  pulmonary mechanics, 177–180
    advanced physiological measurements, 178, 179
    compliance, 179
    lung volumes, 177, 178
    overview, 177, 178f, 178t
    PEEP, 179–180
    WOB, 180
  respiratory muscle testing, 180–182
    invasive tests, 181–182, 183f
    non-invasive tests, 181
    overview, 180
Diaphragm fluoroscopy, 369
Diaphragm pacemaker (DP), 513
Diaphragm pacing, by PNS, 547–552
  alternative treatments, 549
  contraindications, 549
  indications, 548–549
  overview, 547
  practical aspects, 549–550
  preimplantation assessment, 549
  results, 550–551
  techniques, 547
    intramuscular diaphragm pacing, 547–548, 548f
    intrathoracic phrenic nerve stimulation, 547, 548f
Diaphragm paralysis, 180
Diaphragm position, mechanical disadvantage due to, 242, 243f
Diaphragm/extradiaphragmatic respiratory muscles, respiratory pressure and EMG, 442
Diaphragmatic dysfunction, ventilator induced, 584–586, 585t
Diastolic HF, defined, 342
Digestive tubes problems, post-surgery non-invasive ventilation, 498
Digoxin Intervention Group study, 334
Discharge planning, in palliative care, 213
Discharge, HMV in Netherlands, 173
Discharging patient, on home ventilation, 207–214
  organisation of care in HMV, 209–212
    alternatives to home, 210–211
    care coordinator, 209, 210
    networks, strong and weak relationships, 211–212
    team working and coordination of care, 209, 210
  patient safety, 212–213
  planning in HMV, 207–209
  planning in palliative care, 213
  transitional care (TC), 207
Discomfort
  mask, 114, 115
  NIV, 64
Discontinuation
  NIV, 319t
  of IMV, 141–143
    effects of NIV during unsuccessful weaning, 142–143
    pathophysiology of weaning failure, 141–142
Discrepancies in evidence, AHFS, clinical management, 331–332

Distress, 679
Diuretic Optimization Strategies Evaluation trial, 334
Diuretics, in AHFS, 333–334
 evidence base, 333–334
 mechanism of action, 333
 role in management, 334
Diurnal ventilatory insufficiency, 379
DNA trinucleotide CTG, 380
DNA-chip diagnosis, 356
Do-not-intubate/do-not-resuscitate (DNI/DNR) context, 74
Dobutamine, 328, 334, 336
Dopamine, 328
Dose, bronchodilator drugs, 69
Drug dose, 69
Drugs, selection
 analgesic agents, 123–125
  morphine, 124
  remifentanil, 124–125
 benzodiazepines, 126–127
 dexmedetomidine, 125–126
 propofol, 126
Duchenne muscular dystrophy (DMD), 356, 399, 402
 clinical course, 399–400
 complications, in long-term survivors, 403
 components of estimated annual cost, 405
 daytime NIV, 402
 evidence base for NIV, 400–401
 indications for tracheostomy ventilation, 402
 interfaces, 402
 long-term findings
  complications, 402–403
 new therapeutic approaches, 404
  exon skipping drugs, 404
  idebenone, 404
  stop codon gene modification, 404
 new therapeutic possibilities, 404
 newer ventilatory modes, 401–402
 overall IQ, 399
 palliation of symptoms, 403
 pathophysiology, 399
 patient using MPV, 420
 quality of life, 401
 sleep-disordered breathing, 402
 social considerations, 405
 standards of care, 403–404
 supportive care, 403
 survival probability in patients, 401
 tracheostomy ventilation, 402
 transitional care, 402
 ventilator settings, titration of, 401
 ventilators, 401
Dynamic compliance, pulmonary mechanics, 179
Dyspnoea, 102, 113, 117, 123, 134, 366, 372, 587–588
 anxiety component of, 123
Dystrophin gene, 404
Dystrophin–glycoprotein complex, 399
Dystrophinopathies, variability of, 357
Dystrophinopathy, 357

E

E-health, 229
Ear lobe blood gas (ELBG), 176
ECCO2R, *see* Extracorporeal CO_2 removal (ECCO2R)
Echo and electrocardiography (ECG), 403
Echocardiography, AHFS, 327
ECLAIR study, 39
Economic considerations, chronic COPD, 260
Education
 CRF leading to NIV, 77–78
 in-hospital, 169
 patient and caregiver, 200–205
  caregivers, 204
  legal and ethical issues, 200–201
  methodology, 201–203
  overview, 200
  purpose, 201
  setting, 201
Education programmes/assessment, 95–99
 assessing competence, 97
 designing curriculum for learning, 96–97
 developing outcomes for learning, 96
 interprofessional education, 98–99
 overview, 95–96
 simulation-based education for, 97–98
Educational programme, modification of, 202, 203
Elastic recoil, reduced, 242
Elderly, 487
 clinical application, 488–490
  acute hypercapnic exacerbation of chronic pulmonary disease, 488–489
  cardiogenic pulmonary oedema, 489
  NIV in palliative care, 489–490
 clinical impact of comorbidities, 488
 defined, 487
 discharge planning, 213
 epidemiology of ageing population, 487–488
 hypertensive HF in, 344
 NIV for, 487
 NIV failure in, 127
 pathophysiology, 487–489
 patients' prognosis and preferences, 488
 technical considerations, 490–493
  intensity of care, 490–492
  interfaces, 492–493
  NIV initiation, 490
  patients' and relatives' wills, 490
  therapeutic algorithm for NIV, 491f
  three-category approach, 492t
Electrocardiography (ECG), 357
 AHFS, 327
Electromyography, 379
Emergency department (ED)
 HFOT in, 301
 setting, acute NIV, 87–88
 starting NIV, in ARF, 74–75
Emerging modes, for NIV, 30–34
 NAVA, 31–33
 overview, 30
 PAV, 31
 PSV, features of, 30–31
 VAPS modes, 33–34
Emotional health, 680
 ventilator user guidelines for, 679
Emphysema, with alveolar destruction, 239
Enclosures, oxygen delivery systems
 oxygen hat/hood, 312
 oxygen tent, 312
End of life patients, NIV, 319
End-expiratory lung volumes (EELVs), 24, 38–39
End-of-life care
 advance care planning, 574–575
 definitions, duties and ambitions, 571–573
 last days of life, 576–577, 577f
 NIV and, 571–579
 NIV in advanced disease, burdens and benefits, 576
 NIV withdrawal at patient request, 577–579, 578t
 overview, 571
 transitions to, 573–574, 574b
Endothelin antagonists, 336
Endotracheal intubation (ETI), 64, 73, 75, 487
 criteria for NIV discontinuation, 319t
 hypoxaemic ARF, 316–318
 preoxygenation before, 303
 reintubation and, 132–134

COPD exacerbation and hypercapnic respiratory failure, 132
CPO, 132–133
de novo hypoxic respiratory failure, 133–134
risk of, 249
Environmental team factors, in NIV failure, 112
Enzyme replacement therapy, for acid maltase deficiency, 355
EPAP pressure, 465
Equipment; *see also specific entries*
acute NIV, 89
CPAP, 26
CVS
interfaces, 168
ventilators, 168
in children, 519–523
overview, 519
paediatric specificities, 519–520
ventilators for NIV, 521
ventilatory modes, 520–521
NIV failure, 116
Equipment for oxygen therapy, 307–313
high-flow humidified nasal cannulae oxygen therapy systems, 312
liquid oxygen systems, 309
overview, 307
oxygen delivery and NIV systems, 312
oxygen delivery systems, 309–312
mask systems, 310–311
nasal systems, 309–310
overview, 309
OxyArm, 312
oxygen hat/hood, 312
oxygen tent, 312
tracheal systems, 311–312
oxygen safety, 312–313
oxygen-conserving device, 309
oxygen-providing systems, 307–308
cylinders, 307–308
static oxygen concentrators, 308
supply of oxygen at home, 307–308
supply of oxygen in hospital, 307
transportable and portable concentrators, 308–309
Equipment, starting NIV
ARF
interfaces, 76, 77
ventilators, 77
CRF, 79–80
interfaces, 79
ventilator, 79–80
Estimated tidal volume, 218
Ethical issue, patient and caregiver education, 200–201
European Medicines Agency (EMA), 404
European Respiratory Society, 181, 250
Eurovent survey, 56, 57, 211
Evidence base
AHFS, clinical management, 329
diuretics, in AHFS, 333–334
for NIV in chronic HF, 347–349
CSA, 348–349
OSA, 347
hypoxaemic ARF, 315–318
RCTs, 316–318
surveys, 315–316
opiates, 335
vasodilators
nitrates and sodium nitroprusside, 334
Evidence, clinical management of AHFS
discrepancies, 331–332
summary, 332
Evidence-based use, of NIV
in bronchiectasis
chronic respiratory failure, 471
in acute respiratory failure, 471
in CF
chronic respiratory failure, 471
in acute respiratory failure, 471
in SARS, 475–476, 476f
in trauma, 505–506
Exacerbations, asthma, NIV for, 160–161
Exacerbations, COPD, 247–253
ARF
AECOPD, 139–141
prevention, 131
severe, 139–141
clinical applications, 249
endotracheal intubation and reintubation, 132
facilitation, 252
intubation in acute-on-chronic respiratory failure, 249–252
benefit of NIV, 249–250
challenges for NIV, 250–252
invasive ventilation, alternative to, 134
observations using large databases, 159–160
overview, 247
perspectives
CO_2 removal, 253
HFNC, 253
tolerance and patient–ventilator interaction, improving, 253
physiologic effects of, 247–249
arterial blood gases, NIV on, 249
cardiac performance, 249
modality of NIV, 248
obesity hypoventilation and overlap syndrome, 249
overview, 247
reduction of WOB, 247–248
post-extubation respiratory failure
prophylactic NIV, 252
therapeutic NIV, 252
Excessive daytime sleepiness (EDS), 356
Excessive secretions, 115–116
Excessive triggering delay, 105, 106f
Exercise induced oxygen desaturation, 281–282
Exhalation valve
delayed opening of, 107–108
premature opening of, 107
Expiratory asynchrony, 118
Expiratory asynchrony, patient–ventilator asynchrony during, 107–108
exhalation valve
delayed opening of, 107–108
premature opening of, 107
Expiratory flow limitation (EFL), 242, 442
Expiratory positive airway pressure (EPAP), 12f, 14, 15, 17f, 30, 180, 401, 430, 454
Expiratory pressure release, 16, 17f
Expiratory resistance, increased, 242
External nostril mask, 47
Externally applied PEEP ($PEEP_E$), 24
Extracorporeal circuits designed to remove CO_2 ($ECCO_2R$), 253
Extracorporeal CO_2 removal (ECCO2R), 36–40
CO_2 removal technology, principles and circuitry
catheters, 37
membrane 'lung,' 37
pump, 37
future research, 40
in patients with ARDS, 37–38
in patients with COPD, 38–39
other applications, 39
overview, 36–37
Extracorporeal life support (ECLS), 39
Extracorporeal membrane oxygenation (ECMO) systems, 36–37
Extubation failure, 592
clinical application, 603
factors associated with, 592b
future research, 603–604
pathophysiology, 593
post-extubation respiratory failure, NIV to prevent, 601t
evidence base, 600–603

post-extubation respiratory failure, NIV to treat
clinical application, 600
evidence base, 599–600, 600f
prevention, 135
Extubation in COPD patients
facilitation, 252
respiratory failure after
prophylactic NIV, 252
therapeutic NIV, 252
Extubation, importance of facilitating, 591–593, 592b

F

Face masks, 43, 44, 45, 46, 47–49, 50, 66, 76
simple, 310
with reservoir bag, 310
Facilitation, extubation in COPD patients, 252
Failure, NIV
patient-related factors, 114–116
agitation, 115
claustrophobia, 115
excessive secretions, 115–116
intolerance, 114
intolerance of ventilator settings, 115
mask discomfort, 114, 115
mask-related problems, 115
progression of underlying process, 116
predictors, 111–112
predictors of, 320
reasons for, 112–113
environmental/caregiver team factors, 112
proper monitoring, 113
selection of appropriate patients, 112–113
technical factors contributing, 116–117
air leaks, 118–119
oxygenation, 117–118
patient–ventilator asynchrony, 118
proper equipment, 116
ventilation, 116–117
FALLS-protocol, 195
Fat metabolism, 236
FAT-protocol, 195–196
Fatigue, respiratory muscles, 241
Fenestration, tracheostomy, 557
Fentanyl, 125, 126
Fibreoptic bronchoscopy, HFOT during, 303, 304
Fixed CPAP device, 24–25
FKRP gene, 357
Floppy baby, 375
FLORALI study, 298
Flow meters, wall-mounted, 307
Flow tracings, software of home ventilators, 219
Fluid management, weaning outcome, 611
Follow-up system, in home-based care system, 224
Follow-up, HMV in Netherlands, 173
Food and Drug Administration (FDA), 55–56
Forced expiratory volume in one second (FEV1), 459
Forced vital capacity (FVC), 344, 400
pulmonary mechanics, 178
Fraction of inspired oxygen (FiO_2), 14
French Social Security, 170
French survey, hypoxaemic ARF, 316
Full-face masks, 47–49, 76
Functional level, in ventilatory parameters, 63, 64
Functional residual capacity (FRC), 344, 441
acute hypoxaemic respiratory failure, 144
compliance and reduced, 22
CPAP, 23
HFNCO, 145
lung volume, 23
pulmonary mechanics, 177, 178
respiratory muscle testing, 181
Furosemide, 334, 335
Future research
acute oxygen therapy, 292–293
bronchiectasis, 472
bronchoscopy during NIV, 543
chronic COPD, 262
continuity of care, 229–230
cystic fibrosis (CF), 472
ECCO2R, 40, 40
extubation failure, 603–604
for NIV, 3
high-intensity NPPV, 275–276
home oxygen therapy in CRF, 284
HRQL, evidence base and clinical applications, 662
SARS, 479
tracheostomy, 561
trauma, 507
weaning outcomes, 612

G

Gamma aminobutyric acid complex (GABA), in central nervous system, 126
Gas exchange, 102–103
acid–base balance, 177
carbon dioxide, 177
failure, 235
index of, 235
overview, 176
oxygen, 176, 177
pathophysiology of respiratory failure, 234–235
principles, 235
Gastric pressure, measurement, 370
General wards, 88
Generator position, aerosol, 67, 68f
Generators
position, 69
type, 69
German RCT, 260
German Society of Pneumology, 261
Glasgow Coma Scale (GCS), 151–152, 251
Glossopharyngeal breathing (GPB), 421, 637–638
Glyceryl trinitrate (GTN), 334, 335
Glycogen degrading lyosomal enzyme acid alpha-glucosidase (GAA), 381
Glycogen storage disease, 381
definition, 381
pathophysiology, 381
respiratory clinical management, 382
respiratory issues, 381–382
Goal directed learning process, 201
Gower's manoeuvre, 356
Guidelines, for NIV in acute setting, 113
Guillain–Barre syndrome, 240, 354, 361, 372

H

Haematocrit, LTOT on reducing, 281
Haloperidol, 123, 125, 127
Handbag ventilation, 1, 2
Health economics, AHFS, clinical management, 330
Health status, 656–662
Health-related quality of life (HRQL), 219, 259–260, 261, 262, 273, 275, 656
evidence base and clinical applications
clinical studies, 659–660
cross-sectional trials, 660
future research, 662
longitudinal trials, 660–662
side effects, 659, 659t
methodology for assessment, 656–659
COPD-specific questionnaires, 657

Maugeri Foundation Respiratory Failure Item set, 657–658
MOS 36-item Short-Form Health Status Survey, 657
questionnaires, 657, 657t
Severe Respiratory Insufficiency questionnaire, 658–659, 658f
HealthFacts, 161
Healthy normals, sleep-disordered breathing, 342
Heart failure (HF); *see also* Chronic congestive cardiac failure
causes and classifications, 341–342
diastolic, 342
pulmonary effects, 343, 344–349
systolic, 342
Heart failure with reduced ejection fraction (HFrEF), 409
Heat and moisture exchanger filter (HMEF), 63, 64, 66–67
Heat humidifier wire (HHW), 63, 64, 65, 66–67
Heated humidifiers (HH), 67, 77, 80
Helmet ventilation, 46
Helmets, 49–50, 65, 76, 115
Henderson–Hasselbach equation, 177, 241
High altitude, 412
High flow nasal therapy (HFNT), 116
High flow oxygen cannula (HFNC) therapy, 253
High gas flow rate
positive pressure generation by, 296
washout of dead space in airways by, 296
High oxygen flow (HOF), 134
High-dependency unit (HDU), shortage of, 101
High-flow humidified nasal cannulae oxygen therapy systems, 312
High-flow nasal cannula (HFNC), 1
High-flow nasal cannula oxygenation (HFNCO), 145–146, 321–322
High-flow oxygen therapy (HFOT), 295–304
characteristics and physiological effects, 295–296
patient's inspiratory flow rate and oxygen flow rate, 296
positive pressure generation, 296
warming and humidification of delivered gas, 295–296
washout of dead space in airways, 296
clinical effects
decrease in respiratory rate and work of breathing, 297
improvement of oxygenation, 296–297
improvement of patient comfort and breathlessness, 297
clinical evidence, 297–304
acute hypoxaemic respiratory failure, 298–301
during fibreoptic bronchoscopy, 303, 304
emergency department, 301
hypercapnic respiratory failure, 304
preoxygenation before ETI, 303
prevention of postextubation respiratory failure, 301, 302t
overview, 295
High-flow system, defined, 309
High-frequency chest wall oscillation, 638–637, 639f
High-intensity NPPV, 272–276
clinical considerations, 274–275
conflict of interest, 276
defined, 273
description, 273, 274t
future considerations, 275–276
low *vs*., synopsis of differences, 273, 274t
overview, 272–273
physiological considerations, 273, 274
History
CPAP, 22
IMV, 1
mechanical ventilation, 2t
NIV, 1–2
Home care
costs, 170–171
in COPD patients, 224
setting, transition between CVS and home, 170
Home mechanical ventilation (HMV), 2, 5
costs, 200
diagnostic tests in assessment of patients for, 175–187
clinical assessment, 176
gas exchange, 176, 177
overnight physiological monitoring, 184–187
overview, 175, 176f
patient–ventilator interaction, 182, 184, 185f
pulmonary mechanics, 177–180
respiratory muscle testing, 180–182
discharge planning in palliative care, 213
discharging, patient on, *see* Discharging patient, on home ventilation
in Netherlands, 171–173
discharge and follow-up, 173
indication for, 172
organisation, 171, 172
referral and outpatient clinic, 172
start of, 172–173
monitoring patient treated by, 171, 172t
organisation of care in, 209–212
alternatives to home, 210–211
care coordinator, 209, 210
networks, strong and weak relationships, 211–212
team working and coordination of care, 209, 210
permanent supervision by specialised personnel, 55
prevalence in European countries, 224
prevalence of, 165
purpose, 201
rationale for, 202
service and maintenance, 56–57
Home oxygen therapy, in CRF, 279–284
ambulatory, 279–280
assessment
ambulatory oxygen, 283–284
LTOT, 282
future research, 284
indications for ambulatory oxygen therapy, 282–283
indications for LTOT, 280–282
chronic hypoxaemia, 280–281
palliative use, 282
sleep/exercise induced oxygen desaturation, 281–282
LTOT, 279
overview, 279–280
SBOT, 280, 282, 284
Home setting, NIV, 5
Home ventilators
software, data provided by, 217–219
AHI, 218–219
compliance, 218
estimated tidal volume and minute ventilation, 218
flow and pressure tracings, 219
leaks, 218
overview, 217–218
respiratory rate, 218
Home, supply of oxygen at
cylinders, 307–308
static oxygen concentrators, 308
Home-based care system, 223–224
Homefill oxygen delivery systems, 308
Hormone leptin, 458
Hospital setting, CPAP outside, 26–27

Hospital, CVS in, 166–169
 dedicated staff, 167–168
 equipment
  interfaces, 168
  ventilators, 168
 monitoring, 169
 organisation, 166–167
Hospital, supply of oxygen in, 307
Hospitalisation outcomes, COPD subtypes and comorbidities on, 268, 268f, 269
HRQL, *see* Health-related quality of life (HRQL)
Human patient simulator (HPS), 478
Humidification, of delivered gas, 295–296
Humidified nasal cannulae oxygen therapy systems, high-flow, 312
Humidifiers and drug delivery, during NIV, 63–70
 active (HHW) *vs.* passive (HMEF), 66–67
 aerosol therapy, 67–70
  characteristic factors of technique, 67–69
  factors depending on patient, 67
  two factors derived from, 69–70
 anatomy and function of nasal mucosa, 63, 65f
 functional level in ventilatory parameters, 63, 64
 inadequate AH, effects of, 63, 64t
 intolerance, discomfort, low compliance and reduced adherence, 64
 NAWR, increase of, 63, 64f
 overview, 63
 technical considerations, 65–66
  hygrometric values, 65
  interface, 65
  models of NIV ventilators, 65–66
Humivenis Working Group, 66
Hyaline membrane disease (HMD), treatment, 22
Hygrometric values, in NIV, 65
Hyperbaric oxygen therapy, 50
Hypercapnia, 365, 432
 cause of acidosis, 241
 COPD, 259–260
 daytime, 393
Hypercapnic coma, 88, 102
Hypercapnic respiratory failure, 304, 428
 development, 242, 243
 exacerbation of COPD and
  ARF, prevention, 131
  endotracheal intubation and reintubation, 132
Hypercapnic ventilatory, 448
Hypercarbic respiratory failure, 116
Hyperinflation
 dynamic, 139–140
 intrinsic PEEP and, 242
Hyperoxaemia, 290
Hypertensive acute heart failure (H-AHF), defined, 327
Hypnotic/sedative agent, 123
Hypopnoeas, 367
 predominate, 371
Hypoventilation, sleep quality and correction of, 259
Hypoxaemia
 ARF, defined, 315
 chronic, 280–281
 clinical assessment, 287, 288
 in scoliosis, 431
 NIV failure, 116
 respiratory failure, acute, 144
Hypoxaemic respiratory failure
 acute oxygen therapy, *see* Acute oxygen therapy
 equipment for oxygen therapy, *see* Equipment for oxygen therapy
 HFOT, *see* High-flow oxygen therapy (HFOT)
 home oxygen therapy in CRF, *see* Home oxygen therapy, in CRF
 NIV for, 315–322
  application, 319–321
  bronchoscopy, 319
  cardiogenic pulmonary oedema, 318
  CPAP, 315
  end of life, 319
  evidence base, 315–318
  HFNCO, 321–322
  immunocompromission, 318
  lung stretching during, 320–321
  overview, 315
  post-operative patients, 318
  predictors of success/failure, 320
  rationale, 315
  RCTs, 316–318
  surveys, 315–316
  trauma, 319
  weaning, 319
Hypoxemia, 22, 23
Hypoxia, 432, 433
Hypoxia elicits ventilatory acclimatisation, 448
Hypoxic respiratory failure, de novo
 ARF, prevention, 132
 ETI and reintubation, 133–134
 invasive ventilation, alternative to, 134–135

I

Ideal lung, gas exchange in, 236
Idiopathic pulmonary arterial hypertension, 412
Idiopathic pulmonary fibrosis (IPF), 153
Immunocompromission, NIV in, 318
Impaired alveolar capillary diffusion, 239
Impaired gas exchange
 decreased cardiac function, 367–368
 diffuse microatelectasis, 367
 ineffective cough/bronchopneumonia, 367
Impedance plethysmography and magnetometry, 105
Improvement of patient comfort, clinical effects of HFOT, 297
In-hospital education program, continuum of, 169
In-hospital trials, AHFS, clinical management, 329–330
Increased expiratory resistance, 242
Increased static compliance, 242
Incubation period, SARS, 475
Infection control, ventilators, 57–58
Inner cannula, tracheostomy, 557
Inotropes, 336
Insights from surveys, 157–158
Inspiratory muscle weakness, 367
Inspiratory muscles, PTP of, 248
Inspiratory positive airway pressure (IPAP), 12f, 13, 14, 15, 16, 30, 33, 66, 259, 260, 262, 454, 464
 high-intensity NPPV, 272, 273, 274
Inspiratory reserve volume (IRV), 39
Inspiratory resistance, increased, 241–242
Inspired fraction of oxygen (FiO_2), oxygen flow rate and, 296
Inspired oxygen fraction, low, 236
Insulin resistance, 360
Intelligent volume-assured pressure support (IVAPS), 16, 33, 34, 401
Intensive care acquired weakness (ICAW), 586
Intensive Care Delirium Screening Checklist (ICDSC), 127
Intensive care unit (ICU)
 acute NIV service, 86, 87, 88–89
 CAM-ICU, 102, 127
 conventional mechanical ventilators, 65
 delivering NIV outside, 251–252
 shortage of, 101
 starting NIV, 74–75
 stay, costs, 200

stay, duration, 316
with ARF, 315–316
Interaction, patient–ventilator, 182, 184, 185f
Interface(s), 43–51
aerosol therapy, 67, 68f
characteristics, advantages and disadvantages, 43–45
CVS, equipment, 168
for NIV, in children, 521–523, 522f
helmets, 49–50
nasal masks and pillows, 46, 47
oral, 46
oronasal and full-face masks, 47–49
overview, 43
paediatric, 51
patient–ventilator interaction, 182
physiological aspects, 45–46
air leaks, 45
dead space and CO_2 rebreathing, 45–46
starting NIV
ARF, 76, 77
CRF, 79
technological development, 65
Intermediate ventilators, 10, 11
Intermittent negative pressure ventilation (INPV), NIV-INPV, 1, 2
Intermittent positive pressure breathing (IPPB), NIV-IPPB, 2
Intermittent positive pressure ventilation (IPPV), 419
NIV-IPPV, 1, 2, 3
International Task Force, 615
Internet, 694
Interprofessional education, 98–99
Interstitial syndrome, reminder of sign, 191, 193
Interventional lung assist NovaLung (iLA; NovaLung), 39
Intolerance
in NIV, 64, 116, 117
of ventilator settings, 115
Intrapulmonary percussive ventilation, 638
Intrapulmonary shunting, 238–239
Intrathoracic pressure (ITP), 342, 346
Intravenous immunoglobulin (IVIG), 377
Intrinsic PEEP (PEEPi), 23, 24, 25, 31, 139, 140f, 179–180, 241, 242, 247, 248, 259
Intubation in acute-on-chronic respiratory failure, prevention, 249–252
benefit of NIV, 249–250
challenges for NIV, 250–252
as alternative to intubation, 251
continue NIV after acute phase, 251
proportion of patients, receiving NIV, 250
safety reasons, 251–252
success rate, improving, 250–251
Invasive mechanical ventilation (IMV)
asthma exacerbations, 160, 161
complications, 2
COPD exacerbations, 159
discontinuation of, 141–143
effects of NIV during unsuccessful weaning, 142–143
pathophysiology of weaning failure, 141–142
for exacerbations of IPF, 153
history, 1
patients with pneumonia, outcomes, 161
selection of patients, 75
Invasive tests, respiratory muscle testing, 181–182, 183f
Invasive ventilation
alternative to, 134–135
CPO, 134
de novo hypoxic respiratory failure, 134–135
exacerbations of COPD, 134
weaning from, 135–136
Invasive ventilation period, 1
Isothermic saturation boundary, defined, 63
Italian Respiratory high-dependency care unit (RHDCU), 73, 74–75
Italian survey, hypoxaemic ARF, 316
itrated oxygen treatment, 291

J

Japanese pilot study, 125

K

Keyes sign, 193
Kiss trigger, 422
Kugelberg–Welander disease, 376
Kyphoscoliosis, 78, 240, 426

L

Lactate concentration, 289
Large databases, observations using, 159–160
Laser visualisation technique, 476
Last days of life, 576–577, 577f; *see also* End-of-life care
Late failure, defined, 250
Law of Laplace, 346
Leaks
aerosol therapy, 67, 68f
air
for successful NIV, 30, 31
minimisation and comfort, 43
physiological aspects, interfaces, 45
home ventilator software, 218
monitoring, 103–104
non-intentional, 103
positive pressure ventilators, 11–12
Learning
curriculum for, designing, 96–97
outcomes for, 96
Left ventricular afterload, 346
Left ventricular ejection fraction (LVEF), measurement of, 326, 342, 348, 349
Legal issue, patient and caregiver education, 200–201
Leptin
effects of intracerebroventricular administration, 447
resistance, 446
role of, 445
through hypothalamic circuit, 446
Levosimendan, 328, 336
Lidocaine, use, 176
Likert scale measurement, 335
Limb muscle weakness, 366
Limb-girdle dystrophy, 361
Lipseal, 421
Liquid oxygen systems, 309
Location, NIV
acute NIV, 87
for starting NIV
ARF, 74–75
CRF, 78, 79
Long-term NIV, 268, 268f, 269
Long-term oxygen therapy (LTOT), 177, 227t–228t, 258–262
above threshold for, 281–282
assessment for, 282
high-intensity NPPV, 275
home oxygen therapy, 279
indications for, 280–282
chronic hypoxaemia, 280–281
palliative use, 282
sleep/exercise induced oxygen desaturation, 281–282
Long-term ventilation, SCI and, 513
diaphragm pacemaker, 513
phrenic nerve stimulators, 513
Lorazepam, 125, 126–127
Low barometric pressure, 236

Low compliance, in NIV, 64
Low inspired oxygen fraction, 236
Low-flow system, defined, 309
Lower respiratory tract infections (LRTIs), 389
Lumbar spinal deformities, 426
Lung consolidation, reminder of sign, 191, 192f
Lung mechanics, 345
Lung rockets, defined, 193
Lung sliding, 191, 192f
Lung stretching, during NIV, 320–321
Lung transplantation (LT), ECCO2R, 39
Lung ultrasound in critically ill favouring limitation [not *eradication*] of radiations (LUCIFLR) project, 195
Lung ultrasound in the critically ill (LUCI)
    in emergency room, BLUE-protocol, 193
    in ventilated patient with ARDS, Pink-protocol, 194–195
    other potentials, 195–196
        FALLS-protocol, 195
        FAT-protocol, 195–196
        LUCIFLR project, 195
        SESAME-protocol, 195
    principles, 190–191
    technical approach to, 190–191, 192f
    use, 190
Lung volume
    increase in, 345
    pulmonary mechanics, 177, 178
Lung volume recruitment (LVR), 390

M

Magnetic resonance imaging (MRI), 411
Magnetometry, 105
Mandibular movements, assessment, 220
Mask discomfort, 114, 115
Mask systems, 310–311
    face masks with reservoir bag, 310
    simple face masks, 310
    tracheostomy mask, 311
    use of, 311
    Venturi mask, 311
Mask-related problems, 115
Masks, defined, 26
Maugeri Foundation Respiratory Failure Item set, 657–658
Maugeri Foundation Respiratory Failure Questionnaire (MRF-28), 259
Maximal expiratory pressure (MEP), 370
Maximal inspiratory pressure (MIP), 178, 181
Maximum expiratory pressure (MEP), 181
Maximum inspiratory pressures (MIPs), 432
Mechanical disadvantage, due to chest wall and diaphragm position, 242, 243f
Mechanical insufflator-exsufflator (MIE), 377, 390
Mechanical ventilation (MV), 582
    characteristics and performance, 55–56
    evolution of, 1
    future directions, 2t
    history, 2t
    HMV, 2, 5
    IMV, 1
    modern era of, 1
    types, 2t
    weaning from, 607
Mechanically ventilated patient, psychological issues for, 666–671
    empower patients, 666–661
    overview, 666
    patient education, 667
    psychological challenges, 667–670
    strategies for health professionals
        psychological screening tools, 670
        recommend proactive strategies, 670
Mechanism of action
    AHFS, clinical management, 328–329
    diuretics, 333
    opiates, 335
    vasodilators
        nesiritide, 334
        nitrates and sodium nitroprusside, 334
Mechanisms, of NIV in HF, 345–347
    autonomic effects, 347
    bronchodilatation, 345
    cardiac afterload, 346
    increase in lung volume, 345
    lung mechanics, 345
    preload, 346–347
    respiratory muscle strength, 345
    upper airway stabilisation, 345
    ventilatory drive, 345–346
Medical Research Council (MRC) trial, 280
Medical Research Council dyspnoea scale (MRCD), 151
Medicare, 161
Medicare-certified home health agencies, 224
Membrane 'lung,' 37
Mental status, evaluation, 102
Merlin's space, defined, 190
Metered dose inhaler (MDI), nebuliser *vs.*, 69
Mid-oesophageal pressure, 179
Mid-regional pro-atrial natriuretic peptide (MR-proANP), 327, 328
Midazolam, 123, 125, 126–127, 128t
Milrinone, 328, 334, 336
Minute ventilation, 218
Mitochondrial myopathy
    definition, 383
    pathophysiology, 383
    respiratory clinical issues, 383–384
    respiratory management, 384
Modality, of NIV, 248
Models, of NIV ventilators, 65–66
Modes
    emerging, for NIV, *see* Emerging modes, for NIV
    positive pressure ventilators, 14–16
        adaptive pressure support, 16
        CPAP, 14
        NAVA, 15
        PAV, 15
        pressure-controlled ventilation, 15
        PSV, 14–15
        volume-controlled ventilation, 15–16
    VAPS, 30
Monitoring
    acute NIV, 89
    CVS, component, 169
    overnight physiological, 184–187
        advanced sleep studies, 185, 187f
        overview, 184
        oximetry, 184, 186f
        transcutaneous capnography, 185
    patient treated by HMV, 171, 172t
    positive pressure ventilators, 17
    supplementary oxygen therapy, 291–292
    unit, CVS, 166–167
Monitoring during sleep during chronic NIV, 216–220
    basics, 216
    complex assessments, nocturnal ventilatory PG or PSG, 219–220
    data provided by software of home ventilators, 217–219
        AHI, 218–219
        compliance, 218
        estimated tidal volume and minute ventilation, 218
        flow and pressure tracings, 219
        leaks, 218
        overview, 217–218
        respiratory rate, 218

detecting and quantifying nocturnal hypoventilation, 216, 217
HRQL, 219
overview, 216, 217f
systematic approach to monitoring of chronic NIV for CHRF, 220
Monitoring, during acute NIV, 101–108
clinical evaluation, 101–103
conventional vital signs, 102
gas exchange, 102–103
mental and neurological status, 102
patient comfort, 101, 102
WOB, 102
leaks, 103–104
of complications, 108
overview, 101
patient–ventilator asynchrony, 105–108
cycling-off phase (expiratory asynchrony), 107–108
overview, 105
pressure delivery phases, 105, 106
triggering phase, 105
sleep evaluation, 108
tidal volume, 104–105
Morphine, 123, 124, 128t, 335
Mortality rate
AHFR, 150–152
COPD, 150
investigations, 151
observations, 151–152
post initiation, 152
predictive tools, 152
severity and timing of respiratory acidaemia, 151
steady-state variables, 150–151
asthma exacerbations, 160, 161
COPD exacerbations, 159, 160
ICU, 157
in pneumonia, 153
in pulmonary oedema, 153–154
IPF, 153
Mortality, COPD subtypes and comorbidities on, 268, 268f, 269
MOS 36-item Short-Form Health Status Survey, 657
Motor neurone disease (MND), 388
Mouthpiece support arms, 420
Mouthpiece ventilation (MPV), 420
24-year-old DMD patient, 422
advantages, disadvantages and side effects, 421
choice of ventilator, modes, alarms and settings, 421
alarms, 421–422
modes, 421
settings, 422
during walking, 423
indications and protocols for, 420–421
support arms, 420
support to facilitate ambulation, 422–423
Mouthpiece/lip seal NIV, 419
Mucolytics, 116, 395
Mucus and airway clearance techniques, 633–637
instrumental techniques, 634–635, 635f
manually assisted coughing and lung insufflation techniques, 635–636, 636f–637f
positioning, breathing control techniques and CPT, 634, 634f
Mucus hypersecretions and tracheal injury, 402
Multicore myopathy
definition, 383
pathophysiology, 383
respiratory management, of congenital myopathies, 383
Multidisciplinary team
acute NIV, 86–87
providing home care, 224
Multiple inert gas elimination (MIGET) method, 235
Muscle biopsy, 379
Muscle disorders, 354
acquired, 355
Becker muscular dystrophy, 357
clinical aspects, 357–358
molecular aspects, 357
classification of, 354–356
Duchenne muscular dystrophy, 356
clinical features, 356–357
molecular aspects, 356
dystrophies, 360
dystrophinopathies, phenotypic expression of, 357
inherited, 355–356
myotonic dystrophies
additional features, 360
brain, 360
clinical aspects, 359
heart, 360
molecular aspects, 358–359
skeletal muscle, 359–360
with late ventilatory insufficiency, 356
with ventilatory insufficiency
acid maltase deficiency, 360–361
congenital myopathies, 361
Emery–Dreifuss syndrome, 361
LGMD 2I, 361
Muscle immunohistochemistry, 356
Muscle impairment, signs and symptoms of, 368
Muscle strength, respiratory, 345
Muscle sympathetic nerve activity (MSNA), 347
Muscle weakness, 428
Muscular Dystrophy UK, 362
Myasthenia gravis (MG)
Osserman classification, 378
pathophysiology, 377–378
respiratory clinical issues, 378
respiratory management, 378–379
Myocardial infarction
AHFS, clinical management, 330
oxygen therapy, 290, 291
Myocardial ischaemia, oxygen therapy, 290–291
Myotonic dystrophy (MD), 359, 365, 380
additional features, 360
brain, 360
clinical aspects, 359
definition, 380
heart, 360
molecular aspects, 358–359
pathophysiology, 380
respiratory clinical issues, 380–381
skeletal muscle, 359–360
Myotonic dystrophy type 1 (DM1), 358
Myotonic dystrophy type 2 (DM2), 358

N

N-terminal pro-B-type natriuretic peptide (NT-proBNP), 327, 328
Naloxone, 124
Nasal airway resistance (NAWR), increase of, 63, 64f
Nasal cannulae oxygen therapy systems, high-flow humidified, 312
Nasal masks, 11, 43, 44, 45, 46–47, 51, 65, 76, 114–115, 119
Nasal mucosa, anatomy and function of, 63, 66f
Nasal slings, 47
Nasal systems
cannulae, 310
catheter, 309–310
reservoir, 310
use, 310
Nasogastric tube, 44
Nasopharynx, 420
Natriuretic peptides (NPs)
BNP, 327–328
MR-proANP, 327, 328
NT-proBNP, 327, 328
serum, 327
Nebuliser, MDI *vs.*, 69

Negative pressure ventilation (NPV)
  NIV-INPV, 1, 2
  period, 1
Nemaline myopathy
  definition, 382
  pathophysiology, 382
  respiratory clinical issues, 382
Nesiritide, 328, 334–335
  mechanism of action, 334
  role in management, 335
Netherlands, HMV in, 171–173
  discharge and follow-up, 173
  indication for, 172
  organisation, 171, 172
  referral and outpatient clinic, 172
  start of, 172–173
Networks, strong and weak relationships, 211–212
Neurally adjusted ventilatory assistance (NAVA), 15, 30, 31–33, 253
Neurological patients, weaning outcome, 612
Neurological status, evaluation, 102
Neuromuscular disease (NMD), 153, 364, 365, 375, 422
  diagnosis
    arterial blood gas and electrolytes, 372
    bulbar muscle impairment, 368
    expiratory muscle impairment, 370
    inspiratory muscle impairment, 368–370
    sleep studies, 371–372
    tests of inspiratory/expiratory muscle impairment, 370–371
  respiratory failure
    components, 376
  respiratory muscle weakness, 368
  with respiratory failure, 365
Neuromuscular patients, weaning in, 610–611
NeurRx RA/4 diaphragmatic pacing (DP) system, 392
Nicotine abuse, 261
NIV, *see* Non-invasive positive pressure ventilation (NIV)
Nitrates
  evidence base, 334
  mechanism of action, 334
  role in management, 334
Nitroprusside, sodium
  evidence base, 334
  mechanism of action, 334
  role in management, 334
Nocturnal alveolar hypoventilation, 33
Nocturnal hypoventilation, detecting and quantifying, 216, 217
Nocturnal hypoxia, chronic, 430
Nocturnal oxygen saturation (SpO_2), 216
Nocturnal oxygen therapy, 281
Nocturnal Oxygen Therapy Trial (NOTT), 280
Nocturnal ventilatory polygraphy (PG), complex assessments, 219–220
Non-CF bronchiectasis, 470
Non-intentional leaks, 103
Non-invasive CPAP (n-CPAP), 133
Non-invasive mechanical ventilation (NIMV), 67
  benefits and disadvantages, 673–676
  bronchoscopy during, 540–543
    clinical applications, 541
    evidence base, 540–541
    future research, 543
    overview, 540
    rationale, 540
    technical considerations, 541–542, 542f
  carer's journey, 697–703
  end-of-life care and, 571–579
    in advanced disease, burdens and benefits, 576
    NIV withdrawal at patient request, 577–579, 578t
  evidence-based use
    in SARS, 475–476, 476f
  evidence-based use, in bronchiectasis
    chronic respiratory failure, 471
    in acute respiratory failure, 471
  evidence-based use, in CF
    chronic respiratory failure, 471
    in acute respiratory failure, 471
  overview, 471
  patient's journey, 691–694
    challenges accessing NIV, 692–694
    more than 45 years until diagnosis, 691–692
    social media, internet and breathe with MD, 694
    stay mobile, 694
Non-invasive positive pressure ventilation (NIV), 377, 470, 487
  children with SMA, 377
  high-intensity, *see* High-intensity NPPV
  in children with ARF, 533–536
    clinical management, 536
    evidence base, 533–536
    overview, 533
  in obstetric population, 544–545
    respiratory failure in pregnancy, 544
    utilisation of NIV in pregnancy, 544–545, 545t
Non-invasive ventilation (NIV), 1–5, 399, 419, 457
  Acute, *see* Acute NIV
  acute and chronic respiratory failure due to obesity, 457
  AHFS, clinical management, 328–332
    association with myocardial infarction, 330
    discrepancies in evidence, 331–332
    evidence base, 329
    health economics, 330
    in-hospital trials, 329–330
    mechanism of action, 328–329
    place in, 332
    pooled data, 330–331
    practical considerations, 332
    pre-hospital NIV, 330
    summary of evidence, 332
  as 'ceiling' approach, 3, 5
  clinical issues affecting delivery, 454
  criteria for referral, 394
  daytime hypercapnia, 393
  delivery and possible solutions, 454
  emerging modes for, *see* Emerging modes, for NIV
  female patient with spinal muscular atrophy type 2, 378
  high-intensity NPPV, *see* High-intensity NPPV
  history, 1–2
  home setting, 5
  humidifiers and drug delivery, *see* Humidifiers and drug delivery, during NIV
  hypoxaemic respiratory failure, *see* Hypoxaemic respiratory failure
  in COPD, *see* Chronic obstructive pulmonary disease (COPD)
  indications for, 3
  initiation of, 392
  management, 510–511
    acute SCI, 510–511
    chronic SCI, 511
  nocturnal, 419
  nocturnal desaturation, 393
  oxygen delivery and, 312
  present time, 3–5
  quality control, *see* Quality control, for NIV
  RCT of, 393
  respiratory failure, 3, 4t
  starting, *see* Starting NIV
  timing, *see* Timing
  typical interfaces for, 380
  use, *see* Real-life applications, NIV
Noradrenaline, 328
Normal weight control subjects (nOSA control), 448

Nosocomial pneumonia
incidence of, 134
lower rate of, 57
Nottingham Health Profile, 260
NovaLung, 39
Nurses, NIV application, 73

O

Obesity, 365
areas of future research, 445–448
chest radiograph, 453
chest radiograph of obese patient, 453
increases respiratory muscle load, 453
on respiratory physiology, 441–443
respiratory failure, acute/chronic, 457
acute failure, 458, 462
additional oxygen therapy, 463
breathing control, 458
chronic failure, 457, 459–462
clinical applications, 462
continuous positive airway pressure, 464–465
follow-up, of OHS patients, 463
interfaces, 465
length of treatment, 462–463
long-term efficacy, 465
non-invasive ventilation (NIV), 457
non-invasive ventilation/ continuous positive airway pressure, 462
pathogenesis, 466
pathophysiology, 457–458
prophylactic treatment, 466
setting/titration, 464
sleep, 458
technical considerations, 463–464
treatment time, 463, 465
respiratory function alterations, 442
respiratory muscle load, 453
sleep-disordered breathing, 443–445
Obesity hypoventilation syndrome (OHS), 25, 33, 153, 154, 218, 249, 443, 457
AHRF due to, 153
diagnostic criteria, 444
physiologic effect of NIV in COPD, 249
respiratory events in patients with, 218
sleep-induced upper airway obstruction, 445
VAPS modes, indications for, 33
Obesity-related respiratory failure, 452, 454
acute non-invasive ventilation, 452
Obligations, RHCSs, 170–171
Obstacles, acute NIV, set-up, 92
Obstetric population, NIV in, 544–545
respiratory failure in pregnancy, 544
utilisation of NIV in pregnancy, 544–545, 545t
Obstructive sleep apnoea (OSA), 409, 443, 453
bariatric surgery, 162
CPAP
devices, 219
indications for, 25
mode, 14
setting, optimal fixed, 25
evidence base for NIV in chronic HF, 347
opioids in, 124
prevalence of, 267
sleep-disordered breathing, 342
treatment, 2, 15, 23
Obstructive sleep apnoea–hypopnoea syndrome, 249
Oedema, CPO, 316, 318, 319, 329, 331–332, 334, 335
OHS (obesity hypoventilation syndrome), 25, 33, 153, 154, 218, 249
Opiates, 287, 319, 335
Opioids, 122, 123, 124, 126, 412–414
chronic, polysomnogram of, 413
Options, ventilator
to improve tolerance, 16–17
expiratory pressure release, 16, 17f
patient–ventilator synchrony, 17
ramp, 16
rise time, 16
Oral NIV interfaces, 46
Orexin knock-out mice, 448
Organisation
HMV in Netherlands, 171, 172
of care in HMV, 209–212
alternatives to home, 210–211
care coordinator, 209, 210
networks, strong and weak relationships, 211–212
team working and coordination of care, 209, 210
of CVS, 166–167
RHCSs, 170–171
Oronasal interface, for NIV, 44
Oronasal masks, 11, 43, 44, 45, 46, 47–49, 114–115
Oropharyngeal muscle weakness, 380
Orthopnoea, 366, 388, 393
Osserman classification, 377
Osteoporosis, 403
Outcome(s)
for learning, developing, 96
hospitalisation, COPD subtypes and comorbidities on, 268, 268f, 269
predicting, patients with AHFR, *see* Acute hypercapnic respiratory failure (AHFR)
weaning
care facility availability and, 611
fluid management and, 611
future research, 612
neurological patients, 612
rehabilitation and, 611
sedation and, 611
tracheostomised populations, 611–612
Outpatient clinic, HMV in Netherlands, 172
Overlap syndrome, physiologic effect of NIV in COPD, 249
Overnight physiological monitoring, 184–187
advanced sleep studies, 185, 187f
overview, 184
oximetry, 184, 186f
transcutaneous capnography, 185
Oximetry
assessment of hypoxic patient, 288–289
overnight physiological monitoring, 184, 186f
OxyArm, 312
Oxygen cascade
defined, 289
intervention points in, 290t
Oxygen cloud, 312
Oxygen concentrators
static, 308
transportable and portable, 308–309
Oxygen delivery, 176, 177
and NIV systems, 312
positive pressure ventilators, 13–14
Oxygen delivery systems, 309–312
enclosures
oxygen hat/hood, 312
oxygen tent, 312
mask systems, 310–311
face masks with reservoir bag, 310
simple face masks, 310
tracheostomy mask, 311
use of, 311
Venturi mask, 311
nasal systems
cannulae, 310
catheter, 309–310

reservoir, 310
use, 310
overview, 309
OxyArm, 312
tracheal systems
transtracheal catheter, 311–312
Oxygen desaturation, sleep/exercise induced, 281–282
Oxygen flow rate, patient's inspiratory flow rate and, 296
Oxygen fraction, low inspired, 236
Oxygen hat/hood, 312
Oxygen safety, 312–313
Oxygen saturations (SpO2), 389
Oxygen tent, 312
Oxygen therapy
acute, 289–290; *see also* Acute oxygen therapy
equipment for, *see* Equipment for oxygen therapy
HFOT, *see* High-flow oxygen therapy (HFOT)
Oxygen therapy, in CRF
ambulatory
assessment for, 283–284
indications for, 282–283
overview, 279–280
home, *see* Home oxygen therapy, in CRF
LTOT; *see also* Long-term oxygen therapy (LTOT)
assessment for, 282
indications for, 280–282
overview, 279
SBOT, 280, 282, 284
Oxygen, liquid, 309
Oxygen, supply
at home
cylinders, 307–308
static oxygen concentrators, 308
in hospital, 307
Oxygen-conserving device, 309
Oxygen-providing systems, 307–308
supply of oxygen at home
cylinders, 307–308
static oxygen concentrators, 308
supply of oxygen in hospital, 307
Oxygen–haemoglobin dissociation curve, 237, 238f
Oxygenation improvement, clinical effects of HFOT, 296–297
Oxygenation, NIV failure, 117–118

P

Pacemaker recipients, 410
central sleep apnoea (CSA), 410
Paediatric interfaces, 51
Paediatric ventilatory failure
chronic non-invasive ventilation, 525–529
benefits of NIV, 527–528, 528t
clinical applications, 528–529
overview, 525
pathophysiology, 525–526, 526f
equipment and interfaces in children, 519–523
interfaces for NIV, 521–523, 522f
overview, 519
paediatric specificities, 519–520
ventilators for NIV, 521
ventilatory modes, 520–521
NIV in, 533–536
Palliative care, discharge planning in, 213
Palliative use, indications for LTOT, 282
Paralysis, 366
acute/subacute, characteristics, 370
Parkinson's disease, 365, 414
Patient
continuum of in-hospital education program for, 169
education, *see* Education
Patient comfort
improvement, clinical effects of HFOT, 297
monitoring, 101, 102
Patient education, 667
Patient empowerment, 666–661
Patient safety, 212–213
Patient-centered discharge planning, 208
Patient-related factors, NIV failure, 114–116
agitation, 115
claustrophobia, 115
excessive secretions, 115–116
intolerance, 114
intolerance of ventilator settings, 115
mask discomfort, 114, 115
mask-related problems, 115
progression of underlying process, 116
Patient's inspiratory flow rate and oxygen flow rate, mismatch between, 296
Patient's journey, 691–694
challenges accessing NIV, 692–694
more than 45 years until diagnosis, 691–692
social media, internet and breathe with MD, 694
stay mobile, 694
Patient–ventilator asynchrony
cycling-off phase (expiratory asynchrony), 107–108
delayed opening of exhalation valve, 107–108
premature opening of exhalation valve, 107
defined, 105
during triggering phase
auto-triggering, 105, 106f
excessive triggering delay and ineffective effort, 105, 106f
monitoring, 105–108
NIV failure, 118
overview, 105
pressure delivery phases, 105, 106
prevalence, 105
Patient–ventilator interaction, 182, 184, 185f
improving, 253
Patient–ventilator synchrony, 17, 262
Patients, selection
for NIV, 112–113
starting NIV, ARF, 75–76, 77t
Pditw elicited, by phrenic nerve stimulation, 369
Peak cough expiratory flow (PCEF), 371
Peak expiratory flow (PEF), 181, 404
Pendelluft phenomenon, 321
Percutaneous dilational tracheostomy, 559–560
vs. surgical tracheostomy, 560–561
Percutaneous endoscopic gastrostomy (PEG), 388
tube placement, 395
Percutaneous endoscopic gastrostomy (PEG) tube, 202
Percutaneous tracheostomy, QOL after, 558–559, 559t
Perfusion, ventilation–perfusion mismatch, 236, 237, 238, 239, 240
Perprotocol analysis, 349
Personal protective equipment (PPE), 475
Personnel, in ARF, 73, 74f
Perspectives, exacerbation of COPD
CO_2 removal, 253
HFNC, 253
tolerance and patient–ventilator interaction, improving, 253
Pharmacological treatment, AHFS, 333–336; *see also specific entries*
diuretics, 333–334
evidence base, 333–334
mechanism of action, 333
role in management, 334
opiates, 335
other agents, 335–336
vasodilators, nesiritide, 334–335
mechanism of action, 334
role in management, 335

vasodilators, nitrates and sodium nitroprusside
evidence base, 334
mechanism of action, 334
role in management, 334
Phonation
during ventilation, 564–567
tracheostomy and, 555–557
Phosphodiesterase inhibitors, 336
Phrenic nerve stimulation, 369
Phrenic nerve stimulators (PNS), 513
diaphragm pacing by, 547–552
alternative treatments, 549
contraindications, 549
indications, 548–549
intramuscular diaphragm pacing, 547–548, 548f
intrathoracic phrenic nerve stimulation, 547, 548f
overview, 547
practical aspects, 549–550
preimplantation assessment, 549
results, 550–551
techniques, 547
Physiological mismatch, ventilation–perfusion, 236, 237, 238, 239, 240
Physiological shunting, defined, 237
Physiology
aspects, interfaces, 45–46
air leaks, 45
dead space and CO_2 rebreathing, 45–46
CPAP, 23–24
circulatory system, 24
overview, 23
respiratory system, 23–24
Pillows, nasal, 46, 47
Pink-protocol, 194–195
Planning, discharge, 207–209
in palliative care, 213
Plateau exhalation valve, 11
Plethysmography, impedance, 105
Pleural effusions, signs, 191, 192f
Pneumonia
NIV for, 161
occurrence of, 133
predicting outcome in patients with AHFR, 153
ventilator-acquired, 195
Pneumotachograph, 179
Pneumothorax, signs, 193, 194f
Polio, treatment, 1
Poliomyelitis–spinal deformity, 428
Polycythaemia, 281, 287
Polygraphy (PG), nocturnal ventilatory, 219–220
Polysomnographic studies, 371
Polysomnography (PSG), 435, 472
characterization, 167
complex assessments, 219–220
patients with OHS, 219
Pompe disease, 355, 381
Pooled data, 330–331
Portable oxygen concentrators, 308–309
Position of generator, 69
Positive airway pressure (PAP), 341, 342, 419, 457
Positive end-expiratory pressure (PEEP)
application, 23, 24
assessing alveolar recruitment, 194
auto-PEEP, 12, 13, 118, 247
for NIV application, 30
on dead space, 23
$PEEP_E$, 24
PEEPi, 23, 24, 25, 31, 139, 140f, 179–180, 241, 242, 247, 248, 259
PSV and, 315
pulmonary mechanics, 179–180
triggering process, 107
Positive end-expiratory pressure (PEEPi), 442
Positive pressure generation, by high gas flow rate, 296
Positive pressure ventilators, 10–18
bi-level ventilators, 10, 11, 12–13, 14, 15, 16
circuits, 10, 11f
critical care ventilators, 10, 11, 12
cycle, 13
intermediate ventilators, 10, 11
leaks, 11–12
modes, 14–16
adaptive pressure support, 16
CPAP, 14
NAVA, 15
PAV, 15
pressure-controlled ventilation, 15
PSV, 14–15
volume-controlled ventilation, 15–16
options to improve tolerance, 16–17
expiratory pressure release, 16, 17f
patient–ventilator synchrony, 17
ramp, 16
rise time, 16
overview, 10
oxygen delivery, 13–14
rebreathing, 11
safety
alarms and monitoring, 17
battery power, 17, 18f
tidal volume, 12–13
trigger, 12
Positive pressure, level of, 69
Post initiation, AHFR, 152
Post-extubation respiratory failure
NIV to prevent, 601t
evidence base, 600–603
NIV to treat
clinical application, 600
evidence base, 599–600, 600f
prophylactic NIV, 252
therapeutic NIV, 252
Post-extubation respiratory failure/distress, 135
Post-operative NIV, 161–162
Post-operative patients, NIV in, 318
Post-polio syndrome (PPS)
clinical respiratory issues, 379
respiratory management, 379
Post-surgery non-invasive ventilation, 496–502
anaesthesia-induced respiratory alterations, 496–497
bi-level positive airway pressure (BiLevel), 497
continuous positive airway pressure (CPAP), 497
contraindications, 497, 498t
digestive tubes problems, 498
interfaces, 497
limitations, 497
NIV application, 497
overview, 496
rationale for, 496–497
setting up NIV and duration of trial, 497
study results, 499t–500t
abdominal surgery, 501–502
cardiac surgery, 498
thoracic surgery, 501
Posterolateral alveolar and/or pleural syndromes (PLAPS), 191, 192f
Postextubation respiratory failure, prevention of, 301, 302t
Practical part, educational programme, 202
Practical recommendations, chronic COPD, 262–263
Practical skills, on nature of ventilator support, 203
Pre-hospital NIV, 330
Predictive tools, base mortality rate, AHFR, 152
Prednisone, 379
Pregnancy
respiratory failure in, 544
utilisation of NIV in, 544–545, 545t
Preload, mechanism of NIV in HF, 346–347

Premature opening of exhalation valve, 107
Preoxygenation before ETI, 303
Prescription, supplementary oxygen therapy, 291–292
Pressure delivery phases, patient–ventilator asynchrony during, 105, 106
Pressure tracings, software of home ventilators, 219
Pressure-controlled ventilation (PCV), 11, 12, 13, 15, 16, 512
Pressure-support ventilation (PSV)
  features, 30–31
  in ARF, 77
  leaks, 45
  mode, for NIV, 14f, 30–31, 32–34, 45
  PEEP and, 315
Pressure–time product (PTP) of inspiratory muscles (PTPes), 248
Prognostic variables, in AHFS, 333
Prognostication, AHFS, 327–328
Progression, of underlying process, 116
Prolonged mechanical ventilation (PMV), 210
Proper monitoring, of NIV, 113
Prophylactic NIV, post-extubation, 252
Propofol, 123, 124, 125, 126, 128t
Propofol infusion syndrome (PRIS), 126
Proportional assist ventilation (PAV)
  mode, for NIV, 15, 30, 31, 118, 253
Protocols
  for NIV, 92–93
  weaning, 609–610, 610b
Pseudohypertrophy, 356
Psychological screening tools, 670
Pulmonary artery pressure (PAP), 280, 348
Pulmonary capillary wedge pressure (PCWP), 328, 329, 335, 342
Pulmonary effects, chronic congestive cardiac failure, 343, 344–349
  evidence base, 347–349
    CSA, 348–349
    OSA, 347
  mechanisms of NIV, 345–347
    autonomic effects, 347
    bronchodilatation, 345
    cardiac afterload, 346
    increase in lung volume, 345
    lung mechanics, 345
    preload, 346–347
    respiratory muscle strength, 345
    upper airway stabilisation, 345
    ventilatory drive, 345–346
  overview, 343, 344–345
Pulmonary hypertension, 430
Pulmonary mechanics, 177–180
  advanced physiological measurements, 178, 179
  compliance, 179
  lung volumes, 177, 178
  overview, 177, 178f, 178t
  PEEP, 179–180
  WOB, 180
Pulmonary oedema
  CPO, 316, 318, 319, 329, 331–332, 334, 335
  mortality in, 153–154
Pulmonary rehabilitation, 167
Pulse oximetry, monitoring, 103
Pulse transit time (PTT), 219, 220
Pulse wave amplitude (PWA) reductions, 219
Pulsed flow, 308
Pump, CO_2 removal technology, principles and circuitry, 37
Pyridostigmine, 379

Q

QoL, *see* Quality of life (QoL)
Quality assurance, 203
Quality control, for NIV, 55–60
  characteristics and performance of mechanical ventilators, 55–56
  infection control, 57–58
  overview, 55
  procedures, 58–59
  service and maintenance of HMV, 56–57
Quality management, acute NIV, 90–91
Quality of life (QoL), 388, 656–662; *see also* Health-related quality of life (HRQL)
  percutaneous tracheostomy, 558–559, 559t
  rehabilitation and, 647
Quantifying, nocturnal hypoventilation, 216, 217
Questionnaires, HRQL, 657, 657t

R

Ramp, 16
Randomized controlled trials (RCTs), 390
  CPAP, 25
  hypoxaemic ARF, 316–318
  on ECCO2R, use, 38
  survival from randomisation of NIV, 391, 393
  to clinical settings, 250
Rapid eye movement (REM) sleep, 124, 366, 400, 408, 433
  hypoxia suggestive of desaturation, 433
Rapid shallow breathing, 247
Real life, sedation in, 122–123
Real-life applications, NIV, 157–162
  asthma exacerbations, 160–161
  COPD exacerbations, 159–160
  insights from surveys, 157–158
  observations using large databases, 159–160
  overview, 157
  pneumonia, 161
  post-operative use, 161–162
Rebreathing
  CO_2, dead space and, 45–46
  positive pressure ventilators, 11
Reduced adherence, in NIV, 64
Reduced elastic recoil, 242
Referral clinic, HMV in Netherlands, 172
Rehabilitation, 645–651
  functional status, 647
  in critically ill patient, 645
    assessment, 646
    joint mobility, 646
    limb muscle strength testing, 646–647
    respiratory muscle testing, 647
  quality of life, 647
  treatment, 647–651
    cooperative patient, 650–651
    uncooperative critically ill patient, 648–650
  weaning outcome and, 611
Rehabilitation unit, CVS, 167
Relapse of exacerbation of COPD, 251
RELAX-AHF trial, 335
Relaxin-2 (Serelaxin), 335–336
Remifentanil, 124–125
Renin–angiotensin–aldosterone system (RAAS), 333
Reservoir bag, face masks with, 310
Reservoir, nasal system with, 310
Resetting of respiratory centres, 259
ResMed bi-level ventilators, 12
Respiratory acidaemia, severity and timing of, 151
Respiratory assessment, for SMA, 376
Respiratory care, adults with muscle disorders, 361–362
Respiratory centres, resetting of, 259
Respiratory clinical issues, pathophysiology, 383
Respiratory dysfunction, 375
Respiratory events, CO2 loading and unloading, 445

Respiratory exchange ratio, defined, 236
Respiratory failure, 365
acute hypoxaemic, 298–301, 315
acute/acute-on-chronic, development of, 243–244
acute/chronic, 452, 457; *see also* Acute respiratory failure (ARF); Chronic respiratory failure (CRF)
additional oxygen therapy, 463
breathing control, 458
chronic failure, 457, 459–462
clinical applications, 462
continuous positive airway pressure, 464–465
failure, 458, 462
follow-up, of OHS patients, 463
interfaces, 465
length of treatment, 462–463
long-term efficacy, 465
non-invasive ventilation (NIV), 457
non-invasive ventilation/ continuous positive airway pressure, 462
pathogenesis, 466
pathophysiology, 457–458
presentation, outcome, 394
prophylactic treatment, 466
setting/titration, 464
sleep, 458
technical considerations, 463–464
treatment time, 463, 465
chronic hypercapnic, development of, 243
defined, 235–236
evidence-based use of NIV
in chronic respiratory failure, 471
hypercapnic, 304
development of, 242, 243
hypoxaemic
acute, 298–301
acute oxygen therapy, *see* Acute oxygen therapy
equipment for oxygen therapy, *see* Equipment for oxygen therapy
HFOT, *see* High-flow oxygen therapy (HFOT)
home oxygen therapy in CRF, *see* Home oxygen therapy, in CRF
NIV for, *see* Hypoxaemic respiratory failure, NIV for
pathophysiology, 234–244
acid–base balance, 240–241
acute/acute-on-chronic, development of, 243–244
alveolar hypoventilation, 240
barometric pressure, low, 236
chronic hypercapnic, development of, 243
defined, 235–236
gas exchange, 234–235
hypercapnic, development of, 242, 243
impaired alveolar capillary diffusion, 239
inspired oxygen fraction, low, 236
intrapulmonary shunting, 238–239
overview, 234–235
type 1, 236–239
type 2, 235–236, 239–241
ventilation–perfusion mismatch, 236, 237, 238, 239, 240
ventilatory failure in patients with COPD, 241–242
post-extubation
prophylactic NIV, 252
therapeutic NIV, 252
postextubation, prevention of, 301, 302t
type 1, 236–239
impaired alveolar capillary diffusion, 239
intrapulmonary shunting, 238–239
low barometric pressure, 236
low inspired oxygen fraction, 236
overview, 235–236, 237f
ventilation–perfusion mismatch, 236, 237, 238
type 2
acid–base balance, 240–241
alveolar hypoventilation, 240
overview, 235–236
ventilation–perfusion mismatch, 240
ventilatory failure in patients with COPD, 241–242
hyperinflation and intrinsic PEEP, 242
increased expiratory resistance and expiratory flow limitation, 242
increased inspiratory resistance, 241–242
increased static compliance and reduced elastic recoil, 242
mechanical disadvantage due to chest wall and diaphragm position, 242, 243f
overview, 241
Respiratory function, rate of decline, 388
Respiratory home care services (RHCSs)
goals, 169
obligations, organisation and costs, 170–171
role, 169
technicians and nurses of, 169
Respiratory inductance plethysmography (RIP), 185
Respiratory insufficiency, 378
Respiratory intermediate care unit, acute NIV, 88
Respiratory muscle aids, for secretion management, 638–641
high-frequency chest wall oscillation, 638–637, 639f
intrapulmonary percussive ventilation, 638
mechanical insufflation–exsufflation, 639–641, 640f
Respiratory muscle capacity, 453
Respiratory muscle fatigue, 586–587
Respiratory muscle function, 389
Respiratory muscle load, 453
Respiratory muscle strength (RMS), 345
tests of, 178, 180, 181
Respiratory muscle testing, 180–182
invasive tests, 181–182, 183f
non-invasive tests, 181
overview, 180
Respiratory muscle weakness (RMW), 366, 388
symptoms and signs, 389
Respiratory muscle, unloading, 259
Respiratory muscles, 241
Respiratory physiotherapy, 632–641
glossopharyngeal breathing, 637–638
impairment of mucus elimination and clinical indications, 633
mucus and airway clearance techniques, 633–637
instrumental techniques, 634–635, 635f
manually assisted coughing and lung insufflation techniques, 635–636, 636f–637f
positioning, breathing control techniques and CPT, 634, 634f
overview, 632–633
respiratory muscle aids for secretion management, 638–641
high-frequency chest wall oscillation, 638–637, 639f
intrapulmonary percussive ventilation, 638
mechanical insufflation–exsufflation, 639–641, 640f
Respiratory rate
decrease in, 297
home ventilator software, 218

Respiratory special care unit (ReSCU), 620
Respiratory system function
potential clinic measures, 376
pressure-volume curve of, 431
Respiratory system, physiology of CPAP, 23–24
Respiratory therapists (RTs), 73
Respironics bi-level ventilators, 12
Responsibilities
caregivers, 201
hospital/HMV centre, 201
ventilator user, 201
Richmond Agitation Sedation Scale (RASS), 123
Rights and responsibilities, caregivers, 201
Riker Sedation Agitation Scale (RSAS), 125
Rise time (pressurisation rate), 16
Risk factors for NIV failure, 113
Risk variables, in AHFS, 333t
Risperidone, 123
Rolofylline, 336

S

Safety
of ECCO2R, 39
oxygen, 312–313
patient, 212–213
positive pressure ventilators
alarms and monitoring, 17
battery power, 17, 18f
remifentanil, 124
Safety reasons, NIV in COPD exacerbation, 251–252
SARS, *see* Severe acute respiratory syndrome (SARS)
SARS-CoV, 475
SCI, *see* Spinal cord injuries (SCIs)
Scoliosis, 426
cervical and lumbar spinal deformities, 426
classification of, 428
clinical applications, 435
daytime NIV, 436
hypercapnic respiratory failure, 435
nocturnal hypoventilation, 435–436
post-operative, 436
pregnancy, 436
coronal cross section through thorax, 430
embryologically, 428
evidence base, 434
early trials, 434
wider experience, 434–435
idiopathic scoliosis, familial aggregation of, 427
in neuromuscular disorders, 428
loss of vertical height, 426
lower rib cage in patient, 430
mechanisms, 435
drive, 435
muscles, 435
sleep, 435
pathophysiology
compliance, 430–432
hypercapnic respiratory failure, risk, 434
perfusion, 430
post-TB, 434
resistance, 432
respiratory drive, 432–433
respiratory muscle fatigue, 432
respiratory muscle strength, 432
sleep, 433
spinal surgery, respiratory effects of, 434
ventilation, 428–430
work of breathing, 432
risk factors for respiratory failure, 434
technical considerations
inspiratory time, 437
mode, 436
oxygen, 437
pressure, 436
rate, 437
rise time, 437
thoracic scoliosis, 428
chest x-ray, 427
thoracolumbar spine, diagrammatic saggital, 427
tuberculosis, 428
Secondary polycythaemia, 281
Secretion management
respiratory muscle aids for, 638–641
high-frequency chest wall oscillation, 638–637, 639f
intrapulmonary percussive ventilation, 638
Securing system, interfaces, 43
Sedation, 122–128
delirium, 127, 128t
drugs, selection, 123–128
analgesic agents, 123–125
benzodiazepines, 126–127
dexmedetomidine, 125–126
morphine, 124
propofol, 126
remifentanil, 124–125
in real life, 122–123
overview, 122
rationale for using, 123
weaning outcomeand, 611
Sedation–Agitation Scale (SAS) score, 125
Seldinger technique, 37
Selection of candidates, chronic COPD, 260–261
Selling, service, 91–92
Septic shock, incidence of, 316
Sequelae of tuberculosis, 428
Serelaxin (relaxin-2), 335–336
SERVE-HF trial, 348–349
Services
CVS, *see* Chronic ventilator service (CVS)
HMV, 56–57
NIV, 85, 86, 87, 88, 89, 90–91
SESAME-protocol, 195
Setup, acute NIV, 85–93
emergency ward, 87–88
equipment, 89
general wards, 88
ICU, 88–89
instituting change, 91
location, 87
monitoring, 89
multidisciplinary team, 86–87
NIV service, 85, 86, 87, 88, 89, 90–91
overview, 85–86
problems and obstacles, 92
protocols, use, 92–93
quality management, 90–91
respiratory intermediate care unit, 88
selling, service, 91–92
training, 89–90
Severe acute respiratory syndrome (SARS), 474–479
clinical features, 475
evidence base for use of NIV, 475–476, 476f
future research, 479
global outbreak of, 476
implications for healthcare workers, 476–477, 477t
incubation period, 475
Infection control precautions in the ICU, 477t
overview, 474–475
technical considerations, 478–479, 478t
Severe Respiratory Insufficiency (SRI) questionnaire, 219, 658–659, 658f
Severinghaus electrode, 216
Severity, of respiratory acidaemia, 151
SF-36 energy, 391

Short-burst oxygen therapy (SBOT), 280, 282, 284
Shunting, intrapulmonary, 238–239
Simple face masks, 310
Simple Holistic Ultrasound for Low Economy Settings (SHUFLES) program, 196
Simulation-based education, for NIV, 97–98
Sleep
  evaluation, 108
  specialised weaning units and, 618
Sleep studies, overnight physiological monitoring, 185, 187f
Sleep, during chronic NIV
  monitoring during, *see* Monitoring during sleep during chronic NIV
Sleep-breathing disorders, 458
Sleep-disordered breathing (SDB), 342–343, 360, 366, 400, 410, 441, 453, 455
  CSA, 342–343
  healthy normals, 342
  OSA, 342
  post-acute management, 455
Sleep-related oxygen desaturation, 281–282
Sleep-related symptoms, 393
Sleep/breathing disorder, 412
SMN gene, 361
Sniff nasal inspiratory pressure (SNIP), 178, 181
Social considerations, transition between CVS and home, 170
Social media, 694
Sodium nitroprusside
  evidence base, 334
  mechanism of action, 334
  role in management, 334
Software of home ventilators, data provided by, 217–219
  AHI, 218–219
  compliance, 218
  estimated tidal volume and minute ventilation, 218
  flow and pressure tracings, 219
  leaks, 218
  overview, 217–218
  respiratory rate, 218
SomnoNIV, 465
SomnoNIV group, 219
Speaking valve (Passy Muir®), 557f
Speaking, with NIV, 564–566
  and mechanical ventilation, 565–566, 565f
  and respiratory failure, 564–565
Specialised weaning units, 615–621
  early mobility, 616–617, 617f, 617t
  mechanical ventilation strategies in difficult and prolonged weaning, 617
  muscular weakness in ICU, 615–616
  nutritional status and metabolism, 618
  overview, 615
  psychological dysfunction, 618
  respiratory muscle training, 617
  sleep, 618
  speech and swallowing, 618
  units, 616
Spinal cord injuries (SCIs), 414, 509–514
  epidemiology, 509
  global prevalence, 509
  long-term ventilation, 513
    diaphragm pacemaker, 513
    phrenic nerve stimulators, 513
  non-invasive or invasive ventilation management, 510–511
    acute SCI, 510–511
    chronic SCI, 511
  overview, 509
  pathophysiology, 509–510
    chronic central hypoventilation, 510
    decreased strength of respiratory muscles, 510
    dyssynergies of muscles of thorax and abdomen, 510
    patency and reactivity of airways, changes of, 510
    reduced compliance of lungs and thoracic wall, 510
  tidal volumes, 512–513
  ventilation modes, 512
  weaning of patients, 51
    confounding factors, 514
    execution of process, 514
    pathophysiology, 514
Spinal muscular atrophy (SMA), 375, 388
  definition/pathophysiology, 375
  respiratory clinical issues, 376
  respiratory management, 376–377
  type 1, 376
  type 2, 376
  type 3, 376
  type 4, 376
Spinal surgery, 436
Spiral curriculum approach, 96
Spontaneous breathing trials (SBTs), ECCO2R, 39
Spontaneous expiratory threshold, 13
St George's Respiratory Questionnaire (SGRQ), 259, 260, 283
Staff competencies, education programmes/assessment of, *see* Education programmes/assessment
Staff, dedicated, CVS, 167–168
Staffing, 92
Standard care, 229
Starling's law, 329
Starting NIV, 73–80
  case study in chronic ventilatory failure, 80–81
  in ARF, 73–77
    equipment, 76, 77
    location, 74–75
    personnel, 73, 74f
    practical issues, 77
    selection of patients, 75–76, 77t
  in CRF, 77–80
    education, 77–78
    equipment, 79–80
    location, 78, 79
    practical issues, 80
    timing, 78
  overview, 73
Static compliance
  increased, 242
  pulmonary mechanics, 179
Static oxygen concentrators, 308
Steady-state variables, 150–151
Straps, 44
Stroke, oxygen therapy, 290, 291
Subtypes, COPD
  comorbidities
    NIV compliance, tolerance and settings, 269–270
    on mortality and hospitalisation outcomes, 268, 268f, 269
  relevance for NIV management, 267, 267f
Success rate, NIV, COPD exacerbation, 250–251
Success, NIV, predictors of, 320
SUPERNOVA trial, 38
Supplemental oxygen, chronic congestive cardiac failure, 349
Supplementary oxygen therapy, 290–292
  overview, 290–291
  prescription, administration and monitoring, 291–292
  vulnerable to oxygen, patients, 291
Surgical tracheostomy, 560
  vs. percutaneous dilatational tracheostomy, 560–561
Surveys
  hypoxaemic ARF, 315–316
  insights from, 157–158
Survival motor neuron 1 (SMN1), 375

Swallowing
and respiratory failure, 566
during ventilation, 564–567
tracheostomy and, 555
ventilation impact on, 566–567
with NIV, 566–567
Systematic approach, to monitoring of chronic NIV for CHRF, 220
Systolic HF, defined, 342

T

Target-controlled infusion (TCI) technique, 126
Targeted whole-body ultrasound in cardiac arrest, 195
$TcCO_2$ monitoring, 453
Team work, 209, 210
Technical approach, to LUCI, 190–191, 192f
Technical aspects, chronic congestive cardiac failure
CPAP titration in CSA, 349
supplemental oxygen, 349
Technical factors contributing, NIV failure, 116–119
air leaks, 118–119
oxygenation, 117–118
patient–ventilator asynchrony, 118
proper equipment, 116
ventilation, 116–117
Telemonitoring
continuity of care, 226–229
cost, 226
design and acceptance, 229
for chronic respiratory insufficiency, 226
in HMV, 211
rationale for, 226
standard management, 226, 229
summary, 227t–228t
to gold standard, 229
Terminally ill patients, NIV in, 319
Tezosentan, 336
Theoretical part, educational programme, 202
Therapeutic NIV, post-extubation, 252
Thoracic scoliosis, 428
Thoracic surgery, post-surgery non-invasive ventilation, 501
Thoracic ventilatory restrictive disorders, 5
Thorax, diagrammatic representation, 429
Tidal volume
estimated, 218
hypoxaemic ARF, 320
monitoring, 104–105
positive pressure ventilators, 12–13
target, 16
Timing
of respiratory acidaemia, 151
starting NIV, 78
tracheostomy, 556
Timing, NIV, 131–136
ARF, prevention, 131, 132
COPD and hypercapnic respiratory failure, exacerbation, 131
CPO, 131
de novo hypoxic respiratory failure, 132
endotracheal intubation and reintubation, 132–134
COPD exacerbation and hypercapnic respiratory failure, 132
CPO, 132–133
ETI and reintubation
de novo hypoxic respiratory failure, 133–134
extubation failure, prevention, 135
invasive ventilation, alternative to, 134–135
CPO, 134
de novo hypoxic respiratory failure, 134–135
exacerbations of COPD, 134
overview, 131, 132f
post-extubation respiratory failure/distress, 135
weaning from invasive ventilation, process of, 135–136
To Err Is Human, 212
Tolerance
CPAP, 26
improving, 253
NIV, COPD subtypes and comorbidities, 269–270
ventilator options to improve, 16–17
expiratory pressure release, 16, 17f
patient–ventilator synchrony, 17
ramp, 16
rise time, 16
Tolvaptan, 336
Total lung capacity (TLC), 344
Tracheal systems, transtracheal catheter, 311–312
Tracheostomised populations, weaning outcome, 611–612
Tracheostomy (trach), 554–561
additional sources of support, 679–680
and weaning from mechanical ventilation, 556
benefits and disadvantages, 673–676
deciding whether to use, 676
epidemiology, 554–555
exploring option of, 671–672
future research, 561
history, 554
indications, 556
information gathering and insights, 676
learning about pros and cons of, 672–673
living with, 678–679
overview, 554
pathophysiology, 555–556, 556f
airflow resistance, 555
dead space and humidification, 555
indications, 556
phonation, 555–557
swallowing, 555
percutaneous dilatational *vs.* surgical, 560–561
percutaneous dilational tracheostomy, 559–560
practical applications
cannula selection, 556–557, 557f
cuff management, 557–558
fenestration, 557
inner cannula, 557
quality of life after percutaneous, 558–559, 559t
requirement for, 5
support sources for adjusting to, 679
surgical, 560
timing, 556
use, 1
weaning from, 558
Tracheostomy invasive positive pressure support (T-IPPV), 402
Tracheostomy mask, 311
Tracheostomy mechanical ventilation (TMV), 419
Tracheotomy, 419
Tracings, flow and pressure, 219
Training programme, modification of, 202, 203
Training, NIV programme, 89–90
Training, staff, 167–168
Transcutaneous capnography ($TcCO_2$), 185, 372
Transcutaneous carbon dioxide ($tcCO_2$), 452
Transcutaneous CO_2 testing, 383
Transcutaneous measurement, of CO_2 ($PtcCO_2$), 216, 217
Transdiaphragmatic twitch pressure, 369
Transition, between CVS and home, 169–170

continuum of in-hospital education program, 169
home care setting, 170
social considerations, 170
Transitional care (TC), 207
Transoesophageal electromyography, of neural respiratory drive, 31
Transportable oxygen concentrators, 308–309
Transpulmonary pressure, measuring, 320
Transtracheal catheter, 311–312
Trauma, 504–507
clinical applications, 506
evidence base use of NIV, 505–506
future research, 507
NIV in, 319
overview, 504
pathophysiology, 504–505
technical considerations, 506–507
TREAT-MD registry, 405
Trigger efficiency, 182
Trigger, positive pressure ventilators, 12
Triggering delay, excessive, 105, 106f
Triggering phase, patient–ventilator asynchrony during
auto-triggering, 105, 106f
excessive triggering delay and ineffective effort, 105, 106f
Troubleshooting, 111–119
NIV failure
agitation, 115
air leaks, 118–119
claustrophobia, 115
environmental/caregiver team factors, 112
excessive secretions, 115–116
intolerance, 114
intolerance of ventilator settings, 115
mask discomfort, 114, 115
mask-related problems, 115
oxygenation, 117–118
patient-related factors, 114–116
patient–ventilator asynchrony, 118
predictors of, 111–112
progression of underlying process, 116
proper equipment, 116
proper monitoring, 113
reasons for, 112–113
selection of appropriate patients, 112–113
technical factors contributing, 116–119
ventilation, 116–117
overview, 111
Ttitration unit, CVS, 166
Tuberculosis (TB), 428
Type 1 respiratory failure, 236–239
impaired alveolar capillary diffusion, 239
intrapulmonary shunting, 238–239
low barometric pressure, 236
low inspired oxygen fraction, 236
overview, 235–236, 237f
ventilation–perfusion mismatch, 236, 237, 238
Type 2 respiratory failure
acid–base balance, 240–241
alveolar hypoventilation, 240
overview, 235–236
ventilation–perfusion mismatch, 240

U

Ultrasound, 190–199
AHFS, 327
in ventilated patient, 196
LUCI
FALLS-protocol, 195
FAT-protocol, 195–196
in emergency room, BLUE-protocol, 193
in ventilated patient with ARDS, Pink-protocol, 194–195
LUCIFLR project, 195
other potentials, 195–196
SESAME-protocol, 195
technical approach to, 190–191, 192f
overview, 190
reminder of signs, 191, 192–193
interstitial syndrome, 191, 193
lung consolidation, 191, 192f
lung sliding in critically ill, 191
PLAPS, 191, 192f
pleural effusions, 191, 192f
pneumothorax, 193, 194f
various considerations and limitations, 196
WOB, monitoring, 102
Unloading, respiratory muscle, 259
Unsuccessful weaning, effects of NIV during, 142–143
Upper airway obstruction, 365
Upper airway stabilisation, 345
Usual care, 229

V

Variables
prognostic, in AHFS, 333
steady-state, 150–151
Vasodilators
nesiritide, 334–335
mechanism of action, 334
role in management, 335
nitrates and sodium nitroprusside
evidence base, 334
mechanism of action, 334
role in management, 334
Velcro, 44
Ventilated patient
ultrasound in, 196
with ARDS, LUCI, 194–195
Ventilation
handbag, 1, 2
INPV, 1, 2
IPPV, 1, 2, 3
MV, *see* Mechanical ventilation (MV)
NIV, *see* Non-invasive ventilation (NIV)
PAV, 15
PMV, 210
pressure-controlled/support, 12, 13, 15
volume-controlled, 12, 13, 15–16
Ventilation–perfusion (V/Q) mismatching, 470
respiratory failure
type 1, 236, 237, 238
type 2, 240
Ventilation–perfusion imbalance, 437
Ventilator induced diaphragmatic dysfunction, 584–586, 585t
Ventilator rehabilitation unit (VRU), 619
Ventilator user guidelines, for emotional health, 679
connect with people, 683
coping patterns, 681
distress, 679
emotional health, 680
experiences, 683–684
goals identification, 681
guidelines, 680
learning skills and strategies, 681
logistics, 688
personal characteristics, 680
physical support, 681
planning, 681–682
policies and practices, 688
professional assistance, 680
resources, 680
resources and strategies, 682–683
self-acceptance, 681
self-expression, 681
supportive relationships, 681
therapist
decision-making about, 687
finding, 686

interview of, 687
qualities, 686–687
training and background, 687
therapy, 685
therapy approaches, 688
therapy-related guidelines, 684–685
Ventilator(s); *see also specific entries*
bi-level, 10, 11, 12–13, 14, 15, 16
critical care, 10, 11, 12
CVS, *see* Chronic ventilator service (CVS)
features, 10
intermediate, 10, 11
NIV, models of, 65–66
performance, service, maintenance and infection control, *see* Quality control
positive pressure, *see* Positive pressure ventilators
settings, intolerance of, 115
starting NIV, 77
CRF, 79–80
Ventilator-assisted individual (VAI)
alternatives to home, 210–211
caregiver and case manager, 207, 208
discharge plan, 208
education of, 200, 201, 202, 203
Ventilator-associated lung injury (VILI), causes, 38
Ventilator-associated pneumonia (VAP), 57–58
Ventilatory drive, mechanism of NIV in HF, 345–346
Ventilatory failure, 354
Ventilatory failure in patients with COPD, 241–242
hyperinflation and intrinsic PEEP, 242
increased expiratory resistance and expiratory flow limitation, 242
increased inspiratory resistance, 241–242
increased static compliance and reduced elastic recoil, 242
mechanical disadvantage due to chest wall and diaphragm position, 242, 243f
overview, 241
Ventilatory mode, in NIV, 68
Ventilatory parameters, functional level, in, 63, 64
Venturi masks, 290, 298, 311
Visual analogue scale (VAS), 101, 102
Visual analogue scale area under the curve (VAS AUC), 335
Vital capacity (VC), 365
manoeuvre, 370
Vital signs, conventional, 102
Volume-assured modes, 262
Volume-assured pressure support (VAPS) modes, 30, 33–34
Volume-controlled ventilation, 12, 13, 15–16
Vomit aspiration, 46, 47
Vulnerable to oxygen, patients, 291

W

Wall-mounted flow meters, 307
Warming, of delivered gas, 295–296
Washout of dead space in airways, 296
Weakness, muscle disorders, 356
Weaning, 607–612
centres, 210
classification, 615, 616t
failure, pathophysiology of, 141–142
from invasive ventilation, process, 135–136
from mechanical ventilation, 607
importance of facilitating, 591–593, 592b
in neuromuscular patients, 610–611
mental discomfort during mechanical ventilation
dyspnoea, 626
inability to communicate, 626
psychological problems assessment, 626–627
sleep disruption, 626
NIV, 319
clinical application, 598–599, 599t
evidence base, 593–598, 595t, 596f, 597t–598t
outcome, factors influencing
care facility availability, 611
fluid management, 611
future research, 612
neurological patients, 612
rehabilitation, 611
sedation, 611
tracheostomised populations, 611–612
overview, 607
protocols, 609–610, 610b
psychological problems during, 623–627
anxiety, 625
delirium, 624
depression, 623–624, 624f
overview, 623
post-traumatic stress disorder, 624–625, 625f
specialised units, 615–621
early mobility, 616–617, 617f, 617t
mechanical ventilation strategies in difficult and prolonged weaning, 617
muscular weakness in ICU, 615–616
nutritional status and metabolism, 618
overview, 615
psychological dysfunction, 618
respiratory muscle training, 617
sleep, 618
speech and swallowing, 618
strategies to minimising psychological problems, 627
successful, definition of, 607–608, 608f
units, 616
unsuccessful, 142–143
Weaning failure
and life on long-term MV, 618–619, 619t
cardiovascular dysfunction, 587–588
dyspnoea/anxiety (cognitive impairment), 587–588
global experience, 619–620
European perspective, 620
North American perspective, 619–620
intensive care acquired weakness, 586
overview, 582
pathophysiology, 582–588, 593
respiratory muscle fatigue, 586–587
ventilator induced diaphragmatic dysfunction, 584–586, 585t
ventilatory needs and neuromuscular capacity, 582–583, 583f
Werdnig–Hoffman disease, 376
Whilst acute obesity-related respiratory failure, 452
Work of breathing (WOB), 24, 30, 39, 63, 64
clinical effects of HFOT, 297
monitoring, 102
pulmonary mechanics, 180
reduction of, 247–248
Woundcare dressing, 45

X

Xtravent study, 38

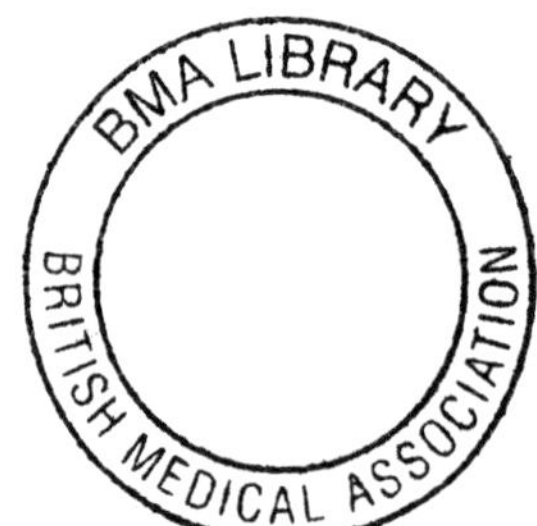
BMA LIBRARY
BRITISH MEDICAL ASSOCIATION